W9-CBX-589

COMPLETE GUIDE TO PRESCRIPTION & NONPRESCRIPTION

DRUGS

By H. WINTER GRIFFITH, M.D.

Revised and Updated by Stephen W. Moore, M.D.

Technical Consultants:
John D. Palmer, M.D., Ph.D.
William N. Jones, B.S., M.S.
Miriam L. Levinson, Pharm.D.

Over 5000 Brand Names
Over 700 Generic Names

A Perigee Book

Notice: The information in this book is true and complete to the best of our knowledge. The book is intended only as a guide to drugs used for medical treatment. It is not intended as a replacement for sound medical advice from a doctor. Only a doctor can include variables of an individual's age, sex and past medical history needed for wise drug prescription. This book does not contain every possible side effect, adverse reaction or interaction with other drugs or substances. Final decision about a drug's safety or effectiveness must be made by the individual and his doctor. All recommendations herein are made without guarantees on the part of the author or the publisher. The author and publisher disclaim all liability in connection with the use of this information.

A Perigee Book
Published by The Berkley Publishing Group
A division of Penguin Putnam Inc.
375 Hudson Street,
New York, New York 10014

Cover photograph by Michael Howell

Copyright © 1983, 1985, 1987, 1988, 1989, 1990, 1991,
1992, 1993, 1994, 1995, 1996, 1997, 1998, 1999, 2000, 2001, 2002
by Penguin Putnam Inc.

All rights reserved. This book, or parts thereof,
may not be reproduced without permission.

First edition: November 2002
ISBN: 0-399-52821-0
ISSN: 1082-2585

Visit our website at www.penguinputnam.com

Printed in the United States of America

10 9 8 7 6 5 4 3 2 1

Contents

About the Author

H. Winter Griffith, M.D., authored 25 medical books, including the *Complete Guide to Symptoms, Illness & Surgery; Complete Guide to Pediatric Symptoms, Illness & Medications*; and *Complete Guide to Sports Injuries*, each now published by The Body Press/Perigee Books. Others include *Instructions for Patients; Drug Information for Patients; Instructions for Dental Patients; Information and Instructions for Pediatric Patients; Vitamins, Minerals and Supplements;* and *Medical Tests—Doctor Ordered and Do-It-Yourself*. Dr. Griffith received his medical degree from Emory University in 1953. After 20 years in private practice, he established and was the first director of a basic medical science program at Florida State University. He then became an associate professor of family and community medicine at the University of Arizona College of Medicine. Until his death in 1993, Dr. Griffith lived in Tucson, Arizona.

Technical Consultants

Stephen Moore, M.D.
Family physician, Tucson, Arizona

John D. Palmer, M.D., Ph.D.
Associate professor of pharmacology, University of Arizona College of Medicine
Associate professor of medicine (clinical pharmacology), University of Arizona College of Medicine

William N. Jones, Pharmacist, B.S., M.S.
Clinical pharmacy coordinator, Veterans Administration Medical Center, Tucson, Arizona
Adjunct assistant professor, Department of Pharmacy Practice, College of Pharmacy, University of Arizona

Miriam L. Levinson, Pharm.D.
Clinical specialist for drug information at Meriter Hospital in Madison, Wisconsin

Drugs and You

A drug cannot "cure." It aids the body's natural defenses to promote recovery. Likewise, a manufacturer or doctor cannot guarantee a drug will be useful for everyone. The complexity of the human body, individual responses in different people and in the same person under different circumstances, past and present health, age and gender influence how well a drug works.

All effective drugs produce desirable changes in the body, but a drug can also cause undesirable adverse reactions or side effects in some people. Despite uncertainties, the drug discoveries of recent years have given us tools to save lives and reduce discomfort. Before you decide whether to take a drug, you or your doctor must ask, "Will the benefits outweigh the risks?"

The purpose of this book is to give you enough information about the most widely used drugs so you can make a wise decision. The information will alert you to potential or preventable problems. You can learn what to do if problems arise.

The information is derived from many authoritative sources and represents the consensus of many experts. Every effort has been made to ensure accuracy and completeness. Where information from different sources conflicts, the majority's opinion is used, coupled with the clinical judgment of the technical consultants. Drug information changes with continuing observations by clinicians and users.

Each year, new drug charts are added and existing charts are updated when appropriate. However, because drug information is constantly changing, you should always talk to your doctor or pharmacist if you have any questions or concerns.

Information in this book applies to generic drugs in both the United States and Canada. Generic names do not vary in these countries, but brand names do.

Be Safe! Tell Your Doctor

Some suggestions for wise drug use apply to all drugs. Always give your doctor, dentist, or health-care provider complete information about the drugs and supplements you take, including your medical history, your medical plans and your progress while under medication.

Medical History

Tell the important facts of your medical history including illness and previous experience with drugs. Include allergic or adverse reactions you have had to any medicine or other substance in the past. Describe the allergic symptoms you have, such as hay fever, asthma, eye watering and itching, throat irritation and reactions to food. People who have allergies to common substances are more likely to develop drug allergies.

List all drugs you take. Don't forget vitamin and mineral supplements; skin, rectal or vaginal medicines; eyedrops and eardrops; antacids; antihistamines; cold and cough remedies; inhalants and nasal sprays; aspirin, aspirin combinations or other pain relievers; motion sickness remedies; weight-loss aids; salt and sugar substitutes; caffeine; oral contraceptives; sleeping pills; laxatives; "tonics" or herbal preparations.

Future Medical Plans

Discuss plans for elective surgery (including dental surgery), pregnancy and breast-feeding. These conditions may require discontinuing or modifying the dosages of medicines you may be taking.

Questions

Don't hesitate to ask questions about a drug. Your doctor, nurse or pharmacist will be able to provide more information if they are familiar with you and your medical history.

Your Role

Learn the generic names and brand names of all your medicines. For example, acetaminophen is the generic name for the brand Tylenol. Write them down to help you remember. If a drug is a combination, learn the names of its generic ingredients.

Filling a Prescription

Once a prescription is written you may purchase the medication from various sources. Pharmacies are usually located in a drug or grocery store. You may need to consider your options: Does the health insurance limit where prescriptions can be filled? Is the location convenient? Does the pharmacy maintain patient records and are the employees helpful and willing to answer drug related questions?

Insurance companies or an HMO (Health Maintenance Organization) may specify certain pharmacies. Some insurance companies have chosen a mail-order pharmacy. Normally a prescription is sent to the mail-order pharmacy or phoned in by the physician. Mail order is best used for maintenance (long-term medications). Short-term medications such as antibiotics should be purchased at a local pharmacy.

Once a pharmacy has been chosen it is best to stay with that one so an accurate drug history can be maintained. The pharmacist can more easily check for drug interactions that may be potentially harmful to the patient or at a minimum decrease the efficacy of one or more of the medications.

You can phone the pharmacy for a refill. Provide the prescription number, name of medication, and name of the patient.

Alcohol & Medications

Alcohol and drugs of abuse defeat the purpose of many medications. For example, alcohol causes depression; if you drink and are depressed, antidepressants will not relieve the depression. If you have a problem with drinking or drugs, discuss it with your doctor. There are many ways to help you conquer such a problem.

Taking A Drug

Never take medicine in the dark! Recheck the label before each use. You could be taking the wrong drug! Tell your doctor about any unexpected new symptoms you have while taking medicine. You may need to change medicines or have a dose adjustment.

Storage

Keep all medicines out of children's reach and in childproof containers. Store drugs in a cool, dry place, such as a kitchen cabinet or bedroom. Avoid medicine cabinets in bathrooms. They get too moist and warm at times.

Keep medicine in its original container, tightly closed. Don't remove the label! If directions call for refrigeration, keep the medicine cool, but don't freeze it.

Discarding

Don't save leftover medicine to use later. Discard it before the expiration date shown on the container. Dispose safely to protect children and pets.

Alertness

Many of the medicines used to treat disorders may alter your alertness. If you drive, work around machinery, or must avoid sedation, discuss the problem with your doctor; usually there are ways (e.g., the time of day you take the medicine) to manage the problem.

Learn About Drugs

Study the information in this book's charts regarding your medications. Read each chart completely. Because of space limitations, most information that fits more than one category appears only once. Any time you are prescribed a new medication, read the information on the chart for that drug, then take the time to review the charts on other medications you already take. Read any instruction sheets or printed warnings provided by your doctor or pharmacist.

Drug Advertising

Ads can cause confusion. Be sure and get sufficient information about any drug you think may help you. Ask your doctor or pharmacist.

Guide to Drug Charts

The drug information in this book is organized in condensed, easy-to-read charts. Each drug is described in a two-page format, as shown in the sample chart below and opposite. Charts are arranged alphabetically by drug generic names, and in some instances, such as *ANTIHISTAMINES*, by drug class name.

A generic name is the official chemical name for a drug. A brand name is a drug manufacturer's registered trademark for a generic drug. Brand names listed on the charts include those from the United States

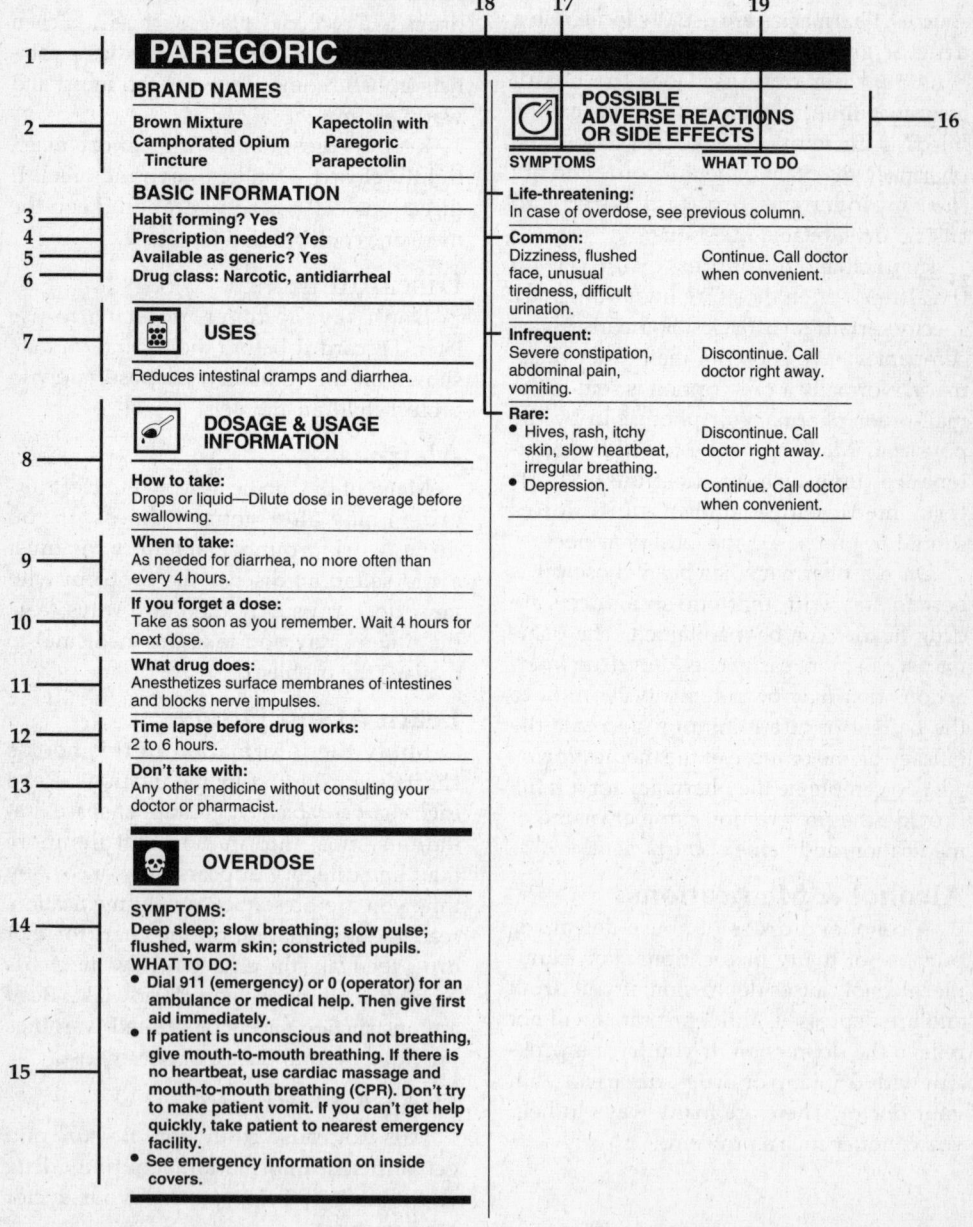

18 17 19

1 **PAREGORIC**

BRAND NAMES

2
Brown Mixture
Camphorated Opium Tincture
Kapectolin with Paregoric
Parapectolin

BASIC INFORMATION

3 **Habit forming? Yes**
4 **Prescription needed? Yes**
5 **Available as generic? Yes**
6 **Drug class: Narcotic, antidiarrheal**

7 **USES**

Reduces intestinal cramps and diarrhea.

8 **DOSAGE & USAGE INFORMATION**

How to take:
Drops or liquid—Dilute dose in beverage before swallowing.

9 **When to take:**
As needed for diarrhea, no more often than every 4 hours.

10 **If you forget a dose:**
Take as soon as you remember. Wait 4 hours for next dose.

11 **What drug does:**
Anesthetizes surface membranes of intestines and blocks nerve impulses.

12 **Time lapse before drug works:**
2 to 6 hours.

13 **Don't take with:**
Any other medicine without consulting your doctor or pharmacist.

OVERDOSE

14 **SYMPTOMS:**
Deep sleep; slow breathing; slow pulse; flushed, warm skin; constricted pupils.

WHAT TO DO:

15
- **Dial 911 (emergency) or 0 (operator) for an ambulance or medical help. Then give first aid immediately.**
- **If patient is unconscious and not breathing, give mouth-to-mouth breathing. If there is no heartbeat, use cardiac massage and mouth-to-mouth breathing (CPR). Don't try to make patient vomit. If you can't get help quickly, take patient to nearest emergency facility.**
- **See emergency information on inside covers.**

POSSIBLE ADVERSE REACTIONS OR SIDE EFFECTS 16

SYMPTOMS	WHAT TO DO
Life-threatening: In case of overdose, see previous column.	
Common: Dizziness, flushed face, unusual tiredness, difficult urination.	Continue. Call doctor when convenient.
Infrequent: Severe constipation, abdominal pain, vomiting.	Discontinue. Call doctor right away.
Rare: • Hives, rash, itchy skin, slow heartbeat, irregular breathing.	Discontinue. Call doctor right away.
• Depression.	Continue. Call doctor when convenient.

and Canada. A generic drug may have one or many brand names.

To find information about a generic drug, look it up in the index. To learn about a brand name, check the index, where each brand name is followed by the name(s) of its generic ingredients and their chart page number(s).

The chart design is the same for every drug. When you are familiar with the chart, you can quickly find information you want to know about a drug.

On the next few pages, each of the numbered chart sections below is explained. This information will guide you in reading and understanding the charts that begin on page 2.

PAREGORIC

20 **WARNINGS & PRECAUTIONS**

21 **Don't take if:**
You are allergic to any narcotic*.

22 **Before you start, consult your doctor:**
If you have impaired liver or kidney function.

23 **Over age 60:**
More likely to be drowsy, dizzy, unsteady or constipated.

24 **Pregnancy:**
Risk factor varies with length of pregnancy. See category list on page xviii and consult doctor.

25 **Breast-feeding:**
Drug filters into milk. May depress infant. Avoid.

26 **Infants & children:**
Use only under medical supervision.

27 **Prolonged use:**
Causes psychological and physical dependence.

28 **Skin & sunlight:**
No problems expected.

29 **Driving, piloting or hazardous work:**
Don't drive or pilot aircraft until you learn how medicine affects you. Don't work around dangerous machinery. Don't climb ladders or work in high places. Danger increases if you drink alcohol or take medicine affecting alertness and reflexes, such as antihistamines, tranquilizers, sedatives, pain medicine, narcotics and mind-altering drugs.

30 **Discontinuing:**
May be unnecessary to finish medicine. Follow doctor's instructions.

31 **Others:**
Great potential for abuse.

POSSIBLE INTERACTION WITH OTHER DRUGS 32

GENERIC NAME OR DRUG CLASS	COMBINED EFFECT
Analgesics*	Increased analgesic effect.
Anticholinergics*	Increased risk of constipation.
Antidepressants*	Increased sedation.
Antidiarrheal preparations*	Increased sedative effect. Avoid.
Antihistamines*	Increased sedation.
Central nervous system (CNS) depressants*	Increased central nerve system depression.
Naloxone	Decreased paregoric effect.
Naltrexone	Decreased paregoric effect.
Narcotics*, other	Increased narcotic effect.

POSSIBLE INTERACTION WITH OTHER SUBSTANCES 33

INTERACTS WITH	COMBINED EFFECT
Alcohol:	Increases alcohol's intoxicating effect. Avoid.
Beverages:	None expected.
Cocaine:	None expected.
Foods:	None expected.
Marijuana:	Impairs physical and mental performance.
Tobacco:	None expected.

1—Generic or Class Name

Each drug chart is titled by generic name or by the name of the drug class, such as DIGITALIS PREPARATIONS.

All drugs have a generic name. Theses generic names are the same worldwide. Sometimes a drug is known by more than one generic name. The chart is titled by the most common one. Less common generic names appear in parentheses following the first. For example, vitamin C is also known as ascorbic acid. Its chart title is VITAMIN C (Ascorbic Acid). The index will include a reference for each name.

Your drug container may show a generic name, a brand name or both. If you have only a brand name, use the index to find the drug's generic name(s) and chart page number(s).

If your drug container shows no name, ask your doctor or pharmacist for the name and record it on the container.

2—Brand Names

A brand name is usually shorter and easier to remember than the generic name. The brand name is selected by the drug manufacturer

The brand names listed for each generic drug in this book may not include all brands available in the United States and Canada. The most common ones are listed. New brands appear on the market, and brands are sometimes removed from the market. No list can reflect every change. In the instances in which the drug chart is titled with a drug class name instead of a generic name, the generic and brand names all appear under the heading GENERIC AND BRAND NAMES. The BRAND NAMES are in lower-case letters, and GENERIC NAMES are in capital letters.

Inclusion of a brand name does not imply recommendation or endorsement. Exclusion does not imply that a missing brand name is less effective or less safe than the ones listed. Some drugs have too many generic and brand names to list on one chart. A complete list is on the page indicated on the chart.

Lists of brand names don't differentiate between prescription and nonprescription drugs. The active ingredients are the same.

If you buy a nonprescription drug, look for generic names of the active ingredients on the container. Common nonprescription drugs are described in this book under their generic components. They are also listed in the index by brand name.

Most drugs contain inert, or inactive, ingredients that are fillers, dyes or solvents for active ingredients. Manufacturers choose inert ingredients that preserve the drug without interfering with the action of the active ingredients.

Inert substances are listed on labels of nonprescription drugs. They do not appear on prescription drugs. Your pharmacist can tell you all active and inert ingredients in a prescription drug.

Occasionally, a tablet, capsule or liquid may contain small amounts of sodium, sugar or potassium. If you are on a diet that severely restricts any of these, ask your pharmacist or doctor to suggest another form.

Some liquid medications contain alcohol. Avoid them if you are susceptible to the adverse effects of alcohol consumption.

BASIC INFORMATION

3—Habit Forming

A drug habit can be physical or psychological. Either leads to drug dependence. Dependence occurs when there is a strong or compelling desire to continue taking the drug to experience its effects or to avoid the symptoms caused by its withdrawal.

Psychological dependence does not cause dangerous withdrawal effects. It may cause stress and unwanted behavior changes until the habit is broken.

4—Prescription Needed?

"Yes" means a doctor must prescribe the drug for you. "No" means you can buy the drug without prescription. Sometimes low strengths of a drug are available without prescription, while high strengths require prescription.

The information about the drug applies

whether it requires prescription or not. If the generic ingredients are the same, nonprescription drugs have the same dangers, warnings, precautions and interactions as prescription drugs. A nonprescription (over-the-counter) drug has dosing and other instructions printed on the container label. Always read them carefully before you take the drug. The information and warnings on containers for nonprescription drugs may not be as complete as the information in this book. Check both sources.

5—Available as Generic?

Some drugs have patent restrictions that protect the manufacturer or distributor of that drug. These drugs may be purchased only by brand name.

Drugs purchased by generic name are usually less expensive than brand names. Once the patent expires, other drug companies can sell that particular drug. They will choose their own brand name

Some states allow pharmacists to fill prescriptions by brand names or generic names. This allows patients to buy the least expensive form of a drug.

A doctor may specify a brand name because he or she trusts a known source more than an unknown manufacturer of generic drugs. You and your doctor should decide together whether you should buy a medicine by generic name or brand name.

Generic drugs manufactured in other countries are not subject to regulation by the U.S. Food and Drug Administration. All drugs manufactured in the United States are subject to regulation.

6—Drug Class

Drugs that possess similar chemical structures or similar therapeutic effects are grouped into classes. Most drugs within a class produce similar benefits, side effects, adverse reactions and interactions with other drugs and substances. For example, all the generic drugs in the narcotic drug class will have similar effects on the body.

Some information on the charts applies to all drugs in a class. For example, a reference may be made to narcotics. The index lists the class—narcotics—and lists drugs in that class.

Names for classes of drugs are not standardized; classes listed in other references may vary from the classes in this book.

7— Uses

This section lists the disease or disorder for which a drug is prescribed.

Most uses listed are approved by the U.S. Food and Drug Administration. Some uses are listed if experiments and clinical trials indicate effectiveness and safety. Still, other uses are included that may not be officially sanctioned, but for which doctors commonly prescribe the drug.

The use for which your doctor prescribes the drug may not appear. You and your doctor should discuss the reason for any prescription medicine you take. You alone will probably decide whether to take a nonprescription drug. This section may help you make a wise decision.

DOSAGE & USAGE INFORMATION

8—How To Take

Drugs are available in tablets, capsules, liquids, suppositories, injections, transdermal patches (See Glossary), aerosol inhalants and topical forms such as drops, sprays, creams, ointments and lotions. This section gives general instructions for taking or using each form.

This information supplements drug label information. If your doctor's instructions differ from the suggestions, follow your doctor's instructions.

Instructions are left out for how much to take. Dose amounts can't be generalized. Dosages of prescription drugs must be individualized for you by your doctor. Be sure the dosage instructions are on the label. Advice to "take as directed" is not helpful if you forget the doctor's instructions or didn't understand them. Nonprescription drugs have instructions on the labels regarding how much to take.

9—When To Take

Dose schedules vary for medicines and for patients.

Drugs prescribed on a schedule should usually be taken at approximately the same times each day. Some must be taken at regular intervals to maintain a steady level of the drug in the body. If the schedule interferes with your sleep, consult your doctor.

Instructions to take on an empty stomach mean the drug is absorbed best in your body this way. Other drugs must be taken with liquid or food because they irritate the stomach.

Instructions for other dose schedules are usually on the label. Variations in standard dose schedules may apply because some medicines interact with others if you take them at the same time.

10—If You Forget a Dose

Suggestions in this section vary from drug to drug. Most tell you when to resume taking the medicine if you forget a scheduled dose.

Establish habits so you won't forget doses. Forgotten doses decrease a drug's therapeutic effect.

11—What Drug Does

This is a simple description of the drug's action in the body. The wording is generalized and may not be a complete explanation of the complex chemical process that takes place. For some drugs, the method of action is unknown.

12—Time Lapse Before Drug Works

The times given are approximations. Times vary a great deal from person to person, and from time to time in the same person. The figures give you some idea of when to expect improvement or side effects.

13—Don't Take With

Some drugs create problems when taken in combination with other substances. Most problems are detailed in the Interaction column of each chart. This section mentions substances that don't appear in the Interaction column.

Occasionally, an interaction is singled out if the combination is particularly harmful.

OVERDOSE

14—Symptoms

The symptoms listed are most likely to develop with accidental or purposeful overdose. Overdosage may not cause all symptoms listed. Sometimes symptoms are identical to ones listed as side effects. The difference is intensity and severity. You will have to judge. Consult a doctor or poison control center if you have any doubt.

15—What To Do

If you suspect an overdose, whether symptoms are apparent or not, follow instructions in this section. Expanded instructions for emergency treatment for overdose are on the inside back cover.

16—Possible Adverse Reactions or Side Effects

Adverse reactions or side effects are symptoms that may occur when you take a drug. They are effects on the body other than the desired therapeutic effect.

The term side effects implies expected and usually unavoidable effects of a drug. Side effects have nothing to do with the drug's intended use.

For example, the generic drug paregoric reduces intestinal cramps and vomiting. It also often causes a flushed face. The flushing is a side effect that is harmless and does not affect the drug's therapeutic potential. Many side effects disappear in a short time without treatment.

The term adverse reaction is more significant. For example, paregoric can cause a serious adverse allergic reaction in some people. This reaction can include hives, rash and severe itch.

Some adverse reactions can be prevented, which is one reason this information is included in the book. Most adverse reactions are minor and last only a short time. With many drugs, adverse reactions that might occur will frequently diminish in intensity as your body adjusts to the medicine.

The majority of drugs, used properly for valid reasons, offer benefits that outweigh potential hazards.

17—Symptoms

Symptoms of commonly known side effects and adverse reactions are listed. Other drug responses may be listed under "Prolonged use," "Skin & sunlight" or "Others." You may experience a symptom that is not listed. It may be a side effect or adverse reaction to the drug, or it may be an additional symptom of the illness. If you are unsure, call your doctor.

18—Frequency

This is an estimation of how often symptoms occur in persons who take the drug. The four most common categories of frequency can be found under the SYMPTOMS heading and are as follows. Life-threatening means exactly what it says; seek emergency treatment immediately. Common means these symptoms are expected and sometimes inevitable. Infrequent means the symptoms occur in approximately 1% to 10% of patients. Rare means symptoms occur in fewer than 1%.

19—What To Do

Follow the guidelines provided opposite the symptoms that apply to you. These are general instructions. If you are concerned or confused, call your doctor.

20— Warnings & Precautions

Read these entries to determine special information that applies to you.

21—Don't Take If

This section lists circumstances when drug use is not safe. On some drug labels and in formal medical literature, these circumstances are called contraindications.

22—Before You Start, Consult Your Doctor

This section lists conditions, especially disease conditions, under which a drug should be used only with caution and medical supervision.

23—Over Age 60

As a person ages, physical changes occur that require special considerations. Liver and kidney functions decrease, metabolism slows and the prostate gland enlarges in men.

Most drugs are metabolized or excreted at a rate dependent on kidney and liver functions. Smaller doses or longer intervals between doses may be necessary to prevent unhealthy concentration of a drug. Toxic effects and adverse reactions occur more frequently and cause more serious problems in older people.

24—Pregnancy

The best rule to follow during pregnancy is to avoid all drugs, including tobacco and alcohol. Any medicine—prescription or nonprescription—requires medical advice and supervision.

This section will alert you if there is evidence that a drug harms the unborn child. Lack of evidence does not guarantee a drug's safety.

The definitions of the pregnancy risk categories of drugs used by the Food and Drug Administration (FDA) are listed on page xviii.

25—Breast-Feeding

Many drugs filter into a mother's milk. Some drugs have dangerous or unwanted effects on the nursing infant. This section suggests ways to minimize harm to the child.

26—Infants & Children

Many drugs carry special warnings and precautions for children because of a child's size and immaturity. In medical terminology, newborns are babies up to 2 weeks old, infants are 2 weeks to 1 year, and children are 1 to 12 years.

27—Prolonged Use

With the exception of immediate allergic reactions, most drugs produce no ill effects during short periods of treatment. However, relatively safe drugs taken for long periods may produce unwanted effects. These are listed. Drugs should be taken in the smallest doses and for the shortest time possible. Nevertheless, some diseases and conditions require a prolonged or even lifelong period of treatment. Therefore, follow-up medical examinations and laboratory tests recommended when a drug is used for long periods are listed. Your doctor may want to change drugs occasionally or alter your treatment regimen to minimize problems.

The words "functional dependence" sometimes appear in this section. This does not mean physical or psychological addiction. Sometimes a body function ceases to work naturally because it has been replaced or interfered with by the drug. The body then becomes dependent on the drug to continue the function.

28—Skin & Sunlight

Many drugs cause photosensitivity, which means increased skin sensitivity to ultraviolet rays from sunlight or artificial rays from a sunlamp. This section will alert you to this potential problem.

29—Driving, Piloting or Hazardous Work

Any drug that alters moods or that decreases alertness, muscular coordination or reflexes may make these activities particularly hazardous. The effects may not appear in all people, or they may disappear after a short exposure to the drug. If this section contains a warning, use caution until you determine how a new drug affects you.

30—Discontinuing

Some patients stop taking a drug when symptoms begin to go away, although complete recovery may require longer treatment.

Other patients continue taking a drug when it is no longer needed. This section gives warnings about prematurely discontinuing. Some drugs cause symptoms days or weeks after they have been discontinued.

31—Others

Warnings and precautions appear here if they don't fit into the other categories. This section includes special instructions, reminders, storage instructions, warnings to persons with chronic illness and other information.

32—Possible Interaction With Other Drugs

People often must take two or more drugs at the same time. Many of these drug combinations have the potential to interact adversely. Fortunately, this adverse reaction occurs in only a small proportion of people who take the interacting combinations. Drugs interact in your body with other drugs, whether prescription or nonprescription. Interactions affect absorption, metabolism, elimination or distribution of either drug. Other factors that can influence drug interactions are the patient's age, state of health and the way the drugs are administered: time taken, how taken, dosage, dosage forms and duration of treatment. The chart lists interactions by generic name, drug class or drug-induced effect. An asterisk (*) in this column reminds you to "See Glossary" in the back of the book, where that entry is further explained.

If a drug class appears, the drug you are looking up may interact with any drug in that class. Drugs in each class that are included in the book are listed in the index. Occasionally drugs that are not included in this book appear in the Interaction column.

Interactions are sometimes beneficial. You may not be able to determine from the chart which interactions are good and which are bad. Don't guess. Consult your doctor or pharmacist if you take drugs that interact. Some combinations can be fatal.

Some drugs have too many interactions to list on one chart. The additional interactions appear on the continuation page indicated at the bottom of the list.

Testing has not been done on all possible drug combinations. It is important to let your doctor or pharmacist know about any drugs you take, both prescription and nonprescription.

33— Possible Interaction With Other Substances

The substances listed here are repeated on every drug chart. All people eat food and drink beverages. Many adults consume alcohol. Many people use cocaine and smoke tobacco or marijuana. This section shows possible interactions between these substances and each drug.

Checklist for Safer Drug Use

- Tell your doctor about *any* drug you take (even aspirin, allergy pills, cough and cold preparations, antacids, laxatives, vitamins, etc.) *before* you take *any* new drug.
- Learn all you can about drugs you may take *before* you take them. Information sources are your doctor, your nurse, your pharmacist, this book, other books in your public library and the Internet.
- Keep an up-to-date list of all the medicines you take in a wallet or purse. Include name, dose and frequency.
- Don't take drugs prescribed for someone else—even if your symptoms are the same.
- Keep your prescription drugs to yourself. Your drugs may be harmful to someone else.
- Tell your doctor about any symptoms you believe are caused by a drug—prescription or nonprescription—that you take.
- Take only medicines that are *necessary*. Avoid taking nonprescription drugs while taking prescription drugs for a medical problem.
- Before your doctor prescribes for you, tell him about your previous experiences with any drug—beneficial results, side effects, adverse reactions or allergies.
- Take medicine in good light after you have identified it. If you wear glasses to read, put them on to check drug labels. It is easy to take the wrong drug at the wrong time.
- Don't keep any drugs that change mood, alertness or judgment—such as sedatives, narcotics or tranquilizers—by your bedside. These cause many accidental deaths

by overdose. You may unknowingly repeat a dose when you are half asleep or confused.

- Know the names of your medicines. These include the generic name, the brand name and the generic names of all ingredients in a combination drug. Your doctor, nurse or pharmacist can give you this information.
- Study the labels on all nonprescription drugs. If the information is incomplete or if you have questions, ask the pharmacist for more details.
- If you must deviate from your prescribed dose schedule, tell your doctor.
- Shake liquid medicines before taking (if directed).
- Store all medicines away from moisture and heat. Bathroom medicine cabinets are usually unsuitable.
- If a drug needs refrigeration, don't freeze.
- Obtain a standard measuring spoon from your pharmacy for liquid medicines. Kitchen teaspoons and tablespoons are not accurate enough.
- Follow diet instructions when you take medicines. Some work better on a full stomach, others on an empty stomach. Some drugs are more useful with special diets. For example, medicine for high blood pressure may be more effective if accompanied by a sodium-restricted diet.
- Tell your doctor about any allergies you have to any substance (e.g., food) or adverse reactions to medicines you've had in the past. A previous allergy to a drug may make it dangerous to prescribe again. People with other allergies, such as eczema, hay fever, asthma, bronchitis and food allergies, are more likely to be allergic to drugs.
- Prior to surgery, tell your doctor, anesthesiologist or dentist about any drug you have taken in the past few weeks. Advise them of any cortisone drugs you have taken within two years.
- If you become pregnant while taking any medicine, including birth control pills, tell your doctor immediately.
- Avoid *all* drugs while you are pregnant, if possible. If you must take drugs during pregnancy, record names, amounts, dates and reasons.
- If you see more than one doctor, tell each one about drugs others have prescribed.
- When you use nonprescription drugs, report it so the information is on your medical record.
- Store all drugs away from the reach of children.
- Note the expiration date on each drug label. Discard outdated ones safely. If no expiration date appears and it has been at least one year since taking the medication, it may be best to discard it.
- Pay attention to the information in the drug charts about safety while driving, piloting or working in dangerous places.
- Alcohol, cocaine, marijuana or other mood-altering drugs, as well as tobacco—mixed with some drugs—can cause a life-threatening interaction, prevent your medicine from being effective or delay your return to health. Common sense dictates that you avoid them during illness.
- Some medications are subject to theft. For example, a repair person in your home who is abusing drugs may ask to use your bathroom, and while there "check out" your medicine cabinet. Sedatives, stimulants and analgesics are especially likely to be stolen, but almost any medication is subject to theft.
- If possible, use the same pharmacy for all your medications. Every pharmacy keeps a "drug profile," and if it is complete, the pharmacist may stop medications that are likely to cause serious interactions. Also, having a record of all your medications in one place helps your doctor or an emergency room doctor get a complete picture in case of an emergency.

- If you have a complicated medical history or a condition that might render you unable to communicate (e.g., diabetes or epilepsy), wear a Medic-Alert identification bracelet or neck tag. Call 888-633-4298, or visit www.medicalert.org for information.
- If you are giving medicine to children, read all instructions carefully. Use the specific dosing device (dropper, cup, etc.) that comes with the product. Don't exceed recommended dose. It does not help and can cause health risks.

Compliance with Doctors' Recommendations

For medical purposes, compliance is defined as the extent to which a patient follows the instructions of a doctor and includes taking medications on schedule, keeping appointments and following directions for changes in lifestyle, such as changing one's diet or exercise.

Although the cost of obtaining medical advice and medication is one of the largest items in a family budget, many people defeat the health-care process by departing from the doctor's recommendations. This failure to carry out the doctor's instructions is the single most common cause of treatment failure. Perhaps the instructions were not presented clearly, or you may not have understood them or realized their importance and benefits.

Factors That Can Cause Problems With Compliance:

- Treatment recommendations that combine two or more actions (such as instructions to take medication, see a therapist and join a support group).
- Recommendations that require lifestyle changes (such as dieting).
- Recommendations that involve long-term regimens (such as taking a medication for life).
- Recommendations for very young patients or for the elderly (another person has to be responsible for following the instructions).

Examples of Noncompliance:

- Medications are forgotten or discontinued too soon. Forgetting to take a medication is the most common of all shortcomings, especially if a medication must be taken more than once a day. If you need to take a medication several times a day, set out a week's supply in an inexpensive pill box that you can carry with you.

- Side effects of medications are a common problem. Almost all medications have some unpleasant side effects. Often these disappear after a few days, but if they don't, let your doctor know right away. Side effects can often be controlled by changing to a similar medication or by adding medications that control the side effects.
- Not taking a drug because it is unpleasant (e.g., bad tasting). Ask your doctor about options.
- Cost is another reason why there are treatment failures; because of a tight budget, a person may take a medication less frequently than prescribed or just not purchase it. If you can't afford a medication, perhaps a less costly one can be prescribed or your doctor can find other ways to provide it.
- Laboratory tests, x-rays or other recommended medical studies are not obtained, perhaps due to concerns about costs or fear of the tests themselves.
- Recommendations about behavioral changes such as diet or exercise are ignored (old habits are difficult for anyone to change).
- Suggested immunizations are not obtained, sometimes due to fear of needles.
- Follow-up visits to the doctor are not made, or appointments are cancelled, perhaps due to problems finding transportation or long waiting times in the doctor's office.

Communicating With Your Doctor:

- If you don't understand something, ask.
- If there are reasons why you cannot follow a recommendation, speak up.
- If you have reservations or fears about treatment, discuss them.

Remember, it is your health and your money that are at issue. You and your doctor are—or should be—working together to make you well and keep you healthy.

Cough and Cold Medicines

Coughs and colds are among humans' most common ailments, and the commercial medicines available for treatment are numerous.

There are hundreds of brands of medicines (each with a registered name) designed to relieve symptoms caused by the common cold, influenza and other minor respiratory illnesses. Most of these medications are over-the-counter (OTC) medicines and can be purchased without a prescription. Cold medicines do not cure the infection or hasten the healing process.

Although these drugs may be safe when taken alone, interactions between these medicines and other nonprescription or prescription drugs, when taken together, may produce undesirable or unsafe results. So, for your own safety, you should study the information in this book with regard to the ingredients of each brand-name cough or cold medicine you are taking. Follow these steps to learn about the safety of your drug:

1. Determine the brand name of your drug.

2. Look on the label for the generic ingredients that are used in your brand of medicine.

3. For each generic ingredient, consult the index or look up each generic drug in the alphabetized drug charts. Read the information about how to use the drug safely, especially regarding its use (interaction) with other drugs you may be taking simultaneously.

The generic ingredients of cough and cold medicines fall into several drug classes:

Antihistamines control allergy symptoms. Antihistamines may cause drowsiness, decreased reflexes and decreased ability to concentrate. Therefore, don't drive vehicles or pilot aircraft until you learn how this medicine affects you. Don't work around dangerous machinery. Don't climb ladders or work in high places. The danger increases if you drink alcohol or take other medicines that affect alertness and reflexes, such as other antihistamines, tranquilizers, sedatives, pain medicines, narcotics or mind-altering drugs. They all may cause other side effects or adverse reactions.

Decongestants relieve symptoms of nasal or bronchial congestion. All decongestants may cause nervousness, irregular heartbeats in some people, dizziness, confusion and other side effects. Conduct your daily activities with these effects in mind. Avoid any product that contains the drug phenylpropanolamine. It is being discontinued as an ingredient in cough/cold drugs due to a risk of stroke in users.

Antitussives reduce frequency and severity of cough. These may be either *narcotic* (codeine and hydrocodone) or *non-narcotic* (dextromethorphan). Narcotic cough suppressants are habit-forming and may cause some of the same mental changes that can take place with antihistamines. The most common non-narcotic antitussive medicine, dextromethorphan, is not habit-forming but has other side effects.

Expectorants loosen secretions to make them easier to cough up. The most common expectorant is guaifenesin, which has very few side effects but doesn't loosen secretions very efficiently.

Analgesics relieve aches and pains. The most common analgesics in cough and cold medicines are aspirin, acetaminophen and ibuprofen.

To learn the details about any cough or cold remedy you may take, look up the brand names in the index of this book. Then consult the generic drug charts listed for each brand name.

Buying Drugs Online

The Food and Drug Administration (FDA) offers these tips to consumers who buy health products online:

- Check with the National Association of Boards of Pharmacy to determine if the site is a licensed pharmacy in good standing (visit their website at www.nabp.net, or call 847-698-6227).
- Don't buy from sites that offer to prescribe a prescription drug for the first time without a physical exam, sell a prescription drug without a prescription, or sell drugs not approved by the FDA.
- Don't purchase from foreign websites at this time, because generally it will be illegal to import the drugs bought from these sites, the risks are greater, and there is very little the U.S. Government can do if you get ripped off.
- Avoid sites that do not identify themselves and do not provide a U.S. address and phone number to contact if there's a problem.
- Beware of sites that advertise a "new cure" for a serious disorder or a quick cure-all for a wide range of ailments.
- Be careful of sites that use impressive sounding terminology to disguise a lack of good science or those that claim the government, the medical profession, or research scientists have conspired to suppress a product.
- Steer clear of sites that include undocumented case histories claiming "amazing" results.
- Talk to your health care practitioner before using any medication for the first time.
- If you suspect a site is illegal, you can report it to the FDA by sending an e-mail to webcomplaints@ora.fda.gov.

Pregnancy Risk Category Information

The pregnancy risk category assigned to a medication identifies the potential risk for that particular drug to cause birth defects or death to an unborn child (fetus). These categories are assigned by applying the definitions of the Food and Drug Administration (FDA) to the available clinical information about the drug. Most drugs are tested only on animals and not on humans for safety during pregnancy, because such testing would subject unborn children to unnecessary risks.

It is best to avoid all drugs during pregnancy, but this rating system can help you and your doctor to assess the risk-to-benefit ratio should drug treatment become necessary. You and your doctor should discuss these benefits and risks carefully before any drug treatment is initiated. You should not take any medications (including nonprescription drugs such as laxatives or cold remedies) without your doctor's approval.

Definitions of the drug categories, labeled A, B, C, D, and X, are listed below:

- A: Adequate studies in pregnant women have failed to show a risk to the fetus in the first trimester of pregnancy, and there is no evidence of risk in later trimesters.

- B: Animal studies have not shown an adverse effect on the fetus, but there are no adequate studies in pregnant women; or animal studies have shown an adverse effect on the fetus, but adequate studies in pregnant women have not shown a risk to the fetus.

- C: Animal studies have shown an adverse effect on the fetus, but there are no adequate studies in humans; or there are no studies in animals or women. The drug may be used by pregnant women because of its benefits and despite its potential risks.

- D: There is evidence of risk to the human fetus, but the potential benefits of use by pregnant women may be acceptable despite the potential risks (e.g., a woman might take such a drug in a life-threatening situation or for a serious disease for which safer drugs cannot be used or are ineffective).

- X: Studies in animals and humans show fetal abnormalities, or reports of adverse reactions indicate evidence of fetal risk. The risks involved clearly outweigh potential benefits, and the drug is contraindicated for pregnant women.

Information about Substances of Abuse

Each of the drug charts beginning on page 2 contains a section listing the interactions of alcohol, marijuana and cocaine with the therapeutic drug in the bloodstream. These three drugs are singled out because of their widespread use and abuse. The information is factual, not judgmental.

The long-term effects of alcohol and tobacco abuse are numerous. They have been well publicized, and information is provided here as a reminder of the inherent dangers of these drugs.

Drugs of potential abuse include those that are addictive and harmful. They usually produce a temporary, false sense of well-being. The long-term effects, however, are harmful and can be devastating to the body and psyche of the addict.

Refresh your memory frequently about the potential harm from prolonged use of any drugs or substances you take. Avoid unwise use of habit-forming drugs.

These are the most common drugs of abuse:

Tobacco (nicotine)

What it does: Tobacco smoke contains noxious, addictive and cancer-producing ingredients. They include nicotine, carbon monoxide, ammonia, and a variety of harmful tars. Carcinogens in smoke probably come from the tars. Most are present in chewing tobacco and snuff as well as smoke from cigarettes, cigars and pipes. Tobacco smoke interferes with the immune mechanisms of the body.

Short-term effects of average amount: Relaxation of mood if you are a steady smoker. Constriction of blood vessels.

Short-term effects of large amount inhaled: Headache, appetite loss, nausea.

Long-term effects: Greatly enhanced chances of developing lung cancer. Impaired breathing and chronic lung disease (asthma, emphysema, chronic bronchitis, lung abscess and others) much more likely. Heart and blood vessel disease more frequent and more severe when they happen. These include myocardial infarction (heart attack), coronary artery disease, heartbeat irregularities, generalized atherosclerosis (hardening of the arteries, making brain, heart, and kidney more vulnerable to disease), peripheral vascular disease such as intermittent claudication, Buerger's disease and others. Tobacco and nicotine lead to an increased incidence of abortion and significantly reduce the birth weight of children brought to term and delivered of women who smoke during pregnancy. Tobacco smoking not only causes higher frequency of lung cancer, but also increases the likelihood of developing cancer of the throat, larynx, mouth, esophagus, bladder and pancreas.

Alcohol

What it does:

- ***Central Nervous System***

Depresses, does not stimulate, the action of all parts of the central nervous system. It depresses normal mental activity and normal muscle function. Short-term effects of an average amount: relaxation, breakdown of inhibitions, euphoria, decreased alertness. Short-term effects of large amounts: nausea, stupor, hangover, unconsciousness, even death. Alcoholism is associated with accidents of all types, marital and family problems, work impairment, legal problems and social problems. Continued abuse of alcohol may result in damage to peripheral nerves and cause various types of brain disorders, including loss of balance and dementia.

- ***Gastrointestinal System***

Increases stomach acid, poisons liver function. Chronic alcoholism frequently leads to permanent damage to the liver.

- ***Heart and Blood Vessels***

Decreased normal function, leading to heart diseases such as cardiomyopathy and disorders of the blood vessels and kidney, such as high blood pressure. Bleeding from the esophagus and stomach frequently accompany liver disease caused by chronic alcoholism.

• ***Unborn Fetus (teratogenicity)***
Alcoholism in the mother carrying a fetus causes *fetal alcohol syndrome (FAS)*, which includes the production of mental deficiency, facial abnormalities, slow growth and other major and minor malformations in the newborn.

Signs of Use:
Early signs: Prominent smell of alcohol on the breath, behavior changes (aggressiveness; passivity; lack of sexual inhibition; poor judgment; outbursts of uncontrolled emotion, such as rage or tearfulness).
Intoxication signs: Unsteady gait, slurred speech, poor performance of any brain or muscle function, stupor or coma in *severe* alcoholic intoxication with slow, noisy breathing, cold and clammy skin, heartbeat faster than usual.

Long-term Effects:
Addiction: Compulsive use of alcohol. Persons addicted to alcohol have severe withdrawal symptoms when alcohol is unavailable. Even with successful treatment, addiction to alcohol (and other drugs that cause addiction) has a high tendency to relapse. (Memories of euphoric feelings plus family, social, emotional, psychological and genetic factors probably are all important factors in producing the addiction.)
Liver disease: Usually cirrhosis; also, deleterious effects on the unborn child of an alcoholic mother.
Loss of sexual function: Impotence, erectile dysfunction, loss of libido.
Increased incidence of cancer: Mouth, pharynx, larynx, esophagus, liver and lung.
Interference with expected or normal actions of many medications: Detailed on every chart in this book, drugs such as sedatives, pain killers, narcotics, antihistamines, anticonvulsants, anticoagulants and others.

Marijuana (cannabis, hashish)
What it does: Heightens perception, causes mood swings, relaxes mind and body.
Signs of use: Red eyes, lethargy, uncoordinated body movements.
Long-term effects: Decreased motivation. Possible brain, heart, lung and reproductive system damage. High dose may initiate symptoms of previously latent schizophrenia.

Amphetamines (including ecstasy)
What they do: Speed up physical and mental processes to cause a false sense of energy and excitement. The moods are temporary and unreal.
Signs of use: Dilated pupils, insomnia, trembling.
Long-term effects or overdose: Violent behavior, paranoia, inflammation of blood vessels, renal failure, possible death from overdose.

Anabolic Steroids
What they do: Enhance strength, increase muscle mass.
Signs of use: Significant mood swings, aggressiveness.
Long-term effects or overdose: Possible heart problems, paranoid delusions and mania, liver and adrenal gland damage, infertility and impotence in men, male characteristics in women.

Barbiturates
What they do: Produce drowsiness and lethargy.
Signs of use: Confused speech, lack of coordination and balance.
Long-term effects or overdose: Disrupt normal sleep pattern. Possible death from overdose, especially in combination with alcohol.

Sedative-hypnotics (benzodiazepines, "party drugs " that include gammahydroxybutyrate and rohypnol)

What they do: Produce drowsiness and lethargy.
Signs of use: Slow breathing, low blood pressure, vomiting, delirium, amnesia, possible coma.
Long-term effects or overdose: Disrupt normal sleep pattern. Possible death from overdose, especially in combination with alcohol.

Cocaine

What it does: Stimulates the nervous system, heightens sensations and may produce hallucinations.
Signs of use: Trembling, intoxication, dilated pupils, constant sniffling.
Long-term effects or overdose: Ulceration of nasal passages where sniffed. Itching all over body, sometimes with open sores. Possible brain damage or heart rhythm disturbance. Possible death from overdose.

Opiates (codeine, heroin, morphine, methadone, opium)

What they do: Relieve pain, create temporary and false sense of well-being.
Signs of use: Constricted pupils, mood swings, slurred speech, sore eyes, lethargy, weight loss, sweating.
Long-term effects or overdose: Malnutrition, extreme susceptibility to infection, the need to increase drug amount to produce the same effects. Possible death from overdose.

Phencyclidine (PCP, angel dust)

What they do: Produce euphoria accompanied by a feeling of numbness.
Signs of use: Psychosis or violent behavior, dizziness, loss of motor skills, disorientation.
Long-term effects or overdose: Seizures, high or low blood pressure, rigid muscles. Possible death from overdose.

Psychedelic Drugs (LSD, mescaline)

What they do: Produce hallucinations, either pleasant or frightening.
Signs of use: Dilated pupils, sweating, trembling, fever, chills.
Long-term effects or overdose: Lack of motivation, unpredictable behavior, narcissism, recurrent hallucinations without drug use ("flashbacks"). Possible death from overdose.

Volatile Substances (glue, solvents, nitrous oxide, other volatile compounds)

What they do: Produce hallucinations, temporary false sense of well-being and possible unconsciousness.
Signs of use: Dilated pupils, flushed face, confusion, respiratory failure, coma.
Long-term effects or overdose: Permanent brain, liver, kidney damage. Possible death from overdose.

Medical Issues and Their Drugs

This list contains the the names of many medical problems and the names of drugs that may be used for their treatment. The drugs are listed either as a generic name (e.g., Acetaminophen) or class name (e.g., Antihistamines). Specific brand or trade names of drugs are not shown. This list of drugs is intended only as a guide and is not meant to be 100% complete. Use it for a general reference.

The inclusion of a drug name does not mean it is necessarily an appropriate treatment for you. Also, your doctor may prescribe a drug for you that is not listed, but is quite appropriate for treatment. Your doctor knows your medical history and can prescribe the drug that should work best for you.

You can find information about the drugs listed by looking up the name in the General Index and referring to the page shown. Do not be alarmed if the drug chart does not list your specific illness in the USES section. For example, that section may state that a drug is used for bacterial infections and not list specific bacterial disorders (such as a vaginal infection or urinary tract infection).

Acid Indigestion & Upset Stomach
- Antacids
- Bismuth Subsalicylate
- Histamine H_2 Receptor Antagonists
- Hyoscyamine
- Proton Pump Inhibitors
- Simethicone
- Sodium Bicarbonate

Acne
- Antiacne Cleansing (Topical)
- Antibacterials for Acne
- Azelaic Acid
- Benzoyl Peroxide
- Erythromycins
- Isotretinoin
- Keratolytics
- Metronidazole
- Retinoids (Topical)
- Tetracyclines

Actinic Keratoses
- Fluorouracil
- Masoprocol

Acute Myocardial Infarction
- Angiotensin Converting Enzyme (ACE) Inhibitors

Addison's Disease
- Adrenocorticoids (Systemic)

Aging
- Dehydroepiandrosterone (DHEA)

AIDS & HIV Infection
- Non-Nucleoside Reverse Transcriptase Inhibitors
- Nucleoside Reverse Transcriptase Inhibitors
- Nucleotide Reverse Transcriptase Inhibitors
- Protease Inhibitors

Alcohol Withdrawal
- Benzodiazepines
- Beta Adrenergic Blocking Agents
- Carbamazepine
- Disulfiram
- Hydroxyzine
- Lithium
- Naltrexone
- Thiamine

Allergies & Allergic Reactions
- Adrenocorticoids (Nasal Inhalation)
- Adrenocorticoids (Oral Inhalation)
- Adrenocorticoids (Systemic)
- Antihistamines
- Antihistamines, Nonsedating
- Antihistamines, Phenothiazine-Derivative
- Azelastine
- Cromolyn
- Decongestants (Ophthalmic)
- Ephedrine
- Hydroxyzine

Alopecia
- Dutasteride
- Finasteride
- Minoxidil

Altitude Illness
- Carbonic Anhydrase Inhibitors

Alzheimer's Disease
- Cholinesterase Inhibitors

Amebiasis
- Chloroquine
- Iodoquinol
- Metronidazole

Amenorrhea
- Bromocriptine
- Progestins

Amyotrophic Lateral Sclerosis (ALS)
- Riluzole

Anemia
- Adrenocorticoids (Systemic)
- Androgens
- Cyclosporine
- Folic Acid
- Iron Supplements
- Leucovorin
- Vitamin B-12

Angina
- Antithyroid Drugs
- Beta Adrenergic Blocking Agents
- Calcium Channel Blockers
- Dipyridamole
- Nitrates

Anorexia
- Antidepressants, Tricyclic
- Progestins
- Selective Serotonin Reuptake Inhibitors (SSRI's)

Anxiety
- Antidepressants, Tricyclic
- Barbiturates
- Benzodiazepines
- Beta Adrenergic Blocking Agents
- Buspirone
- Ergotamine, Belladonna & Phenobarbital
- Haloperidol
- Hydroxyzine
- Loxapine
- Meprobamate
- Phenothiazines
- Selective Serotonin Reuptake Inhibitors (SSRI's)
- Thiothixene
- Venlafaxine

Appetite Stimulant
- Antihistamines
- Dronabinol

Appetite Suppressant
- Appetite Suppressants
- Sibutramine

Arthritis
- Acetaminophen
- Adrenocorticoids (Oral Inhalation)
- Adrenocorticoids (Systemic)
- Antihistamines, Nonsedating
- Anti-Inflammatory Drugs Nonsteroidal, COX-2 Inhibitors
- Anti-Inflammatory Drugs, Nonsteroidal (NSAID's)
- Aspirin
- Azathioprine
- Bronchodilators, Adrenergic
- Bronchodilators, Xanthine
- Capsaicin
- Chloroquine
- Cyclosporine
- Gold Compounds
- Hydroxychloroquine
- Leukotriene Modifiers
- Meloxicam
- Methotrexate
- Salicylates

Asthma
- Adrenocorticoids (Nasal Inhalation)
- Adrenocorticoids (Oral Inhalation)
- Adrenocorticoids (Systemic)
- Bronchodilators, Adrenergic
- Bronchodilators, Xanthine
- Cromolyn
- Ephedrine
- Ipratropium
- Leukotriene Modifiers
- Nedocromil
- Oxtriphylline & Guaifenesin
- Theophylline

Athlete's Foot
- Antibacterials, Antifungals (Topical)
- Antifungals (Topical)

Attention Deficit Hyperactivity Disorder (ADHD)
- Amphetamines
- Dexmethylphenidate
- Methylphenidate
- Pemoline

Autism
- Haloperidol

Bacterial Infections
- Acetohydroxamic Acid (AHA)
- Cephalosporins
- Chloramphenicol
- Clindamycin
- Erythromycins
- Fluoroquinolones
- Kanamycin
- Loracarbef
- Lincomycin
- Linezolid
- Loracarbef
- Macrolide Antibiotics
- Metronidazole
- Neomycin (Oral)
- Nitrofurantoin
- Penicillins
- Penicillins & Beta Lactamase Inhibitors
- Rifamycins
- Sulfonamides
- Tetracyclines
- Trimethoprim
- Vancomycin

Baldness – See Hair Loss

Bedwetting (Enuresis)
- Antidepressants, Tricyclic
- Desmopressin
- Oxybutynin

Benign Prostate Hyperplasia (BPH)
- Alpha Adrenergic Receptor Blockers
- Dutasteride
- Finasteride

Bipolar Disorder
- Carbamazepine
- Lithium
- Divalproex
- Valproate Acid

Birth Control – See Contraceptives

Bites & Stings
- Adrenocorticoids (Topical)
- Anesthetics (Topical)

Bladder Inflammation
- Dimethyl Sulfoxide

Bladder Spasms
- Clidinium
- Propantheline

Bleeding
- Antifibrinolytic Agents
- Vitamin K

Blood Circulation
- Cyclandelate
- Intermittent Claudication Agents
- Isoxsuprine
- Vitamin E

Blood Clots
- Anticoagulants (Oral)
- Dipyridamole
- Ticlopidine

Bronchial Spasms
- Anticholinergics
- Bronchodilators, Adrenergic

Bronchitis
- Bronchodilators, Xanthine
- Cephalosporins
- Dextromethorphan
- Fluoroquinolones
- Ipratropium
- Macrolide Antibiotics
- Sulfonamides
- Tetracyclines

Bulimia
- Antidepressants, Tricyclic
- Lithium
- Selective Serotonin Reuptake Inhibitors (SSRI's)

Burns
- Anesthetics (Topical)
- Zinc Supplements

Bursitis
- Adrenocorticoids (Systemic)
- Anti-Inflammatory Drugs, Nonsteroidal (NSAID's)
- Aspirin
- Salicylates

Cancer
Adrenocorticoids (Systemic)
Aminoglutethimide
Androgens
Antiandrogens, Nonsteroidal
Antifungals, Azoles
Busulfan
Capecitabine
Chlorambucil
Cyclophosphamide
Estramustine
Estrogens
Etoposide
Flutamide
Hydroxyurea
Imatinib
Levamisole
Lomustine
Melphalan
Mercaptopurine
Methotrexate
Mitotane
Paclitaxel
Procarbazine
Progestins
Tamoxifen
Testolactone
Thioguanine
Thyroid Hormones
Toremifene

Cancer Of The Skin
Fluorouracil
Masoprocol
Mechlorethamine (Topical)

Canker Sores
Amlexanox
Anesthetics (Mucosal-Local)

Chickenpox
Acetaminophen
Antihistamines
Antivirals for Herpes Virus

Cholesterol, High - See Hypercholesterolemia

Cirrhosis
Cholestyramine
Colchicine
Cyclosporine
Thiamine (Vitamin B-1)

Colds & Cough
Acetaminophen
Anticholinergics
Antihistamines
Antihistamines, Nonsedating
Anti-Inflammatory Drugs, Nonsteroidal (NSAID's)
Aspirin
Dextromethorphan
Ephedrine
Guaifenesin
Phenylephrine
Phenylephrine (Ophthalmic)
Pseudoephedrine
Terpin Hydrate

Colic
Hyoscyamine
Simethicone

Colitis – See Inflammatory Bowel Disease

Congestion
Bronchodilators, Adrenergic
Ephedrine
Oxtriphylline & Guaifenesin
Oxymetazoline
Phenylephrine
Pseudoephedrine
Xylometazoline

Congestive Heart Failure
Angiotensin-Converting Enzyme (ACE) Inhibitors
Digitalis Preparations
Beta-Adrenergic Blocking Agents
Beta-Adrenergic Blocking Agents & Thiazide

Diuretics
Diuretics, Loop
Diuretics, Potassium-Sparing
Diuretics, Potassium-Sparing & Hydrochlorothiazide
Diuretics, Thiazide
Nitrates

Conjunctivitis (Pink Eye)
Antibacterials (Ophthalmic)
Antivirals (Ophthalmic)

Conjunctivitis, Seasonal Allergic
Anti-Inflammatory Drugs Nonsteroidal (Ophthalmic)
Antiallergic Agents (Ophthalmic)

Constipation
Laxatives, Bulk-Forming
Laxatives, Osmotic
Laxatives, Softener/Lubricant
Laxatives, Stimulant

Contraception
Contraceptives, Oral
Contraceptives, Vaginal
Contraceptives, Vaginal (Spermicides)
Levonorgestrel

Convulsions (Epilepsy; Seizures)
Anticonvulsants, Hydantoin
Anticonvulsants, Succinimide
Barbiturates
Benzodiazepines
Carbamazepine
Divalproex
Felbamate
Gabapentin
Lamotrigine
Levetiracetam
Oxcarbazepine
Paraldehyde
Primidone
Topiramate
Valproic Acid
Zonisamide

Corneal Ulcers
Antibacterials (Ophthalmic)

Crohn's Disease – See Inflammatory Bowel Disease

Cushing's Disease
Adrenocorticoids (Systemic)
Aminoglutethimide
Antifungals, Azoles
Metyrapone
Mitotane
Trilostane

Cystitis
Phenazopyridine
Sulfonamides & Phenazopyridine
See Also – Bacterial Infections

Dandruff
Antifungals (Topical)
Antiseborrheics
Coal Tar

Dementia
Buspirone
Cholinesterase Inhibitors
Ergoloid Mesylates
Haloperidol

Depression
Antidepressants, Tricyclic
Bupropion
Ergoloid Mesylates
Loxapine
Maprotiline
Methylphenidate
Mirtazapine
Monoamine Oxidase Inhibitors
Nefazodone
Selective Serotonin Reuptake Inhibitors (SSRI's)
Selegiline
Trazodone
Venlafaxine

Dermatitis
Adrenocorticoids (Systemic)
Adrenocorticoids (Topical)
Anesthetics (Topical)
Antiseborrheics
Coal Tar

Colchicine
Dapsone
Keratolytics

Dermatomyositis
Aminobenzoate Potassium

Diabetes
Acarbose
Antidiabetic Agents, Sulfonylurea
Insulin
Insulin Analogs
Meglitinides
Metformin
Miglitol
Thiazolidinediones

Diarrhea
Attapulgite
Bismuth Subsalicylate
Charcoal Activated
Difenoxin & Atropine
Diphenoxylate & Atropine
Kaolin & Pectin
Kaolin, Pectin, Belladonna & Opium
Loperamide
Paregoric

Dietary Supplement
Calcium Supplements
Iron Supplements
Niacin
Vitamin A
Vitamin B-12 (Cyanocobalamin)
Vitamin C (Ascorbic Acid)
Vitamin D
Vitamin E
Vitamin K

Digestive Spasms
Clidinium
Difenoxin & Atropine
Dicyclomine
Hyoscyamine
Propantheline

Diverticulitis
Cephalosporins
Clindamycin
Fluoroquinolones
Metronidazole
Penicillins

Drowsiness
Caffeine
Orphenadrine, Aspirin & Caffeine

Dry Eyes
Protectant (Ophthalmic)

Dysmenorrhea – See Menstrual Cramps

Ear Allergies
Anti-Inflammatory Drugs, Steroidal (Otic)

Ear Infections
Antibacterials (Otic)
Anti-Inflammatory Drugs, Steroidal (Otic)
Antipyrine
Phenylephrine
See also – Bacterial Infections

Ear Wax
Antipyrine & Benzocaine (Otic)

Eczema
Adrenocorticoids (Topical)
Antibacterials, Antifungals (Topical)
Coal Tar
Doxepin (Topical)
Keratolytics

Edema – See Fluid Retention

Emphysema
Adrenocorticoids (Systemic)
Bronchodilators, Adrenergic
Bronchodilators, Xanthine
Ipratropium

Endometriosis
Danazol
Nafarelin

Epilepsy – See Convulsions

Erectile Dysfunction
Alprostadil
Papaverine
Sildenafil Citrate
Yohimbine

Esophagitis
Metoclopramide
Histamine H_2 Receptor Antagonists

Estrogen Deficiency
Estrogens

Eye Allergies
Antiallergic Agents (Ophthalmic)

Eye Conditions
Antibacterials (Ophthalmic)
Cromolyn
Cycloplegic, Mydriatic (Ophthalmic)
Cyclopentolate (Ophthalmic)
Decongestants (Ophthalmic)
Natamycin (Ophthalmic)
Phenylephrine (Ophthalmic)

Fatigue
Caffeine

Fever
Acetaminophen
Anti-Inflammatory Drugs, Nonsteroidal (NSAID's)
Aspirin
Barbiturates, Aspirin & Codeine
Chlorzoxazone & Acetaminophen
Narcotic Analgesics & Aspirin
Salicylates

Fibrocystic Breast Disease
Danazol
Vitamin E

Flu – See Influenza

Fluid Retention
Angiotensin Converting Enzyme (Ace) Inhibitors & Hydrochlorothiazide
Carbonic Anhydrase Inhibitors
Clonidine & Chlorthalidone
Diuretics, Loop
Diuretics, Potassium-Sparing
Diuretics, Thiazide
Guanethidine & Hydrochlorothiazide
Hydralazine & Hydrochlorothiazide
Indapamide
Methyldopa & Thiazide Diuretics
Reserpine, Hydralazine & Hydrochlorothiazide

Fungal Infections
Antifungals, Azoles
Antifungals, Topical
Griseofulvin
Nystatin

Gallstones
Ursodiol

Gastroesophageal Reflux
Proton Pump Inhibitors
Sucralfate

Genital Warts
Condyloma Acuminatum Agents

Giardiasis
Furazolidone
Quinacrine

Gingivitis & Gum Disease
Chlorhexidine
Erythromycins
Penicillins
Tetracyclines

Glaucoma
- Antiglaucoma, Adrenergic Agonists
- Antiglaucoma, Anticholinesterases
- Antiglaucoma, Beta Blockers
- Antiglaucoma, Carbonic Anhydrase Inhibitors
- Antiglaucoma, Cholinergic Agonists
- Antiglaucoma, Prostaglandins
- Carbonic Anhydrase Inhibitors

Gonorrhea
- Cephalosporins
- Erythromycins
- Fluoroquinolones
- Macrolide Antibiotics
- Penicillins
- Tetracyclines

Gout
- Adrenocorticoids (Systemic)
- Allopurinol
- Anti-Inflammatory Drugs, Nonsteroidal (NSAID's)
- Colchicine
- Meloxicam
- Probenecid
- Probenecid & Colchicine
- Sulfinpyrazone

Hair Loss
- Anthralin (Topical)
- Finasteride
- Minoxidil (Topical)

Hay Fever
- Antiallergic Agents (Ophthalmic)
- Antihistamines
- Antihistamines, Nonsedating
- Antihistamine, Phenothiazine-Derivative
- Ephedrine
- Hydroxyzine
- Guaifenesin
- Meclizine
- Orphenadrine
- Phenylephrine (Ophthalmic)

Headache (Cluster, Migraine, Sinus, Tension, Vascular)
- Acetaminophen
- Antidepressants, Tricyclic
- Antihistamines
- Anti-Inflammatory Drugs, Nonsteroidal (NSAID's)
- Aspirin
- Barbiturates, Aspirin & Codeine
- Beta Adrenergic Blocking Agents
- Buspirone
- Butorphanol
- Caffeine
- Calcium Channel Blockers
- Clonidine
- Divalproex
- Ergotamine
- Ergotamine, Belladonna & Phenobarbital
- Isometheptene, Dichloralphenazone & Acetaminophen
- Lithium
- Methysergide
- Monoamine Oxidase Inhibitors
- Triptans

Heart Rhythm Disorders
- Amiodarone
- Beta-Adrenergic Blocking Agents
- Calcium Channel Blockers
- Digitalis Preparations
- Disopyramide
- Dofetilide
- Flecainide Acetate
- Mexiletine
- Moricizine
- Procainamide
- Propafenone
- Quinidine
- Tocainide

Heartburn
- Antacids
- Histamine H_2 Receptor Antagonists
- Proton Pump Inhibitors
- Sodium Bicarbonate

Hemorrhoids
- Adrenocorticoids (Topical)
- Anesthetics (Rectal)

Herpes
- Antivirals (Topical)
- Antivirals for Herpes Virus

High Blood Pressure – See Hypertension

HIV Infection – See AIDS

Hives (Urticaria)
- Antihistamines
- Antihistamines, Nonsedating
- Antihistamine, Phenothiazine-Derivative
- Hydroxyzine

Huntington's
- Haloperidol

Hypercalcemia
- Colesevelam
- Colestipol
- Dextrothyroxine
- HMG-CoA Reductase Inhibitors

Hypercholesterolemia
- Cholestyramine
- Colestipol
- Gemfibrozil
- HMG-CoA Reductase Inhibitors
- Neomycin (Oral)
- Niacin
- Raloxifene

Hyperglycemia
- Acarbose
- Metformin

Hypertension
- Alpha Adrenergic Receptor Blockers
- Angiotensin II receptor Antagonists
- Angiotensin-Converting Enzyme (ACE) Inhibitors
- Angiotensin-Converting Enzyme (ACE) Inhibitors & Hydrochlorothiazide
- Calcium Channel Blockers
- Clonidine
- Beta Adrenergic Blocking Agents
- Beta Adrenergic Blocking Agents & Thiazide Diuretics
- Clonidine & Chlorthalidone
- Diuretics, Loop
- Diuretics, Potassium Sparing
- Diuretics, Potassium-Sparing & Hydrochlorothiazide
- Diuretics, Thiazide
- Guanabenz
- Guanadrel
- Guanethidine
- Guanethidine & Hydrochlorothiazide
- Guanfacine
- Hydralazine
- Hydralazine & Hydrochlorothiazide
- Indapamide
- Mecamylamine
- Methyldopa
- Methyldopa & Thiazide Diuretics
- Minoxidil
- Rauwolfia Alkaloids
- Reserpine, Hydralazine & Hydrochlorothiazide

Hyperthyroidism
- Antithyroid Drugs

Hypertriglyceridemia
- HMG-CoA Reductase Inhibitors
- Fibrates
- Gemfibrozil

Hypoglycemia
Glucagon
Miglitol

Hypothyroidism
Dextrothyroxine
Thyroid Hormones

Impotence - See Erectile Dysfunction

Incontinence
Tolterodine

Indigestion – See Heartburn

Infertility
Bromocriptine
Clomiphene
Danazol
Progestins

Inflammation
Acetaminophen & Salicylates
Anti-Inflammatory Drugs, Nonsteroidal (NSAID's)
Anti-Inflammatory Drugs Nonsteroidal, COX-2 Inhibitors
Aspirin
Mesalamine
Narcotic Analgesics & Aspirin
Salicylates

Inflammatory Bowel Disease
Adrenocorticoids (Systemic)
Cyclosporine
Mesalamine
Metronidazole
Olsalazine

Influenza
Antivirals for Influenza
Antivirals for Influenza, Neuraminidase Inhibitors
Ribavirin

Insomnia
Barbiturates
Belladonna Alkaloids & Barbiturates
Benzodiazepines
Chloral Hydrate
Ethchlorvynol
Melatonin
Meprobamate
Meprobamate & Aspirin
Trazodone
Triazolam
Zaleplon
Zolpidem

Intermittent Claudication
Intermittent Claudication Agents

Irregular Heartbeat – See Heart Rhythm Disorders

Irritable Bowel Syndrome – See Crohn's Disease

Itching
Adrenocorticoids (Topical)
Doxepin (Topical)

Jet Lag
Melatonin

Jock Itch
Antifungals (Topical)

Joint Pain
Anti-Inflammatory Drugs, Nonsteroidal (NSAID's)
Anti-Inflammatory Drugs Nonsteroidal, COX-2 Inhibitors
Aspirin
Probenecid & Colchicine

Kidney Stones
Allopurinol
Cellulose Sodium Phosphate
Citrates
Diuretics, Thiazide
Penicillamine
Sodium Bicarbonate
Tiopronin

Labyrinthitis
Antihistamines, Phenothiazine-Derivative
Benzodiazepines
Meclizine

Leg Pain or Cramps
Cyclandelate
Intermittent Claudication Agents
Orphenadrine
Pentoxifylline
Quinine

Leukemia
Thioguanine

Lice
Pediculoides

Lupus (Skin & Systemic)
Anti-Inflammatory Drugs, Nonsteroidal (NSAID's)
Anti-Inflammatory Drugs Nonsteroidal, COX-2 Inhibitors
Adrenocorticoids (Systemic)
Adrenocorticoids (Topical)
Hydroxychloroquine
Methotrexate
Quinacrine

Lyme Disease
Cephalosporins
Erythromycins
Macrolide Antibiotics
Penicillins
Tetracyclines

Malabsorption
Vitamin K
Quinacrine

Malaria
Antimalarial
Atovaquone
Chloroquine
Hydroxychloroquine
Primaquine
Proguanil
Quinidine
Quinine
Sulfadoxine & Pyrimethamine
Tetracyclines

Male Hormone Deficiency
Androgens

Melanoma
Hydroxyurea
Levamisole
Melphalan

Meniere's Disease
Antihistamines
Benzodiazepines
Meclizine
Scopolamine (Hyoscine)

Menopause
Androgens & Estrogens
Estrogens
Progestins

Menstrual Cramps
Anti-Inflammatory Drugs, Nonsteroidal (NSAID's)
Anti-Inflammatory Drugs, Nonsteroidal COX-2 Inhibitors
Contraceptives, Oral

Menstruation, Excessive (Menorrhagia)
Contraceptives, Oral
Danazol
Estrogens
Progestins

Mental & Emotional Disturbances
Loxapine
Molindone
Rauwolfia Alkaloids
Risperidone

Motion Sickness
Antihistamines
Antihistamines, Nonsedating
Antihistamines, Phenothiazine-Derivative
Clotrimazole
Cyclizine
Diphenidol
Meclizine
Scopolamine

Multiple Sclerosis
Adrenocorticoids (Systemic)
Baclofen
Tizanidine

Muscle Cramp, Spasm, Strain
Baclofen
Chlorzoxazone & Acetaminophen
Cyclobenzaprine
Dantrolene
Muscle Relaxants, Skeletal
Orphenadrine
Orphenadrine, Aspirin & Caffeine
Quinine
Tizanidine

Myasthenia Gravis
Adrenocorticoids (Systemic)
Antimyasthenics
Azathioprine
Cyclosporine

Narcolepsy
Amphetamines
Methylphenidate
Modafinil

Narcotic Withdrawal
Clonidine
Naltrexone

Nasal Allergy
Adrenocorticoids (Nasal Inhalation)

Nausea & Vomiting
Antihistamines, Phenothiazine-Derivative
Bismuth Subsalicylate
Diphenidol
Dronabinol
Hydroxyzine
Metoclopramide
Nabilone
Phenothiazines
Scopolamine
Trimethobenzamide

Neural Tube Defects (prevention)
Folic Acid

Night Blindness
Beta Carotene

Obesity
Appetite Suppressants
Orlistat
Selective Serotonin Reuptake Inhibitors (SSRI's)
Sibutramine

Obsessive Compulsive Disorder
Antidepressants, Tricyclic
Selective Serotonin Reuptake Inhibitors (SSRI's)

Ocular Hypertension
Beta Adrenergic Blocking Agents (Ophthalmic)
Dorzolamide

Osteoarthritis – See Arthritis

Osteoporosis
Alendronate
Calcitonin
Calcium Supplements
Estrogens
Raloxifene
Sodium Fluoride
Vitamin D

Otitis Media – See Ear Infection

Overactive Bladder
Tolterodine

Overdose
Ipecac

Paget's Disease
Alendronate
Colchicine
Etidronate

Pain
Acetaminophen
Acetaminophen & Salicylates
Anti-Inflammatory Drugs Nonsteroidal (NSAID's)
Anti-Inflammatory Drugs Nonsteroidal, COX-2 Inhibitors
Aspirin
Barbiturates, Aspirin & Codeine
Butorphanol
Carbamazepine
Chlorzoxazone & Acetaminophen
Meprobamate & Aspirin
Narcotic Analgesics
Narcotic Analgesics & Acetaminophen
Narcotic Analgesics & Aspirin
Orphenadrine, Aspirin & Caffeine
Salicylates
Tramadol
Trazodone

Pain In Mouth
Anesthetics (Mucosal-Local)

Panic Disorder
Antidepressants, Tricyclic
Benzodiazepines
Monoamine Oxidase Inhibitors

Parasites
Anthelmintics
Pentamidine

Parkinson's Disease
Antidyskinetics
Antihistamines
Antivirals for Influenza
Bromocriptine
Carbidopa & Levodopa
Levodopa
Orphenadrine
Pergolide
Selegiline
Tolcapone

Parkinson's Tremors
Antihistamines
Pellagra
Niacin

Peyronie's Disease
Aminobenzoate Potassium

Photosensitivity
Beta Carotene Pneumonia
Cephalosporins
Clindamycin
Erythromycins
Fluoroquinolones
Loracarbef
Lincomycin
Linezolid
Loracarbef
Macrolide Antibiotics
Metronidazole
Penicillins
Penicillins & Beta Lactamase Inhibitors
Sulfonamides
Tetracyclines
Trimethoprim
Vancomycin

Poisoning
Charcoal Activated
Ipecac

Potassium Deficiency
Potassium Supplements

Premature Labor
Isoxsuprine
Ritodrine

Premenstrual Syndrome (PMS)
Antidepressants, Tricyclic
Anti-Inflammatory Drugs, Nonsteroidal (NSAID's)
Buspirone
Calcium Supplements

Contraceptives, Oral
Danazol
Pyridoxine (Vitamin B-6)
Selective Serotonin Reuptake Inhibitors (SSRI's)
Vitamin E

Pressure Sores
Benzoyl Peroxide

Psoriasis
Adrenocorticoids (Topical)
Anthralin
Calcipotriene
Coal Tar
Cyclosporine
Keratolytics
Methotrexate
Psoralens
Retinoids (Topical)
Retinoids (Oral)

Psychosis
Thiothixene

Psychotic Disorders
Carbamazepine
Clozapine
Haloperidol
Loxapine
Molindone
Olanzapine
Phenothiazines
Quetiapine
Risperidone
Thiothixene
Zisprasidone

Rashes – See Skin Disorders

Rectal Fissures
Anesthetics (Rectal)

Respiratory Syncytial Virus (RSV)
Ribavirin

Rheumatoid Arthritis – See Arthritis

Ricketts
Vitamin D

Ringworm – see Fungal Infections

Scabies
Pediculoides

Schizophrenia
Carbamazepine
Clozapine
Haloperidol
Molindone
Olanzapine
Phenothiazines
Quetiapine
Risperidone

Scleroderma
Aminobenzoate Potassium

Seizures – See Convulsions

Shingles
Antivirals (Topical)
Antivirals for Herpes Virus
Capsaicin

Sickle Cell Disease
Hydroxyurea

Sinusitis
Cephalosporins
Erythromycins
Macrolide Antibiotics
Penicillins
Penicillins & Beta Lactamase Inhibitors
Sulfonamides
Tetracyclines
Trimethoprim
Xylometazoline

Skin Disorders
Antibacterials (Topical)
Antibacterials, Antifungals (Topical)
Anesthetics (Topical)
Cyclophosphamide
Isotretinoin
Neomycin (Topical)
Retinoids (Topical)

Sleep Apnea
Antidepressants, Tricyclic
Progestins
Theophylline

Smoking Cessation
Bupropion
Clonidine
Nicotine

Sore Throat
Anesthetics (Mucosal-Local)
See also – Bacterial Infections

Sunburn
Anesthetics (Topical)

Swelling – See Fluid Retention

Thyroid Disorders – See Hyperthyroidism; Hypothyroidism

Tonsilitis
Cephalosporins
Macrolide Antibiotics

Tourette's Syndrome
Antidyskinetics
Haloperidol

Toxoplasmosis
Atovaquone

Transplantation, Organ (Antirejection)
Azathioprine
Cyclosporine
Immunosuppressive Agents

Tremors
Benzodiazepines
Beta-Adrenergic Blocking Agents

Trigeminal Neuralgia
Baclofen
Carbamazepine

Tuberculosis
Cycloserine
Ethionamide
Isoniazid
Rifamycins

Ulcers
Antacids
Anticholinergics
Bismuth Subsalicylate
Glycopyrrolate
Histamine H_2 Receptor Antagonists
Metronidazole
Proton Pump Inhibitors
Sodium Bicarbonate
Sucralfate
Tetracyclines

Ulcerative Colitis
Olsalazine
Sulfasalazine

Urethra Spasms
Clidinium
Propantheline

Urethritis
Erythromycins
Fluoroquinolones
Macrolide Antibiotics
Phenazopyridine
Sulfonamides & Phenazopyridine
Tetracyclines

Urinary Frequency
Oxybutynin
Tolterodine

Urinary Retention
Antimyasthenics
Bethanechol

Urinary Tract Infection
Acetohydroxamic Acid
Atropine, Hyoscyamine, Methenamine
Cephalosporins
Cinoxacin
Cycloserine
Flavoxate
Fluoroquinolones

Loracarbef
Methenamine
Nalidixic Acid
Nitrofurantoin
Penicillins
Penicillins & Beta Lactamase Inhibitors
Nalidixic Acid
Nitrofurantoin
Phenazopyridine
Sulfonamides
Trimethoprim
Tetracyclines

Urine Acidity
Citrates
Vitamin C

Uveitis
Anti-Inflammatory Drugs, Steroidal (Ophthalmic)

Vaginal Infections or Irritation
Clindamycin
Estrogens
Metronidazole
Progestins

Vaginal Yeast Infections
Antifungals (Vaginal)

Vertigo
Meclizine
Niacin

Virus Infections Of The Eye
Antivirals (Ophthalmic)

Vitamin Deficiency
Pantothenic Acid
Riboflavin
Vitamin A
Vitamin B-12
Vitamin C
Vitamin D
Vitamin E
Vitamin K

Vitiligo
Psoralens

Vomiting – See Nausea & Vomiting

Warts
Keratolytics
Retinoids (Topical)

Wilson's Disease
Penicillamine
Zinc Supplements

Worms
Anthelmintics

Zinc Deficiency
Zinc Supplements

Drug Charts

5-ALPHA REDUCTASE INHIBITORS

GENERIC AND BRAND NAMES

FINASTERIDE	DUTASTERIDE
Propecia	Duagen
Proscar	

BASIC INFORMATION

Habit forming? No
Prescription needed? Yes
Available as generic? No
Drug class: Dihydrotestosterone inhibitor

USES

- Treats noncancerous enlargement of the prostate gland in men (benign prostatic hypertrophy or BPH).
- Theoretically, may prevent the development of prostate cancer. Studies are ongoing.
- Treatment of male pattern hair loss in men only.

DOSAGE & USAGE INFORMATION

How to take:
Tablet or capsule—Swallow with liquid. If you can't swallow whole, crumble tablet and take with liquid or food.

When to take:
Once a day or as directed, with or without meals.

If you forget a dose:
Take as soon as you remember up to 2 hours late. If more than 2 hours, wait for next scheduled dose (don't double this dose).

What drug does:
Inhibits the enzyme needed for the conversion of testosterone to dihydrotestosterone. Dihydrotestosterone is required for the development of benign prostatic hypertrophy.

Continued next column

OVERDOSE

SYMPTOMS:
Effects unknown.
WHAT TO DO:
Overdose unlikely to threaten life. If person use much larger amount than prescribed or if accidentally swallowed, call doctor or poison center 1-800-222-1222 for instructions.

Time lapse before drug works:
- May require up to 6 months for full therapeutic effect for BPH.
- For treatment of hair loss, may not see any benefit for 3 months or more.

Don't take with:
Any other medicine without consulting your doctor or pharmacist, especially nonprescription decongestants.

POSSIBLE ADVERSE REACTIONS OR SIDE EFFECTS

SYMPTOMS	WHAT TO DO
Life-threatening:	
None expected.	
Common:	
None expected.	
Infrequent:	
Decreased volume of ejaculation, back or stomach pain, headache.	Continue. Call doctor when convenient.
Rare:	
• Impotence, decreased libido, breast enlargement and tenderness.	Continue. Call doctor when convenient.
• Allergic reaction (skin rash, swelling of lips).	Discontinue. Call doctor right away.

WARNINGS & PRECAUTIONS

Don't take if:

- You are allergic to dutasteride or finasteride.
- You are a female or a child.

Before you start, consult your doctor:

- If you have not had a blood test to check for prostate cancer.
- If your sexual partner is pregnant or may become pregnant.
- If you have a liver disorder.
- If you have reduced urinary flow.
- If you have large residual urinary volume.

Over age 60:
No special problems expected.

Pregnancy:

- Not recommended for women.
- Pregnant women should not handle the crushed tablets.
- Ask your doctor if you should avoid exposure to mate's semen if he takes finasteride.
- Risk category X (see page xviii).

Breast-feeding:
Not recommended for women.

Infants & children:
Not recommended.

Prolonged use:
Talk to your doctor about the need for follow-up medical examinations or laboratory studies to check the effectiveness of the treatment.

Skin & sunlight:
No special problems expected.

Driving, piloting or hazardous work:
No special problems expected.

Discontinuing:
Don't discontinue without medical advice.

Others:

- Advise any doctor or dentist whom you consult that you take this medicine.
- May affect results of some medical tests.
- For those who respond well, the drug must be continued indefinitely.

POSSIBLE INTERACTION WITH OTHER DRUGS

GENERIC NAME OR DRUG CLASS	COMBINED EFFECT
None expected.	

POSSIBLE INTERACTION WITH OTHER SUBSTANCES

INTERACTS WITH	COMBINED EFFECT
Alcohol:	No proven problems.
Beverages:	No proven problems.
Cocaine:	No proven problems.
Foods:	No proven problems.
Marijuana:	No proven problems.
Tobacco:	No proven problems.

ACARBOSE

BRAND NAMES

Precose

BASIC INFORMATION

Habit forming? No
Prescription needed? Yes
Available as generic? No
Drug class: Antihyperglycemic, antidiabetic

USES

Treatment for hyperglycemia (excess sugar in the blood) that cannot be controlled by diet alone in patients with type II non-insulin-dependent diabetes mellitus (NIDDM). May be used alone or in combination with other antidiabetic drugs.

DOSAGE & USAGE INFORMATION

How to take:
Tablet—Swallow with liquid. Take at the very beginning of a meal.

When to take:
Usually 3 times a day or as directed by doctor. Dosage may be increased at 4- to 8-week intervals until maximum benefits are achieved.

Continued next column

OVERDOSE

SYMPTOMS:

- **Symptoms of lactic acidosis (acid in the blood)—chills, diarrhea, severe muscle pain, sleepiness, slow heartbeat, breathing difficulty, unusual weakness.**
- **Symptoms of hypoglycemia (not a problem with acarbose used alone)—stomach pain, anxious feeling, cold sweats, chills, confusion, convulsions, cool pale skin, excessive hunger, nausea or vomiting, rapid heartbeat, nervousness, shakiness, unsteady walk, unusual weakness or tiredness, vision changes, unconsciousness.**

WHAT TO DO:

- **For mild low blood sugar symptoms, drink or eat something containing sugar right away.**
- **For more severe symptoms, dial 911 (emergency) or poison center 1-800-222-1222 for an ambulance or medical help. Then give first aid immediately.**
- **See emergency information on inside covers.**

If you forget a dose:
Take as soon as you remember. If it is almost time for the next dose, then skip the missed dose and wait for your next scheduled dose (don't double this dose).

What drug does:
Impedes the digestion and absorption of carbohydrates and their subsequent conversion into glucose, improving control of blood glucose, and may reduce the complications of diabetes. However, acarbose does not cure diabetes.

Time lapse before drug works:
May take several weeks for full effectiveness.

Don't take with:
Any other prescription or nonprescription drug without consulting your doctor or pharmacist.

POSSIBLE ADVERSE REACTIONS OR SIDE EFFECTS

SYMPTOMS	WHAT TO DO
Life-threatening: In case of overdose or low blood sugar, see previous column.	
Common: Diarrhea, stomach cramps, gas, bloating, feeling of fullness in stomach, nausea.	Continue. Call doctor when convenient.
Infrequent: None expected.	
Rare: Lactic acidosis or severe low blood sugar (see symptoms under Overdose).	Discontinue. Call doctor right away or seek emergency help.

WARNINGS & PRECAUTIONS

Don't take if:
You are allergic to acarbose.

Before you start, consult your doctor:
- If you have any kidney or liver disease or any heart or blood vessel disorder.
- If you have any chronic health problem.
- If you have an infection, illness or any condition that can cause low blood sugar.
- If you have a history of acid in the blood (metabolic acidosis or ketoacidosis).
- If you have inflammatory bowel disease or any other intestinal disorder.
- If you are allergic to any medication, food or other substance.

Over age 60:
No special problems expected. A lower starting dosage may be recommended by your doctor.

Pregnancy:
Decide with your doctor if drug benefits justify risks to unborn child. Risk category B (see page xviii).

Breast-feeding:
It is unknown if drug passes into milk. Avoid drug or discontinue nursing until you finish medicine. Consult doctor for advice on maintaining milk supply.

Infants & children:
Safety and efficacy have not been established. Use only under close medical supervision.

Prolonged use:
- Schedule regular doctor visits to determine if the drug is continuing to be effective in controlling the diabetes and to check for any problems in kidney function.
- You will most likely require an antidiabetic medicine for the rest of your life.
- You will need to test your blood glucose levels several times a day, or for some, once to several times a week.
- Acarbose may reduce absorption of iron, causing anemia. Discuss with your doctor.

Skin & sunlight:
No special problems expected.

Driving, piloting or hazardous work:
No special problems expected.

Discontinuing:
Don't discontinue without consulting your doctor even if you feel well. You can have diabetes without feeling any symptoms. Untreated diabetes can cause serious problems.

Others:
- Advise any doctor or dentist whom you consult that you take this medicine. Drug may interfere with the accuracy of some medical tests.
- Follow any special diet your doctor may prescribe. It can help control diabetes.
- Consult doctor if you become ill with vomiting or diarrhea.
- Use caution when exercising. Ask your doctor about an appropriate exercise program.
- Wear medical identification stating that you have diabetes and take this medication.
- Learn to recognize the symptoms of low blood sugar. You and your family need to know what to do if these symptoms occur.
- Have a glucagon kit and syringe in the event severe low blood sugar occurs.
- High blood sugar (hyperglycemia) may occur with diabetes. Ask your doctor about symptoms to watch for and treatment steps to take.
- Educate yourself about diabetes.

POSSIBLE INTERACTION WITH OTHER DRUGS

GENERIC NAME OR DRUG CLASS	COMBINED EFFECT
Amylase (Pancreatic enzyme)	Decreased acarbose effect.
Charcoal, activated	Decreased acarbose effect.
Hyperglycemia-causing medications*	Increased risk of hyperglycemia.
Metformin	Decreased acarbose effect. Increased risk of side effects.
Pancreatin (Pancreatic enzyme)	Decreased acarbose effect.

POSSIBLE INTERACTION WITH OTHER SUBSTANCES

INTERACTS WITH	COMBINED EFFECT
Alcohol:	May increase effect of acarbose. Avoid excessive amounts.
Beverages:	No special problems.
Cocaine:	No special problems.
Foods:	No special problems.
Marijuana:	No special problems.
Tobacco:	No special problems.

***See Glossary**

ACETAMINOPHEN

BRAND NAMES

See complete list of generic and brand names in the *Generic and Brand Name Directory*, page 862.

BASIC INFORMATION

Habit forming? No
Prescription needed? No
Available as generic? Yes
Drug class: Analgesic, fever reducer

USES

Treatment of mild to moderate pain and fever. Acetaminophen does not relieve redness, stiffness or swelling of joints or tissue inflammation. Use aspirin or other drugs for inflammation.

DOSAGE & USAGE INFORMATION

How to take:

- Tablet or capsule—Swallow with liquid.
- Effervescent granules—Dissolve granules in 4 oz. of cool water. Drink all the water.
- Elixir—Swallow with liquid.
- Suppositories—Remove wrapper and moisten suppository with water. Gently insert larger end into rectum. Push well into rectum with finger.
- Powder—Sprinkle over liquid, then swallow.

When to take:
As needed, no more often than every 3 hours.

If you forget a dose:
Take as soon as you remember. Wait 3 hours for next dose.

Continued next column

OVERDOSE

SYMPTOMS:
Stomach upset, irritability, sweating, diarrhea, loss of appetite, abdominal cramps, convulsions, coma.
WHAT TO DO:

- **Call your doctor or poison center 1-800-222-1222 for advice if you suspect overdose, even if not sure. Symptoms may not appear until damage has occurred.**
- **See emergency information on inside covers.**

What drug does:
May affect hypothalamus—part of brain that helps regulate body heat and receives body's pain messages.

Time lapse before drug works:
15 to 30 minutes. May last 4 hours.

Don't take with:

- Other drugs that contain acetaminophen. Too much acetaminophen can damage liver and kidneys.
- Any other medicine without consulting your doctor or pharmacist.

POSSIBLE ADVERSE REACTIONS OR SIDE EFFECTS

SYMPTOMS	WHAT TO DO
Life-threatening: In case of overdose, see previous column.	
Common: None expected.	
Infrequent: None expected.	
Rare: Extreme fatigue; rash, itch, hives; sore throat and fever; unexplained bleeding or bruising; blood in urine; painful, decreased or frequent urination; yellow skin or eyes.	Discontinue. Call doctor right away.

WARNINGS & PRECAUTIONS

Don't take if:
You are allergic to acetaminophen.

Before you start, consult your doctor:
If you have kidney disease or liver damage.

Over age 60:
Don't exceed recommended dose. You can't eliminate drug as efficiently as younger persons.

Pregnancy:
No proven harm to unborn child. Avoid if possible. Consult doctor. Risk category B (see page xviii).

Breast-feeding:
No proven harm to nursing infant.

Infants & children:
Use only under medical supervision.

Prolonged use:
- May affect blood system and cause anemia. Limit use to 5 days for children 12 and under, and 10 days for adults.
- Talk to your doctor about the need for follow-up medical examinations or laboratory studies to check liver function, kidney function.

Skin & sunlight:
No problems expected.

Driving, piloting or hazardous work:
Avoid if you feel drowsy. Otherwise, no restrictions.

Discontinuing:
Discontinue in 2 days if symptoms don't improve.

Others:
- May interfere with the accuracy of some medical tests.
- Advise any doctor or dentist whom you consult that you take this medicine (if you take it regularly).
- If your symptoms don't improve after 2 days' use. Call your doctor.

POSSIBLE INTERACTION WITH OTHER DRUGS

GENERIC NAME OR DRUG CLASS	COMBINED EFFECT
Anticoagulants, oral*	May increase anticoagulant effect. If combined frequently, prothrombin time should be monitored.
Aspirin and other salicylates*	Prolonged use of high doses of both drugs may lead to kidney disease.
Isoniazid	Increased risk of liver damage.
Nicotine	Increased effect of acetaminophen.

POSSIBLE INTERACTION WITH OTHER SUBSTANCES

INTERACTS WITH	COMBINED EFFECT
Alcohol:	Drowsiness; long-term use may cause toxic effect in liver.
Beverages:	None expected.
Cocaine:	None expected. However, cocaine may slow body's recovery. Avoid.
Foods:	None expected.
Marijuana:	Increased pain relief. However, marijuana may slow body's recovery. Avoid.
Tobacco:	None expected.

*See Glossary

ACETOHYDROXAMIC ACID (AHA)

BRAND NAMES

Lithostat

BASIC INFORMATION

Habit forming? No
Prescription needed? Yes
Available as generic? No
Drug class: Antibacterial (antibiotic), antiurolithic

USES

- Treatment for chronic urinary tract infections.
- Prevents formation of urinary tract stones. Will not dissolve stones already present.

DOSAGE & USAGE INFORMATION

How to take:
Tablet—Swallow with liquid. If you can't swallow whole, crumble tablet and take with liquid or food.

When to take:
At the same time each day, according to instructions on prescription label.

If you forget a dose:
Take as soon as you remember up to 2 hours late. If more than 2 hours, wait for next scheduled dose (don't double this dose).

What drug does:
Stops enzyme action that makes urine too alkaline. Alkaline urine favors bacterial growth and stone formation and growth.

Time lapse before drug works:
1 to 3 weeks.

Don't take with:
- Alcohol or iron.
- Any other medicine without consulting your doctor or pharmacist.

OVERDOSE

SYMPTOMS:
Loss of appetite, tremor, nausea, vomiting.
WHAT TO DO:
Overdose unlikely to threaten life. If person takes much larger amount than prescribed, call doctor, poison center 1-800-222-1222 or hospital emergency room for instructions.

POSSIBLE ADVERSE REACTIONS OR SIDE EFFECTS

SYMPTOMS	WHAT TO DO
Life-threatening:	
In case of overdose, see previous column.	
Common:	
Appetite loss, nausea, vomiting, anxiety, depression, mild headache, unusual tiredness.	Continue. Call doctor when convenient.
Infrequent:	
• Loss of coordination, slurred speech, severe headache, sudden change in vision, shortness of breath, clot or pain over a blood vessel, sudden chest pain, leg pain in calf (deep vein blood clot).	Discontinue. Seek emergency treatment.
• Rash on arms and face.	Continue. Call doctor when convenient.
Rare:	
• Sore throat, fever, unusual bleeding, bruising.	Discontinue. Call doctor right away.
• Hair loss.	Continue. Call doctor when convenient.

ACETOHYDROXAMIC ACID (AHA)

WARNINGS & PRECAUTIONS

Don't take if:
You have severe chronic kidney disease.

Before you start, consult your doctor:
- If you are anemic.
- If you have or have had phlebitis or thrombophlebitis.

Over age 60:
Adverse reactions and side effects may be more frequent and severe than in younger persons.

Pregnancy:
Studies inconclusive on harm to unborn child. Animal studies show fetal abnormalities. Don't use. Risk category X (see page xviii).

Breast-feeding:
Studies inconclusive. May have a potential for adverse reactions in nursing children. Avoid drug or discontinue nursing until you finish medicine. Consult doctor on maintaining milk supply.

Infants & children:
Not recommended. Safety and dosage have not been established.

Prolonged use:
Talk to your doctor about the need for follow-up medical examinations or laboratory studies to check blood pressure, liver function, kidney function, urinary pH.

Skin & sunlight:
No problems expected.

Driving, piloting or hazardous work:
Don't drive or pilot aircraft until you learn how medicine affects you. Don't work around dangerous machinery. Don't climb ladders or work in high places. Danger increases if you drink alcohol or take medicine affecting alertness and reflexes, such as antihistamines, tranquilizers, sedatives, pain medicines, narcotics and mind-altering drugs.

Discontinuing:
Don't discontinue without consulting doctor. Dose may require gradual reduction if you have taken drug for a long time. Doses of other drugs may also require adjustment.

Others:
No problems expected.

POSSIBLE INTERACTION WITH OTHER DRUGS

GENERIC NAME OR DRUG CLASS	COMBINED EFFECT
Iron	Decreased effects of both drugs.

POSSIBLE INTERACTION WITH OTHER SUBSTANCES

INTERACTS WITH	COMBINED EFFECT
Alcohol:	Severe skin rash common in many patients within 30 to 45 minutes after drinking alcohol.
Beverages:	None expected.
Cocaine:	None expected.
Foods:	None expected.
Marijuana:	None expected.
Tobacco:	None expected.

ADRENOCORTICOIDS (Nasal Inhalation)

GENERIC AND BRAND NAMES

BECLOMETHASONE (nasal)
- Beconase
- Beconase AQ
- Vancenase
- Vancenase AQ

BUDESONIDE (nasal)
- Rhinocort Aqua
- Rhinocort Nasal Inhaler
- Rhinocort Turbuhaler

DEXAMETHASONE (nasal)
- Dexacort Turbinaire

FLUNISOLIDE (nasal)
- Nasalide
- Nasarel
- Rhinalar

FLUTICASONE (nasal)
- Flonase
- Advair Diskus

MOMETASONE
- Nasonex

TRIAMCINOLONE
- Nasacort
- Nasacort AQ
- Tri-Nasal

BASIC INFORMATION

Habit forming? No
Prescription needed? Yes
Available as generic? Yes, for some
Drug class: Adrenocorticoid (nasal); anti-inflammatory (steroidal), nasal

USES

- Treats nasal allergy.
- Treats nasal polyps.
- Treats noninfectious inflammatory nasal conditions.

DOSAGE & USAGE INFORMATION

How to take:
- Read patient instruction sheet supplied with your prescription. Usually 1 or 2 sprays into each nostril every 12 hours.
- Save container for possible refills.

When to take:
At the same time each day, according to instructions on prescription label.

Continued next column

OVERDOSE

SYMPTOMS:
None expected.
WHAT TO DO:
Overdose unlikely to threaten life. If person takes much larger amount than prescribed, call doctor, poison center 1-800-222-1222 or hospital emergency room for instructions.

If you forget a dose:
Use as soon as you remember up to an hour late. If you remember more than an hour late, skip this dose. Don't double the next dose.

What drug does:
- Subdues inflammation by decreasing secretion of prostaglandins in cells of the lining of the nose and by inhibiting release of histamine.
- Very little, if any, of the nasal adrenocorticoid gets absorbed into the bloodstream.

Time lapse before drug works:
Usually 5 to 7 days, but may be as long as 2 to 3 weeks.

Don't take with:
Any other medicine without consulting your doctor or pharmacist.

POSSIBLE ADVERSE REACTIONS OR SIDE EFFECTS

SYMPTOMS	WHAT TO DO
Life-threatening: None expected.	
Common: Burning or dryness of nose, sneezing.	Continue. Call doctor when convenient.
Infrequent: Crusting inside the nose, nosebleed, sore throat, ulcers in nose, cough, dizziness, headache, hoarseness, nausea, runny nose, bloody mucus.	Discontinue. Call doctor right away.
Rare:	
• White patches in nose or throat.	Discontinue. Call doctor right away.
• Eye pain, wheezing respiration.	Discontinue. Seek emergency treatment.

WARNINGS & PRECAUTIONS

Don't take if:
You are allergic to cortisone or any cortisone-like medication.

Before you start, consult your doctor:
If you know you are allergic to any of the propellants in the spray. These include benzalkonium chloride, disodium acetate, phenylethanol, fluorocarbons, propylene glycol.

Over age 60:
No special problems expected.

Pregnancy:
Risk factors vary for drugs in this group. See category list on page xviii and consult doctor.

Breast-feeding:
Drug may pass into milk. Avoid drug or discontinue nursing until you finish medicine. Consult doctor on maintaining milk supply.

Infants & children:
Use only under medical supervision.

Prolonged use:
Not recommended.

Skin & sunlight:
No special problems expected.

Driving, piloting or hazardous work:
Don't drive or pilot aircraft until you learn how medicine affects you. Don't work around dangerous machinery. Don't climb ladders or work in high places. Danger increases if you drink alcohol or take medicine affecting alertness and reflexes.

Discontinuing:
No special problems expected.

Others:
Advise any doctor or dentist whom you consult that you use this medicine..

POSSIBLE INTERACTION WITH OTHER DRUGS

GENERIC NAME OR DRUG CLASS	COMBINED EFFECT
None expected.	

POSSIBLE INTERACTION WITH OTHER SUBSTANCES

INTERACTS WITH	COMBINED EFFECT
Alcohol:	None expected.
Beverages:	None expected.
Cocaine:	None expected.
Foods:	None expected.
Marijuana:	None expected.
Tobacco:	None expected.

ADRENOCORTICOIDS (Oral Inhalation)

GENERIC AND BRAND NAMES

BECLOMETHASONE (oral inhalation)
- Beclodisk
- Becloforte
- Beclovent
- Beclovent Rotacaps
- Vanceril

BUDESONIDE (oral inhalation)
- Pulmicort Nebuamp
- Pulmicort Turbuhaler

DEXAMETHASONE (oral inhalation)
- Decadron Respihaler

FLUNISOLIDE (oral inhalation)
- Aerobid
- Aerobid-M
- Bronalide

FLUTICASONE (oral inhalation)
- Flovent

TRIAMCINOLONE (oral inhalation)
- Azmacort

BASIC INFORMATION

Habit forming? No
Prescription needed? Yes
Available as generic? No
Drug class: Anti-inflammatory (inhalation), antiasthmatic

USES

Treatment for prevention of symptoms in patients with chronic bronchial asthma. Does not relieve the symptoms of an acute asthma attack.

DOSAGE & USAGE INFORMATION

How to take:
Oral inhaler—Follow instructions that come with your prescription or take as directed by your doctor. If you don't understand the instructions or have any questions, consult your doctor or pharmacist. Most effective if taken regularly. More effective if taken with a spacer. Talk with your doctor or pharmacist.

Continued next column

When to take:
Your doctor will determine the dosage amount and schedule that will help control the asthma symptoms and lessen risks of side effects. Usually 1 to 2 inhaled puffs 3 to 4 times a day is sufficient.

If you forget a dose:
Take as soon as you remember. Then spread out the remaining doses for that day at regularly spaced intervals.

What drug does:
Helps prevent inflammation in the lungs and breathing passages. May decrease progression of severe disease.

Time lapse before drug works:
1 to 4 weeks for the initial response and up to several months for full benefits.

Don't take with:
Any other medicine without consulting your doctor or pharmacist.

OVERDOSE

SYMPTOMS:
None expected.
WHAT TO DO:
Overdose unlikely to threaten life. If person takes much larger amount than prescribed, call doctor, poison center1-800-222-1222 or hospital emergency room for instructions.

POSSIBLE ADVERSE REACTIONS OR SIDE EFFECTS

SYMPTOMS	WHAT TO DO
Life-threatening: None expected.	
Common: Dry mouth, cough, throat irritation, hoarseness or other voice changes.	Continue. Call doctor when convenient.
Infrequent: Dry throat, headache, nausea, skin bruising, unpleasant taste, white curd-like patches in mouth or throat, pain when eating or swallowing (thrush).	Continue. Call doctor when convenient.
Rare: Increased wheezing; difficulty in breathing; pain, tightness or burning in chest; behavior changes (restlessness, nervousness, depression) with budesonide.	Continue, but call doctor right away.

ADRENOCORTICOIDS (Oral Inhalation)

WARNINGS & PRECAUTIONS

Don't use if:
You are allergic to any corticosteroids*.

Before you start, consult your doctor:
- If you have osteoporosis.
- If you have or have had tuberculosis.
- If you are taking oral corticosteroid drugs.

Over age 60:
No special problems expected.

Pregnancy:
Risk factors may vary for drugs in this group. See category list on page xviii and consult doctor.

Breast-feeding:
Unknown effect. Decide with your doctor if you should continue breast-feeding while using this drug.

Infants & children:
- Should be safe with regular low-dosage regimen. There have been a few reports that long-term use or higher doses may decrease growth rate or cause reduced adrenal gland function. Be sure you and your child's doctor discuss all benefits and risks of the drug.
- Children using large doses of this drug are more susceptible to infectious disease (chicken pox, measles). Avoid exposure to infected people and keep all immunizations up to date.

Prolonged use:
- Talk to your doctor about the need for follow-up medical examinations or laboratory studies to check adrenal function, growth and development in children, pulmonary function, and inhalation technique.
- The drug may lose its effectiveness. If this occurs, consult your doctor.

Skin & sunlight:
No special problems expected.

Driving, piloting or hazardous work:
No special problems expected.

Discontinuing:
Don't discontinue this drug after prolonged use without consulting doctor. Dosage may require a gradual reduction before stopping to avoid any withdrawal symptoms.

Others:
- Advise any doctor or dentist whom you consult that you use this medicine.
- Carry or wear identification to state that you use this medicine.
- Call your doctor if you have any injury, infection or other stress to your body.
- Take medicine only as directed. Do not increase or reduce dosage without doctor's approval.

POSSIBLE INTERACTION WITH OTHER DRUGS

GENERIC NAME OR DRUG CLASS	COMBINED EFFECT
None significant.	

POSSIBLE INTERACTION WITH OTHER SUBSTANCES

INTERACTS WITH	COMBINED EFFECT
Alcohol:	None expected.
Beverages:	None expected.
Cocaine:	Effects not known. Best to avoid.
Foods:	None expected.
Marijuana:	Effects not known. Best to avoid.
Tobacco:	Asthma patients should avoid.

*See Glossary

ADRENOCORTICOIDS (Systemic)

GENERIC AND BRAND NAMES

See complete list of generic and brand names in the *Generic and Brand Name Directory*, page 862.

BASIC INFORMATION

Habit forming? No
Prescription needed? Yes
Available as generic? Yes
Drug class: Corticosteroid, anti-inflammatory (steroidal), immunosuppressant

USES

- Used for their anti-inflammatory and immunosuppressive effect in the treatment of many different medical problems including some cancers.
- Treatment for some allergic diseases, blood disorders, kidney diseases, asthma and emphysema.
- Treatment for mild to moderate active crohn's disease.
- Replaces corticosteroid lost due to adrenal deficiencies.

DOSAGE & USAGE INFORMATION

How to take:
- Tablet, capsules or liquid—Swallow with liquid or food to lessen stomach irritation. If you can't swallow whole, crumble tablet or open capsules.
- Enema—Follow package instructions.

When to take:
At the same times each day. Take once-a-day or once-every-other-day doses in mornings.

If you forget a dose:
Take as soon as you remember up to 2 hours late. If more than 2 hours, wait for next scheduled dose (don't double this dose).

Continued next column

OVERDOSE

SYMPTOMS:
Severe headache or retained fluids, convulsions, heart failure.
WHAT TO DO:
- **Dial 911 (emergency) or poison center 1-800-222-1222 for an ambulance or medical help. Then give first aid immediately.**
- **See emergency information on inside covers.**

What drug does:
Decreases inflammatory responses. Suppresses immune response. Stimulates bone marrow.

Time lapse before drug works:
2 to 4 days.

Don't take with:
Any other prescription or nonpescription drug without consulting your doctor or pharmacist.

POSSIBLE ADVERSE REACTIONS OR SIDE EFFECTS

SYMPTOMS	WHAT TO DO
Life-threatening:	
Hives, rash, intense itching, faintness, swelling soon after a dose (anaphylaxis).	Seek emergency treatment immediately.
Common:	
Acne, indigestion, nausea, vomiting, gaseousness, headache, insomnia, dizziness, increased appetite, weight gain, poor wound healing, swollen legs or feet.	Continue. Call doctor when convenient.
Infrequent:	
• Black, bloody or tarry stool; various infections; decreased or blurred vision; fever.	Continue. Call doctor right away.
• Mood or emotional changes, insomnia, restlessness, frequent urination, round face, irregular menstrual periods, euphoria, muscle cramps or weakness, stomach or hip or shoulder pain, thirstiness, fatigue, loss of appetite (with triamcinolone).	Continue. Call doctor when convenient.
Rare:	
• Irregular heartbeat, convulsions, leg or thigh pain.	Continue. Call doctor right away.
• Skin rash, joint pain, unusual hair growth on face or body, hallucinations, confusion, excitement, darkened or lightened skin color, rectal problems with use of rectal products (irritation, blisters, bleeding).	Continue. Call doctor when convenient.

WARNINGS & PRECAUTIONS

Don't take if:
- You are allergic to any cortisone* drug.
- You have active case of tuberculosis, systemic fungal infection, herpes infection of eyes or peptic ulcer disease.

Before you start, consult your doctor:
If you have, or have had, heart disease, congestive heart failure, diabetes, AIDS, HIV infection, glaucoma, underactive or overactive thyroid, high blood pressure, myasthenia gravis, blood clots in legs or lungs, peptic ulcer disease, tuberculosis, recent or current chickenpox or measles, kidney or liver disease, esophagitis, cold sores, osteoporosis, systemic lupus erythematosus or hyperlipidemia.

Over age 60:
Adverse reactions and side effects may be more frequent and severe than in younger persons. Likely to aggravate edema, diabetes or ulcers. Likely to cause cataracts and osteoporosis (softening of the bones) with long term use.

Pregnancy:
Decide with your doctor if drug benefits justify risk to unborn child. Risk category C (see page xviii).

Breast-feeding:
Drug passes into milk. Avoid drug or discontinue nursing until you finish medicine. Consult doctor for advice on maintaining milk supply.

Infants & children:
Use only under close medical supervision.

Prolonged use:
- May lead to glaucoma, cataracts, diabetes, fragile bones and thin skin, growth retardation in children, functional dependence*.
- Talk to your doctor about the need for follow-up medical examinations or laboratory studies to check progress, blood pressure, serum electrolytes, stools for blood, other blood studies, eyes, growth in children.

Skin & sunlight:
No problems expected.

Driving, piloting or hazardous work:
No problems expected.

Discontinuing:
- Don't discontinue without doctor's advice until you complete prescribed dose, even though symptoms diminish or disappear.
- Drug dose needs to be gradually reduced after long-term therapy. Don't stop drug suddenly.
- Drug can affect your response to surgery, illness, injury or stress for 2 years after discontinuing. Tell anyone who takes medical care of you within 2 years about use of this drug.

Others:
- Avoid immunizations if possible.
- Resistance to infection is less while taking this medicine. Consult doctor if infection occurs.
- Consult doctor about sudden weight gain or swelling.
- Advise any doctor or dentist whom you consult that you take this medicine.
- May cause recurrence of tuberculosis.
- Can interfere with the accuracy of some medical tests.
- Wear or carry medical identification that indicates use of this drug.

POSSIBLE INTERACTION WITH OTHER DRUGS

GENERIC NAME OR DRUG CLASS	COMBINED EFFECT
Antacids*	Decreased effect of prednisone and dexamethasone.
Anticholinergics*	Possible glaucoma.
Anticoagulants*, oral	Decreased anti-coagulant effect.
Anticonvulsants, hydantoin*	Decreased adreno-corticoid effect.
Antidepressants, tricyclic*	Increased risk of mental side effects.
Antidiabetics*, oral	Decreased anti-diabetic effect.
Antihistamines*	Decreased adreno-corticoid effect.
Anti-inflammatory drugs, nonsteroidal (NSAIDs)*	Increased risk of ulcers. Increased adrenocorticoid effect.
Aspirin	Increased adreno-corticoid effect.

Continued on page 894

POSSIBLE INTERACTION WITH OTHER SUBSTANCES

INTERACTS WITH	COMBINED EFFECT
Alcohol:	Risk of stomach ulcers.
Beverages:	No proven problems.
Cocaine:	Overstimulation. Avoid.
Foods:	No proven problems.
Marijuana:	Decreased immunity.
Tobacco:	Increased adreno-corticoid effect.

***See Glossary**

ADRENOCORTICOIDS (Topical)

GENERIC AND BRAND NAMES

See complete list of generic and brand names in the *Generic and Brand Name Directory*, page 862.

BASIC INFORMATION

Habit forming? No
Prescription needed? For some
Available as generic? Yes
Drug class: Adrenocorticoid (topical)

USES

Relieves redness, swelling, itching, skin discomfort of hemorrhoids; insect bites; poison ivy, oak, sumac; soaps, cosmetics; jewelry; burns; sunburn; numerous skin rashes; eczema; discoid lupus erythematosus; swimmers' ear; sun poisoning; hair loss; scars; penphigus; psoriasis; pityriasis rosea.

DOSAGE & USAGE INFORMATION

How to use:

- Cream, lotion, ointment, gel—Apply small amount and rub in gently.
- Topical aerosol—Follow directions on container. Don't breathe vapors.
- Other forms—Follow directions on container.

When to use:
When needed or as directed. Don't use more often than directions allow.

If you forget an application:
Use as soon as you remember.

What drug does:
Reduces inflammation by affecting enzymes that produce inflammation.

Time lapse before drug works:
15 to 20 minutes.

Don't use with:
Any other medicine without consulting your doctor or pharmacist.

OVERDOSE

SYMPTOMS:
None expected.
WHAT TO DO:
If person swallows or inhales drug, call doctor, poison center 1-800-222-1222 or hospital emergency room for instructions.

POSSIBLE ADVERSE REACTIONS OR SIDE EFFECTS

SYMPTOMS	WHAT TO DO
Life-threatening: None expected.	
Common: None expected.	
Infrequent: Infection on skin with pain, redness, blisters, pus; skin irritation with burning, itching, blistering or peeling; acne-like skin eruptions.	Continue. Call doctor when convenient.
Rare: None expected.	

Note: Side effects are unlikely if topical adrenocorticoids are used in low doses for short periods of time. High doses for long periods can possibly cause the adverse reactions of cortisone, listed under ADRENOCORTICOIDS (Systemic).

WARNINGS & PRECAUTIONS

Don't take if:
You are allergic to any topical adrenocorticoid (cortisone) preparation.

Before you start, consult your doctor:
- If you plan pregnancy within medication period.
- If you have diabetes.
- If you have infection at treatment site.
- If you have stomach ulcer.
- If you have tuberculosis.

Over age 60:
Adverse reactions and side effects may be more frequent and severe than in younger persons, especially thinning of the skin.

Pregnancy:
Decide with your doctor whether drug benefits justify risk to unborn child. Risk category C (see page xviii).

Breast-feeding:
No problems expected.

Infants & children:
- Use only under medical supervision. Too much for too long can be absorbed into blood stream through skin and retard growth.
- For infants in diapers, avoid plastic pants or tight diapers.

Prolonged use:
- Increases chance of absorption into blood stream to cause side effects of oral cortisone drugs.
- May thin skin where used.
- Talk to your doctor about the need for follow-up medical examinations or laboratory studies to check complete blood counts (white blood cell count, platelet count, red blood cell count, hemoglobin, hematocrit), adrenal function.

Skin & sunlight:
Desoximetasone may cause rash or intensify sunburn in areas exposed to sun or ultraviolet light (photosensitivity reaction). Avoid overexposure. Notify doctor if reaction occurs.

Driving, piloting or hazardous work:
No problems expected.

Discontinuing:
May be unnecessary to finish medicine. Follow doctor's instructions.

Others:
- Don't use a plastic dressing longer than 2 weeks.
- Aerosol spray—Store in cool place. Don't use near heat or open flame or while smoking. Don't puncture, break or burn container.
- Don't use for acne or gingivitis.

POSSIBLE INTERACTION WITH OTHER DRUGS

GENERIC NAME OR DRUG CLASS	COMBINED EFFECT
Antibacterials* (topical)	Decreased antibiotic effect.
Antifungals* (topical)	Decreased antifungal effect.

POSSIBLE INTERACTION WITH OTHER SUBSTANCES

INTERACTS WITH	COMBINED EFFECT
Alcohol:	None expected.
Beverages:	None expected.
Cocaine:	None expected.
Foods:	None expected.
Marijuana:	None expected.
Tobacco:	None expected.

*See Glossary

ALENDRONATE

BRAND NAMES

Fosamax

BASIC INFORMATION

Habit forming? No
Prescription needed? Yes
Available as generic? No
Drug class: Osteoporosis therapy, bisphosphonate

USES

- Prevention and treatment of postmenopausal osteoporosis (thinning of bones) in females. Osteoporosis is a major cause of bone fractures.
- Treatment for Paget's disease of bone.

DOSAGE & USAGE INFORMATION

How to take:
Tablet—Swallow with a full glass of water (6 to 8 oz.). To help the medicine reach your stomach faster and to prevent throat irritation, don't lie down for 30 minutes after you take it.

When to take:
At the same time each day. Take in the morning at least 30 to 60 minutes before eating, drinking or taking any other medications.

If you forget a dose:
Skip the missed dose entirely, then resume schedule the next morning. Do not double this dose.

What drug does:
Slows down the loss of bone tissue and increases bone mass in women with osteoporosis. Osteoporosis is a progressive disease in which bone breakdown increases faster than bone formation.

Time lapse before drug works:
Up to 6 months or longer.

Continued next column

OVERDOSE

SYMPTOMS:
Increased severity of heartburn, stomach cramps, throat irritation.
WHAT TO DO:
Overdose unlikely to threaten life. If person takes much larger amount than prescribed, call doctor, poison center 1-800-222-1222 or hospital emergency room for instructions.

Don't take with:

- Any other prescription or nonprescription drug without consulting your doctor or pharmacist.
- Any other medication at the same time as alendronate. Wait 30 minutes.

POSSIBLE ADVERSE REACTIONS OR SIDE EFFECTS

SYMPTOMS	WHAT TO DO
Life-threatening: None expected.	
Common: Stomach pain.	Continue. Call doctor when convenient.
Infrequent: Bone or muscle pain, nausea, constipation or diarrhea, gas, bloated feeling, heartburn, throat pain or irritation, swallowing difficulty, headache.	Continue. Call doctor when convenient.
Rare: Skin rash.	Continue. Call doctor when convenient.

WARNINGS & PRECAUTIONS

Don't take if:
You are allergic to alendronate or etidronate.

Before you start, consult your doctor:
- If you are allergic to any medication, food or other substance.
- If you currently have a gastrointestinal problem.
- If you have low blood levels of calcium (hypocalcemia) or vitamin D deficiency.
- If you have kidney problems.

Over age 60:
No special problems expected.

Pregnancy:
Normally not used in premenopausal women. Risk category C (see page xviii).

Breast-feeding:
Unknown if drug passes into milk. Avoid drug or discontinue nursing until you finish medicine. Consult doctor for advice on maintaining milk supply.

Infants & children:
Not recommended for this age group.

Prolonged use:
- No special problems expected. Long-term safety has not been established, and medical studies are continuing.
- Visit your doctor regularly to determine if the drug is continuing to control bone loss and to monitor your calcium levels.

Skin & sunlight:
No special problems expected.

Driving, piloting or hazardous work:
No special problems expected.

Discontinuing:
Don't discontinue without your doctor's approval.

Others:
- In addition to taking the drug, weight-bearing exercise and adequate dietary intake of calcium and vitamin D are essential in preventing bone loss. Dietary supplements of 1000 mg elemental calcium and 400 I.U. vitamin D daily may be recommended by your doctor.
- Advise any doctor or dentist whom you consult that you take this medicine.
- May affect the results of some medical tests.
- Smoking and alcohol consumption are risk factors for osteoporosis and should be discontinued.

POSSIBLE INTERACTION WITH OTHER DRUGS

GENERIC NAME OR DRUG CLASS	COMBINED EFFECT
Antacids*	Decreased effect of alendronate. Take 30 minutes after alendronate.
Aspirin-containing products	Increased risk of stomach irritation.
Calcium supplements*	Decreased effect of alendronate. Take 30 minutes after alendronate.
Hormone replacement therapy*	Unknown effect. Not recommended.
Vitamin supplements	Decreased effect of alendronate. Take 30 minutes after alendronate.

POSSIBLE INTERACTION WITH OTHER SUBSTANCES

INTERACTS WITH	COMBINED EFFECT
Alcohol:	No special problems expected, but alcohol is a risk factor for osteoporosis.
Beverages: Any beverage other than plain water.	Decreased effect of alendronate. Wait 30 minutes after taking alendronate.
Cocaine:	No special problems expected.
Foods: Any food.	Decreased effect of alendronate. Wait 30 minutes after taking alendronate.
Marijuana:	No special problems expected.
Tobacco:	No special problems expected, but smoking is a risk factor for osteoporosis.

*See Glossary

ALLOPURINOL

BRAND NAMES

Alloprin
Apo-Allopurinol
Lopurin
Novopural
Purinol
Zyloprim

BASIC INFORMATION

Habit forming? No
Prescription needed? Yes
Available as generic? Yes
Drug class: Antigout

USES

- Treatment for chronic gout.
- Prevention of kidney stones caused by uric acid.

DOSAGE & USAGE INFORMATION

How to take:
Tablet—Swallow with liquid or food to lessen stomach irritation.

When to take:
At the same times each day.

If you forget a dose:
- 1 dose per day—Take as soon as you remember up to 6 hours late. If more than 6 hours, wait for next scheduled dose (don't double this dose).
- More than 1 dose per day—Take as soon as you remember up to 3 hours late. If more than 3 hours, wait for next scheduled dose (don't double this dose).

What drug does:
Slows formation of uric acid by inhibiting enzyme (xanthine oxidase) activity.

Time lapse before drug works:
Reduces blood uric acid in 1 to 3 weeks. May require 6 months to prevent acute gout attacks.

Don't take with:
Any other medicine without consulting your doctor or pharmacist.

OVERDOSE

SYMPTOMS:
None expected.
WHAT TO DO:
Overdose unlikely to threaten life. If person takes much larger amount than prescribed, call doctor, poison center 1-800-222-1222 or hospital emergency room for instructions.

POSSIBLE ADVERSE REACTIONS OR SIDE EFFECTS

SYMPTOMS	WHAT TO DO
Life-threatening:	
None expected.	
Common:	
Rash, hives, itch.	Discontinue. Call doctor right away.
Infrequent:	
• Jaundice (yellow skin or eyes.)	Discontinue. Call doctor right away.
• Drowsiness, diarrhea, stomach pain, nausea or vomiting without other symptoms, headache.	Continue. Call doctor when convenient.
Rare:	
• Sore throat, fever, unusual bleeding or bruising.	Discontinue. Call doctor right away.
• Numbness, tingling, pain in hands or feet.	Continue. Call doctor when convenient.

WARNINGS & PRECAUTIONS

Don't take if:
You are allergic to allopurinol.

Before you start, consult your doctor:
If you have had liver or kidney problems.

Over age 60:
Adverse reactions and side effects may be more frequent and severe than in younger persons.

Pregnancy:
Decide with your doctor whether drug benefits justify risk to unborn child. Risk category C (see page xviii).

Breast-feeding:
Drug passes into milk. Avoid drug or discontinue nursing. Consult doctor for advice on maintaining milk supply.

Infants & children:
Not recommended.

Prolonged use:
Talk to your doctor about the need for follow-up medical examinations or laboratory studies to check liver function, kidney function, complete blood counts (white blood cell count, platelet count, red blood cell count, hemoglobin, hematocrit), and serum uric-acid determinations.

Skin & sunlight:
No problems expected.

Driving, piloting or hazardous work:
Avoid if you feel drowsy. Use may disqualify you for piloting aircraft.

Discontinuing:
Don't discontinue without doctor's advice until you complete prescribed dose, even though symptoms diminish or disappear.

Others:
Acute gout attacks may increase during first weeks of use. If so, consult doctor about additional medicine.

POSSIBLE INTERACTION WITH OTHER DRUGS

GENERIC NAME OR DRUG CLASS	COMBINED EFFECT
Amoxicillin	Likely skin rash.
Ampicillin	Likely skin rash.
Anticoagulants, oral*	May increase anticoagulant effect.
Antidiabetics, oral*	Increased uric acid elimination.
Azathioprine	Greatly increased azathioprine effect.
Chlorpropamide	May increase chlorpropamide effect.
Chlorthalidone	Decreased all opurinol effect.
Cyclophosphamide	Increased cyclophosphamide toxicity.
Diuretics, thiazide*	Decreased allopurinol effect.
Ethacrynic acid	Decreased allopurinol effect.
Furosemide	Decreased allopurinol effect.
Indapamide	Decreased allopurinol effect.
Iron supplements*	Excessive accumulation of iron in tissues.
Mercaptopurine	Increased mercaptopurine effect.
Metolazone	Decreased allopurinol effect.
Probenecid	Increased allopurinol effect.
Theophylline	May increase theophylline effect.

POSSIBLE INTERACTION WITH OTHER SUBSTANCES

INTERACTS WITH	COMBINED EFFECT
Alcohol:	None expected, but may impair management of gout.
Beverages:	Caffeine drinks. Decreased allopurinol effect.
Cocaine:	Decreased allopurinol effect. Avoid.
Foods:	None expected. Low-purine diet* recommended.
Marijuana:	Occasional use—None expected. Daily use—Possible increase in uric acid level.
Tobacco:	None expected.

*See Glossary

ALPHA ADRENERGIC RECEPTOR BLOCKERS

GENERIC AND BRAND NAMES

DOXAZOSIN	**TAMSULOSIN**
Cardura	Flomax
PRAZOSIN	**TERAZOSIN**
Minipress	Hytrin
Minizide	

BASIC INFORMATION

Habit forming? No
Prescription needed? Yes
Available as generic? Yes, for some
Drug class: Antihypertensive

USES

- Treatment for high blood pressure.
- May improve congestive heart failure.
- Treatment for Raynaud's disease.
- Treatment for benign prostatic hyperplasia.

DOSAGE & USAGE INFORMATION

How to take:
Tablet or capsule—Swallow with liquid. If you can't swallow whole, crumble tablet or open capsule and take with liquid or food.

When to take:
At the same times each day.

If you forget a dose:
Take as soon as you remember up to 2 hours late. If more than 2 hours, wait for next scheduled dose (don't double this dose).

Continued next column

OVERDOSE

SYMPTOMS:
Extreme weakness; rapid or irregular heartbeat; loss of consciousness; cold, sweaty skin; weak, rapid pulse; coma.

WHAT TO DO:
- **Dial 911 (emergency) or poison center 1-800-222-1222 for an ambulance or medical help. Then give first aid immediately.**
- **If patient is unconscious and not breathing, give mouth-to-mouth breathing. If there is no heartbeat, use cardiac massage and mouth-to-mouth breathing (CPR). Don't try to make patient vomit. If you can't get help quickly, take patient to nearest emergency facility.**
- **See emergency information on inside covers.**

What drug does:
Expands and relaxes blood vessel walls to lower blood pressure.

Time lapse before drug works:
30 minutes.

Don't take with:
Any other medicine without consulting your doctor or pharmacist.

POSSIBLE ADVERSE REACTIONS OR SIDE EFFECTS

SYMPTOMS	WHAT TO DO
Life-threatening: In case of overdose, see previous column.	
Common: Headache, dizziness.	Continue. Call doctor when convenient.
Infrequent: • Rash or itchy skin, blurred vision, shortness of breath, difficulty breathing, chest pain, rapid heartbeat.	Discontinue. Call doctor right away.
• Appetite loss, constipation or diarrhea, abdominal pain, nausea, vomiting, fluid retention, joint or muscle aches, tiredness, weakness and faintness when arising from bed or chair.	Continue. Call doctor when convenient.
• Headache, irritability, depression, dry mouth, stuffy nose, increased urination, drowsiness.	Continue. Tell doctor at next visit.
Rare: Decreased sexual function, numbness or tingling in hands or feet.	Continue. Call doctor when convenient.

ALPHA ADRENERGIC RECEPTOR BLOCKERS

WARNINGS & PRECAUTIONS

Don't take if:
You are allergic to alpha adrenergic receptor blockers.

Before you start, consult your doctor:
- If you experience lightheadedness or fainting with other antihypertensive drugs.
- If you are easily depressed.
- If you have impaired brain circulation or have had a stroke.
- If you will have surgery within 2 months, including dental surgery, requiring general or spinal anesthesia.
- If you have coronary heart disease (with or without angina).
- If you have kidney disease or impaired liver function.

Over age 60:
Begin with no more than 1 mg. per day for first 3 days. Increases should be gradual and supervised by your doctor. Don't stand while taking. Sudden changes in position may cause falls. Sit or lie down promptly if you feel dizzy. If you have impaired brain circulation or coronary heart disease, excessive lowering of blood pressure should be avoided. Report problems to your doctor immediately.

Pregnancy:
Risk factors vary for drugs in this group. See category page xviii and consult doctor.

Breast-feeding:
No proven problems. Consult doctor.

Infants & children:
Not recommended.

Prolonged use:
Talk to your doctor about the need for follow-up medical examinations or laboratory studies.

Skin & sunlight:
No problems expected.

Driving, piloting or hazardous work:
Don't drive or pilot aircraft until you learn how medicine affects you. Don't work around dangerous machinery. Don't climb ladders or work in high places.

Discontinuing:
Don't discontinue without doctor's advice until you complete prescribed dose, even though symptoms diminish or disappear.

Others:
- First dose likely to cause dizziness or lightheadedness. Take drug at night and get out of bed slowly next morning.
- Advise any doctor or dentist whom you consult that you take this medicine.
- May affect the results in some medical tests.

POSSIBLE INTERACTION WITH OTHER DRUGS

GENERIC NAME OR DRUG CLASS	COMBINED EFFECT
Amphetamines*	Decreased alpha adrenergic blocker effect.
Antihypertensives, other*	Increased antihypertensive effect. Dosages may require adjustments.
Anti-inflammatory drugs, nonsteroidal (NSAIDs)*	Decreased effect of alpha adrenergic blocker.
Estrogen	Decreased effect of alpha adrenergic blocker.
Sympathomimetics*	Decreased effect of alpha adrenergic blocker.

POSSIBLE INTERACTION WITH OTHER SUBSTANCES

INTERACTS WITH	COMBINED EFFECT
Alcohol:	Excessive blood pressure drop.
Beverages:	None expected.
Cocaine:	Increased risk of heart block and high blood pressure.
Foods:	None expected.
Marijuana:	Possible fainting. Avoid.
Tobacco:	Possible spasm of coronary arteries. Avoid.

ALPROSTADIL

BRAND NAMES

CaverjectMuse

BASIC INFORMATION

Habit forming? No
Prescription needed? Yes
Available as generic? No
Drug class: Impotence therapy

USES

Treatment for impotence in some men who have erectile dysfunction due to neurologic, vascular, psychological or mixed causes.

DOSAGE & USAGE INFORMATION

How to use:

- Injection—The first injection will be given in the doctor's office to determine proper dosage and to train you in preparing and self-injecting the drug. When using it at home, follow the instructions provided with the prescription or use as directed by your doctor to inject drug into the penis.
- Intraurethral—Use as a single dose suppository 10 to 30 minutes prior to intercourse.

When to take:
Usually 10 to 30 minutes prior to sexual intercourse. Do not use injection more than 3 times in one week, and do not use more than once in a 24-hour period. Do not use more than 2 suppositories in one 24-hour period.

If you forget a dose:
Not used on a scheduled basis.

What drug does:
Increases the blood flow into the penis and decreases the blood flow from the penis. The change in blood flow causes the penis to swell and elongate.

Continued next column

OVERDOSE

SYMPTOMS:
Prolonged penile erection.
WHAT TO DO:
Overdose unlikely to threaten life. If someone uses larger amount than prescribed, call doctor, poison center 1-800-222-1222 or hospital emergency room for instructions.

Time lapse before drug works:
5 to 20 minutes. Erections may last up to 60 minutes.

Don't take with:
Any other medication without consulting your doctor or pharmacist.

POSSIBLE ADVERSE REACTIONS OR SIDE EFFECTS

SYMPTOMS	WHAT TO DO
Life-threatening: None expected.	
Common:	
• Pain at site of injection, aching or burning pain during erection.	Discontinue. Call doctor when convenient.
• Pinching sensation at injection site.	Continue. Tell doctor at next visit.
Infrequent: None expected.	
Rare:	
• Erection lasting more than 4 hours is not priapism; (priapism is defined as an erection lasting more than 6 hours). Could cause permanent damage to the penis.	Call doctor right away or seek emergency care.
• Bruising or bleeding at site of injection; redness, swelling, tenderness, lumpiness, itching, rash, irritation, strange feeling, numbness or curving of the erect penis; slight bleeding from urethra, swelling of leg veins, dizziness, fainting, rapid pulse. Female partners may have mild vaginal itching or burning.	Discontinue. Call doctor when convenient.

WARNINGS & PRECAUTIONS

Don't use if:
You are allergic to alprostadil or you have been advised not to have sex.

Before you start, consult your doctor:
- If you have liver disease.
- If you have sickle cell anemia or trait.
- If you have multiple myeloma or leukemia.
- If you have a penile implant or any type of penile malformation.
- If you are allergic to any other medications.
- If you have a history of priapism (prolonged penile erection).

Over age 60:
Effects on this age group are variable. Consult doctor.

Pregnancy:
Not used by females. Men should not use the product to have sexual intercourse with a pregnant woman unless the couple uses a condom barrier.

Breast-feeding:
Not used by females.

Infants & children:
Not used in this age group.

Prolonged use:
Have regular checkups with your doctor while using this drug to determine the effectiveness of the treatment and to check for any penile problems.

Skin & sunlight:
No special problems expected.

Driving, piloting or hazardous work:
No special problems expected.

Discontinuing:
No special problems expected.

Others:
- Don't increase dosage or frequency of use without your doctor's approval.
- Follow label instructions, and dispose of all needles properly after use. Do not reuse or share needles.
- The injection of this drug provides no protection from sexually transmitted diseases. Other protective measures, such as condoms, should be used when necessary to prevent the spread of sexually transmitted diseases.
- Slight bleeding may occur at injection site. Apply pressure if this occurs. If bleeding persists, consult doctor.

POSSIBLE INTERACTION WITH OTHER DRUGS

GENERIC NAME OR DRUG CLASS	COMBINED EFFECT
None significant.	

POSSIBLE INTERACTION WITH OTHER SUBSTANCES

INTERACTS WITH	COMBINED EFFECT
Alcohol:	No special problems expected.
Beverages:	No special problems expected.
Cocaine:	No special problems expected.
Foods:	No special problems expected.
Marijuana:	No special problems expected.
Tobacco:	No special problems expected.

*See Glossary

AMINOBENZOATE POTASSIUM

BRAND NAMES

KPAB
Potaba
Potaba Envules
Potaba Powder
Potassium Aminobenzoate
Potassium Para-aminobenzoate

BASIC INFORMATION

Habit forming? No
Prescription needed? Yes
Available as generic? No
Drug class: Antifibrosis

USES

Reduces inflammation and relieves contractions in tissues lying under the skin that have become tight from such disorders as dermatomyositis, Peyronie's disease, scleroderma, pemphigus, morphea.

DOSAGE & USAGE INFORMATION

How to take:

- Tablets—Dissolve in liquid or take with food to prevent stomach upset.
- Capsules—Take with full glass of liquid.
- Oral solution—Swallow with liquid to lessen stomach upset.
- Powder—Mix with liquid.

When to take:
At the same times each day, according to instructions on prescription label. Usually taken with meals and at bedtime with a snack.

If you forget a dose:
Take as soon as you remember up to 2 hours late. If more than 2 hours, wait for next scheduled dose (don't double this dose).

What drug does:
May increase ability of diseased tissues to use oxygen.

Continued next column

OVERDOSE

SYMPTOMS:
Nausea, vomiting.
WHAT TO DO:
Overdose unlikely to threaten life. If person takes much larger amount than prescribed, call doctor, poison center 1-800-222-1222 or hospital emergency room for instructions.

Time lapse before drug works:
May require 3 to 10 months for improvement to begin.

Don't take with:
Any other medicine without consulting your doctor or pharmacist.

POSSIBLE ADVERSE REACTIONS OR SIDE EFFECTS

SYMPTOMS	WHAT TO DO
Life-threatening: None expected.	
Common: Appetite loss, nausea, rash, fever.	Continue. Call doctor when convenient.
Infrequent:	
• Low blood sugar (hunger, anxiety, cold sweats, rapid pulse).	Discontinue. Seek emergency treatment. (Note: Take sugar or honey on the way to emergency room).
• Sore throat with fever and chills.	Discontinue. Call doctor right away.
Rare: None expected.	

WARNINGS & PRECAUTIONS

Don't take if:
You are allergic to aminobenzoate potassium or para-aminobenzoic acid (PABA).

Before you start, consult your doctor:
- If you have low blood sugar.
- If you have diabetes mellitus.
- If you have kidney disease.

Over age 60:
Adverse reactions and side effects may be more frequent and severe than in younger persons, particularly low blood sugar.

Pregnancy:
Risk factor not designated. See category list on page xviii and consult doctor.

Breast-feeding:
Unknown effect. Consult doctor.

Infants & children:
Not recommended. Safety and dosage have not been established.

Prolonged use:
Talk to your doctor about the need for follow-up medical examinations or laboratory studies to check complete blood counts (white blood cell count, platelet count, red blood cell count, hemoglobin, hematocrit).

Skin & sunlight:
No problems expected.

Driving, piloting or hazardous work:
No problems expected.

Discontinuing:
No problems expected.

Others:
- Advise any doctor or dentist whom you consult that you take this medicine.
- If you become acutely ill and cannot eat well for even a short while, tell your doctor. These circumstances can lead to low blood sugar, and dosage may need adjustment.

POSSIBLE INTERACTION WITH OTHER DRUGS

GENERIC NAME OR DRUG CLASS	COMBINED EFFECT
Dapsone	Decreased dapsone effect.
Salicylates*	May increase salicylate blood level.
Sulfa drugs* (sulfonamides)	Decreased sulfa effect.

POSSIBLE INTERACTION WITH OTHER SUBSTANCES

INTERACTS WITH	COMBINED EFFECT
Alcohol:	None expected.
Beverages:	None expected.
Cocaine:	None expected.
Foods:	None expected.
Marijuana:	None expected.
Tobacco:	None expected.

***See Glossary**

AMINOGLUTETHIMIDE

BRAND NAMES

Cytadren

BASIC INFORMATION

Habit forming? No
Prescription needed? Yes
Available as generic? No
Drug class: Antiadrenal, antineoplastic

USES

- Treats Cushing's syndrome.
- Treats breast malignancies.

DOSAGE & USAGE INFORMATION

How to take:
Tablets—Swallow with liquid. If you can't swallow whole, crumble tablet and take with liquid or food. Instructions to take on empty stomach mean 1 hour before or 2 hours after eating.

When to take:
Follow doctor's instructions exactly.

If you forget a dose:
Take as soon as you remember up to 2 hours late. If more than 2 hours, wait for next scheduled dose (don't double this dose).

What drug does:
Suppresses adrenal cortex.

Time lapse before drug works:
1 to 2 hours.

Don't take with:
Any other medicines (including over-the-counter drugs such as cough and cold medicines, laxatives, antacids, diet pills, caffeine, nose drops or vitamins) without consulting your doctor.

OVERDOSE

SYMPTOMS:
None expected.
WHAT TO DO:
Overdose unlikely to threaten life. If person takes much larger amount than prescribed, call doctor, poison center 1-800-222-1222 or hospital emergency room for instructions.

POSSIBLE ADVERSE REACTIONS OR SIDE EFFECTS

SYMPTOMS	WHAT TO DO
Life-threatening: None expected.	
Common: Skin rash on face and hands.	Continue. Tell doctor at next visit.
Infrequent: • Dizziness, drowsiness, unexplained fatigue, low back pain, pain on urinating, clumsiness, unusual eye movements, appetite loss.	Discontinue. Call doctor right away.
• Vomiting, skin darkening, depression, headache, muscle pain.	Continue. Call doctor when convenient.
Rare: Unusual bleeding or bruising.	Discontinue. Call doctor right away.

WARNINGS & PRECAUTIONS

Don't take if:
- You have recently been exposed to chicken pox.
- You have shingles (herpes zoster).

Before you start, consult your doctor:
- If you have decreased thyroid function (hypothyroidism).
- If you have any form of infection.

Over age 60:
Adverse reactions and side effects may be more frequent and severe than in younger persons. You may need smaller doses for shorter periods of time.

Pregnancy:
Risk category D (see page xviii).

Breast-feeding:
Effect not documented. Consult your doctor.

Infants & children:
Effect not documented. Consult your doctor.

Prolonged use:
Talk to your doctor about the need for follow-up medical examinations or laboratory studies to check thyroid function, liver function, serum electrolytes (sodium potassium, chloride) and blood pressure.

Skin & sunlight:
No problems expected.

Driving, piloting or hazardous work:
No problems expected.

Discontinuing:
No special problems expected.

Others:
- Advise any doctor or dentist whom you consult that you take this medicine.
- May affect results in some medical tests.
- May cause decreased thyroid function.

POSSIBLE INTERACTION WITH OTHER DRUGS

GENERIC NAME OR DRUG CLASS	COMBINED EFFECT
Anticoagulants*	Decreased anti-coagulant effect.
Clozapine	Toxic effect on the central nervous system.
Cortisone-like drugs*	Decreased cortisone effects.
Dexamethasone	Dexamethasone effect decreased by half.
Trilostane	Too much decrease in adrenal function.

POSSIBLE INTERACTION WITH OTHER SUBSTANCES

INTERACTS WITH	COMBINED EFFECT
Alcohol:	Increased stomach irritation.
Beverages: Coffee, tea, cocoa.	Increased stomach irritation.
Cocaine:	No proven problems.
Foods:	No proven problems.
Marijuana:	No proven problems.
Tobacco:	No proven problems.

***See Glossary**

AMIODARONE

BRAND NAMES

Cordarone

BASIC INFORMATION

Habit forming? No
Prescription needed? Yes
Available as generic? No
Drug class: Antiarrhythmic

USES

Prevents and treats life-threatening heartbeat irregularities involving both the large chambers of the heart (auricles and ventricles).

DOSAGE & USAGE INFORMATION

How to take:
Tablets—Swallow whole with liquid or food to lessen stomach irritation. If you can't swallow whole, crumble tablet and take with liquid or food.

When to take:
According to prescription instructions.

If you forget a dose:
Skip this dose and resume regular schedule. Do not double the next dose. If you forget 2 doses or more, consult your doctor.

What drug does:
- Slows nerve impulses in the heart.
- Makes heart muscle fibers less responsive to abnormal electrical impulses arising in the electrical regulatory system of the heart.

Continued next column

OVERDOSE

SYMPTOMS:
Irregular heartbeat, loss of consciousness, seizures.
WHAT TO DO:
- **Dial 911 (emergency) or poison center 1-800-222-1222 for an ambulance or medical help. Then give first aid immediately.**
- **If patient is unconscious and not breathing, give mouth-to-mouth breathing. If there is no heartbeat, use cardiac massage and mouth-to-mouth breathing (CPR). Don't try to make patient vomit. If you can't get help quickly, take patient to nearest emergency facility.**
- **See emergency information on inside covers.**

Time lapse before drug works:
2 to 3 days to 2 to 3 months.

Don't take with:
Any other medicine without consulting your doctor or pharmacist.

POSSIBLE ADVERSE REACTIONS OR SIDE EFFECTS

SYMPTOMS	WHAT TO DO
Life-threatening:	
Shortness of breath, difficulty breathing, cough.	Discontinue. Seek emergency treatment.
Common:	
• Walking difficulty, fever, numbness or tingling in hands or feet, shakiness, weakness in arms and legs.	Discontinue. Call doctor right away.
• Constipation, headache, appetite loss, nausea, vomiting.	Continue. Call doctor when convenient.
Infrequent:	
• Skin color change to blue-gray, blurred vision, cold feeling, dry eyes, nervousness, scrotum swelling or pain, insomnia, swollen feet and ankles, fast or slow heartbeat, eyes hurt in light, weight gain or loss, sweating.	Discontinue. Call doctor right away.
• Bitter or metallic taste, diminished sex drive, dizziness, flushed face, coldness and unusual tiredness.	Continue. Call doctor when convenient.
Rare:	
Jaundice, skin rash.	Discontinue. Call doctor right away.

WARNINGS & PRECAUTIONS

Don't take if:
You are allergic to amiodarone.

Before you start, consult your doctor:
- If you have liver, kidney or thyroid disease.
- If you have heart disease other than coronary artery disease.

Over age 60:
- Adverse reactions and side effects may be more frequent and severe than in younger persons. Ask about smaller doses.
- Pain in legs (while walking) considerably more likely.

Pregnancy:
Risk category D (see page xviii).

Breast-feeding:
Drug passes into milk. Avoid drug or discontinue nursing until you finish medicine. Consult doctor for advice on maintaining milk supply.

Infants & children:
Safety not established. Use only under close medical supervision.

Prolonged use:
- Blue-gray discoloration of skin may appear.
- Don't discontinue without consulting doctor. Dose may require gradual reduction if you have taken drug for a long time. Doses of other drugs may also require adjustment.
- Talk to your doctor about the need for follow-up medical examinations or laboratory studies to check ECG*, SGPT*, serum alkaline phosphatase, SGOT*, thyroid function.

Skin & sunlight:
May cause rash or intensify sunburn in areas exposed to sun or ultraviolet light (photosensitivity reaction). Avoid overexposure. Notify doctor if reaction occurs.

Driving, piloting or hazardous work:
Avoid if you feel dizzy or lightheaded. Otherwise, no problems expected.

Discontinuing:
- Don't discontinue without consulting doctor. Dose may require gradual reduction if you have taken drug for a long time. Doses of other drugs may also require adjustment.
- Notify doctor if cough, fever, breathing difficulty or shortness of breath occur after discontinuing medicine.

Others:
- Learn to check your own pulse. If it drops to lower than 50 or rises to higher than 100 beats per minute, don't take amiodarone until you consult your doctor.
- Advise any doctor or dentist whom you consult that you take this medicine.
- May interfere with the accuracy of some medical tests.

POSSIBLE INTERACTION WITH OTHER DRUGS

GENERIC NAME OR DRUG CLASS	COMBINED EFFECT
Antiarrhythmics, other*	Increased likelihood of heartbeat irregularity.
Anticoagulants*	Increased anti-coagulant effect.
Beta-adrenergic blocking agents*	Increased likelihood of slow heartbeat.
Calcium channel blockers*	Possible heart block.
Cholestyramine	May decrease amio-darone blood levels.
Digitalis	Increased digitalis effect.
Diltiazam	Increased likelihood of slow heartbeat.
Diuretics*	Increased risk of heartbeat irregularity due to low potassium level.
Encainide	Increased effect of toxicity on the heart muscle.
Flecainide	Increased flecainide effect.
Isoniazid	Increased risk of liver damage.
Nicardipine	Possible increased effect and toxicity of each drug.
Nifedipine	Increased likelihood of slow heartbeat.
Phenytoin	Increased effect of phenytoin.
Procainamide	Increased pro-cainamide effect.
Propafenone	Increased effect of both drugs and increased risk of toxicity.
Quinidine	Increased quinidine effect.

POSSIBLE INTERACTION WITH OTHER SUBSTANCES

INTERACTS WITH	COMBINED EFFECT
Alcohol:	Increased risk of heartbeat irregularity. Avoid.
Beverages:	None expected.
Cocaine:	Increased risk of heartbeat irregularity. Avoid.
Foods:	None expected.
Marijuana:	Possible irregular heartbeat. Avoid.
Tobacco:	Possible irregular heartbeat. Avoid.

*See Glossary

AMLEXANOX

BRAND NAMES

Aphthasol

BASIC INFORMATION

Habit forming? No
Prescription needed? Yes
Available as generic? No
Drug class: Antiaphthous ulcer agent

USES

Treatment for severe canker sores (aphthous ulcers) in the mouth.

DOSAGE & USAGE INFORMATION

How to use:
Oral paste—Use fingertips to apply paste directly to each canker sore following oral hygiene.

When to use:
Use as soon as symptoms of a canker sore appear. Apply four times a day—after meals and before bedtime. Wash hands after application.

If you forget a dose:
Use as soon as you remember. If it is almost time for the next dose, wait for the next dose (don't double this dose).

What drug does:
Exact healing mechanism is unknown. Appears to stop the inflammatory process and hypersensitivity reaction.

Time lapse before drug works:
Pain relief may occur within hours or up to 24 hours. Complete healing time will take several days.

Don't use with:
Any other medicine without consulting your doctor or pharmacist.

OVERDOSE

SYMPTOMS:
None expected.
WHAT TO DO:

- **If person accidentally swallows drug, call doctor, poison center 1-800-222-1222 or hospital emergency room for instructions.**
- **See emergency information on inside covers.**

POSSIBLE ADVERSE REACTIONS OR SIDE EFFECTS

SYMPTOMS	WHAT TO DO
Life-threatening: None expected.	
Common: None expected.	
Infrequent: Slight pain, stinging or burning at site of application.	No action necessary.
Rare: Diarrhea, nausea, rash.	Discontinue. Call doctor when convenient.

WARNINGS & PRECAUTIONS

Don't take if:
You are allergic to amlexanox.

Before you start, consult your doctor:
If you are allergic to any medication, food or other substance.

Over age 60:
No problems expected.

Pregnancy:
Decide with your doctor if drug benefits outweigh risks to unborn child. Risk category B (see page xviii).

Breast-feeding:
It is unknown if drug passes into milk. Absorption into the body has occurred with this drug. Avoid drug or discontinue nursing until you finish medicine. Consult doctor for advice on maintaining milk supply.

Infants & children:
Safety and efficacy have not been established. Use only under close medical supervision.

Prolonged use:
Normally only used for up to10 days of treatment.

Skin & sunlight:
No problems expected.

Driving, piloting or hazardous work:
No problems expected.

Discontinuing:
May be unnecessary to finish medicine. Discontinue when canker sores heal.

Others:
- If canker sores do not heal after 10 days, consult your dentist or health-care provider.
- Advise any doctor or dentist whom you consult that you take this medicine.
- Has not been studied in people with weakened immune systems.

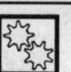

POSSIBLE INTERACTION WITH OTHER DRUGS

GENERIC NAME OR DRUG CLASS	COMBINED EFFECT
None expected.	

POSSIBLE INTERACTION WITH OTHER SUBSTANCES

INTERACTS WITH	COMBINED EFFECT
Alcohol:	None expected.
Beverages:	None expected.
Cocaine:	None expected.
Foods:	None expected.
Marijuana:	None expected.
Tobacco:	None expected.

AMPHETAMINES

GENERIC AND BRAND NAMES

AMPHETAMINE & DEXTRO-AMPHETAMINE
Adderall
Adderall XR
DEXTROAMPHETAMINE
Dexedrine
Dexedrine Spansule
Oxydess
Spancap
METHAMPHETAMINE
Desoxyn
Desoxyn Gradumet

BASIC INFORMATION

Habit forming? Yes
Prescription needed? Yes
Available as generic? Yes
Drug class: Central nervous system stimulant

USES

- Prevents narcolepsy (attacks of uncontrollable sleepiness).
- Controls hyperactivity in children under special circumstances.

DOSAGE & USAGE INFORMATION

How to take:
- Tablet—Swallow with liquid.
- Extended-release capsules and tablets—Swallow each dose whole with liquid; do not crush.

When to take:
- At the same times each day.
- Short-acting form—Don't take later than 6 hours before bedtime.
- Long-acting form—Take on awakening.

If you forget a dose:
- Short-acting form—Take up to 2 hours late. If more than 2 hours, wait for next dose (don't double this dose).

Continued next column

OVERDOSE

SYMPTOMS:
Rapid heartbeat, hyperactivity, high fever, hallucinations, suicidal or homicidal feelings, convulsions, coma.

WHAT TO DO:
- **Dial 911 (emergency) or poison center 1-800-222-1222 for an ambulance or medical help. Then give first aid immediately.**
- **See emergency information at end of book.**

- Long-acting form—Take as soon as you remember. Wait 20 hours for next dose.

What drug does:
- Hyperactivity—Decreases motor restlessness and increases ability to pay attention.
- Narcolepsy—Increases motor activity and mental alertness; diminishes drowsiness.

Time lapse before drug works:
15 to 30 minutes (short-acting).

Don't take with:
Any other medicine without consulting your doctor or pharmacist.

POSSIBLE ADVERSE REACTIONS OR SIDE EFFECTS

SYMPTOMS	WHAT TO DO
Life-threatening: In case of overdose, see previous column.	
Common:	
• Irritability, nervousness, insomnia, euphoria. signs of addiction*.	Continue. Call doctor when convenient.
• Dry mouth.	Continue. Tell doctor at next visit.
• Fast, pounding heartbeat.	Discontinue. Call doctor right away.
Infrequent:	
• Dizziness, reduced alertness, blurred vision, unusual sweating.	Discontinue. Call doctor right away.
• Headache, diarrhea or constipation, appetite loss, stomach pain, nausea, vomiting, weight loss, diminished sex drive, impotence.	Continue. Call doctor when convenient.
Rare:	
• Rash; hives; chest pain or irregular heartbeat; uncontrollable movements of head, neck, arms, legs.	Discontinue. Call doctor right away.
• Mood changes, swollen breasts.	Continue. Call doctor when convenient.

WARNINGS & PRECAUTIONS

Don't take if:
- You are allergic to any amphetamine.
- You will have surgery within 2 months, including dental surgery, requiring general or spinal anesthesia.

Before you start, consult your doctor:

- If you plan to become pregnant within medication period.
- If you have glaucoma.
- If you have diabetes, overactive thyroid, anxiety or tension.
- If you have a history of substance abuse.
- If you have heart or blood vessel disease or high blood pressure.
- If patient has a severe mental illness (especially children).

Over age 60:
Adverse reactions and side effects may be more frequent and severe than in younger persons.

Pregnancy:
Decide with your doctor if drug benefits justify risk to unborn child. Consult doctor. Risk category C (see page xviii).

Breast-feeding:
Drug passes into milk.

Infants & children:
Not recommended for children under 12.

Prolonged use:

- Habit forming.
- Talk to your doctor about the need for follow-up medical examinations or laboratory studies to check blood pressure, growth charts in children, reassessment of need for continued treatment.

Skin & sunlight:
No problems expected.

Driving, piloting or hazardous work:
Don't drive or pilot aircraft until you learn how medicine affects you. Don't work around dangerous machinery. Don't climb ladders or work in high places. Danger increases if you drink alcohol or take medicine affecting alertness and reflexes.

Discontinuing:
May be unnecessary to finish medicine, but don't suddenly stop. Follow doctor's instructions.

Others:

- This is a dangerous drug and must be closely supervised. Don't use for appetite control or depression. Potential for damage and abuse.
- Advise any doctor or dentist whom you consult that you take this medicine.
- During withdrawal phase, may cause prolonged sleep of several days.
- Don't use for fatigue or to replace rest.

POSSIBLE INTERACTION WITH OTHER DRUGS

GENERIC NAME OR DRUG CLASS	COMBINED EFFECT
Antidepressants, tricyclic*	Decreased amphetamine effect.
Antihypertensives*	Decreased anti-hypertensive effect.
Beta-adrenergic blocking agents*	High blood pressure, slow heartbeat.
Carbonic anhydrase inhibitors*	Increased amphetamine effect.
Central nervous system (CNS) stimulants*, other	Excessive CNS stimulation.
Doxazosin	Decreased doxazosin effect.
Furazolidine	Sudden and severe high blood pressure.
Haloperidol	Decreased amphetamine effect.
Monoamine oxidase (MAO) inhibitors*	May severely increase blood pressure.
Phenothiazines*	Decreased amphetamine effect.
Prazosin	Decreased prazosin effect.
Sodium bicarbonate	Increased amphetamine effect.
Sympathomimetics*	Seizures.
Thyroid hormones*	Heartbeat irregularities.

POSSIBLE INTERACTION WITH OTHER SUBSTANCES

INTERACTS WITH	COMBINED EFFECT
Alcohol:	Decreased amphetamine effect. Avoid.
Beverages: Caffeine drinks.	Overstimulation. Avoid.
Cocaine:	Dangerous stimulation of nervous system. Avoid.
Foods:	None expected.
Marijuana:	Frequent use—Severely impaired mental function.
Tobacco:	None expected.

*See Glossary

ANAGRELIDE

BRAND NAMES

Agrylin

BASIC INFORMATION

Habit forming? No
Prescription needed? Yes
Available as generic? No
Drug class: Platelet count–reducing agent, antithrombocythemia

USES

Reduces elevated platelet counts and the risk of thrombosis (formation of a blood clot); also makes symptoms more tolerable in patients with essential thrombocythemia.

DOSAGE & USAGE INFORMATION

How to take:
Capsule—Swallow with liquid. Take with or without food.

When to take:
At the same time each day. Dose may be adjusted to maintain proper platelet count.

If you forget a dose:
Take as soon as you remember. If it is almost time for the next dose, then skip the missed dose and wait for your next scheduled dose (don't double this dose).

What drug does:
Exact mechanism is unknown.

Time lapse before drug works:
One to two weeks.

Don't take with:
Any other prescription or nonprescription drug without consulting your doctor or pharmacist.

OVERDOSE

SYMPTOMS:
None expected immediately. May lower platelet count, leading to increased bleeding.
WHAT TO DO:
Overdose unlikely to threaten life. If person takes much larger amount than prescribed, call doctor, poison center 1-800-222-1222 or hospital emergency room for instructions.

POSSIBLE ADVERSE REACTIONS OR SIDE EFFECTS

SYMPTOMS	WHAT TO DO
Life-threatening:	
Severe headache or weakness; pain or pressure in chest, jaw, neck, back or arms; swelling of feet or legs; severe tiredness or weakness; increased heart rate; difficulty breathing or shortness of breath.	Seek emergency treatment immediately.
Common:	
• Abdominal pain, weakness, dizziness palpitations, shortness of breath.	Continue. Call doctor right away.
• Diarrhea, heartburn, gas, bloating, headache, loss of appetite, general feeling of discomfort or illness, nausea, pain.	Continue. Call doctor if symptoms persist.
Infrequent:	
• Blurred or double vision, painful or difficult urination, blood in urine, tingling in hands or feet, unusual bruising or bleeding, flushing, faintness.	Discontinue. Call doctor right away.
• Canker sore, joint pain, back pain, confusion, constipation, fever or chills, insomnia, leg cramps, depression, nervousness, runny nose, ringing in ears, skin rash, itching, sleepiness, sensitivity to light, vomiting.	Continue. Call doctor if symptoms persist.
Rare:	
Hair loss.	Tell doctor at next visit.

WARNINGS & PRECAUTIONS

Don't take if:
You are allergic to anagrelide.

Before you start, consult your doctor:
- If you have any kidney or liver disease or any heart or blood vessel disorder.
- If you have any chronic health problem.
- If you are pregnant or nursing.

Over age 60:
No problems expected.

Pregnancy:
Decide with your doctor if drug benefits justify risk to unborn child. Risk category C (see page xviii).

Breast-feeding:
It is unknown if drug passes into milk. Avoid drug or discontinue nursing until you finish medicine. Consult doctor for advice on maintaining milk supply.

Infants & children:
Safety and efficacy have not been established in patients under 16. Use only under close medical supervision.

Prolonged use:
Schedule regular visits with your doctor for laboratory examinations to monitor the continued effectiveness of the medication.

Skin & sunlight:
No problems expected.

Driving, piloting or hazardous work:
No problems expected.

Discontinuing:
Don't discontinue without consulting your doctor even if you feel well.

Others:
- Close medical supervision, including frequent platelet counts, required at start of therapy with this drug.
- Advise any doctor or dentist whom you consult that you are using this medicine.

POSSIBLE INTERACTION WITH OTHER DRUGS

GENERIC NAME OR DRUG CLASS	COMBINED EFFECT
Sulcrafate	May interfere with anagrelide absorption. Don't take at the same time.

POSSIBLE INTERACTION WITH OTHER SUBSTANCES

INTERACTS WITH	COMBINED EFFECT
Alcohol:	None expected.
Beverages:	None expected.
Cocaine:	Effects unknown. Avoid.
Foods:	None expected.
Marijuana:	Effects unknown. Avoid.
Tobacco:	None expected.

ANDROGENS

GENERIC AND BRAND NAMES

See complete list of generic and brand names in the *Generic and Brand Name Directory*, page 862.

BASIC INFORMATION

Habit forming? No
Prescription needed? Yes
Available as generic? Yes
Drug class: Androgen

USES

- Corrects male hormone deficiency.
- Reduces "male menopause" symptoms (loss of sex drive, depression, anxiety).
- Decreases calcium loss of osteoporosis (softened bones).
- Blocks growth of breast cancer cells in females.
- Corrects undescended testicles in male children.
- Reduces breast pain and fullness following childbirth.
- Augments treatment of aplastic anemia.
- Stimulates weight gain after illness, injury or for chronically underweight persons.
- Stimulates growth in treatment of dwarfism.

DOSAGE & USAGE INFORMATION

How to take:

- Tablets or capsules—With food to lessen stomach irritation.
- Injection—Once or twice a month.
- Transdermal—Follow instructions provided with prescription.

When to take:
At the same time each day.

If you forget a dose:
Take as soon as you remember up to 2 hours late. If more than 2 hours, wait for next scheduled dose (don't double this dose).

Continued next column

OVERDOSE

SYMPTOMS:
None expected.
WHAT TO DO:
Overdose unlikely to threaten life. If person takes much larger amount than prescribed, call doctor, poison center 1-800-222-1222 or hospital emergency room for instructions.

What drug does:

- Stimulates cells that produce male sex characteristics.
- Replaces hormone deficiencies.
- Stimulates red-blood-cell production.
- Suppresses production of estrogen (female sex hormone).

Time lapse before drug works:
Varies with problems treated. May require 2 or 3 months of regular use for desired effects.

Don't take with:
Any other medicine without consulting your doctor or pharmacist.

POSSIBLE ADVERSE REACTIONS OR SIDE EFFECTS

SYMPTOMS	WHAT TO DO
Life-threatening:	
Intense itching, weakness, loss of consciousness.	Seek emergency treatment immediately.
Common:	
• Acne or oily skin, deep voice, enlarged clitoris in females; frequent erections, swollen breasts in men; mild to moderate redness or itching at site of patch.	Continue. Call doctor when convenient.
• Sore mouth; higher sex drive, decreased testicle size, impotence in men.	Continue. Tell doctor at next visit.
Infrequent:	
• Yellow skin or eyes.	Discontinue. Seek emergency treatment.
• Depression or confusion, flushed face, rash or itch, nausea, vomiting, diarrhea, swollen feet or legs, headache, shortness of breath, rapid weight gain, chills, difficult urination; vaginal bleeding in women; scrotum pain in men.	Discontinue. Call doctor right away.
Rare:	
• Hives, black stool.	Discontinue. Seek emergency treatment.
• Sore throat, fever, abdominal pain.	Discontinue. Call doctor right away.
• Appetite loss, halitosis.	Continue. Call doctor when convenient.

WARNINGS & PRECAUTIONS

Don't take if:
You are allergic to any male hormone.

Before you start, consult your doctor:
- If you might be pregnant.
- If you have cancer of the prostate.
- If you have heart disease or arteriosclerosis.
- If you have kidney or liver disease.
- If you have breast cancer (males).
- If you have high blood pressure.
- If you have migraine attacks.
- If you have a high level of blood calcium.
- If you have epilepsy.

Over age 60:
- May stimulate sexual activity.
- Can make high blood pressure or heart disease worse.
- Can enlarge prostate and cause urinary retention.

Pregnancy:
Risk to unborn child outweighs drug benefits. Don't use. Risk category X (see page xviii).

Breast-feeding:
Drug passes into milk. Avoid drug or discontinue nursing until you finish medicine. Consult doctor for advice on maintaining milk supply.

Infants & children:
Don't give to children younger than 2. Use with older children only under medical supervision.

Prolonged use:
- Reduces sperm count and volume of semen.
- Possible kidney stones.
- Unnatural hair growth and deep voice in women.
- Talk to your doctor about the need for follow-up medical examinations or laboratory studies to check complete blood counts (white blood cell count, platelet count, red blood cell count, hemoglobin, hematocrit).

Skin & sunlight:
No problems expected.

Driving, piloting or hazardous work:
No problems expected.

Discontinuing:
No problems expected.

Others:
- May cause atrophy of testicles.
- Will not increase strength in athletes.
- Advise any doctor or dentist whom you consult that you take this medicine.
- May cause liver cancer.
- In women, may cause male-like changes such as deepened voice, increased hair growth.

POSSIBLE INTERACTION WITH OTHER DRUGS

GENERIC NAME OR DRUG CLASS	COMBINED EFFECT
Anticoagulants*	Increased anti-coagulant effect.
Antidiabetic agents*	Increased antidiabetic effect.
Chlorzoxazone	Decreased androgen effect.
Cyclosporine	Increased cyclosporine effect.
Hepatotoxic drugs* (other)	Increased liver toxicity.
Insulin	Increased antidiabetic effect.
Oxyphenbutazone	Decreased androgen effect.
Phenobarbital	Decreased androgen effect.
Phenylbutazone	Decreased androgen effect.

POSSIBLE INTERACTION WITH OTHER SUBSTANCES

INTERACTS WITH	COMBINED EFFECT
Alcohol:	None expected.
Beverages:	None expected.
Cocaine:	No proven problems.
Foods: Salt.	Excessive fluid retention (edema). Decrease salt intake while taking male hormones.
Marijuana:	Decreased blood levels of androgens.
Tobacco:	No proven problems.

***See Glossary**

ANDROGENS & ESTROGENS

GENERIC AND BRAND NAMES

See complete list of generic and brand names in the *Generic and Brand Name Directory*, page 862.

BASIC INFORMATION

Habit forming? No
Prescription needed? Yes
Available as generic? Yes
Drug class: Androgens-estrogens

USES

- Prevents breast fullness in new mothers after childbirth.
- Relieves menopause symptoms such as unnecessary sweating, hot flashes, chills, faintness and dizziness.

DOSAGE & USAGE INFORMATION

How to take:
- Injection—Given deeply intramuscular.
- Tablets—Swallow with liquid or food to lessen stomach irritation.

When to take:
When directed.

If you forget a dose:
Check with your doctor.

What drug does:
- Restores normal estrogen level in tissues.
- Stimulates cells that produce male sex characteristics.
- Replaces hormones lost due to deficiencies.
- Stimulates red blood cell production.
- Suppresses production of estrogen.

Time lapse before drug works:
10 to 20 days.

Don't take with:
Any other medicine without consulting your doctor or pharmacist.

OVERDOSE

SYMPTOMS:
Headache (severe), coordination loss, vision changes, chest pain, shortness of breath (sudden), speech slurring.
WHAT TO DO:
Overdose unlikely to threaten life. If person takes much larger amount than prescribed, call doctor, poison center 1-800-222-1222 or hospital emergency room for instructions.

POSSIBLE ADVERSE REACTIONS OR SIDE EFFECTS

SYMPTOMS	WHAT TO DO
Life-threatening:	
• In case of overdose, see previous column.	
• Hives, black stool, black or bloody vomit, intense itching, weakness, loss of consciousness.	Discontinue. Seek emergency treatment.
Common:	
• Red or flushed face; rash; swollen, tender breasts.	Discontinue. Call doctor right away.
• Depression, irritability, dizziness, confusion, acne or oily skin, enlarged clitoris, deepened voice, appetite loss, increased sex drive, unnatural hair growth, headache, constipation.	Continue. Call doctor when convenient.
Infrequent:	
• Nausea, vomiting, diarrhea, unusual vaginal bleeding or discharge, uncontrolled muscle movements.	Discontinue. Call doctor right away.
• Swollen feet and ankles, migraine headache.	Continue. Call doctor when convenient.
Rare:	
• Jaundice, abdominal pain.	Discontinue. Call doctor right away.
• Brown blotches on skin; hair loss; sore throat, fever, mouth sores.	Continue. Call doctor when convenient.

WARNINGS & PRECAUTIONS

Don't take if:
- You are allergic to any male hormone or any estrogen-containing drugs.
- You have impaired liver function.
- You have had blood clots, stroke or heart attack.
- You have unexplained vaginal bleeding.

Before you start, consult your doctor:
- If you might be pregnant or plan to become pregnant within 3 months.
- If you have heart disease, arteriosclerosis, diabetes, liver disease, high blood pressure, asthma, congestive heart failure, kidney disease or gallstones.

- If you have a high level of blood calcium.
- If you have had migraine headaches, epilepsy or porphyria.
- If you have had cancer of breast or reproductive organs, fibrocystic breast disease, fibroid tumors of the uterus or endometriosis.

Over age 60:
- May stimulate sexual activity.
- Can make high blood pressure or heart disease worse.
- Controversial. You and your doctor must decide if drug risks outweigh benefits.

Pregnancy:
Risk to unborn child outweighs drug benefits. Don't use. Risk category X (see page xviii).

Breast-feeding:
Drug passes into milk. Avoid drug or discontinue nursing until you finish medicine. Consult doctor for advice on maintaining milk supply.

Infants & children:
Not recommended.

Prolonged use:
- Increased growth of fibroid tumors of uterus.
- Possible kidney stones.
- Unnatural hair growth and deep voice in women.
- Talk to your doctor about the need for follow-up medical examinations or laboratory studies to check pap smear, liver function, mammogram, complete blood counts (white blood cell count, platelet count, red blood cell count, hemoglobin, hematocrit).
- Possible breast lumps, jaundice, sore throat, fever. If any of these occur, call your doctor.

Skin & sunlight:
One or more drugs in this group may cause rash or intensify sunburn in areas exposed to sun or utltraviolet light (photosensitivity reaction). Avoid overexposure. Notify doctor if reaction occurs.

Driving, piloting or hazardous work:
No problems expected.

Discontinuing:
You may need to discontinue estrogens periodically. Consult your doctor.

Others:
- In rare instances, may cause blood clot in lung, brain or leg. Symptoms are *sudden* severe headache, coordination loss, vision change, chest pain, breathing difficulty, slurred speech, pain in legs or groin. Seek emergency treatment immediately.
- Will not increase strength in athletes.
- Advise any doctor or dentist whom you consult that you take this medicine.
- Carefully read the paper delivered with your prescription called "Information for the Patient."
- Don't smoke.

POSSIBLE INTERACTION WITH OTHER DRUGS

GENERIC NAME OR DRUG CLASS	COMBINED EFFECT
Anticoagulants*, oral	Increased effect of anticoagulant.
Anticonvulsants*, hydantoin	Increased seizures.
Antidiabetics*, oral	Unpredictable increase or decrease in blood sugar.
Antifibrinolytic agents*	Increased possibility of blood clotting.
Carbamazepine	Increased seizures.
Chlorzoxazone	Decreased androgen effect.
Cholestyramine	Decreased cholestyramine effect.
Clofibrate	Decreased clofibrate effect.
Colestipol	Decreased colestipol effect.

Continued on page 894

POSSIBLE INTERACTION WITH OTHER SUBSTANCES

INTERACTS WITH	COMBINED EFFECT
Alcohol:	None expected.
Beverages:	None expected.
Cocaine:	None expected.
Foods: Salt.	Excessive fluid retention (edema). Decrease salt intake while taking male hormones.
Marijuana:	Decreased blood levels of androgens. Possible menstrual irregularities and bleeding between periods.
Tobacco:	Increased risk of blood clots leading to stroke or heart attack.

***See Glossary**

ANESTHETICS (Mucosal-Local)

GENERIC AND BRAND NAMES

BENZOCAINE
- Anbesol Baby Gel
- Anbesol Maximum Strength Gel
- Anbesol Maximum Strength Liquid
- Baby Anbesol
- Baby Orabase
- Baby Oragel
- Baby Oragel Nighttime Formula
- Benzodent
- Children's Cloraseptic Lozenges
- Dentapaine
- Dentocaine
- Dent-Zel-Ite
- Hurricaine
- Numzident
- Num-Zit Gel
- Num-Zit Lotion
- Orabase-B with Benzocaine
- Orajel Extra Strength
- Orajel Liquid
- Orajel Maximum Strength
- Oratect Gel
- Rid-A-Pain
- SensoGARD Canker Sore Relief
- Spec-T Sore Throat Anesthetic
- Topicaine

BENZOCAINE & MENTHOL
- Chloraseptic Lozenges Cherry Flavor

BENZOCAINE & PHENOL
- Anbesol Gel
- Anbesol Liquid
- Anbesol Regular Strength Gel
- Anbesol Regular Strength Liquid

DYCLONINE
- Children's Sucrets
- Sucrets Maximum Strength
- Sucrets Regular Strength

LIDOCAINE
- Xylocaine
- Xylocaine Viscous
- Zilactin-L

TETRACAINE
- Supracaine

BASIC INFORMATION

Habit forming? No
Prescription needed? Yes, for some
Available as generic? Yes, for some
Drug class: Anesthetic (mucosal-local)

OVERDOSE

SYMPTOMS:
Overabsorption by body—Dizziness, blurred vision, seizures, drowsiness.
WHAT TO DO:
- **Dial 911 (emergency) for an ambulance or medical help. Then give first aid immediately.**
- **Not for internal use. If child accidentally swallows, call poison center 1-800-222-1222.**
- **See emergency information on inside covers.**

USES

Relieves pain or irritation in mouth caused by toothache, teething, mouth sores, dentures, braces, dental appliances. Also relieves pain of sore throat for short periods of time.

DOSAGE & USAGE INFORMATION

How to use:
- For mouth problems—Apply to sore places with cotton-tipped applicator. Don't swallow.
- For throat—Gargle, but don't swallow.
- For aerosol spray—Don't inhale.

When to use:
As directed by physician or label on package.

If you forget a dose:
Use as soon as you remember.

What drug does:
Blocks pain impulses to the brain.

Time lapse before drug works:
Immediately.

Don't use with:
Any other medicine without consulting your doctor or pharmacist.

POSSIBLE ADVERSE REACTIONS OR SIDE EFFECTS

SYMPTOMS	WHAT TO DO
Life-threatening:	
Unusual anxiety, excitement, nervousness, irregular or slow heartbeat.	Discontinue. Seek emergency treatment.
Common:	
None expected.	
Infrequent:	
Redness, irritation, sores not present before treatment, rash, itchy skin, hives.	Discontinue. Call doctor right away.
Rare:	
None expected.	

WARNINGS & PRECAUTIONS

Don't use if:
You are allergic to any of the products listed.

Before you start, consult your doctor:
- If you are allergic to anything.
- If you have infection, canker sores or other sores in your mouth.
- If you take medicine for myasthenia gravis, eye drops for glaucoma or any sulfa medicine.

Over age 60:
Adverse reactions and side effects may be more frequent and severe than in younger persons. Ask doctor about smaller doses.

Pregnancy:
Risk factors vary for drugs in this group. See category list on page xviii and consult doctor.

Breast-feeding:
No problems expected, but check with doctor.

Infants & children:
No problems expected, but check with doctor.

Prolonged use:
Not intended for prolonged use.

Skin & sunlight:
No problems expected.

Driving, piloting or hazardous work:
Wait to see if causes dizziness, sweating, drowsiness or blurred vision. If not, no problems expected.

Discontinuing:
No problems expected.

Others:
- Keep cool, but don't freeze.
- Don't puncture, break or burn aerosol containers.
- Don't eat, drink or chew gum for 1 hour after use.
- Heat and moisture in bathroom medicine cabinet can cause breakdown of medicine. Store someplace else.
- Before anesthesia, tell dentist about any medicines you take or use.

POSSIBLE INTERACTION WITH OTHER DRUGS

GENERIC NAME OR DRUG CLASS	COMBINED EFFECT

So remote, they are not considered clinically significant.

POSSIBLE INTERACTION WITH OTHER SUBSTANCE

INTERACTS WITH	COMBINED EFFECT
Alcohol:	Adverse reactions more common.
Beverages:	None expected.
Cocaine:	May cause too much nervousness and trembling. Avoid.
Foods:	None expected.
Marijuana:	None expected.
Tobacco:	Avoid. Tobacco makes mouth problems worse.

*See Glossary

ANESTHETICS (Rectal)

GENERIC AND BRAND NAMES

BENZOCAINE
- Americaine Hemorrhoidal
- Ethyl Aminobenzoate

DIBUCAINE
- Nupercainal

PRAMOXINE
- Fleet Relief
- Proctofoam
- Tronolane
- Tronothane

TETRACAINE
- Pontocaine Cream

TETRACAINE & MENTHOL
- Pontocaine Ointment

BASIC INFORMATION

Habit forming? No
Prescription needed? Yes, for some
Available as generic? Yes, Dibucaine. No others, but most brands are available without prescription.
Drug class: Anesthetic (rectal)

USES

- Relieves pain, itching and swelling of hemorrhoids (piles).
- Relieves pain of rectal fissures (breaks in lining membrane of the anus).

DOSAGE & USAGE INFORMATION

How to use:
- Rectal cream or ointment—Apply to surface of rectum with fingers. Insert applicator into rectum no farther than 1/2 and apply inside. Wash applicator with warm soapy water or discard.
- Aerosol foam—Read patient instructions. Don't insert into rectum. Use the special applicator and wash carefully after using.

Continued next column

OVERDOSE

SYMPTOMS:
None expected.
WHAT TO DO:
Not intended for internal use. If child accidentally swallows, call poison center 1-800-222-1222.

- Suppository—Remove wrapper and moisten with water. Lie on side. Push blunt end of suppository into rectum with finger. If suppository is too soft, run cold water over wrapper or put in refrigerator for 15 to 45 minutes before using.
- Pads—For external use only. Follow instructions on label. Do not use for more than 1 week without doctor's approval.

When to use:
As directed.

If you forget a dose:
Use as soon as you remember.

What drug does:
Deadens nerve endings to pain and touch.

Time lapse before drug works:
5 to 15 minutes.

Don't use with:
Any other medicine without consulting your doctor or pharmacist.

POSSIBLE ADVERSE REACTIONS OR SIDE EFFECTS

SYMPTOMS	WHAT TO DO
Life-threatening:	
None expected.	
Common:	
None expected.	
Infrequent:	
• Nervousness, trembling, hives, rash, itch, inflammation or tenderness not present before application, slow heartbeat.	Discontinue. Call doctor right away.
• Dizziness, blurred vision, swollen feet.	Continue. Call doctor when convenient.
Rare:	
• Blood in urine.	Discontinue. Call doctor right away.
• Increased or painful urination.	Continue. Call doctor when convenient.

WARNINGS & PRECAUTIONS

Don't use if:
You are allergic to any topical anesthetic.

Before you start, consult your doctor:
- If you have skin infection at site of treatment.
- If you have had severe or extensive skin disorders such as eczema or psoriasis.
- If you have bleeding hemorrhoids.

Over age 60:
Adverse reactions and side effects may be more frequent and severe than in younger persons.

Pregnancy:
Risk factors vary for drugs in this group. See category list on page xviii and consult doctor.

Breast-feeding:
No problems expected. Consult doctor.

Infants & children:
Use caution. More likely to be absorbed through skin and cause adverse reactions.

Prolonged use:
Possible excess absorption. Don't use longer than 3 days for any one problem.

Skin & sunlight:
No problems expected.

Driving, piloting or hazardous work:
No problems expected.

Discontinuing:
May be unnecessary to finish medicine. Follow doctor's instructions.

Others:
- Report any rectal bleeding to your doctor.
- Keep cool, but don't freeze.

POSSIBLE INTERACTION WITH OTHER DRUGS

GENERIC NAME OR DRUG CLASS	COMBINED EFFECT
Sulfa drugs*	Decreased anti-infective effect of sulfa drugs.

POSSIBLE INTERACTION WITH OTHER SUBSTANCE

INTERACTS WITH	COMBINED EFFECT
Alcohol:	None expected.
Beverages:	None expected.
Cocaine:	Possible nervous system toxicity. Avoid.
Foods:	None expected.
Marijuana:	None expected.
Tobacco:	None expected.

***See Glossary**

ANESTHETICS (Topical)

GENERIC AND BRAND NAMES

See complete list of generic and brand names in the *Generic and Brand Name Directory*, page 862.

BASIC INFORMATION

Habit forming? No
Prescription needed?
High strength: Yes
Low strength: No
Available as generic? Yes
Drug class: Anesthetic (topical)

USES

Relieves pain and itch of sunburn, insect bites, scratches and other minor skin irritations.

DOSAGE & USAGE INFORMATION

How to use:
All forms—Use only enough to cover irritated area. Follow instructions on label or use as directed by doctor. Avoid using on large areas of skin.

When to use:
When needed for discomfort, no more often than every hour.

If you forget an application:
Use as needed.

What drug does:
Blocks pain impulses from skin to brain.

Time lapse before drug works:
3 to 15 minutes.

Don't take with:
Any other medicine without consulting your doctor or pharmacist.

OVERDOSE

SYMPTOMS:
If swallowed or inhaled—Dizziness, nervousness, trembling, seizures.
WHAT TO DO:

- **Dial 911 (emergency) or poison center 1-800-222-1222 for an ambulance or medical help. Then give first aid immediately.**
- **See emergency information on inside covers.**

POSSIBLE ADVERSE REACTIONS OR SIDE EFFECTS

SYMPTOMS	WHAT TO DO
Life-threatening: None expected.	
Common: None expected.	
Infrequent: Hives-like swellings on skin or in mouth or throat; skin problems not present before treatment (rash, burning, stinging, tenderness, redness).	Discontinue. Call doctor right away.
Rare: If too much of drug absorbed into body (very rare)—Nervousness, slow heartbeat, dizziness, blurred or double vision, confusion, convulsions, noises in ears, feeling hot or cold, numbness, trembling, anxiety, paleness, tiredness or weakness.	Discontinue. Call doctor right away.

WARNINGS & PRECAUTIONS

Don't use if:
You are allergic to any topical anesthetic.

Before you start, consult your doctor:
- If you have skin infection at site of treatment.
- If you have had severe or extensive skin disorders such as eczema or psoriasis.
- If you have bleeding hemorrhoids.

Over age 60:
Adverse reactions and side effects may be more frequent and severe than in younger persons.

Pregnancy:
Risk factors vary for drugs in this group. See category list on page xviii and consult doctor.

Breast-feeding:
No problems expected. Consult doctor.

Infants & children:
Use caution. More likely to be absorbed through skin and cause adverse reactions.

Prolonged use:
Possible excess absorption. Don't use longer than 3 days for any one problem.

Skin & sunlight:
May cause rash or intensify sunburn in areas exposed to sun or ultraviolet light (photosensitivity reaction). Avoid overexposure. Notify doctor if reaction occurs.

Driving, piloting or hazardous work:
No problems expected.

Discontinuing:
May be unnecessary to finish medicine. Follow doctor's instructions.

Others:
- Contact doctor if condition being treated doesn't improve within a week. Call sooner if new symptoms develop or pain worsens.
- Wash hands carefully after use.

POSSIBLE INTERACTION WITH OTHER DRUGS

GENERIC NAME OR DRUG CLASS	COMBINED EFFECT
Sulfa drugs*	Decreased effect of sulfa drugs for infection.

POSSIBLE INTERACTION WITH OTHER SUBSTANCE

INTERACTS WITH	COMBINED EFFECT
Alcohol:	None expected.
Beverages:	None expected.
Cocaine:	Possible nervous system toxicity. Avoid.
Foods:	None expected.
Marijuana:	None expected.
Tobacco:	None expected.

*See Glossary

ANGIOTENSIN II RECEPTOR ANTAGONISTS

GENERIC AND BRAND NAMES

CANDESARTAN
- Atacand

EPROSARTAN
- Teveten
- Teveten HCT

IRBESARTAN
- Avalide
- Avapro

LOSARTAN
- Cozaar
- Hyzaar

TELMISARTAN
- Micardis

VALSARTAN
- Diovan
- Diovan HCT
- Diovan Oral

BASIC INFORMATION

Habit forming? No
Prescription needed? Yes
Available as generic? No
Drug class: Antihypertensive, angiotensin II receptor antagonist

USES

Treatment for hypertension (high blood pressure). May be used alone or in combination with other antihypertensive medications.

DOSAGE & USAGE INFORMATION

How to take:
Tablet—Swallow with liquid. May be taken with or without food.

When to take:
Once or twice daily as directed.

If you forget a dose:
Take as soon as you remember. If it is almost time for the next dose, then skip the missed dose and wait for your next scheduled dose (don't double this dose).

What drug does:
Lowers blood pressure by relaxing the blood vessels to allow improved blood flow in the body.

Time lapse before drug works:
May take several weeks for full effectiveness.

Continued next column

OVERDOSE

SYMPTOMS:
Slow or irregular heartbeat, faintness, dizziness, lightheadedness.
WHAT TO DO:
Overdose unlikely to threaten life. If person takes much larger amount than prescribed, call doctor, poison center 1-800-222-1222 or hospital emergency room for instructions.

Don't take with:
Any other prescription or nonprescription drug without consulting your doctor or pharmacist.

POSSIBLE ADVERSE REACTIONS OR SIDE EFFECTS

SYMPTOMS	WHAT TO DO
Life-threatening:	
None expected.	
Common:	
Headache.	Continue. Call doctor when convenient.
Infrequent:	
• Dizziness, fever or sore throat (upper respiratory infection).	Continue, but call doctor right away.
• Diarrhea, back pain, cough, fatigue, stuffy nose.	Continue. Call doctor when convenient.
Rare:	
Dry cough, trouble sleeping, muscle cramps, leg pain.	Continue. Call doctor when convenient.

WARNINGS & PRECAUTIONS

Don't take if:
You are allergic to losartan.

Before you start, consult your doctor:
- If you have any kidney or liver disease.
- If you are allergic to any medication, food or other substance.

Over age 60:
No special problems expected.

Pregnancy:
Decide with your doctor if drug benefits justify risks to unborn child. Risk category C for first trimester and category D for second and third trimesters (see page xviii).

Breast-feeding:
One or more of these drugs pass into milk in laboratory animals. Avoid drug or discontinue nursing until you finish medicine. Consult doctor for advice on maintaining milk supply.

Infants & children:
Not recommended for children under age 18.

Prolonged use:
- No special problems expected. Hypertension usually requires life-long treatment.
- Schedule regular doctor visits to determine if drug is continuing to be effective in controlling the hypertension and to check for any kidney problems.

Skin & sunlight:
No special problems expected.

Driving, piloting or hazardous work:
Don't drive or pilot aircraft until you learn how medicine affects you. Don't work around dangerous machinery. Don't climb ladders or work in high places. Danger increases if you drink alcohol or take other medicines affecting alertness and reflexes.

Discontinuing:
Don't discontinue without consulting your doctor, even if you feel well. You can have hypertension without feeling any symptoms. Untreated high blood pressure can cause serious problems.

Others:
- Advise any doctor or dentist whom you consult that you take this medicine. May interfere with the accuracy of some medical tests.
- Follow any special diet your doctor may prescribe. It can help control hypertension.
- Consult doctor if you become ill with vomiting or diarrhea.
- Use caution when exercising or performing activities in hot weather and with excessive sweating. You may experience dizziness, lightheadedness or faintness.

POSSIBLE INTERACTION WITH OTHER DRUGS

GENERIC NAME OR DRUG CLASS	COMBINED EFFECT
Anti-inflammatory drugs, nonsteroidal (NSAIDs)*	Decreased anti-hypertensive effect.
Cyclosporine	Excess potassium levels in the body.
Diuretics*	Increased anti-hypertensive effect.
Diuretics, potassium-sparing*	Excess potassium levels in the body.
Hypotension-causing drugs*, other	Increased anti-hypertensive effect.
Indomethacin	Decreased anti-hypertensive effect.
Potassium-containing medications	Excess potassium levels in the body.
Potassium supplements*	Excess potassium levels in the body.
Sympathomimetics*	Decreased anti-hypertensive effect.

POSSIBLE INTERACTION WITH OTHER SUBSTANCES

INTERACTS WITH	COMBINED EFFECT
Alcohol:	Unknown effect. Consult doctor.
Beverages: Low-salt milk.	Excess potassium in the body.
Cocaine:	Unknown effect. Consult doctor.
Foods: Salt substitutes containing potassium.	Excess potassium in the body.
Marijuana:	Increased sedation. Avoid.
Tobacco:	No special problems expected.

ANGIOTENSIN-CONVERTING ENZYME (ACE) INHIBITORS

GENERIC AND BRAND NAMES

See complete list of generic and brand names in the *Generic and Brand Name Directory*, page 862.

BASIC INFORMATION

Habit forming? No
Prescription needed? Yes
Available as generic? Yes, for some
Drug class: Antihypertensive, Angiotensin Converting Enzyme (ACE) Inhibitor

USES

- Treatment for high blood pressure and congestive heart failure.
- Used for kidney disease in diabetic patients.
- Treatment for acute myocardial infarction within 24 hours of occurrence.

DOSAGE & USAGE INFORMATION

How to take:
Tablet—Swallow with liquid. Captopril should be taken on an empty stomach 1 hour before or 2 hours after eating.

When to take:
At the same times each day, usually 2-3 times daily. Take first dose at bedtime and lie down immediately.

If you forget a dose:
Take as soon as you remember up to 2 hours late. If more than 2 hours, wait for next scheduled dose (don't double this dose).

What drug does:
- Reduces resistance in arteries.
- Strengthens heartbeat.

Time lapse before drug works:
60 to 90 minutes.

Don't take with:
Any other medicine without consulting your doctor or pharmacist.

OVERDOSE

SYMPTOMS:
Low blood pressure, fever, chills, sore throat, fainting, convulsions, coma.
WHAT TO DO:
- **Dial 911 (emergency) or poison center 1-800-222-1222 for an ambulance or medical help. Then give first aid immediately.**
- **See emergency information on inside covers.**

POSSIBLE ADVERSE REACTIONS OR SIDE EFFECTS

SYMPTOMS	WHAT TO DO
Life-threatening	
Hives, rash, intense itching, faintness soon after a dose (anaphylaxis); difficulty breathing.	Seek emergency treatment immediately.
Common:	
Rash, loss of taste.	Discontinue. Call doctor right away.
Infrequent:	
• Swelling of mouth, face, hands or feet.	Discontinue. Seek emergency treatment.
• Dizziness, fainting, chest pain, fast or irregular heartbeat, confusion, nervousness, numbness and tingling in hands or feet.	Discontinue. Call doctor right away.
• Diarrhea, headache, tiredness, cough.	Continue. Call doctor when convenient.
Rare:	
• Sore throat, cloudy urine, fever, chills.	Discontinue. Call doctor right away.
• Nausea, vomiting, indigestion, abdominal pain.	Continue. Call doctor when convenient.

WARNINGS & PRECAUTIONS

Don't take if:
- You are allergic to any ACE inhibitor*.
- You are receiving blood from a blood bank.
- You will have surgery within 2 months, including dental surgery, requiring general or spinal anesthesia.

Before you start, consult your doctor:
- If you have had a stroke.
- If you have angina or heart or blood vessel disease.
- If you have any autoimmune disease, including AIDS or lupus.
- If you have high level of potassium in blood.
- If you have kidney or liver disease.
- If you are on severe salt-restricted diet.
- If you have a bone marrow disorder.

Over age 60:
Adverse reactions and side effects may be more frequent and severe than in younger persons.

ANGIOTENSIN-CONVERTING ENZYME (ACE) INHIBITORS

Pregnancy:
Risk factors vary for drugs in this group. See category list on page xviii and consult doctor.

Breast-feeding:
Drug passes into milk. Avoid drug or discontinue nursing until you finish medicine. Consult doctor for advice on maintaining milk supply.

Infants & children:
Under close medical supervision only.

Prolonged use:
- May decrease white cells in blood or cause protein loss in urine.
- Request periodic laboratory blood counts and urine tests.

Skin & sunlight:
One or more drugs in this group may cause rash or intensify sunburn in areas exposed to sun or utltraviolet light (photosensitivity reaction). Avoid overexposure. Notify doctor if reaction occurs.

Driving, piloting or hazardous work:
Avoid if you become dizzy or faint. Otherwise, no problems expected.

Discontinuing:
Don't discontinue without consulting doctor. Dose may require gradual reduction if you have taken drug for a long time. Doses of other drugs may also require adjustment.

Others:
- Avoid exercising in hot weather.
- May affect results in some medical tests.
- Advise any doctor or dentist whom you consult that you take this medicine.

POSSIBLE INTERACTION WITH OTHER DRUGS

GENERIC NAME OR DRUG CLASS	COMBINED EFFECT
Amiloride	Possible excessive potassium in blood.
Antihypertensives, other*	Increased anti-hypertensive effect. Dosage of each may require adjustment.
Anti-inflammatory drugs nonsteroidal (NSAIDs), cox-2 inhibitors	May decrease ACE inhibitor effect.
Beta-adrenergic blocking agents*	Increased anti-hypertensive effect. Dosage of each may require adjustment.
Carteolol	Increased anti-hypertensive effects of both drugs. Dosages may require adjustment.
Chloramphenicol	Possible blood disorders.
Diuretics*	Possible severe blood pressure drop with first dose.
Diclofenac	May decrease ACE inhibitor effect.
Guanfacine	Increased effect of both drugs.
Meloxicam	Decreased effect of ACE inhibitor.
Nicardipine	Possible excessive potassium in blood. Dosages may require adjustment.
Nimodipine	Possible excessive potassium in blood. Dangerous blood pressure drop.
Nitrates*	Possible excessive blood pressure drop.
Nonsteroidal anti-inflammatory drugs (NSAIDs)*	Decreased ACE inhibitor effect.

Continued on page 895

POSSIBLE INTERACTION WITH OTHER SUBSTANCES

INTERACTS WITH	COMBINED EFFECT
Alcohol:	Possible excessive blood pressure drop.
Beverages: Low-salt milk.	Possible excessive potassium in blood.
Cocaine	Increased risk of heart block and high blood pressure.
Foods: Salt substitutes.	Possible excessive potassium.
Marijuana:	Increased dizziness.
Tobacco:	May decrease ACE inhibitor effect.

*See Glossary

ANGIOTENSIN-CONVERTING ENZYME (ACE) INHIBITORS & HYDROCHLOROTHIAZIDE

GENERIC AND BRAND NAMES

See complete list of generic and brand names in the *Generic and Brand Names Directory*, page 862.

BASIC INFORMATION

Habit forming? No
Prescription needed? Yes
Available as generic? No
Drug class: Antihypertensive, diuretic (thiazide), ACE inhibitor

USES

- Treatment for high blood pressure and congestive heart failure.
- Reduces fluid retention.

DOSAGE & USAGE INFORMATION

How to take:
Tablet—Swallow with liquid. Instructions to take on empty stomach mean 1 hour before or 2 hours after eating.

When to take:
At the same times each day, usually 2 to 3 times daily. Take first dose at bedtime and lie down immediately.

If you forget a dose:
Take as soon as you remember up to 2 hours late. If more than 2 hours, wait for next scheduled dose (don't double this dose).

What drug does:
- Forces sodium and water excretion, reducing body fluid.
- Relaxes muscle cells of small arteries.
- Reduced body fluid and relaxed arteries lower blood pressure.
- Reduces resistance in arteries.
- Strengthens heartbeat.

Continued next column

OVERDOSE

SYMPTOMS:
Cramps, weakness, drowsiness, weak pulse, low blood pressure.
WHAT TO DO:
- **Dial 911 (emergency) or poison center 1-800-222-1222 for an ambulance or medical help. Then give first aid immediately.**
- **See emergency information on inside covers.**

Time lapse before drug works:
4 to 6 hours. May require several weeks to lower blood pressure.

Don't take with:
Nonprescription drugs without consulting doctor.

POSSIBLE ADVERSE REACTIONS OR SIDE EFFECTS

SYMPTOMS	WHAT TO DO
Life-threatening:	
Irregular heartbeat (fast or uneven); hives, rash, intense itching, faintness soon after a dose (anaphylaxis).	Discontinue. Seek emergency treatment.
Common:	
• Dry mouth, thirst, tiredness, weakness, muscle cramps, vomiting, chest pain, skin rash, coughing, weak pulse.	Discontinue. Call doctor right away.
• Taste loss, dizziness.	Continue. Call doctor when convenient.
Infrequent:	
• Face, mouth, hands swell.	Discontinue. Call doctor right away.
• Nausea, diarrhea.	Continue. Call doctor when convenient.
Rare:	
Jaundice (yellow eyes and skin), bruising, back pain.	Discontinue. Call doctor right away.

WARNINGS & PRECAUTIONS

Don't take if:
- You are allergic to any ACE inhibitor or any thiazide diuretic drug.
- You are receiving blood from a blood bank.
- If you will have surgery within 2 months, including dental surgery, requiring general or spinal anesthesia.

Before you start, consult your doctor:
- If you have had a stroke.
- If you have angina, heart or blood vessel disease, a high level of potassium in blood, lupus, gout, liver, pancreas or kidney disorder.
- If you have any autoimmune disease, including AIDS or lupus.
- If you are on severe salt-restricted diet.
- If you are allergic to any sulfa drug.
- If you have a bone marrow disorder.

ANGIOTENSIN-CONVERTING ENZYME (ACE) INHIBITORS & HYDROCHLOROTHIAZIDE

Over age 60:
Adverse reactions and side effects may be more frequent and severe than in younger persons, especially dizziness and excessive potassium loss.

Pregnancy:
Risk factors vary for drugs in this group. See category list on page xviii and consult doctor.

Breast-feeding:
Drug passes into milk. Avoid drug or discontinue nursing until you finish medicine. Consult doctor for advice on maintaining milk supply.

Infants & children:
Not recommended.

Prolonged use:
Talk to your doctor about the need for follow-up medical examinations or laboratory studies to check blood pressure, ECG*, liver function, kidney function.

Skin & sunlight:
One or more drugs in this group may cause rash or intensify sunburn in areas exposed to sun or ultlraviolet light (photosensitivity reaction). Avoid overexposure. Notify doctor if reaction occurs.

Driving, piloting or hazardous work:
Don't drive or pilot aircraft until you learn how medicine affects you. Don't work around dangerous machinery. Don't climb ladders or work in high places. Danger increases if you drink alcohol or take medicine affecting alertness and reflexes, such as antihistamines, tranquilizers, sedatives, pain medicine, narcotics and mind-altering drugs.

Discontinuing:
Don't discontinue without consulting doctor. Dose may require gradual reduction if you have taken drug for a long time. Doses of other drugs may also require adjustment.

Others:
- Hot weather and fever may cause dehydration and drop in blood pressure. Dose may require temporary adjustment. Weigh daily and report any unexpected weight decreases to your doctor.
- May cause rise in uric acid, leading to gout.
- May cause blood-sugar rise in diabetics.

POSSIBLE INTERACTION WITH OTHER DRUGS

GENERIC NAME OR DRUG CLASS	COMBINED EFFECT
Allopurinol	Decreased allopurinol effect.
Amiloride	Possible excessive potassium in blood.
Antidepressants, tricyclic*	Dangerous drop in blood pressure. Avoid combination unless under medical supervision.
Antihypertensives, other*	Increased anti-hypertensive effect. Dosage of each may require adjustment.
Anti-inflammatory drugs nonsteroidal (NSAIDs)*	Decreased captopril effect.
Barbiturates*	Increased hydro-chlorothiazide effect.
Beta-adrenergic blocking agents*	Increased anti-hypertensive effect. Dosage of each may require adjustments.
Carteolol	Increased antihyper-tensive effects of both drugs. Dosages may require adjustment.
Chloramphenicol	Possible blood disorders.
Cholestyramine	Decreased hydro-chlorothiazide effect.
Digitalis preparations*	Excessive potassium loss that causes dangerous heart rhythms.

Continued on page 895

POSSIBLE INTERACTION WITH OTHER SUBSTANCES

INTERACTS WITH	COMBINED EFFECT
Alcohol:	Dangerous blood pressure drop. Avoid.
Beverages: Low-salt milk.	Possible excessive potassium in blood.
Cocaine	Increased risk of heart block and high blood pressure.
Foods: Salt substitutes.	Possible excessive potassium.
Marijuana:	Increased dizziness; may increase blood-pressure.
Tobacco:	May decrease blood pressure lowering effect.

*See Glossary

ANTACIDS

GENERIC AND BRAND NAMES

See complete list of generic and brand names in the *Generic and Brand Name Directory*, page 862.

BASIC INFORMATION

Habit forming? No
Prescription needed? No
Available as generic? Yes, for some.
Drug class: Antacid

USES

Treatment for hyperacidity in upper gastrointestinal tract, including stomach and esophagus. Symptoms may be heartburn or acid indigestion. Diseases include peptic ulcer, gastritis, esophagitis, hiatal hernia.

DOSAGE & USAGE INFORMATION

How to take:
Follow package instructions.

When to take:
1 to 3 hours after meals unless directed otherwise by your doctor.

If you forget a dose:
Take as soon as you remember, but not simultaneously with any other medicine.

What drug does:
- Neutralizes some of the hydrochloric acid in the stomach.
- Reduces action of pepsin, a digestive enzyme.

Time lapse before drug works:
15 minutes for antacid effect.

Continued next column

OVERDOSE

SYMPTOMS:
Dry mouth, shallow breathing, diarrhea or constipation, headache, mental confusion, weakness, fatigue, stupor, bone pain.
WHAT TO DO:
- **Overdose unlikely to threaten life. Depending on severity of symptoms and amount taken, call doctor, poison center 1-800-222-1222 or hospital emergency room for instructions.**
- **Dial 911 (emergency) for an ambulance or medical help. Then give first aid immediately.**
- **See emergency information on inside covers.**

Don't take with:
Other medicines at the same time. Decreases absorption of other drugs. Wait 2 hours between doses.

POSSIBLE ADVERSE REACTIONS OR SIDE EFFECTS

SYMPTOMS	WHAT TO DO
Life-threatening: None expected.	
Common: Chalky taste.	Continue. Tell doctor at next visit.
Infrequent: Mild constipation, increased thirst, laxative effect, unpleasant taste in mouth, stomach cramps, stool color changes (whitish or speckling).	Continue. Call doctor when convenient.
Rare: Bone pain, frequent or urgent urination, muscle weakness or pain, nausea, weight gain, severe constipation, dizziness, headache, appetite loss, mood changes, vomiting, nervousness, swollen feet and ankles, tiredness or weakness.	Discontinue. Call doctor right away.

Note: Side effects are rare unless too much medicine is taken for a long time.

WARNINGS & PRECAUTIONS

Don't take if:
- You are allergic to any antacid.
- You have a high blood-calcium level.

Before you start, consult your doctor:
If you have kidney disease, chronic constipation, colitis, diarrhea, symptoms of appendicitis, stomach or intestinal bleeding, irregular heartbeat.

Over age 60:
Adverse reactions and side effects may be more frequent and severe than in younger persons. Diarrhea or constipation particularly likely.

Pregnancy:
Risk factors vary for drugs in this group. See category list on page xviii and consult doctor.

Breast-feeding:
Drug passes into milk. Consult doctor.

Infants & children:
Use only under medical supervision.

Prolonged use:
- High blood level of calcium (if your antacid contains calcium) which disturbs electrolyte balance.
- Kidney stones, impaired kidney function.
- Talk to your doctor about the need for follow-up medical examinations or laboratory studies to check kidney function, serum calcium, serum potassium.

Skin & sunlight:
No problems expected.

Driving, piloting or hazardous work:
No problems expected.

Discontinuing:
May be unnecessary to finish medicine. Follow doctor's instructions.

Others:
- Don't take longer than 2 weeks unless under medical supervision.
- Advise any doctor or dentist whom you consult that you take this medicine. May affect results in some medical tests.

POSSIBLE INTERACTION WITH OTHER DRUGS

GENERIC NAME OR DRUG CLASS	COMBINED EFFECT
Alendronate	Decreased alendronate effect. Take antacid 30 minutes after alendronate.
Antifungals, azoles	Decreased azole absorption.
Anti-inflammatory drugs nonsteroidal (NSAIDs), COX-2 inhibitors	Decreased pain relief.
Capecitabine	Increased risk of capecitabine toxicity.
Chlorpromazine	Decreased chlorpromazine effect.
Ciprofloxacin	May cause kidney dysfunction.
Dexamethasone	Decreased dexamethasone effect.
Digitalis preparations*	Decreased digitalis effect.
Iron supplements*	Decreased iron effect.
Isoniazid	Decreased isoniazid effect.
Levodopa	Increased levodopa effect.
Mecamylamine	Increased mecamylamine effect.
Meperidine	Increased meperidine effect.
Methenamine	Reduced methenamine effect.
Nalidixic acid	Decreased nalidixic acid effect.
Nicardipine	Possible decreased nicardipine effect.
Nizatidine	Decreased nizatidine absorption.
Ofloxacin	Decreased ofloxacin effect.
Oxyphenbutazone	Decreased oxyphenbutazone effect.
Para-aminosalicylic acid (PAS)	Decreased PAS effect.
Penicillins*	Decreased penicillin effect.
Prednisone	Decreased prednisone effect.
Pseudoephedrine	Increased pseudoephedrine effect.
Salicylates*	Increased salicylate effect.
Tetracyclines	Decreased tetracycline effect.
Ticlopidine	Decreased ticlopidine effect.

POSSIBLE INTERACTION WITH OTHER SUBSTANCES

INTERACTS WITH	COMBINED EFFECT
Alcohol:	Decreased antacid effect.
Beverages: Milk.	May cause bone discomfort.
Cocaine:	No proven problems.
Foods:	Decreased antacid effect. Wait 1 hour after eating.
Marijuana:	Decreased antacid effect.
Tobacco:	Decreased antacid effect.

*See Glossary

ANTHELMINTICS

GENERIC AND BRAND NAMES

ALBENDAZOLE
Albenza
IVERMECTIN
Stromectol
MEBENDAZOLE
Mebendacin
Mebutar
Nemasole
Vermox
PYRANTEL
Antiminth
Aut
Cobantril
Helmex
Lombriareu
Reese's Pinworm Medicine
Trilombrin
PYRVINIUM
Vanquin
Viprynium
THIABENDAZOLE
Foldan
Mintezol
Mintezol Topical
Minzolum
Triasox

BASIC INFORMATION

Habit forming? No
Prescription needed? Yes
Available as generic? Yes
Drug class: Anthelmintics, antiparasitic

USES

- Treatment of roundworms, pinworms, whipworms, hookworms and other intestinal parasites.
- Treatment of hydatid disease and neurocysticercosis; stronglyoidiasis and onchocerciasis.

DOSAGE & USAGE INFORMATION

How to take or apply:

- Tablet—Swallow with liquid or food to lessen stomach irritation.
- Topical suspension—Apply to end of each tunnel or burrow made by worm.
- Chewable tablets—Chew thoroughly before swallowing.
- Oral suspension—Follow package instructions.

Continued next column

When to take:
Morning and evening with food to increase uptake.

If you forget a dose:
Skip dose and begin treatment again. Often only one or two doses are needed to complete treatment.

What drug does:
Kills or paralyzes the parasites. They then pass out of the body in the feces. Usually the type of worm parasite must be identified so the appropriate drug can be prescribed.

Time lapse before drug works:
Some take only hours, others, 1-3 days.

Don't take with:
Any other medicine without consulting your doctor or pharmacist.

OVERDOSE

SYMPTOMS:
Increased severity of adverse reactions and side effects.
WHAT TO DO:
Overdose unlikely to threaten life. If person takes much larger amount than prescribed, call doctor, poison center 1-800-222-1222 or hospital emergency room for instructions.

POSSIBLE ADVERSE REACTIONS OR SIDE EFFECTS

SYMPTOMS	WHAT TO DO
Life-threatening: None expected.	
Common: None expected.	
Infrequent:	
• Abdominal pain, diarrhea, dizziness, fever, nausea, rectal itching.	Continue. Call doctor when convenient.
• Red stools, asparagus-like urine smell, bad taste in mouth.	No action necessary.
Rare: Skin rash, itching, sore throat and fever, weakness (severe), hair loss, headache, blurred vision, seizures.	Discontinue. Call doctor right away.

WARNINGS & PRECAUTIONS

Don't take if:
You are allergic to any anthelmintics.

Before you start, consult your doctor:
- If you have liver disease.
- If you have Crohn's disease.
- If you have ulcerative colitis.

Over age 60:
Adverse reactions and side effects may be more frequent and severe than in younger persons. You may need smaller doses for shorter periods of time.

Pregnancy:
Risk factors vary for drugs in this group. See category list on page xviii and consult doctor.

Breast-feeding:
Unknown effect. Consult your doctor.

Infants & children:
No problems expected. Don't give to a child under age 2 without doctor's approval.

Prolonged use:
- Not intended for long-term use.
- Talk to your doctor about the need for follow-up medical examinations or laboratory studies to check stools, cellophane tape swabs pressed against rectal area to check for parasite eggs, complete blood counts (white blood cell count, platelet count, red blood cell count, hemoglobin, hematocrit).

Skin & sunlight:
Thiabendazole may cause rash or intensify sunburn in areas exposed to sun or ultraviolet light (photosensitivity reaction). Avoid overexposure. Notify doctor if reaction occurs.

Driving, piloting or hazardous work:
Use caution if the medicine causes you to feel dizzy or weak. Otherwise, no problems expected.

Discontinuing:
No problems expected.

Others:
- Take full course of treatment. Repeat course may be necessary if follow-up examinations reveal persistent infection.
- Advise any doctor or dentist whom you consult that you take this medicine.
- Wash all bedding after treatment to prevent re-infection.

POSSIBLE INTERACTION WITH OTHER DRUGS

GENERIC NAME OR DRUG CLASS	COMBINED EFFECT
Carbamazepine	Decreased effect of mebendazole.
Phenytoin	Decreased effect of mebendazole.
Piperazine	Decreased effect of each drug.
Theophylline	Increased effect of theophylline (with thiabendazole use.)

POSSIBLE INTERACTION WITH OTHER SUBSTANCES

INTERACTS WITH	COMBINED EFFECT
Alcohol:	Decreased mebendazole effect. Avoid.
Beverages:	None expected.
Cocaine:	None expected.
Foods:	None expected.
Marijuana:	None expected.
Tobacco:	None expected.

***See Glossary**

ANTHRALIN (Topical)

BRAND NAMES

Anthra-Derm
Anthraforte
Anthranol
Anthrascalp
Dithranol
Drithocreme
Drithocreme HP
Dritho-Scalp
Lasan
Lasan HP
Lasan Pomade
Lasan Unguent
Micanol

BASIC INFORMATION

Habit forming? No
Prescription needed? Yes
Available as generic? No
Drug class: Antipsoriatic, hair growth stimulant

USES

- Treats quiescent or chronic psoriasis.
- Stimulates hair growth in some people (not an approved use by the FDA).

DOSAGE & USAGE INFORMATION

How to use:

- Wear plastic gloves for all applications.
- If directed, apply at night.
- Cream, lotion, ointment—Bathe and dry area before use. Apply small amount and rub gently.
- If for short contact, same as above for cream.
- Leave on 20 to 30 minutes. Then remove medicine by bathing or shampooing.
- If for scalp overnight—Shampoo before use to remove scales or medicine. Dry hair. Part hair several times and apply to scalp. Wear plastic cap on head. Clean off next morning with petroleum jelly, then shampoo.

When to use:
As directed.

If you forget a dose:
Use as soon as you remember.

Continued next column

OVERDOSE

SYMPTOMS:
None expected.
WHAT TO DO:
Not for internal use. If child accidentally swallows, call poison center 1-800-222-1222.

What drug does:
Reduces growth activity within abnormal cells by inhibiting enzymes.

Time lapse before drug works:
May require several weeks or more.

Don't use with:
Any other medicine without consulting your doctor or pharmacist.

POSSIBLE ADVERSE REACTIONS OR SIDE EFFECTS

SYMPTOMS	WHAT TO DO
Life-threatening:	
None expected.	
Common:	
None expected.	
Infrequent:	
Redness or irritation of skin not present before application, rash.	Discontinue. Call doctor when convenient.
Rare:	
None expected.	

WARNINGS & PRECAUTIONS

Don't use if:
- You are allergic to anthralin.
- You have infected skin.

Before you start, consult your doctor:
- If you have chronic kidney disease.
- If you are allergic to anything.

Over age 60:
No problems expected, but check with doctor.

Pregnancy:
Studies in animals and humans have not been done. Consult doctor. Risk category C (see page xviii).

Breast-feeding:
No problems expected, but check with doctor.

Infants & children:
No problems expected, but check with doctor.

Prolonged use:
No problems expected, but check with doctor.

Skin & sunlight:
May cause rash or intensify sunburn in areas exposed to sun or ultraviolet light (photosensitivity reaction). Avoid overexposure. Notify doctor if reaction occurs.

Driving, piloting or hazardous work:
No problems expected.

Discontinuing:
No problems expected.

Others:
- Keep cool, but don't freeze.
- Apply petroleum jelly to normal skin or scalp to protect areas not being treated.
- Will stain hair, clothing, shower, bathtub or sheets. Wash as soon as possible.
- Advise any doctor or dentist whom you consult that you take this medicine.
- Heat and moisture in bathroom medicine cabinet can cause breakdown of medicine. Store someplace else.

POSSIBLE INTERACTION WITH OTHER DRUGS

GENERIC NAME OR DRUG CLASS	COMBINED EFFECT
Antidiabetic agents*	Increased sensitivity to sun exposure.
Coal tar preparations*	Increased sensitivity to sun exposure.
Diuretics, thiazide*	Increased sensitivity to sun exposure.
Griseofulvin	Increased sensitivity to sun exposure.
Methosalen	Increased sensitivity to sun exposure.
Nalidixic acid	Increased sensitivity to sun exposure.
Phenothiazines*	Increased sensitivity to sun exposure.
Sulfa drugs*	Increased sensitivity to sun exposure.
Tetracyclines*	Increased sensitivity to sun exposure.
Trioxsalen	Increased sensitivity to sun exposure.

POSSIBLE INTERACTION WITH OTHER SUBSTANCES

INTERACTS WITH	COMBINED EFFECT
Alcohol:	None expected.
Beverages:	None expected.
Cocaine:	None expected.
Foods:	None expected.
Marijuana:	None expected.
Tobacco:	None expected.

ANTIACNE, CLEANSING (Topical)

GENERIC AND BRAND NAMES

ALCOHOL & ACETONE
- **Seba-Nil**

ALCOHOL & SULFUR
- **Liquimat**
- **Postacne**

SULFURATED LIME
- **Vlemasque**
- **Vlemickxs Solution**

BASIC INFORMATION

Habit forming? No
Prescription needed? No
Available as generic? Yes
Drug class: Antiacne agent, Cleansing agent

USES

Treats acne or oily skin.

DOSAGE & USAGE INFORMATION

How to use:
- Lotion, gel or pledget—Start with small amount and wipe over face to remove dirt and surface oil. Don't apply to wounds or burns. Don't rinse with water and avoid contact with eyes. Skin may be more sensitive in dry or cold climates.
- Plaster—Follow package instructions.

When to use:
As directed. May increase frequency up to 3 or more times daily as tolerated. Warm, humid weather may allow more frequent use.

If you forget a dose:
Use as soon as you remember and then go back to regular schedule.

Continued next column

OVERDOSE

SYMPTOMS:
None expected.
WHAT TO DO:
- **Not for internal use. If child accidentally swallows, call poison center 1-800-222-1222.**
- **Dial 911 (emergency) for an ambulance or medical help. Then give first aid immediately.**
- **See emergency information on inside covers.**

What drug does:
Helps remove oil from skin's surface.

Time lapse before drug works:
Works immediately.

Don't use with:
Other topical acne treatments unless directed by doctor.

POSSIBLE ADVERSE REACTIONS OR SIDE EFFECTS

SYMPTOMS	WHAT TO DO
Life-threatening: None expected.	
Common: None expected.	
Infrequent:	
• Skin infection, pustules or rash; unusual pain, swelling or redness of treated skin.	Discontinue. Call doctor right away.
• Burning, dryness, stinging, peeling of skin.	Continue. Call doctor when convenient.
Rare: None expected.	

WARNINGS & PRECAUTIONS

Don't use if:
You have to apply over a wounded or burned area.

Before you start, consult your doctor:
If you use benzoyl peroxide, resorcinol, salicylic acid, sulfur or tretinoin (vitamin A acid).

Over age 60:
No problems expected.

Pregnancy:
Risk category not assigned to this drug group. Consult doctor about use.

Breast-feeding:
No problems expected, but check with doctor.

Infants & children:
No problems expected, but check with doctor. Use only under close medical supervision.

Prolonged use:
Excessive drying of skin.

Skin & sunlight:
No special problems expected.

Driving, piloting or hazardous work:
No problems expected, but check with doctor.

Discontinuing:
No problems expected, but check with doctor.

Others:
Some antiacne agents are flammable. Don't use near fire or while smoking.

POSSIBLE INTERACTION WITH OTHER DRUGS

GENERIC NAME OR DRUG CLASS	COMBINED EFFECT
Abrasive or medicated soaps	Irritation or too much drying.
After-shave lotions	Irritation or too much drying.
Antiacne topical preparations (other)	Irritation or too much drying.
"Cover-up" cosmetics	Irritation or too much drying.
Drying cosmetic soaps	Irritation or too much drying.
Isotretinoin	Irritation or too much drying.
Mercury compounds	May stain skin black and smell bad..
Perfumed toilet water	Irritation or too much drying.
Preparations containing skin-peeling agents such as benzoyl peroxide, resorcinol, salicylic acid, sulfur, tretinoin	Irritation or too much drying.

POSSIBLE INTERACTION WITH OTHER SUBSTANCES

INTERACTS WITH	COMBINED EFFECT
Alcohol:	None expected.
Beverages:	None expected.
Cocaine:	None expected.
Foods:	None expected.
Marijuana:	None expected.
Tobacco:	None expected.

***See Glossary**

ANTIALLERGIC AGENTS (Ophthalmic)

GENERIC AND BRAND NAMES

AZELASTINE Optivar	**LODOXAMIDE** Alomide
EMEDASTINE Emadine	**NEDOCROMIL** Alocril
KETOTIFEN Zaditor	**OLOPATADINE** Patanol
LEVOCABASTINE Livostin	**PEMIROLAST** Alamast

BASIC INFORMATION

Habit forming? No
Prescription needed? Yes
Available as generic? No
Drug class: Ophthalmic antiallergic agents, antihistaminic

USES

Prevention and treatment of seasonal allergic (hay fever) eye disorders. May be referred to as seasonal conjunctivitis, vernal conjunctivitis, vernal keratitis and vernal keratoconjunctivitis.

DOSAGE & USAGE INFORMATION

How to use:
Eye solution
- Wash hands.
- Apply pressure to inside corner of eye with middle finger.
- Continue pressure for 1 minute after placing medicine in eye.
- Tilt head backward. Pull lower lid away from eye with index finger of the same hand.
- Drop eye drops into pouch and close eye. Don't blink.
- Keep eyes closed for 1 to 2 minutes.

When to use:
1 to 2 drops 4 times a day or as directed by doctor.

If you forget a dose:
Use as soon as you remember, then return to regular schedule.

Continued next column

OVERDOSE

SYMPTOMS:
None expected.
WHAT TO DO:
Not intended for internal use. If child accidentally swallows, call poison center 1-800-222-1222.

Time lapse before drug works:
Levocabastine—7 days, with confirmed improvement.
Lodoxamide—3 days.
Olopatadine—8 hours.

What drug does:
- Lodoxamide acts as a mast cell* stabilizer to prevent a hypersensitivity reaction to certain allergens such as pollen.
- Levocabastine and olopatadine are histamine H_1 receptor antagonists that block hypersensitivity responses to allergens.

Time lapse before drug works:
Relief of symptoms may begin immediately, but full benefit might take a few days.

Don't use with:
Any other medications without first consulting doctor or pharmacist.

POSSIBLE ADVERSE REACTIONS OR SIDE EFFECTS

SYMPTOMS	WHAT TO DO
Life-threatening: None expected.	
Common: Brief and mild burning or stinging when drops are administered.	No action necessary.
Infrequent: Blurred vision, feeling that something is in the the eye, redness of eye, eye irritation not present before, eye tearing or discharge.	Discontinue. Call doctor right away.
Rare: • Aching in eye, crusting in corner of eye or eyelid, dryness of eyes or nose, drowsiness or sleepiness, feeling of heat in eye or body, nausea, stomach discomfort, sneezing, sticky or tired feeling of eye.	Continue. Call doctor when convenient.
• Redness or irritation of eyelid, swelling of eye, pain in eye, sensitivity to light, headache, dizziness, skin rash.	Discontinue. Call doctor right away.

WARNINGS & PRECAUTIONS

Don't use if:
You are allergic to levocabastine or lodoxamide.

Before you start, consult your doctor:
- If you wear soft contact lenses.
- You are allergic to any other medications, foods or other substances.

Over age 60:
No special problems expected.

Pregnancy:
Risk category C for levocabastine and olopatadine and B for lodoxamide (see page xviii). Consult doctor.

Breast-feeding:
lodoxamide passes into breast milk after administration into the eye. It is unknown if levocabastine or olopatadine pass into breast milk. Consult doctor.

Infants & children:
No information available on safety or effectiveness for children under age 2 for lodoxamide and under age 12 for levocabastine. Consult doctor. Azelastine approved for children 3 years and older.

Prolonged use:
No special problems expected.

Skin & sunlight:
No special problems expected.

Driving, piloting or hazardous work:
Avoid if you feel dizzy or side effects cause vision problems.

Discontinuing:
No special problems expected.

Others:
- Don't use leftover medicine for other eye problems without your doctor's approval.
- If symptoms don't improve after a few days of use, call your doctor.

POSSIBLE INTERACTION WITH OTHER DRUGS

GENERIC NAME OR DRUG CLASS	COMBINED EFFECT
None significant.	

POSSIBLE INTERACTION WITH OTHER SUBSTANCES

INTERACTS WITH	COMBINED EFFECT
Alcohol:	None expected.
Beverages:	None expected.
Cocaine	None expected.
Foods:	None expected.
Marijuana:	None expected.
Tobacco:	None expected.

*See Glossary

ANTIANDROGENS, NONSTEROIDAL

GENERIC AND BRAND NAMES

BICALUTAMIDE
Casodex
FLUTAMIDE
Euflex
Eulexin
NILUTAMIDE
Amandron
Nilandron

BASIC INFORMATION

Habit forming? No
Prescription needed? Yes
Available as generic? No
Drug class: Antineoplastic

USES

Treatment for prostate cancer. Used in combination with a testerone lowering measure such as surgery (removal of the testicles) or use of a special monthly injection of luteinizing hormone-releasing hormone (LHRH).

DOSAGE & USAGE INFORMATION

How to take:
Tablet or capsule—Swallow with liquid. May be taken with or without food.

When to take:
According to doctor's instructions. Normally at the same times each day.

If you forget a dose:
Take as soon as you remember. If it is almost time for your next dose, skip the missed dose and return to your regular dosing schedule (don't double this dose).

What drug does:
Interferes with utilization of androgen (male hormone) testosterone by body cells. Prostate cancer cells require testosterone in order to grow and reproduce.

Continued next column

OVERDOSE

SYMPTOMS:
Diarrhea, nausea, vomiting, tiredness, headache, dizziness, breast tenderness.
WHAT TO DO:
Overdose unlikely to threaten life. If person takes much larger amount than prescribed, call doctor, poison center 1-800-222-1222 or hospital emergency room for instructions.

Time lapse before drug works:
Starts working within two hours, but may take several weeks to be effective.

Don't take with:
Any other medicines (including over-the-counter drugs such as cough and cold medicines, laxatives, antacids, diet pills, caffeine, nose drops or vitamins) without consulting your doctor or pharmacist.

POSSIBLE ADVERSE REACTIONS OR SIDE EFFECTS

SYMPTOMS	WHAT TO DO
Life-threatening: None expected.	
Common:	
• Decreased sex drive, diarrhea, appetite loss, nausea, vomiting, cough or hoarseness, fever, runny nose, sneezing, sore throat, tightness in chest or wheezing, constipation, insomnia.	Continue. Call doctor when convenient.
• Hot flashes with mild sweating.	No action necessary.
Infrequent:	
• Hands and feet tingling or numb, painful or swollen breasts, swollen feet and legs, chest pain, shortness of breath.	Continue. Call doctor right away.
• Bloody or black tarry stools, itching, back or side pain, depression, muscle weakness, unusual tiredness, skin rash, bloated feeling, confusion, dry mouth, nervousness, color vision changes (with nilutamide).	Continue. Call doctor when convenient.
Rare:	
• Jaundice (yellow eyes and skin), pain or tenderness in the stomach.	Continue. Call doctor right away.
• Bluish colored lips, skin or nails; dark urine; dizziness or fainting; unusual bleeding or bruising.	Continue. Call doctor when convenient.

Note: Adverse effects that occur may also be due to use of LHRH or symptoms of prostate cancer.

WARNINGS & PRECAUTIONS

Don't take if:
- You are allergic to any of the antiandrogens.
- You are female.

Before you start, consult your doctor:
- If you have liver disease.
- If you use tobacco.
- If you have lung disease or other breathing problems.
- If you have glucose-6-phosphate dehydrogenase (G6PD) deficiency or hemoglobin M disease.
- If you are planning on starting a family. May decrease sperm count.

Over age 60:
Adverse reactions and side effects may be more frequent and severe than in younger persons. You may need smaller doses for shorter periods of time.

Pregnancy:
These drugs are not intended for use in women. Risk categories vary for each drug. Bicalutamide is risk category X, flutamide is risk category D and nilutamide is risk category C (see page xviii).

Breast-feeding:
Not intended for use in women.

Infants & children:
Not intended for use in infants and children.

Prolonged use:
Talk to your doctor about the need for follow-up medical examinations or laboratory studies to check liver and pulmonary functions, PSA levels, chest x-rays, and other tests as recommended.

Skin & sunlight:
May cause rash or intensify sunburn in areas exposed to sun or ultraviolet light (photosensitivity reaction). Avoid overexposure. Notify doctor if reaction occurs.

Driving, piloting or hazardous work:
You may experience vision problems when going from a dark area to a lighted area and vice versa (such as driving in and out of tunnels). Use caution.

Discontinuing:
No special problems expected. Don't discontinue drug without doctor's approval.

Others:
- Advise any doctor or dentist whom you consult that you take this medicine.
- May affect results in some medical tests.
- May decrease sperm count.

POSSIBLE INTERACTION WITH OTHER DRUGS

GENERIC NAME OR DRUG CLASS	COMBINED EFFECT
Anticoagulants*	Increased effect of anticoagulant.
Phenytoin	Increased effect of phenytoin.
Theophylline	Increased effect of theophylline.

POSSIBLE INTERACTION WITH OTHER SUBSTANCES

INTERACTS WITH	COMBINED EFFECT
Alcohol:	Nilutamide may cause alcohol intolerance reaction. Avoid alcohol while on this drug.
Beverages:	None expected.
Cocaine:	None expected. Best to avoid.
Foods:	None expected.
Marijuana:	None expected. Best to avoid.
Tobacco:	Increased risk of toxicity. Avoid.

*See Glossary

ANTIBACTERIALS, ANTIFUNGALS (Topical)

GENERIC AND BRAND NAMES

CLIOQUINOL & HYDROCORTISONE
- Vioform Hydrocortisone Cream
- Vioform Hydrocortisone Lotion
- Vioform Hydrocortisone Mild Cream
- Vioform Hydrocortisone Mild Ointment
- Vioform Hydrocortisone Ointment

SULFADIAZINE
- Flamazine
- Flint SSD
- Sildamac
- Silvadene
- SSD
- SSD AF
- Thermazene

BASIC INFORMATION

Habit forming? No
Prescription needed? Yes
Available as generic? Yes, some are
Drug class: Antibacterial (topical), antifungal (topical)

USES

Treats eczema, other inflammatory skin conditions, athlete's foot, skin infections.

DOSAGE & USAGE INFORMATION

How to use:
- Cream, lotion, ointment—Bathe and dry area before use. Apply small amount and rub gently.
- Keep away from eyes.

When to use:
2 to 4 times a day.

If you forget a dose:
Use as soon as you remember.

Continued next column

OVERDOSE

SYMPTOMS:
Severe nausea, vomiting, diarrhea.
WHAT TO DO:
- **Not for internal use. If child accidentally swallows, call poison center 1-800-222-1222.**
- **Dial 911 (emergency) for an ambulance or medical help. Then give first aid immediately.**
- **See emergency information on inside covers.**

What drug does:
Kills some types of fungus and bacteria on contact.

Time lapse before drug works:
2 to 4 weeks, sometimes longer.

Don't use with:
Other ointments, creams or lotions without consulting doctor.

POSSIBLE ADVERSE REACTIONS OR SIDE EFFECTS

SYMPTOMS	WHAT TO DO
Life-threatening: None expected.	
Common: May stain skin around nails.	Continue. Tell doctor at next visit.
Infrequent: Stomach cramps; hives; itching, burning, peeling, red, stinging, swelling skin.	Discontinue. Call doctor right away.
Rare: None expected.	

WARNINGS & PRECAUTIONS

Don't use if:
You are allergic to clioquinol, iodine or any iodine-containing preparation.

Before you start, consult your doctor:
If you are allergic to anything that touches your skin.

Over age 60:
No problems expected.

Pregnancy:
Risk factors vary for drugs in this group. See category list on page xviii and consult doctor.

Breast-feeding:
No problems expected, but check with doctor.

Infants & children:
No problems expected, but check with doctor.

Prolonged use:
No problems expected, but check with doctor.

Skin & sunlight:
No special problems expected.

Driving, piloting or hazardous work:
No problems expected, but check with doctor.

Discontinuing:
No problems expected, but check with doctor.

Others:
- If not improved in 2 weeks, check with doctor.
- May stain clothing or bed linens.
- May stain hair, skin and nails yellow.
- If accidentally gets into eyes, flush with clear water immediately.
- Tests of thyroid function may yield inaccurate results if you use clioquinol within 1 month before testing.

POSSIBLE INTERACTION WITH OTHER DRUGS

GENERIC NAME OR DRUG CLASS	COMBINED EFFECT
None expected.	

POSSIBLE INTERACTION WITH OTHER SUBSTANCES

INTERACTS WITH	COMBINED EFFECT
Alcohol:	None expected.
Beverages:	None expected.
Cocaine:	None expected.
Foods:	None expected.
Marijuana:	None expected.
Tobacco:	None expected.

ANTIBACTERIALS FOR ACNE (Topical)

GENERIC AND BRAND NAMES

CHLORTETRACYCLINE (topical)
- Aureomycin

CLINDAMYCIN (topical)
- Cleocin T Gel
- Cleocin T Lotion
- Cleocin T Topical Solution
- Clinda-Derm
- Dalacin T Topical Solution

CLINDAMYCIN & BENZOYL PEROXIDE
- Benzaclin

DOXYCYCLINE
- Adoxa

ERYTHROMYCIN (topical)
- Akne-Mycin
- A/T/S
- Benzamycin
- Erycette
- EryDerm
- EryGel
- EryMax
- ErySol
- Erythro-statin
- ETS
- Sans-Acne
- Staticin
- Theramycin Z
- T-Stat

TETRACYCLINE (topical)
- Achromycin
- Topicycline

BASIC INFORMATION

Habit forming? No
Prescription needed? Yes
Available as generic? Yes
Drug class: Antibacterial (topical)

USES

Treats acne by killing skin bacteria that may be part of the cause of acne.

DOSAGE & USAGE INFORMATION

How to use:
- Pledgets and solutions are flammable. Use away from flame or heat.
- Apply medication to entire area, not just to pimples.
- If you use other acne medicines on skin, wait an hour after using erythromycin before applying other medicine.
- Cream, lotion, ointment—Bathe and dry area before use. Apply small amount and rub gently.

When to use:
2 times a day, morning and evening, or as directed by your doctor.

If you forget a dose:
Use as soon as you remember.

What drug does:
Kills bacteria on skin, skin glands or in hair follicles.

Time lapse before drug works:
3 to 4 weeks to begin improvement.

Don't use with:
Other skin medicine without telling your doctor.

OVERDOSE

SYMPTOMS:
None expected.
WHAT TO DO:
Not for internal use. If child accidentally swallows, call poison center 1-800-222-1222.

POSSIBLE ADVERSE REACTIONS OR SIDE EFFECTS

SYMPTOMS	WHAT TO DO
Life-threatening:	
None expected.	
Common:	
Stinging or burning of skin for a few minutes after application; faint yellow skin color, especially around hair roots (with chlortetracycline, meclocycline or tetracycline).	Continue. Tell doctor at next visit.
Infrequent:	
Red, peeling, itching, irritated or dry skin.	Continue. Call doctor when convenient.
Rare (extremely):	
Symptoms of excess medicine absorbed by body—Abdominal pain, diarrhea, fever, nausea, vomiting, bloating, thirst, weakness, weight loss.	Discontinue. Call doctor right away.

ANTIBACTERIALS FOR ACNE (Topical)

WARNINGS & PRECAUTIONS

Don't use if:
You are allergic to erythromycins, clindamycins or tetracyclines.

Before you start, consult your doctor:
- If you are allergic to any substance that touches your skin.
- If you use benzoyl peroxide, resorcinol, salicylic acid, sulfur or tretinoin (vitamin A acid).

Over age 60:
No problems expected.

Pregnancy:
Risk factors vary for drugs in this group. See category list on page xviii and consult doctor.

Breast-feeding:
No problems expected, but check with doctor.

Infants & children:
No problems expected, but check with doctor.

Prolonged use:
Excess irritation to skin.

Skin & sunlight:
No special problems expected.

Driving, piloting or hazardous work:
No problems expected, but check with doctor.

Discontinuing:
No problems expected, but check with doctor.

Others:
- Use water-base cosmetics.
- Keep medicine away from mouth or eyes.
- If accidentally gets into eyes, flush immediately with clear water.
- Keep away from heat or flame.
- Keep cool, but don't freeze.

POSSIBLE INTERACTION WITH OTHER DRUGS

GENERIC NAME OR DRUG CLASS	COMBINED EFFECT
Abrasive or medicated soaps	Irritation or too much drying.
After-shave lotions	Irritation or too much drying.
Antiacne topical preparations (other)	Irritation or too much drying.
"Cover-up" cosmetics	Irritation or too much drying.
Drying cosmetic soaps	Irritation or too much drying.
Isotretinoin	Irritation or too much drying.
Mercury compounds	May stain skin black and smell bad.
Perfumed toilet water	Irritation or too much drying.
Preparations containing skin peeling agents such as benzoyl peroxide, resorcinol, salicylic acid, sulfur, tretinoin	Irritation or too much drying.

POSSIBLE INTERACTION WITH OTHER SUBSTANCES

INTERACTS WITH	COMBINED EFFECT
Alcohol:	None expected.
Beverages:	None expected.
Cocaine:	None expected.
Foods:	None expected.
Marijuana:	None expected.
Tobacco:	None expected.

*See Glossary

ANTIBACTERIALS (Ophthalmic)

GENERIC AND BRAND NAMES

See complete list of generic and brand names in the *Generic and Brand Name Directory*, page 862.

BASIC INFORMATION

Habit forming? No
Prescription needed? Yes
Available as generic? Yes, for some
Drug class: Antibacterial (ophthalmic)

USES

- Helps body overcome eye infections on surface tissues of the eye.
- Treatment for corneal ulcers, bacterial.

DOSAGE & USAGE INFORMATION

How to use:
Eye drops
- Wash hands.
- Apply pressure to inside corner of eye with middle finger.
- Continue pressure for 1 minute after placing medicine in eye.
- Tilt head backward. Pull lower lid away from eye with index finger of the same hand.
- Drop eye drops into pouch and close eye. Don't blink.
- Keep eyes closed for 1 to 2 minutes.

Eye ointment
- Wash hands.
- Pull lower lid down from eye to form a pouch.
- Squeeze tube to apply thin strip of ointment into pouch.
- Close eye for 1 to 2 minutes.
- Don't touch applicator tip to any surface (including the eye). If you accidentally touch tip, clean with warm soap and water.
- Keep container tightly closed.
- Keep cool, but don't freeze.
- Wash hands immediately after using.

Continued next column

OVERDOSE

SYMPTOMS:
None expected.
WHAT TO DO:
Not intended for internal use. If child accidentally swallows, call poison center 1-800-222-1222.

When to use:
As directed. Don't miss doses.

If you forget a dose:
Use as soon as you remember.

What drug does:
Penetrates bacterial cell membrane and prevents cells from multiplying.

Time lapse before drug works:
Begins in 1 hour. May require 7 to 10 days to control infection.

Don't use with:
Any other eye drops or ointment without checking with your ophthalmologist.

POSSIBLE ADVERSE REACTIONS OR SIDE EFFECTS

SYMPTOMS	WHAT TO DO
Life-threatening: None expected.	
Common: Ointments cause blurred vision for a few minutes.	Continue. Tell doctor at next visit.
Infrequent:	
• Signs of irritation not present before drug use.	Discontinue. Call doctor right away.
• Burning or stinging of the eye.	Continue. Call doctor when convenient.
Rare (with chloramphenicol): Sore throat, pale skin, fever, unusual bleeding or bruising.	Discontinue. Call doctor right away.

WARNINGS & PRECAUTIONS

Don't use if:
You are allergic to any antibiotic used on skin, ears, vagina or rectum.

Before you start, consult your doctor:
If you have had an allergic reaction to any medicine, food or other substances.

Over age 60:
No problems expected.

Pregnancy:
Risk factors vary for drugs in this group. See category list on page xviii and consult doctor.

Breast-feeding:
No problems expected, but check with doctor.

Infants & children:
No problems expected. Use only under medical supervision.

Prolonged use:
Sensitivity reaction may develop.

Skin & sunlight:
No problems expected.

Driving, piloting or hazardous work:
No problems expected.

Discontinuing:
Possible rare adverse reaction of bone marrow depression that leads to aplastic anemia may occur after discontinuing chloramphenicol.

Others:
- Notify doctor if symptoms fail to improve in 2 to 4 days.
- Keep medicine cool, but don't freeze.

POSSIBLE INTERACTION WITH OTHER DRUGS

GENERIC NAME OR DRUG CLASS	COMBINED EFFECT

Clinically significant interactions with oral or injected medicines unlikely.

POSSIBLE INTERACTION WITH OTHER SUBSTANCES

INTERACTS WITH	COMBINED EFFECT
Alcohol:	None expected.
Beverages:	None expected.
Cocaine:	None expected.
Foods:	None expected.
Marijuana:	None expected.
Tobacco:	None expected.

ANTIBACTERIALS (Otic)

GENERIC AND BRAND NAMES

CHLORAMPHENICOL
Chloromycetin
Sopamycetin
COLISTIN, NEOMYCIN & HYDRO-CORTISONE
Coly-Mycin S
GENTAMICIN (otic)
Garamycin Otic Solution
HYDROCORTISONE & ACETIC ACID
Acetasol HC
Otic Tridesilon Solution
Otomycet-HC
VasotateHC
Vosol HC
NEOMYCIN, POLYMIXIN B & HYDROCORTI-SONE
Antibiotic Ear
Cortarigen Modified Ear Drops
Cort-Biotic
Cortisporin
Drotic
Ear-Eze
LazerSporin
Masporin Otic
Octigen
Ortega Otic-M
Oticair
Otimar
Otobione
Otocidin
Otocort
Pediotic

BASIC INFORMATION

Habit forming? No
Prescription needed? Yes
Available as generic? Yes
Drug class: Antibacterial (otic)

USES

Ear infections in external ear canal (not middle ear) caused by susceptible germs (bacteria, virus, fungus).

OVERDOSE

SYMPTOMS:
None expected.
WHAT TO DO:
Not intended for internal use. If child accidentally swallows, call poison center 1-800-222-1222.

DOSAGE & USAGE INFORMATION

How to use:
Ear drops
- Warm ear drops under running water around the unopened bottle.
- Lie down with affected ear up.
- Adults—Pull ear lobe back and up.
- Children—Pull ear lobe down and back.
- Drop medicine into ear canal until canal is full.
- Stay lying down for 2 minutes.
- Gently insert cotton plug into ear to prevent leaking.

Ear ointment
- Apply small amount to skin just inside the ear canal.
- Use finger or piece of sterile gauze.
- Don't use cotton-tipped applicators.

When to use:
As directed on label.

If you forget a dose:
Use as soon as you remember.

What drug does:
Kills germs that infect the skin of the external ear canal.

Time lapse before drug works:
15 minutes.

Don't use with:
Other ear medications unless directed by your doctor.

POSSIBLE ADVERSE REACTIONS OR SIDE EFFECTS

SYMPTOMS	WHAT TO DO
Life-threatening: None expected.	
Common: None expected.	
Infrequent:	
• Itching, redness, swelling.	Discontinue. Call doctor right away.
• Burning or stinging of the ear.	Continue. Call doctor when convenient.
Rare (with chloramphenicol): Pale skin, sore throat, fever, unusual bleeding or bruising, unusual tiredness or weakness.	Discontinue. Call doctor right away.

WARNINGS & PRECAUTIONS

Don't use if:
You are allergic to any of the medicines listed.

Before you start, consult your doctor:
If eardrum is punctured.

Over age 60:
No problems expected.

Pregnancy:
Risk factors vary for drugs in this group. See category list on page xviii and consult doctor.

Breast-feeding:
No problems expected. Consult doctor.

Infants & children:
No problems expected.

Prolonged use:
Not intended for prolonged use. Don't use longer than 7 to 10 days for any one problem.

Skin & sunlight:
No special problems expected.

Driving, piloting or hazardous work:
No problems expected.

Discontinuing:
Possible rare adverse reaction of bone marrow depression that leads to aplastic anemia after discontinuing chloramphenicol.

Others:
Keep cool, but don't freeze.

POSSIBLE INTERACTION WITH OTHER DRUGS

GENERIC NAME OR DRUG CLASS	COMBINED EFFECT
None expected.	

POSSIBLE INTERACTION WITH OTHER SUBSTANCES

INTERACTS WITH	COMBINED EFFECT
Alcohol:	None expected.
Beverages:	None expected.
Cocaine:	None expected.
Foods:	None expected.
Marijuana:	None expected.
Tobacco:	None expected.

*See Glossary

ANTIBACTERIALS (Topical)

GENERIC AND BRAND NAMES

CHLORAMPHENICOL (topical)
- Chloromycetin

GENTAMICIN
- Garamycin
- Gentamar
- G-Myticin Antibiotic

MUPIROCIN
- Bactroban
- Bactroban Nasal

NEOMYCIN & POLYMIXIN B
- Neosporin

NEOMYCIN, POLYMIXIN B & BACITRACIN
- Bactine First Aid
- Foille
- Mycitracin
- Neo-Polycin
- Neosporin Maximum Strength Ointment
- Neosporin Ointment
- Topisporin
- Triple Antibiotic

BASIC INFORMATION

Habit forming? No
Prescription needed? Yes
Available as generic? Yes
Drug class: Antibacterial (topical)

USES

Treats skin infections that may accompany burns, superficial boils, insect bites or stings, skin ulcers, minor surgical wounds.

DOSAGE & USAGE INFORMATION

How to use:
- Cream, lotion, ointment—Bathe and dry area before use. Apply small amount and rub gently. May cover with gauze or bandage if desired.
- Nasal ointment—Follow instructions provided with prescription.

Continued next column

OVERDOSE

SYMPTOMS:
None expected.
WHAT TO DO:
Not for internal use. If child accidentally swallows, call poison center 1-800-222-1222.
- **Dial 911 (emergency) for an ambulance or medical help. Then give first aid immediately.**
- **See emergency information on inside covers.**

When to use:
3 or 4 times daily, or as directed by doctor.

If you forget a dose:
Use as soon as you remember.

What drug does:
Kills susceptible bacteria by interfering with bacterial DNA and RNA.

Time lapse before drug works:
Begins first day. May require treatment for a week or longer to cure infection.

Don't use with:
Any other medicine without consulting your doctor or pharmacist.

POSSIBLE ADVERSE REACTIONS OR SIDE EFFECTS

SYMPTOMS	WHAT TO DO
Life-threatening: None expected.	
Common: None expected.	
Infrequent: Itching, swollen or red skin; rash.	Discontinue. Call doctor right away.
Rare: Any sort of hearing loss (with neomycin products); pale skin, sore throat, fever, unusual bleeding or bruising, unusual tiredness or weakness (with chloramphenicol).	Discontinue. Call doctor right away.

WARNINGS & PRECAUTIONS

Don't use if:
You are allergic to chloramphenicol, gentamicin or related antibiotics (name usually ends with "mycin" or "micin"), mupirocin, neomycin, polymyxins.

Before you start, consult your doctor:
If any of the lesions on the skin are open sores.

Over age 60:
No problems expected.

Pregnancy:
Risk factors vary for drugs in this group. See category list on page xviii and consult doctor.

Breast-feeding:
No problems expected, but check with doctor.

Infants & children:
No problems expected, but check with doctor.

Prolonged use:
No problems expected, but check with doctor.

Skin & sunlight:
No special problems expected.

Driving, piloting or hazardous work:
No problems expected, but check with doctor.

Discontinuing:
No problems expected, but check with doctor.

Others:
- Heat and moisture in bathroom medicine cabinet can cause breakdown of medicine. Store someplace else.
- Keep cool, but don't freeze.

POSSIBLE INTERACTION WITH OTHER DRUGS

GENERIC NAME OR DRUG CLASS	COMBINED EFFECT
Any other topical medication	Hypersensitivity* reactions more likely to occur.

POSSIBLE INTERACTION WITH OTHER SUBSTANCES

INTERACTS WITH	COMBINED EFFECT
Alcohol:	None expected.
Beverages:	None expected.
Cocaine:	None expected.
Foods:	None expected.
Marijuana:	None expected.
Tobacco:	None expected.

*See Glossary

ANTICHOLINERGICS

GENERIC AND BRAND NAMES

See complete list of generic and brand names in the *Generic and Brand Name Directory*, page 862.

BASIC INFORMATION

Habit forming? No
Prescription needed?
Low strength: No
High strength: Yes
Available as generic? Yes
Drug class: Antispasmodic, anticholinergic

USES

- Reduces spasms of digestive system, bladder and urethra.
- Treatment of bronchial spasms.
- Used as a component in some cough and cold preparations.
- Treatment of peptic ulcers.

DOSAGE & USAGE INFORMATION

How to take:
- Tablet—Swallow with liquid or food to lessen stomach irritation.
- Aerosol—Dilute in saline and inhale as nebulizer.

When to take:
30 minutes before meals (unless directed otherwise by doctor).

If you forget a dose:
Take as soon as you remember up to 2 hours late. If more than 2 hours, wait for next scheduled dose (don't double this dose).

What drug does:
Blocks nerve impulses at parasympathetic nerve endings, preventing muscle contractions and gland secretions of organs involved.

Continued next column

OVERDOSE

SYMPTOMS:
Dilated pupils, rapid pulse and breathing, dizziness, fever, hallucinations, confusion, slurred speech, agitation, flushed face, convulsions, coma.
WHAT TO DO:
- **Dial 911 (emergency) or poison center 1-800-222-1222 for an ambulance or medical help. Then give first aid immediately.**
- **See emergency information on inside covers.**

Time lapse before drug works:
15 to 30 minutes.

Don't take with:
- Antacids* or antidiarrheals*.
- Any other medicine without consulting your doctor or pharmacist.

POSSIBLE ADVERSE REACTIONS OR SIDE EFFECTS

SYMPTOMS	WHAT TO DO
Life-threatening: In case of overdose, see previous column.	
Common:	
• Confusion, delirium, rapid heartbeat.	Discontinue. Call doctor right away.
• Nausea, vomiting, decreased sweating.	Continue. Call doctor when convenient.
• Constipation.	Continue. Tell doctor at next visit.
• Dryness in ears, nose, throat, mouth.	No action necessary.
Infrequent:	
• Headache, difficult or painful urination, nasal congestion, altered taste, increased sensitivity to light.	Continue. Call doctor when convenient.
• Lightheadedness.	Discontinue. Call doctor right away.
Rare:	
Rash or hives, eye pain, blurred vision, fever.	Discontinue. Call doctor right away.

WARNINGS & PRECAUTIONS

Don't take if:
- You are allergic to any anticholinergic.
- You have trouble with stomach bloating.
- You have difficulty emptying your bladder completely.
- You have narrow-angle glaucoma.
- You have severe ulcerative colitis.

Before you start, consult your doctor:

- If you have open-angle glaucoma.
- If you have angina or any heart disease or heart rhythm problem.
- If you have chronic bronchitis or asthma.
- If you have liver, kidney or thyroid disease.
- If you have hiatal hernia or esophagitis.
- If you have enlarged prostate or urinary retention.
- If you have myasthenia gravis.
- If you have peptic ulcer.
- If you will have surgery within 2 months, including dental surgery, requiring general or spinal anesthesia.

Over age 60:
Adverse reactions and side effects may be more frequent and severe than in younger persons.

Pregnancy:
Risk factors vary for drugs in this group. See category list on page xviii and consult doctor.

Breast-feeding:
Drug may pass into milk and could affect milk flow. Avoid drug or discontinue nursing until you finish medicine. Consult doctor for advice on maintaining milk supply.

Infants & children:
Use only under medical supervision.

Prolonged use:
Chronic constipation, possible fecal impaction. Consult doctor immediately.

Skin & sunlight:
No special problems expected.

Driving, piloting or hazardous work:
Use disqualifies you for piloting aircraft. Otherwise, no problems expected.

Discontinuing:
May be unnecessary to finish medicine. Follow doctor's instructions.

Others:
Advise any doctor or dentist whom you consult that you take this medicine.

POSSIBLE INTERACTION WITH OTHER DRUGS

GENERIC NAME OR DRUG CLASS	COMBINED EFFECT
Adrenocorticoids, systemic	Possible glaucoma.
Amantadine	Increased anti-cholinergic effect.
Antacids*	Space doses of the drugs 2 to 3 hours apart.
Anticholinergics, other*	Increased anti-cholinergic effect.
Antidepressants, tricyclic*	Increased anti-cholinergic effect. Increased sedation.
Antifungals, azoles	Decreased azole absorption.
Antihistamines*	Increased anti-cholinergic effect.
Attapulgite	Decreased anti-cholinergic effect.
Haloperidol	Increased internal eye pressure.
Methylphenidate	Increased anti-cholinergic effect.
Molindone	Increased anti-cholinergic effect.
Monoamine oxidase (MAO) inhibitors*	Increased anti-cholinergic effect.
Narcotics*	Increased risk of severe constipation.
Orphenadrine	Increased anti-cholinergic effect.
Phenothiazines*	Increased anti-cholinergic effect.
Potassium supplements*	Possible intestinal ulcers with oral potassium tablets.
Quinidine	Increased anti-cholinergic effect.

POSSIBLE INTERACTION WITH OTHER SUBSTANCES

INTERACTS WITH	COMBINED EFFECT
Alcohol:	None expected.
Beverages:	None expected.
Cocaine:	Excessively rapid heartbeat. Avoid.
Foods:	None expected.
Marijuana:	Drowsiness and dry mouth.
Tobacco:	None expected.

ANTICOAGULANTS (Oral)

GENERIC AND BRAND NAMES

ANISINDIONE
Miradon

WARFARIN SODIUM
Coumadin
Panwarfarin
Sofarin
Warfilone

BASIC INFORMATION

Habit forming? No
Prescription needed? Yes
Available as generic? Yes
Drug class: Anticoagulant

USES

Reduces blood clots. Used for abnormal clotting inside blood vessels.

DOSAGE & USAGE INFORMATION

How to take:
Tablet—Swallow with liquid. If you can't swallow whole, crumble tablet and take with liquid or food.

When to take:
At the same time each day.

If you forget a dose:
Take as soon as you remember up to 12 hours late. If more than 12 hours, wait for next scheduled dose (don't double this dose). Inform your doctor of any missed doses.

What drug does:
Blocks action of vitamin K necessary for blood clotting.

Time lapse before drug works:
36 to 48 hours.

Don't take with:
Any other medicine without consulting your doctor or pharmacist.

OVERDOSE

SYMPTOMS:
Bloody vomit, coughing blood, bloody or black stools, red urine.
WHAT TO DO:
- **Dial 911 (emergency) or poison center 1-800-222-1222 for an ambulance or medical help. Then give first aid immediately.**
- **See emergency information on inside covers.**

POSSIBLE ADVERSE REACTIONS OR SIDE EFFECTS

SYMPTOMS	WHAT TO DO
Life-threatening:	
In case of overdose, see previous column.	
Common:	
Bloating, gas.	Continue. Tell doctor at next visit.
Infrequent:	
• Black stools or bloody vomit, coughing up blood.	Discontinue. Seek emergency treatment.
• Rash, hives, itch, blurred vision, sore throat, easy bruising, bleeding, cloudy or red urine, back pain, jaundice, fever, chills, fatigue, weakness, painful urination, decreased amount of urine, heavy menstruation, bleeding gums.	Discontinue. Call doctor right away.
• Diarrhea, cramps, nausea, vomiting, swollen feet or legs, hair loss.	Continue. Call doctor when convenient.
Rare:	
• Bleeding into and under skin.	Discontinue. Seek emergency treatment.
• Dizziness, headache, mouth sores.	Discontinue. Call doctor right away.

WARNINGS & PRECAUTIONS

Don't take if:
- You have been allergic to any oral anticoagulant.
- You have a bleeding disorder.
- You have an active peptic ulcer.
- You have ulcerative colitis.

Before you start, consult your doctor:
- If you take any other drugs, including nonprescription drugs.
- If you have high blood pressure.
- If you have heavy or prolonged menstrual periods.
- If you have diabetes.
- If you have a bladder catheter.
- If you have serious liver or kidney disease.
- If you will have surgery within 2 months, including dental surgery, requiring general or spinal anesthesia.

Over age 60:
Adverse reactions and side effects may be more frequent and severe than in younger persons.

Pregnancy:
Risk factors vary for drugs in this group. See category list on page xviii and consult doctor.

Breast-feeding:
Drug filters into milk. May harm child. Avoid.

Infants & children:
Use only under doctor's supervision.

Prolonged use:
Talk to your doctor about the need for follow-up medical examinations or laboratory studies to check prothorombin time, stool and urine for blood.

Skin & sunlight:
No problems expected.

Driving, piloting or hazardous work:
- Avoid hazardous activities that could cause injury.
- Don't drive if you feel dizzy or have blurred vision.

Discontinuing:
Don't discontinue without consulting doctor. Dose may require gradual reduction if you have taken drug for a long time. Doses of other drugs may also require adjustment.

Others:
- Carry identification to state that you take anticoagulants.
- Advise any doctor or dentist whom you consult that you take this medicine.

POSSIBLE INTERACTION WITH OTHER DRUGS

GENERIC NAME OR DRUG CLASS	COMBINED EFFECT
Acetaminophen	Increased effect of anticoagulant.
Adrenocorticoids, systemic	Decreased anticoagulant effect.
Allopurinol	Increased effect of anticoagulant.
Aminoglutethmide	Decreased effect of anticoagulant.
Amiodarone	Increased effect of anticoagulant.
Androgens*	Increased effect of anticoagulant.
Antacids* (large doses)	Decreased effect of anticoagulant.
Antibiotics*	Increased effect of anticoagulant.
Antidiabetic agents*	Increased effect of anticoagulant.
Antifungals, azoles	Increased anticoagulant effect.
Antihistamines*	Unpredictable increased or decreased effect of anticoagulant.
Anti-inflammatory drugs, nonsteroidal (NSAIDs)*	Increased risk of bleeding.
Anti-inflammatory drugs, nonsteroidal (ophthalmic)*	May increase bleeding tendency.
Aspirin	Possible spontaneous bleeding.
Barbiturates*	Decreased effect of anticoagulant.
Benzodiazepines*	Unpredictable increased or decreased effect of anticoagulant.
Bismuth subsalicylate	Increased risk of bleeding.
Calcium supplements*	Decreased effect of anticoagulant.
Carbamazepine	Decreased effect of anticoagulant.
Cefixime	Increased effect of anticoagulant.
Chloramphenicol	Increased effect of anticoagulant.

Continued on page 896

POSSIBLE INTERACTION WITH OTHER SUBSTANCES

INTERACTS WITH	COMBINED EFFECT
Alcohol:	Can increase or decrease effect of anticoagulant. Use with caution.
Beverages:	None expected.
Cocaine:	None expected.
Foods: High in vitamin K such as fish, liver, spinach, cabbage, cauliflower, Brussels sprouts.	May decrease anticoagulant effect.
Marijuana:	None expected.
Tobacco:	Decreased effect of anticoagulant.

*See Glossary

ANTICONVULSANTS, HYDANTOIN

GENERIC AND BRAND NAMES

ETHOTOIN	PHENYTOIN
Peganone	Dilantin
	Dilantin 30
	Dilantin 125
	Dilantin Infatabs
	Dilantin Kapseals
	Diphenylan

BASIC INFORMATION

Habit forming? No
Prescription needed? Yes
Available as generic? Yes
Drug class: Anticonvulsant (hydantoin)

USES

- Prevents some forms of epileptic seizures.
- Stabilizes irregular heartbeat.

DOSAGE & USAGE INFORMATION

How to take:
- Tablet—Swallow with liquid.
- Chewable tablets—Chew well before swallowing.
- Suspension—Shake solution well before taking with liquid.

When to take:
At the same time each day.

If you forget a dose:
- If drug taken 1 time per day—Take as soon as you remember up to 12 hours late. If more than 12 hours, wait for next scheduled dose (don't double this dose).
- If taken several times per day—Take as soon as possible, then return to regular schedule.

Continued next column

OVERDOSE

SYMPTOMS:
Jerky eye movements; stagger; slurred speech; imbalance; drowsiness; blood pressure drop; slow, shallow breathing; coma.

WHAT TO DO:
- **Dial 911 (emergency) or poison center 1-800-222-1222 for an ambulance or medical help. Then give first aid immediately.**
- **See emergency information on inside covers.**

What drug does:
Promotes sodium loss from nerve fibers. This lessens excitability and inhibits spread of nerve impulses.

Time lapse before drug works:
7 to 10 days continual use.

Don't take with:
Any other medicine without consulting your doctor or pharmacist.

POSSIBLE ADVERSE REACTIONS OR SIDE EFFECTS

SYMPTOMS	WHAT TO DO
Life-threatening:	
Severe allergic reaction (rash, fever, swollen glands, kidney failure).	Seek emergency help.
Common:	
• Bleeding, swollen or tender gums.	Continue, but call doctor right away.
• Mild dizziness or drowsiness, constipation.	Continue. Call doctor when convenient.
Infrequent:	
• Hallucinations, confusion, stagger, fever, uncontrolled eye movements, increase in seizures, rash, change in vision, agitation, sore throat, diarrhea, slurred speech, muscle twitching.	Continue, but call doctor right away.
• Increased body and facial hair, breast swelling, insomnia, enlargement of facial features.	Continue. Call doctor when convenient.
Rare:	
Nausea; vomiting; unusual bleeding or bruising; swollen lymph nodes; stomach pain; yellow skin or eyes; joint pain; light gray stools; loss of appetite; weight loss; trouble breathing; uncontrolled movements of arms, legs, hands, lips, tongue or cheeks; slowed growth; learning problems.	Continue, but call doctor right away.

WARNINGS & PRECAUTIONS

Don't take if:
You are allergic to any hydantoin anticonvulsant.

Before you start, consult your doctor:
- If you have had impaired liver function or disease.
- If you will have surgery within 2 months, including dental surgery, requiring general or spinal anesthesia.
- If you have diabetes.
- If you have a blood disorder.

Over age 60:
Adverse reactions and side effects may be more frequent and severe than in younger persons.

Pregnancy:
Decide with your doctor if drug benefits justify risk to unborn child. Risk category C (see page xviii).

Breast-feeding:
Drug passes into milk. Avoid drug or discontinue nursing until you finish medicine. Consult doctor for advice on maintaining milk supply.

Infants & children:
Use only under medical supervision.

Prolonged use:
- Weakened bones.
- Lymph gland enlargement.
- Possible liver damage.
- Numbness and tingling of hands and feet.
- Continual back-and-forth eye movements.
- Talk to your doctor about the need for follow-up medical examinations or laboratory studies to check complete blood counts (white blood cell count, platelet count, red blood cell count, hemoglobin, hematocrit), liver function, EEG*.

Skin & sunlight:
One or more drugs in this group may cause rash or intensify sunburn in areas exposed to sun or ultraviolet light (photosensitivity reaction). Avoid overexposure. Notify doctor if reaction occurs.

Driving, piloting or hazardous work:
Don't drive or pilot aircraft until you learn how medicine affects you. Don't work around dangerous machinery. Don't climb ladders or work in high places. Danger increases if you drink alcohol or take medicine affecting alertness and reflexes.

Discontinuing:
Don't discontinue without consulting doctor. Dose may require gradual reduction if you have taken drug for a long time. Doses of other drugs may also require adjustment.

Others:
- May cause learning disability.
- Good dental care is important while using this medicine.
- Note: One of the drugs in this group, mephenytoin (brand name Mesantoin), was discontinued in 2001. Talk to your doctor if you have questions about this particular drug.
- Advise any doctor or dentist whom you consult about the use of this drug.

POSSIBLE INTERACTION WITH OTHER DRUGS

GENERIC NAME OR DRUG CLASS	COMBINED EFFECT
Adrenocorticoids, systemic	Decreased adreno-corticoid effect.
Amiodarone	Increased anti-convulsant effect.
Antacids*	Decreased anti-convulsant effect.
Antiandrogens, nonsteroidal	Increased effect of phenytoin.
Anticoagulants*	Increased effect of both drugs.
Antidepressants, tricyclic*	May need to adjust anticonvulsant dose.
Antifungals, azoles	Increased anticoagulant effect.
Antivirals, HIV/AIDS*	Increased risk of peripheral neuropa-thy with phenytoin.
Barbiturates*	Changed seizure pattern.
Calcium	Decreased effects of both drugs.
Carbamazepine	Possible increased anticonvulsant metabolism.
Carbonic anhydrase inhibitors*	Increased chance of bone disease.

Continued on page 897

POSSIBLE INTERACTION WITH OTHER SUBSTANCES

INTERACTS WITH	COMBINED EFFECT
Alcohol:	Possible decreased anticonvulsant effect. Use with caution.
Beverages:	None expected.
Cocaine:	Possible seizures.
Foods:	None expected.
Marijuana:	Drowsiness, unsteadiness, decreased anticonvulsant effect.
Tobacco:	None expected.

*See Glossary

ANTICONVULSANTS, SUCCINIMIDE

GENERIC AND BRAND NAMES

ETHOSUXIMIDE	METHOSUXIMIDE
Zarontin	Celontin

BASIC INFORMATION

Habit forming? No
Prescription needed? Yes
Available as generic? Yes, for some
Drug class: Anticonvulsant (succinimide)

USES

Controls seizures in treatment of some forms of epilepsy.

DOSAGE & USAGE INFORMATION

How to take:
Capsule or syrup—Swallow with liquid or food to lessen stomach irritation.

When to take:
Every day in regularly spaced doses, according to prescription.

If you forget a dose:
Take as soon as you remember up to 2 hours late. If more than 2 hours, wait for next scheduled dose (don't double this dose).

What drug does:
Depresses nerve transmissions in part of brain that controls muscles.

Time lapse before drug works:
3 hours.

Continued next column

OVERDOSE

SYMPTOMS:
Severe drowsiness, slow or irregular breathing, coma.
WHAT TO DO:

- **Dial 911 (emergency) for an ambulance or medical help or poison center 1-800-222-1222. Then give first aid immediately.**
- **If patient is unconscious and not breathing, give mouth-to-mouth breathing. If there is no heartbeat, use cardiac massage and mouth-to-mouth breathing (CPR). Don't try to make patient vomit. If you can't get help quickly, take patient to nearest emergency facility.**
- **See emergency information on inside covers.**

Don't take with:
Any other medicine without consulting your doctor or pharmacist.

POSSIBLE ADVERSE REACTIONS OR SIDE EFFECTS

SYMPTOMS	WHAT TO DO
Life-threatening: In case of overdose, see previous column.	
Common:	
• Nausea, vomiting, appetite loss, dizziness, drowsiness, hiccups, stomach pain, headache, loss of appetite.	Continue. Call doctor when convenient.
• Muscle pain, skin rash or itching, swollen glands, sore throat, fever.	Continue, but call doctor right away.
• Change in urine color (pink, red, red-brown).	No action necessary.
Infrequent:	
Nightmares, irritability, mood changes, tiredness, difficulty concentrating.	Continue, but call doctor right away.
Rare:	
Unusual bleeding or bruising, depression, swollen glands, chills, increased seizures, shortness of breath, wheezing, chest pain, sores in mouth or on lips.	Continue, but call doctor right away.

WARNINGS & PRECAUTIONS

Don't take if:
You are allergic to any succinimide anticonvulsant.

Before you start, consult your doctor:
- If you plan to become pregnant within medication period.
- If you take other anticonvulsants.
- If you have blood disease.
- If you have kidney or liver disease.

Over age 60:
Adverse reactions and side effects may be more frequent and severe than in younger persons.

Pregnancy:
Risk factors vary for drugs in this group. See category list on page xviii and consult doctor.

Breast-feeding:
Drug passes into milk. Avoid drug or discontinue nursing. Consult your doctor about maintaining milk supply.

Infants & children:
Use only under medical supervision.

Prolonged use:
Talk to your doctor about the need for follow-up medical examinations or laboratory studies to check complete blood counts (white blood cell count, platelet count, red blood cell count, hemoglobin, hematocrit), liver function, kidney function, urine.

Skin & sunlight:
No problems expected.

Driving, piloting or hazardous work:
Don't drive or pilot aircraft until you learn how medicine affects you. Don't work around dangerous machinery. Don't climb ladders or work in high places. Danger increases if you drink alcohol or take medicine affecting alertness and reflexes, such as antihistamines, tranquilizers, sedatives, pain medicine, narcotics and mind-altering drugs.

Discontinuing:
Don't discontinue without doctor's advice until you complete prescribed dose, even though symptoms diminish or disappear.

Others:
- Your response to medicine should be checked regularly by your doctor. Dose and schedule may have to be altered frequently to fit individual needs.
- Periodic blood cell counts, kidney and liver function studies recommended.
- May discolor urine pink to red-brown. No action necessary.
- Advise any doctor or dentist whom you consult about the use of this medicine.

POSSIBLE INTERACTION WITH OTHER DRUGS

GENERIC NAME OR DRUG CLASS	COMBINED EFFECT
Anticonvulsants, other*	Increased effect of both drugs.
Antidepressants, tricyclic*	May provoke seizures.
Antipsychotics*	May provoke seizures.
Central nervous system (CNS) depressants*	Decreased anti-convulsant effect.
Haloperidol	Decreased haloperidol effect; changed seizure pattern.
Phenytoin	Increased phenytoin effect.

POSSIBLE INTERACTION WITH OTHER SUBSTANCES

INTERACTS WITH	COMBINED EFFECT
Alcohol:	May provoke seizures.
Beverages:	None expected.
Cocaine:	May provoke seizures.
Foods:	None expected.
Marijuana:	May provoke seizures.
Tobacco:	None expected.

*See Glossary

ANTIDEPRESSANTS, TRICYCLIC

GENERIC AND BRAND NAMES

See complete list of generic and brand names in the *Generic and Brand Name Directory*, page 862.

BASIC INFORMATION

Habit forming? No
Prescription needed? Yes
Available as generic? Yes
Drug class: Antidepressant (tricyclic)

USES

- Gradually relieves symptoms of depression.
- Used to decrease bedwetting in children.
- Pain relief (sometimes).
- Clomipramine is used to treat obsessive-compulsive disorder.
- Treatment for narcolepsy, bulimia, panic attacks, cocaine withdrawal, attention-deficit disorder.
- May be useful for restless leg syndrome.

DOSAGE & USAGE INFORMATION

How to take:
Tablet, capsule or syrup—Swallow with liquid.

When to take:
At the same time each day, usually at bedtime.

Continued next column

OVERDOSE

SYMPTOMS:
Hallucinations, drowsiness, enlarged pupils, respiratory failure, fever, cardiac arrhythmias, convulsions, coma.
WHAT TO DO:

- **Dial 911 (emergency) for an ambulance or medical help or poison center 1-800-222-1222. Then give first aid immediately.**
- **If patient is unconscious and not breathing, give mouth-to-mouth breathing. If there is no heartbeat, use cardiac massage and mouth-to-mouth breathing (CPR). Don't try to make patient vomit. If you can't get help quickly, take patient to nearest emergency facility.**
- **See emergency information at end of book.**

If you forget a dose:
Bedtime dose—If you forget your once-a-day bedtime dose, don't take it more than 3 hours late. If more than 3 hours, wait for next scheduled dose. Don't double this dose.

What drug does:
Probably affects part of brain that controls messages between nerve cells.

Time lapse before drug works:
2 to 4 weeks. May require 4 to 6 weeks for maximum benefit.

Don't take with:
Any prescription or nonprescription drugs without consulting your doctor or pharmacist.

POSSIBLE ADVERSE REACTIONS OR SIDE EFFECTS

SYMPTOMS	WHAT TO DO
Life-threatening:	
In case of overdose, see previous column.	
Common:	
• Tremor.	Discontinue. Call doctor right away.
• Headache, dry mouth or unpleasant taste, constipation or diarrhea, nausea, indigestion, fatigue, weakness, drowsiness, nervousness, anxiety, excessive sweating.	Continue. Call doctor when convenient.
• Insomnia, "sweet tooth."	Continue. Tell doctor at next visit.
Infrequent:	
• Convulsions.	Discontinue. Seek emergency treatment.
• Hallucinations, shakiness, dizziness, fainting, blurred vision, eye pain, vomiting, irregular heartbeat or slow pulse, inflamed tongue, abdominal pain, jaundice, hair loss, rash, fever, chills, joint pain, palpitations, hiccups, visual changes.	Discontinue. Call doctor right away.
• Difficult or frequent urination; decreased sex drive; muscle aches; abnormal dreams; nasal congestion; weakness and faintness when arising from bed or chair; back pain.	Continue. Call doctor when convenient.

Rare:

Itchy skin; sore throat; involuntary movements of jaw, lips and tongue; nightmares; confusion; swollen breasts; swollen testicles.	Discontinue. Call doctor right away.

WARNINGS & PRECAUTIONS

Don't take if:
- You are allergic to any tricyclic antidepressant.
- You drink alcohol in excess.
- You have had a heart attack within 6 weeks.
- You have glaucoma.
- You have taken MAO inhibitors* within 2 weeks.
- Patient is younger than 12.

Before you start, consult your doctor:
- If you will have surgery within 2 months, including dental surgery, requiring general or spinal anesthesia.
- If you have an enlarged prostate or glaucoma.
- If you have heart disease or high blood pressure.
- If you have stomach or intestinal problems.
- If you have an overactive thyroid.
- If you have asthma.
- If you have liver disease.

Over age 60:
More likely to develop urination difficulty and serious side effects such as seizures, hallucinations, shaking, dizziness, fainting, headache, insomnia.

Pregnancy:
Risk factors vary for drugs in this group. See category list on page xviii and consult doctor.

Breast-feeding:
Drug may pass into milk. Avoid drug or discontinue nursing until you finish medicine. Consult doctor about maintaining milk supply.

Infants & children:
Don't give to children younger than 12 except under medical supervision.

Prolonged use:
Talk to your doctor about the need for follow-up medical examinations or laboratory studies to check complete blood counts (white blood cell count, platelet count, red blood cell count, hemoglobin, hematocrit), blood pressure, eyes, teeth.

Skin & sunlight:
One or more drugs in this group may cause rash or intensify sunburn in areas exposed to sun or ultraviolet light (photosensitivity reaction). Avoid overexposure and use sunscreen. Notify doctor if reaction occurs.

Driving, piloting or hazardous work:
Don't drive or pilot aircraft until you learn how medicine affects you. Don't work around dangerous machinery. Don't climb ladders or work in high places. Danger increases if you drink alcohol or take medicine affecting alertness and reflexes.

Discontinuing:
- Don't discontinue without consulting doctor. Dose may require gradual reduction if you have taken drug for a long time. Doses of other drugs may also require adjustment.
- Withdrawal symptoms such as convulsions, muscle cramps, nightmares, insomnia, abdominal pain. Call your physician right away if any of these occur.

Others:
- May affect results in some medical tests.
- Advise any doctor or dentist whom you consult that you take this medicine.

POSSIBLE INTERACTION WITH OTHER DRUGS

GENERIC NAME OR DRUG CLASS	COMBINED EFFECT
Adrenocorticoids, systemic	Increased risk of mental side effects.
Antiçoagulants*, oral	Possible increased anticoagulant effect.
Anticholinergics*	Increased anticholinergic effect.
Antifungals, azoles	Increased effect of antidepressant.
Antiglaucoma agents*	Decreased ocular hypertensive effect.

Continued on page 898

POSSIBLE INTERACTION WITH OTHER SUBSTANCES

Alcohol: Beverages or medicines with alcohol.	Excessive intoxication. Avoid.
Beverages:	None expected.
Cocaine:	Increased risk of heartbeat irregularity.
Foods:	None expected.
Marijuana:	Excessive drowsiness. Increased risk of side effects. Avoid.
Tobacco:	Possible decreased tricyclic antidepressant effect.

***See Glossary**

ANTIDYSKINETICS

GENERIC AND BRAND NAMES

See complete list of generic and brand names in the *Generic and Brand Name Directory*, page 862.

BASIC INFORMATION

Habit forming? No
Prescription needed? Yes
Available as generic? Yes
Drug class: Antidyskinetic, antiparkinsonism, dopamine agonists

USES

- Treatment of Parkinson's disease.
- Treatment of adverse effects of certain central nervous system drugs.
- Treatment for Tourette's syndrome.

DOSAGE & USAGE INFORMATION

How to take:

- Tablets—Swallow with liquid. If you can't swallow whole, crumble tablet and take with liquid or food to lessen stomach irritation.
- Extended-release capsule or elixir—Take with food to lessen stomach irritation.

When to take:
At the same times each day.

If you forget a dose:
Take as soon as you remember up to 2 hours late. If more than 2 hours, wait for next scheduled dose (don't double this dose).

Continued next column

OVERDOSE

SYMPTOMS:
Agitation, dilated pupils, hallucinations, dry mouth, rapid heartbeat, sleepiness.
WHAT TO DO:

- **Dial 911 (emergency) for an ambulance or medical help or poison center 1-800-222-1222. Then give first aid immediately.**
- **If patient is unconscious and not breathing, give mouth-to-mouth breathing. If there is no heartbeat, use cardiac massage and mouth-to-mouth breathing (CPR). Don't try to make patient vomit. If you can't get help quickly, take patient to nearest emergency facility.**
- **See emergency information on inside covers.**

What drug does:

- Balances chemical reactions necessary to send nerve impulses within base of brain.
- Improves muscle control and reduces stiffness.

Time lapse before drug works:
1 to 2 hours. Full effect may take 2 to 3 days.

Don't take with:
Any other medication without consulting your doctor or pharmacist.

POSSIBLE ADVERSE REACTIONS OR SIDE EFFECTS

SYMPTOMS	WHAT TO DO
Life-threatening:	
In case of overdose, see previous column.	
Common:	
• Blurred vision, light sensitivity, unusual body movements, painful or difficult or frequent urination, vomiting, hallucinations.	Continue, but call doctor right away.
• Dry mouth, tiredness, weakness feeling, drowsiness or insomnia, constipation, nausea, lightheadedness.	Continue. Call doctor when convenient.
Infrequent:	
Headache, memory loss, abdominal pain, weakness and faintness when arising from bed or chair, nervousness, impotence, sore throat, cough or wheezing, viral infection, appetite loss, restlessness.	Continue. Call doctor when convenient.
Rare:	
• Rash, hives, eye pain, delusions, amnesia, paranoia, fever, swollen neck glands, vision changes, chest pain, swallowing or breathing difficulty, numbness or tingling or swelling in hands or feet, urine bloody or cloudy, ear buzzing, irregular heartbeat.	Continue. Call doctor right away.
• Confusion, dizziness, sore mouth or tongue, muscle cramps or weakness, depression.	Continue. Call doctor when convenient.

Note: Most symptoms representing side effects either disappear or decrease when dose is reduced. Consult doctor.

WARNINGS & PRECAUTIONS

Don't take if:
You are allergic to any antidyskinetic.

Before you start, consult your doctor:
- If you have glaucoma or retinal problems.
- If you have had high blood pressure, heart disease, impaired liver function.
- If you have hypotension or orthostatic hypotension*.
- If you have had tardive dyskinesia*.
- If you have had kidney disease, urination difficulty, prostatic hypertrophy or intestinal obstruction.
- If you have had myasthenia gravis.

Over age 60:
More sensitive to drug. Aggravates symptoms of enlarged prostate. Causes impaired thinking, hallucinations, nightmares. Consult doctor about any of these.

Pregnancy:
Decide with your doctor whether drug benefits justify risk to unborn child. Risk category C (see page xviii).

Breast-feeding:
Effects unknown. May inhibit lactation. Consult doctor.

Infants & children:
Use only under doctor's supervision.

Prolonged use:
- Possible glaucoma.
- Talk to your doctor about the need for follow-up medical examinations to assess drug's effectiveness and examination to check eye pressure.

Skin & sunlight:
No special problems expected.

Driving, piloting or hazardous work:
Don't drive or pilot aircraft until you learn how medicine affects you. Don't work around dangerous machinery. Don't climb ladders or work in high places. Danger increases if you drink alcohol or take medicine affecting alertness and reflexes, such as antihistamines, tranquilizers, sedatives, pain medicine, narcotics and mind-altering drugs.

Discontinuing:
- Don't discontinue without consulting doctor. Dose may require gradual reduction if you have taken drug for a long time. Doses of other drugs may also require adjustment.
- After discontinuing, if you experience extrapyramidal reaction* recurrence or worsening, orthostatic hypotension, fast heart-beat, trouble in sleeping, consult doctor.

Others:
- Internal eye pressure should be measured regularly.
- Avoid becoming overheated.
- Use caution when arising from a sitting or lying position.
- Advise any doctor or dentist whom you consult that you take this medicine.

POSSIBLE INTERACTION WITH OTHER DRUGS

GENERIC NAME OR DRUG CLASS	COMBINED EFFECT
Antacids*	Possible decreased absorption.
Anticholinergics, others*	Increased anti-cholinergic effect.
Antidepressants, tricyclic*	Increased anti-dyskinetic effect.
Antihistamines*	Increased antidyskinetic effect.
Carbidopa	Increased effect of carbidopa.
Chlorpromazine	Decreased effect of chlorpromazine.
Ciprofloxacin	Increased effect of ropinirole.
Central nervous system (CNS) depressants*	May add to any sedative effect.
Dopamine antagonists*	Decreased effect of pramipexole and ropinirole.
Estrogens	Increased effect of ropinirole.

Continued on page 899

POSSIBLE INTERACTION WITH OTHER SUBSTANCES

INTERACTS WITH	COMBINED EFFECT
Alcohol:	Oversedation. Avoid.
Beverages:	None expected.
Cocaine:	Decreased anti-dyskinetic effect. Avoid.
Foods:	None expected.
Marijuana:	None expected.
Tobacco:	Decreased effect of ropinirole.

ANTIFIBRINOLYTIC AGENTS

GENERIC AND BRAND NAMES

AMINOCAPROIC ACID	TRANEXAMIC ACID
Amicar	Cyclokapron

BASIC INFORMATION

Habit forming? No
Prescription needed? Yes
Available as generic? Yes
Drug class: Antifibrinolytic, antihemorrhagic

USES

- Treats serious bleeding, especially occurring after surgery, dental or otherwise.
- Sometimes used before surgery in hopes of preventing excessive bleeding in patients with disorders that increase the chance of serious bleeding.

DOSAGE & USAGE INFORMATION

How to take:
- Tablet—Swallow with liquid or food to lessen stomach irritation. If you can't swallow whole, crumble tablet and take with liquid or food.
- Syrup—Take as directed on label.

When to take:
As directed by your doctor.

If you forget a dose:
Take as soon as you remember. Don't double this dose.

What drug does:
Inhibits activation of plasminogen to cause blood clots to disintegrate.

Time lapse before drug works:
Within 2 hours.

Don't take with:
- Thrombolytic chemicals such as streptokinase, urokinase.
- Any other medicine without consulting your doctor or pharmacist.

OVERDOSE

SYMPTOMS:
None expected for oral forms. Injectable forms may cause drop in blood pressure or slow heartbeat.
WHAT TO DO:
Follow doctor's instructions.

POSSIBLE ADVERSE REACTIONS OR SIDE EFFECTS

SYMPTOMS	WHAT TO DO
Life-threatening:	
Shortness of breath, slurred speech, leg or arm numbness.	Seek emergency treatment.
Common:	
Diarrhea, nausea, vomiting, severe menstrual cramps.	Continue. Call doctor when convenient.
Infrequent:	
Dizziness; headache; muscular pain and weakness; red eyes; ringing in ears; skin rash; abdominal pain; stuffy nose; decreased urine; swelling of feet, face, legs; rapid weight gain.	Continue. Call doctor when convenient.
Rare:	
• Unusual tiredness, blurred vision, clotting of menstrual flow.	Continue. Call doctor when convenient.
• Signs of thrombosis (sudden, severe head-ache; pains in chest, groin or legs; loss of coordination; shortness of breath; slurred speech; vision changes; weakness or numbness in arms or leg).	Seek emergency treatment.

WARNINGS & PRECAUTIONS

Don't take if:
- You are allergic to aminocaproic acid or tranexamic acid.
- You have a diagnosis of disseminated intravascular coagulation (DIC).

Before you start, consult your doctor:
- If you have heart disease.
- If you have bleeding from the kidney.
- If you have had impaired liver function.
- If you have had kidney disease or urination difficulty.
- If you have blood clots in parts of the body.

Over age 60:
No changes from other age groups expected.

Pregnancy:
Risk factors vary for drugs in this group. See category list on page xviii and consult doctor.

Breast-feeding:
No problems documented. Consult doctor.

Infants & children:
Use for children only under doctor's supervision.

Prolonged use:
Talk to your doctor about the need for follow-up medical examinations or laboratory studies to check eyes.

Skin & sunlight:
No problems expected.

Driving, piloting or hazardous work:
Don't drive or pilot aircraft until you learn how medicine affects you. Don't work around dangerous machinery. Don't climb ladders or work in high places. Danger increases if you drink alcohol or take medicine affecting alertness and reflexes, such as antihistamines, tranquilizers, sedatives, pain medicine, narcotics and mind-altering drugs.

Discontinuing:
Don't discontinue without consulting doctor. Dose may require gradual reduction if you have taken drug for a long time. Doses of other drugs may also require adjustment.

Others:
- Should not be used in patients with disseminated intravascular coagulation.
- Advise any doctor or dentist whom you consult that you take this medicine.
- Have eyes checked frequently.

POSSIBLE INTERACTION WITH OTHER DRUGS

GENERIC NAME OR DRUG CLASS	COMBINED EFFECT
Contraceptives, oral*	Increased possibility of blood clotting.
Estrogens*	Increased possibility of blood clotting.
Thrombolytic agents* (alteplase, streptokinase, urokinase)	Decreased effects of both drugs.

POSSIBLE INTERACTION WITH OTHER SUBSTANCES

INTERACTS WITH	COMBINED EFFECT
Alcohol:	Decreases effectiveness. Avoid.
Beverages:	No problems expected.
Cocaine:	Combined effect unknown. Avoid.
Foods:	No problems expected.
Marijuana:	Combined effect unknown. Avoid.
Tobacco:	Combined effect unknown. Avoid.

*See Glossary

ANTIFUNGALS, AZOLES

GENERIC AND BRAND NAMES

FLUCONAZOLE
Diflucan
ITRACONAZOLE
Sporanox
KETOCONAZOLE
Nizoral
Nizoral A-D

BASIC INFORMATION

Habit forming? No
Prescription needed? Yes, for some
Available as generic? No
Drug class: Antifungal

USES

- Treatment for fungal infections.
- Treatment for meningitis (fluconazole).
- Treatment for prostate cancer (ketoconazole).

DOSAGE & USAGE INFORMATION

How to take:
- Capsule or tablet—Swallow with liquid. If you can't swallow whole, crumble tablet or open capsule and take with liquid or food.
- Oral suspension—Shake well before using; follow instructions supplied with medication.
- Shampoo or cream—Follow instructions supplied with medication.

When to take:
At the same time each day.

If you forget a dose:
- Take as soon as you remember up to 2 hours late. If more than 2 hours, wait for next scheduled dose (don't double this dose).
- Itraconazole may come in one-a-day or twice daily dosages. Follow instructions for proper usage (don't double this dose).

What drug does:
Prevents fungi from growing and reproducing. In treating prostate cancer, ketoconazole decreases male hormone (testosterone) levels.

Continued next column

OVERDOSE

SYMPTOMS:
None expected.
WHAT TO DO:
Overdose is unlikely to threaten life. If person takes much larger amount than prescribed, call doctor, poison center 1-800-222-1222 or hospital emergency room for instructions.

Time lapse before drug works:
For fluconazole, 1-2 hours, several weeks or months for full benefit and for all other azoles.

Don't take with:
Any other medicine without consulting your doctor or pharmacist.

POSSIBLE ADVERSE REACTIONS OR SIDE EFFECTS

SYMPTOMS	WHAT TO DO
Life-threatening: None expected.	
Common: None expected.	
Infrequent:	
• Skin rash.	Discontinue. Call doctor right away.
• Diarrhea, nausea, vomiting, appetite loss, constipation, headache, abdominal pain.	Continue. Call doctor when convenient.
Rare:	
• Pale stools, yellow skin or eyes, dark or amber urine, unusual tiredness or weakness.	Discontinue. Call doctor right away.
• Diminished sex drive in males, swollen breasts in males, increased sensitivity to light, drowsiness, dizziness, insomnia.	Continue. Call doctor when convenient.

WARNINGS & PRECAUTIONS

Don't take if:
You have had an allergic reaction to any of the azoles.

Before you start, consult your doctor:
- If you have impaired kidney or liver function.
- If you have been diagnosed with reduced stomach acidity.

Over age 60:
Adverse reactions and side effects may be more frequent and severe than in younger persons. Dosage may need adjustment if there is age-related kidney impairment.

Pregnancy:
Decide with your doctor whether drug benefits justify risk to unborn child. Risk category C (see page xviii).

Breast-feeding:
Drug passes into milk. Avoid drug or discontinue nursing until you finish medicine. Consult doctor for advice on maintaining milk supply.

Infants & children:
Use only under close medical supervision.

Prolonged use:
Request periodic liver function studies.

Skin & sunlight:
No problems expected.

Driving, piloting or hazardous work:
Don't drive or pilot aircraft until you learn how medicine affects you. Don't work around dangerous machinery. Don't climb ladders or work in high places. Danger increases if you drink alcohol or take medicine affecting alertness and reflexes, such as antihistamines, tranquilizers, sedatives, pain medicine, narcotics and mind-altering drugs.

Discontinuing:
Don't discontinue without consulting doctor. Dose may require gradual reduction if you have taken drug for a long time. Doses of other drugs may also require adjustment.

Others:
- Advise any doctor or dentist whom you consult that you take this medicine.
- May affect the results of some medical tests.

POSSIBLE INTERACTION WITH OTHER DRUGS

GENERIC NAME OR DRUG CLASS	COMBINED EFFECT
Adrenocorticoids, systemic	Decreased azole effect.
Antacids*	Decreased azole absorption.
Anticholinergics*	Decreased azole absorption.
Anticoagulants, oral*	Increased effect of anticoagulant.
Antidepressants, tricyclic*	Increased effect of antidepressant.
Antidiabetics, oral*	Increased risk of hypoglycemia.
Antihistamines, nonsedating	Serious heart ryhthm problems with astemizole or terfenadine. Avoid.
Antivirals, HIV/AIDS*	Reduced absorption of both drugs. Increased risk of pancreatitis.
Astemizole	Heart problems. Never combine.
Atropine	Decreased azole absorption.
Belladonna	Decreased azole absorption.
Carbamazepine	Decreased azole effect.
Cimetidine	Decreased azole absorption.
Cisapride	Heartbeat irregularities. Avoid.
Clidinium	Decreased azole absorption.
Contraceptives, oral*	Decreased effect of contraceptive.
Cyclosporine	Increased risk of toxicity to kidney.
Digoxin	Possible toxic levels of digoxin.
Famotidine	Reduced absorption of azole. Take famotidine at least 2 hours after any dose of ketoconazole.
Glycopyrrolate	Decreased azole absorption.
Hepatotoxic medications*	Increased risk of toxicity to kidney.
Histamine H_2 receptor antagonists	Decreased azole absorption.
HMG-CoA reductase inhibitors	Risk of muscle toxicity.
Hyoscyamine	Decreased azole effect.
Hypoglycemics, oral	Increased effect of oral hypoglycemics.

Continued on page 900

POSSIBLE INTERACTION WITH OTHER SUBSTANCES

INTERACTS WITH	COMBINED EFFECT
Alcohol:	Increased chance of liver damage and disulfiram reaction.*
Beverages:	None expected.
Cocaine:	Decreased azole effect. Avoid.
Foods:	None expected.
Marijuana:	Decreased azole effect. Avoid.
Tobacco:	Decreased azole effect. Avoid.

*See Glossary

ANTIFUNGALS (Topical)

GENERIC AND BRAND NAMES

See complete list of generic and brand names in the *Generic and Brand Name Directory*, page 862.

BASIC INFORMATION

Habit forming? No
Prescription needed? Yes, for some
Available as generic? Yes, for some
Drug class: Antifungal (topical)

USES

Fights fungus infections such as ringworm of the scalp, athlete's foot, jockey itch, "sun fungus," nail fungus and others.

DOSAGE & USAGE INFORMATION

How to use:

- Solution—Apply to affected area once daily for one week.
- Cream, lotion, ointment, gel—Bathe and dry area before use. Apply small amount and rub gently.
- Powder—Apply lightly to skin.
- Shampoo—Follow package instructions.
- Don't bandage or cover treated areas with plastic wrap.
- Follow other instructions from manufacturer listed on label.

When to use:
Twice a day, morning and evening, unless otherwise directed by your doctor.

If you forget a dose:
Use as soon as you remember.

What drug does:
Kills fungi by damaging the fungal cell wall.

Continued next column

OVERDOSE

SYMPTOMS:
None expected.
WHAT TO DO:

- **Not for internal use. If child accidentally swallows, call poison control center.**
- **Dial 911 (emergency) for an ambulance or medical help or poison center 1-800-222-1222. Then give first aid immediately.**
- **See emergency information on inside covers.**

Time lapse before drug works:
May require 6 to 8 weeks for cure.

Don't use with:
Other skin medicines without telling your doctor.

POSSIBLE ADVERSE REACTIONS OR SIDE EFFECTS

SYMPTOMS	WHAT TO DO
Life-threatening: None expected.	
Common: None expected.	
Infrequent: Itching, redness, swelling of treated skin not present before treatment.	Discontinue. Call doctor right away.
Rare: None expected.	

WARNINGS & PRECAUTIONS

Don't use if:
You are allergic to any topical antifungal medicine listed.

Before you start, consult your doctor:
If you are allergic to anything that touches your skin.

Over age 60:
No problems expected.

Pregnancy:
Risk factors vary for drugs in this group. See category list on page xviii and consult doctor.

Breast-feeding:
No problems expected, but check with doctor.

Infants & children:
No problems expected, but check with doctor. Some drugs in this group have not been studied in children under 12.

Prolonged use:
No problems expected, but check with doctor.

Skin & sunlight:
No special problems expected.

Driving, piloting or hazardous work:
No problems expected, but check with doctor.

Discontinuing:
No problems expected, but check with doctor.

Others:
- Avoid contact with eyes.
- Heat and moisture in bathroom medicine cabinet can cause breakdown of medicine. Store someplace else.
- Keep medicine cool, but don't freeze.
- Store away from heat or sunlight.
- Don't use on other members of the family without consulting your doctor.
- If using for jock itch, avoid wearing tight underwear.
- If using for athlete's foot, dry feet carefully after bathing, wear clean cotton socks with sandals or well-ventilated shoes.

POSSIBLE INTERACTION WITH OTHER DRUGS

GENERIC NAME OR DRUG CLASS	COMBINED EFFECT
None expected.	

POSSIBLE INTERACTION WITH OTHER SUBSTANCES

INTERACTS WITH	COMBINED EFFECT
Alcohol:	None expected.
Beverages:	None expected.
Cocaine:	None expected.
Foods:	None expected.
Marijuana:	None expected.
Tobacco:	None expected.

*See Glossary

ANTIFUNGALS (Vaginal)

GENERIC AND BRAND NAMES

See complete list of generic and brand names in the *Generic and Brand Name Directory*, page 862.

BASIC INFORMATION

Habit forming? No
Prescription needed? Yes, for some
Available as generic? Yes, some
Drug class: Antifungal (vaginal)

USES

Treats fungus infections of the vagina.

DOSAGE & USAGE INFORMATION

How to use:

- Vaginal creams—Insert into vagina with applicator as illustrated in patient instructions that come with prescription.
- Vaginal tablets—Insert with applicator as illustrated in instructions.
- Vaginal suppositories—Insert as illustrated in instructions.

When to use:
According to instructions. Usually once or twice daily.

If you forget a dose:
Use as soon as you remember.

What drug does:
Destroys fungus cells membrane causing loss of essential elements to sustain fungus cell life.

Time lapse before drug works:
Begins immediately. May require 2 weeks of treatment to cure vaginal fungus infections. Recurrence common.

Don't use with:
Other vaginal preparations or douches unless otherwise instructed by your doctor.

OVERDOSE

SYMPTOMS:
None expected.
WHAT TO DO:
Overdose unlikely to threaten life.

POSSIBLE ADVERSE REACTIONS OR SIDE EFFECTS

SYMPTOMS	WHAT TO DO
Life-threatening: None expected.	
Common: None expected.	
Infrequent: Vaginal burning, itching, irriation, swelling of labia, redness, increased discharge (not present before starting medicine).	Discontinue. Call doctor right away.
Rare: Skin rash, hives, irritation of sex partner's penis.	Discontinue. Call doctor right away.

WARNINGS & PRECAUTIONS

Don't use if:
- You are allergic to any of the products listed.
- You have pre-existing liver disease.

Before you start, consult your doctor:
If you are pregnant.

Over age 60:
No problems expected.

Pregnancy:
Risk factors vary for drugs in this group. See category list on page xviii and consult doctor.

Breast-feeding:
No problems expected. Consult doctor.

Infants & children:
Use only under close medical supervision.

Prolonged use:
No problems expected.

Skin & sunlight:
No problems expected.

Driving, piloting or hazardous work:
No problems expected.

Discontinuing:
Recurrence likely if you stop before time suggested.

Others:
- Gentian Violet and some of the other products can stain clothing. Sanitary napkins may protect against staining.
- Keep the genital area clean. Use plain unscented soap.
- Take showers rather than tub baths.
- Wear cotton underpants or pantyhose with a cotton crotch. Avoid underpants made from non-ventilating materials. Wear freshly laundered underpants.
- Don't sit around in wet clothing—especially a wet bathing suit.
- If you will take antibiotics in the future, ask your doctor about eating yogurt, sour cream, buttermilk or taking acidophilus tablets.
- After urination or bowel movements, cleanse by wiping or washing from front to back (vagina to anus).
- Don't douche unless your doctor recommends it.
- If urinating causes burning, urinate through a tubular device, such as a toilet-paper roll or plastic cup with the end cut out.

POSSIBLE INTERACTION WITH OTHER DRUGS

GENERIC NAME OR DRUG CLASS	COMBINED EFFECT
Warfarin	May cause bleeding with miconazole vaginal cream.

POSSIBLE INTERACTION WITH OTHER SUBSTANCES

INTERACTS WITH	COMBINED EFFECT
Alcohol:	None expected.
Beverages:	None expected.
Cocaine:	None expected.
Foods:	None expected.
Marijuana:	None expected.
Tobacco:	None expected.

*See Glossary

ANTIGLAUCOMA, ADRENERGIC AGONISTS

GENERIC AND BRAND NAMES

APRACLONIDINE
- **Iopidine**

BRIMONIDINE
- **Alphagan**

DIPIVEFRIN
- **AKPro**
- **DPE**
- **Ophtho-Dipivefrin**
- **Propine**
- **Propine C Cap**

EPINEPHRINE
- **Epifren**
- **Epinal**
- **Eppy/N**
- **Glaucon**

BASIC INFORMATION

Habit forming? No
Prescription needed? Yes
Available as generic? Yes, for some
Drug class: Antiglaucoma

USES

Treats open-angle glaucoma, secondary glaucoma and ocular hypertension. May be used with eye surgery.

DOSAGE & USAGE INFORMATION

How to use:
Eye drops
- Wash hands.
- Apply pressure to inside corner of eye with middle finger.
- Continue pressure for 1 minute after placing medicine in eye.
- Tilt head backward. Pull lower lid away from eye with index finger of the same hand.
- Drop eye drops into pouch and close eye. Don't blink.
- Keep eyes closed for 1 to 2 minutes.
- If using more than one eye solutions, wait at least 10 minutes between instillations to avoid a "wash-out" effect.

When to use:
As directed on label.

Continued next column

OVERDOSE

SYMPTOMS:
Effects unknown.
WHAT TO DO:
Overdose unlikely to threaten life. If person use much larger amount than prescribed or if accidentally swallowed, call doctor or poison center 1-800-222-1222 for instructions.

If you forget a dose:
Apply as soon as you remember. If almost time for next dose, wait and apply at regular time (don't double this dose).

What drug does:
Inactivates enzyme and facilitates movement of fluid (aquemous humor) into and out of the eye.

Time lapse before drug works:
30 minutes to 4 hours.

Don't use with:
Any other medicine without consulting your doctor or pharmacist.

POSSIBLE ADVERSE REACTIONS OR SIDE EFFECTS

SYMPTOMS	WHAT TO DO
Life-threatening:	
None expected.	
Common:	
• Allergic reaction (itching, redness, tearing of eye).	Discontinue. Call doctor right away.
• Headache, eye discomfort, dry mouth.	Continue. Call doctor when convenient.
Infrequent:	
Eye symptoms: pain, changes in vision, blurred vision, discharge or swelling, color change in white of eye, feeling of something in the eye, stinging, burning, watering, light sensitivity, crusting on eyelid, paleness of eye or inner eyelid.	Continue. Call doctor right away.
Rare:	
• Symptoms of too much drug absorbed in body: faintness, skin paleness, chest pain, increased or fast or irregular heartbeat, swelling (face, hands, or feet), dizziness, numbness or tingling in fingers or toes, wheezing, troubled breathing.	Discontinue. Call doctor right away.
• Other symptoms of drug absorbed in body: sore throat, muscle aches, nausea, smell or taste changes, anxiety, nervousness, depression, constipation, insomnia or drowsiness.	Continue. Call doctor when convenient.

ANTIGLAUCOMA, ADRENERGIC AGONISTS

WARNINGS & PRECAUTIONS

Don't use if:
You are allergic to any of the adrenergic agonist antiglaucoma drugs.

Before you start, consult your doctor:
- If you suffer from depression.
- If you have any eye disease.
- If you have heart problems, high or low blood pressure or thromboangiitis obliterans.
- If you have Raynaud's disease.
- If you have a history of vasovagal attacks* (if using apraclonidine).
- If you have liver or kidney problems.

Over age 60:
No problems expected.

Pregnancy:
Risk factors vary for drugs in this group. See category list on page xviii and consult doctor.

Breast-feeding:
It is not known if drugs pass into milk. Avoid drugs or discontinue nursing until you finish medicine. Consult doctor for advice on maintaining milk supply.

Infants & children:
Use only under close medical supervision.

Prolonged use:
May be necessary.

Skin & sunlight:
No problems expected.

Driving, piloting or hazardous work:
Your vision may be blurred or there may be a change in your near or far vision or night vision for a short time after drug use. Don't drive or pilot aircraft until you learn how medicine affects you. Don't work around dangerous machinery. Don't climb ladders or work in high places.

Discontinuing:
Don't discontinue without consulting your doctor. Dose may require gradual reduction if you have used drug for a long time. Doses of other drugs may also require adjustment.

Others:
- Advise any doctor or dentist whom you consult that you use this medicine.
- Drugs may cause your eyes to become more sensitive to light. Wear sunglasses and avoid too much exposure to bright light.
- Brimonidine contains a preservative that could be absorbed by soft contact lenses. Wait at least 15 minutes after putting eye drops in before you put in your soft contact lenses.
- If you have any eye infection, injury or wound, consult doctor before using this medicine.
- Keep appointments for regular eye examinations to measure pressure in the eye.

POSSIBLE INTERACTION WITH OTHER DRUGS

GENERIC NAME OR DRUG CLASS	COMBINED EFFECT
Antidepressants, tricyclic	May decrease ocular hypertensive effect. Dipivefrin may cause heart rhythm problem, high blood pressure.
Antiglaucoma, beta blockers	May help decrease eye pressure.
Antihypertensives*	May decrease blood pressure.
Central nervous system (CNS) depressants*	May increase CNS depressant effect.
Digitalis preparations*	Increased risk of heart problems.
Maprotiline	Heart rhythm problems, high blood pressure.
Monoamine oxidase (MAO) inhibitors*	Separate use by at least 14 days.

POSSIBLE INTERACTION WITH OTHER SUBSTANCES

INTERACTS WITH	COMBINED EFFECT
Alcohol:	None expected.
Beverages:	None expected.
Cocaine:	None expected. Best to avoid.
Foods:	None expected.
Marijuana:	Unknown effect. Consult doctor.
Tobacco:	None expected.

*See Glossary

ANTIGLAUCOMA, ANTICHOLINESTERASES

BRAND NAMES

DEMECARIUM	ECHOTHIOPHATE
Humorsol	Phospholine Iodide

BASIC INFORMATION

Habit forming? No
Prescription needed? Yes
Available as generic? No
Drug class: Antiglaucoma

USES

- Treatment for certain types of glaucoma.
- Used for diagnosis and treatment for other eye conditions.

DOSAGE & USAGE INFORMATION

How to use:
Eye drops
- Wash hands.
- Apply pressure to inside corner of eye with middle finger.
- Continue pressure for 1 minute after placing medicine in eye.
- Tilt head backward. Pull lower lid away from eye with index finger of the same hand.
- Drop eye drops into pouch and close eye. Don't blink.
- Keep eyes closed for 1 to 2 minutes.
- Press finger to tear duct in corner of eye for 2 minutes to prevent possible absorption by body.
- If using more than one eye solutions, wait at least 10 minutes between instillations to avoid a "wash-out" effect.

Continued next column

When to use:
As directed on label.

If you forget a dose:
Apply as soon as you remember. If almost time for next dose, wait and apply at regular time (don't double this dose).

What drug does:
Inactivates an enzyme to reduce pressure inside the eye.

Time lapse before drug works:
5 to 60 minutes.

Don't use with:
Any other medicine without consulting your doctor or pharmacist.

OVERDOSE

SYMPTOMS:
Fast heartbeat, diarrhea, heavy sweating, breathing difficulty, unable to control bladder, shock.
WHAT TO DO:
- **For overdose in the eye, flush with warm tap water and call doctor immediately.**
- **For accidentally ingested overdose or signs of system toxicity, dial 911 (emergency) for an ambulance or medical help or poison center 1-800-222-1222. Then give first aid immediately.**
- **See emergency information on inside covers.**

POSSIBLE ADVERSE REACTIONS OR SIDE EFFECTS

SYMPTOMS	WHAT TO DO
Life-threatening: None expected.	
Common: Stinging, burning watery eyes.	Continue. Call doctor when convenient.
Infrequent: Blurred vision, change in vision, change in night vision, eyelids twitch, headache, ache in brow area	Continue. Call doctor when convenient.
Rare: Decreased vision with veil or curtain appearing in part of vision, eye redness, symptoms of too much of drug absorbed in body (loss of bladder control, slow heartbeat, increased sweating, weakness, difficult breathing, vomiting, nausea, diarrhea, stomach pain or cramping).	Discontinue. Call doctor right away.

WARNINGS & PRECAUTIONS

Don't use if:
You are allergic to demecarium or echothiophate.

Before you start, consult your doctor:

- If you have eye infection or other eye disease.
- If you have ulcers in stomach or duodenum or other stomach disorder.
- If you have myasthenia gravis, overactive thyroid or urinary tract blockage.
- If you have asthma, epilepsy, Down syndrome, heart disease, high or low blood pressure, Parkinson's disease.

Over age 60:
Adverse reactions and side effects may be more frequent and severe than in younger persons.

Pregnancy:
Risk factors vary for drugs in this group. See category list on page xviii and consult doctor.

Breast-feeding:
It is not known if drug passes into milk. Avoid drugs or discontinue nursing until you finish medicine. Consult doctor for advice on maintaining milk supply.

Infants & children:
Use under medical supervision only. Children are more susceptible to adverse effects.

Prolonged use:
Cataracts or other eye problems may occur. Be sure to see your doctor for regular eye examinations.

Skin & sunlight:
No problems expected.

Driving, piloting or hazardous work:
Your vision may be blurred or there may be a change in your near or far vision or night vision for a short time after drug use. Don't drive or pilot aircraft until you learn how medicine affects you. Don't work around dangerous machinery. Don't climb ladders or work in high places.

Discontinuing:
Don't discontinue without consulting your doctor. Dose may require gradual reduction if you have used drug for a long time. Doses of other drugs may also require adjustment.

Others:

- Advise any doctor or dentist whom you consult that you use this medicine.
- Keep appointments for regular eye examinations to measure pressure in the eye.
- If you have any eye infection, injury or wound, consult doctor before using this medicine.

POSSIBLE INTERACTION WITH OTHER DRUGS

GENERIC NAME OR DRUG CLASS	COMBINED EFFECT
Anticholinergics*	Increased risk of toxicity.
Antimyasthenics*	Increased risk of side effects.
Cholinesterase inhibitors*	Increased risk of toxicity.
Insecticides or pesticides with organic phosphates	Increased toxic absorption of pesticides.
Topical anesthetics	Increased risk of toxic effects of antiglaucoma eye medicines.

POSSIBLE INTERACTION WITH OTHER SUBSTANCES

INTERACTS WITH	COMBINED EFFECT
Alcohol:	None expected.
Beverages:	None expected.
Cocaine:	None expected. Best to avoid.
Foods:	None expected.
Marijuana:	Unknown effect. Consult doctor.
Tobacco:	None expected.

*See Glossary

ANTIGLAUCOMA, BETA BLOCKERS

GENERIC AND BRAND NAMES

BETAXOLOL (ophthalmic)
Betoptic
Betoptic S
CARTEOLOL (ophthalmic)
Ocupress
LEVOBUNOLOL (ophthalmic)
AKBeta
Betagen C Cap B.I.D.
Betagen C Cap Q.D.
Betagen Standard Cap
METIPRANOLOL (ophthalmic)
OptiPranolol
TIMOLOL (ophthalmic)
Apo-Timop
Beta-Tim
Betimol
Cosopt
Gen-Timolol
Med Timolol
Novo-Timolol
Nu-Timolol
Timodal
Timoptic
Timoptic in Ocudose
Timoptic-XE
Xalcom

BASIC INFORMATION

Habit forming? No
Prescription needed? Yes
Available as generic? Yes, for some
Drug class: Antiglaucoma

USES

Treatment for glaucoma and ocular hypertension. May be used in eye surgery.

DOSAGE & USAGE INFORMATION

How to take:
Eye drops—Follow directions on prescription.

Continued next column

OVERDOSE

SYMPTOMS:
Slow heartbeat, low blood pressure, broncho-spasm, heart failure (these symptoms are what might be expected if similar drugs were taken orally).
WHAT TO DO:
- **For overdose in the eye, flush with warm tap water and call doctor immediately.**
- **For accidentally ingested overdose or signs of system toxicity, dial 911 (emergency) for an ambulance or medical help or poison center 1-800-222-1222. Then give first aid immediately.**
- **See emergency information on inside covers.**

When to take:
At the same time each day usually in the morning. Follow your doctor's instructions.

If you forget a dose:
- Once-a-day dose—Apply as soon as you remember. If almost time for next dose, wait and apply at regular time (don't double this dose).
- More than once-a-day dose—Apply as soon as you remember. If close to time for next dose, wait and apply at regular time (don't double this dose).

What drug does:
Appears to reduce production of aqueous humor (fluid inside eye), thereby reducing pressure inside eye.

Time lapse before drug works:
30 minutes to 1 hour.

Don't take with:
Any other prescription or nonprescription drug without consulting your doctor or pharmacist.

POSSIBLE ADVERSE REACTIONS OR SIDE EFFECTS

SYMPTOMS	WHAT TO DO
Life-threatening:	
In case of overdose, see previous column.	
Common:	
• Redness of eyes or inside of eyelids.	Continue. Call doctor right away.
• Temporary blurred vision, night vision decreased, eye irritation or discomfort when drug is used.	Continue. Call doctor when convenient.
Infrequent:	
Ongoing blurred vision, other vision changes, different size pupils, eyeball discolored, droopy eyelid, eye pain, or swelling or irritation.	Continue. Call doctor when convenient.
Rare:	
• Increased sensitivity to light; sensation of foreign body in eye; dryness, discharge or pain in eye; crusty eyelids; inflammation.	Continue. Call doctor when convenient.
• Symptoms of body absorbing too much of drug include problems with heart, stomach, lungs (breathing difficulties), skin, nervous system, hair loss, and others.	Discontinue. Call doctor right away.

WARNINGS & PRECAUTIONS

Don't take if:
You are allergic to any beta-adrenergic blocking agent taken orally or used in the eye.

Before you start, consult your doctor:
- If you have asthma, a bronchial disorder or pulmonary disease.
- If you have any heart disease or heart problem.
- If you suffer from depression.
- If you have diabetes or low blood sugar, overactive thyroid or myasthenia gravis.

Over age 60:
Adverse reactions and side effects may be more frequent and severe than in younger persons.

Pregnancy:
Decide with your doctor whether drug benefits justify risk to unborn child. Risk category C (see page xviii).

Breast-feeding:
Some of these drugs pass into milk; others are unknown. Avoid drugs or discontinue nursing until you finish medicine. Consult doctor for advice on maintaining milk supply.

Infants & children:
Give only under close medical supervision. Children may be more sensitive to drug and side effects.

Prolonged use:
Talk to your doctor about the need for follow-up medical examinations to check pressure inside eye.

Skin & sunlight:
No special problems expected.

Driving, piloting or hazardous work:
Your vision may be blurred or there may be a change in your near or far vision or night vision for a short time after drug use. Don't drive or pilot aircraft until you learn how medicine affects you. Don't work around dangerous machinery. Don't climb ladders or work in high places.

Discontinuing:
- Don't discontinue without doctor's approval.
- May need to discontinue drug temporarily before major surgery. Your doctor will provide instructions.

Others:
- Advise any doctor or dentist whom you consult that you take this medicine.
- These drugs may affect blood sugar levels in diabetic patients.
- Keep appointments for regular eye examinations to measure pressure in the eye.
- If you have any eye infection, injury or wound, consult doctor before using this medicine.

POSSIBLE INTERACTION WITH OTHER DRUGS

GENERIC NAME OR DRUG CLASS	COMBINED EFFECT

Drug interactions are unlikely unless a significant amount of the eye medication is absorbed into the system. Potential interactions that may occur are similar to those listed in Possible Interactions With Other Drugs under Beta-Adrenergic Blocking Agents.

POSSIBLE INTERACTION WITH OTHER SUBSTANCES

INTERACTS WITH	COMBINED EFFECT
Alcohol:	None expected.
Beverages:	None expected.
Cocaine:	Decreased anti-glaucoma effect; heart problems. Avoid.
Foods:	None expected.
Marijuana:	Unknown effect. Consult doctor.
Tobacco:	None expected.

*See Glossary

ANTIGLAUCOMA, CARBONIC ANHYDRASE INHIBITORS

RAND NAMES

BRINZOLAMIDE	DORZOLAMIDE
Azopt	Cosopt
	Trusopt

BASIC INFORMATION

Habit forming? No
Prescription needed? Yes
Available as generic? No
Drug class: Antiglaucoma

USES

- Treatment for open-angle glaucoma (increased pressure in the eye).
- Treatment for ocular hypertension.

DOSAGE & USAGE INFORMATION

How to use:

Eye drops

- Wash hands. Tilt head back.
- Press finger gently on the skin right under the lower eyelid; pull the eyelid away from the eye to make a space or small pocket.
- Drop the medicine into this pocket, then let go of the skin and gently close the eyes; don't blink.
- Keep the eyes closed and apply pressure to the inner corner of the eye with your finger for 1 to 2 minutes.
- Wash hands again after using the drops.
- To keep the solution germ-free, do not allow the applicator tip to touch the skin or eye.
- If using more than one eye solutions, wait at least 10 minutes between instillations to avoid a "wash-out" effect.

When to use:
Normally used 3 times a day (about 8 hours apart). Always use as directed by your doctor.

Continued next column

OVERDOSE

SYMPTOMS:
Unknown effect.
WHAT TO DO:
Overdose unlikely to threaten life. If person use much larger amount than prescribed or if accidentally swallowed, call doctor, poison center 1-800-222-1222 or hospital emergency room for instructions.

If you forget a dose:
Use as soon as you remember. If it is almost time for the next dose, wait for next dose (don't double this dose).

What drug does:
This medicine is a topically applied carbonic anhydrase inhibitor that helps decrease production of aqueous humor (the fluid in the eye) and lowers the pressure inside the eye.

Time lapse before drug works:
30 to 60 minutes.

Don't take with:
Any other medicine (oral or topical) without consulting your doctor or pharmacist.

POSSIBLE ADVERSE REACTIONS OR SIDE EFFECTS

SYMPTOMS	WHAT TO DO
Life-threatening:	
None expected.	
Common:	
• Allergic reaction (redness, itching or swelling of eye or eyelid); feeling of something in the eye; continued or severe sensitivity to light.	Discontinue. Call doctor right away.
• Bitter taste; burning, stinging or discomfort when medicine is used; mild sensitivity to light.	Continue. Call doctor when convenient.
Infrequent:	
Blurred vision, dryness or mild tearing of eyes, tiredness or weakness, headache hair loss.	Continue. Call doctor when convenient.
Rare:	
Blood in urine; continued nausea or vomiting; hives; pain in chest, back, side or abdomen; eye pain; severe or continued tearing; seeing double; skin rash; shortness of breath.	Discontinue. Call doctor right away.

ANTIGLAUCOMA, CARBONIC ANHYDRASE INHIBITORS

WARNINGS & PRECAUTIONS

Don't use if:
You are allergic to ophthalmic carbonic anhydrase inhibitors or any sulfonamide* medications.

Before you start, consult your doctor:
- If you have kidney or liver disease.
- If you are allergic to any medication, food, or other substances.

Over age 60:
No special problems expected.

Pregnancy:
Decide with your doctor whether drug benefits justify risk to unborn child. Risk category C (see page xviii).

Breast-feeding:
It is not known if drug passes into milk. Avoid drugs or discontinue nursing until you finish medicine. Consult doctor for advice on maintaining milk supply.

Infants & children:
Safety and dosage have not been established. Use only under medical supervision.

Prolonged use:
Schedule regular appointments with your doctor for eye examinations to be sure the medication is controlling the glaucoma.

Skin & sunlight:
No special problems expected.

Driving, piloting or hazardous work:
Your vision may be blurred or there may be a change in your near or far vision or night vision for a short time after drug use. Don't drive or pilot aircraft until you learn how medicine affects you. Don't work around dangerous machinery. Don't climb ladders or work in high places.

Discontinuing:
Don't discontinue without consulting your doctor.

Others:
- If you have any eye infection, injury or wound, consult doctor before using this medicine.
- Advise any doctor or dentist whom you consult that you use this medicine.
- Keep appointments for regular eye examinations to measure pressure in the eye.
- Wear sunglasses when outside in sunlight.

POSSIBLE INTERACTION WITH OTHER DRUGS

GENERIC NAME OR DRUG CLASS	COMBINED EFFECT
Amphetamines	Increased risk of side effects.
Carbonic anhydrase inhibitors (oral)	Increased effect of both drugs. Avoid.
Mecamylamine	Increased risk of side effects.
Quinidine	Increased risk of side effects.

POSSIBLE INTERACTION WITH OTHER SUBSTANCES

INTERACTS WITH	COMBINED EFFECT
Alcohol:	None expected.
Beverages:	None expected.
Cocaine:	None expected. Best to avoid.
Foods:	None expected.
Marijuana:	Unknown effect. Consult doctor.
Tobacco:	None expected.

***See Glossary**

ANTIGLAUCOMA, CHOLINERGIC AGONISTS

GENERIC AND BRAND NAMES

CARBACHOL
- **Carbastat**
- **Carboptic**
- **Isopto Carbachol**
- **Miostat**

PILOCARPINE
- **Adsorbocarpine**
- **Akarpine**
- **Almocarpine**
- **Isopto Carpine**
- **Minims**
- **Miocarpine**
- **Ocu-Carpine**
- **Ocusert Pilo**
- **Pilocarpine Pilocar**
- **Pilopine HS**
- **Piloptic**
- **Pilostat**
- **P.V. Carpine Liquifilm**

BASIC INFORMATION

Habit forming? No
Prescription needed? Yes
Available as generic? Yes, for some
Drug class: Antiglaucoma

USES

Treatment for glaucoma and other eye conditions. May be used in eye surgery.

DOSAGE & USAGE INFORMATION

How to take:
- Drops—Apply to eyes. Close eyes for 1 or 2 minutes to absorb medicine.
- Eye insert system—Follow label directions.
- Gel—Follow label directions.

When to use:
As directed on label.

Continued next column

OVERDOSE

SYMPTOMS:
If accidental overdose in eye, flush with water. If swallowed—nausea, vomiting, diarrhea, sweating.
WHAT TO DO:
Overdose unlikely to threaten life. If person or a child accidentally swallows, call doctor, poison center 1-800-222-1222 or hospital emergency room for instructions.

If you forget a dose:
- For eye drops or gel, use as soon as possible. If it is almost time for your next dose, skip the missed dose and return to regular schedule (don't double this dose).
- For eye insert, replace it as soon as possible. Then return to your regular schedule.

What drug does:
Reduces internal eye pressure.

Time lapse before drug works:
75 minutes to 4 hours.

Don't take with:
Any other medicine without consulting your doctor or pharmacist.

POSSIBLE ADVERSE REACTIONS OR SIDE EFFECTS

SYMPTOMS	WHAT TO DO
Life-threatening: None expected.	
Common: Blurred or altered vision (near or distant vision), eye stinging or burning.	Continue. Call doctor when convenient.
Infrequent: Headache, eye irritation, redness, of eye, eyelid twitching.	Continue. Call doctor when convenient.
Rare: Eye pain, a veil or curtain appears across part of vision, symptoms of too much of drug absorbed in the body (increased sweating, muscle trembling, nausea, vomiting, diarrhea, troubled breathing or wheezing, mouth watering, stomach cramps, fainting, flushing or redness of face, urge to urinate).	Discontinue. Call doctor right away.

ANTIGLAUCOMA, CHOLINERGIC AGONISTS

WARNINGS & PRECAUTIONS

Don't take if:
You are allergic to carbachol or pilocarpine.

Before you start, consult your doctor:
- If you have other eye problems
- If you have heart disease, overactive thyroid, Parkinson's disease, ulcers, or urinary blockage problems.
- If you have asthma.

Over age 60:
No special problems expected.

Pregnancy:
Decide with your doctor if drug benefits justify risk to unborn child. Risk category C (see page xviii).

Breast-feeding:
It is not known if drugs pass into milk. Avoid drugs or discontinue nursing until you finish medicine. Consult doctor for advice on maintaining milk supply.

Infants & children:
Not recommended.

Prolonged use:
- You may develop tolerance* for drug, making it ineffective. Your doctor may switch antiglaucoma drugs for a period of time to return effectiveness.
- Talk to your doctor about the need for follow-up medical examinations to check eye pressure.

Skin & sunlight:
No problems expected.

Driving, piloting or hazardous work:
Your vision may be blurred or there may be a change in your near or far vision or night vision for a short time after drug use. Don't drive or pilot aircraft until you learn how medicine affects you. Don't work around dangerous machinery. Don't climb ladders or work in high places.

Discontinuing:
Don't discontinue without consulting your doctor.

Others:
- Advise any doctor or dentist whom you consult that you use this medicine.
- Keep appointments for regular eye examinations to measure pressure in the eye.
- If you have any eye infection, injury or wound, consult doctor before using this medicine.

POSSIBLE INTERACTION WITH OTHER DRUGS

GENERIC NAME OR DRUG CLASS	COMBINED EFFECT
Belladonna (ophthalmic)	Decreased antiglaucoma effect.
Flurbiprofen (ophthalmic)	Decreased antiglaucoma effect.
Cyclopentolate	Decreased antiglaucoma effect.

POSSIBLE INTERACTION WITH OTHER SUBSTANCES

INTERACTS WITH	COMBINED EFFECT
Alcohol:	None expected.
Beverages:	None expected.
Cocaine:	None expected. Best to avoid.
Foods:	None expected.
Marijuana:	Unknown effect. Consult doctor.
Tobacco:	None expected.

*See Glossary

ANTIGLAUCOMA, PROSTAGLANDINS

GENERIC AND BRAND NAMES

BIMATOPROST
Lumigan
Xalcom
ISOPROPYL UNOPROSTONE
Rescula
LATANOPROST
Xalatan
TRAVOPROST
Travatan

BASIC INFORMATION

Habit forming? No
Prescription needed? Yes
Available as generic? No
Drug class: Antiglaucoma

USES

Treats diseases of the eye like glaucoma and hypertension of the eye.

DOSAGE & USAGE INFORMATION

How to use:
Eye drops

- Wash hands.
- Apply pressure on the skin just beneath the lower eyelid. Pull the lower eyelid away from the eye to make a space.
- Drop the medicine into this space.
- Release eyelid and gently close eyes
- Don't blink.
- Keep eyes closed for 1 to 2 minutes.
- Remove excess solution from around the eye with a clean tissue, being careful not to touch the eye.
- Don't touch applicator tip to any surface (including the eye). If you accidentally touch tip, clean with warm soap and water.
- Keep container tightly closed.
- Wash hands immediately after using.

When to use:
As directed on label.

Continued next column

OVERDOSE

SYMPTOMS:
Unknown effect.
WHAT TO DO:
Overdose unlikely to threaten life. If person use much larger amount than prescribed or if accidentally swallowed, call doctor, poison center 1-800-222-1222 or hospital emergency room for instructions.

If you forget a dose:
Use as soon as you remember. If it is almost time for the next dose; wait for next dose (don't double this dose).

What drug does:
Inactivates enzyme and facilitates movement of fluid (aquemous humor) into and out of the eye.

Time lapse before drug works:
10-30 minutes.

Don't use with:
Any other medicine without consulting your doctor or pharmacist.

POSSIBLE ADVERSE REACTIONS OR SIDE EFFECTS

SYMPTOMS	WHAT TO DO
Life-threatening:	
None expected.	
Common:	
Eye symptoms: itching, discomfort, mild pain, redness, feeling of something in eye, vision decreased.	Continue. Call doctor when convenient.
Infrequent:	
Eye tearing or dry, crusting on eyelid, eyes more sensitivity to light, eye discharge, color vision or other vision changes, hair growth increased.	Continue. Call doctor when convenient.
Rare:	
• Faintness, increased sweating, irregular or fast heartbeat, chest pain or tightness, shortness of breath, wheezing, unusual tiredness, paleness, heartburn, indigestion, coughing up mucus, fainting, chills or fever, dizziness, pain and stiffness in muscles or joints, headache, urination problems, cold symptoms, back pain, mental and mood changes.	Discontinue. Call doctor right away.

• May cause changes in the treated eye only (color of the iris and eyelid). It may change eyelashes (thicker, longer, color). Changes may take months or years and may be permanent.	Continue. Call doctor when convenient.

WARNINGS & PRECAUTIONS

Don't take if:
You are allergic to any prostaglandin eye medicine.

Before you start, consult your doctor:
- If you plan to have eye or dental surgery.
- If you have any eye disease.
- If you have heart problems or high blood pressure.
- If you have liver or kidney problems.

Over age 60:
Adverse reactions and side effects may be more frequent and severe than in younger persons. Ask doctor about smaller doses.

Pregnancy:
Risk factors vary for drugs in this group. See category list on page xviii and consult doctor.

Breast-feeding:
It is not known if drugs pass into milk. Avoid drugs or discontinue nursing until you finish medicine. Consult doctor for advice on maintaining milk supply.

Infants & children:
Safety and efficacy not established in this age group.

Prolonged use:
May be necessary.

Skin & sunlight:
No problems expected.

Driving, piloting or hazardous work:
Your vision may be blurred or there may be a change in your near or far vision or night vision for a short time after drug use. Don't drive or pilot aircraft until you learn how medicine affects you. Don't work around dangerous machinery. Don't climb ladders or work in high places.

Discontinuing:
Don't discontinue without consulting your doctor. Dose may require gradual reduction if you have used drug for a long time. Doses of other drugs may also require adjustment.

Others:
- If you have any eye infection, injury or wound, consult doctor before using this medicine.
- Advise any doctor or dentist whom you consult that you use this medicine.
- Keep appointments for regular eye examinations to measure pressure in the eye.

POSSIBLE INTERACTION WITH OTHER DRUGS

GENERIC NAME OR DRUG CLASS	COMBINED EFFECT
None specific	Other drugs may increase or decrease antiglaucoma effect. Consult doctor.

POSSIBLE INTERACTION WITH OTHER SUBSTANCES

INTERACTS WITH	COMBINED EFFECT
Alcohol:	None expected.
Beverages:	None expected.
Cocaine:	None expected. Best to avoid.
Foods:	None expected.
Marijuana:	Unknown effect. Consult doctor.
Tobacco:	None expected.

ANTIHISTAMINES

GENERIC AND BRAND NAMES

See complete list of generic and brand names in the *Generic and Brand Name Directory*, page 862.

BASIC INFORMATION

Habit forming? No
Prescription needed?
High strength: Yes
Low strength: No
Available as generic? Yes
Drug class: Antihistamine

USES

- Reduces allergic symptoms such as hay fever, hives, rash or itching.
- Prevents motion sickness, nausea, vomiting.
- Relieves symptoms associated with the common cold.
- Induces sleep.
- Reduces stiffness and tremors of Parkinson's disease.

DOSAGE & USAGE INFORMATION

How to take:
Follow label directions.

When to take:
Varies with form. Follow label directions.

If you forget a dose:
Take as soon as you remember up to 2 hours late. If more than 2 hours, wait for next scheduled dose (don't double this dose).

What drug does:
- Blocks action of histamine after an allergic response triggers histamine release in sensitive cells. Histamines cause itching, sneezing, runny nose and eyes and other symptoms.
- Appears to work in the vomiting center of the brain to control nausea and vomiting and help prevent motion sickness.

Time lapse before drug works:
15 minutes to 1 hour.

Continued next column

OVERDOSE

SYMPTOMS:
Convulsions, red face, hallucinations, coma.
WHAT TO DO:
- **Dial 911 (emergency) for an ambulance or medical help or poison center 1-800-222-1222. Then give first aid immediately.**
- **See emergency information on inside covers.**

Don't take with:
Any other medicine without consulting your doctor or pharmacist.

POSSIBLE ADVERSE REACTIONS OR SIDE EFFECTS

SYMPTOMS	WHAT TO DO
Life-threatening: In case of overdose, see previous column.	
Common:	
Drowsiness (less likely with cetirizine, loratadine or astemizole); dizziness; dryness of mouth, nose or throat.	Continue. Tell doctor at next visit.
Infrequent:	
• Change in vision, clumsiness, rash.	Discontinue. Call doctor right away.
• Less tolerance for contact lenses, painful or difficult urination.	Continue. Call doctor when convenient.
• Appetite loss.	Continue. Tell doctor at next visit.
Rare:	
Nightmares, agitation, irritability, sore throat, fever, rapid heartbeat, unusual bleeding or bruising, fatigue, weakness, confusion, fainting, seizures.	Discontinue. Call doctor right away.

WARNINGS & PRECAUTIONS

Don't take if:
You are allergic to any antihistamine.

Before you start, consult your doctor:
- If you have glaucoma.
- If you have enlarged prostate.
- If you have asthma.
- If you have kidney disease.
- If you have peptic ulcer.
- If you will have surgery within 2 months, including dental surgery, requiring general or spinal anesthesia.

Over age 60:
Don't exceed recommended dose. Adverse reactions and side effects may be more frequent and severe than in younger persons, especially urination difficulty, diminished alertness and other brain and nervous-system symptoms.

Pregnancy:
Risk factors vary for drugs in this group. See category list on page xviii and consult doctor.

Breast-feeding:
Drug passes into milk. Avoid drug or discontinue nursing until you finish medicine. Consult doctor for advice on maintaining milk supply.

Infants & children:
Not recommended for premature or newborn infants. Otherwise, no problems expected.

Prolonged use:
Avoid. May damage bone marrow and nerve cells.

Skin & sunlight:
May cause rash or intensify sunburn in areas exposed to sun or sunlamp.

Driving, piloting or hazardous work:
Don't drive or pilot aircraft until you learn how medicine affects you. Don't work around dangerous machinery. Don't climb ladders or work in high places. Danger increases if you drink alcohol or take medicine affecting alertness and reflexes, such as antihistamines, tranquilizers, sedatives, pain medicine, narcotics and mind-altering drugs.

Discontinuing:
No problems expected.

Others:
- May mask symptoms of hearing damage from aspirin, other salicylates, cisplatin, paromomycin, vancomycin or anticonvulsants. Consult doctor if you use these.
- Advise any doctor or dentist whom you consult that you take this medicine.

POSSIBLE INTERACTION WITH OTHER DRUGS

GENERIC NAME OR DRUG CLASS	COMBINED EFFECT
Adrenocorticoids, systemic	Decreased adreno-corticoid effect.
Anticholinergics*	Increased anti-cholinergic effect.
Anticoagulants, oral*	Decreased anti-histamine effect.
Antidepressants*	Excess sedation. Avoid.
Antihistamines, other*	Excess sedation. Avoid.
Carteolol	Decreased anti-histamine effect.
Central nervous system (CNS) depressants*	May increase sedation.
Clozapine	Toxic effect on the central nervous system.
Dirithromycin	Serious heart rhythm problems with astemizole. Avoid.
Dronabinol	Increased effects of both drugs. Avoid.
Erythromycins*	Increased risk of cardiac toxicity with astemizole.
Fluvoxamine	Serious heart rhythm problems with astemizole. Avoid.
Hypnotics*	Excess sedation. Avoid.
Itraconazole	Increased risk of cardiac toxicity and death with astemizole.
Ketocanazole	Increased risk of cardiac toxicity and death with astemizole.
Mind-altering drugs*	Excess sedation. Avoid.
Molindone	Increased sedative and antihistamine effect.
Monoamine oxidase (MAO) inhibitors*	Increased antihistamine effect.
Nabilone	Greater depression of central nervous system.
Narcotics*	Excess sedation. Avoid.
Nefazodone	Serious heart rhythm problems with astemizole. Avoid.

Continued on page 900

POSSIBLE INTERACTION WITH OTHER SUBSTANCES

INTERACTS WITH	COMBINED EFFECT
Alcohol:	Excess sedation. Avoid.
Beverages: Caffeine drinks.	Less antihistamine sedation.
Cocaine:	Decreased antihista-mine effect. Avoid.
Foods:	None expected.
Marijuana:	Excess sedation. Avoid.
Tobacco:	None expected.

*See Glossary

ANTIHISTAMINES, NONSEDATING

GENERIC AND BRAND NAMES

CETIRIZINE
- Reactine
- Zyrtec

CETIRIZINE & PSEUDOEPHEDRINE
- Zyrtec-D

FEXOFENADINE
- Allegra
- Allegra-D

LORATADINE
- Claritin
- Claritin Extra
- Claritin RediTabs
- Claritin-D
- Claritin-D 12 Hour
- Claritin-D 24 Hour

BASIC INFORMATION

Habit forming? No
Prescription needed? Yes, for some
Available as generic? Yes, for some
Drug class: Antihistamine

USES

- Reduces allergic symptoms caused by hay fever (seasonal allergic rhinitis), such as sneezing, runny nose, itchy nose or throat, itchy and watery eyes.
- Treatment for chronic idiopathic urticaria (hives).
- Used to help relieve some asthma symptoms.
- Other uses as recommended by your doctor.

DOSAGE & USAGE INFORMATION

How to take:
Capsule, tablet, suspension, syrup—Swallow with liquid. Most may be taken with food or milk to lessen stomach irritation. Astemizole needs to be taken on an empty stomach, 1 hour before or 2 hours after eating.

When to take:
Varies with form. Follow label directions.

If you forget a dose:
Take as soon as you remember up to 2 hours late. If more than 2 hours, wait for next scheduled dose (don't double this dose).

Continued next column

OVERDOSE

SYMPTOMS:
Serious irregular heartbeat, convulsions, severe headache, nausea.
WHAT TO DO:
- **Dial 911 (emergency) for an ambulance or medical help or poison center 1-800-222-1222. Then give first aid immediately.**
- **See emergency information on inside covers.**

What drug does:
- Blocks action of histamine after an allergic response triggers histamine release in sensitive cells. Histamines cause itching, sneezing, runny nose and eyes and other symptoms.

Time lapse before drug works:
1 to 2 hours.

Don't take with:
Any other medicine without consulting your doctor or pharmacist.

POSSIBLE ADVERSE REACTIONS OR SIDE EFFECTS

SYMPTOMS	WHAT TO DO
Life-threatening:	
In case of overdose, see previous column.	
Common:	
Dryness of mouth, nose or throat.	Continue. Tell doctor at next visit.
Infrequent:	
Increased appetite, weight gain, mild stomach or intestinal problems, cold or flu-like symptoms.	Continue. Call doctor when convenient.
Rare:	
• Heart rhythm disturbances, fainting.	Discontinue. Call doctor right away or get emergency care.
• Allergic reaction such as mild skin rash, headache, nausea, dizziness, nervousness, fatigue, muscle aches. Drowsiness may occur even though these drugs are nonsedating.	Discontinue. Call doctor when. convenient.

WARNINGS & PRECAUTIONS

Don't take if:
You are allergic to any antihistamine.

Before you start, consult your doctor:
- If you have any type of heart disorder.
- If you have glaucoma.
- If you have enlarged prostate or urinary retention problems.
- If you have asthma or a respiratory disease.
- If you have liver or kidney disease.
- If you have peptic ulcer.
- If you have electrolyte abnormality, such as low potassium (hypokalemia).

Over age 60:
Adverse reactions and side effects may be more frequent and severe than in younger persons.

Pregnancy:
Risk factors vary for drugs in this group. See category list on page xviii and consult doctor.

Breast-feeding:
Drug may pass into milk. Avoid drug or discontinue nursing until you finish medicine. Consult doctor for advice on maintaining milk supply.

Infants & children:
- Use cetirizine only under close medical supervision.
- All others are not recommended for children under age 12.

Prolonged use:
Antihistamines are normally taken during the hay fever season. They are not intended for long-term uninterrupted use.

Skin & sunlight:
Rarely, may cause rash or intensify sunburn in areas exposed to sun or ultraviolet light (photosensitivity reaction). Avoid overexposure. Notify doctor if reaction occurs.

Driving, piloting or hazardous work:
No problems expected.

Discontinuing:
No problems expected.

Others:
- Claritin-D 24 Hour Extended Release round-shaped tablets have been replaced by oval-shaped tablets due to reports of throat obstruction. You should replace the old round-shaped tablets with the new oval-shaped tablets and be sure to swallow them with a full glass of water.
- Don't exceed recommended dose. This can increase the risk of adverse reactions.
- Advise any doctor or dentist whom you consult that you take this medicine.

POSSIBLE INTERACTION WITH OTHER DRUGS

GENERIC NAME OR DRUG CLASS	COMBINED EFFECT
Anticholinergics	Increased anticholinergic effect.
Central nervous system (CNS) depressants*	May add to any sedative effect.
Erythromycins*	Heart rhythm problems. Avoid.
Fluvoxamine	Increased antihistamine effect.
Itraconazole	Heart rhythm problems with astemizole. Avoid.
Ketocanazole	Heart rhythm problems with astemizole. Avoid.
Leukotriene modifiers	Effects unknown. Consult doctor.
Macrolide antibiotics	Increased risk of adverse reactions.
Metronidazole	Heart rhythm problems with astemizole. Avoid.
Monoamine oxidase (MAO) inhibitors	Increased sedation. Avoid.
Nefazodone	Heart rhythm problems with astemizole. Avoid.
QT interval prolongation-causing drugs*	Heart rhythm problems. Avoid.
Zafirlukast	May increase effect of astemizole.

POSSIBLE INTERACTION WITH OTHER SUBSTANCES

INTERACTS WITH	COMBINED EFFECT
Alcohol:	May cause sedation. Avoid.
Beverages:	None expected.
Cocaine:	Decreased antihistamine effect. Avoid.
Foods:	None expected.
Marijuana:	May cause sedation. Avoid.
Tobacco:	None expected.

*See Glossary

ANTIHISTAMINES, PHENOTHIAZINE-DERIVATIVE

GENERIC AND BRAND NAMES

See complete list of generic and brand names in the *Generic and Brand Name Directory*, page 862.

BASIC INFORMATION

Habit forming? No
Prescription needed? Yes
Available as generic? Yes
Drug class: Tranquilizer (phenothiazine), antihistamine

USES

- Relieves itching of hives, skin allergies, chickenpox.
- Treatment for hay fever, motion sickness, vertigo.
- Treatment for nausea and vomiting.

DOSAGE & USAGE INFORMATION

How to take:
- Tablet or syrup—Swallow with liquid or food to lessen stomach irritation.
- Extended-release capsules—Swallow each dose whole. If you take regular tablets, you may chew or crush them.

When to take:
At the same times each day.

If you forget a dose:
Take as soon as you remember up to 2 hours late. If more than 2 hours, wait for next scheduled dose (don't double this dose).

CoContinued next column

OVERDOSE

SYMPTOMS:
Fast heartbeat, flushed face, shortness of breath, clumsiness, drowsiness, muscle spasms, jerking movements of head and face.
WHAT TO DO:
- **Dial 911 (emergency) for an ambulance or medical help or poison center 1-800-222-1222. Then give first aid immediately.**
- **See emergency information on inside covers.**

What drug does:
- Blocks action of histamine after an allergic response triggers histamine release in sensitive cells. Histamines cause itching, sneezing, runny nose and eyes and other symptoms.
- Appears to work in the vomiting center of the brain to control nausea and vomiting and help prevent motion sickness.

Time lapse before drug works:
15 minutes to 1 hour.

Don't take with:
- Antacid or medicine for diarrhea.
- Nonprescription drug for cough, cold or allergy.
- Any other medicine without consulting your doctor or pharmacist.

POSSIBLE ADVERSE REACTIONS OR SIDE EFFECTS

SYMPTOMS	WHAT TO DO
Life-threatening: In case of overdose, see previous column.	
Common:	
Drowsiness; dryness of mouth, nose or throat; nasal congestion.	Continue. Call doctor when convenient.
Infrequent:	
• Nightmares, unusual excitement, nervousness, irritability, loss of appetite, sweating.	Continue. Call doctor when convenient.
• Difficult urination; blurred or changed vision; dizziness; ringing in ears; skin rash; uncontrolled, jerky movements (with high doses); slow, snakelike movement of arms; spasm of neck muscles; stiffening of tongue; eyes rolling upward.	Discontinue. Call doctor right away.
Rare:	
Sore throat, fever, confusion, yellow skin or eyes, fast heartbeat, feeling faint, unusual tiredness or weakness, unusual bleeding or bruising.	Discontinue. Call doctor right away.

WARNINGS & PRECAUTIONS

Don't take if:
- You are allergic to any phenothiazine.
- You have a blood or bone marrow disease.

Before you start, consult your doctor:
- If you will have surgery within 2 months, including dental surgery, requiring general or spinal anesthesia.
- If you have asthma, emphysema or other lung disorder.
- If you take nonprescription ulcer medicine, asthma medicine or amphetamines.

Over age 60:
Adverse reactions and side effects may be more frequent and severe than in younger persons. More likely to develop tardive dyskinesia (involuntary movement of jaws, lips, tongue, chewing). Report this to your doctor immediately. Early treatment can help.

Pregnancy:
Decide with your doctor if drug benefits justify risk to unborn child. Risk category C (see page xviii).

Breast-feeding:
Drug passes into milk. Avoid drug or discontinue nursing until you finish medicine. Consult doctor for advice on maintaining milk supply.

Infants & children:
Don't give to children younger than 2.

Prolonged use:
- May lead to tardive dyskinesia (involuntary movement of jaws, lips, tongue; chewing).
- Talk to your doctor about the need for follow-up medical examinations or laboratory studies to check complete blood counts (white blood cell count, platelet count, red blood cell count, hemoglobin, hematocrit), liver function, eyes.

Skin & sunlight:
One or more drugs in this group may cause rash or intensify sunburn in areas exposed to sun or ultraviolet light (photosensitivity reaction). Avoid overexposure. Notify doctor if reaction occurs.

Driving, piloting or hazardous work:
Don't drive or pilot aircraft until you learn how medicine affects you. Don't work around dangerous machinery. Don't climb ladders or work in high places. Danger increases if you drink alcohol or take medicine affecting alertness and reflexes.

Discontinuing:
May be unnecessary to finish medicine. Follow doctor's instructions.

Others:
May affect results in some medical tests.

POSSIBLE INTERACTION WITH OTHER DRUGS

GENERIC NAME OR DRUG CLASS	COMBINED EFFECT
Antacids*	Decreased antihistamine effect.
Anticholinergics*	Increased anticholinergic effect.
Anticonvulsants, hydantoin*	Increased anticonvulsant effect.
Antidepressants, tricyclic*	Increased antihistamine effect.
Antihistamines*, other	Increased antihistamine effect.
Antithyroid drugs*	Increased risk of bone marrow depression.
Appetite suppressants*	Decreased appetite suppressant effect.
Barbiturates*	Oversedation.
Carteolol	Decreased antihistamine effect.
Central nervous system (CNS) depressants*	Dangerous degree of sedation.
Cisapride	Decreased antihistamine effect.
Clozapine	Toxic effect on the central nervous system.

Continued on page 900

POSSIBLE INTERACTION WITH OTHER SUBSTANCES

INTERACTS WITH	COMBINED EFFECT
Alcohol:	Dangerous oversedation.
Beverages:	None expected.
Cocaine:	Decreased trimeprazine effect. Avoid.
Foods:	None expected.
Marijuana:	Drowsiness.
Tobacco:	None expected.

***See Glossary**

ANTI-INFLAMMATORY DRUGS, NONSTEROIDAL (NSAIDs)

GENERIC AND BRAND NAMES

See complete list of generic and brand names in the *Generic and Brand Name Directory*, page 862.

BASIC INFORMATION

Habit forming? No
Prescription needed? Yes, for some.
Available as generic? Yes, for some.
Drug class: Anti-inflammatory (nonsteroidal), analgesic, antigout agent, fever-reducer

USES

- Treatment for joint pain, stiffness, inflammation and swelling of arthritis and gout.
- Treatment for pain, fever and inflammation.
- Treatment for dysmenorrhea (painful or difficult menstruation).
- Treats juvenile rheumatoid arthritis.

DOSAGE & USAGE INFORMATION

How to take:

- Tablet or capsule—Swallow with liquid or food to lessen stomach irritation. If you can't swallow whole, crumble tablet and take with liquid or food. Don't crumble delayed release tablet.
- Liquid—Take as directed on bottle. Don't freeze.
- Rectal suppositories—Remove wrapper and moisten suppository with water. Gently insert into rectum, large end first. If suppository is too soft, chill in refrigerator or cool water before removing wrapper.

When to take:
At the same times each day.

If you forget a dose:
Take as soon as you remember up to 2 hours late. If more than 2 hours, wait for next scheduled dose (don't double this dose).

Continued next column

OVERDOSE

SYMPTOMS:
Confusion, agitation, severe headache, incoherence, convulsions, possible hemorrhage from stomach or intestine, coma.
WHAT TO DO:

- **Dial 911 (emergency) for an ambulance or medical help or poison center 1-800-222-1222. Then give first aid immediately.**
- **See emergency information on inside covers.**

What drug does:
Reduces tissue concentration of prostaglandins (hormones which produce inflammation and pain).

Time lapse before drug works:
Begins in 4 to 24 hours. May require 3 weeks regular use for maximum benefit.

Don't take with:
Any other medicine without consulting your doctor or pharmacist.

POSSIBLE ADVERSE REACTIONS OR SIDE EFFECTS

SYMPTOMS	WHAT TO DO
Life-threatening:	
Hives, rash, intense itching, faintness soon after a dose (anaphylaxis in aspirin-sensitive persons).	Seek emergency treatment immediately.
Common:	
• Dizziness, nausea, stomach cramps, headache.	Continue. Call doctor when convenient.
• Diarrhea, skin rash, bleeding from rectum (with suppositories).	Discontinue. Call doctor right away.
Infrequent:	
• Depression; drowsiness; ringing in ears; swollen feet, face or legs; constipation or diarrhea; vomiting; gaseousness; dry mouth; tremors; insomnia.	Continue. Call doctor when convenient.
• Muscle cramps, numbness or tingling in hands or feet, mouth ulcers, rapid weight gain.	Discontinue. Call doctor right away.
Rare:	
• Convulsions; confusion; rash, hives or itch; blurred vision; black, bloody, tarry stool; difficult breathing; tightness in chest; rapid heartbeat; unusual bleeding or bruising; blood in urine; jaundice; psychosis; frequent, painful urination; fainting; sore throat; fever; chills; diminished hearing; eye pain; nose bleeds; severe abdominal pain.	Discontinue. Call doctor right away.
• Fatigue, weakness, menstrual irregularities.	Continue. Call doctor when convenient.

WARNINGS & PRECAUTIONS

Don't take if:
- You are allergic to aspirin or any nonsteroidal, anti-inflammatory drug.
- You have gastritis, peptic ulcer, enteritis, ileitis, ulcerative colitis, asthma, heart failure, high blood pressure or bleeding problems.
- Patient is younger than 15.

Before you start, consult your doctor:
- If you have epilepsy.
- If you have Parkinson's disease.
- If you have been mentally ill.
- If you have impaired kidney or liver function.

Over age 60:
Adverse reactions and side effects may be more frequent and severe than in younger persons.

Pregnancy:
Risk factors vary for drugs in this group. See category list on page xviii and consult doctor.

Breast-feeding:
May harm child. Avoid.

Infants & children:
Not recommended for anyone younger than 15. Use only under medical supervision.

Prolonged use:
- Eye damage.
- Reduced hearing.
- Sore throat, fever.
- Weight gain.
- Talk to your doctor about the need for follow-up medical examinations or laboratory studies to check complete blood counts (white blood cell count, platelet count, red blood cell count, hemoglobin, hematocrit), liver function, stools for blood, eyes.

Skin & sunlight:
One or more drugs in this group may cause rash or intensify sunburn in areas exposed to sun or ultraviolet light (photosensitivity reaction). Avoid overexposure. Notify doctor if reaction occurs.

Driving, piloting or hazardous work:
Don't drive or pilot aircraft until you learn how medicine affects you. Don't work around dangerous machinery. Don't climb ladders or work in high places. Danger increases if you drink alcohol or take medicine affecting alertness and reflexes, such as antihistamines, tranquilizers, sedatives, pain medicine, narcotics and mind-altering drugs.

Discontinuing:
No problems expected. If drug has been taken for a long time, consult doctor before discontinuing.

Others:
Advise any doctor or dentist whom you consult that you take this medicine.

POSSIBLE INTERACTION WITH OTHER DRUGS

GENERIC NAME OR DRUG CLASS	COMBINED EFFECT
Adrenocorticoids, systemic	Increased risk of ulcers. Increased adrenocorticoid effect.
Angiotensin-converting enzyme (ACE) inhibitors*	May decrease ACE inhibitor effect.
Antacids*	Decreased pain relief.
Anticoagulants, oral*	Increased risk of bleeding.
Anticonvulsants, hydantoin*	Increased anti-convulsant effect.
Anti-inflammatory pain relievers (any combination of)	Danger of increased side effects such as stomach bleeding.
Aspirin	Increased risk of stomach ulcer.
Beta-adrenergic blocking agents*	Decreased anti-hypertensive effect.
Carteolol	Decreased anti-hypertensive effect.
Cephalosporins*	Increased risk of bleeding.
Didanosine	Increased risk of pancreatitis (sulindac only).

Continued on page 901

POSSIBLE INTERACTION WITH OTHER SUBSTANCES

INTERACTS WITH	COMBINED EFFECT
Alcohol:	Possible stomach ulcer or bleeding.
Beverages:	None expected.
Cocaine:	None expected.
Foods:	None expected.
Marijuana:	Increased pain relief from NSAIDs.
Tobacco:	None expected.

***See Glossary**

ANTI-INFLAMMATORY DRUGS, NONSTEROIDAL (NSAIDs) COX-2 INHIBITORS

GENERIC AND BRAND NAMES

CELECOXIB
Celebrex
ROFECOXIB
Vioxx
VALDECOXIB
Bextra

BASIC INFORMATION

Habit forming? No
Prescription needed? Yes
Available as generic? No
Drug class: Anti-inflammatory (nonsteroidal), analgesic, antigout agent, fever-reducer

USES

- Treatment for joint pain, stiffness, inflammation and swelling of rheumatoid arthritis, osteoarthritis and gout.
- Treatment for pain, fever and inflammation.
- Treatment for dysmenorrhea (painful or difficult menstruation).
- Treatment for colorectal polyps.

DOSAGE & USAGE INFORMATION

How to take:
- Tablet or capsule—Swallow with liquid. If you can't swallow whole, open capsule or crumble tablet and take with liquid or food.
- Suspension—Shake the bottle well before use. Carefully measure dose with measuring spoon or cup.

When to take:
At the same times each day.

If you forget a dose:
Take as soon as you remember up to 2 hours late. If more than 2 hours, wait for next scheduled dose (don't double this dose).

Continued next column

OVERDOSE

SYMPTOMS:
Breathing problems, tightness in chest, decreased urine amount, swelling, thirst, tiredness or weakness, stomach pain, bloody or black stools, dizziness, headache, nausea or vomiting.
WHAT TO DO:
If person takes much larger amount than prescribed, call doctor, poison center 1-800-222-1222 or hospital emergency room for instructions.

What drug does:
Reduces tissue concentration of prostaglandins (hormones which produce inflammation and pain).

Time lapse before drug works:
Begins in 2 to 3 hours. May require 3 weeks of regular use for maximum benefit.

Don't take with:
Any other medicine without consulting your doctor or pharmacist.

POSSIBLE ADVERSE REACTIONS OR SIDE EFFECTS

SYMPTOMS	WHAT TO DO
Life-threatening:	
Hives, rash, intense itching, faintness soon after a dose (anaphylaxis in aspirin-sensitive persons).	Seek emergency treatment immediately.
Common:	
• Cough, fever, skin rash, swelling of face, fingers, feet and/or lower legs.	Discontinue. Call doctor right away.
• Back pain, dizziness, gas, headache, nausea, heartburn, burning in throat, sleeplessness, stuffy or runny nose.	Continue. Call doctor when convenient.
Infrequent:	
• Bloody or tarry stools, chills, congestion, diarrhea, fatigue, loss of appetite, muscle pains,blood in urine, pale skin, shortness of breath, severe stomach pain, weight gain, vomiting.	Discontinue. Call doctor right away.
• Anxiety, vision changes, noises in ears, changes in sense of taste, difficulty swallowing, dry mouth, constipation, depression, rapid heartbeat, increased sweating, numbness in fingers or toes, sleepiness.	Continue. Call doctor when convenient.
Rare:	
None expected.	

WARNINGS & PRECAUTIONS

Don't take if:
- You are allergic to aspirin or any nonsteroidal, anti-inflammatory drug.
- You are in the third trimester of your pregnancy.

Before you start, consult your doctor:
- If you have a history of alcohol abuse.
- If you have bleeding problems or ulcers.
- If you have used tobacco recently.
- If you have impaired kidney or liver function.
- If you have anemia, asthma, dehydration or fluid retention.
- If you have high blood pressure or heart disease.

Over age 60:
Adverse reactions and side effects may be more frequent and severe than in younger persons.

Pregnancy:
Decide with your doctor whether drug benefits justify risk to unborn child. Risk category C (see page xviii).

Breast-feeding:
May harm child. Avoid drug or discontinue nursing until you finish medicine. Consult doctor for advice on maintaining milk supply.

Infants & children:
Not recommended for anyone younger than 18.

Prolonged use:
- Eye damage; reduced hearing.
- Sore throat, fever.
- Weight gain.
- Talk to your doctor about the need for follow-up medical exams or laboratory studies to check complete blood counts, liver function, stools for blood, eyes.

Skin & sunlight:
No problems expected.

Driving, piloting or hazardous work:
Don't drive or pilot aircraft until you learn how medicine affects you. Don't work around dangerous machinery. Don't climb ladders or work in high places. Danger increases if you drink alcohol or take medicine affecting alertness and reflexes, such as antihistamines, tranquilizers, sedatives, pain medicine, narcotics and mind-altering drugs.

Discontinuing:
No problems expected. If drug has been taken for a long time, consult doctor before discontinuing.

Others:
- May affect results in some medical tests.
- Advise any doctor or dentist whom you consult that you take this medicine.

POSSIBLE INTERACTION WITH OTHER DRUGS

GENERIC NAME OR DRUG CLASS	COMBINED EFFECT
Angiotensin-converting enzyme (ACE) inhibitors*	May decrease ACE inhibitor effect.
Antacids*	Decreased pain relief.
Anti-inflammatory drugs, nonsteroidal (NSAID's)* other	Increased risk of side effects.
Aspirin	Increased risk of stomach ulcer.
Dextromethorphan	Increased effect of dextromethorphan.
Diuretics	Decreased diuretic effect.
Fluconazole	Increased risk of side effects from NSAID.
Lithium	Increased lithium effect.
Methotrexate	Increased methotrexate effect.
Rifampin	Decreased rifampin effect.
Warfarin	Increased risk of bleeding problems.

POSSIBLE INTERACTION WITH OTHER SUBSTANCES

INTERACTS WITH	COMBINED EFFECT
Alcohol:	Possible stomach ulcer or bleeding.
Beverages:	None expected.
Cocaine:	None expected.
Foods:	None expected.
Marijuana:	Increased pain relief from NSAIDs.
Tobacco:	Possible stomach ulcer or bleeding.

*See Glossary

ANTI-INFLAMMATORY DRUGS, NONSTEROIDAL (NSAIDs) (Ophthalmic)

GENERIC AND BRAND NAMES

DICLOFENAC
Solaraze
Voltaren Ophtha
Voltaren Ophthalmic
FLURBIPROFEN
Ocufen
INDOMETHACIN
Indocid
KETOROLAC
Acular
SUPROFEN
Profenal

BASIC INFORMATION

Habit forming? No
Prescription needed? Yes
Available as generic? Yes, for some
Drug class: Ophthalmic anti-inflammatory agents, nonsteroidal

USES

- Used to prevent problems during and following eye surgery, such as cataract removal.
- Treatment for eye itching caused by seasonal allergic conjunctivitis.

DOSAGE & USAGE INFORMATION

How to use:
Eye solution
- Wash hands.
- Apply pressure to inside corner of eye with middle finger.
- Continue pressure for 1 minute after placing medicine in eye.
- Tilt head backward. Pull lower lid away from eye with index finger of the same hand.
- Drop eye drops into pouch and close eye. Don't blink.
- Keep eyes closed for 1 to 2 minutes.

When to use:
As directed by your doctor or on the label. Your doctor or nurse may instill the drug before an eye operation.

If you forget a dose:
Use as soon as you remember.

Continued next column

OVERDOSE

SYMPTOMS:
None expected.
WHAT TO DO:
Not intended for internal use. If child accidentally swallows, call poison center 1-800-222-1222.

What drug does:
Blocks prostaglandin production. Prostaglandins cause inflammatory responses and constriction of the pupil.

Time lapse before drug works:
Immediately.

Don't use with:
Any other medications without first consulting doctor or pharmacist.

POSSIBLE ADVERSE REACTIONS OR SIDE EFFECTS

SYMPTOMS	WHAT TO DO
Life-threatening:	
None expected.	
Common:	
Brief and mild burning or stinging when drops are administered.	No action necessary.
Infrequent:	
None expected.	
Rare:	
Allergic reaction (itching, tearing); redness, swelling or bleeding in eye not present before; eye pain; sensitivity to light.	Discontinue. Call doctor right away.

ANTI-INFLAMMATORY DRUGS, NONSTEROIDAL (NSAIDs) (Ophthalmic)

WARNINGS & PRECAUTIONS

Don't use if:
- You are allergic to any eye medication.
- You are allergic to any nonsteroidal anti-inflammatory drugs taken orally, e.g., aspirin.

Before you start, consult your doctor:
- If you have any bleeding disorder such as hemophilia.
- If you have or have had herpes simplex keratitis (an inflammation of the cornea).
- If you have allergies to any medications, foods or other substances.

Over age 60:
No special problems expected.

Pregnancy:
Risk category C (see page xviii). Decide with your doctor whether drug benefit justifies risk to unborn child.

Breast-feeding:
Unknown if drug passes into breast milk after administration into the eye. Consult doctor.

Infants & children:
No information available on safety or effectiveness. Consult doctor.

Prolonged use:
Not intended for long-term use.

Skin & sunlight:
No special problems expected.

Driving, piloting or hazardous work:
No special problems expected.

Discontinuing:
No special problems expected.

Others:
Don't use leftover medicine for other eye problems without your doctor's approval. Some eye infections could be made worse.

POSSIBLE INTERACTION WITH OTHER DRUGS

GENERIC NAME OR DRUG CLASS	COMBINED EFFECT
Anticoagulants*, oral	May increase bleeding tendency.
Antiglaucoma drugs*	May decrease antiglaucoma effect (with flubiprofen).
Carbachol	Decreased carbachol effect.

POSSIBLE INTERACTION WITH OTHER SUBSTANCES

INTERACTS WITH	COMBINED EFFECT
Alcohol:	None expected.
Beverages:	None expected.
Cocaine:	None expected.
Foods:	None expected.
Marijuana:	None expected.
Tobacco:	None expected.

***See Glossary**

ANTI-INFLAMMATORY DRUGS, STEROIDAL (Ophthalmic)

GENERIC AND BRAND NAMES

See complete list of generic and brand names in the *Generic and Brand Name Directory*, page 862.

BASIC INFORMATION

Habit forming? No
Prescription needed? Yes
Available as generic? Yes
Drug class: Adrenocorticoid (ophthalmic); anti-inflammatory, steroidal (ophthalmic)

USES

- Relieves redness and irritation due to allergies or other irritants.
- Prevents damage to eye.
- Treatment for anterior uveitis (a type of eye infection).

DOSAGE & USAGE INFORMATION

How to use:

Eye drops

- Wash hands.
- Apply pressure to inside corner of eye with middle finger.
- Continue pressure for 1 minute after placing medicine in eye.
- Tilt head backward. Pull lower lid away from eye with index finger of the same hand.
- Drop eye drops into pouch and close eye. Don't blink.
- Keep eyes closed for 1 to 2 minutes.

Eye ointment

- Wash hands.
- Pull lower lid down from eye to form a pouch.
- Squeeze tube to apply thin strip of ointment into pouch.
- Close eye for 1 to 2 minutes.
- Don't touch applicator tip to any surface (including the eye). If you accidentally touch tip, clean with warm soap and water.
- Keep container tightly closed.

Continued next column

- Keep cool, but don't freeze.
- Wash hands immediately after using.

When to use:
As directed.

If you forget a dose:
Use as soon as you remember.

What drug does:
Affects cell membranes and decreases response to irritating substances.

Time lapse before drug works:
Immediately.

Don't use with:
Medicines for abdominal cramps or glaucoma without first consulting doctor.

OVERDOSE

SYMPTOMS:
None expected.
WHAT TO DO:
Not intended for internal use. If child accidentally swallows, call poison center 1-800-222-1222.

POSSIBLE ADVERSE REACTIONS OR SIDE EFFECTS

SYMPTOMS	WHAT TO DO
Life-threatening: None expected.	
Common: None expected.	
Infrequent: Watery, stinging, burning eyes.	Continue. Call doctor when convenient.
Rare:	
• Eye pain, blurred vision, drooping eyelid, halos around lights, enlarged pupils, flashes of light.	Discontinue. Call doctor right away.
• Eye symptoms (discharge, dryness, irritation, tearing, sensation of foreign body); sore throat; runny or stuffy nose.	Continue. Call doctor when convenient.

ANTI-INFLAMMATORY DRUGS, STEROIDAL (Ophthalmic)

WARNINGS & PRECAUTIONS

Don't use if:
You are allergic to any cortisone medicine.

Before you start, consult your doctor:
- If you have or ever have had any eye infection, glaucoma, virus (herpes) or fungus infection of the eye, tuberculosis of the eye.
- If you wear contact lenses (may need to discontinue wearing temporarily).

Over age 60:
No problems expected.

Pregnancy:
Risk factors vary for drugs in this group. See category list on page xviii and consult doctor.

Breast-feeding:
Safety unestablished. Avoid if possible. Consult doctor.

Infants & children:
Use for short periods of time only.

Prolonged use:
- Recheck with eye doctor at regular intervals.
- May develop glaucoma, hypertension of the eye, damage to optic nerve, vision changes, cataracts or infections due to suppressive effects of drug.

Skin & sunlight:
No problems expected.

Driving, piloting or hazardous work:
No problems expected.

Discontinuing:
No problems expected.

Others:
- Cortisone eye medicines should not be used for bacterial, viral, fungal or tubercular infections.
- Keep cool, but don't freeze.
- Notify doctor if condition doesn't improve within 3 days.
- Contact lens wearers have increased risk of infection.

POSSIBLE INTERACTION WITH OTHER DRUGS

GENERIC NAME OR DRUG CLASS	COMBINED EFFECT
Antiglaucoma drugs*, long- and short-acting	Decreased antiglaucoma effect.

POSSIBLE INTERACTION WITH OTHER SUBSTANCES

INTERACTS WITH	COMBINED EFFECT
Alcohol:	None expected.
Beverages:	None expected.
Cocaine:	None expected.
Foods:	None expected.
Marijuana:	None expected.
Tobacco:	None expected.

*See Glossary

ANTI-INFLAMMATORY DRUGS, STEROIDAL (Otic)

GENERIC AND BRAND NAMES

BETAMETHASONE (otic)
Betnesol
DEXAMETHASONE (otic)
Ak-Dex
Decadron
I-Methasone
HYDROCORTISONE (otic)
Cortamed
Cortisol

BASIC INFORMATION

Habit forming? No
Prescription needed? Yes
Available as generic? No
Drug class: Anti-inflammatory, steroidal (otic); adrenocorticoid (otic)

USES

- Treats allergic conditions involving external ear.
- Used together with antibiotics to treat ear infections.
- Treats seborrheic and eczematoid dermatitis involving the ear.

DOSAGE & USAGE INFORMATION

How to use:
Ear drops
- Warm ear drops under running water around the unopened bottle.
- Lie down with affected ear up.
- Adults—Pull ear lobe back and up.
- Children—Pull ear lobe down and back.
- Drop medicine into ear canal until canal is full.
- Stay lying down for 2 minutes.
- Gently insert cotton plug into ear to prevent leaking.

Continued next column

Ear ointment
- Apply small amount to skin just inside the ear canal.
- Use finger or piece of sterile gauze.
- Don't use cotton-tipped applicators.

When to use:
As directed by your doctor.

If you forget a dose:
Use as soon as you remember.

What drug does:
Decreases tissue inflammation, decreases scarring.

Time lapse before drug works:
15 minutes.

Don't use with:
Other ear medications unless directed by your doctor.

OVERDOSE

SYMPTOMS:
None expected.
WHAT TO DO:
Not intended for internal use. If child accidentally swallows, call poison center 1-800-222-1222.

POSSIBLE ADVERSE REACTIONS OR SIDE EFFECTS

SYMPTOMS	WHAT TO DO
Life-threatening: None expected.	
Common: None expected.	
Infrequent: Itching, burning, redness, swelling.	Discontinue. Call doctor right away.
Rare: None expected.	

ANTI-INFLAMMATORY DRUGS, STEROIDAL (Otic)

WARNINGS & PRECAUTIONS

Don't use if:
You are allergic to any of the medications listed under Brand and Generic Names.

Before you start, consult your doctor:
- If eardrum is punctured.
- If you have a viral infection.
- If you have a fungal ear infection.

Over age 60:
No problems expected.

Pregnancy:
Risk factors vary for drugs in this group. See category list on page xviii and consult doctor.

Breast-feeding:
No problems expected. Consult doctor.

Infants & children:
Use small amounts only.

Prolonged use:
Not intended for prolonged use.

Skin & sunlight:
No problems expected.

Driving, piloting or hazardous work:
No problems expected.

Discontinuing:
No problems expected.

Others:
Keep cool, but don't freeze.

POSSIBLE INTERACTION WITH OTHER DRUGS

GENERIC NAME OR DRUG CLASS	COMBINED EFFECT
None expected.	

POSSIBLE INTERACTION WITH OTHER SUBSTANCES

INTERACTS WITH	COMBINED EFFECT
Alcohol:	None expected.
Beverages:	None expected.
Cocaine:	None expected.
Foods:	None expected.
Marijuana:	None expected.
Tobacco:	None expected.

ANTIMALARIAL

GENERIC AND BRAND NAMES

HALOFANTRINE
Halfan

MEFLOQUINE
Lariam

BASIC INFORMATION

Habit forming? No
Prescription needed? Yes
Available as generic? No
Drug class: Antiprotozoal, antimalarial, antiparasitic

USES

- Treats malaria caused by *plasmodium falciparum* (either chloroquine-sensitive or chloroquine-resistant).
- Treats malaria caused by *plasmodium vivax.*
- Mefloquine helps prevent malaria in people traveling into areas where malaria is prevalent.

DOSAGE & USAGE INFORMATION

How to take:
- Mefloquine tablet—Swallow with food, milk or water to lessen stomach irritation.
- Halofantrine tablet—Take on an empty stomach.
- Halofantrine suspension—Varies by age and weight; follow physician's directions.

When to take:
- Mefloquine treatment is usually given as 5 tablets in a single dose, while prevention with mefloquine should start a week prior to travel.
- Halofantrine tablets and suspension are taken every 6 hours, 3 times a day for one day on an empty stomach, 1 hour before or 2 hours after a meal.

Continued next column

OVERDOSE

SYMPTOMS:
Seizures, heart rhythm disturbances.
WHAT TO DO:
- **Dial 911 (emergency) for an ambulance or medical help or poison center 1-800-222-1222. Then give first aid immediately.**
- **Induce vomiting and see a doctor immediately because of the potential cardiotoxic effect. Treat vomiting or diarrhea with standard fluid therapy.**
- **See emergency information on inside covers.**

If you forget a dose:
Take as soon as you remember, then return to regular dosing schedule.

What drug does:
Exact mechanism unknown. Mefloquine kills parasite in one of its developmental stages, while halofantrine treats malaria in its acute stage.

Time lapse before drug works:
6 to 24 hours.

Don't take with:
- Sulfadoxine and pyrimethamine combination (Fansidar).
- Any other medicines (including over-the-counter drugs such as cough and cold medicines, laxatives, antacids, diet pills, caffeine, nose drops or vitamins) without consulting your doctor or pharmacist.

POSSIBLE ADVERSE REACTIONS OR SIDE EFFECTS

SYMPTOMS	WHAT TO DO
Life-threatening:	
Seizures.	Seek emergency treatment immediately.
Common:	
• Dizziness, headache, lightheadedness, abdominal pain, diarrhea, nausea or vomiting, rash, visual disturbances.	Discontinue. Call doctor right away.
• Insomnia, appetite loss.	Continue. Call doctor when convenient.
Infrequent:	
None expected.	
Rare:	
Change in heart rate, confusion, anxiety, depression, hallucinations, psychosis, black urine or decrease in urine amount, chest or lower back pain, rapid breathing.	Discontinue. Call doctor right away.

WARNINGS & PRECAUTIONS

Don't take if:
You are allergic to mefloquine, halofantrine, quinine, quinidine or related medications.

Before you start, consult your doctor:
- If you plan to become pregnant within the medication period or 2 months after.
- If you have heart trouble, especially heart block.
- If you have depression or other emotional problems.
- If you are giving this to a child under 40 pounds of body weight.
- If you have epilepsy or a seizure disorder.

Over age 60:
Adverse reactions and side effects may be more frequent and severe than in younger persons.

Pregnancy:
Not recommended. If traveling to an area where malaria is endemic, consult your doctor about prophylaxis. Risk category C (see page xviii).

Breast-feeding:
One or more of these drugs may pass into mother's milk. Avoid drug or discontinue nursing.

Infants & children:
- For halofantrine pediatric use, consult your doctor.
- Mefloquine is not recommended for children under 2.

Prolonged use:
Not recommended.

Skin & sunlight:
No problems expected.

Driving, piloting or hazardous work:
Don't drive or pilot aircraft until you learn how medicine affects you. Don't work around dangerous machinery. Don't climb ladders or work in high places. Danger increases if you drink alcohol or take medicine affecting alertness and reflexes.

Discontinuing:
Don't discontinue without doctor's advice until you complete the prescribed dosage.

Others:
- Periodic physical (including eye) examinations and blood studies recommended.
- Resistance to one or more of these drugs by some strains of malaria has been reported, so prevention and treatment of malaria may not be uniformly effective.

POSSIBLE INTERACTION WITH OTHER DRUGS

GENERIC NAME OR DRUG CLASS	COMBINED EFFECT
Antiseizure medications	Possible lowered seizure control.
Beta-adrenergic blocking agents*	Heartbeat irregularities or cardiac arrest. Avoid.
Calcium channel blockers*	Heartbeat irregularities.
Chloroquine	Increased chance of seizures. Avoid.
Divalproex	Increased risk of seizures.
Propranolol	Heartbeat irregularities.
Quinidine	Increased chance of seizures and heart rhythm disturbances.
Quinine	Increased chance of seizures and heart rhythm disturbances.
Typhoid vaccine (oral)	Concurrent use may decrease effectiveness of vaccine.
Valproic acid	Decreased valproic acid effect.

POSSIBLE INTERACTION WITH OTHER SUBSTANCES

INTERACTS WITH	COMBINED EFFECT
Alcohol:	Possible liver toxicity. Avoid.
Beverages: Any alcoholic beverage.	Possible liver toxicity. Avoid.
Cocaine:	No problems expected.
Foods:	No problems expected.
Marijuana:	No problems expected.
Tobacco:	No problems expected.

*See Glossary

ANTIMYASTHENICS

GENERIC AND BRAND NAMES

AMBENONIUM	**PYRIDOSTIGMINE**
Mytelase Caplets	**Mestinon**
NEOSTIGMINE	**Mestinon Timespans**
Prostigmin	**Regonol**

BASIC INFORMATION

Habit forming? No
Prescription needed? Yes
Available as generic? No
Drug class: Cholinergic, antimyasthenic

USES

- Diagnosis and treatment of myasthenia gravis.
- Treatment of urinary retention and abdominal distention.
- Antidote to adverse effects of muscle relaxants used in surgery.

DOSAGE & USAGE INFORMATION

How to take:
- Tablet or syrup—Swallow with liquid or food to lessen stomach irritation.
- Extended-release tablets—Swallow each dose whole. If you take regular tablets, you may chew or crush them.

When to take:
As directed, usually 3 or 4 times a day.

Continued next column

OVERDOSE

SYMPTOMS:
Muscle weakness or paralysis, cramps, twitching or clumsiness; severe diarrhea, nausea, vomiting, stomach cramps or pain; breathing difficulty; confusion, irritability, nervousness, restlessness, fear; unusually slow heartbeat; seizures; blurred vision; extreme fatigue.
WHAT TO DO:
- **Dial 911 (emergency) for an ambulance or medical help or poison center 1-800-222-1222. Then give first aid immediately.**
- **See emergency information on inside covers.**

If you forget a dose:
Take as soon as you remember up to 2 hours late. If more than 2 hours, wait for next scheduled dose (don't double this dose).

What drug does:
Inhibits the chemical activity of an enzyme (cholinesterase) so nerve impulses can cross the junction of nerves and muscles.

Time lapse before drug works:
Usually takes 10 to 14 days to determine if drug helps relieve symptoms.

Don't take with:
Any other medicine without consulting your doctor or pharmacist.

POSSIBLE ADVERSE REACTIONS OR SIDE EFFECTS

SYMPTOMS	WHAT TO DO
Life-threatening: In case of overdose, see previous column.	
Common:	
Excess saliva, unusual sweating, mild diarrhea, nausea, vomiting, stomach cramps or pain.	Continue. Call doctor when convenient.
Infrequent:	
Constricted pupils, watery eyes, lung congestion, frequent urge to urinate, confusion, slurred speech.	Continue. But call doctor right away.
Rare:	
Other symptoms.	Continue. Call doctor when convenient.

WARNINGS & PRECAUTIONS

Don't take if:
You are allergic to any cholinergic* or bromide.

Before you start, consult your doctor:
- If you plan to become pregnant within medication period.
- If you have bronchial asthma.
- If you have heartbeat irregularities.
- If you have urinary obstruction or urinary tract infection.

Over age 60:
Adverse reactions and side effects may be more frequent and severe than in younger persons.

Pregnancy:
Decide with your doctor if drug benefits justify risk to unborn child. Risk category C (see page xviii).

Breast-feeding:
Pyridostigmine passes into milk. It is unknown if others pass into milk. Avoid drug or discontinue nursing until you finish medicine. Consult doctor for advice on maintaining milk supply.

Infants & children:
Use only under close medical supervision.

Prolonged use:
Medication may lose effectiveness. Ask your doctor about discontinuing drug for a few days to possibly help restore effect.

Skin & sunlight:
No problems expected.

Driving, piloting or hazardous work:
Don't drive or pilot aircraft until you learn how medicine affects you. Don't work around dangerous machinery. Don't climb ladders or work in high places. Danger increases if you drink alcohol or take medicine affecting alertness and reflexes, such as antihistamines, tranquilizers, sedatives, pain medicine, narcotics and mind-altering drugs.

Discontinuing:
Don't discontinue without doctor's advice until you complete prescribed dose, even though symptoms diminish or disappear.

Others:
- Advise any doctor or dentist whom you consult that you take this medicine.
- Be cautious about participating in hot weather activities since drug may cause excessive sweating.

POSSIBLE INTERACTION WITH OTHER DRUGS

GENERIC NAME OR DRUG CLASS	COMBINED EFFECT
Anesthetics, local or general*	Decreased effect of antimyasthenic.
Antiarrhythmics*	Decreased effect of antimyasthenic.
Anticholinergics*	May mask severe side effects.
Cholinergics*, other	Possible brain and nervous system toxicity.
Guanadrel	Decreased effect of antimyasthenic.
Guanethidine	Decreased effect of antimyasthenic.
Mecamylamine	Decreased effect of antimyasthenic.
Procainamide	Decreased effect of antimyasthenic.
Quinidine	Decreased effect of antimyasthenic.

POSSIBLE INTERACTION WITH OTHER SUBSTANCES

INTERACTS WITH	COMBINED EFFECT
Alcohol:	No proven problems with small doses.
Beverages:	None expected.
Cocaine:	Decreased antimyasthenic effect. Avoid.
Foods:	None expected.
Marijuana:	No proven problems.
Tobacco:	No proven problems.

*See Glossary

ANTIPYRINE & BENZOCAINE (Otic)

BRAND NAMES

A/B Otic
Allergen
Analgesic Ear Drops
Antiben
Aurafair
Auralgan
Aurodex
Dolotic
Earache Drops
Earocol
Otiprin
Oto
Otocalm

BASIC INFORMATION

Habit forming? No
Prescription needed? Yes
Available as generic? Yes
Drug class: Analgesic (otic), anesthetic

USES

- Relieves pain of middle ear infections (otitis media). It does not treat the infection itself.
- Used to soften earwax so it can be removed.

DOSAGE & USAGE INFORMATION

How to use:
- Warm ear drops under running water around the unopened bottle.
- Lie down with affected ear up.
- Adults—Pull ear lobe back and up.
- Children—Pull ear lobe down and back.
- Drop medicine into ear canal until canal is full.
- Stay lying down for 2 minutes.
- Gently insert cotton plug into ear to prevent leaking.

When to use:
Every 1 to 2 hours for 4 hours, then 4 times a day when needed for pain.

If you forget a dose:
Use as soon as you remember.

What drug does:
Functions as a topical anesthetic/analgesic on the eardrum.

Time lapse before drug works:
10 minutes.

Continued next column

OVERDOSE

SYMPTOMS:
None expected.
WHAT TO DO:
Not intended for internal use. If child accidentally swallows, call poison center 1-800-222-1222.

Don't use with:
Any other medicine without consulting your doctor or pharmacist.

POSSIBLE ADVERSE REACTIONS OR SIDE EFFECTS

SYMPTOMS	WHAT TO DO
Life-threatening: None expected.	
Common: None expected.	
Infrequent: Itching or burning in ear (probably represents allergic reaction).	Discontinue. Call doctor right away.
Rare: None expected.	

ANTIPYRINE & BENZOCAINE (Otic)

WARNINGS & PRECAUTIONS

Don't use if:
You are allergic to any local anesthetic (name usually ends with "caine").

Before you start, consult your doctor:
If eardrum is ruptured.

Over age 60:
No problems expected.

Pregnancy:
Consult doctor. Risk category C (see page xviii).

Breast-feeding:
No problems expected. Consult doctor.

Infants & children:
No problems expected.

Prolonged use:
Not intended for prolonged use.

Skin & sunlight:
No problems expected.

Driving, piloting or hazardous work:
No problems expected.

Discontinuing:
No problems expected.

Others:
- Keep cool, but don't freeze.
- Don't touch tip of dropper to any other surface.
- Don't rinse the dropper. Wipe with clean cloth and close tightly.

POSSIBLE INTERACTION WITH OTHER DRUGS

GENERIC NAME OR DRUG CLASS	COMBINED EFFECT
None expected.	

POSSIBLE INTERACTION WITH OTHER SUBSTANCES

INTERACTS WITH	COMBINED EFFECT
Alcohol:	None expected.
Beverages:	None expected.
Cocaine:	None expected.
Foods:	None expected.
Marijuana:	None expected.
Tobacco:	None expected.

ANTISEBORRHEICS (Topical)

GENERIC AND BRAND NAMES

See complete list of generic and brand names in the *Generic and Brand Name Directory*, page 862.

BASIC INFORMATION

Habit forming? No
Prescription needed? Yes
Available as generic? Yes
Drug class: Antiseborrheic

USES

Treats dandruff or seborrheic dermatitis of scalp.

DOSAGE & USAGE INFORMATION

How to use:

- Wet hair and scalp.
- Apply enough medicine to form lather.
- Rub in well. Keep away from eyes.
- Allow to remain on scalp 3 to 5 minutes then rinse.
- Repeat above steps once.

Continued next column

OVERDOSE

SYMPTOMS:
None expected.
WHAT TO DO:

- **Not for internal use. If child accidentally swallows, call poison control center.**
- **Dial 911 (emergency) for an ambulance or medical help or poison center 1-800-222-1222. Then give first aid immediately.**
- **See emergency information on inside covers.**

When to use:
As directed by doctor. Twice a week for shampoo is average.

If you forget a dose:
Use as soon as you remember.

What drug does:
Slows cell growth in scales on scalp.

Time lapse before drug works:
Varies a great deal. If no improvement in 2 weeks, notify doctor.

Don't use with:

- Other scalp preparations without notifying doctor.
- Any other medicine without consulting your doctor or pharmacist.

POSSIBLE ADVERSE REACTIONS OR SIDE EFFECTS

SYMPTOMS	WHAT TO DO
Life-threatening: None expected.	
Common: None expected.	
Infrequent:	
• Irritation not present before using, rash.	Discontinue. Call doctor when convenient.
• Dryness or itching scalp.	Continue. Call doctor when convenient.
Rare: None expected.	

WARNINGS & PRECAUTIONS

Don't use if:

- You have had an allergic reaction to chloroxine, clioquinol (iodochlorhydroxyquin), iodoquinol (diiodohydroxyquin) or edate sodium.
- Scalp is blistered or infected with oozing or raw areas.

Before you start, consult your doctor:
If you are allergic to anything.

Over age 60:
No problems expected.

Pregnancy:
Risk factors vary for drugs in this group. See category list on page xviii and consult doctor.

Breast-feeding:
No problems expected, but check with doctor.

Infants & children:
No problems expected, but check with doctor.

Prolonged use:
No problems expected, but check with doctor.

Skin & sunlight:
No special problems expected.

Driving, piloting or hazardous work:
No problems expected, but check with doctor.

Discontinuing:
No problems expected, but check with doctor.

Others:

- If medicine accidentally gets into eyes, flush them immediately with cool water.
- Heat and moisture in bathroom medicine cabinet can cause breakdown of medicine. Store someplace else.
- Keep cool, but don't freeze.

POSSIBLE INTERACTION WITH OTHER DRUGS

GENERIC NAME OR DRUG CLASS	COMBINED EFFECT
Other medicated shampoos	May increase adverse reactions of each medicine.

POSSIBLE INTERACTION WITH OTHER SUBSTANCES

INTERACTS WITH	COMBINED EFFECT
Alcohol:	None expected.
Beverages:	None expected.
Cocaine:	None expected.
Foods:	None expected.
Marijuana:	None expected.
Tobacco:	None expected.

ANTITHYROID DRUGS

GENERIC AND BRAND NAMES

METHIMAZOLE
Tapazole
Thiamazole

PROPYLTHIOURACIL
Propyl-Thyracil

BASIC INFORMATION

Habit forming? No
Prescription needed? Yes
Available as generic? Yes
Drug class: Antihyperthyroid

USES

- Treatment of overactive thyroid (hyperthyroidism).
- Treatment of angina in patients who have overactive thyroid.

DOSAGE & USAGE INFORMATION

How to take:
Tablet—Swallow with liquid or food to lessen stomach irritation. If you can't swallow whole, crumble tablet and take with liquid or food.

When to take:
At the same times each day.

If you forget a dose:
Take as soon as you remember up to 2 hours late. If more than 2 hours, wait for next scheduled dose (don't double this dose).

What drug does:
Prevents thyroid gland from producing excess thyroid hormone.

Time lapse before drug works:
10 to 20 days.

Don't take with:
- Anticoagulants
- Any other medicine without consulting your doctor or pharmacist.

OVERDOSE

SYMPTOMS:
Bleeding, spots on skin, jaundice (yellow eyes and skin), loss of consciousness.
WHAT TO DO:
Overdose unlikely to threaten life. If person takes much larger amount than prescribed, call doctor, poison center 1-800-222-1222 or hospital emergency room for instructions.

POSSIBLE ADVERSE REACTIONS OR SIDE EFFECTS

SYMPTOMS	WHAT TO DO
Life-threatening: In case of overdose, see previous column.	
Common:	
Skin rash, itching, dryness.	Continue. Call doctor right away.
Infrequent:	
• Dizziness, sore throat with chills and fever, abdominal pain.	Continue. Call doctor right away.
• Taste loss, constipation, diarrhea.	Continue. Call doctor when convenient.
Rare:	
Headache; enlarged lymph glands; irregular or rapid heartbeat; unusual bruising or bleeding; backache; numbness or tingling in toes, fingers or face; joint pain; muscle aches; menstrual irregularities; jaundice; tired, weak, sleepy, listless; swollen eyes or feet; black stools; excessive cold feeling; puffy skin; irritability.	Continue. Call doctor right away.

WARNINGS & PRECAUTIONS

Don't take if:
You are allergic to antithyroid medicines.

Before you start, consult your doctor:
- If you have liver disease.
- If you have blood disease.
- If you have an infection.
- If you take anticoagulants.

Over age 60:
Adverse reactions and side effects may be more frequent and severe than in younger persons.

Pregnancy:
Consult doctor. Risk category D (see page xviii).

Breast-feeding:
Drug filters into milk. Consult doctor.

Infants & children:
Use only under special medical supervision by experienced clinician.

Prolonged use:
- Adverse reactions and side effects more common.
- Talk to your doctor about the need for follow-up medical examinations or laboratory studies to check thyroid function, complete blood counts (white blood cell count, platelet count, red blood cell count, hemoglobin, hematocrit).

Skin & sunlight:
No problems expected.

Driving, piloting or hazardous work:
Don't drive or pilot aircraft until you learn how medicine affects you. Don't work around dangerous machinery. Don't climb ladders or work in high places. Danger increases if you drink alcohol or take medicine affecting alertness and reflexes, such as antihistamines, tranquilizers, sedatives, pain medicine, narcotics and mind-altering drugs.

Discontinuing:
Don't discontinue without consulting doctor. Dose may require gradual reduction if you have taken drug for a long time. Doses of other drugs may also require adjustment.

Others:
- Advise any doctor or dentist whom you consult that you take this medicine.
- Ask your doctor about the symptoms of overactive or underactive thyroid and what to do if they occur.

POSSIBLE INTERACTION WITH OTHER DRUGS

GENERIC NAME OR DRUG CLASS	COMBINED EFFECT
Amiodarone	Decreased antithyroid effect.
Anticoagulants*	Increased effect of anticoagulants.
Antineoplastic drugs*	Increased chance to suppress bone marrow.
Chloramphenicol	Increased chance to suppress bone marrow.
Clozapine	Toxic effect on bone marrow.
Digitalis preparations*	Increased digitalis effect.
Iodine	Decreased antithyroid effect.
Levamisole	Increased risk of bone marrow depression.
Lithium	Decreased thyroid activity.
Potassium iodide	Decreased antithyroid effect.
Tiopronin	Increased risk of toxicity to bone marrow.

POSSIBLE INTERACTION WITH OTHER SUBSTANCES

INTERACTS WITH	COMBINED EFFECT
Alcohol:	Increased possibility of liver toxicity. Avoid.
Beverages:	No problems expected.
Cocaine:	Increased toxicity potential of medicines. Avoid.
Foods:	No problems expected.
Marijuana:	Increased rapid or irregular heartbeat. Avoid.
Tobacco:	Increased chance of rapid heartbeat. Avoid.

*See Glossary

ANTIVIRALS FOR HERPES VIRUS

GENERIC AND BRAND NAMES

ACYCLOVIR
Avirax
DOCOSANOL
Abreva
FAMCICLOVIR
Famvir
GANCICLOVIR
Cytovene
VALACYCLOVIR
Valtrex

BASIC INFORMATION

Habit forming? No
Prescription needed? Yes
Available as generic? Yes, for some
Drug class: Antiviral

USES

- Treatment for symptoms of herpes virus infections (does not cure the disorders). These infections include herpes simplex, genital herpes and herpes zoster (also known as shingles). Herpes infections may occur on the lips and mouth, genitals, skin and the brain.
- May be used to treat chickenpox and other viral infections as prescribed by your doctor.
- Docosanol is a topical drug for treatment of cold sores (herpes simplex virus).
- Ganciclovir is used for treatment of cytomegalovirus (CMV) eye infection in persons whose immune system is impaired.

DOSAGE & USAGE INFORMATION

How to take:

- Tablet, capsule or oral suspension—Swallow with liquid. If you can't swallow whole, open capsule or crumble tablet and take with liquid or food. Take ganciclovir with food and do not open capsule. Other drugs may be taken with or without food. Measure oral suspension with specially marked measuring device.

Continued next column

OVERDOSE

SYMPTOMS:
Unknown effects.
WHAT TO DO:
Overdose unlikely to threaten life. If person takes much larger amount than prescribed or accidentally swallows topical form of drug, call doctor, poison center 1-800-222-1222 or hospital emergency room for instructions.

- Docosanol cream—Apply directly to the affected area at the first sign of a cold sore. It should be used five times daily until the cold sore or fever blister is completely healed.

When to take:

- At the same times each day and night. Drugs work best if started within 48 hours of diagnosis (or when symptoms first appear).
- Use docosanol cream as soon as symptoms appear (pain, blister, burning).

If you forget a dose:
Take as soon as you remember up to 2 hours late. If more than 2 hours, wait for next dose (don't double this dose). Use docosanol as soon as you remember.

What drug does:
Inhibits the growth and spread of the virus thereby decreasing length of infection and lessening the severity of the symptoms.

Time lapse before drug works:
Begins the first day, but may take several days for symptoms (pain, burning and blisters) to improve.

Don't take with:
Any other medicine without consulting your doctor or pharmacist.

POSSIBLE ADVERSE REACTIONS OR SIDE EFFECTS

SYMPTOMS	WHAT TO DO
Life-threatening:	
Hives, rash, intense itching, faintness soon after a dose (anaphylaxis); difficulty breathing.	Seek emergency treatment immediately.
Common:	
General feeling of illness or discomfort.	Continue. Call doctor when convenient.
Infrequent:	
• Headache, nausea, diarrhea, vomiting, tiredness, dizziness; with ganciclovir—sore throat and fever, unusual bleeding or bruising, mood changes.	Continue. Call doctor when convenient.
• Docosanol cream may cause acne, rash, soreness, swelling, dryness, redness.	Discontinue if symptoms persist.

Rare:	
Vision changes, eyes irritated, swelling agitation, confusion, fever, hallucinations, chills, fever, sore throat or mouth, skin (rash, blister, itch, peel), muscle cramps.	Discontinue. Call doctor right away.

WARNINGS & PRECAUTIONS

Don't take if:
You are allergic to antiviral agents.

Before you start, consult your doctor:
- If you have kidney disease or neurological problems.
- If you have any disease of the blood.
- If you are allergic to any medication, food or other substance.

Over age 60:
No special problems expected.

Pregnancy:
Risk factors vary for drugs in this group. See category page xviii and consult doctor.

Breast-feeding:
Drugs may pass into milk. Avoid nursing until you finish medicine. Consult doctor for advice on maintaining milk supply.

Infants & children:
Use only under medical supervision.

Prolonged use:
See your doctor for regular visits to check effectiveness of the drug and to check for any blood problems.

Skin & sunlight:
No special problems expected.

Driving, piloting or hazardous work:
Avoid if you experience dizziness after taking drug, otherwise no problems expected.

Discontinuing:
Don't discontinue without doctor's advice until you complete prescribed dose, even though symptoms diminish or disappear.

Others:
- Advise any doctor or dentist whom you consult that you take this medicine.
- If symptoms don't improve within a few days, or if they worsen, consult doctor.
- See your eye doctor regularly if you are taking the drug for eye infection
- If drug is prescribed for genital herpes, be sure you use proper precautions to prevent spreading the disorder to your sexual partner. If unsure, ask your doctor for information.
- Keep affected skin area clean and dry.
- Decrease blister irritation by wearing loose-fitting clothing.

POSSIBLE INTERACTION WITH OTHER DRUGS

GENERIC NAME OR DRUG CLASS	COMBINED EFFECT
Bone marrow depressants*	Increased risk of bone marrow depression with ganciclovir.
Cimetidine	Increased antiviral effect.
Didanosine	Increased didanosine effect with ganciclovir.
Probenecid	Increased effect of antivirals.
Nephrotoxic medications*	Increased risk of nephrotoxicity.
Nucleotide reverse transcriptase inhibitors	Increased effect of nucleotide reverse transcriptase inhibitor.
Zidovudine	Increased risk of. adverse effects.

POSSIBLE INTERACTION WITH OTHER SUBSTANCES

INTERACTS WITH	COMBINED EFFECT
Alcohol:	None expected.
Beverages:	None expected.
Cocaine:	None expected. Best to avoid.
Foods:	None expected.
Marijuana:	None expected. Best to avoid.
Tobacco:	None expected.

*See Glossary

ANTIVIRALS FOR INFLUENZA

GENERIC AND BRAND NAMES

AMANTIDINE	RIMANTIDINE
Symadine	Flumadine
Symmetrel	

BASIC INFORMATION

Habit forming? No
Prescription needed? Yes
Available as generic? Yes
Drug class: Antiviral, antiparkinsonism

USES

- Prevention and treatment for Type-A flu infections.
- Relief for symptoms of Parkinson's disease (amantidine).

DOSAGE & USAGE INFORMATION

How to take:
- Capsule—Swallow with liquid or food to lessen stomach irritation.
- Syrup—Dilute dose in beverage before swallowing.

When to take:
At the same times each day. For Type-A flu it is especially important to take regular doses as prescribed.

If you forget a dose:
Take as soon as you remember. Wait 4 hours for next dose. Return to schedule.

What drug does:
- Type-A flu—May block penetration of tissue cells by infectious material from virus cells.
- Parkinson's disease and drug-induced extrapyramidal* reactions—Improves muscular condition and coordination.

Continued next column

OVERDOSE

SYMPTOMS:
Heart rhythm disturbances, blood pressure drop, convulsions, hallucinations, violent behavior, confusion, slurred speech, rolling eyes.

WHAT TO DO:
- **Dial 911 (emergency) for an ambulance or medical help or poison center 1-800-222-1222. Then give first aid immediately.**
- **See emergency information on inside covers.**

Time lapse before drug works:
- Type-A flu—48 hours.
- Parkinson's disease—2 days to 2 weeks.

Don't take with:
- Alcohol
- Any other medicine without consulting your doctor or pharmacist.

POSSIBLE ADVERSE REACTIONS OR SIDE EFFECTS

SYMPTOMS	WHAT TO DO
Life-threatening:	
In case of overdose, see previous column.	
Common:	
Headache, difficulty in concentrating, dizziness or lightheadedness, insomnia, irritability, nervousness, nightmares (these side effects infrequent with rimantadine).	Continue. Call doctor when convenient.
Infrequent:	
• With amantadine—Blurred or changed vision, confusion, difficult urination, hallucinations, fainting.	Discontinue. Call doctor right away.
• Constipation; dry mouth, nose or throat; vomiting, appetite loss, nausea.	Continue. Call doctor when convenient.
Rare:	
• With amantadine—Swelling or irritated eyes; depression; swelling of hands, legs or feet; skin rash.	Discontinue. Call doctor right away.
• Seizures (may occur in persons with a history of seizures).	Discontinue. Seek emergency help.

WARNINGS & PRECAUTIONS

Don't take if:
You are allergic to amantadine or rimantadine.

Before you start, consult your doctor:
- If you have had epilepsy or other seizures.
- If you have had heart disease or heart failure.
- If you have had liver or kidney disease.
- If you have had peptic ulcers.
- If you have had eczema or skin rashes.
- If you have had emotional or mental disorders or taken drugs for them.

Over age 60:
Adverse reactions and side effects may be more frequent and severe than in younger persons.

Pregnancy:
Decide with your doctor whether benefits justify risk to unborn child. Risk category C (see page xviii).

Breast-feeding:
Drug may pass into milk. Avoid drug or discontinue nursing until you finish medicine. Consult doctor for advice on maintaining milk supply.

Infants & children:
Use only under medical supervision.

Prolonged use:
Skin splotches, feet swelling, rapid weight gain, shortness of breath. Consult doctor.

Skin & sunlight:
One or more drugs in this group may cause rash or intensify sunburn in areas exposed to sun or ultraviolet light (photosensitivity reaction). Avoid overexposure. Notify doctor if reaction occurs.

Driving, piloting or hazardous work:
Don't drive or pilot aircraft until you learn how medicine affects you. Don't work around dangerous machinery. Don't climb ladders or work in high places. Danger increases if you drink alcohol or take medicine affecting alertness and reflexes.

Discontinuing:
- Parkinson's disease—Don't discontinue without doctor's advice until you complete prescribed dose, even though symptoms diminish or disappear.
- Type-A flu—Discontinue 48 hours after symptoms disappear.

Others:
- Parkinson's disease—May lose effectiveness in 3 to 6 months. Consult doctor.
- These drugs are not effective for influenza-B virus.
- Drug-resistant strains of the virus may occur within the same household.

POSSIBLE INTERACTION WITH OTHER DRUGS

GENERIC NAME OR DRUG CLASS	COMBINED EFFECT
Acetaminophen	With rimantadine—Decreased antiviral effect.
Anticholinergics*	With amantadine—Increased benefit, but excessive anticholinergic dose produces mental confusion, hallucinations, delirium.
Antidepressants, tricyclic*	With amantadine—Increased risk of confusion, hallucinations, nightmares.
Antidyskinetics*	With amantadine—Increased risk of confusion, hallucinations, nightmares.
Antihistamines*	With amantadine—Increased risk of confusion, hallucinations, nightmares.
Aspirin	With rimantadine—Decreased antiviral effect.
Central nervous system (CNS) stimulants*	With amantadine—Increased risk of adverse reactions.
Levodopa	With amantadine—Increased benefit of levodopa. Can cause agitation.

POSSIBLE INTERACTION WITH OTHER SUBSTANCES

INTERACTS WITH	COMBINED EFFECT
Alcohol:	Increased alcohol effect. Possible fainting.
Beverages:	None expected.
Cocaine:	Dangerous overstimulation.
Foods:	None expected.
Marijuana:	None expected.
Tobacco:	None expected.

*See Glossary

ANTIVIRALS FOR INFLUENZA, NEURAMINIDASE INHIBITORS

GENERIC AND BRAND NAMES

OSELTAMIVIR	ZANAMIVIR
Tamiflu	Relenza

BASIC INFORMATION

Habit forming? No
Prescription needed? Yes
Available as generic? No
Drug class: Anti-influenza

USES

Shortens the duration of influenza types A and B. It is best to start using this medicine within 2 days of onset of symptoms. Oseltamivir helps prevent influenza types A and B.

DOSAGE & USAGE INFORMATION

How to take:

- Capsule—Swallow with liquid. If you can't swallow whole, open capsule and take with liquid or food.
- Oral Solution—Take as directed on label.
- Powder—This medication is to be used with a device called a Diskhaler. Read and carefully follow the instructions provided with the device. If you are still unsure, consult your pharmacist for detailed instructions.

When to take:

- For oseltamivir, take two doses daily at the same times.
- For zanamavir, take two doses on the first day separated by 2 hours and then two doses daily for 5 days separated by 12 hours.

If you forget a dose:
Take or use the missed dose as soon as possible. You can use your next dose 2 hours after taking the missed dose, then return to your normal dosing schedule. Do not double dose.

Continued next column

OVERDOSE

SYMPTOMS:
There has been very little experience with overdose; however, relatively large doses have resulted in nausea and vomiting.
WHAT TO DO:

- **Dial 911 (emergency) for an ambulance or medical help or poison center 1-800-222-1222. Then give first aid immediately.**
- **See emergency information on inside covers.**

What drug does:
Inhibits the spread of the virus by preventing release of the cells within the respiratory tract.

Time lapse before drug works:
Begins in 2 to 3 days.

Don't take with:
Any other medicine without consulting your doctor or pharmacist.

POSSIBLE ADVERSE REACTIONS OR SIDE EFFECTS

SYMPTOMS	WHAT TO DO
Life-threatening:	
Hives, rash, intense itching, faintness soon after a dose (anaphylaxis in aspirin-sensitive persons).	Seek emergency treatment immediately.
Common:	
• Cough, fever, skin, rash, swelling of face, fingers, feet and/or lower legs.	Discontinue. Call doctor right away.
• Back pain, dizziness, gas, headache, nausea, heartburn, burning in throat, sleeplessness, stuffy or runny nose.	Continue. Call doctor when convenient.
Infrequent:	
• Bloody or tarry stools, chills, congestion, cough, diarrhea, fatigue, fever, loss of appetite, muscle pains, shortness of breath, severe stomach pain, weight gain, vomiting.	Discontinue. Call doctor right away.
• Anxiety, vision changes, noises in ears, change in sense of taste, difficulty swallowing, dry mouth, constipation, depression, rapid heartbeat, increased sweating, numbness in fingers or toes, sleepiness.	Continue. Call doctor if symptoms persist.
Rare:	
None expected.	

WARNINGS & PRECAUTIONS

Don't take if:
You are allergic to zanamivir or oseltamavir.

Before you start, consult your doctor:
- If you have a history of asthma or chronic obstructive pulmonary disease (zanamivir).
- If you have kidney disease (oseltamivir).

Over age 60:
Adverse reactions and side effects may be more frequent and severe than in younger persons.

Pregnancy:
Decide with your doctor whether drug benefits justify risk to unborn child. Risk category B for zanamivir, risk category C for oseltamivir (see page xviii).

Breast-feeding:
It is unknown if oseltamivir or zanamivir passes into milk. Avoid drug or discontinue nursing until you finish medicine. Consult doctor for advice on maintaining milk supply.

Infants & children:
- Oseltamivir capsules are not recommended for anyone younger than 18. Oseltamivir solution is approved for children over 1 year.
- Zanamivir is not recommended for children under 7 years of age.

Prolonged use:
Not intended for long-term use.

Skin & sunlight:
No problems expected.

Driving, piloting or hazardous work:
Don't drive or pilot aircraft until you learn how medicine affects you. Don't work around dangerous machinery. Don't climb ladders or work in high places. Danger increases if you drink alcohol or take medicine affecting alertness and reflexes, such as antihistamines, tranquilizers, sedatives, pain medicine, narcotics and mind-altering drugs.

Discontinuing:
Do not discontinue until you finish all of your medicine; otherwise, symptoms may return.

Others:
- You should continue receiving an annual flu shot according to guidelines on immunization practices or as recommended by your doctor.
- Does not reduce the risk of influenza transmission to others.
- Advise any doctor or dentist whom you consult that you take this medicine.

POSSIBLE INTERACTION WITH OTHER DRUGS

GENERIC NAME OR DRUG CLASS	COMBINED EFFECT
None expected.	

POSSIBLE INTERACTION WITH OTHER SUBSTANCES

INTERACTS WITH	COMBINED EFFECT
Alcohol:	None expected.
Beverages:	None expected.
Cocaine:	None expected.
Foods:	None expected.
Marijuana:	None expected.
Tobacco:	None expected.

ANTIVIRALS (Ophthalmic)

GENERIC AND BRAND NAMES

IDOXURIDINE
Herplex Eye Drops
Stoxil Eye Ointment

TRIFLURIDINE
Trifluorothymidine
Viroptic

BASIC INFORMATION

Habit forming? No
Prescription needed? Yes
Available as generic? No
Drug class: Antiviral (ophthalmic)

USES

Treats virus infections of the eye (usually herpes simplex virus).

DOSAGE & USAGE INFORMATION

How to use:
Eye drops
- Wash hands.
- Apply pressure to inside corner of eye with middle finger.
- Continue pressure for 1 minute after placing medicine in eye.
- Tilt head backward. Pull lower lid away from eye with index finger of the same hand.
- Drop eye drops into pouch and close eye. Don't blink.
- Keep eyes closed for 1 to 2 minutes.

Eye ointment
- Wash hands.
- Pull lower lid down from eye to form a pouch.
- Squeeze tube to apply thin strip of ointment into pouch.
- Close eye for 1 to 2 minutes.
- Don't touch applicator tip to any surface (including the eye). If you accidentally touch tip, clean with warm soap and water.
- Keep container tightly closed.
- Keep cool, but don't freeze.
- Wash hands immediately after using.

Continued next column

OVERDOSE

SYMPTOMS:
None expected.
WHAT TO DO:
Not intended for internal use. If child accidentally swallows, call poison center 1-800-222-1222.

When to use:
As directed. Usually 1 drop every 2 hours up to maximum of 9 drops daily.

If you forget a dose:
Use as soon as you remember.

What drug does:
Destroys reproductive capacity of virus.

Time lapse before drug works:
Begins to work immediately. Usual course of treatment is 7 days.

Don't use with:
Other eye drops, boric acid or ointment without consulting doctor.

POSSIBLE ADVERSE REACTIONS OR SIDE EFFECTS

SYMPTOMS	WHAT TO DO
Life-threatening	
None expected.	
Common	
Stinging or burning eyes.	Continue. Tell doctor at next visit.
Infrequent	
Blurred vision for a few minutes (with ointment).	No action necessary.
Rare	
Itchy, red eyes; swollen eyelid or eye; excess flow of tears; dimming or haziness of vision.	Discontinue. Call doctor right away.

WARNINGS & PRECAUTIONS

Don't use if:
You are allergic to trifluridine or idoxuridine.

Before you start, consult your doctor:
- If you have had any other eye problems.
- If you use eye drops for glaucoma.

Over age 60:
No problems expected.

Pregnancy:
Risk factors vary for drugs in this group. See category list on page xviii and consult doctor.

Breast-feeding:
No problems expected, but safety not established. Consult doctor.

Infants & children:
Use only under close medical supervision.

Prolonged use:
Avoid unless directed by your eye doctor.

Skin & sunlight:
No problems expected.

Driving, piloting or hazardous work:
No problems expected.

Discontinuing:
Don't discontinue without consulting doctor.

Others:
- Don't use more often or longer than prescribed.
- Keep cool, but don't freeze.
- If problem doesn't improve within a week, notify your doctor.

POSSIBLE INTERACTION WITH OTHER DRUGS

GENERIC NAME OR DRUG CLASS	COMBINED EFFECT
Eye products containing boric acid	Increased risk of toxicity to eye.

POSSIBLE INTERACTION WITH OTHER SUBSTANCES

INTERACTS WITH	COMBINED EFFECT
Alcohol:	None expected.
Beverages:	None expected.
Cocaine:	None expected.
Foods:	None expected.
Marijuana:	None expected.
Tobacco:	None expected.

***See Glossary**

ANTIVIRALS (Topical)

GENERIC AND BRAND NAMES

ACYCLOVIR
Zovirax Ointment

PENCICLOVIR
Denavir

BASIC INFORMATION

Habit forming? No
Prescription needed? Yes
Available as generic? No
Drug class: Antiviral

USES

- Treatment of symptoms of herpes infections of the skin, mucous membranes, lips, mouth and genitals.
- May be used for other skin disorders as prescribed by your doctor.

DOSAGE & USAGE INFORMATION

How to take:
- Acyclovir ointment—Apply to skin and mucous membranes every 3 hours (6 times a day) for 7 days. Use rubber glove when applying. Apply 1/2-inch strip to each sore or blister. Wash before using.
- Penciclovir cream—Use only on lips and face. Avoid eye area. Use every 2 hours, while awake, for 4 days.

When to use:
Use as soon as symptoms begin to appear (burning, pain or blisters).

If you forget a dose:
Apply as soon as you remember, then continue with regular schedule.

What drug does:
- Inhibits reproduction of virus in cells without killing normal cells.
- Does not cure. Herpes breakout often recurs.

Time lapse before drug works:
2 hours.

Don't take with:
Any other topical medicine without consulting your doctor or pharmacist.

OVERDOSE

SYMPTOMS:
None expected.
WHAT TO DO:
If person accidentally swallows topical form of drug, call doctor, poison center 1-800-222-1222 or hospital emergency room for instructions.

POSSIBLE ADVERSE REACTIONS OR SIDE EFFECTS

SYMPTOMS	WHAT TO DO
Life-threatening: None expected.	
Common: May cause mild pain, burning, itching or stinging.	Continue. Call doctor when convenient.
Infrequent: None expected.	
Rare: Skin rash.	Continue. Call doctor when convenient.

WARNINGS & PRECAUTIONS

Don't take if:
You are allergic to topical acyclovir or penciclovir.

Before you start, consult your doctor:
If you are allergic to any medication, food or other substance.

Over age 60:
Adverse reactions and side effects may be more frequent and severe than in younger persons.

Pregnancy:
Decide with your doctor whether drug benefits justify risk to unborn child. Risk category C (see page xviii).

Breast-feeding:
Is is unknown if topical antivirals are absorbed and then pass into breast milk. Consult doctor.

Infants & children:
Use only under special medical supervision.

Prolonged use:
Don't use longer than prescribed time.

Skin & sunlight:
No problems expected.

Driving, piloting or hazardous work:
No problems expected.

Discontinuing:
May be unnecessary to finish medicine. Follow doctor's instructions.

Others:
- Women: Get pap smear every 6 months because those with herpes infections are possibly at increased risk to develop cancer of the cervix. Avoid sexual activity until all blisters or sores heal.
- Don't get topical medicine in eyes.
- Check with doctor if no improvement in 1 week.

POSSIBLE INTERACTION WITH OTHER DRUGS

GENERIC NAME OR DRUG CLASS	COMBINED EFFECT
None expected.	

POSSIBLE INTERACTION WITH OTHER SUBSTANCES

INTERACTS WITH	COMBINED EFFECT
Alcohol:	None expected.
Beverages:	None expected.
Cocaine:	None expected.
Foods:	None expected.
Marijuana:	None expected.
Tobacco:	None expected.

***See Glossary**

APPETITE SUPPRESSANTS

GENERIC AND BRAND NAMES

See complete list of generic and brand names in the *Generic and Brand Name Directory*, page 862.

BASIC INFORMATION

Habit forming? Yes
Prescription needed? Yes
Available as generic? Yes
Drug class: Appetite suppressant

USES

Suppresses appetite. Temporary treatment for obesity.

DOSAGE & USAGE INFORMATION

How to take:

- Tablet or capsule—Swallow with liquid. You may chew or crush tablet.
- Extended-release tablets or capsules—Swallow each dose whole with liquid; do not crush.
- Elixir—Swallow with liquid.

When to take:

- Long-acting forms—10 to 14 hours before bedtime.
- Short-acting forms—1 hour before meals. Last dose no later than 4 to 6 hours before bedtime.

If you forget a dose:

- Long-acting form—Take as soon as you remember up to 2 hours late. If more than 2 hours, wait for next scheduled dose (don't double this dose).
- Short-acting form—Wait for next scheduled dose. Don't double this dose.

Continued next column

OVERDOSE

SYMPTOMS:
Irritability, overactivity, trembling, insomnia, mood changes, fever, rapid heartbeat, confusion, disorientation, hallucinations, convulsions, coma.
WHAT TO DO:

- **Dial 911 (emergency) for an ambulance or medical help or poison center 1-800-222-1222. Then give first aid immediately.**
- **See emergency information on inside covers.**

What drug does:
Apparently stimulates brain's appetite control center.

Time lapse before drug works:
Begins in 1 hour. Short-acting form lasts 4 hours. Long-acting form lasts 14 hours.

Don't take with:
Nonprescription drugs without consulting doctor.

POSSIBLE ADVERSE REACTIONS OR SIDE EFFECTS

SYMPTOMS	WHAT TO DO
Life-threatening: In case of overdose, see previous column.	
Common:	
Irritability, nervousness, insomnia, false sense of well-being.	Continue. Call doctor when convenient.
Infrequent:	
• Irregular or pounding heartbeat, urgent or difficult urination.	Discontinue. Call doctor right away.
• Blurred vision, unpleasant taste or dry mouth, constipation or diarrhea, nausea, vomiting, cramps, changes in sex drive, increased sweating, headache, nightmares, weakness.	Continue. Call doctor when convenient.
Rare:	
• Rash or hives, breathing difficulty.	Discontinue. Call doctor right away.
• Hair loss.	Continue. Call doctor when convenient.

WARNINGS & PRECAUTIONS

Don't take if:

- You are allergic to any sympathomimetic or phenylpropanolamine.
- You have glaucoma.
- You have taken MAO inhibitors within 2 weeks.
- You plan to become pregnant within medication period.
- You have a history of drug or alcohol abuse.
- You have irregular or rapid heartbeat.

Before you start, consult your doctor:
- If you have high blood pressure or heart disease.
- If you have an overactive thyroid, nervous tension or anxiety.
- If you have epilepsy.
- If you will have surgery within 2 months, including dental surgery, requiring general or spinal anesthesia.
- If you take any other nonprescription medicine.

Over age 60:
Adverse reactions and side effects may be more frequent and severe than in younger persons.

Pregnancy:
Risk factors vary for drugs in this group. See category list on page xviii and consult doctor.

Breast-feeding:
Safety not established. Consult doctor.

Infants & children:
Don't give to children younger than 12.

Prolonged use:
- Loses effectiveness. Avoid.
- Talk to your doctor about the need for follow-up medical examinations or laboratory studies.

Skin & sunlight:
No problems expected.

Driving, piloting or hazardous work:
Don't drive or pilot aircraft until you learn how medicine affects you. Don't work around dangerous machinery. Don't climb ladders or work in high places. Danger increases if you drink alcohol or take medicine affecting alertness and reflexes, such as antihistamines, tranquilizers, sedatives, pain medicine, narcotics and mind-altering drugs.

Discontinuing:
- Don't discontinue without consulting doctor. Dose may require gradual reduction if you have taken drug for a long time. Doses of other drugs may also require adjustment.
- Consult doctor if following symptoms occur after stopping the drug—depression, nausea and vomiting, stomach cramps, insomnia, nightmares, extreme tiredness or weakness.

Others:
- Don't increase dose without doctor's approval.
- Advise any doctor or dentist whom you consult that you take this medicine.

POSSIBLE INTERACTION WITH OTHER DRUGS

GENERIC NAME OR DRUG CLASS	COMBINED EFFECT
Antidiabetic agents*, oral or insulin	May require dosage adjustment of antidiabetic agent.
Antihypertensives*	Decreased antihypertensive effect.
Appetite suppressants, other*	Dangerous overstimulation.
Caffeine	Increased stimulant effect.
Central nervous system (CNS) depressants*	Increased depressive effects of both drugs.
Central nervous system (CNS) stimulants*	Increased stimulant effects of both drugs.
Guanethidine	Decreased guanethidine effect.
Methyldopa	Decreased methyldopa effect.
Monoamine oxidase (MAO) inhibitors*	Dangerous blood pressure rise.
Phenothiazines*	Decreased appetite suppressant effect.
Rauwolfia alkaloids*	Decreased effect of rauwolfia alkaloids.

POSSIBLE INTERACTION WITH OTHER SUBSTANCES

INTERACTS WITH	COMBINED EFFECT
Alcohol:	Increased sedation.
Beverages: Caffeine drinks.	Excessive stimulation.
Cocaine:	Convulsions or excessive nervousness.
Foods:	None expected.
Marijuana:	Frequent use—Irregular heartbeat.
Tobacco:	None expected.

*See Glossary

ASPIRIN

BRAND NAMES

See complete list of brand names in the *Generic and Brand Name Directory*, page 862.

BASIC INFORMATION

Habit forming? No
Prescription needed? No
Available as generic? Yes
Drug class: Analgesic, anti-inflammatory (nonsteroidal)

USES

- Reduces pain, fever, inflammation.
- Relieves swelling, stiffness, joint pain of arthritis or rheumatism.
- Antiplatelet effect to reduce chances of heart attack and/or stroke.

DOSAGE & USAGE INFORMATION

How to take:

- Tablet or capsule—Swallow with liquid or food to lessen stomach irritation.
- Extended-release tablets or capsules—Swallow each dose whole.
- Effervescent tablets—Dissolve in water.
- Chewing gum tablets—Chew completely. Don't swallow whole.
- Dispersible tablets—Dissolve in the mouth before swallowing.
- Chewable tablets—Chew before swallowing or dissolve in small amount of liquid before swallowing.

Continued next column

- Suppositories—Remove wrapper and moisten suppository with water. Gently insert into rectum, large end first.

When to take:
Pain, fever, inflammation—As needed, no more often than every 4 hours.

If you forget a dose:

- Pain, fever—Take as soon as you remember. Wait 4 hours for next dose.
- Arthritis—Take as soon as you remember up to 2 hours late. Return to regular schedule.

What drug does:

- Affects hypothalamus, the part of the brain which regulates temperature by dilating small blood vessels in skin.
- Prevents clumping of platelets (small blood cells) so blood vessels remain open.
- Decreases prostaglandin effect.
- Suppresses body's pain messages.

Time lapse before drug works:
30 minutes for pain, fever, arthritis.

Don't take with:

- Tetracyclines. Space doses 1 hour apart.
- Any other medicine without consulting your doctor or pharmacist.

OVERDOSE

SYMPTOMS:

- **Mild overdose—Confusion, severe diarrhea, stomach pain, increased thirst, vision problems, ringing or buzzing in ears, dizziness, lightheadedness, severe headache.**
- **Severe overdose—Bloody urine; hallucinations; severe nervousness, excitement or confusion; shortness of breath; trouble breathing; convulsions.**
- **In some children—The only symptoms may be behavior changes, severe drowsiness or tiredness, fast or deep breathing.**

WHAT TO DO:

- **Dial 911 (emergency) for an ambulance or medical help or poison center 1-800-222-1222. Then give first aid immediately.**
- **See emergency information on inside covers.**

POSSIBLE ADVERSE REACTIONS OR SIDE EFFECTS

SYMPTOMS	WHAT TO DO
Life-threatening:	
Black or bloody vomit; blood in urine; difficulty breathing; hives, rash, intense itching, faintness soon after a dose (anaphylaxis).	Seek emergency treatment immediately.
Common:	
Heartburn, indigestion, mild nausea or vomiting.	Continue. Call doctor when convenient.
Infrequent:	
Trouble sleeping; rectal irritation (with suppository).	Continue. Call doctor when convenient.
Rare:	
Severe headache, convulsions, extreme drowsiness, flushing or other change in skin color, any loss of hearing, severe vomiting, swelling of face, vision problems, bloody or black stools, ringing in ears, severe stomach cramps or pain (all symptoms more likely with repeated doses for long periods since aspirin can build up in the body).	Discontinue. Call doctor right away or seek emergency treatment.

WARNINGS & PRECAUTIONS

Don't take if:

- You need to restrict sodium in your diet. Buffered effervescent tablets and sodium salicylate are high in sodium.
- You are sensitive to aspirin or aspirin has a strong vinegar-like odor, which means it has decomposed.
- You have a peptic ulcer of stomach or duodenum or a bleeding disorder.

Before you start, consult your doctor:

- If you have had stomach or duodenal ulcers.
- If you have had gout.
- If you have asthma or nasal polyps.
- If you have kidney or liver disease.

Over age 60:
More likely to cause hidden bleeding in stomach or intestines. Watch for dark stools.

Pregnancy:
Risk category C; D in third trimester (see page xviii). Consult doctor.

Breast-feeding:
Drug passes into milk. Avoid drug or discontinue nursing until you finish medicine. Consult doctor for advice on maintaining milk supply.

Infants & children:

- Overdose frequent and severe. Keep bottles out of children's reach.
- Do not give to persons under age 18 who have fever and discomfort of viral illness, especially chicken pox and influenza. Probably increases risk of Reye's syndrome.

Prolonged use:

- Talk to your doctor about the need for follow-up medical examinations or laboratory studies to check liver function, complete blood counts (white blood cell count, platelet count, red blood cell count, hemoglobin, hematocrit).
- Kidney damage may result. Periodic kidney function tests recommended.

Skin & sunlight:
No special problems expected.

Driving, piloting or hazardous work:
No restrictions unless you feel drowsy.

Discontinuing:
For chronic illness—Don't discontinue without doctor's advice until you complete prescribed dose, even though symptoms diminish or disappear.

Others:

- Aspirin can complicate surgery, pregnancy, labor and delivery, and illness.
- For arthritis—Don't change dose without consulting doctor.
- Urine tests for blood sugar may be inaccurate.
- Don't take if pills have vinegar-like odor.

*See Glossary

POSSIBLE INTERACTION WITH OTHER DRUGS

GENERIC NAME OR DRUG CLASS	COMBINED EFFECT
Acebutolol	Decreased anti-hypertensive effect of acebutolol.
Adrenocorticoids, systemic	Increased adreno-corticoid effect.
Alendronate	Increased risk of stomach irritation.
Allopurinol	Decreased allopurinol effect.
Angiotensin-converting enzyme (ACE) inhibitors*	Decreased ACE inhibitor effect.
Antacids*	Decreased aspirin effect.
Anticoagulants*	Increased anti-coagulant effect. Abnormal bleeding.
Antidiabetic agents, oral*	Low blood sugar.
Anti-inflammatory drugs nonsteroidal (NSAIDs)*	Risk of stomach bleeding and ulcers.
Bumetanide	Possible aspirin toxicity.
Carteolol	Decreased anti-hypertensive effect of carteolol.

Continued on page 901

POSSIBLE INTERACTION WITH OTHER SUBSTANCES

INTERACTS WITH	COMBINED EFFECT
Alcohol:	Possible stomach irritation and bleeding. Avoid.
Beverages:	None expected.
Cocaine:	None expected.
Foods:	None expected.
Marijuana:	Possible increased pain relief, but mari-juana may slow body's recovery. Avoid.
Tobacco:	None expected.

ATOVAQUONE

BRAND NAMES

Mepron
Malarone

BASIC INFORMATION

Habit forming? No
Prescription needed? Yes
Available as generic? No
Drug class: Antiprotozoal, antimalarial.

USES

- Treats mild to moderate pneumocystis carinii pneumonia.
- May be effective for other parasitic infections such as toxoplasmosis and malaria.

DOSAGE & USAGE INFORMATION

How to take:
Tablet–Swallow with liquid. If you cannot swallow whole, crumble tablet and take with liquid or food.

When to take:
At the same times each day. Take with meals that are high in fat (eggs, cheese, butter, milk, meat, pizza, nuts) to increase absorption.

If you forget a dose:
Take as soon as you remember up to 2 hours late. If more than 2 hours, wait for next scheduled dose (don't double this dose).

What drug does:
Stops harmful growth of susceptible organisms.

Time lapse before drug works:
3 weeks.

Don't take with:
Any other prescription or nonprescription drug without consulting your doctor or pharmacist.

OVERDOSE

SYMPTOMS:
None expected.
WHAT TO DO:
Overdose unlikely to threaten life. If person takes much larger amount than prescribed, call doctor, poison center 1-800-222-1222 or hospital emergency room for instructions.

POSSIBLE ADVERSE REACTIONS OR SIDE EFFECTS

SYMPTOMS	WHAT TO DO
Life-threatening: None expected.	
Common:	
• Fever, skin rash.	Discontinue. Call doctor right away.
• Nausea or vomiting, diarrhea, headache, cough, trouble sleeping.	Continue. Call doctor when convenient.
Infrequent: None expected.	
Rare: None expected.	

WARNINGS & PRECAUTIONS

Don't take if:
You are allergic to atovaquone.

Before you start, consult your doctor:
If you have any gastrointestinal disorder.

Over age 60:
No problems expected.

Pregnancy:
Discuss with your doctor whether drug benefits justify risk to unborn child. Risk category C (see page xviii).

Breast-feeding:
Not known if drug passes into breast milk. Avoid drug or discontinue nursing until you finish medicine. Consult doctor for advice on maintaining milk supply.

Infants & children:
Give only under close medical supervision.

Prolonged use:
Not intended for long-term use.

Skin & sunlight:
No problems expected.

Driving, piloting or hazardous work:
No problems expected.

Discontinuing:
No problems expected.

Others:
- Advise any doctor or dentist whom you consult that you take this medicine.
- May affect the results in some medical tests.
- Talk to your doctor about the need for follow-up medical examinations or laboratory studies to check blood counts and liver function.

POSSIBLE INTERACTION WITH OTHER DRUGS

GENERIC NAME OR DRUG CLASS	COMBINED EFFECT
None significant.	

POSSIBLE INTERACTION WITH OTHER SUBSTANCES

INTERACTS WITH	COMBINED EFFECT
Alcohol:	None expected.
Beverages:	None expected.
Cocaine:	None expected.
Foods:	None expected.
Marijuana:	None expected.
Tobacco:	None expected.

ATROPINE, HYOSCYAMINE, METHENAMINE, METHYLENE BLUE, PHENYLSALICYLATE & BENZOIC ACID

BRAND NAMES

Atrosept	Urinary Antiseptic No. 2
Dolsed	Urised
Hexalol	Uriseptic
Prosed/DS	Uritab
Trac Tabs 2X	Uritin
UAA	Uro-Ves
Uridon Modified	U-Tract
Urimed	

BASIC INFORMATION

Habit forming? No
Prescription needed? Yes
Available as generic? No
Drug class: Analgesic (urinary), antispasmodic, anti-infective (urinary)

USES

A combination medicine to control infection, spasms and pain caused by urinary tract infections.

DOSAGE & USAGE INFORMATION

How to take:
Tablet—Swallow with liquid or food to lessen stomach irritation.

When to take:
30 minutes before meals (unless directed otherwise by doctor).

Continued next column

OVERDOSE

SYMPTOMS:
Dilated pupils, rapid pulse and breathing, dizziness, fever, hallucinations, confusion, slurred speech, agitation, flushed face, convulsions, coma.

WHAT TO DO:
- **Dial 911 (emergency) for an ambulance or medical help or poison center 1-800-222-1222. Then give first aid immediately.**
- **See emergency information on inside covers.**

If you forget a dose:
Take as soon as you remember up to 2 hours late. If more than 2 hours, wait for next scheduled dose (don't double this dose).

What drug does:
Makes urine acid. Blocks nerve impulses at parasympathetic nerve endings, preventing muscle contractions and gland secretions of organs involved. Methenamine destroys some germs.

Time lapse before drug works:
15 to 30 minutes.

Don't take with:
- Antacids* or antidiarrheals*.
- Any other medicine without consulting your doctor or pharmacist.

POSSIBLE ADVERSE REACTIONS OR SIDE EFFECTS

SYMPTOMS	WHAT TO DO
Life-threatening:	
Heartbeat irregularity, shortness of breath or difficulty breathing.	Seek emergency treatment immediately.
Common:	
Dry mouth, throat, ears, nose.	Continue. Call doctor when convenient.
Infrequent:	
• Flushed, red face; drowsiness; difficult urination; nausea and vomiting; abdominal pain; ringing or buzzing in ears; severe drowsiness; back pain; lightheadedness.	Discontinue. Call doctor right away.
• Headache, nasal congestion, altered taste.	Continue. Call doctor when convenient.
Rare:	
Blurred vision; pain in eyes; skin rash, hives.	Discontinue. Seek emergency treatment.

WARNINGS & PRECAUTIONS

Don't take if:
- You are allergic to any of the ingredients or aspirin.
- Brain damage in child.
- You have glaucoma.

ATROPINE, HYOSCYAMINE, METHENAMINE, METHYLENE BLUE, PHENYLSALICYLATE & BENZOIC ACID

Before you start, consult your doctor:

- If you are on any special diet such as low-sodium.
- If you have had a hiatal hernia, bronchitis, asthma, liver disease, stomach or duodenal ulcers.
- If you have asthma, nasal polyps, bleeding disorder, glaucoma or enlarged prostate.
- If you will have any surgery within 2 months.
- If you have heart disease.

Over age 60:

- Adverse reactions and side effects may be more frequent and severe than in younger persons.
- More likely to cause hidden bleeding in stomach or intestines. Watch for dark stools.

Pregnancy:
Risk factors vary for drugs in this group. See category list on page xviii and consult doctor.

Breast-feeding:
Drug passes into milk. Avoid or discontinue nursing until you finish medicine.

Infants & children:
Side effects more likely. Not recommended in children under 12.

Prolonged use:
May lead to constipation or kidney damage. Request lab studies to monitor effects of prolonged use.

Skin & sunlight:
No problems expected.

Driving, piloting or hazardous work:
May disqualify for piloting aircraft during time you take medicine.

Discontinuing:
May be unnecessary to finish medicine. Follow your symptoms and doctor's advice.

Others:

- Salicylates can complicate surgery, pregnancy, labor and delivery, and illness.
- Urine tests for blood sugar may be inaccurate.
- Drink cranberry juice or eat prunes or plums to help make urine more acid.

POSSIBLE INTERACTION WITH OTHER DRUGS

GENERIC NAME OR DRUG CLASS	COMBINED EFFECT
Allopurinol	Decreased allopurinol effect.
Amantadine	Increased atropine and belladonna effect.
Antacids*	Decreased salicylate and methenamine effect.
Anticoagulants*	Increased anti-coagulant effect. Abnormal bleeding.
Anticholinergics, other*	Increased atropine and belladonna effect.
Antidepressants, other*	Increased sedation.
Antidiabetics, oral*	Low blood sugar.
Antifungals, azoles	Reduced azole effect.
Antihistamines*	Increased atropine and hyoscyamine effect.
Anti-inflammatory drugs, nonsteroidal (NSAIDs)*	Risk of stomach bleeding and ulcers.
Aspirin	Likely salicylate toxicity.
Beta-adrenergic blocking agents*	Decreased anti-hypertensive effect.
Carbonic anhydrase inhibitors*	Decreased methenamine effect.
Cortisone drugs*	Increased internal eye pressure, increased cortisone effect. Risk of ulcers and stomach bleeding.

Continued on page 902

POSSIBLE INTERACTION WITH OTHER SUBSTANCES

INTERACTS WITH	COMBINED EFFECT
Alcohol:	Excessive sedation. Possible stomach irritation and bleeding. Avoid.
Beverages:	None expected.
Cocaine:	Excessively rapid heartbeat. Avoid.
Foods:	None expected.
Marijuana:	Drowsiness and dry mouth. May slow body's recovery.
Tobacco:	Dry mouth.

***See Glossary**

ATTAPULGITE

BRAND NAMES

Diar-Aid
Diasorb
Fowlers Diarrhea Tablets
Kaopectate
Kaopectate Advanced Formula
Kaopectate Maximum Strength
Rheaban
St. Joseph Antidiarrheal

BASIC INFORMATION

Habit forming? No
Prescription needed? No
Available as generic? Yes
Drug class: Antidiarrheal

USES

Treats diarrhea. Used in conjunction with fluids, appropriate diet and rest. Treats symptoms only. Does not cure any disorder that causes diarrhea.

DOSAGE & USAGE INFORMATION

How to take:

- Tablets—Swallow with liquid. If you can't swallow whole, crumble tablet and take with liquid or food. Instructions to take on empty stomach mean 1 hour before or 2 hours after eating.
- Chewable tablets—Chew well before swallowing.
- Oral suspension—Follow label instructions.

When to take:
2 hours before or 3 hours after taking any other oral medications. Outside of this restriction, take a dose after each loose bowel movement until diarrhea is controlled.

If you forget a dose:
Take as soon as you remember, then resume regular schedule.

Continued next column

OVERDOSE

SYMPTOMS:
None expected.
WHAT TO DO:
Overdose unlikely to threaten life. If person takes much larger amount than prescribed, call doctor, poison center 1-800-222-1222 or hospital emergency room for instructions.

What drug does:
Absorbs bacteria and toxins and reduces water loss. Attapulgite does not get absorbed into the body.

Time lapse before drug works:
5 to 8 hours.

Don't take with:
Any other medicine without consulting your doctor or pharmacist.

POSSIBLE ADVERSE REACTIONS OR SIDE EFFECTS

SYMPTOMS	WHAT TO DO
Life-threatening: None expected.	
Common: None expected.	
Infrequent: Constipation (usually mild and of short duration).	Continue. Call doctor when convenient.
Rare: None expected.	

WARNINGS & PRECAUTIONS

Don't take if:
- You are allergic to attapulgite.
- You or your doctor suspects intestinal obstruction.

Before you start, consult your doctor:
If you are dehydrated (signs are a dry mouth, loose skin, sunken eyes and parched lips).

Over age 60:
- Dehydration is more likely in this age group.
- Side effects of constipation are more likely.

Pregnancy:
Risk category not designated. See list on page xviii and consult doctor.

Breast-feeding:
No problems expected, but consult doctor.

Infants & children:
Use only under close medical supervision for children up to 3 years of age. This age group is quite susceptible to fluid and electrolyte loss.

Prolonged use:
Not intended for prolonged use.

Skin & sunlight:
No special problems expected.

Driving, piloting or hazardous work:
No special problems expected.

Discontinuing:
May be unnecessary to finish medicine. Follow doctor's instructions.

Others:
No special problems expected.

POSSIBLE INTERACTION WITH OTHER DRUGS

GENERIC NAME OR DRUG CLASS	COMBINED EFFECT
Digitalis	May decrease effectiveness of digitalis.
Lincomycin*	May decrease effectiveness of lincomycins.
Any other medicine taken by mouth	When taken at the same time, neither drug may be as effective. Take other medicines 2 hours before or 3 hours after attapulgite.

POSSIBLE INTERACTION WITH OTHER SUBSTANCES

INTERACTS WITH	COMBINED EFFECT
Alcohol:	None expected.
Beverages:	None expected.
Cocaine:	None expected.
Foods: Prunes, prune juice and other fruits or foods that may cause diarrhea.	Decreased effect of attapulgite.
Marijuana:	None expected.
Tobacco:	None expected.

***See Glossary**

AZATHIOPRINE

BRAND NAMES

Imuran

BASIC INFORMATION

Habit forming? No
Prescription needed? Yes
Available as generic? Yes
Drug class: Immunosuppressant, antirheumatic

USES

- Protects against rejection of transplanted organs (e.g., kidney, heart).
- Treats severe active rheumatoid arthritis and other immunologic diseases if simpler treatment plans have been ineffective.

DOSAGE & USAGE INFORMATION

How to take:
Tablets—Swallow with liquid. If you can't swallow whole, crumble tablet and take with liquid or food. Instructions to take on empty stomach mean 1 hour before or 2 hours after eating.

When to take:
Follow your doctor's instructions. Usually once a day.

If you forget a dose:
Take as soon as you remember up to 2 hours late. If more than 2 hours, wait for next scheduled dose (don't double this dose).

What drug does:
Unknown; probably inhibits synthesis of DNA and RNA.

Time lapse before drug works:
6 to 8 weeks.

Don't take with:
Any other medicines (including over-the-counter drugs such as cough and cold medicines, laxatives, antacids, diet pills, caffeine, nose drops or vitamins) without consulting your doctor.

OVERDOSE

SYMPTOMS:
None expected.
WHAT TO DO:
Overdose unlikely to threaten life. If person takes much larger amount than prescribed, call doctor, poison center 1-800-222-1222 or hospital emergency room for instructions.

POSSIBLE ADVERSE REACTIONS OR SIDE EFFECTS

SYMPTOMS	WHAT TO DO
Life-threatening:	
Rapid heart rate, sudden fever, muscle or joint pain, cough, shortness of breath.	Seek emergency treatment immediately.
Common:	
• Infection or low blood count causing fever and chills, back pain cough, painful urination; anemia (tiredness or weakness); nausea; vomiting.	Discontinue. Call doctor right away.
• Appetite loss.	Continue. Call doctor when convenient.
Infrequent:	
Jaundice (yellow eyes, skin), skin rash.	Discontinue. Call doctor right away.
Rare:	
Low platelet count causing bleeding or bruising, tarry or black stools, bloody urine, red spots under skin; severe abdominal pain; mouth sores.	Discontinue. Call doctor right away.

WARNINGS & PRECAUTIONS

Don't take if:
- You are allergic to azathioprine
- You have chicken pox.
- You have shingles (herpes zoster).

Before you start, consult your doctor:
- If you have gout.
- If you have liver or kidney disease.
- If you have an infection.

Over age 60:
Adverse reactions and side effects may be more frequent and severe than in younger persons. You may need smaller doses for shorter periods of time.

Pregnancy:
Risk to unborn child outweighs drug benefits. Don't use. Risk category D (see page xviii).

Breast-feeding:
Drug passes into milk. Avoid drug or discontinue nursing until you finish medicine. Consult doctor for advice on maintaining milk supply.

Infants & children:
No special problems expected.

Prolonged use:
- May increase likelihood of problems upon discontinuing.
- Talk to your doctor about the need for follow-up medical examinations or laboratory studies to check thyroid function, liver function, electrolytes (sodium potassium, chloride), blood pressure and complete blood counts (white blood count, platelet count, red blood cell count, hemoglobin, hematocrit) every week during first two months, then once a month.

Skin & sunlight:
No special problems expected.

Driving, piloting or hazardous work:
Avoid if you feel confused, drowsy or dizzy.

Discontinuing:
May still experience symptoms of bone marrow depression, such as: blood in stools, fever or chills, blood spots under the skin, back pain, hoarseness, bloody urine. If any of these occur, call your doctor right away.

Others:
- Advise any doctor or dentist whom you consult that you take this medicine.
- May affect results in some medical tests.

POSSIBLE INTERACTION WITH OTHER DRUGS

GENERIC NAME OR DRUG CLASS	COMBINED EFFECT
Allopurinol	Greatly increased azathioprine activity.
Antivirals, HIV/AIDS*	Increased risk of pancreatitis.
Clozapine	Toxic effect on bone marrow.
Tiopronin	Increased risk of toxicity to bone marrow.
Immunosuppressants, other*	Higher risk of developing infection or malignancies.
Levamisole	Increased risk of bone marrow depression.
Vaccines	May decrease effectiveness or cause disease itself.

POSSIBLE INTERACTION WITH OTHER SUBSTANCES

INTERACTS WITH	COMBINED EFFECT
Alcohol:	No special problems expected.
Beverages:	No special problems expected.
Cocaine:	Increased likelihood of adverse reactions. Avoid.
Foods:	No special problems expected.
Marijuana:	Increased likelihood of adverse reactions. Avoid.
Tobacco:	No special problems expected.

*See Glossary

AZELAIC ACID

BRAND NAMES

Azelex
Finevin

BASIC INFORMATION

Habit forming? No
Prescription needed? Yes
Available as generic? No
Drug class: Antiacne agent, hypopigmentation agent

USES

- Topical treatment for mild to moderate acne vulgaris.
- May be used for treatment of melasma (chloasma), a skin condition in which brownish patches of pigmentation appear on the face.

DOSAGE & USAGE INFORMATION

How to use:
Cream—Wash the affected skin area and then apply the prescribed amount of cream and rub it into the skin. Rub it in thoroughly, but gently, to avoid irritation. Wash hands after applying.

When to use:
Usually twice a day (morning and evening).

If you forget a dose:
Use as soon as you remember.

What drug does:
The drug helps prevents the development of new acne lesions (whiteheads), but the exact mechanism is unknown. It appears to have some antibacterial and anti-inflammatory effect, and also helps in skin renewal.

Time lapse before drug works:
Results should be visible in about 4 weeks, but full benefits may take months.

Don't use with:
Other topical medications without consulting your doctor or pharmacist.

OVERDOSE

SYMPTOMS:
None expected.
WHAT TO DO:
If person accidently swallows drug, call doctor, poison center 1-800-222-1222 or hospital emergency room for instructions.

POSSIBLE ADVERSE REACTIONS OR SIDE EFFECTS

SYMPTOMS	WHAT TO DO
Life-threatening: None expected.	
Common: Peeling, itching, redness or dryness of skin; tingling, burning or stinging may occur when medicine first used.	Continue. Call doctor when convenient.
Infrequent: None expected.	
Rare: Lightening of skin or white spots in persons with darker complexions.	Discontinue. Call doctor when. convenient.

WARNINGS & PRECAUTIONS

Don't use if:
You are sensitive to azelaic acid.

Before you start, consult your doctor:
- If you are allergic to any medicine, food or other substance, or have a family history of allergies.
- If you have a dark complexion.

Over age 60:
No special problems expected, however the drug has not been tested extensively in this age group.

Pregnancy:
Consult doctor. Risk category B (see page xviii).

Breast-Feeding:
No special problems expected. Consult doctor.

Infants & children:
Normally not used in this age group. Safety and effectiveness in children under age 12 has not been established.

Prolonged use:
No problems expected.

Skin & sunlight:
No problems expected.

Driving, piloting or hazardous work:
No problems expected.

Discontinuing:
No problems expected.

Others:
- Use as directed. Don't increase or decrease dosage without doctor's approval. Using more of the cream or using it more frequently than prescribed won't improve results and may cause excessive skin irritation.
- The side effects involving skin irritation usually go away with continued use. If they continue beyond 4 weeks, or are severe, consult doctor about reducing the dosage to once a day.
- You may use water-based cosmetics while undergoing treatment with this drug.

POSSIBLE INTERACTION WITH OTHER DRUGS

GENERIC NAME OR DRUG CLASS	COMBINED EFFECT
None expected.	

POSSIBLE INTERACTION WITH OTHER SUBSTANCES

INTERACTS WITH	COMBINED EFFECT
Alcohol:	None expected.
Beverages:	None expected.
Cocaine:	None expected.
Foods:	None expected.
Marijuana:	None expected.
Tobacco:	None expected.

AZELASTINE

BRAND NAMES

Astelin

BASIC INFORMATION

Habit forming? No
Prescription needed? Yes
Available as generic? No
Drug class: Antihistamine (H_1 receptor)

USES

Reduces allergic symptoms caused by hay fever (seasonal allergic rhinitis), such as sneezing, runny nose, stuffy nose, itchy and watery eyes.

DOSAGE & USAGE INFORMATION

How to use:
Nasal spray—Blow nose before using. Prime the pump per package instructions. Spray in nostrils (2 sprays per nostril).

When to take:
Usually once or twice a day according to doctor's instructions.

If you forget a dose:
Take as soon as you remember. If it is almost time for next dose, wait for next scheduled dose (don't double this dose).

What drug does:
Blocks action of histamine after an allergic response triggers histamine release in sensitive cells. Histamines cause itching, sneezing, runny nose and eyes and other symptoms.

Time lapse before drug works:
1 to 3 hours.

Don't take with:
Any other medicine or herbal remedy without consulting your doctor or pharmacist.

OVERDOSE

SYMPTOMS:
May increase sleepiness, but an overdose with this dosage form is unlikely to occur.
WHAT TO DO:
If person uses much larger amount than prescribed, call doctor, poison center 1-800-222-1222 or hospital emergency room for instructions.

POSSIBLE ADVERSE REACTIONS OR SIDE EFFECTS

SYMPTOMS	WHAT TO DO
Life-threatening: None expected.	
Common: Sleepiness, bitter taste.	Usually no action needed. If symptoms continue, call doctor.
Infrequent: Dry mouth, weight gain, headache, sore throat, mild burning in the nose, nausea, sneezing, muscle aches, small amount of bloody mucus from nose.	Continue. Call doctor when convenient.
Rare: Allergic reaction, skin rash, shortness of breath, changes in vision, eye pain, bloody urine, mouth or lip sores, fast heartbeat, wheezing.	Discontinue. Call doctor right away.

WARNINGS & PRECAUTIONS

Don't take if:
You are allergic to azelastine.

Before you start, consult your doctor:
- If you have kidney problems.
- If you are allergic to any medication, food or other substance.

Over age 60:
No problems expected.

Pregnancy:
Decide with your doctor if drug benefits justify risks to unborn child. Risk category C (see page xviii).

Breast-feeding:
It is not known if drugs pass into milk. Avoid drug or discontinue nursing until you finish medicine. Consult doctor for advice on maintaining milk supply.

Infants & children:
Not recommended for children under age 12.

Prolonged use:
Antihistamines are normally taken during the hay fever season. They are not intended for long-term uninterrupted use.

Skin & sunlight:
No problems expected.

Driving, piloting or hazardous work:
Don't drive or pilot aircraft until you learn how medicine affects you. Don't work around dangerous machinery. Don't climb ladders or work in high places. Danger increases if you drink alcohol or take other medicines affecting alertness and reflexes such as antihistamines, tranquilizers, sedatives, pain medicine, narcotics and mind-altering drugs.

Discontinuing:
No problems expected.

Others:
- Don't exceed recommended dose. It could increase the risk of adverse reactions.
- Advise any doctor or dentist whom you consult that you take this medicine.
- Avoid getting the spray in your eyes.
- Pump must be "primed" before first use if unused 3-4 days before. To prime pump, activate for 3-4 sprays or until a fine mist appears.

POSSIBLE INTERACTION WITH OTHER DRUGS

GENERIC NAME OR DRUG CLASS	COMBINED EFFECT
Central nervous system (CNS) depressants*	May add to any sedative effect.
Cimetidine	Increased azelastine effect. May see increased sedation.

POSSIBLE INTERACTION WITH OTHER SUBSTANCES

INTERACTS WITH	COMBINED EFFECT
Alcohol:	May cause excessive sedation. Avoid.
Beverages:	None expected.
Cocaine:	Decreased antihistamine effect. Avoid.
Foods:	None expected.
Marijuana:	May cause sedation. Avoid.
Tobacco:	None expected.

*See Glossary

BACLOFEN

BRAND NAMES

Lioresal

BASIC INFORMATION

Habit forming? No
Prescription needed? Yes
Available as generic? Yes
Drug class: Muscle relaxant for multiple sclerosis

USES

- Relieves spasms, cramps and spasticity of muscles caused by medical problems, including multiple sclerosis and spine injuries.
- Reduces number and severity of trigeminal neuralgia attacks.

DOSAGE & USAGE INFORMATION

How to take:
Tablet—Swallow with liquid or food to lessen stomach irritation.

When to take:
3 or 4 times daily as directed.

If you forget a dose:
Take as soon as you remember up to 2 hours late. If more than 2 hours, wait for next scheduled dose (don't double this dose).

What drug does:
Blocks body's pain and reflex messages to brain.

Time lapse before drug works:
Variable. Few hours to weeks.

Continued next column

OVERDOSE

SYMPTOMS:
Blurred vision, blindness, difficult breathing, vomiting, drowsiness, muscle weakness, convulsive seizures.
WHAT TO DO:

- **Dial 911 (emergency) for an ambulance or medical help or poison center 1-800-222-1222. Then give first aid immediately.**
- **If patient is unconscious and not breathing, give mouth-to-mouth breathing. If there is no heartbeat, use cardiac massage and mouth-to-mouth breathing (CPR). Don't try to make patient vomit. If you can't get help quickly, take patient to nearest emergency facility.**
- **See emergency information on inside covers.**

Don't take with:
Any other medicine without consulting your doctor or pharmacist.

POSSIBLE ADVERSE REACTIONS OR SIDE EFFECTS

SYMPTOMS	WHAT TO DO
Life-threatening:	
In case of overdose, see previous column.	
Common:	
Dizziness, lightheadedness, confusion, drowsiness, nausea.	Continue. Call doctor when convenient.
Infrequent:	
• Rash with itching, numbness or tingling in hands or feet.	Discontinue. Call doctor right away.
• Headache, abdominal pain, diarrhea or constipation, appetite loss, muscle weakness, difficult or painful urination, male sex problems, nasal congestion, clumsiness, slurred speech, insomnia.	Continue. Call doctor when convenient.
Rare:	
• Fainting, weakness, hallucinations, depression, chest pain, muscle pain, pounding heatbeat.	Discontinue. Call doctor right away.
• Ringing in ears, lowered blood pressure, dry mouth, taste disturbance, euphoria, weight gain.	Continue. Call doctor when convenient.

WARNINGS & PRECAUTIONS

Don't take if:

- You are allergic to any muscle relaxant.
- Muscle spasm due to strain or sprain.

Before you start, consult your doctor:

- If you have Parkinson's disease.
- If you have cerebral palsy.
- If you have had a recent stroke.
- If you have had a recent head injury.
- If you have arthritis.
- If you have diabetes.
- If you have epilepsy.
- If you have psychosis.
- If you have kidney disease.
- If you will have surgery within 2 months, including dental surgery, requiring general or spinal anesthesia.

Over age 60:
Adverse reactions and side effects may be more frequent and severe than in younger persons.

Pregnancy:
Decide with your doctor if drug benefits justify risk to unborn child. Risk category C (see page xviii).

Breast-feeding:
Avoid nursing or discontinue until you finish medicine. Consult doctor about maintaining milk supply.

Infants & children:
Not recommended.

Prolonged use:
Epileptic patients should be monitored with EEGs. Diabetics should more closely monitor blood sugar levels. Obtain periodic liver function tests.

Skin & sunlight:
No problems expected.

Driving, piloting or hazardous work:
Don't drive or pilot aircraft until you learn how medicine affects you. Don't work around dangerous machinery. Don't climb ladders or work in high places. Danger increases if you drink alcohol or take medicine affecting alertness and reflexes, such as antihistamines, tranquilizers, sedatives, pain medicine, narcotics and mind-altering drugs.

Discontinuing:
Don't discontinue without consulting doctor. Dose may require gradual reduction if you have taken drug for a long time. Doses of other drugs may also require adjustment.

Others:
Advise any doctor or dentist whom you consult that you take this medicine.

POSSIBLE INTERACTION WITH OTHER DRUGS

GENERIC NAME OR DRUG CLASS	COMBINED EFFECT
Anesthetics, general*	Increased sedation. Low blood pressure. Avoid.
Antidiabetic drugs*, insulin or oral	Need to adjust diabetes medicine dosage.
Central nervous system (CNS) depressants* (antidepressants,* antihistamines,* narcotics,* other muscle relaxants,* sedatives,* sleeping pills,* tranquilizers*)	Increased sedation Low blood pressure. Avoid.
Clozapine	Toxic effect on the central nervous system.
Ethinamate	Dangerous increased effects of ethinamate. Avoid combining.
Fluoxetine	Increased depressant effects of both drugs.
Guanfacine	May increase depressant effects of either drug.
Leucovorin	High alcohol content of leucovorin may cause adverse effects.
Methyprylon	Increased sedative effect, perhaps to dangerous level. Avoid.
Nabilone	Greater depression of the central nervous system.
Sertraline	Increased depressive effects of both drugs.

POSSIBLE INTERACTION WITH OTHER SUBSTANCES

INTERACTS WITH	COMBINED EFFECT
Alcohol:	Increased sedation. Low blood pressure. Avoid.
Beverages:	None expected.
Cocaine:	Increased spasticity. Avoid.
Foods:	None expected.
Marijuana:	Increased spasticity. Avoid.
Tobacco:	May interfere with absorption of medicine.

*See Glossary

BARBITURATES

GENERIC AND BRAND NAMES

See complete list of generic and brand names in the *Generic and Brand Name Directory*, page 862.

BASIC INFORMATION

Habit forming? Yes
Prescription needed? Yes
Available as generic? Yes, for some
Drug class: Sedative-hypnotic agent, anticonvulsant

USES

- Reduces likelihood of seizures (tonic-clonic seizure pattern and simple partial) in epilepsy.
- Preventive treatment for febrile seizures.
- Reduces anxiety or nervous tension.
- As an ingredient in combination drugs to treat gastrointestinal disorders, headaches and asthma.
- Aids sleep at night (on a short-term basis).

DOSAGE & USAGE INFORMATION

How to take:
- Capsule—Swallow with liquid. If you can't swallow whole, open capsule and take with liquid or food. Instructions to take on empty stomach mean 1 hour before or 2 hours after eating.
- Elixir—Swallow with liquid.
- Rectal suppositories—Remove wrapper and moisten suppository with water. Gently insert into rectum, pointed end first. If suppository is too soft, chill in refrigerator or cool water before removing wrapper.
- Tablet—Swallow with liquid or food to lessen stomach irritation. If you can't swallow whole, crumble tablet and take with liquid or food.

Continued next column

OVERDOSE

SYMPTOMS:
Deep sleep, trouble breathing, weak pulse, coma.
WHAT TO DO:
- **Dial 911 (emergency) for an ambulance or medical help or poison center 1-800-222-1222. Then give first aid immediately.**
- **If patient is unconscious and not breathing, give mouth-to-mouth breathing. If there is no heartbeat use cardiac massage and mouth-to-mouth breathing (CPR). Don't try to make patient vomit. If you can't get help quickly, take patient to emergency facility. See emergency facts at end of book.**

When to take:
At the same times each day.

If you forget a dose:
Take as soon as you remember up to 2 hours late. If more than 2 hours, wait for next scheduled dose (don't double this dose).

What drug does:
May partially block nerve impulses at nerve-cell connections.

Time lapse before drug works:
60 minutes; will take several weeks for maximum antiepilepsy effect.

Don't take with:
Nonprescription drugs without consulting doctor or pharmacist.

POSSIBLE ADVERSE REACTIONS OR SIDE EFFECTS

SYMPTOMS	WHAT TO DO
Life-threatening:	
In case of overdose, see previous column.	
Common:	
Dizziness, drowsiness, clumsiness, unsteadiness, signs of addiction*.	Continue. Call doctor when convenient.
Infrequent:	
Confusion, headache, irritability, feeling faint, nausea, vomiting, depression, nightmares, trouble sleeping.	Continue, but call doctor right away.
Rare:	
Agitation, slow heartbeat, difficult breathing, bleeding sores on lips, fever, chest pain, unexplained bleeding or bruising, muscle or joint pain, skin rash or hives, thickened or scaly skin, white spots in mouth, tightness in chest, face swelling, sore throat, yellow eyes or skin, hallucinations, unusual tiredness or weakness.	Continue, but call doctor right away.

WARNINGS & PRECAUTIONS

Don't take if:
- You are allergic to any barbiturate.
- You have porphyria.

Before you start, consult your doctor:
- If you have epilepsy.
- If you have kidney or liver damage.
- If you have asthma.
- If you have anemia.
- If you have chronic pain.
- If you will have surgery within 2 months, including dental surgery, requiring general or spinal anesthesia.

Over age 60:
Adverse reactions and side effects may be more frequent and severe than in younger persons. Use small doses.

Pregnancy:
Risk to unborn child outweighs drug benefits. Don't use. Risk category D (see page xviii).

Breast-feeding:
Drug passes into milk. Avoid drug or discontinue nursing until you finish medicine. Consult doctor for advice on maintaining milk supply.

Infants & children:
Use only under doctor's supervision.

Prolonged use:
- May cause addiction, anemia, chronic intoxication. Unlikely to occur with the usual anticonvulsant or sedative dosage levels.
- May lower body temperature, making exposure to cold temperatures hazardous.
- Talk to your doctor about the need for follow-up medical examinations or laboratory studies to check blood sugar, kidney function.

Skin and sunlight:
No problems expected.

Driving, piloting or hazardous work:
Don't drive or pilot aircraft until you learn how medicine affects you. Don't work around dangerous machinery. Don't climb ladders or work in high places. Danger increases if you drink alcohol or take medicine affecting alertness and reflexes.

Discontinuing:
If you become addicted, don't stop taking barbiturates suddenly. Seek medical help for safe withdrawal.

Others:
- May affect results in some medical tests.
- Barbiturate addiction is common. Withdrawal effects may be fatal.
- Advise any doctor or dentist whom you consult that you take this medicine.

POSSIBLE INTERACTION WITH OTHER DRUGS

GENERIC NAME OR DRUG CLASS	COMBINED EFFECT
Adrenocorticoids, systemic	Decreased prednisone effect. Oversedation.
Anticoagulants, oral*	Decreased effect of anticoagulant.
Anticonvulsants*	Changed seizure patterns.
Antidepressants, tricyclic*	Decreased antidepressant effect. Possible dangerous oversedation.
Antidiabetic, agents, oral*	Increased effect of barbiturate.
Antihistamines*	Dangerous sedation. Avoid.
Aspirin	Decreased aspirin effect.
Beta-adrenergic blocking agents*	Decreased effect of beta-adrenergic blocker.
Carbamazepine	Decreased carbamazepine effect.
Carteolol	Increased barbiturate effect. Dangerous sedation.
Clozapine	Toxic effect on the central nervous system.
Contraceptives, oral*	Decreased contraceptive effect.
Dextrothyroxine	Decreased barbiturate effect.
Divalproex	Dangerous sedation. Avoid.
Doxycycline	Decreased doxycycline effect.
Griseofulvin	Decreased griseofulvin effect.

Continued on page 903

POSSIBLE INTERACTION WITH OTHER SUBSTANCES

INTERACTS WITH	COMBINED EFFECT
Alcohol:	Possible fatal oversedation. Avoid.
Beverages:	None expected.
Cocaine:	Decreased barbiturate effect.
Foods:	None expected.
Marijuana:	Excessive sedation. Avoid.
Tobacco:	None expected.

*See Glossary

BARBITURATES, ASPIRIN & CODEINE (Also contains caffeine)

GENERIC AND BRAND NAMES

See complete list of generic and brand names in the *Generic and Brand Name Directory*, page 862.

BASIC INFORMATION

Habit forming? Yes
Prescription needed? Yes
Available as generic? Yes
Drug class: Narcotic, analgesic

USES

- Reduces anxiety or nervous tension (low dose).
- Reduces pain, fever, inflammation.

DOSAGE & USAGE INFORMATION

How to take:

- Tablet or capsule—Swallow with liquid or food to lessen stomach irritation. If you can't swallow whole, crumble tablet or open capsule and take with liquid or food.
- Extended-release tablets or capsules—Swallow each dose whole.

When to take:
When needed. No more often than every 4 hours.

If you forget a dose:
Take as soon as you remember. Wait 4 hours for next dose.

Continued next column

OVERDOSE

SYMPTOMS:
Deep sleep, slow and weak pulse, ringing in ears, nausea, vomiting, dizziness, fever, deep and rapid breathing, hallucinations, convulsions, coma.
WHAT TO DO:

- **Dial 911 (emergency) for an ambulance or medical help or poison center 1-800-222-1222. Then give first aid immediately.**
- **If patient is unconscious and not breathing, give mouth-to-mouth breathing. If there is no heartbeat, use cardiac massage and mouth-to-mouth breathing (CPR). Don't try to make patient vomit. If you can't get help quickly, take patient to nearest emergency facility.**
- **See emergency information on inside covers.**

What drug does:

- May partially block nerve impulses at nerve-cell connections.
- Affects hypothalamus, the part of the brain which regulates temperature by dilating small blood vessels in skin.
- Prevents clumping of platelets (small blood cells) so blood vessels remain open.
- Decreases prostaglandin effect.
- Blocks pain messages to brain and spinal cord.
- Reduces sensitivity of brain's cough-control center.

Time lapse before drug works:
30 minutes.

Don't take with:
Nonprescription drugs without consulting doctor.

POSSIBLE ADVERSE REACTIONS OR SIDE EFFECTS

SYMPTOMS	WHAT TO DO
Life-threatening:	
Wheezing, tightness in chest, pinpoint pupils.	Seek emergency treatment immediately.
Common:	
Dizziness, drowsiness, heartburn, flushed face, depression, false sense of well-being, increased urination.	Continue. Call doctor when convenient.
Infrequent:	
Jaundice; vomiting blood; easy bruising; skin rash, hives; confusion; depression; sore throat, fever, mouth sores; difficult urination; hearing loss; slurred speech; blood in urine; decreased vision.	Discontinue. Call doctor right away.
Rare:	
Insomnia, nightmares, constipation, headache, nervousness, flushed face, increased sweating, unusual tiredness.	Continue. Call doctor when convenient.

WARNINGS & PRECAUTIONS

Don't take if:
You are allergic to any barbiturate or narcotic.

Before you start, consult your doctor:
- If you have had stomach or duodenal ulcers.
- If you have asthma, epilepsy, kidney or liver damage, anemia, chronic pain, gout.
- If you will have surgery within 2 months, including dental surgery, requiring general or spinal anesthesia.

Over age 60:
- Adverse reactions and side effects may be more frequent and severe than in younger persons.
- More likely to cause hidden bleeding in stomach or intestines. Watch for dark stools.
- More likely to be drowsy, dizzy, unsteady or constipated. Use only if absolutely necessary.

Pregnancy:
Risk factors vary for drugs in this group. See category list on page xviii and consult doctor.

Breast-feeding:
Drug passes into milk. Avoid drug or discontinue nursing until you finish medicine. Consult doctor for advice on maintaining milk supply.

Infants & children:
- Overdose frequent and severe. Keep bottles out of children's reach.
- Use only under doctor's supervision.
- Do not give to persons under age 18 who have fever and discomfort of viral illness, especially chicken pox and influenza. Probably increases risk of Reye's syndrome*.

Prolonged use:
- Kidney damage. Periodic kidney function test recommended.
- May cause addiction, anemia, chronic intoxication.
- May lower body temperature, making exposure to cold temperatures hazardous.

Skin & sunlight:
One or more drugs in this group may cause rash or intensity sunburn in areas exposed to sun or ultraviolet light (photosensitivity reaction). Avoid overexposure. Notify doctor if reaction occurs.

Driving, piloting or hazardous work:
Don't drive or pilot aircraft until you learn how medicine effects you. Don't work around dangerous machinery. Don't climb ladders or work in high places. Danger increases if you drink alcohol or take medicine affecting alertness and reflexes, such as antihistamines, tranquilizers, sedatives, pain medicine, narcotics and mind-altering drugs.

Discontinuing:
May be unnecessary to finish medicine. Follow doctor's instructions. If you develop withdrawal symptoms of hallucinations, agitation or sleeplessness after discontinuing, call doctor right away.

Others:
- Aspirin can complicate surgery; illness; pregnancy, labor and delivery.
- For arthritis—Don't change dose without consulting doctor.
- Advise any doctor or dentist whom you consult that you take this medicine.
- Urine tests for blood sugar may be inaccurate.
- Great potential for abuse.

POSSIBLE INTERACTION WITH OTHER DRUGS

GENERIC NAME OR DRUG CLASS	COMBINED EFFECT
Adrenocorticoids, systemic	Increased risk of ulcers.
Allopurinol	Decreased allopurinol effect.
Analgesics, other*	Increased analgesic effect.
Antacids*	Decreased aspirin effect.
Anticoagulants, oral*	Increased anticoagulant effect. Abnormal bleeding.

Continued on page 903

POSSIBLE INTERACTION WITH OTHER SUBSTANCES

INTERACTS WITH	COMBINED EFFECT
Alcohol:	Possible stomach irritation and bleeding, possible fatal oversedation. Avoid.
Beverages:	None expected.
Cocaine:	Increased cocaine toxic effects. Avoid.
Foods:	None expected.
Marijuana:	Possible increased pain relief, but marijuana may slow body's recovery. Impairs physical and mental performance. Avoid.
Tobacco:	None expected.

*See Glossary

BECAPLERMIN

BRAND NAMES

Regranex

BASIC INFORMATION

Habit forming? No
Prescription needed? Yes
Available as generic? No
Drug class: Platelet-derived growth factor.

USES

Treatment of skin ulcers in patients with diabetes mellitus.

DOSAGE & USAGE INFORMATION

How to use:
Gel—Apply to the affected area. Follow all instructions provided with the prescription. Dosage may change as wound heals.

When to use:
At the same time each day. Change the wound dressing between applications of the medication.

If you forget a dose:
Apply it as soon as possible. If it is almost time for your next dose, skip the missed dose and go back to your regular dosing schedule. Do not double doses.

What drug does:
Stimulates growth of cells involved in wound repair.

Time lapse before drug works:
Up to six months.

Don't use with:
Any other prescription or nonprescription drug without consulting your doctor.

OVERDOSE

SYMPTOMS:
None expected.
WHAT TO DO:
Overdose unlikely to threaten life. If person uses much larger amount than prescribed, call doctor, poison center 1-800-222-1222 or hospital emergency room for instructions.

POSSIBLE ADVERSE REACTIONS OR SIDE EFFECTS

SYMPTOMS	WHAT TO DO
Life-threatening:	
None expected.	
Common:	
None expected.	
Infrequent:	
Rash in area of skin ulcer.	Discontinue. Call doctor right away.
Rare:	
None expected.	

WARNINGS & PRECAUTIONS

Don't take if:
- You are allergic to becaplermin, parabens or metacresol.
- You have any new growths or wounds in the application area.

Before you start, consult your doctor:
- If you have any other medical problem.
- If you are allergic to any other substances, such as food preservatives or dyes.

Over age 60:
No problems expected.

Pregnancy:
Decide with your doctor if drug benefits justify risk to unborn child. Risk category C (see page xviii).

Breast-feeding:
It is not known if drug passes into milk. Avoid drugs or discontinue nursing until you finish medicine. Consult doctor for advice on maintaining milk supply.

Infants & children:
Safety and efficacy in children under age 16 has not been established.

Prolonged use:
No problems expected. Your doctor should periodically evaluate your response to the drug and adjust the dose according to the rate of change in the width and length of the diabetic ulcer.

Skin & sunlight:
No problems expected.

Driving, piloting or hazardous work:
No problems expected.

Discontinuing:
Don't discontinue without consulting doctor.

Others:
- Do not place tip of tube onto ulcer or any other object; it may contaminate the medication.
- Be sure you follow application instructions carefully.
- Avoid bearing weight on the affected extremity.
- Wash hands carefully before preparing your dose.
- Keep this medication in refrigerator; do not freeze.
- Advise any doctor or dentist whom you consult that you take this medicine.

POSSIBLE INTERACTION WITH OTHER DRUGS

GENERIC NAME OR DRUG CLASS	COMBINED EFFECT
None expected.	

POSSIBLE INTERACTION WITH OTHER SUBSTANCES

INTERACTS WITH	COMBINED EFFECT
Alcohol:	None expected.
Beverages:	None expected.
Cocaine:	Effects unknown. Avoid.
Foods:	None expected.
Marijuana:	Effects unknown. Avoid.
Tobacco:	None expected.

BELLADONNA ALKALOIDS & BARBITURATES

GENERIC AND BRAND NAMES

See complete list of generic and brand names in the *Generic and Brand Name Directory*, page 862.

BASIC INFORMATION

Habit forming? Yes
Prescription needed? Yes
Available as generic? Some yes, some no
Drug class: Antispasmodic, anticholinergic, sedative

USES

- Reduces spasms of digestive system, bladder and urethra.
- Reduces anxiety or nervous tension (low dose).
- Relieves insomnia (higher bedtime dose).

DOSAGE & USAGE INFORMATION

How to take:
- Tablet, liquid or capsule—Swallow with liquid or food to lessen stomach irritation. If you can't swallow whole, crumble tablet or open capsule and take with liquid or food.
- Extended-release tablets or capsules—Swallow each dose whole.
- Chewable tablets—Chew well before swallowing.
- Drops—Dilute dose in beverage before swallowing.

When to take:
At the same times each day.

If you forget a dose:
Take as soon as you remember up to 2 hours late. If more than 2 hours, wait for next scheduled dose (don't double this dose).

Continued next column

What drug does:
- May partially block nerve impulses at nerve cell connections.
- Blocks nerve impulses at parasympathetic nerve endings, preventing muscle contractions and gland secretions of organs involved.

Time lapse before drug works:
15 to 30 minutes.

Don't take with:
- Antacids* or antidiarrheals*.
- Any other medicine without consulting your doctor or pharmacist.

OVERDOSE

SYMPTOMS:
Blurred vision, confusion, convulsions, irregular heartbeat, hallucinations, coma.
WHAT TO DO:
- **Dial 911 (emergency) for an ambulance or medical help or poison center 1-800-222-1222. Then give first aid immediately.**
- **See emergency information on inside covers.**

POSSIBLE ADVERSE REACTIONS OR SIDE EFFECTS

SYMPTOMS	WHAT TO DO
Life-threatening:	
Unusual excitement, restlessness, fast heartbeat, breathing difficulty.	Seek emergency treatment immediately.
Common:	
• Dry mouth, throat, nose; drowsiness; constipation; dizziness; nausea; vomiting; "hangover" effect; depression; confusion.	Discontinue. Call doctor right away.
• Reduced sweating, slurred speech, agitation, nasal congestion, altered taste.	Continue. Call doctor when convenient.
Infrequent:	
Difficult urination; difficult swallowing; rash or hives; face, lip or eyelid swelling; joint or muscle pain; lightheadedness.	Discontinue. Call doctor right away.
Rare:	
Jaundice; unusual bruising or bleeding; hives, skin rash; pain in eyes; blurred vision; sore throat, fever, mouth sores; unexplained bleeding or bruising.	Discontinue. Call doctor right away.

BELLADONNA ALKALOIDS & BARBITURATES

WARNINGS & PRECAUTIONS

Don't take if:
- You are allergic to any barbiturate or any anticholinergic.
- You have prophyria, trouble with stomach bloating, difficulty emptying your bladder completely, narrow-angle glaucoma, severe ulcerative colitis.

Before you start, consult your doctor:
- If you have open-angle glaucoma, angina, chronic bronchitis or asthma, hiatal hernia, liver disease, enlarged prostate, myasthenia gravis, peptic ulcer, epilepsy, kidney or liver damage, anemia, chronic pain, thyroid disease.
- If you will have surgery within 2 months, including dental surgery, requiring general or spinal anesthesia.

Over age 60:
Adverse reactions and side effects may be more frequent and severe than in younger persons. Ask your doctor about small doses.

Pregnancy:
Risk factors vary for drugs in this group. See category list on page xviii and consult doctor.

Breast-feeding:
Drug passes into milk. Avoid drug or discontinue nursing until you finish medicine.

Infants & children:
Use only under doctor's supervision.

Prolonged use:
- May cause addiction, anemia, chronic intoxication.
- May lower body temperature, making exposure to cold temperatures hazardous.

Skin & sunlight:
One or more drugs in this group may cause rash or intensity sunburn in areas exposed to sun or ultraviolet light (photosensitivity reaction). Avoid overexposure. Notify doctor if reaction occurs.

Driving, piloting or hazardous work:
Don't drive or pilot aircraft until you learn how medicine affects you. Don't work around dangerous machinery. Don't climb ladders or work in high places. Danger increases if you drink alcohol or take medicine affecting alertness and reflexes.

Discontinuing:
May be unnecessary to finish medicine. Follow doctor's instructions. If you develop withdrawal symptoms of hallucinations, agitation or sleeplessness after discontinuing, call doctor right away.

Others:
- Great potential for abuse.
- Advise any doctor or dentist whom you consult that you take this medicine.

POSSIBLE INTERACTION WITH OTHER DRUGS

GENERIC NAME OR DRUG CLASS	COMBINED EFFECT
Acetaminophen	Possible decreased barbiturate effect.
Adrenocorticoids, systemic	Possible glaucoma.
Amantadine	Increased belladonna effect.
Antacids*	Decreased belladonna effect.
Anticoagulants, oral*	Decreased anti-coagulant effect.
Anticholinergics, other*	Increased belladonna effect.
Anticonvulsants*	Changed seizure patterns.
Antidepressants, tricyclic*	Possible dangerous oversedation. Avoid.
Antidiabetics, oral*	Increased barbiturate effect.
Antihistamines*	Dangerous sedation. Avoid.
Anti-inflammatory drugs nonsteroidal (NSAIDs)*	Decreased anti-inflammatory effect.
Aspirin	Decreased aspirin effect.

Continued on page 904

POSSIBLE INTERACTION WITH OTHER SUBSTANCES

INTERACTS WITH	COMBINED EFFECT
Alcohol:	Possible fatal oversedation. Avoid.
Beverages:	None expected.
Cocaine:	Excessively rapid heartbeat. Avoid.
Foods:	None expected.
Marijuana:	Drowsiness and dry mouth. Avoid.
Tobacco:	Decreased effectiveness of acid reduction in stomach.

***See Glossary**

BENZODIAZEPINES

GENERIC AND BRAND NAMES

See complete list of generic and brand names in the *Generic and Brand Name Directory*, page 862.

BASIC INFORMATION

Habit forming? Yes
Prescription needed? Yes
Available as generic? Yes, for most
Drug class: Tranquilizer (benzodiazepine), anticonvulsant

USE

- Treatment for anxiety disorders and panic disorders.
- Treatment for muscle spasm.
- Treatment for seizure disorders.
- Treatment for alcohol withdrawal.
- Treatment for insomnia (short-term).

DOSAGE & USAGE INFORMATION

How to take:
- Tablet or capsule—Swallow with liquid. If you can't swallow whole, crumble tablet or open capsule and take with liquid or small amount of food.
- Extended-release capsule—Swallow capsule whole. Do not open or chew.
- Oral suspension—Dilute dose in water, soda or sodalike beverage or small amount of food such as applesauce or pudding.
- Sublingual tablet—Do not chew or swallow. Place under tongue until dissolved.
- Rectal gel—Follow instructions provided with prescription or as directed by the doctor.

Continued next column

OVERDOSE

SYMPTOMS:
Drowsiness, weakness, tremor, stupor, coma.
WHAT TO DO:
- **Dial 911 (emergency) for an ambulance or medical help or poison center 1-800-222-1222. Then give first aid immediately.**
- **If patient is unconscious and not breathing, give mouth-to-mouth breathing. If there is no heartbeat, use cardiac massage and mouth-to-mouth breathing (CPR). Don't try to make patient vomit. If you can't get help quickly, take patient to nearest emergency facility.**
- **See emergency information at end of book.**

When to take:
At the same time each day, according to instructions on prescription label.

If you forget a dose:
Take as soon as you remember up to 2 hours late. If more than 2 hours, wait for next scheduled dose (don't double this dose).

What drug does:
Affects limbic system of brain, the part that controls emotions.

Time lapse before drug works:
May take 6 weeks for full benefit; depends on drug when treating anxiety.

Don't take with:
Any other medicine without consulting your doctor or pharmacist.

POSSIBLE ADVERSE REACTIONS OR SIDE EFFECTS

SYMPTOMS	WHAT TO DO
Life-threatening:	
In case of overdose, see previous column.	
Common:	
Clumsiness, drowsiness, dizziness. signs of addiction*.	Continue. Call doctor when convenient.
Infrequent:	
• Hallucinations, confusion, depression, irritability, rash, itch, vision changes, sore throat, fever, chills.	Discontinue. Call doctor right away.
• Constipation or diarrhea, nausea, vomiting, difficult urination, vivid dreams, behavior changes, abdominal pain, headache, dry mouth.	Continue. Call doctor when convenient.
Rare:	
• Slow heartbeat, breathing difficulty.	Discontinue. Seek emergency treatment.
• Mouth, throat ulcers; jaundice.	Discontinue. Call doctor right away.
• Decreased sex drive.	Continue. Call doctor when convenient.

WARNINGS & PRECAUTIONS

Don't take if:
- You are allergic to any benzodiazepine.
- You have myasthenia gravis.
- You are an active or recovering alcoholic.
- Patient is younger than 6 months.

Before you start, consult your doctor:
- If you have liver, kidney or lung disease.
- If you have diabetes, epilepsy or porphyria.
- If you have glaucoma.

Over age 60:
Adverse reactions and side effects may be more frequent and severe than in younger persons. You may need smaller doses for shorter periods of time. You may develop increased sedation or agitation or difficulty walking.

Pregnancy:
Risk factors vary for drugs in this group. See category list on page xviii and consult doctor.

Breast-feeding:
Drug passes into milk. Avoid drug or discontinue nursing until you finish medicine. Consult doctor for advice on maintaining milk supply.

Infants & children:
Use only under medical supervision.

Prolonged use:
May impair liver function.

Skin & sunlight:
- One or more drugs in this group may cause rash or intensify sunburn in areas exposed to sun or ultraviolet light (photosensitivity reaction). Avoid overexposure and use sunscreen. Notify doctor if reaction occurs.
- Hot weather, heavy exercise and sweating may reduce excretion and cause overdose in some people with one or more of these drugs.

Driving, piloting or hazardous work:
Don't drive or pilot aircraft until you learn how medicine affects you. Don't work around dangerous machinery. Don't climb ladders or work in high places. Danger increases if you drink alcohol or take medicine affecting alertness and reflexes.

Discontinuing:
Don't discontinue without consulting doctor. Dose may require gradual reduction if you have taken drug for a long time. Doses of other drugs may also require adjustment.

Others:
- Blood sugar may rise in diabetics, requiring insulin adjustment.
- Don't use for insomnia more than 4-7 days.
- Caution—Keep in safe secure place to avoid theft.
- Advise any doctor or dentist whom you consult that you take this medicine.

POSSIBLE INTERACTION WITH OTHER DRUGS

GENERIC NAME OR DRUG CLASS	COMBINED EFFECT
Anticonvulsants*	Change in seizure pattern.
Antidepressants, tricyclic*	Increased sedative effect of both drugs.
Antihistamines*	Increased sedative effect of both drugs.
Central nervous system (CNS) depressants*	Increased sedative effect.
Cimetidine	Increased benzodiazepine effect.
Clozapine	Toxic effect on the central nervous system.
Contraceptives, oral*	Increased benzodiazepine effect.
Disulfiram	Increased benzodiazepine effect.
Erythromycins*	Increased benzodiazepine effect.
Fluoxetine	Increased sedative effect.
Fluvoxamine	Increased sedative effect.
Ketoconazole	Increased benzodiazepine effect.
Levodopa	Possible decreased levodopa effect.
Mirtazapine	Increased sedative effect. Avoid.
Modafinil	Possible decreased modafinil effect.
Molindone	Increased tranquilizer effect.
Monoamine oxidase (MAO) inhibitors*	Convulsions, deep sedation, rage.

Continued on page 905

POSSIBLE INTERACTION WITH OTHER SUBSTANCES

INTERACTS WITH	COMBINED EFFECT
Alcohol:	Heavy sedation. Avoid.
Beverages:	None expected.
Cocaine:	Decreased benzodiazepine effect.
Foods:	None expected.
Marijuana:	Heavy sedation. Avoid.
Tobacco:	Decreased benzodiazepine effect.

***See Glossary**

BENZOYL PEROXIDE

BRAND NAMES

See complete list of brand names in the *Generic and Brand Name Directory*, page 862.

BASIC INFORMATION

Habit forming? No
Prescription needed? No
Available as generic? Yes
Drug class: Antiacne (topical)

USES

- Treatment for acne.
- Treats pressure sores.

DOSAGE & USAGE INFORMATION

How to use:
Cream, gel, pads, sticks, lotion, cleansing bar or facial mask—Wash affected area with plain soap and water. Dry gently with towel. Rub medicine into affected areas. Keep away from eyes, nose, mouth. Wash hands after using.

When to use:
Apply 1 or more times daily. If you have a fair complexion, start with single application at bedtime.

If you forget an application:
Use as soon as you remember.

What drug does:
Slowly releases oxygen from skin, which controls some skin bacteria. Also causes peeling and drying, helping control blackheads and whiteheads.

Time lapse before drug works:
1 to 2 weeks.

Don't use with:
Any other medicine without consulting your doctor or pharmacist.

OVERDOSE

SYMPTOMS:
None expected.
WHAT TO DO:
- **If person swallows drug, call doctor, poison center 1-800-222-1222 or hospital emergency room for instructions.**
- **See emergency information on inside covers.**

POSSIBLE ADVERSE REACTIONS OR SIDE EFFECTS

SYMPTOMS	WHAT TO DO
Life-threatening: None expected.	
Common: Mild redness and chapping of skin during first few weeks of use.	No action necessary.
Infrequent:	
• Rash, excessive dryness, peeling skin.	Discontinue. Call doctor right away.
• Painful skin irritation.	Continue. Call doctor when convenient.
Rare: None expected.	

WARNINGS & PRECAUTIONS

Don't take if:
You are allergic to benzoyl peroxide.

Before you start, consult your doctor:
- If you plan to become pregnant within medication period.
- If you take oral contraceptives.
- If you are using any other prescription or nonprescription medicine for acne.
- If you are using abrasive skin cleansers or medicated cosmetics.

Over age 60:
No problems expected.

Pregnancy:
Consult doctor. Risk category C (see page xviii.

Breast-feeding:
No proven problems. Consult doctor.

Infants & children:
Not recommended.

Prolonged use:
Permanent rash or scarring.

Skin & sunlight:
May cause rash or intensify sunburn in areas exposed to sun or ultraviolet light (photosensitivity reaction). Avoid overexposure. Notify doctor if reaction occurs.

Driving, piloting or hazardous work:
No problems expected.

Discontinuing:
- May be unnecessary to finish medicine. Discontinue when acne improves.
- If acne doesn't improve in 2 weeks, call doctor.

Others:
- Drug may bleach hair or dyed fabrics, including clothing or carpet.
- Store away from heat in cool, dry place.
- Avoid contact with eyes, lips, nose and sensitive areas of the neck.

POSSIBLE INTERACTION WITH OTHER DRUGS

GENERIC NAME OR DRUG CLASS	COMBINED EFFECT
Antiacne topical preparations, other	Excessive skin irritation.
Skin-peeling agents (salicylic acid, sulfur, resorcinol, tretinoin)	Excessive skin irritation.

POSSIBLE INTERACTION WITH OTHER SUBSTANCES

INTERACTS WITH	COMBINED EFFECT
Alcohol:	None expected.
Beverages:	None expected.
Cocaine:	None expected.
Foods: Cinnamon, foods with benzoic acid.	Skin rash.
Marijuana:	None expected.
Tobacco:	None expected.

*See Glossary

BETA CAROTENE

BRAND NAMES

Solatene
Numerous multiple vitamin and mineral supplements. Check labels.

BASIC INFORMATION

Habit forming? No
Prescription needed? No
Available as generic? Yes
Drug class: Nutritional supplement

USES

- Used as a nutritional supplement.
- Prevents night blindness.
- Used as an adjunct to the treatment of steatorrhea, chronic fever, obstructive jaundice, pancreatic insufficiency, protein deficiency, total parenteral nutrition and photosensitivity in photo porphyria.

DOSAGE & USAGE INFORMATION

How to take:
Tablet or capsule—Swallow with liquid. If you can't swallow whole, crumble tablet or open capsule and take with liquid or food.

When to take:
At the same time each day, according to directions on package or prescription label.

If you forget a dose:
Take as soon as you remember (don't double this dose).

What drug does:
Enables the body to manufacture vitamin A, which is essential for the normal functioning of the retina, normal growth and development and normal testicular and ovarian function.

Time lapse before drug works:
Total effect may take several weeks.

Don't take with:
No restrictions.

OVERDOSE

SYMPTOMS:
Yellow skin
WHAT TO DO:
Overdose unlikely to threaten life. If person takes much larger amount than prescribed, call doctor, poison center 1-800-222-1222 or hospital emergency room for instructions.

POSSIBLE ADVERSE REACTIONS OR SIDE EFFECTS

SYMPTOMS	WHAT TO DO
Life-threatening: None expected.	
Common: Yellow palms, hands, soles of feet.	Continue. Call doctor when convenient.
Infrequent: None expected.	
Rare:	
• Joint pain, unusual bleeding or bruising.	Discontinue. Call doctor right away.
• Diarrhea, dizziness.	Continue. Call doctor when convenient.

WARNINGS & PRECAUTIONS

Don't take if:
You are hypersensitive to beta carotene.

Before you start, consult your doctor:
- If you have liver or kidney disease.
- If you have hypervitaminosis*.

Over age 60:
No problems expected.

Pregnancy:
Consult doctor. Risk category C (see page xviii).

Breast-feeding:
No problems expected.

Infants & children:
No problems expected.

Prolonged use:
No problems expected.

Skin & sunlight:
No special problems expected.

Driving, piloting or hazardous work:
No special problems expected.

Discontinuing:
No special problems expected.

Others:
- Some researchers claim that beta carotene may reduce the occurrence of some cancers. There is insufficient data to substantiate this claim.
- Advise any doctor or dentist whom you consult that you take this medicine.
- May affect results of some medical tests.

POSSIBLE INTERACTION WITH OTHER DRUGS

GENERIC NAME OR DRUG CLASS	COMBINED EFFECT
Cholestyramine	Decreased absorption of beta carotene.
Colestipol	Decreased absorption of beta carotene.
Mineral oil	Decreased absorption of beta carotene.
Neomycin	Decreased absorption of beta carotene.

POSSIBLE INTERACTION WITH OTHER SUBSTANCES

INTERACTS WITH	COMBINED EFFECT
Alcohol:	None expected.
Beverages:	None expected.
Cocaine:	None expected.
Foods:	None expected.
Marijuana:	None expected.
Tobacco:	None expected.

***See Glossary**

BETA-ADRENERGIC BLOCKING AGENTS

GENERIC AND BRAND NAMES

See complete list of generic and brand names in the *Generic and Brand Name Directory*, page 862.

BASIC INFORMATION

Habit forming? No
Prescription needed? Yes
Available as generic? Yes, for some.
Drug class: Antiadrenergic, antianginal, antiarrhythmic, antihypertensive

USES

- Treats high blood pressure (hypertension).
- Some beta-blockers are used to relieve angina (chest pain).
- May be used to treat irregular heartbeat.
- May be used to treat anxiety disorders and other conditions as determined by your doctor.
- Treats tremors (some types).
- Reduces frequency of vascular headaches (does not relieve headache pain).

DOSAGE & USAGE INFORMATION

How to take:
Tablet, liquid or extended-release capsule—Swallow with liquid. If you can't swallow whole, crumble tablet or open capsule and take with liquid or food. Don't crush capsule or extended-release tablet.

When to take:
With meals or immediately after.

If you forget a dose:
Take as soon as you remember. Return to regular schedule, but allow 3 hours between doses.

Continued next column

OVERDOSE

SYMPTOMS:
Weakness, slow or weak pulse, blood pressure drop, fainting, difficulty breathing, convulsions, cold and sweaty skin.
WHAT TO DO:
- **Dial 911 (emergency) for an ambulance or medical help or poison center 1-800-222-1222. Then give first aid immediately.**
- **See emergency information at end of book.**

What drug does:
- Blocks certain actions of sympathetic nervous system.
- Lowers heart's oxygen requirements.
- Slows nerve impulses through heart.
- Reduces blood vessel contraction in heart, scalp and other body parts.

Time lapse before drug works:
1 to 4 hours.

Don't take with:
Nonprescription drugs or drugs in Interaction column without consulting doctor or pharmacist.

POSSIBLE ADVERSE REACTIONS OR SIDE EFFECTS

SYMPTOMS	WHAT TO DO
Life-threatening:	
Congestive heart failure (severe shortness of breath, rapid heartbeat); severe asthma.	Discontinue. Seek emergency treatment.
Common:	
• Pulse slower than 50 beats per minute.	Discontinue. Call doctor right away.
• Drowsiness, fatigue, numbness or tingling of fingers or toes, dizziness, diarrhea, nausea, weakness.	Continue. Call doctor when convenient.
• Cold hands or feet; dry mouth, eyes and skin.	Continue. Tell doctor at next visit.
Infrequent:	
• Hallucinations, nightmares, insomnia, headache, difficult breathing, joint pain, anxiety, chest pain.	Discontinue. Call doctor right away.
• Confusion, reduced alertness, depression, impotence, abdominal pain.	Continue. Call doctor when convenient.
• Constipation.	Continue. Tell doctor at next visit.
Rare:	
• Rash, sore throat, fever.	Discontinue. Call doctor right away.
• Unusual bleeding and bruising; dry, burning eyes.	Continue. Call doctor when convenient.

BETA-ADRENERGIC BLOCKING AGENTS

WARNINGS & PRECAUTIONS

Don't take if:
- You are allergic to any beta-adrenergic blocker.
- You have asthma.
- You have hay fever symptoms.
- You have taken a monoamine oxidase (MAO) inhibitor* in the past 2 weeks.

Before you start, consult your doctor:
- If you have heart disease or poor circulation to the extremities.
- If you have hay fever, asthma, chronic bronchitis, emphysema.
- If you have overactive thyroid function.
- If you have impaired liver or kidney function.
- If you will have surgery within 2 months, including dental surgery, requiring general or spinal anesthesia.
- If you have diabetes or hypoglycemia.

Over age 60:
Adverse reactions and side effects may be more frequent and severe than in younger persons.

Pregnancy:
Risk factors vary for drugs in this group. See category list on page xviii and consult doctor.

Breast-feeding:
Drug passes into milk. Avoid drug or discontinue nursing until you finish medicine. Consult doctor for advice on maintaining milk supply.

Infants & children:
Not recommended.

Prolonged use:
Talk to your doctor about the need for follow-up medical examinations or laboratory studies to check blood pressure, ECG*, kidney function, blood sugar.

Skin & sunlight:
No problems expected.

Driving, piloting or hazardous work:
Don't drive or pilot aircraft until you learn how medicine affects you. Don't work around dangerous machinery. Don't climb ladders or work in high places. Danger increases if you drink alcohol or take medicine affecting alertness and reflexes.

Discontinuing
Don't discontinue without consulting doctor. Dose may require gradual reduction if you have taken drug for a long time. Doses of other drugs may also require adjustment. Angina may result from abrupt discontinuing.

Others:
- May mask diabetic hypoglycemia symptoms.
- May affect results in some medical tests.
- Advise any doctor or dentist whom you consult that you take this medicine.

***See Glossary**

POSSIBLE INTERACTION WITH OTHER DRUGS

GENERIC NAME OR DRUG CLASS	COMBINED EFFECT
Angiotensin-converting (ACE) inhibitors*	Increased anti-hypertensive effects of both drugs. Dosages may require adjustment.
Antidiabetics*	Increased anti-diabetic effect.
Antihistamines*	Decreased antihistamine effect.
Antihypertensives*	Increased anti-hypertensive effect.
Anti-inflammatory drugs, nonsteroidal (NSAIDs)*	Decreased anti-hypertensive effect of beta blocker.
Betaxolol eyedrops	Possible increased beta blocker effect.
Calcium channel blockers*	Additional blood pressure drop.
Clonidine	Additional blood pressure drop. High blood pressure if clonidine stopped abruptly.
Dextrothyroxine	Possible decreased beta blocker effect.

Continued on page 905

POSSIBLE INTERACTION WITH OTHER SUBSTANCES

INTERACTS WITH	COMBINED EFFECT
Alcohol:	Excessive blood pressure drop. Avoid.
Beverages:	None expected.
Cocaine:	Irregular heartbeat; decreased beta-adrenergic effect. Avoid.
Foods:	None expected.
Marijuana:	Daily use—Impaired circulation to hands and feet.
Tobacco:	Possible irregular heartbeat.

BETA-ADRENERGIC BLOCKING AGENTS & THIAZIDE DIURETICS

GENERIC AND BRAND NAMES

See complete list of generic and brand names in the *Generic and Brand Name Directory*, page 862.

BASIC INFORMATION

Habit forming? No
Prescription needed? Yes
Available as generic? Yes
Drug class: Beta-adrenergic blocker, diuretic (thiazide)

USES

- Controls, but doesn't cure, high blood pressure.
- Reduces fluid retention (edema).
- Reduces angina attacks.
- Stabilizes irregular heartbeat.
- Lowers blood pressure.
- Reduces frequency of migraine headaches. (Does not relieve headache pain.)
- Other uses prescribed by your doctor.

DOSAGE & USAGE INFORMATION

How to take:
Extended-release capsules—Swallow with liquid. If you can't swallow whole, open capsule and take with liquid or food.

When to take:
At the same time each day.

If you forget a dose:
Take as soon as you remember up to 4 hours late. If more than 4 hours, wait for next scheduled dose (don't double this dose).

What drug does:
- Forces sodium and water excretion, reducing body fluid.
- Relaxes muscle cells of small arteries.

Continued next column

- Reduced body fluid and relaxed arteries lower blood pressure.
- Blocks some of the actions of sympathetic nervous system.
- Lowers heart's oxygen requirements.
- Slows nerve impulses through heart.
- Reduces blood vessel contraction in heart, scalp and other body parts.

Time lapse before drug works:
- 1 to 4 hours for beta-blocker effect.
- May require several weeks to lower blood pressure.

Don't take with:
Any other medicines, even over-the-counter drugs such as cough/cold medicines, diet pills, nose drops, caffeine, without consulting your doctor.

OVERDOSE

SYMPTOMS:
Irregular heartbeat (usually too slow), seizures, confusion, fainting, convulsions, coma.
WHAT TO DO:
- **Dial 911 (emergency) for an ambulance or medical help or poison center 1-800-222-1222. Then give first aid immediately.**
- **See emergency information on inside covers.**

POSSIBLE ADVERSE REACTIONS OR SIDE EFFECTS

SYMPTOMS	WHAT TO DO
Life-threatening:	
Wheezing, chest pain, seizures, irregular heartbeat.	Seek emergency treatment immediately.
Common:	
• Dry mouth, weak pulse, vomiting, muscle cramps, increased thirst, mood changes, nausea.	Discontinue. Call doctor right away.
• Weakness, tiredness, dizziness, mental depression, diminished sex drive, constipation, nightmares, insomnia.	Continue. Call doctor when convenient.
Infrequent:	
• Cold feet and hands, chest pain, breathing difficulty, anxiety, nervousness, headache, appetite loss, abdominal pain, numbness and tingling in fingers and toes, slow heartbeat.	Discontinue. Call doctor right away.
• Confusion, diarrhea.	Continue. Call doctor when convenient.
Rare:	
• Hives, skin rash; joint pain; jaundice; fever, sore throat, mouth ulcers.	Discontinue. Call doctor right away.
• Impotence, back pain.	Continue. Call doctor when convenient.

BETA-ADRENERGIC BLOCKING AGENTS & THIAZIDE DIURETICS

WARNINGS & PRECAUTIONS

Don't take if:
- You are allergic to any beta-adrenergic blocker or any thiazide diuretic drug.
- You have asthma or hay fever symptoms.
- You have taken MAO inhibitors in past two weeks.

Before you start, consult your doctor:
- If you have heart disease or poor circulation to the extremities.
- If you have hay fever, asthma, chronic bronchitis, emphysema, overactive thyroid function, impaired liver or kidney function, gout, diabetes, hypoglycemia, pancreas disorder, systemic lupus erythematosus.
- If you are allergic to any sulfa drug or tartrazine dye.
- If you will have surgery within 2 months, including dental surgery, requiring general or spinal anesthesia.

Over age 60:
Adverse reactions and side effects may be more frequent and severe than in younger persons, especially dizziness and excessive potassium loss.

Pregnancy:
Risk factors vary for drugs in this group. See category list on page xviii and consult doctor.

Breast-feeding:
Drug passes into milk. Avoid drug or discontinue nursing until you finish medicine. Consult doctor for advice on maintaining milk supply.

Infants & children:
Not recommended.

Prolonged use:
- Weakens heart muscle contractions.
- You may need medicine to treat high blood pressure for the rest of your life.
- Talk to your doctor about the need for follow-up medical examinations or laboratory studies.

Skin & sunlight:
One or more drugs in this group may cause rash or intensify sunburn in areas exposed to sun or ultraviolet light (photosensitivity reaction). Avoid overexposure. Notify doctor if reaction occurs.

Driving, piloting or hazardous work:
Don't drive or pilot aircraft until you learn how medicine affects you. Don't work around dangerous machinery. Don't climb ladders or work in high places. Danger increases if you drink alcohol or take medicine affecting alertness and reflexes, such as antihistamines, tranquilizers, sedatives, pain medicine, narcotics and mind-altering drugs.

Discontinuing:
Don't discontinue without consulting doctor. Dose may require gradual reduction if you have taken drug for a long time. Doses of other drugs may also require adjustment.

Others:
- May mask hypoglycemia symptoms.
- Hot weather and fever may cause dehydration and drop in blood pressure. Dose may require temporary adjustment. Weigh daily and report any unexpected weight decreases to your doctor.
- May cause rise in uric acid, leading to gout.
- May cause blood sugar rise in diabetics.

POSSIBLE INTERACTION WITH OTHER DRUGS

GENERIC NAME OR DRUG CLASS	COMBINED EFFECT
Allopurinol	Decreased allopurinol effect.
Aminophylline	Decreased effectiveness of both.
Antidepressants, tricyclic*	Dangerous drop in blood pressure. Avoid combination unless under medical supervision.

Continued on page 906

POSSIBLE INTERACTION WITH OTHER SUBSTANCES

INTERACTS WITH	COMBINED EFFECT
Alcohol:	Dangerous blood pressure drop. Avoid.
Beverages:	None expected.
Cocaine:	Irregular heartbeat, decreased beta blocker effect. Avoid.
Foods: Licorice.	Excessive potassium loss that causes dangerous heart rhythms.
Marijuana:	May increase blood pressure.
Tobacco:	May increase blood pressure and make heart work harder. Avoid.

***See Glossary**

BETHANECHOL

BRAND NAMES

Duvoid
Urabeth
Urecholine

BASIC INFORMATION

Habit forming? No
Prescription needed? Yes
Available as generic? Yes
Drug class: Cholinergic

USES

- Helps initiate urination following surgery, or for persons with urinary infections or enlarged prostate.
- Treats reflux esophagitis.

DOSAGE & USAGE INFORMATION

How to take:
Tablet—Swallow with liquid, 1 hour before or 2 hours after eating.

When to take:
At the same times each day.

If you forget a dose:
Take as soon as you remember up to 2 hours late. If more than 2 hours, wait for next scheduled dose (don't double this dose).

What drug does:
Affects chemical reactions in the body that strengthen bladder muscles.

Continued next column

OVERDOSE

SYMPTOMS:
Shortness of breath, wheezing or chest tightness, unconsciousness, coma.
WHAT TO DO:

- **Dial 911 (emergency) for an ambulance or medical help or poison center 1-800-222-1222. Then give first aid immediately.**
- **If patient is unconscious and not breathing, give mouth-to-mouth breathing. If there is no heartbeat, use cardiac massage and mouth-to-mouth breathing (CPR). Don't try to make patient vomit. If you can't get help quickly, take patient to nearest emergency facility.**
- **See emergency information on inside covers.**

Time lapse before drug works:
30 to 90 minutes.

Don't take with:
Any other medicine without consulting your doctor or pharmacist.

POSSIBLE ADVERSE REACTIONS OR SIDE EFFECTS

SYMPTOMS	WHAT TO DO
Life-threatening: In case of overdose, see previous column.	
Common: None expected.	
Infrequent: Dizziness, headache, faintness, blurred or changed vision, diarrhea, nausea, vomiting, stomach discomfort, belching, excessive urge to urinate.	Continue. Call doctor when convenient.
Rare: Shortness of breath, wheezing, tightness in chest.	Discontinue. Call doctor right away.

WARNINGS & PRECAUTIONS

Don't take if:
You are allergic to any cholinergic.

Before you start, consult your doctor:
- If you plan to become pregnant within medication period.
- If you have asthma.
- If you have epilepsy.
- If you have heart or blood vessel disease.
- If you have high or low blood pressure.
- If you have overactive thyroid.
- If you have intestinal blockage.
- If you have Parkinson's disease.
- If you have stomach problems (including ulcer).
- If you have had bladder or intestinal surgery within 1 month.

Over age 60:
Adverse reactions and side effects may be more frequent and severe than in younger persons.

Pregnancy:
Decide with your doctor if drug benefits justify risk to unborn child. Risk category C (see page xviii).

Breast-feeding:
Unknown effect. Consult doctor.

Infants & children:
Use only under medical supervision.

Prolonged use:
No problems expected.

Skin & sunlight:
No problems expected.

Driving, piloting or hazardous work:
Don't drive or pilot aircraft until you learn how medicine effects you. Don't work around dangerous machinery. Don't climb ladders or work in high places. Danger increases if you drink alcohol or take medicine affecting alertness and reflexes, such as antihistamines, tranquilizers, sedatives, pain medicine, narcotics and mind-altering drugs.

Discontinuing:
May be unnecessary to finish medicine. Follow doctor's instructions.

Others:
- Be cautious about standing up suddenly.
- Advise any doctor or dentist whom you consult that you take this medicine.
- Interferes with laboratory studies of liver and pancreas function.
- Side effects more likely with injections.

POSSIBLE INTERACTION WITH OTHER DRUGS

GENERIC NAME OR DRUG CLASS	COMBINED EFFECT
Cholinergics, other*	Increased effect of both drugs. Possible toxicity.
Ganglionic blockers*	Decreased blood pressure.
Nitrates*	Decreased bethanechol effect.
Procainamide	Decreased bethanechol effect.
Quinidine	Decreased bethanechol effect.

POSSIBLE INTERACTION WITH OTHER SUBSTANCES

INTERACTS WITH	COMBINED EFFECT
Alcohol:	None expected.
Beverages:	None expected.
Cocaine:	None expected.
Foods:	None expected.
Marijuana:	None expected.
Tobacco:	None expected.

*See Glossary

BISMUTH SUBSALICYLATE

BRAND NAMES

Helidac
Pepto-Bismol

BASIC INFORMATION

Habit forming? No
Prescription needed? No
Available as generic? Yes
Drug class: Antidiarrheal, antacid

USES

- Treats symptoms of diarrhea, heartburn, nausea, acid indigestion.
- Helps prevent traveler's diarrhea.
- Treats ulcers.
- Used with other medications to treat a stomach infected by the bacteria *H. Pylori*.

DOSAGE & USAGE INFORMATION

How to take:
- Tablets—Swallow with water.
- Chewable tablets—Chew well before swallowing.
- Liquid—Take as directed on label.

When to take:
As directed on label or by your doctor.

If you forget a dose:
Take as soon as you remember. Don't double this dose.

What drug does:
- Binds toxin of some bacteria.
- Stimulates absorption of fluid and electrolytes across the intestinal wall.
- Decreases inflammation and increased motility of the intestinal muscles and lining.

Time lapse before drug works:
30 minutes to 1 hour.

Continued next column

OVERDOSE

SYMPTOMS:
Hearing loss, ringing or buzzing in the ears, severe drowsiness or tiredness, severe excitement or nervousness, fast or deep breathing.
WHAT TO DO:
- **Dial 911 (emergency) for an ambulance or medical help or poison center 1-800-222-1222. Then give first aid immediately.**
- **See emergency information on inside covers.**

Don't take with:
Any other medicine without consulting your doctor or pharmacist.

POSSIBLE ADVERSE REACTIONS OR SIDE EFFECTS

SYMPTOMS	WHAT TO DO
Life-threatening: In case of overdose, see previous column.	
Common: Black stools, dark tongue. (These symptoms are normal and medically insignificant.)	No action necessary.
Infrequent: None expected.	
Rare: Abdominal pain, increased sweating, muscle weakness, drowsiness, anxiety, trembling, hearing loss, ringing or buzzing in ears, confusion, dizziness, headache, increased thirst, vision problems, severe constipation, continuing diarrhea, trouble breathing (all more likely to occur with high doses or chronic use).	Discontinue. Call doctor right away.

WARNINGS & PRECAUTIONS

Don't take if:
- You are allergic to aspirin, salicylates or other nonsteroidal anti-inflammatory drugs.
- You have stomach ulcers that have ever bled.
- The patient is a child with fever.

Before you start, consult your doctor:
- If you are on a low-sodium, low-sugar or other special diet.
- If you have had diarrhea for more than 24 hours. This is especially applicable to infants, children and those over 60.
- If you have had kidney disease.

Over age 60:
- Consult doctor before using.
- May cause severe constipation.

Pregnancy:
Decide with your doctor if drug benefits justify risk to unborn child. Risk category C; D in third trimester (see page xviii).

Breast-feeding:
- Drug passes into milk. Avoid or discontinue nursing until you finish medicine.
- May harm baby if mother takes large amounts.

Infants & children:
Not recommended for children 3 and younger. May cause constipation.

Prolonged use:
May cause constipation.

Skin & sunlight:
No problems expected.

Driving, piloting or hazardous work:
Don't drive or pilot aircraft if you take high or prolonged dose until you learn how medicine affects you. Don't work around dangerous machinery. Don't climb ladders or work in high places. Danger increases if you drink alcohol or take medicine affecting alertness and reflexes, such as antihistamines, tranquilizers, sedatives, pain medicine, narcotics and mind-altering drugs.

Discontinuing:
No problems expected.

Others:
- Pepto-Bismol contains salicylates. When given to children with flu or chicken pox, salicylates may cause a serious illness called Reye's syndrome*. An overdose in children can cause the same problems as aspirin poisoning.
- May cause false urine sugar tests.
- Dehydration can develop if too much body fluid has been lost. Consult doctor if any of the following symptoms occur: decreased urination, dizziness or lightheadedness, dryness of mouth, increased thirst, wrinkled skin.
- Don't store tablet form of drug in bathroom or near kitchen sink. Heat and moisture can cause it to break down.
- Consult doctor if diarrhea doesn't improve within 2 days.
- Read labels of any other drugs being used, such as for pain or inflammation. They may contain salicylates* and can lead to increased risk of side effects and overdose.

POSSIBLE INTERACTION WITH OTHER DRUGS

GENERIC NAME OR DRUG CLASS	COMBINED EFFECT
Anticoagulants*	Increased risk of bleeding.
Insulin or oral antidiabetic drugs*	Increased insulin effect. May require dosage adjustment.
Probenecid	Decreased effect of probenecid.
Salicylates*, other	Increased risk of salicylate toxicity.
Sulfinpyrazone	Decreased effect of sulfinpyrazone.
Tetracylines*	Decreased absorption of tetracycline.
Thrombolytic agents*	Increased risk of bleeding.

POSSIBLE INTERACTION WITH OTHER SUBSTANCES

INTERACTS WITH	COMBINED EFFECT
Alcohol:	None expected.
Beverages:	None expected.
Cocaine:	Decreased Pepto-Bismol effect. Avoid.
Foods:	None expected.
Marijuana:	None expected.
Tobacco:	None expected.

***See Glossary**

BROMOCRIPTINE

BRAND NAMES

Alti-Bromocriptine
Apo-Bromocriptine
Parlodel
Parlodel Snaptabs

BASIC INFORMATION

Habit forming? No
Prescription needed? Yes
Available as generic? Yes
Drug class: Antiparkinsonism

USES

- Controls Parkinson's disease symptoms such as rigidity, tremors and unsteady gait.
- Treats male and female infertility.
- Treats acromegaly (an overproduction of growth hormone).
- Treats some pituitary tumors.

DOSAGE & USAGE INFORMATION

How to take:
Tablet or capsule—Swallow with liquid or food to lessen stomach irritation. If you can't swallow whole, crumble tablet or open capsule and take with liquid or food.

When to take:
At the same times each day.

If you forget a dose:
Take as soon as you remember up to 2 hours late. If more than 2 hours, wait for next scheduled dose (don't double this dose).

Continued next column

OVERDOSE

SYMPTOMS:
Muscle twitch, spastic eyelid closure, nausea, vomiting, diarrhea, irregular and rapid pulse, weakness, fainting, confusion, agitation, hallucination, coma.
WHAT TO DO:
- **Dial 911 (emergency) for an ambulance or medical help or poison center 1-800-222-1222. Then give first aid immediately.**
- **If patient is unconscious and not breathing, give mouth-to-mouth breathing. If there is no heartbeat, use cardiac massage and mouth-to-mouth breathing (CPR). Don't try to make patient vomit. If you can't get help quickly, take patient to nearest emergency facility.**
- **See emergency information on inside covers.**

What drug does:
Restores chemical balance necessary for normal nerve impulses.

Time lapse before drug works:
2 to 3 weeks to improve; several months or longer for maximum benefit.

Don't take with:
Any other medicine without consulting your doctor or pharmacist.

POSSIBLE ADVERSE REACTIONS OR SIDE EFFECTS

SYMPTOMS	WHAT TO DO
Life-threatening: In case of overdose, see previous column.	
Common: Dizziness, mild nausea, lightheadedness when getting up, headache.	Continue. Call doctor when convenient.
Infrequent: Constipation, diarrhea, tiredness, drowsiness, dry mouth, depression, tingling and numbness of hands and feet.	Continue. Call doctor when convenient.
Rare: • Severe nausea and vomiting (may be bloody), vision changes, nervousness, sudden weakness, unusual headache, excess sweating, seizures, fainting, chest pain, black or tarry stools, uncontrollable body movements.	Discontinue. Call doctor right away.
• Stomach or back pain, runny nose, urinary frequency.	Continue. Call doctor when convenient.

WARNINGS & PRECAUTIONS

Don't take if:
- You are allergic to bromocriptine or ergotamine.
- You have taken a monoamine oxidase (MAO) inhibitor* in the past 2 weeks.
- You have glaucoma (narrow-angle type).

Before you start, consult your doctor:
- If you have diabetes or epilepsy.
- If you have had high blood pressure, heart or lung disease.
- If you have had liver or kidney disease.
- If you have a peptic ulcer.
- If you have a history of mental problems.
- If you will have surgery within 2 months, requiring general or spinal anesthesia.

Over age 60:
Adverse reactions and side effects may be more frequent and severe than in younger persons.

Pregnancy:
Decide with your doctor if drug benefits justify risk to unborn child. Risk category B (see page xviii).

Breast-feeding:
Drug inhibits milk production. Avoid.

Infants & children:
Not recommended if under 15 years old.

Prolonged use:
- May lead to uncontrolled movements of head, face, mouth, tongue, arms or legs.
- Changes in lung tissue and excess fluid in chest cavity may occur.
- Talk to your doctor about the need for follow-up medical examinations or laboratory studies to check blood pressure, x-rays, growth hormone levels.

Skin & sunlight:
No problems expected.

Driving, piloting or hazardous work:
Don't drive or pilot aircraft until you learn how medicine effects you. Don't work around dangerous machinery. Don't climb ladders or work in high places. Danger increases if you drink alcohol or take medicine affecting alertness and reflexes, such as antihistamines, tranquilizers, sedatives, pain medicine, narcotics and mind-altering drugs.

Discontinuing:
Don't discontinue without doctor's advice until you complete prescribed dose, even though symptoms diminish or disappear.

Others:
- Expect to start with small doses and increase gradually to lessen frequency and severity of adverse reactions.
- Advise any doctor or dentist whom you consult that you take this medicine.

POSSIBLE INTERACTION WITH OTHER DRUGS

GENERIC NAME OR DRUG CLASS	COMBINED EFFECT
Antihypertensives*	May decrease blood pressure.
Antiparkinsonism drugs, other*	Increased bromocriptine effect.
Ergot alkaloids, other	Increased risk of high blood pressure.
Erythromycin	Increased bromocriptine effect.
Haloperidol	Decreased bromocriptine effect.
Levodopa	Decreased antiparkinson effect.
Methyldopa	Decreased bromocriptine effect.
Papaverine	Decreased bromocriptine effect.
Phenothiazines*	Decreased bromocriptine effect.
Risperidone	Increased bromocriptine effect.
Ritonavir	Increased bromocriptine effect.

POSSIBLE INTERACTION WITH OTHER SUBSTANCES

INTERACTS WITH	COMBINED EFFECT
Alcohol:	Decreased alcohol tolerance. Avoid.
Beverages:	None expected.
Cocaine:	Decreased bromocriptine effect. Avoid.
Foods:	None expected.
Marijuana:	Increased fatigue, lethargy, fainting. Avoid.
Tobacco:	Interferes with absorption. Avoid.

*See Glossary

BRONCHODILATORS, ADRENERGIC

GENERIC AND BRAND NAMES

See complete list of generic and brand names in the *Generic and Brand Name Directory*, page 862.

BASIC INFORMATION

Habit forming? No
Prescription needed? Yes, for most
Available as generic? Yes, for some
Drug class: Sympathomimetic

USES

- Relieves bronchial asthma.
- Decreases congestion of breathing passages.
- Suppresses allergic reactions.
- Treats bronchoconstriction in COPD*.
- Relieves exercise-induced bronchospasm.

DOSAGE & USAGE INFORMATION

How to take:
- Tablet or capsule—Swallow with liquid. You may chew or crush tablet.
- Extended-release tablets—Swallow each dose whole.
- Syrup—Take as directed on bottle.
- Drops—Dilute dose in beverage.
- Aerosol inhaler—Follow directions in package.

When to take:
As needed, no more often than every 4 hours.

If you forget a dose:
Take up to 2 hours late. If more than 2 hours, wait for next dose (don't double this dose).

What drug does:
- Prevents cells from releasing allergy-causing chemicals (histamines).
- Relaxes muscles of bronchial tubes.
- Decreases blood-vessel size and blood flow, thus causing decongestion.

Continued next column

OVERDOSE

SYMPTOMS:
Severe anxiety, confusion, delirium, muscle tremors, rapid and irregular pulse, severe weakness.
WHAT TO DO:
- **Dial 911 (emergency) for an ambulance or medical help or poison center 1-800-222-1222. Then give first aid immediately.**
- **See emergency information on inside covers.**

Time lapse before drug works:
30 to 60 minutes.

Don't take with:
- Nonprescription drugs with ephedrine, pseudoephedrine or epinephrine.
- Nonprescription drugs for cough, cold, allergy or asthma without consulting doctor.
- Any other medicine without consulting your doctor or pharmacist.

POSSIBLE ADVERSE REACTIONS OR SIDE EFFECTS

SYMPTOMS	WHAT TO DO
Life-threatening: In case of overdose, see previous column.	
Common:	
• Nervousness, restlessness, trembling.	Continue. Call doctor when convenient.
• Dry mouth or throat.	Continue. Tell doctor at next visit.
Infrequent:	
• Fast heartbeat, nausea, vomiting, headache, dizziness, lightheadedness.	Discontinue. Call doctor right away.
• Trouble sleeping, appetite loss, coughing.	Continue. Call doctor when convenient.
Rare:	
• Increased wheezing, difficulty breathing, chest discomfort or pain, irregular heartbeat, painful or difficult urination, allergic reaction (bluish, reddish or flushed skin; rash; itching; hives; swelling of face area; wheezing).	Discontinue. Call doctor right away.
• Smell or taste changes.	No action necessary.

WARNINGS & PRECAUTIONS

Don't take if:
You are allergic to ephedrine, any bronchodilator* drug or sulfites used in some preparations.

Before you start, consult your doctor:
- If you have high blood pressure.
- If you have diabetes.
- If you have cardiovascular disease.
- If you have overactive thyroid gland.
- If you have difficulty urinating.
- If you have taken any monoamine oxidase(MAO) inhibitor* in past 2 weeks.
- If you have taken digitalis preparations* in the last 7 days.

- If you will have surgery within 2 months, including dental surgery, requiring general or spinal anesthesia.
- If you have pheochromocytoma.

Over age 60:
More likely to develop high blood pressure, heart rhythm disturbances, angina and to feel drug's stimulant effects.

Pregnancy:
Risk factors vary for drugs in this group. See category list on page xviii and consult doctor.

Breast-feeding:
Drug passes into milk. Avoid drug or discontinue nursing until you finish medicine. Consult doctor for advice on maintaining milk supply.

Infants & children:
No problems expected for most. Use only under close medical supervision. Xopenex is not recommended for children under 12.

Prolonged use:
- Excessive doses—Rare toxic psychosis.
- Men with enlarged prostate gland may have more urination difficulty.
- Talk to your doctor about the need for follow-up medical examinations or laboratory studies to check ECG*, blood pressure.

Skin & sunlight:
No problems expected.

Driving, piloting or hazardous work:
Avoid if you feel dizzy. Otherwise, no problems expected.

Discontinuing:
May be unnecessary to finish medicine. Follow doctor's instructions.

Others:
- May affect results in some medical tests.
- Advise any doctor or dentist whom you consult that you take this medicine.
- Complications increase if you use more than prescribed. If you need to use more frequently, consult your doctor.

POSSIBLE INTERACTION WITH OTHER DRUGS

GENERIC NAME OR DRUG CLASS	COMBINED EFFECT
Antidepressants, tricyclic*	Increased effect of bronchodilator. Excessive stimulation of heart and blood pressure.
Antihypertensives*	Decreased antihypertensive effect.
Beta-adrenergic blocking agents*	Decreased effects of both drugs.
Digitalis preparations*	Serious heart rhythm disturbances.
Epinephrine	Increased bronchodilator effect.
Ergot preparations*	Serious blood-pressure rise.
Finasteride	Decreased finasteride effect.
Furazolidine	Sudden severe increase in blood pressure.
Maprotiline	Increased heart stimulation.
Methyldopa	Possible increased blood pressure.
Monoamine oxidase (MAO) inhibitors*	Increased bronchodilator effect. Dangerous blood pressure rise.
Nicotine	Decreased effect of isoproterenol.
Nitrates*	Possible decreased effects of both drugs.
Phenothiazines*	Possible increased bronchodilator toxicity. Possible decreased bronchodilator effect.
Pseudoephedrine	Increased bronchodilator effect.

Continued on page 907

POSSIBLE INTERACTION WITH OTHER SUBSTANCES

INTERACTS WITH	COMBINED EFFECT
Alcohol:	None expected.
Beverages: Caffeine drinks.	Nervousness or insomnia.
Cocaine:	High risk of heartbeat irregularities and high blood pressure.
Foods:	None expected.
Marijuana:	Rapid heartbeat, possible heart rhythm disturbance.
Tobacco:	None expected.

*See Glossary

BRONCHODILATORS, XANTHINE

GENERIC AND BRAND NAMES

See complete list of generic and brand names in the *Generic and Brand Name Directory*, page 862.

BASIC INFORMATION

Habit forming? No
Prescription needed? Yes
Available as generic? Yes
Drug class: Bronchodilator (xanthine)

USES

- Treatment for bronchial asthma symptoms.
- Treatment for chronic bronchitis, emphysema and other pulmonary diseases.

DOSAGE & USAGE INFORMATION

How to take:

- Tablet or capsule—Swallow with liquid.
- Extended-release tablets or capsules—Swallow each dose whole. If you take regular tablets, you may chew or crush them.
- Suppositories—Remove wrapper and moisten suppository with water. Gently insert larger end into rectum. Push well into rectum with finger.
- Syrup, elixir or oral solution—Take as directed on bottle.
- Enema—Use as directed on label.

When to take:
Most effective taken on empty stomach 1 hour before or 2 hours after eating. However, may take with food to lessen stomach upset.

If you forget a dose:
Take as soon as you remember up to 2 hours late. If more than 2 hours, wait for next scheduled dose (don't double this dose).

What drug does:
Relaxes and expands bronchial tubes.

Continued next column

OVERDOSE

SYMPTOMS:
Restlessness, irritability, confusion, black or tarry stool, breathing difficulty, pounding and irregular heartbeat, vomiting blood, delirium, convulsions, rapid pulse, coma.

WHAT TO DO:

- **Dial 911 (emergency) for an ambulance or medical help or poison center 1-800-222-1222. Then give first aid immediately.**
- **See emergency information on inside covers.**

Time lapse before drug works:
15 to 30 minutes.

Don't take with:
Any other medicine without consulting your doctor or pharmacist.

POSSIBLE ADVERSE REACTIONS OR SIDE EFFECTS

SYMPTOMS	WHAT TO DO
Life-threatening: In case of overdose, see previous column.	
Common: Headache, irritability, nervousness, nausea, restlessness, insomnia, vomiting, stomach pain.	Continue. Call doctor when convenient.
Infrequent:	
• Rash or hives, flushed face, diarrhea, rapid breathing, irregular heartbeat.	Discontinue. Call doctor right away.
• Dizziness or light-headedness, appetite loss, trembling, fatigue, weakness.	Continue. Call doctor when convenient.
Rare: Frequent urination.	Continue. Call doctor when convenient.

WARNINGS & PRECAUTIONS

Don't take if:

- You are allergic to any bronchodilator.
- You have an active peptic ulcer.

Before you start, consult your doctor:

- If you have had impaired kidney or liver function.
- If you have gastritis.
- If you have a peptic ulcer.
- If you have high blood pressure or heart disease.
- If you take medication for gout.

Over age 60:
Adverse reactions and side effects may be more frequent and severe than in younger persons.

Pregnancy:
Decide with your doctor if drug benefits justify risk to unborn child. Risk category C (see page xviii).

Breast-feeding:
Drug passes into milk. Avoid drug or discontinue nursing until you finish medicine. Consult doctor for advice on maintaining milk supply.

Infants & children:
Use only under medical supervision.

Prolonged use:
Stomach irritation may occur.

Skin & sunlight:
No problems expected.

Driving, piloting or hazardous work:
Avoid if lightheaded or dizzy. Otherwise, no problems expected.

Discontinuing:
May be unnecessary to finish medicine. Follow doctor's instructions.

Others:
Advise any doctor or dentist whom you consult that you take this medicine.

POSSIBLE INTERACTION WITH OTHER DRUGS

GENERIC NAME OR DRUG CLASS	COMBINED EFFECT
Allopurinol	Increased theophylline effect.
Aminoglutethimide	Possible decreased bronchodilator effect.
Beta-agonists*	Increased effect of both drugs.
Beta-adrenergic blocking agents*	Decreased bronchodilator effect.
Cimetidine	Increased bronchodilator effect.
Clarithromycin	Increased concentration of theophylline.
Clindamycin	May increase bronchodilator effect.
Corticosteroids*	Possible increased bronchodilator effect.
Erythromicin	Increased bronchodilator effect.
Finasteride	Decreased finasteride effect.
Fluoroquinolones	Increased xanthine bronchodilator in blood. May need dose adjustment.
Fluvoxamine	Increased theophylline effect.
Furosemide	Increased furosemide effect.
Lansoprazole	May require dosage adjustment of theophylline.
Leukotriene modifiers	Unknown effects. Consult doctor.
Lincomycins*	May increase bronchodilator effect.
Lithium	Decreased lithium effect.
Modafinil	Decreased bronchodilator effect.
Moricizine	Decreased bronchodilator effect.
Nicotine	Possible increased bronchodilator effect.
Phenobarbital	Decreased bronchodilator effect.
Phenytoin	Decreased effect of both drugs.
Probenecid	Increased effect of dyphylline.
Ranitidine	Possible increased bronchodilator effect and toxicity.
Rauwolfia alkaloids*	Rapid heartbeat.
Rifampin	Decreased bronchodilator effect.
Sulfinpyrazone	Increased effect of dyphylline.
Sympathomimetics*	Possible increased bronchodilator effect.

Continued on page 907

POSSIBLE INTERACTION WITH OTHER SUBSTANCES

INTERACTS WITH	COMBINED EFFECT
Alcohol:	None expected.
Beverages: Caffeine drinks.	Nervousness and insomnia.
Cocaine:	Excess stimulation. Avoid.
Foods:	None expected.
Marijuana:	Slightly increased antiasthmatic effect of bronchodilator. Decreased effect with chronic use.
Tobacco:	Decreased bronchodilator effect.

***See Glossary**

BUPROPION

BRAND NAMES

Wellbutrin	Wellbutrin SR
	Zyban

BASIC INFORMATION

Habit forming? No
Prescription needed? Yes
Available as generic? No
Drug class: Antidepressant

USES

- Relieves severe depression. (Has less effect on sexual functioning than some other antidepressants and may be more acceptable to some patients.)
- May be used in combination with other therapy for smoking cessation.

DOSAGE & USAGE INFORMATION

How to take:
- Tablets—Swallow with liquid. If you can't swallow whole, crumble tablet and take with liquid or food (but drug does have a bitter taste). May take with food to lessen stomach irritation.
- Sustained-release tablets—Swallow with liquid. Do not crumble sustained release tablet.

When to take:
At the same times each day, according to instructions on prescription label.

If you forget a dose:
Take as soon as you remember up to 4 hours late. If more than 4 hours, wait for next scheduled dose (don't double this dose). Do not take more often than every 6 hours.

What drug does:
Blocks certain chemicals that are necessary for nerve transmission in the brain. Boosts dopamine and norepinephrine (two brain chemicals) that are also boosted by nicotine.

Continued next column

OVERDOSE

SYMPTOMS:
Confusion, agitation, seizures, coma.
WHAT TO DO:
- **Dial 911 (emergency) for an ambulance or medical help or poison center 1-800-222-1222. Then give first aid immediately. Do not induce vomiting.**
- **See emergency information at end of book.**

Time lapse before drug works:
3 to 4 weeks.

Don't take with:
Any other medicine without consulting your doctor or pharmacist.

POSSIBLE ADVERSE REACTIONS OR SIDE EFFECTS

SYMPTOMS	WHAT TO DO
Life-threatening: In case of overdose, see previous column.	
Common:	
• Excitement, anxiety, insomnia, restlessness. constipation, loss of appetite, dry mouth, dizziness, nausea or vomiting, unusual weight loss.	Continue. Call doctor when convenient.
• Confusion, heartbeat irregularity, severe headache.	Discontinue. Call doctor right away.
Infrequent:	
Rash, blurred vision, drowsiness, chills, fever, hallucinations, fatigue, nightmares.	Discontinue. Call doctor right away
Rare:	
Fainting, seizures.	Discontinue. Call doctor right away.

WARNINGS & PRECAUTIONS

Don't take if:
- You are allergic to bupropion.
- You have anorexia nervosa or bulimia.
- You have had recent head injury.
- You have a brain or spinal cord tumor.

Before you start, consult your doctor:
- If you have manic phases to your illness.
- If you abuse drugs.
- If you have seizures.
- If you have liver, kidney or heart disease.

Over age 60:
No problems expected.

Pregnancy:
No proven harm to unborn child, but avoid if possible. Risk category B (see page xviii).

Breast-feeding:
Drug passes into milk. May cause adverse reactions. Avoid drug or discontinue breast-feeding. Consult doctor about maintaining milk supply.

Infants & children:
Effect not documented. Consult your doctor.

Prolonged use:
Talk to your doctor about the need for follow-up medical examinations or laboratory studies to check kidney function, liver function and serum bupropion levels in blood.

Skin & sunlight:
No problems expected.

Driving, piloting or hazardous work:
Don't drive or pilot aircraft until you learn how medicine affects you. Don't work around dangerous machinery. Don't climb ladders or work in high places. Danger increases if you drink alcohol or take medicine affecting alertness and reflexes.

Discontinuing:
Don't discontinue without doctor's approval. Dose may require gradual reduction to avoid adverse effects.

Others:
- May affect results in some medical tests.
- Advise any doctor or dentist whom you consult that you take this medicine.

POSSIBLE INTERACTION WITH OTHER DRUGS

GENERIC NAME OR DRUG CLASS	COMBINED EFFECT
Antidepressants, tricyclic*	Increased risk of seizures.
Carbamazepine	Decreased carbamazepine effect. Risk of seizures.
Cimetidine	Increased bupropion effect.
Clozapine	Increased risk of seizures.
Fluoxetine	Increased risk of seizures.
Haloperidol	Increased risk of seizures.
Levodopa	Increased levodopa effect.
Lithium	Increased risk of seizures.
Loxapine	Increased risk of seizures.
Maprotiline	Increased risk of seizures.
Molindone	Increased risk of seizures.
Monoamine oxidase (MAO) inhibitors*	Increased risk of side effects.
Phenothiazines*	Increased risk of seizures.
Phenytoin	Increased phenytoin effect and risk of seizures.
Thioxanthenes*	Increased risk of seizures.
Trazodone	Increased risk of seizures.

POSSIBLE INTERACTION WITH OTHER SUBSTANCES

INTERACTS WITH	COMBINED EFFECT
Alcohol:	Increased risk of seizures. Avoid.
Beverages: Coffee, tea, cocoa.	Increased side effects such as restlessness, insomnia.
Cocaine:	Increased risk of seizures. Avoid.
Foods:	None expected.
Marijuana:	Increased risk of seizures. Avoid.
Tobacco:	None expected.

*See Glossary

BUSPIRONE

BRAND NAMES

BuSpar

BASIC INFORMATION

Habit forming? Probably not
Prescription needed? Yes
Available as generic? Yes
Drug class: Antianxiety agent

USES

- Treats chronic anxiety disorders with nervousness or tension. Not intended for treatment of ordinary stress of daily living. Causes less sedation than some antianxiety drugs. Not useful for acute anxiety.
- Useful in agitation associated with dementia.
- Reduces agggression and irritability in patients with dementia, brain injury, mental retardation.
- Used for anxiety in alcoholics or substance abusers (buspirone has low abuse potential).
- Reduces frequency of vascular headaches (does not relieve headache pain).
- Not useful in withdrawal from sedatives.

DOSAGE & USAGE INFORMATION

How to take:
Tablets—Take with food.

When to take:
As directed. Usually 3 times daily. Food increases absorption.

If you forget a dose:
Take as soon as you remember, but skip this dose and don't double the next dose if it is almost time for the next dose.

What drug does:
Chemical family azaspirodecanedione; *not* a benzodiazepine. Probably has an effect on neurotransmitter systems.

Continued next column

OVERDOSE

SYMPTOMS:
Severe drowsiness or nausea, vomiting, small pupils, unconsciousness.
WHAT TO DO:
- **Dial 911 (emergency) for an ambulance or medical help or poison center 1-800-222-1222. Then give first aid immediately.**
- **See emergency information at end of book.**

Time lapse before drug works:
1 to 2 weeks before beneficial effects may be observed.

Don't take with:
- Alcohol, other tranquilizers, antihistamines, muscle relaxants, sedatives or narcotics
- Any other medicine without consulting your doctor or pharmacist..

POSSIBLE ADVERSE REACTIONS OR SIDE EFFECTS

SYMPTOMS	WHAT TO DO
Life-threatening:	
Chest pain; pounding, fast heartbeat (rare).	Discontinue. Seek emergency treatment.
Common:	
Lightheadedness, headache, nausea, restlessness, dizziness (if these side effects continue).	Discontinue. Call doctor right away.
Infrequent:	
Drowsiness, dry mouth, ringing in ears, nightmares or vivid dreams, unusual fatigue.	Continue. Call doctor when convenient.
Rare:	
Numbness or tingling in feet or hands; sore throat; fever; depression or confusion; uncontrollable movements of tongue, lips, arms and legs; slurred speech; psychosis; blurred vision.	Discontinue. Call doctor right away.

WARNINGS & PRECAUTIONS

Don't take if:
You are allergic to buspirone.

Before you start, consult your doctor:
- If you have ever been addicted to any substance.
- If you have chronic kidney or liver disease.
- If you are already taking any medicine.

Over age 60:
Adverse reactions and side effects may be more frequent and severe than in younger persons.

Pregnancy:
No problems expected, but better to avoid if possible. Consult doctor. Risk category B (see page xviii).

Breast-feeding:
Unknown if drug passes into milk. Avoid nursing until you finish medicine. Consult doctor for advice on maintaining milk supply.

Infants & children:
Safety and efficacy not established for under 18 years old.

Prolonged use:
- Not recommended for prolonged use. Adverse side effects more likely.
- Request follow-up studies to check kidney function, blood counts, and platelet counts.

Skin & sunlight:
No problems expected.

Driving, piloting or hazardous work:
Don't drive or pilot aircraft until you learn how medicine affects you. Don't work around dangerous machinery. Don't climb ladders or work in high places. Danger increases if you drink alcohol or take medicine affecting alertness and reflexes, such as antihistamines, tranquilizers, sedatives, pain medicine, narcotics and mind-altering drugs.

Discontinuing:
No problems expected.

Others:
- Before elective surgery requiring local or general anesthesia, tell your dentist, surgeon or anesthesiologist that you take buspirone.
- Advise any doctor or dentist whom you consult that you take this medicine.

POSSIBLE INTERACTION WITH OTHER DRUGS

GENERIC NAME OR DRUG CLASS	COMBINED EFFECT
Antihistamines*	Increased sedative effect of both drugs.
Barbiturates*	Excessive sedation. Sedative effect of both drugs may be increased.
Benzodiazepines*	Recent use of benzodiazepines may lessen effect of buspirone.
Central nervous system (CNS) depressants*	Increased sedative effect.
Monoamine oxidase MAO inhibitors*	May increase blood pressure.
Narcotics*	Excessive sedation. Sedative effect of both drugs may be increased.

POSSIBLE INTERACTION WITH OTHER SUBSTANCES

INTERACTS WITH	COMBINED EFFECT
Alcohol:	Excess sedation. Use caution.
Beverages: Caffeine-containing drinks.	Avoid. Decreased antianxiety effect of buspirone.
Cocaine:	Avoid. Decreased antianxiety effect of buspirone.
Foods:	None expected.
Marijuana:	Avoid. Decreased antianxiety effect of buspirone.
Tobacco:	Avoid. Decreased antianxiety effect of buspirone.

BUSULFAN

BRAND NAMES

Myleran

BASIC INFORMATION

Habit forming? No
Prescription needed? Yes
Available as generic? No
Drug class: Antineoplastic, immunosuppressant

USES

- Treatment for some kinds of cancer.
- Suppresses immune response after transplant and in immune disorders.

DOSAGE & USAGE INFORMATION

How to take:
Tablet—Swallow with liquid after light meal. Don't drink fluids with meals. Drink extra fluids between meals. Avoid sweet or fatty foods.

When to take:
At the same time each day.

If you forget a dose:
Take as soon as you remember. Never double dose.

What drug does:
Inhibits abnormal cell reproduction. May suppress immune system.

Time lapse before drug works:
Up to 6 weeks for full effect.

Continued next column

OVERDOSE

SYMPTOMS:
Bleeding, chills, fever, collapse, stupor, seizure.
WHAT TO DO:

- **Dial 911 (emergency) for an ambulance or medical help or poison center 1-800-222-1222. Then give first aid immediately.**
- **If patient is unconscious and not breathing, give mouth-to-mouth breathing. If there is no heartbeat, use cardiac massage and mouth-to-mouth breathing (CPR). Don't try to make patient vomit. If you can't get help quickly, take patient to nearest emergency facility.**
- **See emergency information on inside covers.**

Don't take with:
Any other medicine without consulting your doctor or pharmacist.

POSSIBLE ADVERSE REACTIONS OR SIDE EFFECTS

SYMPTOMS	WHAT TO DO
Life-threatening: In case of overdose, see previous column.	
Common:	
• Unusual bleeding or bruising, mouth sores with sore throat, chills and fever, black stools, lip sores, menstrual irregularities.	Discontinue. Call doctor right away.
• Hair loss.	Continue. Call doctor when convenient.
• Nausea, vomiting, diarrhea (almost always occurs), tiredness, weakness.	Continue. Tell doctor at next visit.
Infrequent:	
• Mental confusion, shortness of breath.	Continue. Call doctor when convenient.
• Cough, joint pain, dizziness, appetite loss.	Continue. Tell doctor at next visit.
Rare:	
• Jaundice, cataracts, symptoms of myasthenia gravis.*	Discontinue. Call doctor right away.
• Swollen breasts.	Continue. Call doctor when convenient.

WARNINGS & PRECAUTIONS

Don't take if:
- You have had hypersensitivity to alkylating antineoplastic drugs.
- Your physician has not explained the serious nature of your medical problem and risks of taking this medicine.

Before you start, consult your doctor:
- If you have gout.
- If you have had kidney stones.
- If you have active infection.
- If you have impaired kidney or liver function.
- If you have taken other antineoplastic drugs or had radiation treatment in last 3 weeks.

Over age 60:
Adverse reactions and side effects may be more frequent and severe than in younger persons.

Pregnancy:
Consult doctor. Risk to child is significant. Risk category D (see page xviii).

Breast-feeding:
Drug passes into milk. Don't nurse.

Infants & children:
Use only under care of medical supervisors who are experienced in anticancer drugs.

Prolonged use:
- Adverse reactions more likely the longer drug is required.
- Talk to your doctor about the need for follow-up medical examinations or laboratory studies to check complete blood counts (white blood cell count, platelet count, red blood cell count, hemoglobin, hematocrit), serum uric acid.

Skin & sunlight:
No problems expected.

Driving, piloting or hazardous work:
No problems expected.

Discontinuing:
Don't discontinue without doctor's advice until you complete prescribed dose, even though symptoms diminish or disappear. Some side effects may follow discontinuing. Report to doctor blurred vision, convulsions, confusion, persistent headache.

Others:
- Advise any doctor or dentist whom you consult that you take this medicine.
- May increase chance of developing lung or blood problems.

POSSIBLE INTERACTION WITH OTHER DRUGS

GENERIC NAME OR DRUG CLASS	COMBINED EFFECT
Antigout drugs*	Decreased antigout effect.
Antineoplastic drugs, other*	Increased effect of all drugs (may be beneficial).
Chloramphenicol	Increased likelihood of toxic effects of both drugs.
Clozapine	Toxic effect on bone marrow.
Lovastatin	Increased heart and kidney damage.
Tiopronin	Increased risk of toxicity to bone marrow.
Vaccines, live or killed	Increased risk of toxicity or reduced effectiveness of vaccine.

POSSIBLE INTERACTION WITH OTHER SUBSTANCES

INTERACTS WITH	COMBINED EFFECT
Alcohol:	May increase chance of intestinal bleeding.
Beverages:	None expected.
Cocaine:	Increases chance of toxicity.
Foods:	Reduces irritation in stomach.
Marijuana:	None expected.
Tobacco:	Increases lung toxicity.

*See Glossary

BUTORPHANOL

BRAND NAMES

Stadol NS

BASIC INFORMATION

Habit forming? Yes
Prescription needed? Yes
Available as generic? No
Drug class: Narcotic analgesic

USES

- Treatment for migraine headache pain and postoperative pain.
- Treatment for other types of pain for which a narcotic analgesic is appropriate.

DOSAGE & USAGE INFORMATION

How to take:
Nasal spray—Spray in one nostril using the metered-dose pump.

When to take:
For pain as directed by your doctor. Usual treatment consists of one dose in one nostril followed by a second dose in 60 to 90 minutes if pain persists. Your doctor may direct that the initial 2-dose sequence may be repeated in 3 to 4 hours as needed.

If you forget a dose:
Unlikely to be a problem since the drug is taken for pain and not routinely.

What drug does:
Blocks the pain impulses at specific sites in the brain and spinal cord.

Time lapse before drug works:
Within 15 minutes of the first dose.

Don't take with:
Any other medicine without consulting your doctor or pharmacist.

OVERDOSE

SYMPTOMS:
Heartbeat irregularities, breathing difficulty, coma.
WHAT TO DO:
- **Dial 911 (emergency) for an ambulance or medical help or poison center 1-800-222-1222. Then give first aid immediately.**
- **See emergency information on inside covers.**

POSSIBLE ADVERSE REACTIONS OR SIDE EFFECTS

SYMPTOMS	WHAT TO DO
Life-threatening: In case of overdose, see previous column.	
Common: Drowsiness, dizziness, nausea or vomiting, nasal congestion or irritation.	Discontinue. Call doctor when convenient.
Infrequent: Constipation (with continued use), faintness, high or low blood pressure.	Discontinue. Call doctor when convenient.
Rare:	
• Taste changes, ear ringing, dry mouth.	No action necessary.
• Difficult breathing, heart palpitations.	Discontinue. Call doctor right away.

WARNINGS & PRECAUTIONS

Don't take if:
You are allergic to butorphanol or the preservative benzethonium chloride*, which is used in the manufacture of the drug.

Before you start, consult your doctor:
- If you have a respiratory disorder or a central nervous system disease.
- If you have had adverse reactions to other narcotics*.
- If you have a history of emotional problems.
- If you have heart, kidney or liver disease.

Over age 60:
Adverse reactions and side effects (particularly dizziness) may be more frequent and severe than in younger persons.

Pregnancy:
Risk category C (see page xviii). Decide with your doctor if drug benefits justify any possible risk to unborn child.

Breast-feeding:
Drug may pass into milk. Decide with your doctor if you should continue breast-feeding while taking this drug.

Infants & children:
Not recommended for children under age 18. Safety and effectiveness have not been established.

Prolonged use:
Long-term use effects are unknown. Probably habit forming. Consult with your doctor on a regular basis while using this drug.

Skin & sunlight:
No special problems expected.

Driving, piloting or hazardous work:
Don't drive or pilot aircraft until you learn how medicine affects you. Don't work around dangerous machinery. Don't climb ladders or work in high places. Danger increases if you drink alcohol or take medicine affecting alertness and reflexes.

Discontinuing:
Don't discontinue this drug after prolonged use without consulting doctor. Dosage may require a gradual reduction before stopping to avoid any withdrawal symptoms.

Others:
- When first using this drug, get up slowly from a sitting or lying position to avoid any dizziness, faintness or lightheadedness.
- Advise any doctor or dentist whom you consult that you take this medicine.
- Take medicine only as directed. Do not increase or reduce dosage without doctor's approval.

POSSIBLE INTERACTION WITH OTHER DRUGS

GENERIC NAME OR DRUG CLASS	COMBINED EFFECT
Central nervous system (CNS) depressants*, other	Increased sedative effect.
Oxymetazoline	Delays start of butorphanol effect.

POSSIBLE INTERACTION WITH OTHER SUBSTANCES

INTERACTS WITH	COMBINED EFFECT
Alcohol:	Increased sedative affect. Avoid.
Beverages:	None expected.
Cocaine:	Effect not known. Best to avoid.
Foods:	None expected.
Marijuana:	Effect not known. Best to avoid.
Tobacco:	None expected.

*See Glossary

CAFFEINE

BRAND NAMES

See complete list of brand names in the *Generic and Brand Name Directory*, page 862.

BASIC INFORMATION

Habit forming? Yes
Prescription needed? No
Available as generic? Yes
Drug class: Stimulant (xanthine), vasoconstrictor

USES

- Treatment for drowsiness and fatigue (occasional use only).
- Treatment for migraine and other vascular headaches in combination with ergot.

DOSAGE & USAGE INFORMATION

How to take:
- Tablet or liquid—Swallow with liquid or food to lessen stomach irritation. If you can't swallow whole, crumble tablet and take with liquid or food.
- Extended-release capsules—Swallow whole with liquid.
- Powder—Stir powder into water or other liquid. The powder may also be placed on the tongue and then followed by liquid.

When to take:
At the same times each day.

If you forget a dose:
Take as soon as you remember up to 2 hours late. If more than 2 hours, wait for next scheduled dose (don't double this dose).

What drug does:
- Constricts blood vessel walls.
- Stimulates central nervous system.

Continued next column

OVERDOSE

SYMPTOMS:
Excitement, insomnia, rapid heartbeat (infants can have slow heartbeat), confusion, fever, hallucinations, convulsions, coma.
WHAT TO DO:
- **Dial 911 (emergency) for an ambulance or medical help or poison center 1-800-222-1222. Then give first aid immediately.**
- **See emergency information at end of book.**

Time lapse before drug works:
30 minutes.

Don't take with:
Nonprescription drugs without consulting your doctor or pharmacist.

POSSIBLE ADVERSE REACTIONS OR SIDE EFFECTS

SYMPTOMS	WHAT TO DO
Life-threatening:	
In case of overdose, see previous column.	
Common:	
• Rapid heartbeat, low blood sugar (hunger, anxiety, cold sweats, rapid pulse) with tremor, irritability (mild).	Discontinue. Call doctor right away.
• Nervousness, insomnia.	Continue. Tell doctor at next visit.
• Increased urination.	No action necessary.
Infrequent:	
• Confusion, irritability (severe).	Discontinue. Call doctor right away.
• Nausea, indigestion, burning feeling in stomach.	Continue. Call doctor when convenient.
Rare:	
None expected.	

WARNINGS & PRECAUTIONS

Don't take if:
- You are allergic to any stimulant.
- You have heart disease.
- You have active peptic ulcer of stomach or duodenum.

Before you start, consult your doctor:
- If you have irregular heartbeat.
- If you have hypoglycemia (low blood sugar).
- If you have epilepsy.
- If you have a seizure disorder.
- If you have high blood pressure.
- If you have insomnia.

Over age 60:
Adverse reactions and side effects may be more frequent and severe than in younger persons.

Pregnancy:
Decide with your doctor if drug benefits justify risk to unborn child. Risk category C (see page xviii).

Breast-feeding:
Drug passes into milk. Avoid drug or discontinue nursing until you finish medicine. Consult doctor for advice on maintaining milk supply.

Infants & children:
Not recommended.

Prolonged use:
Stomach ulcers.

Skin & sunlight:
No problems expected.

Driving, piloting or hazardous work:
No problems expected.

Discontinuing:
Will cause withdrawal symptoms of headache, irritability, drowsiness. Discontinue gradually if you use caffeine for a month or more.

Others:
Consult your doctor if drowsiness or fatigue continues, recurs or is not relieved by caffeine.

POSSIBLE INTERACTION WITH OTHER DRUGS

GENERIC NAME OR DRUG CLASS	COMBINED EFFECT
Caffeine-containing drugs, other	Increased risk of overstimulation.
Central nervous system (CNS) stimulants*	Increased risk of overstimulation.
Cimetidine	Increased caffeine effect.
Contraceptives, oral*	Increased caffeine effect.
Isoniazid	Increased caffeine effect.
Monoamine oxidase (MAO) inhibitors*	Dangerous blood pressure rise.
Sympathomimetics*	Overstimulation.
Xanthines*	Increased risk of overstimulation.

POSSIBLE INTERACTION WITH OTHER SUBSTANCES

INTERACTS WITH	COMBINED EFFECT
Alcohol:	Decreased alcohol effect.
Beverages: Caffeine drinks (coffee, tea or soft drinks).	Increased caffeine effect. Use caution.
Cocaine	Convulsions or excessive nervousness.
Foods:	None expected.
Marijuana:	Increased effect of both drugs. May lead to dangerous, rapid heartbeat. Avoid.
Tobacco:	Increased heartbeat. Avoid. Decreased caffeine effect.

*See Glossary

CALCIPOTRIENE

BRAND NAMES

Dovonex

BASIC INFORMATION

Habit forming? No
Prescription needed? Yes
Available as generic? No
Drug class: Antipsoriatic

USES

Treats discoid or "plaque" psoriasis, the most common form of the disorder.

DOSAGE & USAGE INFORMATION

How to use:
Cream, ointment or topical solution—Apply a thin layer to the affected skin. Rub in gently and completely. It should not be used on the face.

When to use:
Twice a day.

If you forget a dose:
Apply ointment as soon as you remember, then return to regular schedule.

What drug does:
Calcipotriene is a vitamin D product that helps regulate skin cell production and development.

Time lapse before drug works:
2 weeks. May take up to 8 weeks for maximum benefits that can include marked improvement in symptoms for most patients or complete clearing for others.

Don't use with:
Other topical or systemic drugs without consulting with your doctor or pharmacist.

OVERDOSE

SYMPTOMS:
May be absorbed into the system through excessive topical application and increase the levels of calcium, which could cause muscle weakness, excess fatigue, depression, loss of appetite and nausea.
WHAT TO DO:
Overdose unlikely to threaten life. If symptoms occur, call doctor for instructions. If child accidentally swallows, call poison center 1-800-222-1222.

POSSIBLE ADVERSE REACTIONS OR SIDE EFFECTS

SYMPTOMS	WHAT TO DO
Life-threatening:	
None expected.	
Common:	
Irritation, burning, itching of the skin.	Discontinue. Call doctor when convenient.
Infrequent:	
Redness, dryness, peeling or skin rash, worsening of psoriasis.	Discontinue. Call doctor when convenient.
Rare:	
None expected.	

WARNINGS & PRECAUTIONS

Don't use if:
- You are allergic to calcipotriene or any of its components.
- You have hypercalcemia (excess of calcium in the system).

Before you start, consult your doctor:
If you have had allergic reactions to other topical drugs.

Over age 60:
Adverse reactions and side effects may be more frequent and severe than in younger persons.

Pregnancy:
Decide with your doctor if drug benefits justify any possible risk to unborn child. Risk category C (see page xviii).

Breast-feeding:
Unknown if drug passes into milk. Avoid nursing until you finish medicine. Consult doctor for advice on maintaining milk supply.

Infants & children:
Safety in children has not been established. Use only under close medical supervision. Adverse reactions and side effects may be more frequent and severe.

Prolonged use:
Not intended for long-term use. Usual length of treatment is 8 weeks. If your doctor recommends continued treatment with calcipotriene, discuss the need for follow-up laboratory studies to check calcium levels.

Skin & sunlight:
No special problems expected.

Driving, piloting or hazardous work:
No special problems expected.

Discontinuing:
No special problems expected.

Others:
Wash hands after applying the drug.

POSSIBLE INTERACTION WITH OTHER DRUGS

GENERIC NAME OR DRUG CLASS	COMBINED EFFECT
None expected.	

POSSIBLE INTERACTION WITH OTHER SUBSTANCES

INTERACTS WITH	COMBINED EFFECT
Alcohol:	None expected.
Beverages:	None expected.
Cocaine:	None expected.
Foods:	None expected.
Marijuana:	None expected.
Tobacco:	None expected.

CALCITONIN

BRAND NAMES

Miacalcin

BASIC INFORMATION

Habit forming? No
Prescription needed? Yes
Available as generic? No
Drug class: Osteoporosis therapy

USES

Treatment for postmenopausal osteoporosis (thinning of bones) in females. Osteoporosis is a major cause of bone fractures.

DOSAGE & USAGE INFORMATION

How to take:
Nasal spray—One spray per day in a nostril, alternating nostrils daily. Follow directions on label about activating and using the pump supplied with the medication.

When to take:
At the same time each day.

If you forget a dose:
Take as soon as you remember up to 12 hours late. If more than 12 hours, wait for next scheduled dose (don't double this dose).

What drug does:
The exact mechanism is not fully understood. It slows down the loss of bone tissue and increases bone mass in women with osteoporosis.

Time lapse before drug works:
Up to 6 months or longer.

Don't take with:
Any other prescription or nonprescription drug without consulting your doctor or pharmacist.

OVERDOSE

SYMPTOMS:
None reported.
WHAT TO DO:
Overdose unlikely to threaten life. If person takes much larger amount than prescribed, call doctor, poison center 1-800-222-1222 or hospital emergency room for instructions.

POSSIBLE ADVERSE REACTIONS OR SIDE EFFECTS

SYMPTOMS	WHAT TO DO
Life-threatening:	
Rare allergic reaction—Breathing difficulty; swelling of hands, feet, face, mouth, neck; skin rash.	Discontinue. Seek emergency treatment.
Common:	
Nasal inflammation, dryness, crusting, sores, irritation, itching, redness; swollen, runny, stuffy nose; small amount of nasal bleeding, discomfort, tenderness.	Continue. Call doctor when convenient.
Infrequent:	
Back pain, joint pain, headache, mild bloody nose, flushing, nausea, sinus infection.	Continue. Call doctor when convenient.
Rare:	
None expected.	

WARNINGS & PRECAUTIONS

Don't take if:
You are allergic to calcitonin.

Before you start, consult your doctor:
If you are allergic to any medication, food or other substance. A skin test may be performed before beginning treatment with calcitonin.

Over age 60:
No special problems expected.

Pregnancy:
Not normally used in premenopausal women. Risk category C (see page xviii).

Breast-feeding:
Not normally used in premenopausal women.

Infants & children:
Not recommended for this age group.

Prolonged use:
- No special problems expected.
- Visit your doctor regularly to determine if the drug is continuing to control bone loss and to have periodic nasal examinations to check for ulceration or irritation.

Skin & sunlight:
No special problems expected.

Driving, piloting or hazardous work:
No special problems expected.

Discontinuing:
Don't discontinue without your doctor's approval.

Others:
- In addition to taking the drug, weight-bearing exercise and adequate dietary intake of calcium and vitamin D are essential in preventing bone loss. Dietary supplements of 1000 mg elemental calcium and 400 I.U. vitamin D daily may be recommended by your doctor.
- Advise any doctor or dentist whom you consult that you take this medicine.
- May affect the results of some medical tests.

POSSIBLE INTERACTION WITH OTHER DRUGS

GENERIC NAME OR DRUG CLASS	COMBINED EFFECT
None significant.	

POSSIBLE INTERACTION WITH OTHER SUBSTANCES

INTERACTS WITH	COMBINED EFFECT
Alcohol:	None expected.
Beverages:	None expected.
Cocaine:	None expected.
Foods:	None expected.
Marijuana:	None expected.
Tobacco:	None expected.

CALCIUM CHANNEL BLOCKERS

GENERIC AND BRAND NAMES

See complete list of generic and brand names in *Generic and Brand Name Directory*, page 862.

BASIC INFORMATION

Habit forming? No
Prescription needed? Yes
Available as generic? Yes
Drug class: Calcium channel blocker, antiarrhythmic, antianginal

USES

- Used for angina attacks, irregular heartbeat, high blood pressure.
- Treats migraine.

DOSAGE & USAGE INFORMATION

How to take:
- Tablet or capsule—Swallow with liquid. You may chew or crush tablet.
- Extended-release tablets or capsules—Swallow each dose whole with liquid; do not crush tablet or open capsule.

When to take:
At the same times each day. Take verapamil with food.

If you forget a dose:
Take as soon as you remember up to 2 hours late. If more than 2 hours, wait for next scheduled dose (don't double this dose).

What drug does:
- Reduces work that heart must perform.
- Reduces normal artery pressure.
- Increases oxygen to heart muscle.

Continued next column

OVERDOSE

SYMPTOMS:
Unusually fast or unusually slow heartbeat, loss of consciousness, cardiac arrest.
WHAT TO DO:
- **Dial 911 (emergency) for an ambulance or medical help or poison center 1-800-222-1222. Then give first aid immediately.**
- **If patient is unconscious and not breathing, give mouth-to-mouth breathing. If there is no heartbeat, use cardiac massage and mouth-to-mouth breathing (CPR). Don't try to make patient vomit. If you can't get help quickly, take patient to nearest emergency facility.**
- **See emergency information at end of book.**

Time lapse before drug works:
1 to 2 hours.

Don't take with:
Any other medicine without consulting your doctor or pharmacist.

POSSIBLE ADVERSE REACTIONS OR SIDE EFFECTS

SYMPTOMS	WHAT TO DO
Life-threatening: In case of overdose, see previous column.	
Common:	
Tiredness.	Continue. Tell doctor at next visit.
Infrequent:	
• Unusually fast or unusually slow heartbeat, wheezing, cough, shortness of breath.	Discontinue. Call doctor right away.
• Dizziness; numbness or tingling in hands and feet; swollen feet, ankles or legs; difficult urination.	Continue. Call doctor when convenient.
• Nausea, constipation.	Continue. Tell doctor at next visit.
Rare:	
• Fainting, depression, psychosis, rash, jaundice.	Discontinue. Call doctor right away.
• Headache, insomnia, vivid dreams, hair loss.	Continue. Tell doctor at next visit.

WARNINGS & PRECAUTIONS

Don't take if:
- You are allergic to calcium channel blockers.
- You have very low blood pressure.

Before you start, consult your doctor:
- If you have kidney or liver disease.
- If you have high blood pressure.
- If you have heart disease other than coronary artery disease.

Over age 60:
Adverse reactions and side effects may be more frequent and severe than in younger persons.

Pregnancy:
Decide with your doctor if drug benefits justify risk to unborn child. Risk category C (see page xviii).

Breast-feeding:
Safety not established. Avoid if possible. Consult doctor.

Infants & children:
Not recommended.

Prolonged use:
Talk to your doctor about the need for follow-up medical examinations or laboratory studies to check blood pressure, liver function, kidney function, ECG*.

Skin & sunlight:
One or more drugs in this group may cause rash or intensity sunburn in areas exposed to sun or ultraviolet light (photosensitivity reaction). Avoid overexposure. Notify doctor if reaction occurs.

Driving, piloting or hazardous work:
Avoid if you feel dizzy. Otherwise, no problems expected.

Discontinuing:
Don't discontinue without doctor's advice until you complete prescribed dose, even though symptoms diminish or disappear.

Others:
- Learn to check your own pulse rate. If it drops to 50 beats per minute or lower, don't take drug until your consult your doctor.
- Advise any doctor or dentist whom you consult that you take this medicine.

POSSIBLE INTERACTION WITH OTHER DRUGS

GENERIC NAME OR DRUG CLASS	COMBINED EFFECT
Angiotensin-converting enzyme (ACE) inhibitors*	Possible excessive potassium in blood. Dosages may require adjustment.
Antiarrhythmics*	Possible increased effect and toxicity of each drug.
Anticoagulants, oral*	Possible increased anticoagulant effect.
Anticonvulsants, hydantoin*	Increased anti-convulsant effect.
Antihypertensives*	Blood pressure drop. Dosages may require adjustment.
Beta-adrenergic blocking agents*	Possible irregular heartbeat and con-gestive heart failure.
Calcium (large doses)	Possible decreased effect of calcium channel blocker.
Carbamazepine	May increase carba-mazepine effect and toxicity.
Cimetidine	Possible increased effect of calcium channel blocker.
Colesevelam	Unknown effect consult doctor.
Cyclosporine	Increased cyclosporine toxicity.
Digitalis preparations*	Increased digitalis effect. May need to reduce dose.
Disopyramide	May cause danger-ously slow, fast or irregular heartbeat.
Diuretics*	Dangerous blood pressure drop. Dosages may require adjustment.
Dofetilide	Increased risk of heart problems.
Encainide	Increased effect of toxicity on heart muscle.
Fluvoxamine	Slow heartbeat (with diltiazem).
HMG-CoA reductase inhibitors	Increased effect of HMG-CoA reductase inhibitor.
Hypokalemia-causing medications*	Increased anti-hypertensive effect.
Leukotriene modifiers	Increased effect of calcium channel blocker.
Lithium	Possible decreased lithium effect.

Continued on page 907

POSSIBLE INTERACTION WITH OTHER SUBSTANCES

INTERACTS WITH	COMBINED EFFECT
Alcohol:	Dangerously low blood pressure. Avoid.
Beverages: Grapefruit juice.	Possible increased drug effect.
Cocaine:	Possible irregular heartbeat. Avoid.
Foods:	None expected.
Marijuana:	Possible irregular heartbeat. Avoid.
Tobacco:	Possible rapid heart-beat. Avoid.

*See Glossary

CALCIUM SUPPLEMENTS

GENERIC AND BRAND NAMES

See complete list of generic and brand names in the *Generic and Brand Name Directory*, page 862.

BASIC INFORMATION

Habit forming? No
Prescription needed? For some
Available as generic? Yes
Drug class: Antihypocalcemic, dietary replacement

USES

- Treats or prevents osteoporosis (thin, porous, easily fractured bones). Frequently prescribed with estrogen beginning at menopause.
- Helps heart, muscle and nervous system to work properly.
- Dietary supplement when calcium ingestion is insufficient or there is a deficiency such as osteomalacia or rickets.

DOSAGE & USAGE INFORMATION

How to take:
- Take in addition to foods high in calcium (milk, yogurt, sardines, cheese, canned salmon, turnip greens, broccoli, shrimp, tofu).
- Tablet—Swallow with liquid or food to lessen stomach irritation. If you can't swallow whole, crumble tablet and take with food or liquid.
- Syrup—Take before meals.
- Suspension—Swallow with liquid or food to lessen stomach irritation.

When to take:
As directed. Don't take within 2 hours of any other medicine you take by mouth.

If you forget a dose:
Use as soon as you remember.

Continued next column

OVERDOSE

SYMPTOMS:
Confusion, irregular heartbeat, depression, bone pain, coma.
WHAT TO DO:
- **Dial 911 (emergency) for an ambulance or medical help or poison center 1-800-222-1222. Then give first aid immediately.**
- **See emergency information on inside covers.**

What drug does:
- Participates in metabolism of all activities essential for normal life and function of cells.
- Provides calcium necessary for bone, nerve function.

Time lapse before drug works:
15 to 30 minutes.

Don't take with:
- Any other medicine until 2 hours have passed since taking calcium.
- Any other medicine without consulting your doctor or pharmacist.

POSSIBLE ADVERSE REACTIONS OR SIDE EFFECTS

SYMPTOMS	WHAT TO DO
Life-threatening:	
Irregular or very slow heart rate.	Discontinue. Seek emergency treatment.
Common:	
None expected.	
Infrequent:	
Constipation, diarrhea, drowsiness, headache, appetite loss, dry mouth, weakness.	Discontinue. Call doctor right away.
Rare:	
Frequent, painful or difficult urination; increased thirst; nausea, vomiting; rash; urine frequency increased and volume larger; confusion; high blood pressure; eyes sensitive to light.	Discontinue. Call doctor right away.

WARNINGS & PRECAUTIONS

Don't take if:
- You are allergic to calcium.
- You have a high blood calcium level.

Before you start, consult your doctor:
If you have diarrhea, heart disease, kidney stones, kidney disease, sarcoidosis, malabsorption.

Over age 60:
No problems expected.

Pregnancy:
Consult doctor. Risk category C (see page xviii).

Breast-feeding:
No problems expected. Consult doctor.

Infants & children:
Use only under close medical supervision.

Prolonged use:
- Side effects more likely.
- Talk to your doctor about the need for follow-up medical examinations or laboratory studies to check serum calcium determinations, blood pressure, urine.

Skin & sunlight:
No problems expected.

Driving, piloting or hazardous work:
No problems expected.

Discontinuing:
No problems expected.

Others:
- Exercise, along with vitamin D from sunshine and calcium, helps prevent osteoporosis.
- Don't use bone meal or dolomite as a source for calcium supplement (they may contain lead).

POSSIBLE INTERACTION WITH OTHER DRUGS

GENERIC NAME OR DRUG CLASS	COMBINED EFFECT
Alendronate	Decreased alendronate effect. Take calcium 30 minutes after alendronate.
Anticoagulants, oral*	Decreased anticoagulant effect.
Calcitonin	Decreased calcitonin effect.
Calcium-containing medicines, other	Increased calcium effect.
Chlorpromazine	Decreased chlorpromazine effect.
Contraceptives, oral*	May increase absorption of calcium—frequently a desirable combined effect.
Corticosteroids*	Decreased calcium absorption and effect.
Digitalis preparations*	Decreased digitalis effect.
Diuretics, thiazide*	Increased calcium in blood.
Estrogens*	May increase absorption of calcium—frequently a desirable combined effect.
Etidronate	Decreased etidronate absorption. Take drugs 2 hours apart.
Iron supplements*	Decreased iron effect.
Meperidine	Increased meperidine effect.
Mexiletine	May slow elimination of mexiletine and cause need to adjust dosage.
Nalidixic acid	Decreased effect of nalidixic acid.
Nicardipine	Possible decreased nicardipine effect.
Nimodipine	Possible decreased nimodipine effect.
Oxyphenbutazone	Decreased oxyphenbutazone effect.
Para-aminosalicylic acid (PAS)	Decreased PAS effect.
Penicillins*	Decreased penicillin effect.
Pentobarbital	Decreased pentobarbital effect.
Phenylbutazone	Decreased phenylbutazone effect.
Phenytoin	Decreased phenytoin absorption.
Propafenone	Increased effects of both drugs and increased risk of toxicity.
Pseudoephedrine	Increased pseudoephedrine effect.

Continued on page 908

POSSIBLE INTERACTION WITH OTHER SUBSTANCES

INTERACTS WITH	COMBINED EFFECT
Alcohol:	Decreased absorption of calcium.
Beverages:	None expected.
Cocaine:	No proven problems.
Foods: Don't take within 1 or 2 hours of eating.	Decreased absorption of calcium.
Marijuana:	Decreased absorption of calcium.
Tobacco:	Decreased absorption of calcium.

***See Glossary**

CAPECITABINE

BRAND NAMES

Xeloda

BASIC INFORMATION

Habit forming? No
Prescription needed? Yes
Available as generic? No
Drug class: Antineoplastic

USES

Treats metastatic breast cancer in patients resistant to both paclitaxel and an anthracycline containing chemotherapy regimen.

DOSAGE & USAGE INFORMATION

How to take:
Tablets—Swallow with water. If you can't swallow whole, crumble tablet and take with liquid or food.

When to take:
Take in two divided doses every 12 hours after a meal and with water.

If you forget a dose:
Do not take missed dose or double next dose. Continue your regular dosing schedule and consult your doctor.

What drug does:
Capecitabine is converted in the body to the substance 5-fluorouracil. In some patients, this substance kills cancer cells and decreases the size of the tumor.

Time lapse before drug works:
Results may not show for several months.

Don't take with:
Any other prescription or nonprescription drug without consulting your doctor.

OVERDOSE

SYMPTOMS:
Nausea, vomiting, diarrhea, gastrointestinal irritation and bleeding, and bone marrow depression.
WHAT TO DO:
Overdose unlikely to threaten life. If person takes much larger amount than prescribed, call doctor, poison center 1-800-222-1222 or hospital emergency room for instructions.

POSSIBLE ADVERSE REACTIONS OR SIDE EFFECTS

SYMPTOMS	WHAT TO DO
Life-threatening:	
None expected.	
Common:	
• Diarrhea (if you have more than 4 bowel movements in a day or any diarrhea at night); vomiting (more than once a day); nausea; loss of appetite; stomatitis (pain, redness or swelling in mouth); hand and foot syndrome (pain, redness or swelling in hands or feet); fever (100.5 or higher).	Discontinue. Call doctor right away.
• Diarrhea, nausea and vomiting, rash, dry or itchy skin, tiredness, weakness, dizziness, headache.	Continue. Call doctor when convenient.
Infrequent:	
Jaundice.	Continue. Call doctor right away.
Rare:	
None expected.	

WARNINGS & PRECAUTIONS

Don't take if:
You are allergic to capecitabine.

Before you start, consult your doctor:
- If you have an infection or any other medical problem.
- If you have heart problems.
- If you are taking folic acid.
- If you are pregnant or if you plan to become pregnant.
- If you have had liver problems.

Over age 60:
Adverse reactions and side effects, especially gastrointestinal, may be more severe and frequent than in younger patients.

Pregnancy:
Animal studies show fetal abnormalities and increased risk of abortion. Discuss with your doctor whether drug benefits justify risk to unborn child. Risk category D (see page xviii).

Breast-feeding:
Not known if drug passes into milk. Avoid drug or discontinue nursing until you finish medicine. Consult doctor for advice on maintaining milk supply.

Infants & children:
Safety and effectiveness of use in children not established.

Prolonged use:
Talk to your doctor about the need for follow-up medical examinations or laboratory studies.

Skin & sunlight:
No problems expected.

Driving, piloting or hazardous work:
Avoid if you feel side effects such as nausea and vomiting.

Discontinuing:
Your doctor will determine the schedule.

Others:
Advise any doctor or dentist whom you consult that you take this medicine.

POSSIBLE INTERACTION WITH OTHER DRUGS

GENERIC NAME OR DRUG CLASS	COMBINED EFFECT
Antacids	Increased risk of capecitabine toxicity.
Leucovorin	Increased risk of capecitabine toxicity.

POSSIBLE INTERACTION WITH OTHER SUBSTANCES

INTERACTS WITH	COMBINED EFFECT
Alcohol:	None expected.
Beverages:	None expected.
Cocaine:	Effects unknown. Avoid.
Foods:	None expected.
Marijuana:	Effects unknown. Avoid.
Tobacco:	None expected.

CAPSAICIN

BRAND NAMES

ArthriCare
ARTH-RX
Axsain
Capsagel
Dura-Patch
Dura Patch Joint
Methacin
Zotrix
Zotrix-HP

BASIC INFORMATION

Habit forming? No
Prescription needed? No
Available as generic? Yes
Drug class: Analgesic (topical)

USES

- Treats neuralgias, such as pain that occurs following shingles (herpes zoster) or neuropathy of the feet, ankles and fingers (common in diabetes).
- Treats discomfort caused by arthritis.

DOSAGE & USAGE INFORMATION

How to use:
- Cream—Apply a small amount and rub carefully on the affected areas. Use every day. Wash hands after applying. Don't apply to irritated skin. Don't bandage over treated areas.
- Patch—Follow package instructions for proper application.

When to use:
Apply 3 or 4 times a day.

If you forget a dose:
Use as soon as you remember.

What drug does:
Depletes the nerves of the substance that triggers pain sensation.

Time lapse before drug works:
Begins to work immediately. Frequently takes 2 to 3 weeks for full benefit, but may take up to 6 or 8 weeks.

Don't use with:
No problems expected.

OVERDOSE

SYMPTOMS:
None expected.
WHAT TO DO:
Not intended for internal use. If child accidentally swallows, call poison center 1-800-222-1222.

POSSIBLE ADVERSE REACTIONS OR SIDE EFFECTS

SYMPTOMS	WHAT TO DO
Life-threatening: None expected.	
Common: Stinging or burning sensation at application site.	Nothing. It usually improves in 2 to 3 days or becomes less severe the longer you use the drug.
Infrequent: None expected.	
Rare: None expected.	

WARNINGS & PRECAUTIONS

Don't use if:
You are allergic to capsaicin or to the fruit of capsaicin plants (for example, hot peppers).

Before you start, consult your doctor:
If you have any allergies.

Over age 60:
No problems expected.

Pregnancy:
Consult doctor. Risk category C (see page xviii).

Breast-feeding:
No problems expected. Consult doctor.

Infants & children:
Not recommended for children under age 2.

Prolonged use:
No problems expected.

Skin & sunlight:
No problems expected.

Driving, piloting or hazardous work:
No problems expected.

Discontinuing:
Discontinue if there are no signs of improvement within a month.

Others:
- Capsaicin is not a local anesthetic*.
- Although capsaicin may help relieve the pain of neuropathy, it does not cure any disorder.
- If you accidently get some capsaicin in your eye, flush with water.

POSSIBLE INTERACTION WITH OTHER DRUGS

GENERIC NAME OR DRUG CLASS	COMBINED EFFECT
None expected.	

POSSIBLE INTERACTION WITH OTHER SUBSTANCES

INTERACTS WITH	COMBINED EFFECT
Alcohol:	None expected.
Beverages:	None expected.
Cocaine:	None expected.
Foods:	None expected.
Marijuana:	None expected.
Tobacco:	None expected.

***See Glossary**

CARBAMAZEPINE

BRAND NAMES

Apo-Carbamazepine
Epitol
Mazepine
Novocarbamaz
PMS Carbamazepine
Taro-Carbamazepine
Tegretol
Tegretol Chewtabs
Tegretol CR

BASIC INFORMATION

Habit forming? No
Prescription needed? Yes
Available as generic? Yes
Drug class: Analgesic, anticonvulsant, antimanic agent

USES

- Decreases frequency, severity and duration of attacks of tic douloureux*.
- Treats bipolar (manic-depressive) disorder.
- Prevents seizures.
- Used for pain relief, alcohol withdrawal.

DOSAGE & USAGE INFORMATION

How to take:
Regular or chewable tablet—Swallow with liquid or food to lessen stomach irritation.

When to take:
At the same times each day.

If you forget a dose:
Take as soon as you remember up to 2 hours late. If more than 2 hours, wait for next scheduled dose (don't double this dose).

Continued next column

OVERDOSE

SYMPTOMS:
Involuntary movements, drowsiness, irregular heartbeat, irregular bleeding, decreased urination, decreased blood pressure, dilated pupils, flushed skin, stupor, coma.
WHAT TO DO:

- **Dial 911 (emergency) for an ambulance or medical help or poison center 1-800-222-1222. Then give first aid immediately.**
- **If patient is unconscious and not breathing, give mouth-to-mouth breathing. If there is no heartbeat, use cardiac massage and mouth-to-mouth breathing (CPR). Don't try to make patient vomit. If you can't get help quickly, take patient to nearest emergency facility.**
- **See emergency information at end of book.**

What drug does:
Reduces excitability of nerve fibers in brain, thus inhibiting repetitive spread of nerve impulses. Reduces transmission of pain messages at certain nerve terminals.

Time lapse before drug works:
- Tic douloureux—24 to 72 hours.
- Bipolar disorder—Unknown.
- Seizures—1 to 2 weeks.

Don't take with:
Any other medicine without consulting your doctor or pharmacist. May inactiviate other medications, such as birth control pills.

POSSIBLE ADVERSE REACTIONS OR SIDE EFFECTS

SYMPTOMS	WHAT TO DO
Life-threatening: In case of overdose, see previous column.	
Common:	
• Blurred vision.	Continue. Call doctor when convenient.
• Back-and-forth eye movements.	Discontinue. Call doctor right away.
Infrequent:	
• Confusion, slurred speech, fainting, depression, headache, hallucinations, hives, rash, mouth sores, sore throat, fever, unusual bleeding or bruising, unusual fatigue, jaundice.	Discontinue. Call doctor right away.
• Diarrhea, nausea, vomiting, constipation, dry mouth, impotence.	Continue. Call doctor when convenient.
Rare:	
• Breathing difficulty; irregular, pounding or slow heartbeat; chest pain; uncontrollable body jerks; numbness, weakness or tingling in hands and feet; tender, bluish legs or feet; less urine; swollen lymph glands, blood disorder (symptoms of anemia, bleeding, frequent infections).	Discontinue. Call doctor right away.
• Frequent urination, muscle pains, joint aches.	Continue. Call doctor when convenient.

WARNINGS & PRECAUTIONS

Don't take if:
- You are allergic to carbamazepine or any tricyclic antidepressant*.
- You have had liver or bone marrow disease.
- You have taken a monoamine oxidase (MAO) inhibitor* in the past 2 weeks.

Before you start, consult your doctor:
- If you have high blood pressure, thrombophlebitis or heart disease.
- If you have glaucoma.
- If you have emotional or mental problems.
- If you have liver or kidney disease.
- If you have a history of blood disorders.
- If you are taking any other medications.
- If you drink more than 2 alcoholic drinks per day.

Over age 60:
Adverse reactions and side effects may be more frequent and severe than in younger persons.

Pregnancy:
Decide with your doctor whether drug benefits justify risk to unborn child. Risk category C (see page xviii).

Breast-feeding:
Drug passes into milk. Avoid drug or discontinue nursing until you finish medicine. Consult doctor for advice on maintaining milk supply.

Infants & children:
Approved for children under age 6 with epilepsy for treatment of seizures and for trigeminal neuralgia.

Prolonged use:
- Lowers sex drive.
- Talk to your doctor about the need for follow-up medical examinations or laboratory studies to check complete blood counts (white blood cell count, platelet count, red blood cell count, hemoglobin, hematocrit), serum iron and serum levels.

Skin & sunlight:
May cause rash or intensity sunburn in areas exposed to sun or ultraviolet light (photosensitivity reaction). Avoid overexposure and use sunscreen. Notify doctor if reaction occurs.

Driving, piloting or hazardous work:
Don't drive or pilot aircraft until you learn how medicine effects you. Don't work around dangerous machinery. Don't climb ladders or work in high places. Danger increases if you drink alcohol or take medicine affecting alertness and reflexes.

Discontinuing:
Don't discontinue without doctor's advice until you complete prescribed dose, even though symptoms diminish or disappear.

Others:
- Use only if less hazardous drugs are not effective. Stay under medical supervision.
- Periodic blood tests are needed.
- Advise any doctor or dentist whom you consult that you take this medicine.

POSSIBLE INTERACTION WITH OTHER DRUGS

GENERIC NAME OR DRUG CLASS	COMBINED EFFECT
Adrenocorticoids, systemic	Decreased adreno-corticoid effect.
Anticoagulants, oral*	Decreased anti-coagulant effect.
Anticonvulsants, hydantoin* or succinimide*	Decreased effect of both drugs.
Antidepressants, tricyclic*	Confusion. Possible psychosis.
Barbiturates*	Possible increased barbiturate metabolism.
Bupropion	Decreased carba-mazepine effect. Seizure risk.
Cimetidine	Increased carba-mazepine effect.
Cisapride	Decreased carba-mazepine effect.
Citalopram	May lessen effect of citalopram.

Continued on page 908

POSSIBLE INTERACTION WITH OTHER SUBSTANCES

INTERACTS WITH	COMBINED EFFECT
Alcohol:	Increased sedative effect of alcohol. Avoid.
Beverages:	None expected.
Cocaine:	Increased adverse effects of carba-mazepine. Avoid.
Foods:	None expected.
Marijuana:	Increased adverse effects of carba-mazepine. Avoid.
Tobacco:	None expected.

***See Glossary**

CARBIDOPA & LEVODOPA

BRAND NAMES

Sinemet **Sinemet CR**

BASIC INFORMATION

Habit forming? No
Prescription needed? Yes
Available as generic? Yes
Drug class: Antiparkinsonism

USES

Controls Parkinson's disease symptoms such as rigidity, tremor and unsteady gait.

DOSAGE & USAGE INFORMATION

How to take:
- Tablet—Swallow with liquid or food to lessen stomach irritation. If you can't swallow whole, crumble tablet and take with liquid or food.
- Extended-release tablet—Swallow each dose whole; do not crumble.

When to take:
At the same times each day.

If you forget a dose:
Take as soon as you remember up to 2 hours late. If more than 2 hours, wait for next scheduled dose (don't double this dose).

What drug does:
Restores chemical balance necessary for normal nerve impulses.

Continued next column

OVERDOSE

SYMPTOMS:
Muscle twitch, spastic eyelid closure, nausea, vomiting, diarrhea, irregular and rapid pulse, weakness, fainting, confusion, agitation, hallucination, coma.

WHAT TO DO:
- **Dial 911 (emergency) for an ambulance or medical help or poison center 1-800-222-1222. Then give first aid immediately.**
- **If patient is unconscious and not breathing, give mouth-to-mouth breathing. If there is no heartbeat, use cardiac massage and mouth-to-mouth breathing (CPR). Don't try to make patient vomit. If you can't get help quickly, take patient to nearest emergency facility.**
- **See emergency information on inside covers.**

Time lapse before drug works:
2 to 3 weeks to improve; 6 weeks or longer for maximum benefit.

Don't take with:
Any other medicine without consulting your doctor or pharmacist.

POSSIBLE ADVERSE REACTIONS OR SIDE EFFECTS

SYMPTOMS	WHAT TO DO
Life-threatening:	
In case of overdose, see previous column.	
Common:	
• Mood changes, uncontrollable body movements, diarrhea.	Continue. Call doctor when convenient.
• Dry mouth, body odor.	No action necessary.
Infrequent:	
• Fainting, severe dizziness, headache, insomnia, nightmares, rash, itch, nausea, vomiting, irregular heartbeat.	Discontinue. Call doctor right away.
• Flushed face, blurred vision, muscle twitching, discolored or dark urine, difficult urination.	Continue. Call doctor when convenient.
• Constipation, tiredness.	Continue. Tell doctor at next visit.
Rare:	
• High blood pressure.	Discontinue. Call doctor right away.
• Upper abdominal pain, anemia.	Continue. Call doctor when convenient.

WARNINGS & PRECAUTIONS

Don't take if:
- You are allergic to levodopa or carbidopa.
- You have taken MAO inhibitors in past 2 weeks.
- You have glaucoma (narrow-angle type).

Before you start, consult your doctor:
- If you have diabetes or epilepsy.
- If you have had high blood pressure, heart or lung disease.
- If you have had liver or kidney disease.
- If you have a peptic ulcer.
- If you have malignant melanoma.
- If you will have surgery within 2 months, including dental surgery, requiring general or spinal anesthesia.

Over age 60:
Adverse reactions and side effects may be more frequent and severe than in younger persons.

Pregnancy:
Decide with your doctor whether drug benefits justify risk to unborn child. Risk category C (see page xviii).

Breast-feeding:
Drug filters into milk. May harm child. Avoid.

Infants & children:
Not recommended.

Prolonged use:
- May lead to uncontrolled movements of head, face, mouth, tongue, arms or legs.
- Talk to your doctor about the need for follow-up medical examinations or laboratory studies to check complete blood counts (white blood cell count, platelet count, red blood cell count, hemoglobin, hematocrit), liver function, eyes, kidney function.

Skin & sunlight:
No problems expected.

Driving, piloting or hazardous work:
Don't drive or pilot aircraft until you learn how medicine affects you. Don't work around dangerous machinery. Don't climb ladders or work in high places. Danger increases if you drink alcohol or take medicine affecting alertness and reflexes, such as antihistamines, tranquilizers, sedatives, pain medicine, narcotics and mind-altering drugs.

Discontinuing:
Don't discontinue without doctor's advice until you complete prescribed dose, even though symptoms diminish or disappear.

Others:
- Expect to start with small dose and increase gradually to lessen frequency and severity of adverse reactions.
- Advise any doctor or dentist whom you consult that you take this medicine.

POSSIBLE INTERACTION WITH OTHER DRUGS

GENERIC NAME OR DRUG CLASS	COMBINED EFFECT
Anticonvulsants*, hydantoin	Decreased effect of carbidopa and levodopa.
Antidepressants*	Weakness or faintness when arising from bed or chair.
Antihypertensives*	Decreased blood pressure and effect of carbidopa and levodopa.
Antiparkinsonism drugs, other*	Increased effect of carbidopa and levodopa.
Bupropion	Increased levodopa effect.
Haloperidol	Decreased effect of carbidopa and levodopa.
Methyldopa	Decreased effect of carbidopa and levodopa.
Monoamine oxidase (MAO) inhibitors*	Dangerous rise in blood pressure.
Papaverine	Decreased effect of carbidopa and levodopa.
Phenothiazines*	Decreased effect of carbidopa and levodopa.
Phenytoin	Decreased effect of carbidopa and levodopa.
Pyridoxine (Vitamin B-6)	Decreased effect of carbidopa and levodopa.
Rauwolfia alkaloids*	Decreased effect of carbidopa and levodopa.
Selegiline	May require adjustment in dosage of carbidopa and levodopa.

POSSIBLE INTERACTION WITH OTHER SUBSTANCES

INTERACTS WITH	COMBINED EFFECT
Alcohol:	None expected.
Beverages:	None expected.
Cocaine:	Decreased cabidopa and levodopa effect. High rise of hearbeat irregularities. Avoid.
Foods:	None expected.
Marijuana:	Increased fatigue, lethargy, fainting.
Tobacco:	None expected.

CARBONIC ANHYDRASE INHIBITORS

GENERIC AND BRAND NAMES

ACETAZOLAMIDE
- Acetazolam
- Ak-Zol
- Apo Acetazolamide
- Dazamide
- Diamox
- Storzolamide

BRINZOLAMIDE
- Azopt

DICHLORPHENAMIDE
- Daranide

METHAZOLAMIDE
- MZM
- Neptazane

BASIC INFORMATION

Habit forming? No
Prescription needed? Yes
Available as generic? Yes
Drug class: Carbonic anhydrase inhibitor

USES

- Treatment of glaucoma.
- Treatment of epileptic seizures.
- Treatment of body fluid retention.
- Treatment for shortness of breath, insomnia and fatigue at high altitudes.
- Treatment for prevention of altitude illness.

DOSAGE & USAGE INFORMATION

How to take:
- Sustained-release tablets—Swallow whole with liquid or food to lessen stomach irritation.
- Extended-release capsules—Swallow whole with liquid.
- Topical—1 drop in the affected eye 3 times a day.

When to take:
- 1 dose per day—At the same time each morning.
- More than 1 dose per day—Take last dose several hours before bedtime.

Continued next column

OVERDOSE

SYMPTOMS:
Drowsiness, confusion, excitement, nausea, vomiting, numbness in hands and feet, coma.
WHAT TO DO:
- **Call your doctor or poison center 1-800-222-1222 for advice if you suspect overdose, even if not sure. Symptoms may not appear until damage has occurred.**
- **See emergency information on inside covers.**

If you forget a dose:
Take as soon as you remember. Continue regular schedule.

What drug does:
- Inhibits action of carbonic anhydrase, an enzyme. This lowers the internal eye pressure by decreasing fluid formation in the eye.
- Forces sodium and water excretion, reducing body fluid.

Time lapse before drug works:
2 hours.

Don't take with:
Nonprescription drugs without consulting doctor.

POSSIBLE ADVERSE REACTIONS OR SIDE EFFECTS

SYMPTOMS	WHAT TO DO
Life-threatening:	
Convulsions.	Seek emergency treatment immediately.
Common:	
None expected.	
Infrequent:	
Back pain, sedation, fatigue, weakness, tingling or burning in feet or hands.	Continue. Call doctor when convenient.
Rare:	
• Headache; mood changes; nervousness; clumsiness; trembling; confusion; hives, itch, rash; sores; ringing in ears; hoarseness; dry mouth; thirst; sore throat; fever; appetite change; nausea; vomiting; black, tarry stool; breathing difficulty; irregular or weak heartbeat; easy bleeding or bruising; muscle cramps; painful or frequent urination; blood in urine.	Continue. Call doctor right away.
• Depression, loss of libido.	Continue. Call doctor when convenient.

CARBONIC ANHYDRASE INHIBITORS

WARNINGS & PRECAUTIONS

Don't take if:
You are allergic to any carbonic anhydrase inhibitor.

Before you start, consult your doctor:
- If you have gout or lupus.
- If you are allergic to any sulfa drug.
- You have liver or kidney disease.
- You have Addison's disease (adrenal gland failure).
- You have diabetes.
- If you will have surgery within 2 months, including dental surgery, requiring general or spinal anesthesia.

Over age 60:
- Don't exceed recommended dose.
- If you take a digitalis preparation, eat foods high in potassium content or take a potassium supplement.

Pregnancy:
Avoid if possible, especially first 3 months. Consult doctor. Risk category C (see page xviii).

Breast-feeding:
Avoid drug or don't nurse your infant. Consult doctor about maintaining milk supply.

Infants & children:
Not recommended for children younger than 12.

Prolonged use:
May cause kidney stones, vision change, loss of taste and smell, jaundice or weight loss.

Skin & sunlight:
One or more drugs in this group may cause rash or intensity sunburn in areas exposed to sun or ultraviolet light (photosensitivity reaction). Avoid overexposure. Notify doctor if reaction occurs.

Driving, piloting or hazardous work:
Avoid if you feel drowsy or dizzy. Otherwise, no problems expected.

Discontinuing:
Don't discontinue without medical advice.

Others:
- Medicine may increase sugar levels in blood and urine. Diabetics may need insulin adjustment.
- Advise any doctor or dentist whom you consult that you take this medicine.

POSSIBLE INTERACTION WITH OTHER DRUGS

GENERIC NAME OR DRUG CLASS	COMBINED EFFECT
Adrenocorticoids, systemic	Increased loss of calcium.
Amphetamines*	Increased amphetamine effect.
Anticonvulsants*	Increased loss of bone minerals.
Antiglaucoma, carbonic anhydrase inhibitors	Increased effect of both drugs. Avoid.
Antidiabetics, oral*	Increased potassium loss.
Aspirin	Decreased aspirin effect.
Ciprofloxacin	May cause kidney dysfunction.
Digitalis preparations*	Possible digitalis toxicity.
Diuretics*	Increased potassium loss.
Lithium	Decreased lithium effect.
Mecamylamine	Increased mecamylamine effect.
Methenamine	Decreased methenamine effect.
Mexiletene	May slow elimination of mexilitene and cause need to adjust dosage.
Quinidine	Increased quinidine effect.
Salicylates*	Salicylate toxicity.
Sympathomimetics*	Increased sympathomimetic effect.

POSSIBLE INTERACTION WITH OTHER SUBSTANCES

INTERACTS WITH	COMBINED EFFECT
Alcohol:	None expected.
Beverages:	None expected.
Cocaine:	Avoid. Decreased carbonic anhydrase inhibitor effect.
Foods: Potassium-rich foods.*	Eat these to decrease potassium loss.
Marijuana:	Avoid. Increased carbonic anhydrase inhibitor effect.
Tobacco:	May decrease effect of carbonic anhydrase inhibitors.

*See Glossary

CELLULOSE SODIUM PHOSPHATE

BRAND NAMES

Calcibind

BASIC INFORMATION

Habit forming? No
Prescription needed? Yes
Available as generic? No
Drug class: Antiurolithic

USES

Prevents formation of calcium kidney stones.

DOSAGE & USAGE INFORMATION

How to take:
Oral suspension—Dissolve in full glass of liquid and swallow. Note: Drink 8 ounces of water or other liquid every hour while you are awake.

When to take:
- According to instructions on prescription label. Usually 3 times a day with meals.
- Don't take within 1-1/2 hours of taking any laxative or antacid containing magnesium.

If you forget a dose:
Take as soon as you remember up to 2 hours late. If more than 2 hours, wait for next scheduled dose (don't double this dose).

What drug does:
Combines with calcium in food to prevent absorption into the bloodstream.

Time lapse before drug works:
None. Works right away.

Don't take with:
Any other medicines (including over-the-counter drugs such as cough and cold medicines, laxatives, antacids, diet pills, caffeine, nose drops or vitamins) without consulting your doctor.

OVERDOSE

SYMPTOMS:
Drowsiness, mental changes, muscle spasms, seizures.
WHAT TO DO:
- **Dial 911 (emergency) for an ambulance or medical help or poison center 1-800-222-1222. Then give first aid immediately.**
- **See emergency information on inside covers.**

POSSIBLE ADVERSE REACTIONS OR SIDE EFFECTS

SYMPTOMS	WHAT TO DO
Life-threatening:	
In case of overdose, see previous column.	
Common:	
Loose bowel movements.	Continue. Call doctor when convenient.
Infrequent:	
Abdominal pain.	Discontinue. Call doctor right away.
Rare:	
None expected.	

WARNINGS & PRECAUTIONS

Don't take if:
- You have bone disease.
- You have hyperparathyroidism.
- You have too little calcium in your blood.

Before you start, consult your doctor:
- If you have heart disease.
- If you have kidney disease.

Over age 60:
No special problems expected.

Pregnancy:
Decide with your doctor if drug benefits justify risk to unborn child. Risk category C (see page xviii).

Breast-feeding:
No special problems expected. Consult doctor.

Infants & children:
Not recommended up to age 16.

Prolonged use:
Talk to your doctor about the need for follow-up medical examinations or laboratory studies to check serum calcium and magnesium concentrations (every 6 months), serum parathyroid hormone, urinary calcium and urinary oxalate levels (occasionally).

Skin & sunlight:
No problems expected.

Driving, piloting or hazardous work:
Avoid if you feel confused, drowsy or dizzy.

Discontinuing:
No special problems expected.

Others:
Advise any doctor or dentist whom you consult that you take this medicine.

POSSIBLE INTERACTION WITH OTHER DRUGS

GENERIC NAME OR DRUG CLASS	COMBINED EFFECT
Calcium-containing medications	Decreased effect of cellulose sodium phosphate.
Magnesium-containing medicines (includes many laxatives* and antacids*)	Decreased magnesium effect.
Vitamin C (ascorbic acid)	Decreased vitamin C effect.

POSSIBLE INTERACTION WITH OTHER SUBSTANCES

INTERACTS WITH	COMBINED EFFECT
Alcohol:	None expected.
Beverages: Milk or other dairy products or tea.	Decreases effectiveness of cellulose sodium phosphate.
Cocaine:	None expected.
Foods: Spinach, broccoli, rhubarb.	Decreases effectiveness of cellulose sodium phosphate.
Marijuana:	None expected.
Tobacco:	None expected.

*See Glossary

CEPHALOSPORINS

GENERIC AND BRAND NAMES

CEFACLOR
Ceclor
Ceclor CD
CEFADROXIL
Duricef
Ultracef
CEFDINIR
Omnicef
CEFDITOREN
Spectracef
CEFIXIME
Suprax
CEFOTETAN
Cefotan
CEFPODOXIME
Vantin
CEFPROZIL
Cefzil
CEFTIBUTEN
Cedax
CEFUROXIME
Ceftin
CEPHALEXIN
Apo-Cephalex
Cefanex
Ceporex
C-Lexin
Keflex
Keftab
Novolexin
Nu-Cephalex
CEPHRADINE
Anspor
Velosef

BASIC INFORMATION

Habit forming? No
Prescription needed? Yes
Available as generic? Yes
Drug class: Antibacterial

USES

Treatment of bacterial infections. Will not cure viral infections such as cold and flu.

DOSAGE & USAGE INFORMATION

How to take:
- Tablet or capsule—Swallow with liquid. If you can't swallow whole, crumble tablet or open capsule and take with liquid or food.
- Extended-release tablet—Swallow with liquid. Do not open capsule.
- Liquid—Use measuring spoon. Mix according to package instructions.

Continued next column

When to take:
- At same times each day, 1 hour before or 2 hours after eating.
- Take until gone or as directed.

If you forget a dose:
Take as soon as you remember or double next dose. Return to regular schedule.

What drug does:
Kills susceptible bacteria.

Time lapse before drug works:
May require several days to affect infection.

Don't take with:
Any other medicine without consulting your doctor or pharmacist.

OVERDOSE

SYMPTOMS:
Abdominal cramps, nausea, vomiting, severe diarrhea with mucus or blood in stool, convulsions.
WHAT TO DO:
Overdose unlikely to threaten life. If person takes much larger amount than prescribed, call doctor, poison center 1-800-222-1222 or hospital emergency room for instructions.

POSSIBLE ADVERSE REACTIONS OR SIDE EFFECTS

SYMPTOMS	WHAT TO DO
Life-threatening:	
Hives, rash, intense itching, faintness soon after a dose (anaphylaxis); difficulty breathing.	Seek emergency treatment immediately.
Common:	
Mild diarrhea, nausea, vomiting, sore mouth or tongue, mild stomach cramps (all less common with some cephalosporins).	Continue. Call doctor when convenient.
Infrequent:	
None expected.	
Rare:	
• Severe stomach cramps, severe diarrhea with mucus or blood in stool, fever, unusual weakness or tiredness, weight loss, bleeding or bruising, increased thirst, decreased urine, dizziness, joint pain, appetite loss, skin symptoms (rash, itching, redness, swelling), yellow skin or eyes.	Discontinue. Call doctor right away.
• Genital itching or vaginal discharge.	Continue. Call doctor when convenient.

WARNINGS & PRECAUTIONS

Don't take if:
You are allergic to any cephalosporin antibiotic.

Before you start, consult your doctor:
- If you are allergic to any penicillin antibiotic.
- If you have a kidney disorder.
- If you have colitis or enteritis.

Over age 60:
Adverse reactions and side effects may be more frequent and severe than in younger persons. More likely to itch around rectum and genitals.

Pregnancy:
No proven harm to unborn child. Avoid if possible. Consult doctor. Risk category B (see page xviii).

Breast-feeding:
Drug passes into milk. Avoid drug or discontinue nursing until you finish medicine. Consult doctor for advice on maintaining milk supply.

Infants & children:
No special warnings.

Prolonged use:
- Kills beneficial bacteria that protect body against other germs. Unchecked germs may cause secondary infections.
- Talk to your doctor about the need for follow-up medical examinations or laboratory studies to check prothrombin time.

Skin & sunlight:
No problems expected.

Driving, piloting or hazardous work:
No problems expected.

Discontinuing:
Don't discontinue without doctor's advice until you complete prescribed dose, even though symptoms diminish or disappear.

Others:
- Don't use drug for other medical problems without doctor's approval.
- Advise any doctor or dentist whom you consult that you take this medicine.
- If diarrhea occurs, consult doctor.

POSSIBLE INTERACTION WITH OTHER DRUGS

GENERIC NAME OR DRUG CLASS	COMBINED EFFECT
Anticoagulants*	Increased anticoagulant effect.
Anti-inflammatory drugs, nonsteroidal (NSAIDs)*	Increased risk of peptic ulcer.
Erythromycins*	Decreased antibiotic effect of cephalosporin.
Chloramphenicol	Decreased antibiotic effect of cephalosporin.
Probenecid	Increased cephalosporin effect.
Tetracyclines*	Decreased antibiotic effect of cephalosporin.

POSSIBLE INTERACTION WITH OTHER SUBSTANCES

INTERACTS WITH	COMBINED EFFECT
Alcohol:	Increased kidney toxicity, likelihood of disulfiram-like* effect.
Beverages:	None expected.
Cocaine:	None expected, but cocaine may slow body's recovery. Avoid.
Foods:	Slow absorption. Take with liquid 1 hour before or 2 hours after eating.
Marijuana:	None expected, but marijuana may slow body's recovery. Avoid.
Tobacco:	None expected.

*See Glossary

CHARCOAL, ACTIVATED

BRAND NAMES

Acta-Char
Acta-Char Liquid
Actidose with Sorbitol
Actidose-Aqua
Aqueous Charcodote
Charac-50
Charac-tol 50
Charcoaid
Charcocaps
Charcodote
Charcodote TFS
Insta-Char
Liqui-Char
Pediatric Aqueous Charcodote
Pediatric Charcodote
SuperChar

BASIC INFORMATION

Habit forming? No
Prescription needed? No
Available as generic? Yes
Drug class: Antidote (adsorbent)

USES

- Treatment of poisonings from medication.
- Treatment (infrequent) for diarrhea or excessive gaseousness.

DOSAGE & USAGE INFORMATION

How to take:
- Tablet or capsule—Swallow with liquid. If you can't swallow whole, crumble tablet or open capsule and take with liquid or food.
- Liquid—Take as directed on label. Don't mix with chocolate syrup, ice cream or sherbet.

When to take:
- For poisoning—Take immediately after poisoning. If your doctor or emergency poison control center has also recommended syrup of ipecac, don't take charcoal for 30 minutes or until vomiting from ipecac stops.
- For diarrhea or gas—Take at same times each day.
- Take 2 or more hours after taking other medicines.

Continued next column

OVERDOSE

SYMPTOMS:
None expected.
WHAT TO DO:
Overdose unlikely to threaten life. If person takes much larger amount than prescribed, call doctor, poison center 1-800-222-1222 or hospital emergency room for instructions.

If you forget a dose:
- For poisonings—Not applicable.
- For diarrhea or gas—Take as soon as you remember up to 2 hours late. If more than 2 hours, wait for next scheduled dose (don't double this dose).

What drug does:
- Helps prevent poison from being absorbed from stomach and intestines.
- Helps absorb gas in intestinal tract.

Time lapse before drug works:
Begins immediately.

Don't take with:
Ice cream or sherbet.

POSSIBLE ADVERSE REACTIONS OR SIDE EFFECTS

SYMPTOMS	WHAT TO DO
Life-threatening: None expected.	
Always: Black bowel movements.	No action necessary.
Infrequent: None expected.	
Rare: Unless taken with cathartic, can cause constipation when taken for overdose of other medicine.	Take a laxative after crisis is over.

WARNINGS & PRECAUTIONS

Don't take if:
The poison was lye or other strong alkali, strong acids (such as sulfuric acid), cyanide, iron, ethyl alcohol or methyl alcohol. Charcoal will not prevent these poisons from causing ill effects.

Before you start, consult your doctor:
If you are taking it as an antidote for poison.

Over age 60:
No problems expected.

Pregnancy:
Consult doctor. Risk category C (see page xviii).

Breast-feeding:
No problems expected. Consult doctor.

Infants & children:
Don't give to children for more than 3 or 4 days for diarrhea. Continuing for longer periods can interfere with normal nutrition.

Prolonged use:
No problems expected.

Skin & sunlight:
No problems expected.

Driving, piloting or hazardous work:
No problems expected.

Discontinuing:
No problems expected.

Others:
No problems expected.

POSSIBLE INTERACTION WITH OTHER DRUGS

GENERIC NAME OR DRUG CLASS	COMBINED EFFECT
Any medicine taken at the same time	May decrease absorption of medicine. Take drugs 2 hours apart.

POSSIBLE INTERACTION WITH OTHER SUBSTANCES

INTERACTS WITH	COMBINED EFFECT
Alcohol:	None expected.
Beverages:	None expected.
Cocaine:	None expected.
Foods: Chocolate syrup, ice cream or sherbet.	Decreased charcoal effect.
Marijuana:	None expected.
Tobacco:	None expected.

CHLORAL HYDRATE

BRAND NAMES

Aquachloral
Noctec
Novochlorhydrate

BASIC INFORMATION

Habit forming? Yes
Prescription needed? Yes
Available as generic? Yes
Drug class: Sedative-hypnotic agent

USES

Short term treatment to relieve insomnia.

DOSAGE & USAGE INFORMATION

How to take:
- Syrup or capsule—Swallow with liquid or food to lessen stomach irritation.
- Suppositories—Remove wrapper and moisten suppository with water. Gently insert smaller end into rectum. Push well into rectum with finger.

When to take:
At the same time each day.

If you forget a dose:
Take as soon as you remember up to 2 hours late. If more than 2 hours, wait for next scheduled dose (don't double this dose).

Continued next column

OVERDOSE

SYMPTOMS:
Confusion, weakness, breathing difficulty, throat irritation, jaundice, stagger, slow or irregular heartbeat, unconsciousness, convulsions, coma.
WHAT TO DO:
- **Dial 911 (emergency) for an ambulance or medical help or poison center 1-800-222-1222. Then give first aid immediately.**
- **If patient is unconscious and not breathing, give mouth-to-mouth breathing. If there is no heartbeat, use cardiac massage and mouth-to-mouth breathing (CPR). Don't try to make patient vomit. If you can't get help quickly, take patient to nearest emergency facility.**
- **See emergency information at end of book.**

What drug does:
Affects brain centers that control wakefulness and alertness.

Time lapse before drug works:
30 to 60 minutes.

Don't take with:
Any other medicine without consulting your doctor or pharmacist.

POSSIBLE ADVERSE REACTIONS OR SIDE EFFECTS

SYMPTOMS	WHAT TO DO
Life-threatening: In case of overdose, see previous column.	
Common: Nausea, stomach pain, vomiting.	Discontinue. Call doctor right away.
Infrequent: "Hangover" effect, clumsiness or unsteadiness, drowsiness, dizziness, lightheadedness, diarrhea.	Continue. Call doctor when convenient.
Rare: • Hallucinations, agitation, confusion. leukopenia (white blood cells causing sore throat and fever).	Discontinue. Call doctor right away.
• Hives, rash.	Continue. Call doctor when convenient.

WARNINGS & PRECAUTIONS

Don't take if:
You are allergic to chloral hydrate or you have porphyria.

Before you start, consult your doctor:
- If you have had liver, kidney or heart trouble.
- If you are prone to stomach upsets (if medicine is in oral form).
- If you are allergic to tartrazine dye.
- If you have colitis or a rectal inflammation (if medicine is in suppository form).

Over age 60:
Adverse reactions and side effects may be more frequent and severe than in younger persons. More likely to have "hangover" effect.

Pregnancy:
Decide with your doctor if drug benefits justify risk to unborn child. Risk category C (see page xviii).

Breast-feeding:
Small amounts may filter into breast milk. Best to avoid.

Infants & children:
Use only under medical supervision.

Prolonged use:
- Drug loses its effectiveness as an antianxiety agent or sleep aid after about 2 weeks. Not recommended for longer use.
- Addiction and possible kidney damage may result if used long-term.

Skin & sunlight:
No problems expected.

Driving, piloting or hazardous work:
Don't drive or pilot aircraft until you learn how medicine affects you. Don't work around dangerous machinery. Don't climb ladders or work in high places. Danger increases if you drink alcohol or take medicine affecting alertness and reflexes, such as antihistamines, tranquilizers, sedatives, pain medicine, narcotics and mind-altering drugs.

Discontinuing:
Don't discontinue without consulting doctor. Dose may require gradual reduction if you have taken drug for a long time. Doses of other drugs may also require adjustment.

Others:
- Frequent kidney function tests recommended when drug is used for long time.
- Advise any doctor or dentist whom you consult that you take this medicine.

POSSIBLE INTERACTION WITH OTHER DRUGS

GENERIC NAME OR DRUG CLASS	COMBINED EFFECT
Anticoagulants, oral*	Possible hemorrhaging.
Antidepressants*	Increased chloral hydrate effect.
Antihistamines*	Increased chloral hydrate effect.
Central nervous system (CNS) depressants*	Increased sedative effect.
Clozapine	Toxic effect on the central nervous system.
Fluoxetine	Increased depressant effects of both drugs.
Guanfacine	May increase depressant effects of either drug.
Leucovorin	High alcohol content of leucovorin may cause adverse effects.
Mind-altering drugs*	Increased chloral hydrate effect.
Molindone	Increased tranquilizer effect.
Monoamine oxidase (MAO) inhibitors*	Increased chloral hydrate effect.
Narcotics*	Increased chloral hydrate effect.
Phenothiazines*	Increased chloral hydrate effect.
Sertraline	Increased depressive effects of both drugs.

POSSIBLE INTERACTION WITH OTHER SUBSTANCES

INTERACTS WITH	COMBINED EFFECT
Alcohol:	Increased sedative effects of both. Avoid.
Beverages:	None expected.
Cocaine:	Decreased chloral hydrate effect. Avoid.
Foods:	None expected.
Marijuana:	May severely impair mental and physical functioning. Avoid.
Tobacco:	None expected.

***See Glossary**

CHLORAMBUCIL

BRAND NAMES

Leukeran

BASIC INFORMATION

Habit forming? No
Prescription needed? Yes
Available as generic? No
Drug class: Antineoplastic, immuno-suppressant

USES

- Treatment for some kinds of cancer.
- Suppresses immune response after transplant and in immune disorders.

DOSAGE & USAGE INFORMATION

How to take:
Tablet—Swallow with liquid after light meal. Don't drink fluids with meals. Drink extra fluids between meals. Avoid sweet or fatty foods.

When to take:
At the same time each day.

If you forget a dose:
Take as soon as you remember. Don't ever double dose.

What drug does:
Inhibits abnormal cell reproduction. May suppress immune system.

Time lapse before drug works:
Up to 6 weeks for full effect.

Don't take with:
Any other medicine without consulting your doctor or pharmacist.

OVERDOSE

SYMPTOMS:
Bleeding, chills, fever, vomiting, abdominal pain, ataxia, collapse, stupor, seizure.
WHAT TO DO:

- **Dial 911 (emergency) for an ambulance or medical help or poison center 1-800-222-1222. Then give first aid immediately.**
- **If patient is unconscious and not breathing, give mouth-to-mouth breathing. If there is no heartbeat, use cardiac massage and mouth-to-mouth breathing (CPR). Don't try to make patient vomit. If you can't get help quickly, take patient to nearest emergency facility.**
- **See emergency information on inside covers.**

POSSIBLE ADVERSE REACTIONS OR SIDE EFFECTS

SYMPTOMS	WHAT TO DO
Life-threatening: In case of overdose, see previous column.	
Common:	
• Unusual bleeding or bruising, mouth sores with sore throat, chills and fever, black stools, mouth and lip sores, menstrual irregularities, back pain.	Discontinue. Call doctor right away.
• Hair loss, joint pain.	Continue. Call doctor when convenient.
• Nausea, vomiting, diarrhea, tiredness, weakness.	Continue. Tell doctor at next visit.
Infrequent:	
• Mental confusion, shortness of breath.	Continue. Call doctor when convenient.
• Cough, rash, foot swelling.	Continue. Tell doctor at next visit.
Rare:	
Jaundice, convulsions, hallucinations, muscle twitching.	Discontinue. Call doctor right away.

WARNINGS & PRECAUTIONS

Don't take if:
- You have had hypersensitivity to alkylating antineoplastic drugs.
- Your physician has not explained serious nature of your medical problem and risks of taking this medicine.

Before you start, consult your doctor:
- If you have gout.
- If you have had kidney stones.
- If you have active infection.
- If you have impaired kidney or liver function.
- If you have taken other antineoplastic drugs or had radiation treatment in last 3 weeks.

Over age 60:
Adverse reactions and side effects may be more frequent and severe than in younger persons.

Pregnancy:
Consult doctor. Risk to unborn child is significant. Risk category D (see page xviii).

Breast-feeding:
Safety not established. Consult doctor.

Infants & children:
Use only under care of medical supervisors who are experienced in anticancer drugs.

Prolonged use:
- Adverse reactions more likely the longer drug is required.
- Talk to your doctor about the need for follow-up medical examinations or laboratory studies to check complete blood counts (white blood cell count, platelet count, red blood cell count, hemoglobin, hematocrit).

Skin & sunlight:
No problems expected.

Driving, piloting or hazardous work:
No problems expected.

Discontinuing:
Don't discontinue without doctor's advice until you complete prescribed dose, even though symptoms diminish or disappear. Some side effects may follow discontinuing. Report to doctor blurred vision, convulsions, confusion, persistent headache.

Others:
- May cause blood problems or cancer.
- Advise any doctor or dentist whom you consult that you take this medicine.
- Consult your doctor before you or a household member gets any immunization.

POSSIBLE INTERACTION WITH OTHER DRUGS

GENERIC NAME OR DRUG CLASS	COMBINED EFFECT
Antigout drugs*	Decreased antigout effect.
Antineoplastic drugs, other*	Increased effect of all drugs (may be beneficial).
Chloramphenicol	Increased likelihood of toxic effects of both drugs.
Clozapine	Toxic effect on bone marrow.
Cyclosporine	May increase risk of infection.
Immuno-suppressants*	Increased chance of infection.
Lovastatin	Increased heart and kidney damage.
Tiopronin	Increased risk of toxicity to bone marrow.

POSSIBLE INTERACTION WITH OTHER SUBSTANCES

INTERACTS WITH	COMBINED EFFECT
Alcohol:	May increase chance of intestinal bleeding.
Beverages:	No problems expected.
Cocaine:	Increases chance of toxicity.
Foods:	Reduces irritation in stomach.
Marijuana:	No problems expected.
Tobacco:	Increases lung toxicity.

*See Glossary

CHLORAMPHENICOL

BRAND NAMES

Chloromycetin
Novochlorocap

BASIC INFORMATION

Habit forming? No
Prescription needed? Yes
Available as generic? Yes
Drug class: Antibacterial

USES

Treatment of infections susceptible to chloramphenicol. Will not treat viral infections such as cold or flu.

DOSAGE & USAGE INFORMATION

How to take:
Suspension or capsule—Take with a full glass of water.

When to take:
Capsule or suspension—1 hour before or 2 hours after eating.

If you forget a dose:
Take as soon as you remember up to 2 hours late. If more than 2 hours, wait for next scheduled dose (don't double this dose).

What drug does:
Prevents bacteria from growing and reproducing. Will not kill viruses.

Time lapse before drug works:
2 to 5 days, depending on type and severity of infection.

Don't take with:
Any other medicine without consulting your doctor or pharmacist.

OVERDOSE

SYMPTOMS:
Nausea, vomiting, diarrhea.
WHAT TO DO:
Overdose unlikely to threaten life. If person takes much larger amount than prescribed, call doctor, poison center 1-800-222-1222 or hospital emergency room for instructions.

POSSIBLE ADVERSE REACTIONS OR SIDE EFFECTS

SYMPTOMS	WHAT TO DO
Life-threatening:	
Hives, rash, intense itching, faintness soon after a dose (anaphylaxis).	Seek emergency treatment immediately.
Common:	
None expected.	
Infrequent:	
• Swollen face or extremities; diarrhea; nausea; vomiting; numbness, tingling, burning pain or weakness in hands and feet; pale skin; unusual bleeding or bruising.	Discontinue. Call doctor right away.
• Headache, confusion.	Continue. Call doctor when convenient.
Rare:	
• Pain, blurred vision, possible vision loss, delirium, rash, sore throat, fever, jaundice, anemia.	Discontinue. Call doctor right away.
• In babies: Bloated stomach, uneven breathing, drowsiness, low temperature, gray skin.	Discontinue. Call doctor right away.

WARNINGS & PRECAUTIONS

Don't take if:
- You are allergic to chloramphenicol.
- It is prescribed for a minor disorder such as flu, cold or mild sore throat.

Before you start, consult your doctor:
- If you have had a blood disorder or bone-marrow disease.
- If you have had kidney or liver disease.
- If you have diabetes.

Over age 60:
Adverse reactions and side effects may be more frequent and severe than in younger persons, particularly skin irritation around rectum.

Pregnancy:
Decide with your doctor if drug benefits justify risk to unborn child. Risk category C (see page xviii).

Breast-feeding:
Drug passes into milk. Avoid drug or discontinue nursing until you finish medicine. Consult doctor for advice on maintaining milk supply.

Infants & children:
Use only under close medical supervision, especially in infants younger than 2.

Prolonged use:
- You may become more susceptible to infections caused by germs not responsive to chloramphenicol.
- Talk to your doctor about the need for follow-up medical examinations or laboratory studies to check complete blood counts (white blood cell count, platelet count, red blood cell count, hemoglobin, hematocrit), chloramphenicol serum levels.

Skin & sunlight:
No problems expected.

Driving, piloting or hazardous work:
Don't drive or pilot aircraft until you learn how medicine affects you. Don't work around dangerous machinery. Don't climb ladders or work in high places. Danger increases if you drink alcohol or take medicine affecting alertness and reflexes.

Discontinuing:
Don't discontinue without doctor's advice until you complete prescribed dose, even though symptoms diminish or disappear.

Others:
- Chloramphenicol can cause serious anemia. Frequent laboratory blood studies, liver and kidney tests recommended.
- Advise any doctor or dentist whom you consult that you take this medicine.
- Second medical opinion recommended before starting.

POSSIBLE INTERACTION WITH OTHER DRUGS

GENERIC NAME OR DRUG CLASS	COMBINED EFFECT
Anticoagulants*	Increased anti-coagulant effect.
Antidiabetics, oral*	Increased antidiabetic effect.
Anticonvulsants*	Increased chance of toxicity to bone marrow.
Antivirals, HIV/AIDS*	Increased risk of peripheral neuropathy.
Cefiximine	Decreased antibiotic effect of cefiximine.
Cephalosporins*	Decreased chloramphenicol effect.
Clindamycin	Decreased clindamycin effect.
Clozapine	Toxic effect on bone marrow.
Cyclophosphamide	Increased cyclophosphamide effect.
Erythromycins	Decreased erythromycin effect.
Flecainide	Possible decreased blood cell production in bone marrow.
Levamisole	Increased risk of bone marrow depression.
Lincomycin	Decreased lincomycin effect.
Lisinopril	Possible blood disorders.
Penicillins*	Decreased penicillin effect.
Phenobarbital	Increased phenobarbital effect.
Phenytoin	Increased phenytoin effect.
Rifampin	Decreased chloramphenicol effect.
Thioguanine	More likelihood of toxicity of both drugs.
Tiopronin	Increased risk of toxicity to bone marrow.
Tocainide	Possible decreased blood cell production in bone marrow.

POSSIBLE INTERACTION WITH OTHER SUBSTANCES

INTERACTS WITH	COMBINED EFFECT
Alcohol:	Possible liver problems. Possible disulfiram reaction.*
Beverages:	None expected.
Cocaine:	No proven problems.
Foods:	None expected.
Marijuana:	None expected.
Tobacco:	None expected.

*See Glossary

CHLORHEXIDINE

BRAND NAMES

Peridex
Periochip
Periogard

BASIC INFORMATION

Habit forming? No
Prescription needed? Yes
Available as generic? Yes
Drug class: Antibacterial (dental)

USES

Treatment for gingivitis (inflammation of the gums), periodontal disease and other infections of the mouth.

DOSAGE & USAGE INFORMATION

How to use:

- Oral rinse—Swish in mouth for 30 seconds, then spit out. Do not swallow the solution, and do not rinse mouth with water after using. Use product at full strength; do not dilute.
- Implants—Inserted by dentist.

When to use:
Twice a day after brushing and flossing teeth.

If you forget a dose:
Use as soon as you remember, then return to regular schedule.

What drug does:
Kills or prevents growth of susceptible bacteria.

Time lapse before drug works:
Antibacterial action begins within an hour, but full benefit may take several weeks.

Don't use with:
Other mouthwashes without consulting your dentist or pharmacist.

OVERDOSE

SYMPTOMS:
None expected. If a child swallows several ounces of the solution, may have slurred speech, staggering or stumbling walk, sleepiness.
WHAT TO DO:
If symptoms occur, call doctor for instructions. If child weighing under 22 pounds accidentally swallows more than 4 ounces, seek emergency help. Dial 911 (emergency) for an ambulance or medical help or poison center 1-800-222-1222. Then give first aid immediately.

POSSIBLE ADVERSE REACTIONS OR SIDE EFFECTS

SYMPTOMS	WHAT TO DO
Life-threatening: None expected.	
Common: Staining of teeth and other oral surfaces, increased tartar, taste changes, minor mouth irritation.	Continue. Call dentist when convenient.
Infrequent: None expected.	
Rare: Allergic reaction (stuffy nose, shortness of breath, skin rash, hives, itching, face swelling); swollen glands on side of face or neck.	Discontinue. Call doctor right away.

WARNINGS & PRECAUTIONS

Don't take if:
You are allergic to chlorhexidine or skin cleaners that contain chlorhexidine.

Before you start, consult your dentist:
- If you have front tooth fillings (may become discolored).
- If you have periodontitis.

Over age 60:
No special problems expected.

Pregnancy:
Consult doctor. Risk category B (see page xviii).

Breast-feeding:
It is unknown if drug passes into milk. Consult doctor.

Infants & children:
Safety in children under age 18 has not been established.

Prolonged use:
See your dentist every 6 months.

Skin & sunlight:
No special problems expected.

Driving, piloting or hazardous work:
No special problems expected.

Discontinuing:
No special problems expected.

Others:
Brush teeth with a tartar-control toothpaste, and floss daily to help reduce tartar buildup.

POSSIBLE INTERACTION WITH OTHER DRUGS

GENERIC NAME OR DRUG CLASS	COMBINED EFFECT
None expected.	

POSSIBLE INTERACTION WITH OTHER SUBSTANCES

INTERACTS WITH	COMBINED EFFECT
Alcohol:	None expected.
Beverages:	Avoid drinking any fluids for several hours after using mouthwash.
Cocaine:	None expected.
Foods:	Avoid eating any foods for several hours after using mouthwash.
Marijuana:	None expected.
Tobacco:	None expected.

CHLOROQUINE

BRAND NAMES

Aralen

BASIC INFORMATION

Habit forming? No
Prescription needed? Yes
Available as generic? Yes
Drug class: Antiprotozoal, antirheumatic

USES

- Treatment for protozoal infections, such as malaria and amebiasis.
- Treatment for some forms of arthritis and lupus.

DOSAGE & USAGE INFORMATION

How to take:
Tablet—Swallow with food or milk to lessen stomach irritation.

When to take:
- Depends on condition. Is adjusted during treatment.
- Malaria prevention—Begin taking medicine 2 weeks before traveling to areas where malaria is present and until 8 weeks after return.

If you forget a dose:
- 1 or more doses a day—Take as soon as you remember up to 2 hours late. If more than 2 hours, wait for next scheduled dose (don't double this dose).
- 1 dose weekly—Take as soon as possible, then return to regular dosing schedule.

What drug does:
- Inhibits parasite multiplication.
- Decreases inflammatory response in diseased joint.

Continued next column

OVERDOSE

SYMPTOMS:
Severe breathing difficulty, drowsiness, faintness, headache, seizures.
WHAT TO DO:
- **Dial 911 (emergency) for an ambulance or medical help or poison center 1-800-222-1222. Then give first aid immediately.**
- **See emergency information on inside covers.**

Time lapse before drug works:
1 to 2 hours. For treatment of arthritis symptoms, may take up to 6 months for maximum effectiveness.

Don't take with:
Any other medicine without consulting your doctor or pharmacist.

POSSIBLE ADVERSE REACTIONS OR SIDE EFFECTS

SYMPTOMS	WHAT TO DO
Life-threatening: In case of overdose, see previous column.	
Common: Headache, appetite loss, abdominal pain.	Continue. Tell doctor at next visit.
Infrequent:	
• Blurred or changed vision.	Discontinue. Call doctor right away.
• Rash or itch, diarrhea, nausea, vomiting, decreased blood pressure, hair loss, blue-black skin or mouth, dizziness, nervousness.	Continue. Call doctor when convenient.
Rare:	
• Mood or mental changes, seizures, sore throat, fever, unusual bleeding or bruising, muscle weakness, convulsions.	Discontinue. Call doctor right away.
• Ringing or buzzing in ears, hearing loss.	Continue. Call doctor when convenient.

WARNINGS & PRECAUTIONS

Don't take if:
You are allergic to chloroquine or hydroxychloroquine.

Before you start, consult your doctor:
- If you plan to become pregnant within the medication period.
- If you have blood disease.
- If you have eye or vision problems.
- If you have a G6PD deficiency.
- If you have liver disease.
- If you have nerve or brain disease (including seizure disorders).
- If you have porphyria.
- If you have psoriasis.
- If you have stomach or intestinal disease.
- If you drink more than 3 oz. of alcohol daily.

Over age 60:
Adverse reactions and side effects may be more frequent and severe than in younger persons.

Pregnancy:
Decide with your doctor if drug benefits justify risk to unborn child. Risk category C (see page xviii).

Breast-feeding:
Drug passes into milk. Avoid drug or discontinue nursing. Consult doctor about maintaining milk supply.

Infants & children:
Not recommended. Dangerous.

Prolonged use:
- Permanent damage to the retina (back part of the eye) or nerve deafness.
- Talk to your doctor about the need for follow-up medical examinations or laboratory studies to check complete blood counts (white blood cell count, platelet count, red blood cell count, hemoglobin, hematocrit), eyes.

Skin & sunlight:
May cause rash or intensify sunburn in areas exposed to sun or ultraviolet light (photosensitivity reaction). Avoid overexposure. Notify doctor if reaction occurs.

Driving, piloting or hazardous work:
Don't drive or pilot aircraft until you learn how medicine affects you. Don't work around dangerous machinery. Don't climb ladders or work in high places. Danger increases if you drink alcohol or take medicine affecting alertness and reflexes.

Discontinuing:
Don't discontinue without doctor's advice until you complete prescribed dose, even though symptoms diminish or disappear.

Others:
- Periodic physical and blood examinations recommended.
- Advise any doctor or dentist whom you consult that you take this medicine.
- If you are in a malaria area for a long time, you may need to change to another preventive drug every 2 years.

POSSIBLE INTERACTION WITH OTHER DRUGS

GENERIC NAME OR DRUG CLASS	COMBINED EFFECT
Penicillamine	Possible blood or kidney toxicity.

POSSIBLE INTERACTION WITH OTHER SUBSTANCES

INTERACTS WITH	COMBINED EFFECT
Alcohol:	Possible liver toxicity. Avoid.
Beverages:	None expected.
Cocaine:	None expected.
Foods:	None expected.
Marijuana:	None expected.
Tobacco:	None expected.

CHLORZOXAZONE & ACETAMINOPHEN

BRAND NAMES

Parafon Forte

BASIC INFORMATION

Habit forming? Possibly
Prescription needed? Yes
Available as generic? Yes
Drug class: Muscle relaxant, analgesic, fever-reducer

USES

- Adjunctive treatment to rest, analgesics and physical therapy for muscle spasms.
- Treatment of mild to moderate pain and fever.

DOSAGE & USAGE INFORMATION

How to take:
Tablet—Swallow with liquid.

When to take:
As needed, no more often than every 3 hours.

If you forget a dose:
Take as soon as you remember. Wait 3 hours for next dose.

What drug does:
- Blocks body's pain messages to brain. Also causes sedation.
- May affect hypothalamus, the part of the brain that helps regulate body heat and receives body's pain messages.

Time lapse before drug works:
15 to 30 minutes. May last 4 hours.

Continued next column

OVERDOSE

SYMPTOMS:
Nausea, vomiting, diarrhea, anorexia, headache, severe weakness, unusual increase in sweating, fainting, breathing difficulty, irritability, convulsions, sensation of paralysis, coma.
WHAT TO DO:
- **Overdose unlikely to threaten life. Depending on severity of symptoms and amount taken, call doctor, poison center 1-800-222-1222 or hospital emergency room for instructions.**
- **Dial 911 (emergency) for an ambulance or medical help. Then give first aid immediately.**
- **See emergency information on inside covers.**

Don't take with:
- Other drugs with acetaminophen. Too much acetaminophen can damage liver and kidneys.
- Any other medicine without consulting your doctor or pharmacist.

POSSIBLE ADVERSE REACTIONS OR SIDE EFFECTS

SYMPTOMS	WHAT TO DO
Life-threatening:	
Hives, rash, intense itching, faintness soon after a dose (anaphylaxis); extreme weakness, transient paralysis, temporary loss of vision.	Seek emergency treatment immediately.
Common:	
Dizziness, lightheadedness, drowsiness.	Discontinue. Call doctor right away.
Infrequent:	
• Difficult or frequent urination, severe back pain, cloudy urine.	Discontinue. Call doctor right away.
• Nervousness, restlessness, irritability, headache, indigestion, depression, agitation, constipation, tiredness, weakness.	Continue. Call doctor when convenient.
Rare:	
• Sudden decrease in urine output; swelling of lips, face or tongue.	Discontinue. Seek emergency treatment.
• Bloody or black stools, jaundice, unusual bleeding or bruising, sore mouth or throat, fever, hiccups, skin rash, hives.	Discontinue. Call doctor right away.

WARNINGS & PRECAUTIONS

Don't take if:
- You are allergic to any skeletal muscle relaxant or acetaminophen.
- Your symptoms don't improve after 2 days use. Call your doctor.

Before you start, consult your doctor:
- If you have had liver disease.
- If you have kidney disease or liver damage.
- If you plan pregnancy within medication period.
- If you are allergic to tartrazine dye*.

Over age 60:
- Adverse reactions and side effects may be more frequent and severe than in younger persons.
- Don't exceed recommended dose. You can't eliminate drug as efficiently as younger persons.

Pregnancy:
Safety not proven. Avoid if possible. Consult doctor. Risk category C (see page xviii).

Breast-feeding:
Drug passes into milk. Avoid drug or discontinue nursing until you finish medicine. Consult doctor for advice on maintaining milk supply.

Infants & children:
Not recommended.

Prolonged use:
- May affect blood system and cause anemia. Limit use to 5 days for children 12 and under, and 10 days for adults.
- Talk to your doctor about the need for follow-up medical examinations or laboratory studies to check complete blood counts (white blood cell count, platelet count, red blood cell count, hemoglobin, hematocrit), liver function.

Skin & sunlight:
No problems expected.

Driving, piloting or hazardous work:
Don't drive or pilot aircraft until you learn how medicine affects you. Don't work around dangerous machinery. Don't climb ladders or work in high places. Danger increases if you drink alcohol or take medicine affecting alertness and reflexes, such as antihistamines, tranquilizers, sedatives, pain medicine, narcotics and mind-altering drugs.

Discontinuing:
Don't discontinue without consulting your doctor. Dose may require gradual reduction if you have taken drug for a long time. Doses of other drugs may also require adjustment.

Others:
- Advise any doctor or dentist whom you consult that you take this medicine.
- Periodic liver-function tests recommended if you use this drug for a long time.

POSSIBLE INTERACTION WITH OTHER DRUGS

GENERIC NAME OR DRUG CLASS	COMBINED EFFECT
Anticoagulants, oral*	May increase anticoagulant effect.
Antidepressants*	Increased sedation.
Antihistamines*	Increased sedation.
Clozapine	Toxic effect on the central nervous system.
Dronabinol	Increased effect of dronabinol on central nervous system. Avoid combination.
Mind-altering drugs*	Increased sedation.
Monoamine oxidase (MAO) inhibitors*	Increased effect of both drugs (but safety not established).
Muscle relaxants, others*	Increased sedation.
Narcotics*	Increased sedation.
Phenobarbital	Quicker elimination and decreased effects of acetaminophen.
Sedatives*	Increased sedation.
Sertraline	Increased depressive effects of both drugs.
Sleep inducers*	Increased sedation.
Tetracyclines* (effervescent granules or tablets)	May slow tetracycline absorption. Space doses 2 hours apart.

Continued on page 909

POSSIBLE INTERACTION WITH OTHER SUBSTANCES

INTERACTS WITH	COMBINED EFFECT
Alcohol:	Drowsiness, increased sedation. Long-term use may cause toxic effect in liver.
Beverages:	None expected.
Cocaine:	Lack of coordination. May slow body's recovery. Avoid.
Foods:	None expected.
Marijuana:	Increased pain relief, lack of coordination, drowsiness, fainting. May slow body's recovery. Avoid.
Tobacco:	None expected.

CHOLESTYRAMINE

BRAND NAMES

Cholybar
Questran
Questran Light

BASIC INFORMATION

Habit forming? No
Prescription needed? Yes
Available as generic? Yes
Drug class: Antihyperlipidemic, antipruritic

USES

- Removes excess bile acids that occur with some liver problems. Reduces persistent itch caused by bile acids.
- Lowers cholesterol level.
- Treatment of one form of colitis (rare).

DOSAGE & USAGE INFORMATION

How to take:
Powder, granules—Sprinkle into 8 oz. liquid. Let stand for 2 minutes, then mix with liquid before swallowing. Or mix with cereal, soup or pulpy fruit. Don't swallow dry.

When to take:
- 3 or 4 times a day on an empty stomach, 1 hour before or 2 hours after eating.
- If taking other medicines, take 1 hour before or 4 to 6 hours after taking cholestyramine.

If you forget a dose:
Take as soon as you remember up to 2 hours late. If more than 2 hours, wait for next scheduled dose (don't double this dose).

What drug does:
Binds with bile acids to prevent their absorption.

Time lapse before drug works:
- Cholesterol reduction—1 day.
- Bile-acid reduction—3 to 4 weeks.

Continued next column

OVERDOSE

SYMPTOMS:
Increased side effects and adverse reactions.
WHAT TO DO:
Overdose unlikely to threaten life. Depending on severity of symptoms and amount taken, call doctor, poison center 1-800-222-1222 or hospital emergency room for instructions.

Don't take with:
- Any drug or vitamin simultaneously. Space doses 2 hours apart.
- Any other medicine without consulting your doctor or pharmacist.

POSSIBLE ADVERSE REACTIONS OR SIDE EFFECTS

SYMPTOMS	WHAT TO DO
Life-threatening: In case of overdose, see previous column.	
Common:	
Constipation.	Continue. Call doctor when convenient.
Infrequent:	
• Belching, bloating, diarrhea, mild nausea, vomiting, stomach pain, rapid weight gain.	Discontinue. Call doctor when convenient.
• Heartburn (mild).	Continue. Call doctor when convenient.
Rare:	
• Severe stomach pain, black, tarry stool.	Discontinue. Seek emergency treatment.
• Rash, hives, hiccups.	Discontinue. Call doctor right away.
• Sore tongue.	Continue. Call doctor when convenient.

WARNINGS & PRECAUTIONS

Don't take if:
You are allergic to cholestyramine.

Before you start, consult your doctor:
- If you plan to become pregnant within medication period.
- If you have angina, heart or blood-vessel disease.
- If you have stomach problems (including ulcer).
- If you have tartrazine sensitivity.
- If you have constipation or hemorrhoids.
- If you have kidney disease.

Over age 60:
Adverse reactions and side effects may be more frequent and severe than in younger persons.

Pregnancy:
Decide with your doctor whether drug benefits justify risk to unborn child. Risk category C (see page xviii).

Breast-feeding:
No problems expected, but consult doctor.

Infants & children:
Not recommended.

Prolonged use:
- May decrease absorption of folic acid.
- Talk to your doctor about the need for follow-up medical examinations or laboratory studies to check serum cholesterol and triglycerides.

Skin & sunlight:
No problems expected.

Driving, piloting or hazardous work:
No problems expected.

Discontinuing:
Don't discontinue without doctor's advice until you complete prescribed dose, even though symptoms diminish or disappear.

Others:
Advise any doctor or dentist whom you consult that you take this medicine.

POSSIBLE INTERACTION WITH OTHER DRUGS

GENERIC NAME OR DRUG CLASS	COMBINED EFFECT
Adrenocorticoids, systemic	Decreased adrenocorticoid effect.
Anticoagulants, oral*	Increased anticoagulant effect.
Beta carotene	Decreased absorption of beta carotene.
Dexfenfluramine	May require dosage change as weight loss occurs.
Dextrothyroxine	Decreased dextrothyroxine effect.
Digitalis preparations*	Decreased digitalis effect.
Indapamide	Decreased indapamide effect.
Penicillins*	May decrease penicillin effect.
Raloxifene	Decreased effect of raloxifene.
Thiazides*	Decreased absorption of cholestyramine.
Thyroid hormones*	Decreased thyroid effect.
Trimethoprim	Decreased absorption of cholestyramine.
Troglitazone	Decreased effect of troglitazone. Avoid.
Ursodiol	Decreased absorption of ursodiol.
Vancomycin	Increased chance of hearing loss or kidney damage. Decreased therapeutic effect of vancomycin.
Vitamins	Decreased absorption of fat-soluble vitamins (A,D,E,K).
All other medicines	Decreased absorption, so dosages or dosage intervals may require adjustment.

POSSIBLE INTERACTION WITH OTHER SUBSTANCES

INTERACTS WITH	COMBINED EFFECT
Alcohol:	None expected.
Beverages:	None expected.
Cocaine:	None expected.
Foods:	Absorption of vitamins in foods decreased. Take vitamin supplements, particularly A, D, E & K.
Marijuana:	None expected.
Tobacco:	None expected.

***See Glossary**

CHOLINESTERASE INHIBITORS

GENERIC AND BRAND NAMES

DONEPEZIL
Aricept
GALANTAMINE
Reminyl
RIVASTIGMINE
Exelon
TACRINE
Cognex

BASIC INFORMATION

Habit forming? No
Prescription needed? Yes
Available as generic? No
Drug class: Cholinesterase inhibitor

USES

Treats symptoms of mild to moderate Alzheimer's disease. May improve memory, reasoning and other cognitive functions slightly in some patients or slow the progress of the disease. It will not reverse the disease.

DOSAGE & USAGE INFORMATION

How to take:
- Capsule or tablet–Swallow with liquid. If unable to swallow whole, open capsule or crumble tablet and take with liquid or food.
- Oral solution–Take as directed on label.

When to take:
- Donepezil–Once a day at bedtime.
- Rivastigmine and Tacrine–At the same times each day.

Continued next column

OVERDOSE

SYMPTOMS:
Severe nausea and vomiting, excessive saliva, sweating, blood pressure decrease, slow heartbeat, collapse, convulsions, muscle weakness (including respiratory muscles, which could lead to death).
WHAT TO DO:
- **Dial 911 (emergency) for an ambulance or medical help or poison center 1-800-222-1222. Then give first aid immediately.**
- **If patient is unconscious and not breathing, use cardiac massage and mouth-to-mouth breathing (CPR). Don't try to make patient vomit. If you can't get help quickly, take patient to nearest emergency facility.**
- **See emergency information at end of book.**

What drug does:
Slows breakdown of a brain chemical (acetylcholine) that gradually disappears from the brains of people with Alzheimer's disease.

If you forget a dose:
- Donepezil–Skip missed dose. Do not double dose.
- Others–Take as soon as you remember up to 2 hours late. If more than 2 hours, wait for next scheduled dose (do not double this dose).

Time lapse before drug works:
May take several weeks or months before beneficial results are observed. Dosage is normally increased over a period of time to help prevent adverse reactions.

Don't take with:
Any other medication without consulting your doctor or pharmacist.

POSSIBLE ADVERSE REACTIONS OR SIDE EFFECTS

SYMPTOMS	WHAT TO DO
Life-threatening:	
In case of overdose, see previous column.	
Common:	
Nausea, vomiting, diarrhea, lack of coordination.	Continue. Call doctor when convenient.
Infrequent:	
Rash, indigestion, headache, muscle aches, loss of appetite, stomach pain, nervousness, chills, dizziness, drowsiness, dry or itching eyes, increased sweating, joint pain, runny nose, sore throat, swelling of feet or legs, insomnia, weight loss, unusual tiredness or weakness, flushing of face.	Continue. Call doctor when convenient.
Rare:	
Changes in liver function (yellow skin or eyes; black, very dark or light stool color); lack of coordination, convulsions, speech problems, irregular heartbeat, vision changes, increased libido, changes in blood pressure, hot flashes, breathing difficulty.	Continue. Call doctor right away.

WARNINGS & PRECAUTIONS

Don't take if:
You are allergic to cholinesterase inhibitors.

Before you start, consult your doctor:
- If you have heart rhythm problems.
- If you have a history of ulcer disease or are at risk of developing ulcers.
- If you have a history of liver disease.
- If you have a history of urinary tract problems.
- If you have epilepsy or seizure disorder.
- If you have a history of asthma.
- If you have had a head injury with loss of consciousness.
- If you have had previous treatment with any cholinesterase inhibitor that caused jaundice (yellow skin and eyes) or elevated bilirubin.

Over age 60:
No problems expected.

Pregnancy:
Unknown effect. Drug is usually not prescribed for women of childbearing age. Risk category C (see page xviii).

Breast-feeding:
Unknown effect. Not recommended for women of childbearing age.

Infants & children:
Not used in this age group.

Prolonged use:
- Drug may lose its effectiveness.
- Talk to your doctor about the need for follow-up medical examinations or laboratory studies to check blood chemistries and liver function.

Skin & sunlight:
No problems expected.

Driving, piloting or hazardous work:
Don't drive or pilot aircraft until you learn how medicine affects you. Don't work around dangerous machinery. Don't climb ladders or work in high places. Danger increases if you drink alcohol or take other medicines affecting alertness and reflexes such as antihistamines, tranquilizers, sedatives, pain medicine, narcotics and mind-altering drugs.

Discontinuing:
Do not discontinue drug unless advised by doctor. Abrupt decreases in dosage may cause a cognitive decline.

Others:
- Advise any doctor or dentist whom you consult that you take this medicine.
- May affect the results in some medical tests.
- Do not increase dosage without doctor's approval.
- Treatment may need to be discontinued or the dosage lowered if weekly blood tests indicate a sensitivity to the drug or liver toxicity develops.

POSSIBLE INTERACTION WITH OTHER DRUGS

GENERIC NAME OR DRUG CLASS	COMBINED EFFECT
Anticholinergics*	Decreased anti-cholinergic effect.
Anti-inflammatories, nonsteroidal (NSAIDs)	May increase gastric acid secretions
Cimetidine	Increased tacrine effect, especially adverse effects.
Enzyme inducers* nonsedating*	May decrease effect of cholinesterase inhibitor.
Ketoconazole	May interact, but effect unknown.
Quinidine	May interact, but effect unknown.
Theophylline	Increased theophylline effect or toxicity.

POSSIBLE INTERACTION WITH OTHER SUBSTANCES

INTERACTS WITH	COMBINED EFFECT
Alcohol:	None expected.
Beverages:	None expected.
Cocaine:	None expected.
Foods:	None expected.
Marijuana:	None expected.
Tobacco:	May decrease tacrine effect.

CINOXACIN

BRAND NAMES

Cinobac

BASIC INFORMATION

Habit forming? No
Prescription needed? Yes
Available as generic? Yes
Drug class: Anti-infective (urinary)

USES

Treatment for urinary tract infections.

DOSAGE & USAGE INFORMATION

How to take:
Capsules—Swallow with food or milk to lessen stomach irritation. If you can't swallow whole, open capsule and take with liquid or food.

When to take:
At the same times each day.

If you forget a dose:
Take as soon as you remember up to 2 hours late. If more than 2 hours, wait for next scheduled dose (don't double this dose).

What drug does:
Destroys bacteria susceptible to cinoxacin.

Time lapse before drug works:
1 to 2 weeks.

Don't take with:
Any other medicine without consulting your doctor or pharmacist.

OVERDOSE

SYMPTOMS:
Lethargy, stomach upset, behavioral changes, convulsions and stupor.
WHAT TO DO:
- **Dial 911 (emergency) for an ambulance or medical help or poison center 1-800-222-1222. Then give first aid immediately.**
- **If patient is unconscious and not breathing, give mouth-to-mouth breathing. If there is no heartbeat, use cardiac massage and mouth-to-mouth breathing (CPR). Don't try to make patient vomit. If you can't get help quickly, take patient to nearest emergency facility.**
- **See emergency information on inside covers.**

POSSIBLE ADVERSE REACTIONS OR SIDE EFFECTS

SYMPTOMS	WHAT TO DO
Life-threatening:	
Hives, rash, intense itching, faintness soon after a dose (anaphylaxis).	Seek emergency treatment immediately.
Common:	
Rash, itch; decreased, blurred or double vision; halos around lights or excess brightness; changes in color vision; nausea, vomiting, diarrhea.	Discontinue. Call doctor right away.
Infrequent:	
Dizziness, drowsiness, headache, ringing in ears, insomnia, appetite loss.	Continue. Call doctor when convenient.
Rare:	
Severe stomach pain, seizures, psychosis, joint pain, numbness or tingling in hands or feet (infants and children).	Discontinue. Call doctor right away.

WARNINGS & PRECAUTIONS

Don't take if:
- You are allergic to cinoxacin or nalidixic acid.
- You have a seizure disorder (epilepsy, convulsions).

Before you start, consult your doctor:
- If you plan to become pregnant during medication period.
- If you have or have had kidney or liver disease.
- If you have impaired circulation to the brain (hardened arteries).

Over age 60:
Adverse reactions and side effects may be more frequent and severe than in younger persons.

Pregnancy:
Decide with your doctor if drug benefits justify risk to unborn child. Risk category C (see page xviii).

Breast-feeding:
Unknown effect. Avoid drug or discontinue nursing until you finish medicine. Consult doctor for advice on maintaining milk supply.

Infants & children:
Give only under close medical supervision.

Prolonged use:
Talk to your doctor about the need for follow-up medical examinations or laboratory studies to check kidney function, liver function.

Skin & sunlight:
No special problems expected.

Driving, piloting or hazardous work:
Avoid if you feel drowsy, dizzy or have vision problems. Otherwise, no problems expected.

Discontinuing:
Don't discontinue without consulting doctor. Dose may require gradual reduction if you have taken drug for a long time. Doses of other drugs may also require adjustment.

Others:
- May interfere with the accuracy of some medical tests.
- Advise any doctor or dentist whom you consult that you take this medicine.

POSSIBLE INTERACTION WITH OTHER DRUGS

GENERIC NAME OR DRUG CLASS	COMBINED EFFECT
Probenecid	Decreased cinoxacin effect.

POSSIBLE INTERACTION WITH OTHER SUBSTANCES

INTERACTS WITH	COMBINED EFFECT
Alcohol:	Impaired alertness, judgment and coordination.
Beverages:	None expected.
Cocaine:	Impaired judgment and coordination.
Foods:	None expected.
Marijuana:	Impaired alertness, judgment and coordination.
Tobacco:	None expected.

CITRATES

BRAND AND GENERIC NAMES

POTASSIUM CITRATE
- Citra Forte
- Urocit-K

POTASSIUM CITRATE & CITRIC ACID
- Phanadex
- Polycitra-K

POTASSIUM CITRATE & SODIUM CITRATE
- Citrolith

SODIUM CITRATE & CITRIC ACID
- Albright's Solution
- Bicitra
- Lanatuss Expectorant
- Modified Shohl's Solution
- Oracit
- Tussirex with Codeine Liquid

TRICITRATES
- Polycitra
- Polycitra LC

BASIC INFORMATION

Habit forming? No
Prescription needed? Yes
Available as generic? No
Drug class: Urinary alkalizer, antiurolithic

USES

- To make urine more alkaline (less acid).
- To treat or prevent recurrence of some types of kidney stones.

DOSAGE & USAGE INFORMATION

How to take:
Tablets or liquid—Take right after a meal or with a bedtime snack.

When to take:
On full stomach, usually after meals or with food.

If you forget a dose:
Take as soon as you remember up to 2 hours late. If more than 2 hours, wait for next scheduled dose (don't double this dose).

Continued next column

OVERDOSE

SYMPTOMS:
Convulsions, coma.
WHAT TO DO:
- **Dial 911 (emergency) for an ambulance or medical help or poison center 1-800-222-1222. Then give first aid immediately.**
- **See emergency information on inside covers.**

What drug does:
Increases urinary alkalinity by excretion of bicarbonate ions.

Time lapse before drug works:
1 hour.

Don't take with:
Any medicine that will decrease mental alertness or reflexes, such as alcohol, other mind-altering drugs, cough/cold medicines, antihistamines, allergy medicine, sedatives, tranquilizers (sleeping pills or "downers"), barbiturates, seizure medicine, narcotics, other prescription medicine for pain, muscle relaxants, anesthetics.

POSSIBLE ADVERSE REACTIONS OR SIDE EFFECTS

SYMPTOMS	WHAT TO DO
Life-threatening:	
Black, tarry stools; vomiting blood; severe abdominal cramps; irregular heartbeat; shortness of breath.	Discontinue. Seek emergency treatment.
Common:	
Nausea or vomiting.	Continue. Call doctor when convenient.
Infrequent:	
Confusion, dizziness, swollen feet and ankles, irritability, depression, muscle pain, nervousness, numbness or tingling in hands or feet, unpleasant taste, weakness.	Discontinue. Call doctor right away.
Rare:	
Slow breathing, tiredness.	Discontinue. Call doctor right away.

WARNINGS & PRECAUTIONS

Don't take if:
You are allergic to any citrate.

Before you start, consult your doctor:
- If you have any disease involving the adrenal glands, diabetes, chronic diarrhea, heart problems, hypertension, kidney disease, stomach ulcer or gastritis, urinary tract infection, toxemia of pregnancy.
- If you plan strenuous exercise.

Over age 60:
Adverse reactions and side effects may be more frequent and severe than in younger persons. Ask doctor about smaller doses.

Pregnancy:
Avoid if possible. Consult doctor. Risk category C (see page xviii).

Breast-feeding:
Safety during lactation not established. Consult doctor.

Infants & children:
Use only under close medical supervision.

Prolonged use:
- Adverse reactions more likely.
- Talk to your doctor about the need for follow-up medical examinations or laboratory studies to check complete blood counts (white blood cell count, platelet count, red blood cell count, hemoglobin, hematocrit), serum electrolytes, urine.

Skin & sunlight:
No problems expected.

Driving, piloting or hazardous work:
Don't drive or pilot aircraft until you learn how medicine affects you. Don't work around dangerous machinery. Don't climb ladders or work in high places. Danger increases if you drink alcohol or take medicine affecting alertness and reflexes, such as antihistamines, tranquilizers, sedatives, pain medicine, narcotics and mind-altering drugs.

Discontinuing:
Don't discontinue without consulting doctor. Dose may require gradual reduction if you have taken drug for a long time. Doses of other drugs may also require adjustment.

Others:
- Drink at least 8 ounces of water or other liquid (except milk) every hour while awake.
- Liquid may be chilled (don't freeze) to improve taste.
- Monitor potassium in blood with frequent laboratory studies.

POSSIBLE INTERACTION WITH OTHER DRUGS

GENERIC NAME OR DRUG CLASS	COMBINED EFFECT
Amphetamines*	Increased amphetamine effect.
Antacids*	Toxic effect of citrates (alkalosis).
Calcium supplements*	Increased risk of kidney stones.
Digitalis preparations*	Increased risk of too much potassium in blood.
Methenamine	Decreased effects of methenamine.
Mexiletine	May slow elimination of mexiletine and cause need to adjust dosage.
Quinidine	Prolonged quinidine effect.

POSSIBLE INTERACTION WITH OTHER SUBSTANCES

INTERACTS WITH	COMBINED EFFECT
Alcohol:	Decreased mental alertness.
Beverages: Salt-free milk.	May cause potassium toxicity.
Cocaine:	None expected.
Foods: Milk, cheese, ice cream, yogurt, buttermilk, salty foods, salt, salt substitutes.	May increase likelihood of kidney stones.
Marijuana:	None expected.
Tobacco:	Increased likelihood of stomach irritation.

*See Glossary

CLIDINIUM

BRAND NAMES

Apo-Chlorax
Clindex
Clinoxide
Corium
Librax
Lidox
Lodoxide
Quarzan
Zebrax

BASIC INFORMATION

Habit forming? No
Prescription needed?
Low strength: No
High strength: Yes
Available as generic? No
Drug class: Antispasmodic, anticholinergic

USES

Reduces spasms of digestive system, bladder and urethra.

DOSAGE & USAGE INFORMATION

How to take:
Capsule—Swallow with liquid or food to lessen stomach irritation.

When to take:
30 minutes before meals (unless directed otherwise by doctor).

If you forget a dose:
Take as soon as you remember up to 2 hours late. If more than 2 hours, wait for next scheduled dose (don't double this dose).

What drug does:
Blocks nerve impulses at parasympathetic nerve endings, preventing muscle contractions and gland secretions of organs involved.

Time lapse before drug works:
15 to 30 minutes.

Continued next column

OVERDOSE

SYMPTOMS:
Dilated pupils, rapid pulse and breathing, dizziness, fever, hallucinations, confusion, slurred speech, agitation, flushed face, convulsions, coma.
WHAT TO DO:

- **Dial 911 (emergency) for an ambulance or medical help or poison center 1-800-222-1222. Then give first aid immediately.**
- **See emergency information on inside covers.**

Don't take with:
Any other medicine without consulting your doctor or pharmacist.

POSSIBLE ADVERSE REACTIONS OR SIDE EFFECTS

SYMPTOMS	WHAT TO DO
Life-threatening:	
In case of overdose, see previous column.	
Common:	
• Confusion, delirium, rapid heartbeat.	Discontinue. Call doctor right away.
• Nausea, vomiting, decreased sweating.	Continue. Call doctor when convenient.
• Constipation.	Continue. Tell doctor at next visit.
• Dryness in ears, nose, throat, mouth.	No action necessary.
Infrequent:	
• Nasal congestion, altered taste, difficult urination, headache, impotence.	Continue. Call doctor when convenient.
• Lightheadedness.	Discontinue. Call doctor right away.
Rare:	
Rash or hives, eye pain, blurred vision.	Discontinue. Call doctor right away.

WARNINGS & PRECAUTIONS

Don't take if:

- You are allergic to any anticholinergic.
- You have trouble with stomach bloating.
- You have difficulty emptying your bladder completely (enlarged prostate).
- You have narrow-angle glaucoma.
- You have severe ulcerative colitis.

Before you start, consult your doctor:

- If you have open-angle glaucoma.
- If you have angina, chronic bronchitis or asthma, kidney or thyroid disease, hiatal hernia, liver disease, enlarged prostate, myasthenia gravis, peptic ulcer.
- If you will have surgery within 2 months, including dental surgery, requiring general or spinal anesthesia.

Over age 60:
Adverse reactions and side effects may be more frequent and severe than in younger persons.

Pregnancy:
Decide with your doctor whether drug benefits justify risk to unborn child. Risk category C (see page xviii).

Breast-feeding:
Drug passes into milk and decreases milk flow. Avoid drug or discontinue nursing until you finish medicine. Consult doctor for advice on maintaining milk supply.

Infants & children:
Use only under medical supervision.

Prolonged use:
Chronic constipation, possible fecal impaction. Consult doctor immediately.

Skin & sunlight:
No problems expected.

Driving, piloting or hazardous work:
Don't drive or pilot aircraft until you learn how medicine affects you. Don't work around dangerous machinery. Don't climb ladders or work in high places. Danger increases if you drink alcohol or take medicine affecting alertness and reflexes, such as antihistamines, tranquilizers, sedatives, pain medicine, narcotics, or mind-altering drugs.

Discontinuing:
May be unnecessary to finish medicine. Follow doctor's instructions.

Others:
Advise any doctor or dentist whom you consult that you take this medicine.

POSSIBLE INTERACTION WITH OTHER DRUGS

GENERIC NAME OR DRUG CLASS	COMBINED EFFECT
Amantadine	Increased clidinium effect.
Antacids*	Decreased clidinium effect.
Anticholinergics, other*	Increased clidinium effect.
Antidepressants, tricyclic*	Increased clidinium effect. Increased sedation.
Antidiarrheals*	Increased clidinium effect.
Antihistamines*	Increased clidinium effect.
Attapulgite	Decreased clidinium effect.
Haloperidol	Increased internal eye pressure.
Ketoconazole	Decreased ketoconazole effect.
Meperidine	Increased clidinium effect.
Methylphenidate	Increased clidinium effect.
Molindone	Increased anti-cholinergic effect.
Monoamine oxidase (MAO) inhibitors*	Increased clidinium effect.
Nitrates*	Increased internal eye pressure.
Nizatidine	Increased nizatidine effect.
Orphenadrine	Increased clidinium effect.
Pilocarpine	Loss of pilocarpine effect in glaucoma treatment.
Potassium supplements*	Possible intestinal ulcers with oral potassium tablets.
Tranquilizers*	Increased clidinium effect.
Vitamin C	Decreased clidinium effect. Avoid large doses of vitamin C.

POSSIBLE INTERACTION WITH OTHER SUBSTANCES

INTERACTS WITH	COMBINED EFFECT
Alcohol:	None expected.
Beverages:	None expected.
Cocaine:	Excessively rapid heartbeat. Avoid.
Foods:	None expected.
Marijuana:	Drowsiness and dry mouth.
Tobacco:	None expected.

*See Glossary

CLINDAMYCIN

BRAND NAMES

Cleocin
Cleocin Pediatric
Cleocin (Vaginal)
Dalacin C
Dalacin C Palmitate
Dalacin C Phosphate

BASIC INFORMATION

Habit forming? No
Prescription needed? Yes
Available as generic? Yes
Drug class: Antibacterial

USES

Treatment of bacterial infections that are susceptible to clindamycin.

DOSAGE & USAGE INFORMATION

How to take:
- Capsule or liquid—Swallow with liquid. Take with a full glass of water or a meal to avoid gastric irritation.
- Vaginal cream—Use applicator supplied with product to insert cream into vagina. Wash hands immediately after using.

When to take:
- Oral—At the same times each day.
- Vaginal cream—Apply at bedtime unless directed differently by your doctor.

If you forget a dose:
Take as soon as you remember up to 2 hours late. If more than 2 hours, wait for next scheduled dose (don't double this dose).

What drug does:
Destroys susceptible bacteria. Does not kill viruses.

Time lapse before drug works:
3 to 5 days.

Don't take with:
Any other medicine without consulting your doctor or pharmacist.

OVERDOSE

SYMPTOMS:
Severe nausea, vomiting, diarrhea.
WHAT TO DO:
Overdose unlikely to threaten life. If person takes much larger amount than prescribed, call doctor, poison center 1-800-222-1222 or hospital emergency room for instructions.

POSSIBLE ADVERSE REACTIONS OR SIDE EFFECTS

SYMPTOMS	WHAT TO DO
Life-threatening:	
Hives, wheezing, faintness, itching, coma.	Seek emergency treatment immediately.
Common:	
Bloating.	Discontinue. Call doctor right away.
Infrequent:	
• Unusual thirst; vomiting; stomach cramps; severe and watery diarrhea with blood or mucus; painful, swollen joints; fever; jaundice; tiredness; weakness.	Discontinue. Call doctor right away.
• White patches in mouth; rash, itch around groin, rectum or armpits; vaginal discharge, itching; dizziness; nausea; mild diarrhea; pain during intercourse.	Continue. Call doctor when convenient.
Rare:	
None expected.	

WARNINGS & PRECAUTIONS

Don't take if:
- You are allergic to lincomycins, clindamycin or doxorubicin.
- You have had ulcerative colitis.

Before you start, consult your doctor:
- If you have had yeast infections of mouth, skin or vagina.
- If you will have surgery within 2 months, including dental surgery, requiring general or spinal anesthesia.
- If you have kidney or liver disease.
- If you have allergies of any kind.
- If you have a history of gastrointestinal disorders.

Over age 60:
Adverse reactions and side effects may be more frequent and severe than in younger persons.

Pregnancy:
Decide with your doctor if drug benefits justify risk to unborn child. Risk category B (see page xviii).

Breast-feeding:
Drug passes into milk. Avoid drug or discontinue nursing until you finish medicine. Consult doctor for advice on maintaining milk supply.

Infants & children:
Don't give to infants younger than 1 month. Use for children only under medical supervision.

Prolonged use:
- Severe colitis with diarrhea and bleeding.
- You may become more susceptible to infections caused by germs not responsive to clindamycin.
- Talk to your doctor about the need for follow-up medical examinations or laboratory studies to check stool exams and perform proctosigmoidoscopy.

Skin & sunlight:
No problems expected.

Driving, piloting or hazardous work:
No problems expected.

Discontinuing:
- Don't discontinue without doctor's advice until you complete prescribed dose, even though symptoms diminish or disappear.
- If vaginal discharge, itching or pain occurs after discontinuing medicine, consult doctor.

Others:
- May interfere with the accuracy of some medical tests. Advise any doctor or dentist whom you consult that you take this medicine.
- Vaginal cream product may decrease the effectiveness of condoms, cervical caps or diaphragms. Wait 72 hours after treatment to use any of these devices.

POSSIBLE INTERACTION WITH OTHER DRUGS

GENERIC NAME OR DRUG CLASS	COMBINED EFFECT
Antidiarrheal preparations*	Decreased clindamycin effect.
Antimyasthenics*	Decreased anti-myasthenic effect.
Chloramphenicol	Decreased clindamycin effect.
Erythromycins*	Decreased clindamycin effect.
Muscle blockers*	Increased actions of muscle blockers to unsafe degree. Avoid.
Narcotics*	Increased risk of respiratory problems.

POSSIBLE INTERACTION WITH OTHER SUBSTANCES

INTERACTS WITH	COMBINED EFFECT
Alcohol:	None expected.
Beverages:	None expected.
Cocaine:	None expected.
Foods:	None expected.
Marijuana:	None expected.
Tobacco:	None expected.

***See Glossary**

CLOMIPHENE

BRAND NAMES

Clomid
Milophene
Serophene

BASIC INFORMATION

Habit forming? No
Prescription needed? Yes
Available as generic? Yes
Drug class: Gonad stimulant

USES

- Treatment for men with low sperm counts.
- Treatment for ovulatory failure in women who wish to become pregnant.

DOSAGE & USAGE INFORMATION

How to take:
Tablet—Swallow with liquid.

When to take:
- Men—Take at the same time each day.
- Women—Follow physician's instructions carefully.

If you forget a dose:
Take as soon as you remember. If you forget a day, double next dose. If you miss 2 or more doses, consult doctor.

What drug does:
Antiestrogen effect stimulates ovulation and sperm production.

Time lapse before drug works:
Usually 3 to 6 months. Ovulation may occur 6 to 10 days after last day of treatment in any cycle.

Don't take with:
No restrictions.

OVERDOSE

SYMPTOMS:
Increased severity of adverse reactions and side effects.
WHAT TO DO:
Overdose unlikely to threaten life. If person takes much larger amount than prescribed, call doctor, poison center 1-800-222-1222 or hospital emergency room for instructions.

POSSIBLE ADVERSE REACTIONS OR SIDE EFFECTS

SYMPTOMS	WHAT TO DO
Life-threatening:	
Sudden shortness of breath.	Seek emergency treatment.
Common:	
• Bloating, abdominal pain, pelvic pain.	Discontinue. Call doctor right away.
• Hot flashes.	Continue. Tell doctor at next visit.
Infrequent:	
• Rash, itch, vomiting, jaundice.	Discontinue. Call doctor right away.
• Constipation, diarrhea, increased appetite, heavy menstrual flow, frequent urination, breast discomfort, weight change, hair loss, nausea, eyes sensitive to light.	Continue. Call doctor when convenient.
Rare:	
• Vision changes.	Discontinue. Call doctor right away.
• Dizziness, headache, tiredness, depression, nervousness.	Continue. Call doctor when convenient.

WARNINGS & PRECAUTIONS

Don't take if:
You are allergic to clomiphene.

Before you start, consult your doctor:
- If you have an ovarian cyst, fibroid uterine tumors or unusual vaginal bleeding.
- If you have inflamed veins caused by blood clots.
- If you have liver disease.
- If you are depressed.

Over age 60:
Not recommended.

Pregnancy:
Stop taking at first sign of pregnancy. Consult doctor. Risk category C (see page xviii).

Breast-feeding:
Not used.

Infants & children:
Not used.

Prolonged use:
- Not recommended.
- Talk to your doctor about the need for follow-up medical examinations or laboratory studies to check basal body temperature, endometrial biopsy, kidney function, eyes.

Skin & sunlight:
No special problems expected.

Driving, piloting or hazardous work:
- Avoid if you feel dizzy.
- May cause blurred vision.

Discontinuing:
May be unnecessary to finish medicine. Follow doctor's instructions.

Others:
- Have a complete pelvic examination before treatment.
- Advise any doctor or dentist whom you consult that you take this medicine.
- If you become pregnant, twins or triplets are possible.

POSSIBLE INTERACTION WITH OTHER DRUGS

GENERIC NAME OR DRUG CLASS	COMBINED EFFECT
Thyroglobulin	May increase serum thyroglobulin.
Thyroxine (T-4)	May increase serum thyroxine.

POSSIBLE INTERACTION WITH OTHER SUBSTANCES

INTERACTS WITH	COMBINED EFFECT
Alcohol:	None expected.
Beverages:	None expected.
Cocaine:	None expected.
Foods:	None expected.
Marijuana:	None expected.
Tobacco:	None expected.

CLONIDINE

BRAND NAMES

Catapres
Catapres-TTS
Dixarit

BASIC INFORMATION

Habit forming? No
Prescription needed? Yes
Available as generic? Yes
Drug class: Antihypertensive

USES

- Treatment of narcotic withdrawal syndrome.
- May be used for nicotine withdrawal.
- Prevention of migraine headaches.
- Control of overactivity and tics in children.
- Treatment of high blood pressure.

DOSAGE & USAGE INFORMATION

How to take:
- Tablet—Swallow with liquid.
- Transdermal patch (attaches to skin)—Apply to clean, dry, hairless skin on arm or trunk. Follow all prescription instructions carefully.

When to take:
- Tablet—Once or twice a day as directed.
- Transdermal patch—Replace as directed, usually once a week.

Continued next column

OVERDOSE

SYMPTOMS:
Vomiting, fainting, slow heartbeat, feeling cold, coma, diminished reflexes, shortness of breath, dizziness, extreme tiredness.
WHAT TO DO:
- **Dial 911 (emergency) for an ambulance or medical help or poison center 1-800-222-1222. Then give first aid immediately.**
- **If patient is unconscious and not breathing, give mouth-to-mouth breathing. If there is no heartbeat, use cardiac massage and mouth-to-mouth breathing (CPR). Don't try to make patient vomit. If you can't get help quickly, take patient to nearest emergency facility.**
- **See emergency information at end of book.**

If you forget a dose:
- Take tablet as soon as you remember. If it is almost time for the next dose, wait for the next scheduled dose (don't double this dose). If you miss more than 2 doses in a row, call your doctor.
- If the once-a-week patch change is 3 days late, call your doctor.

What drug does:
- Reduces nervous system overactivity.
- Relaxes and allows expansion of blood vessel walls.

Time lapse before drug works:
2 to 3 weeks for full benefit.

Don't take with:
- Medicines containing alcohol; read labels carefully.
- Any other medicine without consulting your doctor or pharmacist.

POSSIBLE ADVERSE REACTIONS OR SIDE EFFECTS

SYMPTOMS	WHAT TO DO
Life-threatening: In case of overdose, see previous column.	
Common: Dizziness, constipation, drowsiness, irritated skin (with skin patch), dry mouth, tiredness, headache.	Continue. Call doctor when convenient.
Infrequent: • Depression, swollen hands or feet.	Discontinue. Call doctor right away.
• Darkened skin (with skin patch), light-headedness upon rising from sitting or lying, nausea, vomiting, dry or burning eyes, diminished sex drive or ability, appetite loss, nervousness.	Continue. Call doctor when convenient.
Rare: Cold fingers and toes, nightmares, slow heart rate.	Discontinue. Call doctor right away.

WARNINGS & PRECAUTIONS

Don't take if:
You are allergic to clonidine.

Before you start, consult your doctor:
- If you will have surgery within 2 months, including dental surgery, requiring general or spinal anesthesia.
- If you have heart disease or kidney disease.
- If you have a peripheral circulation disorder (intermittent claudication, Raynaud's syndrome, Buerger's disease).
- If you have history of depression.
- If you have a disorder affecting the skin or any skin irritation (with use of transdermal patch).

Over age 60:
Adverse reactions and side effects may be more frequent and severe than in younger persons.

Pregnancy:
Decide with your doctor whether drug benefits justify risk to unborn child. Risk category C (see page xviii).

Breast-feeding:
Unknown whether safe or not. Consult doctor.

Infants & children:
Useful for controlling overactivity or tics.

Prolonged use:
- Don't discontinue without consulting doctor. Dose may require gradual reduction if you have taken drug for a long time. Doses of other drugs may also require adjustment.
- Request yearly eye examinations.
- Talk to your doctor about the need for follow-up medical examinations or laboratory studies.

Skin & sunlight:
Use with caution in hot weather.

Driving, piloting or hazardous work:
Don't drive or pilot aircraft until you learn how medicine affects you. Don't work around dangerous machinery. Don't climb ladders or work in high places. Danger increases if you drink alcohol or take medicine affecting alertness and reflexes.

Discontinuing:
Don't discontinue abruptly. May cause a withdrawal syndrome including anxiety, chest pain, insomnia, headache, nausea, irregular heartbeat, flushed face, sweating. Consult doctor if any symptoms occur after discontinuing the medication.

Others:
- Advise any doctor or dentist whom you consult that you take this medicine.
- For dry mouth, suck sugarless hard candy or chew sugarless gum. If dry mouth continues, consult your dentist.

POSSIBLE INTERACTION WITH OTHER DRUGS

GENERIC NAME OR DRUG CLASS	COMBINED EFFECT
Antidepressants, tricyclic*	Decreased clonidine effect.
Antihypertensives*, other	Excessive blood pressure drop.
Appetite suppressants*	Decreased clonidine effect.
Beta-adrenergic blocking agents*	Possible precipitous change in blood pressure.
Central nervous system (CNS) depressants*	Increased depressive effects of both drugs.

POSSIBLE INTERACTION WITH OTHER SUBSTANCES

INTERACTS WITH	COMBINED EFFECT
Alcohol:	Increased sensitivity to sedative effect of alcohol and very low blood pressure. Avoid.
Beverages:	None expected.
Cocaine:	Increased risk of heart block and high blood pressure.
Foods:	None expected.
Marijuana:	Weakness on standing.
Tobacco:	None expected.

*See Glossary

CLONIDINE & CHLORTHALIDONE

BRAND NAMES

Combipres

BASIC INFORMATION

Habit forming? No
Prescription needed? Yes
Available as generic? Yes
Drug class: Antihypertensive, diuretic

USES

- Treatment of high blood pressure.
- Reduces fluid retention (edema) caused by conditions such as heart disorders and liver disease.

DOSAGE & USAGE INFORMATION

How to take:
Tablet—Swallow with liquid. If you can't swallow whole, crumble tablet and take with liquid or food. Don't exceed dose.

When to take:
At the same time each day.

If you forget a dose:
Take as soon as you remember up to 2 hours late. If more than 2 hours, wait for next scheduled dose (don't double this dose).

What drug does:
- Relaxes and allows expansion of blood vessel walls.
- Forces sodium and water excretion, reducing body fluid.
- Reduced body fluid and relaxed arteries lower blood pressure.

Time lapse before drug works:
4 to 6 hours. May require several weeks to lower blood pressure.

Don't take with:
Any medicine that will decrease mental alertness such as alcohol, antihistamines, cold/cough medicines, sedatives, tranquilizers, narcotics, prescription pain medicine, barbiturates, seizure medicine, anesthetics.

OVERDOSE

SYMPTOMS:
Vomiting; fainting; rapid, irregular, slow heartbeat; diminished reflexes; cramps; shortness of breath; weakness; drowsiness; weak pulse; coma.

WHAT TO DO:
- **Dial 911 (emergency) for an ambulance or medical help or poison center 1-800-222-1222. Then give first aid immediately.**
- **If patient is unconscious and not breathing, give mouth-to-mouth breathing. If there is no heartbeat, use cardiac massage and mouth-to-mouth breathing (CPR). Don't try to make patient vomit. If you can't get help quickly, take patient to nearest emergency facility.**
- **See emergency information at end of book.**

POSSIBLE ADVERSE REACTIONS OR SIDE EFFECTS

SYMPTOMS	WHAT TO DO
Life-threatening:	
Irregular heartbeat, weak pulse.	Discontinue. Seek emergency treatment.
Common:	
Dry mouth, increased thirst, muscle cramps, nausea or vomiting, mood changes, drowsiness.	Discontinue. Call doctor right away.
Infrequent:	
Vomiting, diminished sex desire and performance, insomnia, dizziness, diarrhea, constipation, appetite loss.	Continue. Call doctor when convenient.
Rare:	
• Jaundice; easy bruising or bleeding; sore throat, fever, mouth ulcers; rash or hives; joint pain; flank pain; abdominal pain.	Discontinue. Call doctor right away.
• Cold fingers and toes, nightmares.	Continue. Call doctor when convenient.

WARNINGS & PRECAUTIONS

Don't take if:
- You are allergic to any thiazide diuretic drug or alpha-adrenergic blocker.
- You are under age 12.

Before you start, consult your doctor:
- If you are allergic to any sulfa drug.
- If you have gout, liver, pancreas or kidney disorder, a peripheral circulation disorder (intermittent claudication, Buerger's disease), history of depression, heart disease.
- If you will have surgery within 2 months, including dental surgery, requiring general or spinal anesthesia.

Over age 60:
Adverse reactions and side effects may be more frequent and severe than in younger persons, especially dizziness and excessive potassium loss.

Pregnancy:
Decide with your doctor if drug benefits justify risk to unborn child. Risk category C (see page xviii).

Breast-feeding:
Drug passes into milk. Avoid drug or discontinue nursing until you finish medicine. Consult doctor for advice on maintaining milk supply.

Infants & children:
Use only after careful medical supervision after age 12. Avoid before age 12.

Prolonged use:
- Don't discontinue without consulting doctor. Dose may require gradual reduction if you have taken drug for a long time. Doses of other drugs may also require adjustment.
- Request yearly eye examinations.
- Talk to your doctor about the need for follow-up medical examinations or laboratory studies.

Skin & sunlight:
No special problems expected.

Driving, piloting or hazardous work:
Don't drive or pilot aircraft until you learn how medicine affects you. Don't work around dangerous machinery. Don't climb ladders or work in high places. Danger increases if you drink alcohol or take medicine affecting alertness and reflexes.

Discontinuing:
Don't discontinue abruptly. May cause rebound high blood pressure, anxiety, chest pain, insomnia, headache, nausea, irregular heartbeat, flushed face, sweating.

Others:
- Hot weather and fever may cause dehydration and drop in blood pressure. Dose may require temporary adjustment. Weigh daily and report any unexpected weight decreases to your doctor.
- Advise any doctor or dentist whom you consult that you take this medicine.
- May cause rise in uric acid, leading to gout.
- May cause blood-sugar rise in diabetics.

POSSIBLE INTERACTION WITH OTHER DRUGS

GENERIC NAME OR DRUG CLASS	COMBINED EFFECT
Allopurinol	Decreased allopurinol effect.
Angiotensin-converting enzyme (ACE) inhibitors*	Possible excessive potassium in blood.
Antidepressants, tricyclic*	Dangerous drop in blood pressure. Avoid combination unless under medical supervision.
Antihypertensives, other*	Excessive blood pressure drop.
Appetite suppressants*	Decreased clonidine effect.
Barbiturates*	Increased chlorthalidone effect.
Beta-adrenergic blocking agents*	Possible precipitous change in blood pressure.
Carteolol	Increased anti-hypertensive effect.
Central nervous system (CNS) depressants*	Increased sedative effect.
Cholestyramine	Decreased chlorthalidone effect.
Digitalis preparations*	Excessive potassium loss that causes dangerous heart rhythms.
Diuretics*	Excessive blood pressure drop.

Continued on page 909

POSSIBLE INTERACTION WITH OTHER SUBSTANCES

INTERACTS WITH	COMBINED EFFECT
Alcohol:	Increased sensitivity to sedative effect of alcohol and very low blood pressure. Avoid.
Beverages: Caffeine-containing drinks.	Decreased clonidine effect.
Cocaine:	Increased risk of heart block and high blood pressure.
Foods: Licorice.	Excessive potassium loss that causes dangerous heart rhythm.
Marijuana:	Weakness on standing. May increase blood pressure.
Tobacco:	None expected.

***See Glossary**

CLOTRIMAZOLE (Oral-Local)

BRAND NAMES

Mycelex Troches

BASIC INFORMATION

Habit forming? No
Prescription needed? Yes
Available as generic? No
Drug class: Antifungal

USES

- Treats thrush, white mouth (candidiasis).
- Used primarily in immunosuppressed patients to treat and prevent mouth infection.

DOSAGE & USAGE INFORMATION

How to take:
Lozenges—Dissolve slowly and completely in the mouth, 5 times a day. Swallow saliva during this time. Don't swallow lozenge whole and don't chew.

When to take:
14 days or longer.

If you forget a dose:
Take as soon as you remember up to 2 hours late. If more than 2 hours, wait for next scheduled dose (don't double this dose).

What drug does:
Kills fungus by interfering with cell wall membrane and its permeability.

Time lapse before drug works:
1 to 3 hours.

Don't take with:
Any other medicine without consulting your doctor or pharmacist.

OVERDOSE

SYMPTOMS:
None expected, but if large dose has been taken, follow instructions below.
WHAT TO DO:
- **Dial 911 (emergency) for an ambulance or medical help or poison center 1-800-222-1222. Then give first aid immediately.**
- **See emergency information on inside covers.**

POSSIBLE ADVERSE REACTIONS OR SIDE EFFECTS

SYMPTOMS	WHAT TO DO
Life-threatening: None expected.	
Common: None expected.	
Infrequent: Abdominal pain, diarrhea, nausea, vomiting.	Discontinue. Call doctor right away.
Rare: None expected.	

WARNINGS & PRECAUTIONS

Don't take if:
You have severe liver disease.

Before you start, consult your doctor:
If you have had a recent organ transplant.

Over age 60:
Adverse reactions and side effects may be more frequent and severe than in younger persons. You may need smaller doses for shorter periods of time.

Pregnancy:
Decide with your doctor if drug benefits justify risk to unborn child. Risk category C (see page xviii).

Breast-feeding:
Unknown effect. Consult doctor.

Infants & children:
Use only under medical supervision for children younger than 4 or 5 years.

Prolonged use:
No problems expected.

Skin & sunlight:
No problems expected.

Driving, piloting or hazardous work:
Don't drive or pilot aircraft until you learn how medicine affects you. Don't work around dangerous machinery. Don't climb ladders or work in high places. Danger increases if you drink alcohol or take medicine affecting alertness and reflexes.

Discontinuing:
Don't discontinue without consulting doctor. Dose may require gradual reduction if you have taken drug for a long time. Doses of other drugs may also require adjustment.

Others:
- Continue for full term of treatment. May require several months.
- Check with physician if not improved in 1 week.

POSSIBLE INTERACTION WITH OTHER DRUGS

GENERIC NAME OR DRUG CLASS	COMBINED EFFECT
None expected.	

POSSIBLE INTERACTION WITH OTHER SUBSTANCES

INTERACTS WITH	COMBINED EFFECT
Alcohol:	Decreased effects of clotrimazole.
Beverages:	None expected.
Cocaine:	Decreased effects of clotrimazole.
Foods:	None expected.
Marijuana:	Decreased effects of clotrimazole.
Tobacco:	Decreased effects of clotrimazole.

***See Glossary**

CLOZAPINE

BRAND NAMES

Clozaril
Leponex

BASIC INFORMATION

Habit forming? No
Prescription needed? Yes. Prescribed only through a special program.
Available as generic? Yes
Drug class: Antipsychotic

USES

Treats severe schizophrenia in patients not helped by other medicines.

DOSAGE & USAGE INFORMATION

How to take:
Tablet—Swallow with liquid. If you can't swallow whole, crumble tablet and take with liquid or food.

When to take:
Once or twice daily as directed.

If you forget a dose:
Take as soon as you remember up to 2 hours late. If more than 2 hours, wait for next scheduled dose (don't double this dose).

What drug does:
Interferes with binding of dopamine. May produce significant improvement, but may at times also make schizophrenia worse.

Time lapse before drug works:
Weeks to months before improvement is evident. Your doctor may increase the dosage to obtain optimal effectiveness..

Don't take with:
Any other prescription drug, nonprescription drug or alcohol without first checking with your doctor or pharmacist.

OVERDOSE

SYMPTOMS:
Heartbeat fast, slow, irregular; hallucinations; restlessness; excitement; drowsiness; breathing difficulty.
WHAT TO DO:
- **Dial 911 (emergency) for an ambulance or medical help or poison center 1-800-222-1222. Then give first aid immediately.**
- **See emergency information at end of book.**

POSSIBLE ADVERSE REACTIONS OR SIDE EFFECTS

SYMPTOMS	WHAT TO DO
Life-threatening:	
High fever, rapid pulse, profuse sweating, muscle rigidity, confusion and irritability, seizures; fever, chills, mouth sores.	Discontinue. Seek emergency treatment.
Common:	
Dry mouth, blurred vision, constipation, difficulty urinating; sedation, low blood pressure, dizziness.	Continue. Call doctor when convenient.
Infrequent:	
None expected.	
Rare:	
• Jerky or involuntary movements, especially of the face, lips, jaw, tongue; slow-frequency tremor of head or limbs, especially while moving; muscle rigidity, lack of facial expression and slow inflexible movements; seizures.	Discontinue. Call doctor right away.
• Pacing or restlessness; (akathisia); intermittent spasms of muscles of face, eyes, tongue, jaw, neck, body or limbs.	Continue. Call doctor when convenient.

WARNINGS & PRECAUTIONS

Don't take if:
- You are significantly mentally depressed.
- You have bone marrow depression from other drugs.
- You have an enlarged prostate.
- You have glaucoma.

Before you start, consult your doctor:
- If you have ever had seizures from any cause.
- If you have liver, heart or gastrointestinal disease or any type of blood disorder.

Over age 60:
Possible greater risk of weakness or dizziness upon standing after sitting or lying down. Greater risk of excitement, confusion. Great risk of difficulty in urination.

Pregnancy:
Risk category B (see page xviii).

Breast-feeding:
May cause sedation, restlessness or irritability in the nursing infant. Avoid.

Infants & children:
Safety not established. Consult doctor.

Prolonged use:
Effects unknown.

Skin & sunlight:
No problems expected.

Driving, piloting or hazardous work:
Don't drive or pilot aircraft until you learn how medicine affects you. Don't work around dangerous machinery. Don't climb ladders or work in high places. Danger increases if you drink alcohol or take medicine affecting alertness and reflexes.

Discontinuing:
Don't discontinue without consulting doctor. Dose may require gradual reduction if you have taken drug for a long time. Doses of other drugs may also require adjustment.

Others:
- This medicine is available only through a special management program for monitoring and distributing this drug.
- You will need laboratory studies each week for white blood cell and differential counts.

POSSIBLE INTERACTION WITH OTHER DRUGS

GENERIC NAME OR DRUG CLASS	COMBINED EFFECT
Antihypertensives*	Lower than expected blood pressure.
Bone marrow depressants*	Toxic bone marrow depression.
Bupropion	Increased risk of seizures.
Carbamazepine	Decreased clozapine effect.
Central nervous system (CNS) depressants*	Toxic effects on the central nervous system.
Fluoxetine	Increased risk of adverse reactions.
Fluvoxamine	Increased risk of adverse reactions.
Haloperidol	Increased risk of seizures.
Lithium	Increased risk of seizures.
Phenytoin	Decreased clozapine effect.
Risperidone	Increased risperidone effect.
Valproic acid	Increased clozapine effect.

POSSIBLE INTERACTION WITH OTHER SUBSTANCES

INTERACTS WITH	COMBINED EFFECT
Alcohol:	Avoid. Increases toxic effect on the central nervous system.
Beverages: Caffeine drinks.	Excess (more than 3 cups of coffee or equivalent) increases risk of heartbeat irregularities.
Cocaine:	Increased risk of heartbeat irregularities.
Foods:	None expected.
Marijuana:	Increased risk of heartbeat irregularities.
Tobacco:	Decreased serum concentration of clozapine. Avoid.

*See Glossary

COAL TAR (Topical)

BRAND NAMES

See complete list of brand names in the *Generic and Brand Name Directory*, page 862.

BASIC INFORMATION

Habit forming? No
Prescription needed? No (for most)
Available as generic? Yes
Drug class: Antiseborrheic, antipsoriatic, keratolytic

USES

Applied to the skin to treat dandruff, seborrhea, dermatitis, eczema and other skin diseases.

DOSAGE & USAGE INFORMATION

How to use:

- Follow package instructions.
- Don't apply to blistered, oozing, infected or raw skin.
- Keep away from eyes.
- Protect treated area from sunshine for 72 hours.

When to use:
According to package instructions.

If you forget a dose:
Use as soon as you remember.

What drug does:

- Kills bacteria and fungus organisms on contact.
- Suppresses overproduction of skin cells.

Time lapse before drug works:
None. Works immediately. May take several days before maximum effect.

Don't take with:
Any other medicine without consulting your doctor or pharmacist.

OVERDOSE

SYMPTOMS:
None expected.
WHAT TO DO:
Overdose unlikely to threaten life. If person takes much larger amount than prescribed, call doctor, poison center 1-800-222-1222 or hospital emergency room for instructions.

POSSIBLE ADVERSE REACTIONS OR SIDE EFFECTS

SYMPTOMS	WHAT TO DO
Life-threatening:	
None expected.	
Common:	
Skin stinging.	Continue. Call doctor when convenient.
Infrequent:	
Skin more irritated.	Continue. Call doctor when convenient.
Rare:	
Pus forms in lesions on skin.	Continue. Call doctor when convenient.

WARNINGS & PRECAUTIONS

Don't use if:
You have intolerance to coal tar.

Before you start, consult your doctor:
If you have infected skin or open wounds.

Over age 60:
No special problems expected.

Pregnancy:
Consult doctor. Risk category C (see page xviii).

Breast-feeding:
No special problems expected. Consult doctor.

Infants & children:
Don't use on infants.

Prolonged use:
No special problems expected.

Skin & sunlight:
One or more drugs in this group may cause rash or intensify sunburn in areas exposed to sun or ultraviolet light (photosensitivity reaction). Avoid overexposure. Notify doctor if reaction occurs.

Driving, piloting or hazardous work:
No problems expected.

Discontinuing:
No special problems expected.

Others:
- May affect results in some medical tests.
- Protect treated area from direct sunlight for 72 hours.

POSSIBLE INTERACTION WITH OTHER DRUGS

GENERIC NAME OR DRUG CLASS	COMBINED EFFECT
Psoralens (methoxsalen, trioxsalen)	Excess sensitivity to sun.

POSSIBLE INTERACTION WITH OTHER SUBSTANCES

INTERACTS WITH	COMBINED EFFECT
Alcohol:	None expected.
Beverages:	None expected.
Cocaine:	None expected.
Foods:	None expected.
Marijuana:	None expected.
Tobacco:	None expected.

***See Glossary**

COLCHICINE

GENERIC NAMES

COLCHICINE

BASIC INFORMATION

Habit forming? No
Prescription needed? Yes
Available as generic? Yes
Drug class: Antigout

USES

- Relieves joint pain, inflammation, swelling of gout.
- Also used for familial Mediterranean fever, dermatitis herpetiformis, calcium pyrophosphate deposition disease, amyloidosis, Paget's disease of bone, recurrent pericarditis, Behcet's syndrome.

DOSAGE & USAGE INFORMATION

How to take:
Tablet—Swallow with liquid or food to lessen stomach irritation.

When to take:
- As prescribed. Stop taking when pain stops or at first sign of digestive upset. Wait at least 3 days between treatments.
- Don't take more than 8 doses.

If you forget a dose:
Don't double next dose. Consult doctor.

What drug does:
Decreases acidity of joint tissues and prevents deposits of uric-acid crystals.

Time lapse before drug works:
12 to 48 hours.

Don't take with:
Any other medicine without consulting your doctor or pharmacist.

OVERDOSE

SYMPTOMS:
Bloody urine; diarrhea; burning feeling in the throat, skin or stomach; nausea or vomiting; muscle weakness; fever; shortness of breath; stupor; convulsions; coma.
WHAT TO DO:
- **Dial 911 (emergency) for an ambulance or medical help or poison center 1-800-222-1222. Then give first aid immediately.**
- **See emergency information on inside covers.**

POSSIBLE ADVERSE REACTIONS OR SIDE EFFECTS

SYMPTOMS	WHAT TO DO
Life-threatening:	
In case of overdose, see previous column.	
Common:	
Diarrhea, nausea, vomiting, abdominal pain.	Discontinue. Call doctor right away.
Infrequent:	
Hair loss with long-term use.	Continue. Call doctor when convenient.
Rare:	
Jaundice, black or tarry stool, blood in urine, breathing difficulty, fever, chills, headache, hives, mouth or lip sores, sore throat, unusual bruising or bleeding, unusual tiredness or weakness.	Discontinue. Call doctor right away.

WARNINGS & PRECAUTIONS

Don't take if:
You are allergic to colchicine.

Before you start, consult your doctor:
- If you have had peptic ulcers or ulcerative colitis.
- If you have heart, liver or kidney disease.
- If you will have surgery within 2 months, including dental surgery, requiring general or spinal anesthesia.
- If you have a gastrointestinal disorder.
- If you drink large amounts of alcohol.

Over age 60:
Adverse reactions and side effects may be more frequent and severe than in younger persons. Colchicine has a narrow margin of safety for people in this age group.

Pregnancy:
Consult doctor. Risk category D (see page xviii).

Breast-feeding:
Drug passes into breast milk. Effect unknown. Consult doctor.

Infants & children:
Not recommended.

Prolonged use:
- Hair loss.
- Numbness or tingling in hands and feet.
- Talk to your doctor about the need for follow-up medical examinations or laboratory studies to check complete blood counts (white blood cell count, platelet count, red blood cell count, hemoglobin, hematocrit).

Skin & sunlight:
No problems expected.

Driving, piloting or hazardous work:
Don't drive or pilot aircraft until you learn how medicine affects you. Don't work around dangerous machinery. Don't climb ladders or work in high places. Danger increases if you drink alcohol or take medicine affecting alertness and reflexes, such as antihistamines, tranquilizers, sedatives, pain medicine, narcotics and mind-altering drugs.

Discontinuing:
- May be unnecessary to finish medicine. Follow doctor's instructions.
- Stop taking if digestive upsets occur before symptoms are relieved.

Others:
- Limit each course of treatment to 8 mg. Don't exceed 3 mg. per 24 hours.
- May cause decreased sperm production in males.
- May interfere with the accuracy of some medical tests.

POSSIBLE INTERACTION WITH OTHER DRUGS

GENERIC NAME OR DRUG CLASS	COMBINED EFFECT
Anticoagulants*	Increased anticoagulant effect.
Anti-inflammatory drugs, nonsteroidal (NSAIDs)*	Increased risk of gastrointestinal problems.
Blood dyscrasia-causing medications*	Increased bone marrow depressant effect.
Bone marrow depressants,* other	Increased bone marrow depressant effect.
Phenylbutazone	Increased chance of ulcers in gastrointestinal tract.
Thioguanine	May need increased dosage of colchicine.
Vitamin B-12	Decreased absorption of vitamin B-12.

POSSIBLE INTERACTION WITH OTHER SUBSTANCES

INTERACTS WITH	COMBINED EFFECT
Alcohol:	Increased risk of gastrointestinal toxicity.
Beverages: Herbal teas.	Increased colchicine effect. Avoid.
Cocaine:	Overstimulation Avoid.
Foods:	None expected.
Marijuana:	Decreased colchicine effect.
Tobacco:	None expected.

*See Glossary

COLESEVELAM

BRAND NAMES

Welchol

BASIC INFORMATION

Habit forming? No
Prescription needed? Yes
Available as generic? No
Drug class: Antihyperlipidemic

USES

Reduces low density lipoprotein (LDL) cholesterol. Should be used in addition to diet and exercise.

DOSAGE & USAGE INFORMATION

How to take:
Tablets—Take with food and a full glass of water. If you can't swallow whole, crumble tablet and take with liquid and food.

When to take:
As directed by your doctor. Usually once or twice daily with meals.

If you forget a dose:
Skip the missed dose and go back to your regular dosing schedule (don't double this dose).

What drug does:
Attaches to cholesterol and bile fluid in the intestine and passes out of the body without being absorbed.

Time lapse before drug works:
2 to 4 weeks.

Don't take with:
Any other medicine without consulting your doctor or pharmacist.

OVERDOSE

SYMPTOMS:
None expected.
WHAT TO DO:
Overdose unlikely to threaten life. If person takes much larger amount than prescribed, call doctor, poison center 1-800-222-1222 or hospital emergency room for instructions.

POSSIBLE ADVERSE REACTIONS OR SIDE EFFECTS

SYMPTOMS	WHAT TO DO
Life-threatening: None expected.	
Common: Acid or sour stomach, belching, constipation, indigestion, stomach upset or pain.	Continue. Call doctor if condition persists.
Infrequent: Congestion, cough, dry or sore throat, hoarseness, muscle aches or pain, trouble swallowing.	Continue. Call doctor when convenient.
Rare: None expected.	

WARNINGS & PRECAUTIONS

Don't take if:
You are allergic to colesevelam.

Before you start, consult your doctor:
- If you have been diagnosed with a bowel obstruction.
- You have had recent gastrointestinal surgery.
- You have had gastrointestinal motility disorders.
- If you have a vitamin deficiency.
- If you have difficulty swallowing.

Over age 60:
Colesevelam has not been shown to cause different side effects in older adults.

Pregnancy:
No proven harm to unborn child. Decide with your doctor if drug benefits justify risk to unborn child. Risk category B. (see page xviii).

Breast-feeding:
Drug may pass into milk. Avoid drug or discontinue nursing until you finish medicine. Consult doctor for advice on maintaining milk supply.

Infants & children:
Safety and efficacy not established.

Prolonged use:
Talk to your doctor about the need for follow-up medical examinations to determine the effect of colesevelam on your body.

Skin & sunlight:
No problems expected.

Driving, piloting or hazardous work:
No problems expected.

Discontinuing:
Don't discontinue without consulting your doctor.

Others:
- Advise any doctor or dentist whom you consult that you take this medicine.
- May affect the results in some medical tests.

POSSIBLE INTERACTION WITH OTHER DRUGS

GENERIC NAME OR DRUG CLASS	COMBINED EFFECT
Verapamil	May decrease effect of verapamil.

POSSIBLE INTERACTION WITH OTHER SUBSTANCES

INTERACTS WITH	COMBINED EFFECT
Alcohol:	Unknown effect Avoid.
Beverages:	None expected.
Cocaine:	Unknown effect. Avoid.
Foods:	None expected.
Marijuana:	Unknown effect. Avoid.
Tobacco:	None expected.

COLESTIPOL

BRAND NAMES

Colestid

BASIC INFORMATION

Habit forming? No
Prescription needed? Yes
Available as generic? No
Drug class: Antihyperlipidemic

USES

- Reduces cholesterol level in blood in patients with type IIa hyperlipidemia.
- Treats overdose of digitalis.
- Reduces skin itching associated with some forms of liver disease.
- Treats diarrhea after some surgical operations.
- Treatment of one form of colitis (rare).

DOSAGE & USAGE INFORMATION

How to take:
Oral suspension—Mix well with 6 ounces or more or water or liquid, or in soups, pulpy fruits, with milk or in cereals. Will not dissolve.

When to take:
- Before meals.
- If taking other medicine, take it 1 hour before or 4 to 6 hours after taking colestipol.

If you forget a dose:
Take as soon as you remember up to 2 hours late. If more than 2 hours, wait for next scheduled dose (don't double this dose).

What drug does:
Binds with bile acids in intestines, preventing reabsorption.

Time lapse before drug works:
3 to 12 months.

Don't take with:
Any other medicine without consulting your doctor or pharmacist.

OVERDOSE

SYMPTOMS:
Fecal impaction.
WHAT TO DO:
Overdose unlikely to threaten life. If person takes much larger amount than prescribed, call doctor, poison center 1-800-222-1222 or hospital emergency room for instructions.

POSSIBLE ADVERSE REACTIONS OR SIDE EFFECTS

SYMPTOMS	WHAT TO DO
Life-threatening:	
None expected.	
Common:	
None expected.	
Infrequent:	
• Black, tarry stools from gastrointestinal bleeding.	Discontinue. Seek emergency treatment.
• Severe abdominal pain.	Discontinue. Call doctor right away.
• Constipation, belching, diarrhea, nausea, unexpected weight loss.	Continue. Call doctor when convenient.
Rare:	
Hives, skin rash, hiccups.	Discontinue. Call doctor right away.

WARNINGS & PRECAUTIONS

Don't take if:
You are allergic to colestipol.

Before you start, consult your doctor:
- If you have liver disease such as cirrhosis.
- If you are jaundiced.
- If you will have surgery within 2 months, including dental surgery, requiring general or spinal anesthesia.
- If you are constipated.
- If you have peptic ulcer.
- If you have coronary artery disease.

Over age 60:
Constipation more likely. Other adverse effects more likely.

Pregnancy:
Safety not established. Consult doctor. Risk category C (see page xviii).

Breast-feeding:
No proven harm to child. Consult doctor.

Infants & children:
Only under expert medical supervision.

Prolonged use:
- Request lab studies to determine serum cholesterol and serum triglycerides.
- May decrease absorption of folic acid.

Skin & sunlight:
No problems expected.

Driving, piloting or hazardous work:
No problems expected.

Discontinuing:
Don't discontinue without consulting doctor. Dose may require gradual reduction if you have taken drug for a long time. Doses of other drugs may also require adjustment, particularly digitalis.

Others:
- This medicine does not cure disorders, but helps to control them.
- May interfere with the accuracy of some medical tests.

POSSIBLE INTERACTION WITH OTHER DRUGS

GENERIC NAME OR DRUG CLASS	COMBINED EFFECT
Anticoagulants, oral*	Decreased anti-coagulant effect.
Beta carotene	Decreased absorption of beta carotene.
Dexfenfluramine	May require dosage change as weight loss occurs.
Dextrothyroxine	Decreased dextrothyroxine effect.
Digitalis preparations*	Decreased absorption of digitalis preparations.
Diuretics, thiazide*	Decreased absorption of thiazide diuretics.
Penicillins*	Decreased absorption of penicillins.
Tetracyclines*	Decreased absorption of tetracyclines.
Thiazides*	Decreased absorption of colestipol.
Thyroid hormones*	Decreased thyroid effect.
Trimethoprim	Decreased absorption of colestipol.
Ursodiol	Decreased absorption of ursodiol.
Vancomycin	Increased chance of hearing loss or kidney damage. Decreased therapeutic effect of vancomycin.
Vitamins	Decreased absorption of fat-soluble vitamins (A,D,E,K).
Other medicines	May delay or reduce absorption.

POSSIBLE INTERACTION WITH OTHER SUBSTANCES

INTERACTS WITH	COMBINED EFFECT
Alcohol:	None expected.
Beverages:	None expected.
Cocaine:	None expected.
Foods:	Interferes with absorption of vitamins. Take supplements.
Marijuana:	None expected.
Tobacco:	None expected.

***See Glossary**

CONDYLOMA ACUMINATUM AGENTS

GENERIC AND BRAND NAMES

IMIQUIMOD
Aldara
PODOFILOX
Condylox
PODOPHYLLUM
Podofin

BASIC INFORMATION

Habit forming? No
Prescription needed? Yes
Available as generic? No
Drug class: Cytotoxic (topical)

USES

- Treatment for *condylomata acuminata*—external genital and perianal warts.
- May be used for other skin disorders as prescribed by your doctor.

DOSAGE & USAGE INFORMATION

How to use:
For all treatments—Always follow instructions provided with prescription. Wash hands before and after applying medicine. Let the solution dry before allowing other skin surfaces to touch the treated area.

- Imiquimod—Apply a thin film of cream to the wart and rub in well. Leave cream on the treated skin 6 to 10 hours, then wash with soap and water.

Continued next column

OVERDOSE

SYMPTOMS:

- **Imiquimod: Overdose unlikely. It may increase adverse skin reactions.**
- **Podofilox or podophyllum: The following symptoms may occur when the body absorbs too much—painful urination, breathing difficulty, dizziness, severe nausea or vomiting, fever, heartbeat irregularity, numbness and tingling of hands and feet, abdominal pain, excitement, irritability, seizures, coma.**

WHAT TO DO:

- **Dial 911 (emergency) for an ambulance or medical help or poison center 1-800-222-1222. Then give first aid immediately.**
- **See emergency information on inside covers.**

- Podofilox—Apply drug to warts with cotton applicator (supplied with drug). Allow drug to remain on warts for 1 to 6 hours, then remove with soap and water.
- Podophyllum—Apply petroleum jelly on normal skin surrounding warts. With a glass applicator or cotton swab, carefully apply podophyllum to the warts. Allow drug to remain on warts for 1 to 6 hours after application, then remove with soap and water.

When to use:

- Imiquimod cream—Once every other day 3 times a week. Apply at bedtime for up to 16 weeks.
- Podofilox topical solution—Apply twice a day (12 hours apart) for 3 consecutive days, then discontinue use for 4 consecutive days. May repeat this cycle of treatment 4 times (4 weeks).
- Podophyllum topical solution—Once at 1 week intervals for up to 6 weeks.

If you forget a dose:
Apply it as soon as you remember, then return to regular schedule.

What drug does:
Kills cells and erodes tissue.

Time lapse before drug works:
Several weeks.

Don't use with:
Any other medicines without consulting your doctor or pharmacist.

POSSIBLE ADVERSE REACTIONS OR SIDE EFFECTS

SYMPTOMS	WHAT TO DO
Life-threatening: In case of overdose, see previous column.	
Common: Mild skin reactions (slight stinging, mild redness, tenderness or slight swelling in treated area).	No action necessary. If they continue, call doctor.
Infrequent: Skin rash, burning, red skin, severe skin reaction. If too much of drug absorbed into body: hallucinations, diarrhea, nausea and vomiting, unusual bleeding, fever, muscle pain, flu-like symptoms.	Discontinue. Call doctor right away.
Rare: Lightening of normal skin at application site.	Continue. Call doctor when convenient.

WARNINGS & PRECAUTIONS

Don't use if:
- Warts are crumbled and bleeding.
- If warts have just been biopsied or had other surgery performed on them.
- If you are allergic to condyloma acuminatum agents.

Before you start, consult your doctor:
If you have used one of these drugs previously and have a new outbreak of warts.

Over age 60:
No special problems expected.

Pregnancy:
Consult doctor. Pregnancy risk factor not designated for podophyllum. Imiquimod is risk category B and podofilox is risk category C. See category list on page xviii.

Breast-feeding:
It is not known if drugs pass into milk. Avoid drugs or discontinue nursing until you finish medicine. Consult doctor for advice on maintaining milk supply.

Infants & children:
Efficacy and safety have not been established.

Prolonged use:
Increased risk of adverse reactions.

Skin & sunlight:
No problems expected.

Driving, piloting or hazardous work:
No problems expected.

Discontinuing:
No problems expected. Discontinue medicine once warts are healed.

Others:
- Advise any doctor whom you consult that you are using this medicine.
- Keep medicine away from unaffected skin, eyes, nose and mouth. Wash hands before and after using.
- Don't bandage or cover the treated warts with material that is occlusive. If covering is needed, use cotton gauze or cotton underwear.
- Don't use medicine on moles or birthmarks.
- Don't use near heat or open flame.
- Do not apply more of the medicine than prescribed. It will increase risk of side effects.
- Avoid sexual contact while medicine is on the warts.
- Imiquimod may weaken contraceptive devices such as cervical caps, condoms and diaphragms and reduce their contraceptive effect.
- Recurrence of genital warts is common after treatment.

POSSIBLE INTERACTION WITH OTHER DRUGS

GENERIC NAME OR DRUG CLASS	COMBINED EFFECT
Other topical medicines used in same skin area.	Increases risk of side effects. Avoid.

POSSIBLE INTERACTION WITH OTHER SUBSTANCES

INTERACTS WITH	COMBINED EFFECT
Alcohol:	None expected.
Beverages:	None expected.
Cocaine:	None expected.
Foods:	None expected.
Marijuana:	None expected.
Tobacco:	None expected.

CONTRACEPTIVES, ORAL & SKIN

GENERIC AND BRAND NAMES

See complete list of generic and brand names in the *Generic and Brand Name Directory*, page 862.

BASIC INFORMATION

Habit forming? No
Prescription needed? Yes
Available as generic? No
Drug class: Female sex hormone, contraceptive (oral)

USES

- Prevents pregnancy.
- Regulates menstrual periods.
- May be used to treat acne vulgaris in females.

DOSAGE & USAGE INFORMATION

How to take:
- Tablet—Swallow with liquid or food to lessen stomach irritation.
- Skin patch—Follow instructions on package.

When to take:
At same time each day according to prescribed instructions, usually for 21 days of 28-day cycle.

If you forget a dose:
Call doctor's office for advice about additional protection against pregnancy.

What drug does:
- Alters mucus at cervix entrance to prevent sperm entry.
- Alters uterus lining to resist implantation of fertilized egg.
- Creates same chemical atmosphere in blood that exists during pregnancy, suppressing pituitary hormones which stimulate ovulation.

Time lapse before drug works:
10 days or more to provide contraception.

Don't take with:
Any other medicine without consulting your doctor or pharmacist.

OVERDOSE

SYMPTOMS:
Drowsiness, nausea, vomiting, vaginal bleeding.
WHAT TO DO:
Overdose unlikely to threaten life. If person takes much larger amount than prescribed, call doctor, poison center 1-800-222-1222 or hospital emergency room for instructions.

POSSIBLE ADVERSE REACTIONS OR SIDE EFFECTS

SYMPTOMS	WHAT TO DO
Life-threatening:	
Stroke, chest pain, coughing blood, sudden severe headache, severe leg pain, shortness of breath.	Seek emergency treatment immediately.
Common:	
Brown blotches on skin; vaginal discharge, itch; fluid retention; break-through bleeding; acne.	Continue. Call doctor when convenient.
Infrequent:	
• Headache; pain, swelling in leg (possible blood clots in leg vein); muscle, joint pain; depression; severe abdominal pain; bulging eyes; fainting; frequent urination; breast lumps.	Discontinue. Call doctor right away.
• Blue tinge to objects, lights; appetite change; nausea; bloating; vomiting; pain; changed sex drive.	Continue. Call doctor when convenient.
Rare:	
• Jaundice, rash, hives, itch, fever, hyper-calcemia in breast cancer, intolerance of contact lenses, excess hair growth, voice change, enlarged clitoris in women.	Discontinue. Call doctor right away.
• Amenorrhea, insom-nia, hair loss, skin. irritation from patch.	Continue. Call doctor when convenient.

WARNINGS & PRECAUTIONS

Don't take if:
- You are allergic to any female hormone.
- You have had heart disease, blood clots or stroke.
- You have liver disease.
- You have cancer of breast, uterus or ovaries.
- You have unexplained vaginal bleeding.
- You smoke cigarettes.

Before you start, consult your doctor:
- If you have fibrocystic disease of breast.
- If you have migraine headaches.
- If you have fibroid tumors of uterus.
- If you have epilepsy.

- If you have asthma.
- If you have high blood pressure.
- If you will have surgery within 2 months, including dental surgery, requiring general or spinal anesthesia.
- If you have endometriosis.
- If you have diabetes.
- If you have sickle-cell anemia.
- If you are over age 35.

Over age 60:
Not used.

Pregnancy:
Discontinue at first sign of pregnancy. Risk category X (see page xviii).

Breast-feeding:
Drug passes into milk. Avoid drug or discontinue nursing.

Infants & children:
Not recommended.

Prolonged use:
- possibly cause gallstones or gradual blood pressure rise.
- Possible difficulty becoming pregnant after discontinuing.
- Talk to your doctor about the need for follow-up medical examinations or laboratory studies to check blood pressure, liver function, pap smear.

Skin & sunlight:
One or more drugs in this group may cause rash or intensify sunburn in areas exposed to sun or ultraviolet light (photosensitivity reaction). Avoid overexposure. Notify doctor if reaction occurs.

Driving, piloting or hazardous work:
No problems expected.

Discontinuing:
Don't become pregnant for 6 months after discontinuing.

Others:
- Failure to take oral contraceptives for 1 day may cancel pregnancy protection. If you forget a dose, use other contraceptive measures and call doctor for instructions on re-starting oral contraceptive.
- Advise any doctor you consult that you take this drug. May interfere with the accuracy of some medical tests.
- May cause some vitamin deficiencies.

POSSIBLE INTERACTION WITH OTHER DRUGS

GENERIC NAME OR DRUG CLASS	COMBINED EFFECT
Ampicillin	Decreased contraceptive effect.
Anticoagulants*	Decreased anticoagulant effect.
Anticonvulsants, hydantoin*	Decreased contraceptive effect.
Antidepressants, tricyclic*	Increased toxicity of antidepressants.
Antidiabetics* oral	Decreased antidiabetic effect.
Antifibronolytic agents*	Increased possibility of blood clotting.
Anti-inflammatory drugs nonsteroidal (NSAIDs)*	Decreased contraceptive effect.
Antihistamines*	Decreased contraceptive effect.
Barbiturates*	Decreased contraceptive effect.
Chloramphenicol	Decreased contraceptive effect.
Clofibrate	Decreased clofibrate effect.
Dextrothyroxine	Decreased dextrothyroxine effect.
Guanethidine	Decreased guanethidine effect.
Hypoglycemics, oral*	Decreased effect of hypoglycemics.
Insulin	Possibly decreased insulin effect.
Insulin lispro	May need increased dosage of insulin.
Meperidine	Increased meperidine effect.

Continued on page 909

POSSIBLE INTERACTION WITH OTHER SUBSTANCES

INTERACTS WITH	COMBINED EFFECT
Alcohol:	None expected.
Beverages:	None expected.
Cocaine:	None expected.
Foods: Salt.	Increased edema (fluid retention).
Marijuana:	Increased bleeding between periods. Avoid.
Tobacco:	Possible heart attack, blood clots and stroke. If you take "the pill," *don't smoke.*

CONTRACEPTIVES, VAGINAL

GENERIC AND BRAND NAMES

See complete list of generic and brand names in the *Generic and Brand Name Directory*, page 862.

BASIC INFORMATION

Habit forming? No
Prescription needed? Not for most
Available as generic? Most aren't
Drug class: Contraceptive (vaginal)

USES

- Provides a degree of protection against pregnancy.
- Spermicides may help to protect against some sexually transmitted diseases, such as those caused by chlamydia, gardnerella, mycoplasma, neisseria, trichomonas, ureaplasma and possibly herpes virus, but not HIV.

DOSAGE & USAGE INFORMATION

How to take:
- Read package insert carefully. Some cautions to remember:
- Do not douche for 6 to 8 hours after intercourse.
- Do not remove sponge, cervical cap or diaphragm for 6 to 8 hours after intercourse.
- Follow product label instructions for storage.
- Plastic ring device—Follow special patient brochure instructions.

When to take:
For barrier forms, use consistently with every sexual exposure. The plastic ring device is replaced every month.

If you forget to use:
Contact your doctor to consider using another form of pregnancy protection, such as the "morning-after" pill.

What drug does:
- Spermicides form a chemical barrier between sperm in semen and the mucous membranes in the vagina. The chemical acts to inactivate viable sperm and also kills some bacteria, viruses, yeast and fungus.

Continued next column

OVERDOSE

SYMPTOMS:
None expected.

- The plastic ring device releases hormones that go into the bloodstream and provide the same protection as birth control pills.

Time lapse before vaginal contraceptive works:
- Immediate for foam, gels, jellies and sponges.
- 5 to 15 minutes for film and suppositories.
- Plastic ring device takes 7 days to be effective. Use another form of birth control during that time.

Don't use with:
Not applicable.

POSSIBLE ADVERSE REACTIONS OR SIDE EFFECTS

SYMPTOMS	WHAT TO DO
Life-threatening:	
Toxic shock syndrome (chills; fever; skin rash; muscle aches; extreme weakness; confusion; redness of vagina, inside of mouth, nose, throat or eyes). (Very rare).	Seek emergency treatment immediately.
Common:	
None expected.	
Infrequent:	
None expected.	
Rare:	
Vaginal discharge, irritation or rash; painful urination; cloudy or bloody urine.	Discontinue. Call doctor right away.

WARNINGS & PRECAUTIONS

Don't take if:
You are allergic to any form of octoxynol, nonoxynol or benzalkonium chloride or female hormones.

Before you start, consult your doctor:
If you desire complete protection against pregnancy, a combination of methods gives better protection than vaginal contraceptives alone.

Over age 60:
Adverse reactions and side effects may be more frequent and severe than in younger persons.

Pregnancy:
Risk factor not designated. See categories on page xviii and consult doctor.

Breast-feeding:
Safety not established. Consult doctor.

Infants & children:
Not recommended.

Prolonged use:
Allergic reactions and irritation more likely.

Skin & sunlight:
No problems expected.

Driving, piloting or hazardous work:
No special problems expected.

Discontinuing:
No special problems expected.

Others:
- Failure rate when used alone is relatively high. Therefore a vaginal cream, sponge, suppository, foam, gel, jelly or other product should be used with a mechanical barrier, such as a condom, cervical cap, vaginal diaphragm or other form of pregnancy protection.
- Don't use a cervical cap, sponge or diaphragm during menstruation. Consider using a condom instead if additional protection is desired.
- Vaginal contraceptives usually also have spermicidal effects and may partially protect against sexually transmitted diseases.

POSSIBLE INTERACTION WITH OTHER DRUGS

GENERIC NAME OR DRUG CLASS	COMBINED EFFECT
Topical vaginal medications that include any of the following: sulfa drugs, soaps or disinfectants, nitrates*, permanganates, lanolin, hydrogen peroxide, iodides, cotton dressings, aluminum citrates, salicylates*	Spermicidal activity may be reduced or negated. Avoid combinations.
Vaginal douche products	May prevent spermicidal effect. Avoid until 8 hours following intercourse.

POSSIBLE INTERACTION WITH OTHER SUBSTANCES

INTERACTS WITH	COMBINED EFFECT
Alcohol:	None expected.
Beverages:	None expected.
Cocaine:	None expected.
Foods:	None expected.
Marijuana:	None expected.
Tobacco:	None expected.

***See Glossary**

CROMOLYN

BRAND NAMES

Crolom
Fivent
Gastrocrom
Intal
Nalcrom
Nasalcrom
Novo-Cromolyn
Opticrom
PMS-Sodium Cromoglycate
Rynacrom
Sodium Cromoglycate
Vistacrom

BASIC INFORMATION

Habit forming? No
Prescription needed? Yes, for some
Available as generic? Yes, for some
Drug class: Nasal decongestant, anti-inflammatory (nonsteroidal)

USES

- Powdered form and nebulizer solution prevent asthma attacks. Will not stop an active asthma attack.
- Eye drops treat inflammation of covering to eye and cornea.
- Nasal spray reduces nasal allergic symptoms.
- Capsules may help prevent allergic symptoms.

DOSAGE & USAGE INFORMATION

How to take:

Inhaler

Follow instructions enclosed with inhaler. Don't swallow cartridges for inhaler. Gargle and rinse mouth after inhalations.

Eye drops

- Wash hands.
- Apply pressure to inside corner of eye with middle finger.
- Continue pressure for 1 minute after placing medicine in eye.
- Tilt head backward. Pull lower lid away from eye with index finger of the same hand.
- Drop eye drops into pouch and close eye. Don't blink.

Continued next column

- Keep eyes closed for 1 to 2 minutes.
- Don't touch applicator tip to any surface (including the eye). If you accidentally touch tip, clean with warm soap and water.
- Keep container tightly closed.
- Keep cool, but don't freeze.
- Wash hands immediately after using.

Nasal solution

Follow prescription instructions.

Capsules

Open capsule and dissolve contents in 4 ounces of hot water, then add equal amount of cold water. Drink all the liquid.

When to take:

At the same times each day. If you also use a bronchodilator inhaler, use the bronchodilator before the cromolyn.

If you forget a dose:

Take as soon as you remember up to 2 hours late. If more than 2 hours, wait for next scheduled dose (don't double this dose).

What drug does:

Blocks histamine release from mast cells.

Time lapse before drug works:

- For inhaler forms: 4 weeks for prevention of asthma attacks. However, if taken 10-15 minutes after exercise or exposure to known allergens, may prevent wheezing.
- 1 to 2 weeks for nasal symptoms; only a few days for eye symptoms.

Don't take with:

Any other medicine without consulting your doctor or pharmacist.

OVERDOSE

SYMPTOMS:

Increased side effects and adverse reactions listed.

WHAT TO DO:

Overdose unlikely to threaten life. If person inhales much larger amount than prescribed, call doctor, poison center 1-800-222-1222 or hospital emergency room for instructions.

POSSIBLE ADVERSE REACTIONS OR SIDE EFFECTS

SYMPTOMS	WHAT TO DO
Life-threatening:	
Hives, rash, intense itching, faintness soon after a dose (anaphylaxis).	Seek emergency treatment immediately.
Common:	
Inhaler—cough, stuffy nose, dry mouth or throat; nasal—burning or stinging inside nose, increased sneezing; oral—diarrhea, headache.	Continue. Call doctor when convenient.
Infrequent:	
Inhaler—hoarseness, watery eyes; nasal—headache, bad taste, postnasal drip; oral—stomach pain, nausea, insomnia, rash.	Continue. Call doctor when convenient.

Rare:

Inhaler—rash, hives, swallowing difficulty, increased wheezing, joint pain or swelling, weakness, muscle pain, difficult or painful urination, difficulty breathing; nasal—difficulty swallowing, hives, itching, skin rash, facial swelling, wheezing, nosebleed; oral—cough, difficulty swallowing, facial swelling, wheezing, breathing difficulty.	Discontinue. Call doctor right away.

WARNINGS & PRECAUTIONS

Don't take if:
You use the dry powder form of cromolyn and if you are allergic to cromolyn, lactose, milk or milk products.

Before you start, consult your doctor:
- If you plan to become pregnant within medication period.
- If you have kidney or liver disease.

Over age 60:
Adverse reactions and side effects may be more frequent and severe than in younger persons.

Pregnancy:
No proven harm to unborn child, but avoid if possible. Consult doctor. Risk category B (see page xviii).

Breast-feeding:
Effects unknown. Confer with your doctor.

Infants & children:
Do not use for children under age two..

Prolonged use:
Consult doctor on a regular basis while using this drug.

Skin & sunlight:
No problems expected.

Driving, piloting or hazardous work:
No problems expected.

Discontinuing:
Don't discontinue without doctor's approval if drug is used to prevent asthma symptoms. Dosages of other drugs may need to be adjusted.

Others:
- Inhaler must be cleaned and work well for drug to be effective.
- Treatment with inhalation cromolyn does not stop an acute asthma attack and may aggravate it.
- Advise any doctor or dentist whom you consult about the use of this medicine.
- Be sure you and the doctor discuss benefits and risks of this drug before starting.
- Call doctor if symptoms worsen or new symptoms develop with use of this medicine.
- Wear a medical identification that indicates the use of this medicine.
- Use medicine only as directed. Don't increase or decrease dosage without doctor's approval.

POSSIBLE INTERACTION WITH OTHER DRUGS

GENERIC NAME OR DRUG CLASS	COMBINED EFFECT
None significant.	

POSSIBLE INTERACTION WITH OTHER SUBSTANCES

INTERACTS WITH	COMBINED EFFECT
Alcohol:	None expected.
Beverages:	None expected.
Cocaine:	None expected.
Foods:	None expected.
Marijuana:	None expected.
Tobacco:	None expected, but tobacco smoke aggravates asthma and eye irritation. Avoid.

CYCLANDELATE

BRAND NAMES

Cyclospasmol
Cyraso-400

BASIC INFORMATION

Habit forming? No
Prescription needed?
U.S.: Yes
Canada: No
Available as generic? Yes
Drug class: Vasodilator

USES

May improve poor blood flow to extremities.

DOSAGE & USAGE INFORMATION

How to take:
Tablet or capsule—Swallow with liquid. If you can't swallow whole, crumble tablet or open capsule and take with liquid or food.

When to take:
At the same time each day.

If you forget a dose:
Take as soon as you remember up to 2 hours late. If more than 2 hours, wait for next scheduled dose (don't double this dose).

What drug does:
Increases blood flow by relaxing and expanding blood-vessel walls.

Time lapse before drug works:
3 weeks.

Don't take with:
Any other medicine without consulting your doctor or pharmacist.

OVERDOSE

SYMPTOMS:
Severe headache, dizziness; nausea, vomiting; flushed, hot face.
WHAT TO DO:
Overdose unlikely to threaten life. If person takes much larger amount than prescribed, call doctor, poison center 1-800-222-1222 or hospital emergency room for instructions.

POSSIBLE ADVERSE REACTIONS OR SIDE EFFECTS

SYMPTOMS	WHAT TO DO
Life-threatening: In case of overdose, see previous column.	
Common: None expected.	
Infrequent:	
• Rapid heartbeat.	Discontinue. Call doctor right away.
• Dizziness; headache; weakness; flushed face; tingling in face, fingers or toes; unusual sweating.	Continue. Call doctor when convenient.
• Belching, heartburn, nausea or stomach pain.	Continue. Tell doctor at next visit.
Rare: None expected.	

WARNINGS & PRECAUTIONS

Don't take if:
You have had allergic reaction to cyclandelate.

Before you start, consult your doctor:
- If you have glaucoma.
- If you have had heart attack or stroke.

Over age 60:
Adverse reactions and side effects may be more frequent and severe than in younger persons.

Pregnancy:
Consult doctor. Risk category C (see page xviii).

Breast-feeding:
No proven problems. Consult doctor.

Infants & children:
Not recommended.

Prolonged use:
No problems expected.

Skin & sunlight:
No problems expected.

Driving, piloting or hazardous work:
Avoid if you feel dizzy or weak. Otherwise, no problems expected.

Discontinuing:
Don't discontinue without doctor's advice until you complete prescribed dose, even though symptoms diminish or disappear.

Others:
Response to drug varies. If your symptoms don't improve after 3 weeks of use, consult doctor.

POSSIBLE INTERACTION WITH OTHER DRUGS

GENERIC NAME OR DRUG CLASS	COMBINED EFFECT
None expected.	

POSSIBLE INTERACTION WITH OTHER SUBSTANCES

INTERACTS WITH	COMBINED EFFECT
Alcohol:	None expected.
Beverages:	None expected.
Cocaine:	Decreased cyclandelate effect. Avoid.
Foods:	None expected.
Marijuana:	None expected.
Tobacco:	May decrease cyclandelate effect.

*See Glossary

CYCLIZINE

BRAND NAMES

Marezine
Marzine

BASIC INFORMATION

Habit forming? No
Prescription needed?
U.S.: No
Canada: Yes
Available as generic? No
Drug class: Antiemetic, antimotion sickness

USES

Prevention and treatment for motion sickness.

DOSAGE & USAGE INFORMATION

How to take:
Tablet—Swallow with liquid or food to lessen stomach irritation. If you can't swallow whole, crumble tablet and chew or take with liquid or food.

When to take:
30 minutes to 1 hour before traveling.

If you forget a dose:
Take as soon as you remember. Wait 4 hours for next dose.

What drug does:
Reduces sensitivity of nerve endings in inner ear, blocking messages to brain's vomiting center.

Time lapse before drug works:
30 to 60 minutes.

Don't take with:
Any other medicine without consulting your doctor or pharmacist.

OVERDOSE

SYMPTOMS:
Drowsiness, confusion, incoordination, stupor, coma, weak pulse, shallow breathing, hallucinations.
WHAT TO DO:
- **Dial 911 (emergency) for an ambulance or medical help or poison center 1-800-222-1222. Then give first aid immediately.**
- **See emergency information on inside covers.**

POSSIBLE ADVERSE REACTIONS OR SIDE EFFECTS

SYMPTOMS	WHAT TO DO
Life-threatening: In case of overdose, see previous column.	
Common: Drowsiness.	Continue. Tell doctor at next visit.
Infrequent:	
• Headache, diarrhea or constipation, nausea, fast heartbeat.	Continue. Call doctor when convenient.
• Dry mouth, nose, throat; dizziness.	Continue. Tell doctor at next visit.
Rare:	
• Rash or hives, jaundice.	Discontinue. Call doctor right away.
• Restlessness, excitement, insomnia, blurred vision, frequent or difficult urination, hallucinations.	Continue. Call doctor when convenient.
• Appetite loss, nausea.	Continue. Tell doctor at next visit.

WARNINGS & PRECAUTIONS

Don't take if:
- You are allergic to meclizine, buclizine or cyclizine.
- You have taken a monoamine oxidase (MAO) inhibitor* in the past 2 weeks.

Before you start, consult your doctor:
- If you have glaucoma.
- If you have prostate enlargement.
- If you have reacted badly to any antihistamine
- If you have asthma.

Over age 60:
Adverse reactions and side effects may be more frequent and severe than in younger persons, especially impaired urination from enlarged prostate gland.

Pregnancy:
Consult doctor. Risk category B (see page xviii).

Breast-feeding:
Drug passes into milk. Avoid drug or discontinue nursing until you finish medicine. Consult doctor for advice on maintaining milk supply.

Infants & children:
Avoid if under age 6.

Prolonged use:
No problems expected.

Skin & sunlight:
No problems expected.

Driving, piloting or hazardous work:
Don't fly aircraft. Don't drive until you learn how medicine affects you. Don't work around dangerous machinery. Don't climb ladders or work in high places. Danger increases if you drink alcohol or take medicine affecting alertness and reflexes, such as antihistamines, tranquilizers, sedatives, pain medicine, narcotics and mind-altering drugs.

Discontinuing:
No problems expected.

Others:
- Some products contain tartrazine dye. Avoid if allergic (especially aspirin hypersensitivity).
- May interfere with the accuracy of some medical tests.

POSSIBLE INTERACTION WITH OTHER DRUGS

GENERIC NAME OR DRUG CLASS	COMBINED EFFECT
Amphetamines*	May decrease drowsiness caused by cyclizine.
Anticholinergics*	Increased effect of both drugs.
Antidepressants, tricyclic*	Increased effect of both drugs.
Carteolol	Decreased antihistamine effect.
Clozapine	Toxic effect on the central nervous system.
Dronabinol	Increased cyclizine effect.
Ethinamate	Dangerous increased effects of ethinamate. Avoid combining.
Fluoxetine	Increased depressant effects of both drugs.
Guanfacine	May increase depressant effects of either drug.
Leucovorin	High alcohol content of leucovorin may cause adverse effects.
Methyprylon	Increased sedative effect, perhaps to dangerous level. Avoid.
Monoamine oxidase (MAO) inhibitors*	Increased cyclizine effect.
Nabilone	Greater depression of central nervous system.
Narcotics*	Increased effect of both drugs.
Pain relievers*	Increased effect of both drugs.
Sedatives*	Increased effect of both drugs.
Sertraline	Increased depressive effect of both drugs.
Sleep inducers*	Increased effect of both drugs.
Sotalol	Increased antihistamine effect.
Tranquilizers*	Increased effect of both drugs.

POSSIBLE INTERACTION WITH OTHER SUBSTANCES

INTERACTS WITH	COMBINED EFFECT
Alcohol:	Increased sedation. Avoid.
Beverages: Caffeine drinks.	May decrease drowsiness.
Cocaine:	None expected.
Foods:	None expected.
Marijuana:	Increased drowsiness, dry mouth.
Tobacco:	None expected.

*See Glossary

CYCLOBENZAPRINE

BRAND NAMES

Cycoflex
Flexeril

BASIC INFORMATION

Habit forming? No
Prescription needed? Yes
Available as generic? Yes
Drug class: Muscle relaxant

USES

Treatment for pain and limited motion caused by spasms in voluntary muscles.

DOSAGE & USAGE INFORMATION

How to take:
Tablet—Swallow with liquid.

When to take:
At the same time each day or according to label instructions.

If you forget a dose:
Take as soon as you remember. Wait 4 hours for next dose.

What drug does:
Blocks body's pain messages to brain. May also sedate.

Time lapse before drug works:
30 to 60 minutes.

Continued next column

OVERDOSE

SYMPTOMS:
Drowsiness, confusion, difficulty concentrating, visual problems, vomiting, blood pressure drop, low body temperature, weak and rapid pulse, convulsions, coma.
WHAT TO DO:
- **Dial 911 (emergency) for an ambulance or medical help or poison center 1-800-222-1222. Then give first aid immediately.**
- **If patient is unconscious and not breathing, give mouth-to-mouth breathing. If there is no heartbeat, use cardiac massage and mouth-to-mouth breathing (CPR). Don't try to make patient vomit. If you can't get help quickly, take patient to nearest emergency facility.**
- **See emergency information on inside covers.**

Don't take with:
Nonprescription drugs without consulting doctor.

POSSIBLE ADVERSE REACTIONS OR SIDE EFFECTS

SYMPTOMS	WHAT TO DO
Life-threatening:	
In case of overdose, see previous column.	
Common:	
Drowsiness, dizziness, dry mouth.	Continue. Call doctor when convenient.
Infrequent:	
• Blurred vision, fast heartbeat.	Discontinue. Call doctor right away.
• Insomnia, numbness in extremities, bad taste in mouth, fatigue, nausea, sweating.	Continue. Call doctor when convenient.
Rare:	
• Unsteadiness, confusion, depression, hallucinations, rash, itch, swelling, breathing difficulty.	Discontinue. Call doctor right away.
• Difficult urination, rash.	Continue. Call doctor when convenient.

WARNINGS & PRECAUTIONS

Don't take if:
- You are allergic to any skeletal muscle relaxant*.
- You have taken a monoamine oxidase (MAO) inhibitor* in last 2 weeks.
- You have had a heart attack within 6 weeks, or suffer from congestive heart failure.
- You have an overactive thyroid.

Before you start, consult your doctor:
- If you have a heart problem.
- If you have reacted to tricyclic anti-depressants.
- If you have glaucoma.
- If you have a prostate condition and urination difficulty.
- If you intend to pilot aircraft.

Over age 60:
Adverse reactions and side effects may be more frequent and severe than in younger persons. Avoid extremes of heat and cold.

Pregnancy:
No problems expected. Consult doctor. Risk category B (see page xviii).

Breast-feeding:
Drug may pass into milk. Avoid drug or discontinue nursing until you finish medicine. Consult doctor for advice on maintaining milk supply.

Infants & children:
Don't use for children younger than 15.

Prolonged use:
Do not take for longer than 2 to 3 weeks.

Skin & sunlight:
No special problems expected.

Driving, piloting or hazardous work:
Don't drive or pilot aircraft until you learn how medicine affects you. Don't work around dangerous machinery. Don't climb ladders or work in high places. Danger increases if you drink alcohol or take medicine affecting alertness and reflexes.

Discontinuing:
May be unnecessary to finish medicine. Follow doctor's instructions.

Others:
No problems expected.

POSSIBLE INTERACTION WITH OTHER DRUGS

GENERIC NAME OR DRUG CLASS	COMBINED EFFECT
Anticholinergics*	Increased anticholinergic effect.
Antidepressants*	Increased sedation.
Antihistamines*	Increased antihistamine effect.
Barbiturates*	Increased sedation.
Central nervous system (CNS) depressants*	Increased sedation.
Cimetidine	Possible increased cyclobenzaprine effect.
Cisapride	Decreased cyclobenzaprine effect.
Clonidine	Decreased clonidine effect.
Dronabinol	Increased effect of dronabinol on central nervous system. Avoid combination.
Guanethidine	Decreased guanethidine effect.
Methyldopa	Decreased methyldopa effect.
Mind-altering drugs*	Increased mind-altering effect.
Monoamine oxidase (MAO) inhibitors*	High fever, convulsions, possible death.
Narcotics*	Increased sedation.
Pain relievers*	Increased pain reliever effect.
Procainamide	Possible increased conduction disturbance.
Quinidine	Possible increased conduction disturbance.
Rauwolfia alkaloids*	Decreased effect of rauwolfia alkaloids.
Sedatives*	Increased sedative effect.
Sleep inducers*	Increased sedation.
Tranquilizers*	Increased tranquilizer effect.

POSSIBLE INTERACTION WITH OTHER SUBSTANCES

INTERACTS WITH	COMBINED EFFECT
Alcohol:	Depressed brain function. Avoid.
Beverages:	None expected.
Cocaine:	Decreased cyclobenzaprine effect.
Foods:	None expected.
Marijuana:	Occasional use—Drowsiness. Frequent use—Severe mental and physical impairment.
Tobacco:	None expected.

*See Glossary

CYCLOPENTOLATE (Ophthalmic)

BRAND NAMES

Ak-Pentolate
Cyclogyl
I-Pentolate
Minims
  Cyclopentolate
Ocu-Pentolate
Pentolair
Spectro-Pentolate

BASIC INFORMATION

Habit forming? No
Prescription needed? Yes
Available as generic? Yes
Drug class: Cycloplegic, mydriatic

USES

- Enlarges (dilates) pupil.
- Temporarily paralyzes the normal pupil accommodation to light before eye examinations and to treat some eye conditions.

DOSAGE & USAGE INFORMATION

How to use:
Eye drops
- Wash hands.
- Apply pressure to inside corner of eye with middle finger.
- Continue pressure for 1 minute after placing medicine in eye.
- Tilt head backward. Pull lower lid away from eye with index finger of the same hand.
- Drop eye drops into pouch and close eye. Don't blink.
- Keep eyes closed for 1 to 2 minutes.
- Don't touch applicator tip to any surface (including the eye). If you accidentally touch tip, clean with warm soap and water.
- Keep container tightly closed.
- Keep cool, but don't freeze.
- Wash hands immediately after using.

When to use:
As directed on bottle.

Continued next column

OVERDOSE

SYMPTOMS:
None expected.
WHAT TO DO:
Not intended for internal use. If child accidentally swallows, call poison center 1-800-222-1222.

If you forget a dose:
Use as soon as you remember.

What drug does:
Blocks sphincter muscle of the iris and ciliary body.

Time lapse before drug works:
Within 30 to 60 minutes. Effects usually disappear in 24 hours.

Don't use with:
Other eye medicines such as carbachol, demecarium, echothiopate, isoflurophate, physostigmine, pilocarpine without doctor's approval.

POSSIBLE ADVERSE REACTIONS OR SIDE EFFECTS

SYMPTOMS	WHAT TO DO
Life-threatening: None expected.	
Common:	
• Increased sensitivity to light.	Continue. Call doctor when convenient.
• Burning eyes.	Continue. Tell doctor at next visit.
Infrequent: None expected.	
Rare (extremely):	
Symptoms of excess medicine absorbed by the body—Clumsiness, confusion, fever, flushed face, hallucinations, rash, slurred speech, swollen stomach (children), drowsiness, fast heartbeat.	Discontinue. Call doctor right away.

WARNINGS & PRECAUTIONS

Don't use if:
You are allergic to cyclopentolate.

Before you start, consult your doctor:
- If medicine is for a brain-damaged child or child with Down syndrome.
- If prescribed for a child with spastic paralysis.

Over age 60:
No problems expected.

Pregnancy:
Avoid if possible. Consult doctor. Risk category C (see page xviii).

Breast-feeding:
Safety unestablished. Avoid if possible. Consult doctor.

Infants & children:
Use only under close medical supervision.

Prolonged use:
Avoid. May increase absorption into body.

Skin & sunlight:
No special problems expected.

Driving, piloting or hazardous work:
Don't drive or pilot aircraft until you learn how medicine affects you. Don't work around dangerous machinery. Don't climb ladders or work in high places. Danger increases if you drink alcohol or take medicine affecting alertness and reflexes, such as antihistamines, tranquilizers, sedatives, pain medicine, narcotics and mind-altering drugs.

Discontinuing:
If effects last longer than 36 hours after last drops, consult doctor.

Others:
Wear sunglasses to protect eyes from sunlight and bright light.

POSSIBLE INTERACTION WITH OTHER DRUGS

GENERIC NAME OR DRUG CLASS	COMBINED EFFECT
Antiglaucoma agents*	Decreased antiglaucoma effect.

POSSIBLE INTERACTION WITH OTHER SUBSTANCES

INTERACTS WITH	COMBINED EFFECT
Alcohol:	None expected.
Beverages:	None expected.
Cocaine:	None expected.
Foods:	None expected.
Marijuana:	None expected.
Tobacco:	None expected.

***See Glossary**

CYCLOPHOSPHAMIDE

BRAND NAMES

Cytoxan
Neosar
Procytox

BASIC INFORMATION

Habit forming? No
Prescription needed? Yes
Available as generic? No
Drug class: Immunosuppressant, antineoplastic

USES

- Treatment for cancer.
- Treatment for severe rheumatoid arthritis.
- Treatment for blood-vessel disease.
- Treatment for skin disease.

DOSAGE & USAGE INFORMATION

How to take:
Tablet or liquid—Swallow with liquid. If you can't swallow whole, crumble tablet and take with liquid or food.

When to take:
Works best if taken first thing in morning. Should be taken on an empty stomach. However, may take with food to lessen stomach irritation. Don't take at bedtime.

If you forget a dose:
Take as soon as you remember up to 12 hours late. If more than 12 hours, wait for next scheduled dose (don't double this dose).

What drug does:
- Kills cancer cells.
- Suppresses spread of cancer cells.
- Suppresses immune system.

Time lapse before drug works:
7 to 10 days continual use.

Don't take with:
Any other medicine without consulting your doctor or pharmacist.

OVERDOSE

SYMPTOMS:
Bloody urine, water retention, weight gain, severe infection.
WHAT TO DO:
Overdose unlikely to threaten life. If person takes much larger amount than prescribed, call doctor, poison center 1-800-222-1222 or hospital emergency room for instructions.

POSSIBLE ADVERSE REACTIONS OR SIDE EFFECTS

SYMPTOMS	WHAT TO DO
Life-threatening:	
Hives, rash, intense itching, faintness soon after a dose (anaphylaxis).	Seek emergency treatment immediately.
Common:	
• Sore throat, fever.	Continue, but call doctor right away.
• Dark skin, nails; nausea; appetite loss; vomiting; missed menstrual period.	Continue. Call doctor when convenient.
Infrequent:	
• Rash, hives, itch; shortness of breath; rapid heartbeat; cough; blood in urine, painful urination; pain in side; bleeding, bruising; increased sweating; hoarseness; foot or ankle swelling.	Continue, but call doctor right away.
• Confusion, agitation, headache, dizziness, flushed face, stomach pain, joint pain, fatigue, weakness, diarrhea.	Continue. Call doctor when convenient.
Rare:	
• Mouth, lip sores; black stool; unusual thirst; jaundice.	Continue, but call doctor right away.
• Blurred vision, increased urination, hair loss.	Continue. Call doctor when convenient.

WARNINGS & PRECAUTIONS

Don't take if:
- You are allergic to any alkylating agent.
- You have an infection.
- You have bloody urine.
- You will have surgery within 2 months, including dental surgery, requiring general or spinal anesthesia.

Before you start, consult your doctor:
- If you have impaired liver or kidney function.
- If you have impaired bone marrow or blood cell production.
- If you have had chemotherapy or x-ray therapy.
- If you have taken cortisone drugs in the past year.
- If you plan to become pregnant.

Over age 60:
Adverse reactions and side effects may be more frequent and severe than in younger persons. To reduce risk of chemical bladder inflammation, drink 8 to 10 glasses of water daily.

Pregnancy:
Risk to unborn child outweighs drug benefits. Don't use. Risk category D (see page xviii).

Breast-feeding:
Drug passes into milk. Avoid drug or discontinue nursing until you finish medicine. Consult doctor for advice on maintaining milk supply.

Infants & children:
Use only under medical supervision.

Prolonged use:
- Development of fibrous lung tissue.
- Possible jaundice.
- Swelling of feet, lower legs.
- Cancer.
- Infertility in men.
- Talk to your doctor about the need for follow-up medical examinations or laboratory studies to check complete blood counts (white blood cell count, platelet count, red blood cell count, hemoglobin, hematocrit), urine, liver function.

Skin & sunlight:
No problems expected.

Driving, piloting or hazardous work:
Avoid if you feel dizzy or have blurred vision. Otherwise, no problems expected.

Discontinuing:
Don't discontinue without consulting doctor. Dose may require gradual reduction if you have taken drug for a long time. Doses of other drugs may also require adjustment.

Others:
- Frequently causes hair loss. After treatment ends, hair should grow back.
- Avoid vaccinations.

POSSIBLE INTERACTION WITH OTHER DRUGS

GENERIC NAME OR DRUG CLASS	COMBINED EFFECT
Allopurinol or other medicines to treat gout	Possible anemia; decreased antigout effect.
Antidiabetics, oral*	Increased antidiabetic effect.
Bone marrow depressants,* other	Increased bone marrow depressant effect.
Clozapine	Toxic effect on bone marrow.
Cyclosporine	May increase risk of infection.
Digoxin	Possible decreased digoxin absorption.
Immuno-suppressants,* other	Increased risk of infection.
Insulin	Increased insulin effect.
Levamisole	Increased risk of bone marrow depression.
Lovastatin	Increased heart and kidney damage.
Phenobarbital	Increased cyclophosphamide effect.
Probenecid	Increased blood uric acid.
Sulfinpyrazone	Increased blood uric acid.
Tiopronin	Increased risk of toxicity to bone marrow.

POSSIBLE INTERACTION WITH OTHER SUBSTANCES

INTERACTS WITH	COMBINED EFFECT
Alcohol:	None expected.
Beverages:	None expected. Drink at least 2 quarts fluid every day.
Cocaine:	Increased danger of brain damage.
Foods:	None expected.
Marijuana:	Increased impairment of immunity.
Tobacco:	None expected.

*See Glossary

CYCLOPLEGIC, MYDRIATIC (Ophthalmic)

GENERIC AND BRAND NAMES

ATROPINE
- **Atropair**
- **Atropine Care Eye Drops and Ointment**
- **Atropine Sulfate S.O.P.**
- **Atropisol**
- **Atrosulf**
- **Isopto Atropine**
- **I-Tropine**
- **Minims Atropine**
- **Ocu-Tropine**

HOMATROPINE
- **AK Homatropine**
- **I-Homatrine**
- **I-Homatropine**
- **Isopto Homatropine**
- **Minims Homatropine**
- **Spectro-Homatropine**

SCOPOLAMINE
- **Isopto Hyoscine**

BASIC INFORMATION

Habit forming? No
Prescription needed? Yes
Available as generic? Yes, some
Drug class: Cycloplegic, mydriatic

USES

- Dilates pupil of the eye.
- Used before some eye examinations, before and after some eye surgical procedures and, rarely, to treat some eye problems such as glaucoma.

DOSAGE & USAGE INFORMATION

How to use:
Eye drops
- Wash hands.
- Apply pressure to inside corner of eye with middle finger.
- Continue pressure for 1 minute after placing medicine in eye.
- Tilt head backward. Pull lower lid away from eye with index finger of the same hand.
- Drop eye drops into pouch and close eye. Don't blink.
- Keep eyes closed for 1 to 2 minutes.

Continued next column

OVERDOSE

SYMPTOMS:
None expected.
WHAT TO DO:
Not intended for internal use. If child accidentally swallows, call poison center l1-800-222-1222.

Eye ointment
- Wash hands.
- Pull lower lid down from eye to form a pouch.
- Squeeze tube to apply thin strip of ointment into pouch.
- Close eye for 1 to 2 minutes.
- Don't touch applicator tip to any surface (including the eye). If you accidentally touch tip, clean with warm soap and water.
- Keep container tightly closed.
- Keep cool, but don't freeze.
- Wash hands immediately after using.

When to use:
As directed on label.

If you forget a dose:
Use as soon as you remember.

What drug does:
Blocks normal response to sphincter muscle of the iris of the eye and the accommodative muscle of the ciliary body.

Time lapse before drug works:
Begins within 1 minute. Residual effects may last up to 14 days.

Don't use with:
Other eye medicines such as carbachol, demecarium, echothiopate, isoflurophate, physostigmine, pilocarpine.

POSSIBLE ADVERSE REACTIONS OR SIDE EFFECTS

SYMPTOMS	WHAT TO DO
Life-threatening:	
None expected.	
Common:	
• Increased sensitivity to light.	Continue. Call doctor when convenient.
• Burning eyes.	Continue. Tell doctor at next visit.
Infrequent:	
None expected.	
Rare (extremely):	
Symptoms of excess medicine absorbed by the body—Clumsiness, confusion, fever, flushed face, hallucinations, rash, slurred speech, swollen stomach (children), unusual drowsiness, fast heartbeat.	Discontinue. Call doctor right away.

CYCLOPLEGIC, MYDRIATIC (Ophthalmic)

WARNINGS & PRECAUTIONS

Don't use if:
You are allergic to cyclopentolate.

Before you start, consult your doctor:
- If medicine is for a brain-damaged child or child with Down's syndrome.
- If prescribed for a child with spastic paralysis.

Over age 60:
No problems expected.

Pregnancy:
Decide with your doctor if drug benefits justify risk to unborn child. Risk category C (see page xviii).

Breast-feeding:
Safety unestablished. Avoid if possible.

Infants & children:
Use only under close medical supervision.

Prolonged use:
Avoid. May increase absorption into body.

Skin & sunlight:
No special problems expected.

Driving, piloting or hazardous work:
Don't drive or pilot aircraft until you learn how medicine affects you. Don't work around dangerous machinery. Don't climb ladders or work in high places. Danger increases if you drink alcohol or take medicine affecting alertness and reflexes, such as antihistamines, tranquilizers, sedatives, pain medicine, narcotics and mind-altering drugs.

Discontinuing:
Effects may last up to 14 days later.

Others:
Wear sunglasses to protect eyes from sunlight and bright light.

POSSIBLE INTERACTION WITH OTHER DRUGS

GENERIC NAME OR DRUG CLASS	COMBINED EFFECT

Clinically significant interactions with oral or injected medicines unlikely.

POSSIBLE INTERACTION WITH OTHER SUBSTANCES

INTERACTS WITH	COMBINED EFFECT
Alcohol:	None expected.
Beverages:	None expected.
Cocaine:	None expected.
Foods:	None expected.
Marijuana:	None expected.
Tobacco:	None expected.

*See Glossary

CYCLOSERINE

BRAND NAMES

Seromycin

BASIC INFORMATION

Habit forming? No
Prescription needed? Yes
Available as generic? No
Drug class: Antibacterial

USES

- Treats urinary tract infections.
- Treats tuberculosis.

DOSAGE & USAGE INFORMATION

How to take:
Capsules—Swallow with liquid or food to lessen stomach irritation. If you can't swallow whole, open capsule and take with liquid or food.

When to take:
- Once or twice daily.
- At the same time each day after meals to prevent stomach irritation.

If you forget a dose:
Take as soon as you remember up to 2 hours late. If more than 2 hours, wait for next scheduled dose (don't double this dose).

What drug does:
Interferes with bacterial wall synthesis and keeps germs from multiplying.

Time lapse before drug works:
3 to 4 hours.

Don't take with:
Any other medicine without consulting your doctor or pharmacist.

OVERDOSE

SYMPTOMS:
Seizures.
WHAT TO DO:
- **Dial 911 (emergency) for an ambulance or medical help or poison center 1-800-222-1222. Then give first aid immediately.**
- **See emergency information on inside covers.**

POSSIBLE ADVERSE REACTIONS OR SIDE EFFECTS

SYMPTOMS	WHAT TO DO
Life-threatening:	
Seizures, muscle twitching or trembling.	Seek emergency treatment immediately.
Common:	
Gum inflammation, pale skin, depression, confusion, dizziness, restlessness, anxiety, nightmares, severe headache, drowsiness.	Continue, but call doctor right away.
Infrequent:	
Visual changes; skin rash; numbness, tingling or burning in hands and feet; jaundice; eye pain.	Continue. Call doctor when convenient.
Rare:	
Seizures, thoughts of suicide.	Discontinue. Seek emergency treatment.

WARNINGS & PRECAUTIONS

Don't take if:
- You are a frequent user of alcohol.
- You have a convulsive disorder.

Before you start, consult your doctor:
- If you are depressed.
- If you have kidney disease.
- If you have severe anxiety.

Over age 60:
Adverse reactions and side effects may be more frequent and severe than in younger persons. You may need smaller doses for shorter periods of time.

Pregnancy:
Decide with your doctor if drug benefits justify risk to unborn child. Risk category C (see page xviii).

Breast-feeding:
Drug passes into milk. Avoid drug or discontinue nursing until you finish medicine. Consult doctor for advice on maintaining milk supply.

Infants & children:
Use only under close medical supervision.

Prolonged use:
- May cause liver or kidney damage.
- May cause anemia.

Skin & sunlight:
No special problems expected.

Driving, piloting or hazardous work:
Don't drive or pilot aircraft until you learn how medicine affects you. Don't work around dangerous machinery. Don't climb ladders or work in high places. Danger increases if you drink alcohol or take medicine affecting alertness and reflexes.

Discontinuing:
Don't discontinue without consulting doctor. Dose may require gradual reduction if you have taken drug for a long time. Doses of other drugs may also require adjustment.

Others:
- May have to take anticonvulsants, sedatives and/or pyridoxine to prevent or minimize toxic effects on the brain.
- If you must take more than 500 mg per day, toxicity is much more likely to occur.
- Talk to your doctor about taking pyridoxine as a supplement.

POSSIBLE INTERACTION WITH OTHER DRUGS

GENERIC NAME OR DRUG CLASS	COMBINED EFFECT
Ethionamide	Increased risk of seizures.
Isoniazid	Increased risk of central nervous system effects.
Pyridoxine	Reduces effects of pyridoxine. Since pyridoxine is a vital vitamin, patients on cycloserine require pyridoxine supplements to prevent anemia or peripheral neuritis.

POSSIBLE INTERACTION WITH OTHER SUBSTANCES

INTERACTS WITH	COMBINED EFFECT
Alcohol:	Toxic. May increase risk of seizures. Avoid.
Beverages:	None expected. All beverages except those with alcohol.
Cocaine:	Toxic. Avoid.
Foods:	None expected.
Marijuana:	May increase risk of seizures.
Tobacco:	May decrease effect of cycloserine.

*See Glossary

CYCLOSPORINE

BRAND NAMES

Neoral
Sandimmune

BASIC INFORMATION

Habit forming? No
Prescription needed? Yes
Available as generic? No
Drug class: Immunosuppressant

USES

- Suppresses the immune response in patients who have transplants of the heart, lung, kidney, liver, pancreas. Cyclosporine treats rejection as well as helps prevent it.
- Treatment for severe psoriasis when regular treatment is ineffective or not appropriate.

DOSAGE & USAGE INFORMATION

How to take:
- Oral solution—Take after meals with liquid to decrease stomach irritation. May mix with milk, chocolate milk or orange juice. Don't mix in styrofoam cups. Use special dropper for exact dosage.
- Capsules—Take with water or other fluid. Don't break capsule open.

When to take:
At the same time each day, according to instructions on prescription label.

If you forget a dose:
Take as soon as you remember up to 2 hours late. If more than 2 hours, wait for next scheduled dose (don't double this dose).

What drug does:
Exact mechanism is unknown, but believed to inhibit interluken II to affect T-lymphocytes.

Time lapse before drug works:
3 to 3-1/2 hours.

Don't take with:
Any other medicine without consulting your doctor or pharmacist.

OVERDOSE

SYMPTOMS:
Irregular heartbeat, seizures, coma.
WHAT TO DO:
- **Dial 911 (emergency) for an ambulance or medical help or poison center 1-800-222-1222. Then give first aid immediately.**
- **See emergency information on inside covers.**

POSSIBLE ADVERSE REACTIONS OR SIDE EFFECTS

SYMPTOMS	WHAT TO DO
Life-threatening:	
Seizures, wheezing with shortness of breath, convulsions.	Discontinue. Seek emergency treatment.
Common:	
• Gum inflammation, blood in urine, jaundice, tremors.	Continue. Call doctor when convenient.
• Increased hair growth.	Continue. Tell doctor at next visit.
Infrequent:	
• Fever, chills, sore throat, shortness of breath.	Call doctor right away.
• Frequent urination, headache, leg cramps.	Continue. Call doctor when convenient.
Rare:	
• Confusion, irregular heartbeat, numbness of hands and feet, nervousness, face flushing, severe abdominal pain, weakness.	Call doctor right away.
• Acne, headache.	Continue. Call doctor when convenient.

WARNINGS & PRECAUTIONS

Don't take if:
- You have chicken pox.
- You have shingles (herpes zoster).

Before you start, consult your doctor:
- If you have liver problems.
- If you have an infection.
- If you have kidney disease.

Over age 60:
No special problems expected.

Pregnancy:
Decide with your doctor if drug benefits justify risk to unborn child. Risk category C (see page xviii).

Breast-feeding:
Drug passes into milk. Avoid drug or discontinue nursing until you finish medicine. Consult doctor for advice on maintaining milk supply.

Infants & children:
No problems expected.

Prolonged use:
- Can cause reduced function of kidney.
- Talk to your doctor about the need for follow-up medical examinations or laboratory studies to check blood pressure, kidney function, liver function.

Skin & sunlight:
No problems expected.

Driving, piloting or hazardous work:
Don't drive or pilot aircraft until you learn how medicine affects you. Don't work around dangerous machinery. Don't climb ladders or work in high places. Danger increases if you drink alcohol or take medicine affecting alertness and reflexes.

Discontinuing:
Don't discontinue without consulting doctor. You probably will require this medicine for the remainder of your life.

Others:
- Request regular laboratory studies to measure levels of potassium and cyclosporine in blood and to evaluate liver and kidney function.
- Check blood pressure. Cyclosporine sometimes causes hypertension.
- Don't store solution in the refrigerator.
- Avoid any immunizations except those specifically recommended by your doctor.
- Maintain good dental hygiene. Cyclosporine can cause gum problems.
- Kidney toxicity occurs commonly after 12 months of taking cyclosporine.
- Don't mix in styrofoam cups.

POSSIBLE INTERACTION WITH OTHER DRUGS

GENERIC NAME OR DRUG CLASS	COMBINED EFFECT
Androgens	Increased effect of cyclosporine.
Anticonvulsants*	Decreased effect of cyclosporine.
Cimetidine	Increased effect of cyclosporine.
Danazol	Increased effect of cyclosporine.
Diltiazem	Increased effect of cyclosporine.
Diuretics, potassium-sparing	Increased effect of cyclosporine.
Erythromycin	Increased effect of cyclosporine.
Estrogens	Increased effect of cyclosporine.
Fluconazole	Increased effect of cyclosporine. Cyclosporine dosage must be adjusted.
HMG-CoA reductase inhibitors	Increased risk of muscle and kidney problems.
Imatinib	Increased effect of cyclosporine.
Immuno-suppressants* (adrenocorticoids, azathioprine, chlorambucil, cyclophosphamide, mercaptopurine, muromonab-CD3)	May increase risk of infection.
Itraconazole	Increased cyclosporine toxicity.
Ketoconazole	Increased risk of toxicity to kidney.
Leukotriene modifiers	Increased effect of cyclosporine.
Losartan	Increased potassium levels.
Lovastatin	Increased heart and kidney damage.
Medicines that may be toxic to kidneys (gold*, NSAIDs*, sulfonamides*)	Increased risk of toxicity to kidneys.

Continued on page 910

POSSIBLE INTERACTION WITH OTHER SUBSTANCES

INTERACTS WITH	COMBINED EFFECT
Alcohol:	May increase possibility of toxic effects. Avoid.
Beverages: Grapefruit juice.	Increased cyclosporine effect.
Cocaine:	May increase possibility of toxic effects. Avoid.
Foods:	None expected.
Marijuana:	May increase possibility of toxic effects. Avoid.
Tobacco:	May increase possibility of toxic effects. Avoid.

***See Glossary**

DANAZOL

BRAND NAMES

Cyclomen
Danocrine

BASIC INFORMATION

Habit forming? No
Prescription needed? Yes
Available as generic? No
Drug class: Gonadotropin inhibitor

USES

Treatment of endometriosis, fibrocystic breast disease, angioneurotic edema except in pregnant women, gynecomastia, infertility, excessive menstruation, precocious puberty.

DOSAGE & USAGE INFORMATION

How to take:
Capsule—Swallow with liquid or food to lessen stomach irritation. If you can't swallow whole, open capsule and take with liquid or food.

When to take:
At the same times each day.

If you forget a dose:
Take as soon as you remember (don't double dose).

What drug does:
Partially prevents output of pituitary follicle-stimulating hormone and lutenizing hormone reducing estrogen production.

Time lapse before drug works:
- 2 to 3 months to treat endometriosis.
- 1 to 2 months to treat other disorders.

Don't take with:
- Birth control pills.
- Any other medicine without consulting your doctor or pharmacist.

OVERDOSE

SYMPTOMS:
None expected.
WHAT TO DO:
Overdose unlikely to threaten life. If person takes much larger amount than prescribed, call doctor, poison center 1-800-222-1222 or hospital emergency room for instructions.

POSSIBLE ADVERSE REACTIONS OR SIDE EFFECTS

SYMPTOMS	WHAT TO DO
Life-threatening: None expected.	
Common: Menstrual irregularities.	Continue. Call doctor when convenient.
Infrequent:	
• Unnatural hair growth in women, nosebleeds, bleeding gums, sore throat and chills.	Discontinue. Call doctor right away.
• Dizziness; deepened voice; hoarseness; flushed or red skin; muscle cramps; enlarged clitoris; decreased testicle size; vaginal burning, itching; swollen feet; decreased breast size; increased or decreased sex drive.	Continue. Call doctor when convenient.
• Headache, acne, weight gain, vision changes.	Continue. Tell doctor at next visit.
Rare: Jaundice, flushing, sweating, vaginitis, rash, nausea, vomiting, constipation, abdominal pain.	Discontinue. Call doctor right away.

WARNINGS & PRECAUTIONS

Don't take if:
- You become pregnant.
- You have breast cancer.

Before you start, consult your doctor:
- If you take birth control pills.
- If you have diabetes.
- If you have heart disease.
- If you have epilepsy.
- If you have kidney disease.
- If you have liver disease.
- If you have migraine headaches.

Over age 60:
Adverse reactions and side effects may be more frequent and severe than in younger persons.

Pregnancy:
Risk to unborn child outweighs drug benefits. Don't use. Stop if you get pregnant. Risk category X (see page xviii).

Breast-feeding:
Unknown whether medicine filters into milk. Consult doctor.

Infants & children:
Not recommended.

Prolonged use:
- Required for full effect. Don't discontinue without consulting doctor.
- Talk to your doctor about the need for follow-up medical examinations or laboratory studies to check liver function, mammogram.

Skin & sunlight:
No problems expected.

Driving, piloting or hazardous work:
No problems expected.

Discontinuing:
Don't discontinue without consulting doctor. Menstrual periods may be absent for 2 to 3 months after discontinuation.

Others:
- May alter blood sugar levels in diabetic persons.
- May interfere with the accuracy of some medical tests.

POSSIBLE INTERACTION WITH OTHER DRUGS

GENERIC NAME OR DRUG CLASS	COMBINED EFFECT
Anticoagulants, oral*	Increased anti-coagulant effect.
Antidiabetic agents, oral*	Decreased anti-diabetic effect.
Cyclosporine	Increased risk of kidney damage.
Insulin	Decreased insulin effect.

POSSIBLE INTERACTION WITH OTHER SUBSTANCES

INTERACTS WITH	COMBINED EFFECT
Alcohol:	Excessive nervous system depression. Avoid.
Beverages:	
Caffeine.	Rapid, irregular heartbeat. Avoid.
Cocaine:	May interfere with expected action of danazol. Avoid.
Foods:	None expected.
Marijuana:	May interfere with expected action of danazol. Avoid.
Tobacco:	Rapid, irregular heartbeat. Avoid. Increased leg cramps.

*See Glossary

DANTROLENE

BRAND NAMES

Dantrium

BASIC INFORMATION

Habit forming? No
Prescription needed? Yes
Available as generic? No
Drug class: Muscle relaxant, antispastic

USES

- Relieves muscle spasticity caused by diseases such as multiple sclerosis, cerebral palsy, stroke.
- Relieves muscle spasticity caused by injury to spinal cord.
- Relieves or prevents excess body temperature brought on by some surgical procedures.

DOSAGE & USAGE INFORMATION

How to take:
Capsules—Swallow with liquid.

When to take:
Once a day for muscle spasticity during first 6 days. Later, every 6 hours. For excess body temperature, follow label instructions.

If you forget a dose:
Take as soon as you remember up to 2 hours late. If more than 2 hours, wait for next scheduled dose (don't double this dose).

Continued next column

What drug does:
Acts directly on muscles to prevent excess contractions.

Time lapse before drug works:
1 or more weeks.

Don't take with:
Any other medicine without consulting your doctor or pharmacist.

OVERDOSE

SYMPTOMS:
Shortness of breath, bloody urine, chest pain, convulsions.
WHAT TO DO:

- **Dial 911 (emergency) for an ambulance or medical help or poison center 1-800-222-1222. Then give first aid immediately.**
- **If patient is unconscious and not breathing, give mouth-to-mouth breathing. If there is no heartbeat, use cardiac massage and mouth-to-mouth breathing (CPR). Don't try to make patient vomit. If you can't get help quickly, take patient to nearest emergency facility.**
- **See emergency information on inside covers.**

POSSIBLE ADVERSE REACTIONS OR SIDE EFFECTS

SYMPTOMS	WHAT TO DO
Life-threatening:	
Seizure.	Seek emergency treatment immediately.
Common:	
Drowsiness, dizziness, weakness.	Discontinue. Call doctor right away.
Infrequent:	
• Rash, hives; black or bloody stools; chest pain; fast heartbeat; backache; blood in urine; painful, swollen feet; chills; fever; shortness of breath.	Discontinue. Call doctor right away.
• Depression, confusion, headache, slurred speech, insomnia, nervousness, diarrhea, blurred vision, difficult swallowing, appetite loss, difficult urination, decreased sexual function in males.	Continue. Call doctor when convenient.
Rare:	
• Jaundice, abdominal cramps, double vision.	Discontinue. Call doctor right away.
• Constipation.	Continue. Call doctor when convenient.

WARNINGS & PRECAUTIONS

Don't take if:
You are allergic to dantrolene or any muscle relaxant or antispastic medication.

Before you start, consult your doctor:
- If you have liver disease.
- If you have heart disease.
- If you have lung disease (especially emphysema).
- If you are over age 35.
- If you will have surgery within 2 months, including dental surgery, requiring general or spinal anesthesia.

Over age 60:
Adverse reactions and side effects may be more frequent and severe than in younger persons.

Pregnancy:
Decide with your doctor if drug benefits justify risk to unborn child. Risk category C (see page xviii).

Breast-feeding:
Avoid nursing or discontinue until you finish drug. Consult doctor.

Infants & children:
Only under close medical supervision.

Prolonged use:
Recommended periodically during prolonged use—Blood counts, G6PD* tests, liver function studies.

Skin & sunlight:
No special problems expected.

Driving, piloting or hazardous work:
Don't drive or pilot aircraft until you learn how medicine affects you. Don't work around dangerous machinery. Don't climb ladders or work in high places. Danger increases if you drink alcohol or take medicine affecting alertness and reflexes, such as antihistamines, tranquilizers, sedatives, pain medicine, narcotics and mind-altering drugs.

Discontinuing:
Don't discontinue without consulting doctor. Dose may require gradual reduction if you have taken drug for a long time. Doses of other drugs may also require adjustment.

Others:
- No problems expected.
- Advise any doctor or dentist whom you consult that you take this medicine.

POSSIBLE INTERACTION WITH OTHER DRUGS

GENERIC NAME OR DRUG CLASS	COMBINED EFFECT
Central nervous system (CNS) depressants *	Increased sedation, low blood pressure. Avoid.
Dronabinol	Increased effect of dronabinol on central nervous system. Avoid.

POSSIBLE INTERACTION WITH OTHER SUBSTANCES

INTERACTS WITH	COMBINED EFFECT
Alcohol:	Increased sedation, low blood pressure. Avoid.
Beverages:	None expected.
Cocaine:	Increased spasticity. Avoid.
Foods:	None expected.
Marijuana:	Increased spasticity. Avoid.
Tobacco:	May interfere with absorption of medicine.

*See Glossary

DAPSONE

BRAND NAMES

Avlosulfon **DDS**

BASIC INFORMATION

Habit forming? No
Prescription needed? Yes
Available as generic? Yes
Drug class: Antibacterial (antileprosy), sulfone

USES

- Treatment of dermatitis herpetiformis.
- Treatment of leprosy.
- Prevention and treatment of pneumocystis carnii pneumonia.
- Other uses include granuloma annulare, pemphigoid, pyoderma gangrenosum, polychondritis, eye ulcerations, systemic lupus erythematosus.

DOSAGE & USAGE INFORMATION

How to take:
Tablet—Swallow with liquid or food to lessen stomach irritation.

When to take:
Once a day at same time.

If you forget a dose:
Take as soon as you remember up to 2 hours late. If more than 2 hours, wait for next scheduled dose (don't double this dose).

Continued next column

OVERDOSE

SYMPTOMS:
Bleeding, vomiting, seizures, cyanosis, coma.
WHAT TO DO:

- **Dial 911 (emergency) for an ambulance or medical help or poison center 1-800-222-1222. Then give first aid immediately.**
- **If patient is unconscious and not breathing, give mouth-to-mouth breathing. If there is no heartbeat, use cardiac massage and mouth-to-mouth breathing (CPR). Don't try to make patient vomit. If you can't get help quickly, take patient to nearest emergency facility.**
- **See emergency information on inside covers.**

What drug does:
Inhibits enzymes. Kills leprosy germs.

Time lapse before drug works:

- 3 years for leprosy.
- 1 to 2 weeks for dermatitis herpetiformis.

Don't take with:
Any other medicine without consulting your doctor or pharmacist.

POSSIBLE ADVERSE REACTIONS OR SIDE EFFECTS

SYMPTOMS	WHAT TO DO
Life-threatening:	
In case of overdose, see previous column.	
Common:	
• Rash, abdominal pain.	Discontinue. Call doctor right away.
• Appetite loss.	Continue. Call doctor when convenient.
Infrequent:	
Pale.	Discontinue. Call doctor right away.
Rare:	
• Dizziness; mental changes; sore throat; fever; difficult breathing; bleeding; jaundice; numbness, tingling, pain or burning in hands or feet; swelling of feet, hands, eyelids; blurred vision; anemia; peeling skin.	Discontinue. Call doctor right away.
• Headache; itching; nausea; vomiting; blue fingernails, lips.	Continue. Call doctor when convenient.

WARNINGS & PRECAUTIONS

Don't take if:

- You have G6PD* deficiency.
- You are allergic to furosemide, thiazide diuretics, sulfonureas, carbonic anhydrase inhibitors, sulfonamides.

Before you start, consult your doctor:
- If you take any other medicine.
- If you are anemic.
- If you have liver or kidney disease.
- If you are Negro or Caucasian with Mediterranean heritage.
- If you will have surgery within 2 months, including dental surgery, requiring general or spinal anesthesia.

Over age 60:
Adverse reactions and side effects may be more frequent and severe than in younger persons.

Pregnancy:
Decide with your doctor if drug benefits justify risk to unborn child. Risk category C (see page xviii).

Breast-feeding:
Consult doctor. Avoid drug or discontinue nursing.

Infants & children:
Under close medical supervision only.

Prolonged use:
- Request liver function studies.
- Talk to your doctor about the need for follow-up medical examinations or laboratory studies to check complete blood counts (white blood cell count, platelet count, red blood cell count, hemoglobin, hematocrit).

Skin & sunlight:
May cause rash or intensify sunburn in areas exposed to sun or ultraviolet light photosensitivity reaction). Avoid overexposure. Notify doctor if reaction occurs.

Driving, piloting or hazardous work:
Don't drive or pilot aircraft until you learn how medicine affects you. Don't work around dangerous machinery. Don't climb ladders or work in high places. Danger increases if you drink alcohol or take medicine affecting alertness and reflexes, such as antihistamines, tranquilizers, sedatives, pain medicine, narcotics and mind-altering drugs.

Discontinuing:
Don't discontinue without consulting doctor. Dose may require gradual reduction if you have taken drug for a long time. Doses of other drugs may also require adjustment.

Others:
- Dapsone may rarely cause liver damage.
- For full effect you may need to take dapsone for many months or years.

POSSIBLE INTERACTION WITH OTHER DRUGS

GENERIC NAME OR DRUG CLASS	COMBINED EFFECT
Aminobenzoic acid (PABA)	Decreased dapsone effect. Avoid.
Antivirals, HIV/AIDS*	Increased risk of peripheral neuropathy. Reduced absorption of both drugs.
Dideoxyinosine (ddl)	Decreased dapsone effect.
Hemolytics*	May increase adverse effects on blood cells.
Methotrexate	May increase blood toxicity.
Probenecid	Increased toxicity of dapsone.
Pyrimethamine	May increase blood toxicity.
Rifampin	Decreased effect of dapsone.
Trimethoprim	May increase blood toxicity.

POSSIBLE INTERACTION WITH OTHER SUBSTANCES

INTERACTS WITH	COMBINED EFFECT
Alcohol:	Increased chance of toxicity to liver.
Beverages:	None expected.
Cocaine:	Increased chance of toxicity. Avoid.
Foods:	None expected.
Marijuana:	Increased chance of toxicity. Avoid.
Tobacco:	May interfere with absorption of medicine.

DECONGESTANTS (Ophthalmic)

GENERIC AND BRAND NAMES

ANTAZOLINE
- Vasocon-A

NAPHAZOLINE
- Ak-Con
- Albalon
- Albalon Liquifilm
- Allerest
- Allergy Drops
- Clear Eyes
- Comfort Eye Drops
- Degest 2
- Estivin II
- I-Naphline
- Murine Plus
- Muro's Opcon
- Nafazair
- Naphcon
- Naphcon A
- Naphcon Forte
- Ocu-Zoline
- Vasoclear
- Vasoclear A
- Vasocon
- Vasocon Regular

OXYMETAZOLINE
- OcuClear
- Visine L.R.

TETRAHYDROZILINE
- Visine

BASIC INFORMATION

Habit forming? No
Prescription needed? Yes, for some
Available as generic? Yes
Drug class: Decongestant (ophthalmic)

USES

Treats eye redness, itching, burning or other irritation due to dust, colds, allergies, rubbing eyes, wearing contact lenses, swimming or eye strain from close work, watching TV, reading.

OVERDOSE

SYMPTOMS:
None expected.
WHAT TO DO:
Not intended for internal use. If child accidentally swallows, call poison center 1-800-222-1222.

DOSAGE & USAGE INFORMATION

How to use:
Eye drops
- Wash hands.
- Apply pressure to inside corner of eye with middle finger.
- Tilt head backward. Pull lower lid away from eye with index finger of the same hand.
- Drop eye drops into pouch and close eye. Don't blink.
- Keep eyes closed for 1 to 2 minutes.
- Continue pressure for 1 minute after placing medicine in eye.
- Don't touch applicator tip to any surface (including the eye). If you accidentally touch tip, clean with warm soap and water.
- Keep container tightly closed.
- Keep cool, but don't freeze.
- Wash hands immediately after using.

When to use:
As directed. Usually every 3 or 4 hours.

If you forget a dose:
Use as soon as you remember.

What drug does:
Acts on small blood vessels to make them constrict or become smaller.

Time lapse before drug works:
2 to 10 minutes.

Don't use with:
Other eye drops without consulting your doctor.

POSSIBLE ADVERSE REACTIONS OR SIDE EFFECTS

SYMPTOMS	WHAT TO DO
Life-threatening:	
None expected.	
Common:	
Increased eye irritation.	Discontinue. Call doctor right away.
Infrequent:	
None expected.	
Rare:	
Blurred vision, large pupils, weakness, drowsiness, decreased body temperature, slow heartbeat, dizziness, headache, nervousness, nausea.	Discontinue. Call doctor right away.

WARNINGS & PRECAUTIONS

Don't use if:
You are allergic to any decongestant eye drops.

Before you start, consult your doctor:
- If you take antidepressants or maprolitine.
- If you have glaucoma, eye disease, infection or injury.
- If you have heart disease, high blood pressure, thyroid disease.

Over age 60:
No problems expected.

Pregnancy:
Decide with your doctor if drug benefits justify risk to unborn child. Risk category C (see page xviii).

Breast-feeding:
No problems expected, but check with doctor.

Infants & children:
Don't use.

Prolonged use:
Don't use for more than 3 or 4 days.

Skin & sunlight:
No problems expected.

Driving, piloting or hazardous work:
No problems expected.

Discontinuing:
May not need all the medicine in container. If symptoms disappear, stop using.

Others:
Check with your doctor if eye irritation continues or becomes worse.

POSSIBLE INTERACTION WITH OTHER DRUGS

GENERIC NAME OR DRUG CLASS	COMBINED EFFECT

Clinically significant interactions with oral or injected medicines unlikely.

POSSIBLE INTERACTION WITH OTHER SUBSTANCES

INTERACTS WITH	COMBINED EFFECT
Alcohol:	None expected.
Beverages:	None expected.
Cocaine:	None expected.
Foods:	None expected.
Marijuana:	None expected.
Tobacco:	Smoke may increase eye irritation. Avoid.

DEHYDROEPIANDROSTERONE (DHEA)

BRAND NAMES

Numerous brand names are available

BASIC INFORMATION

Habit forming? No
Prescription needed? No
Available as generic? Yes
Drug class: Adrenal steroid

USES

DHEA is a steroid produced in the human body by the adrenal glands (which sit on top of each kidney). DHEA concentration peaks at about age 20 and then decreases progressively with age. Supplements are sold as an antiaging remedy claimed by some, to improve energy, strength, and immunity. DHEA is also said to increase muscle and decrease fat. Studies to date do not provide a clear picture of the risks and benefits of DHEA.

DOSAGE & USAGE INFORMATION

How to take:
For tablet or capsule—Follow instructions on the label or consult your doctor or pharmacist. Different brands supply different doses. DHEA, as a product, is marketed as a dietary supplement and is not reviewed by the U.S. Food & Drug Administration (FDA) for effectiveness and safety. The best dosage amounts are unknown. Use with caution.

When to take:
At the same times each day according to label directions.

If you forget a dose:
Follow label instructions for your particular brand of DHEA. Usually you can take a medication as soon as you remember up to 2 hours late. If more than 2 hours, wait for the next scheduled dose (don't double this dose).

Continued next column

OVERDOSE

SYMPTOMS:
It is unknown what symptoms may occur.
WHAT TO DO:
If person takes much larger amount than prescribed, call doctor, poison center 1-800-222-1222 or hospital emergency room for instructions.

What drug does:

- Although it is not known whether DHEA itself causes hormonal effects, the body breaks DHEA down into two hormones—estrogen and testosterone. Some people's bodies make large amounts of estrogen and testosterone from DHEA, while others make smaller amounts.
- Hormone supplements may not have the same effects on the body as naturally produced hormones have, because the body processes them differently. Higher doses of supplements may result in higher amounts of hormones in the blood than are healthy.

Time lapse before drug works:
Effectiveness will vary from person to person and will also depend on the reason for taking DHEA, such as for a chronic health problem.

Don't take with:
Any prescription or nonprescription medicine without consulting your doctor or pharmacist.

POSSIBLE ADVERSE REACTIONS OR SIDE EFFECTS

SYMPTOMS	WHAT TO DO
Life-threatening: None expected.	
Common: Unknown.	
Infrequent: In women: acne, hair loss, facial hair growth (hirsutism), deepening of voice (the last two may be irreversible).	Discontinue. Call doctor when convenient.
Rare: Unknown. If symptoms occur that you are concerned about, talk to your doctor or pharmacist. Further research may uncover other side effects.	

DEHYDROEPIANDROSTERONE (DHEA)

WARNINGS & PRECAUTIONS

Don't use if:
You are allergic to DHEA.

Before you start, consult your doctor:
- If you have any chronic health problem.
- If you have a family history of cancer.
- If you are allergic to any medication, food or other substance.
- If you have or have had prostate, ovarian, breast, cervical or uterine cancer.

Over age 60:
A lower starting dosage may be recommended until a response is determined.

Pregnancy:
Decide with your doctor if any possible benefits of DHEA justify risk to unborn child. Risk category is unknown since DHEA is not regulated by the FDA (see page xviii).

Breast-feeding:
It is unknown if DHEA passes into milk. Avoid it or discontinue nursing until you finish medicine. Consult doctor for advice on maintaining milk supply.

Infants & children:
Not recommended for children.

Prolonged use:
Effects are unknown. More research is needed to determine long-term effects of DHEA use.

Skin & sunlight:
No problems expected.

Driving, piloting or hazardous work:
No problems expected.

Discontinuing:
No problems expected, but effects after long-term use are unknown.

Others:
- Advise any doctor or dentist whom you consult that you take DHEA.
- DHEA is not researched carefully as yet for use in humans. Most research has been performed on animals. Studies are ongoing to find more definite answers about its effect on aging, muscles, and the immune system. Studies in men and women have shown an improvement in the feeling of well being. Studies in AIDS patients and those with multiple sclerosis also have shown improvement in well being, but without an outcome change.
- Researchers are concerned that DHEA supplements may cause high levels of estrogen or testosterone in some people. The body's own testosterone plays a role in prostate cancer and high levels of naturally produced estrogen are suspected of increasing breast cancer risk. The effect of DHEA is unknown.

POSSIBLE INTERACTION WITH OTHER DRUGS

GENERIC NAME OR DRUG CLASS	COMBINED EFFECT
All medications	Effects are unknown. Talk to your doctor or pharmacist.

POSSIBLE INTERACTION WITH OTHER SUBSTANCES

INTERACTS WITH	COMBINED EFFECT
Alcohol:	Unknown.
Beverages:	None expected.
Cocaine:	Problems not known. Best to avoid.
Foods:	None expected.
Marijuana:	Problems not known. Best to avoid.
Tobacco:	Unknown.

DESMOPRESSIN

BRAND NAMES

DDAVP
Stimate

BASIC INFORMATION

Habit forming? No
Prescription needed? Yes
Available as generic? No
Drug class: Antidiuretic, antihemorrhagic

USES

- Prevents and controls symptoms associated with central diabetes insipidus.
- Treats primary nocturnal enuresis (bedwetting during sleep).

DOSAGE & USAGE INFORMATION

How to take:

- Nasal spray—Fill the rhinyle (a flexible, calibrated catheter) with a measured dose of the nasal spray. Blow on the other end of the catheter to deposit the solution deep in the nasal cavity. For infants and children, an air-filled syringe may be used.
- Tablet—Swallow with liquid.

When to take:
At the same time each day, according to instructions on prescription label.

If you forget a dose:
Take as soon as you remember up to 2 hours late. If more than 2 hours, wait for next scheduled dose. Don't double this dose.

What drug does:
Increases water reabsorption in the kidney and decreases urine output.

Time lapse before drug works:
Within 1 hour. Effect may last from 6 to 24 hours.

Don't take with:
Any other medicine without consulting your doctor or pharmacist.

OVERDOSE

SYMPTOMS:
Confusion, coma, seizures.
WHAT TO DO:
Overdose unlikely to threaten life. If person takes much larger amount than prescribed, call doctor, poison center 1-800-222-1222 or hospital emergency room for instructions.

POSSIBLE ADVERSE REACTIONS OR SIDE EFFECTS

SYMPTOMS	WHAT TO DO
Life-threatening: None expected.	
Common: None expected.	
Infrequent: Flushing or redness of skin, headache, nausea, nasal congestion.	Continue. Call doctor when convenient.
Rare: Water intoxication—confusion, drowsiness, headache, seizures, rapid weight gain, decreased urination (very rare).	Discontinue. Seek emergency treatment.

WARNINGS & PRECAUTIONS

Don't take if:
You know that you are sensitive to desmopressin.

Before you start, consult your doctor:
- If you have allergic rhinitis.
- If you have nasal congestion.
- If you have a cold or other upper respiratory infection or are dehydrated.
- If you have heart disease or high blood pressure.
- If you have had cystic fibrosis.

Over age 60:
Increased risk of water intoxication.

Pregnancy:
No proven harm to unborn child, but avoid if possible. Consult doctor. Risk category B (see page xviii).

Breast-feeding:
Drug passes into milk. Avoid drug or discontinue nursing until you finish medicine. Consult doctor for advice on maintaining milk supply.

Infants & children:
More sensitive to effect. Use only under close medical supervision.

Prolonged use:
May require increasing dosage for same effect.

Skin & sunlight:
No special problems expected.

Driving, piloting or hazardous work:
Don't drive or pilot aircraft until you learn how medicine affects you. Don't work around dangerous machinery. Don't climb ladders or work in high places. Danger increases if you drink alcohol or take medicine affecting alertness and reflexes.

Discontinuing:
No special problems expected.

Others:
- Advise any doctor or dentist whom you consult that you take this medicine.
- Fluid intake may need to be adjusted.

POSSIBLE INTERACTION WITH OTHER DRUGS

GENERIC NAME OR DRUG CLASS	COMBINED EFFECT
Carbamazepine	May increase desmopressin effect.
Chlorpropamide	May increase desmopressin effect.
Clofibrate	May increase desmopressin effect.
Demeclocycline	May decrease desmopressin effect.
Lithium	May decrease desmopressin effect.
Norepinephrine	May decrease desmopressin effect.

POSSIBLE INTERACTION WITH OTHER SUBSTANCES

INTERACTS WITH	COMBINED EFFECT
Alcohol:	May decrease desmopressin effect.
Beverages:	
Caffeine drinks.	May decrease desmopressin effect.
Cocaine:	May decrease desmopressin effect.
Foods:	None expected.
Marijuana:	May decrease desmopressin effect.
Tobacco:	May decrease desmopressin effect.

*See Glossary

DEXTROMETHORPHAN

BRAND NAMES

See complete list of brand names in the *Generic and Brand Name Directory*, page 862.

BASIC INFORMATION

Habit forming? No
Prescription needed? No
Available as generic? Yes
Drug class: Cough suppressant, antitussive

USES

Suppresses cough associated with allergies or infections such as colds, bronchitis, flu and lung disorders. Used in many cough, cold and allergy combination medicines.

DOSAGE & USAGE INFORMATION

How to take:

- Chewable tablet—Chew well before swallowing.
- Oral suspension, lozenges or syrups—Take as directed on label.
- Capsules—Swallow with liquid.

When to take:
As needed, no more often than every 4 hours.

If you forget a dose:
Take as soon as you remember. Wait 4 hours for next dose.

What drug does:
Reduces sensitivity of brain's cough control center, suppressing urge to cough.

Time lapse before drug works:
15 to 30 minutes.

Don't take with:
Any other medicine without consulting your doctor or pharmacist.

OVERDOSE

SYMPTOMS:
Euphoria, overactivity, sense of intoxication, visual and auditory hallucinations, lack of coordination, stagger, stupor, shallow breathing.
WHAT TO DO:

- **Dial 911 (emergency) for an ambulance or medical help or poison center 1-800-222-1222. Then give first aid immediately.**
- **See emergency information on inside covers.**

POSSIBLE ADVERSE REACTIONS OR SIDE EFFECTS

SYMPTOMS	WHAT TO DO
Life-threatening: None expected.	
Common: None expected.	
Infrequent: Mild dizziness or drowsiness, nausea, stomach cramps.	Continue. Call doctor when convenient.
Rare: None expected.	

WARNINGS & PRECAUTIONS

Don't take if:
You are allergic to any cough syrup containing dextromethorphan.

Before you start, consult your doctor:
- If you have asthma attacks.
- If you have impaired liver function.

Over age 60:
Adverse reactions and side effects may be more frequent and severe than in younger persons. You may require smaller doses for shorter periods of time.

Pregnancy:
Decide with your doctor if drug benefits justify risk to unborn child. Risk category C (see page xviii).

Breast-feeding:
No proven problems. Consult doctor.

Infants & children:
Use only as label directs.

Prolonged use:
No problems expected.

Skin & sunlight:
No problems expected.

Driving, piloting or hazardous work:
Don't drive or pilot aircraft until you learn how medicine affects you. Don't work around dangerous machinery. Don't climb ladders or work in high places. Danger increases if you drink alcohol or take medicine affecting alertness and reflexes, such as antihistamines, tranquilizers, sedatives, pain medicine, narcotics and mind-altering drugs.

Discontinuing:
May be unnecessary to finish medicine. Follow doctor's instructions.

Others:
- If cough persists or if you cough blood or brown-yellow, thick mucus, call your doctor.
- Excessive use may lead to functional dependence.

POSSIBLE INTERACTION WITH OTHER DRUGS

GENERIC NAME OR DRUG CLASS	COMBINED EFFECT
Doxepin (topical)	Increased risk of toxicity of both drugs.
Monozmine oxidase (MAO) inhibitors*	Disorientation, high fever, drop in blood pressure and loss of consciousness.
Sedatives* and other central nervous system (CNS) depressants*	Increased sedative effect of both drugs.

POSSIBLE INTERACTION WITH OTHER SUBSTANCES

INTERACTS WITH	COMBINED EFFECT
Alcohol:	None expected.
Beverages:	None expected.
Cocaine:	Decreased dextromethorphan effect. Avoid.
Foods:	None expected.
Marijuana:	None expected.
Tobacco:	None expected.

DEXTROTHYROXINE

BRAND NAMES

Choloxin

BASIC INFORMATION

Habit forming? No
Prescription needed? Yes
Available as generic? No
Drug class: Antihyperlipidemic, thyroid hormone

USES

- Lowers blood cholesterol and low-density lipoproteins in patients who don't respond to low-fat diet and weight loss alone.
- Treats hypothyroidism in patients with heart disease.

DOSAGE & USAGE INFORMATION

How to take:
Tablets—Swallow with liquid. If you can't swallow whole, crumble tablet and take with liquid or food. Instructions to take on empty stomach mean 1 hour before or 2 hours after eating.

When to take:
According to your doctor's instructions.

If you forget a dose:
Take as soon as you remember up to 2 hours late. If more than 2 hours, wait for next scheduled dose (don't double this dose).

What drug does:
Increases breakdown of LDL (low-density lipoprotein).

Time lapse before drug works:
1 to 2 months.

Don't take with:
Any other medicines (including over-the-counter drugs such as cough and cold medicines, laxatives, antacids, diet pills, caffeine, nose drops or vitamins) without consulting your doctor.

OVERDOSE

SYMPTOMS:
None expected.
WHAT TO DO:
Overdose unlikely to threaten life. If person takes much larger amount than prescribed, call doctor, poison center 1-800-222-1222 or hospital emergency room for instructions.

POSSIBLE ADVERSE REACTIONS OR SIDE EFFECTS

SYMPTOMS	WHAT TO DO
Life-threatening:	
None expected.	
Common:	
• Tremor, headache, irritability, insomnia.	Discontinue. Call doctor right away.
• Appetite change, diarrhea, leg cramps, menstrual irregularities, fever, heat sensitivity, unusual sweating, weight loss.	Continue. Call doctor when convenient.
Infrequent:	
Hives, rash, vomiting, chest pain, rapid and irregular heartbeat, shortness of breath.	Discontinue. Call doctor right away.
Rare:	
None expected.	

WARNINGS & PRECAUTIONS

Don't take if:
- You have had a heart attack within 6 weeks.
- You have no thyroid deficiency, but want to use this to lose weight.

Before you start, consult your doctor:
- If you have heart disease or high blood pressure.
- If you have diabetes.
- If you have Addison's disease, have had adrenal gland deficiency or use epinephrine, ephedrine or isoproterenol for asthma.

Over age 60:
More sensitive to thyroid hormone. May need smaller doses.

Pregnancy:
Consult doctor. Risk category B (see page xviii).

Breast-feeding:
Present in milk. Considered safe if dose is correct.

Infants & children:
Use only under medical supervision.

Prolonged use:
- No problems expected, if dose is correct.
- Talk to your doctor about the need for follow-up medical examinations or laboratory studies to check serum cholesterol and triglycerides.

Skin & sunlight:
No problems expected.

Driving, piloting or hazardous work:
No problems expected.

Discontinuing:
Don't discontinue without consulting doctor. Dose may require gradual reduction if you have taken drug for a long time. Doses of other drugs may also require adjustment.

Others:
- Digestive upsets, tremors, cramps, nervousness, insomnia or diarrhea may indicate need for dose adjustment.
- Advise any doctor or dentist whom you consult that you take this medicine.
- May affect results in some medical tests.
- Stay on a low-fat diet.

POSSIBLE INTERACTION WITH OTHER DRUGS

GENERIC NAME OR DRUG CLASS	COMBINED EFFECT
Adrenocorticoids, systemic	Requires dose adjustment to prevent adreno-corticoid deficiency.
Amphetamines*	Increased amphetamine effect.
Anticoagulants, oral*	Increased anticoagulant effect.
Antidepressants, tricyclic*	Increased anti-depressant effect. Irregular heartbeat.
Antidiabetics*	Antidiabetic may require adjustment.
Aspirin (large doses, continuous use)	Increased dextrothyroxine effect.
Barbiturates*	Decreased barbiturate effect.
Beta-adrenergic blocking agents*	Possible decreased beta blocker effect.
Cholestyramine	Decreased dextrothyroxine effect.
Colestipol	Decreased dextrothyroxine effect.
Contraceptives, oral*	Decreased dextrothyroxine effect.
Dexfenfluramine	May require dosage change as weight loss occurs.
Digitalis preparations*	Decreased digitalis effect.
Ephedrine	Increased ephedrine effect.
Epinephrine	Increased epinephrine effect.
Estrogens*	Decreased dextrothyroxine effect.
Methylphenidate	Increased methylphenidate effect.
Phenytoin	Possible decreased dextrothyroxine effect.

POSSIBLE INTERACTION WITH OTHER SUBSTANCES

INTERACTS WITH	COMBINED EFFECT
Alcohol:	None expected.
Beverages:	None expected.
Cocaine:	Excess stimulation. Avoid.
Foods: Soybeans.	Heavy consumption interferes with thyroid function.
Marijuana:	None expected.
Tobacco:	None expected.

*See Glossary

DICYCLOMINE

BRAND NAMES

See complete list of brand names in the *Generic and Brand Name Directory*, page 306.

BASIC INFORMATION

Habit forming? No
Prescription needed? Yes
Available as generic? Yes
Drug class: Antispasmodic, anticholinergic

USES

- Reduces spasms of digestive system, bladder and urethra.
- Treats irritable bowel syndrome.

DOSAGE & USAGE INFORMATION

How to take:
Tablet, syrup or capsule—Swallow with liquid or food to lessen stomach irritation.

When to take:
30 minutes before meals (unless directed otherwise by doctor).

If you forget a dose:
Take as soon as you remember up to 2 hours late. If more than 2 hours, wait for next scheduled dose (don't double this dose).

What drug does:
Blocks nerve impulses at parasympathetic nerve endings, preventing muscle contractions and gland secretions of organs involved.

Time lapse before drug works:
15 to 30 minutes.

Don't take with:
Any other medicine without consulting your doctor or pharmacist.

OVERDOSE

SYMPTOMS:
Dilated pupils, blurred vision, rapid pulse and breathing, dizziness, fever, hallucinations, confusion, slurred speech, agitation, flushed face, convulsions, coma.
WHAT TO DO:
- **Dial 911 (emergency) for an ambulance or medical help or poison center 1-800-222-1222. Then give first aid immediately.**
- **See emergency information on inside covers.**

POSSIBLE ADVERSE REACTIONS OR SIDE EFFECTS

SYMPTOMS	WHAT TO DO
Life-threatening:	
Hives, rash, intense itching, faintness soon after a dose (anaphylaxis).	Seek emergency treatment immediately.
Common:	
• Confusion, delirium, rapid heartbeat.	Discontinue. Call doctor right away.
• Nausea, vomiting.	Discontinue. Call doctor when convenient.
• Constipation, loss of taste, decreased sweating.	Continue. Tell doctor at next visit.
• Dry ears, nose, throat, mouth.	No action necessary.
Infrequent:	
• Headache, difficult urination, nasal congestion, altered taste.	Continue. Call doctor when convenient.
• Lightheadedness.	Discontinue. Call doctor right away.
Rare:	
Rash or hives, eye pain, blurred vision.	Discontinue. Call doctor right away.

WARNINGS & PRECAUTIONS

Don't take if:
- You are allergic to any anticholinergic.
- You have trouble with stomach bloating.
- You have difficulty emptying your bladder completely.
- You have narrow-angle glaucoma.
- You have severe ulcerative colitis.

Before you start, consult your doctor:
- If you have open-angle glaucoma.
- If you have angina, chronic bronchitis or asthma.
- If you have hiatal hernia, liver disease, kidney or thyroid disease, enlarged prostate, myasthenia gravis, peptic ulcer.
- If you will have surgery within 2 months, including dental surgery, requiring general or spinal anesthesia.

Over age 60:
Adverse reactions and side effects may be more frequent and severe than in younger persons.

Pregnancy:
Decide with your doctor whether drug benefits justify risk to unborn child. Risk category C (see page xviii).

Breast-feeding:
Drug passes into milk and decreases milk flow. Avoid drug or discontinue nursing until you finish medicine. Consult doctor for advice on maintaining milk supply.

Infants & children:
Use only under medical supervision.

Prolonged use:
Chronic constipation, possible fecal impaction. Consult doctor immediately.

Skin & sunlight:
No problems expected.

Driving, piloting or hazardous work:
Use disqualifies you for piloting aircraft. Otherwise, no problems expected.

Discontinuing:
May be unnecessary to finish medicine. Follow doctor's instructions.

Others:
Advise any doctor or dentist whom you consult that you take this medicine.

POSSIBLE INTERACTION WITH OTHER DRUGS

GENERIC NAME OR DRUG CLASS	COMBINED EFFECT
Adrenocorticoids, systemic	Possible glaucoma.
Amantadine	Increased dicyclomine effect.
Antacids*	Decreased dicyclomine effect.
Anticholinergics, other*	Increased dicyclomine effect.
Antidepressants, tricyclic*	Increased dicyclomine effect. Increased sedation.
Antidiarrheals*	Decreased dicyclomine effect.
Antihistamines*	Increased dicyclomine effect.
Attapulgite	Decreased dicyclomine effect.
Buclizine	Increased dicyclomine effect.
Digitalis	Possible decreased absorption of digitalis.
Haloperidol	Increased internal eye pressure.
Ketoconazole	Decreased ketoconazole effect.
Meperidine	Increased dicyclomine effect.
Methylphenidate	Increased dicyclomine effect.
Monoamine oxidase (MAO) inhibitors*	Increased dicyclomine effect.
Nitrates*	Increased internal eye pressure.
Nizatidine	Increased nizatidine effect.
Orphenadrine	Increased dicyclomine effect.
Phenothiazines*	Increased dicyclomine effect.
Pilocarpine	Loss of pilocarpine effect in glaucoma treatment.
Potassium supplements*	Possible intestinal ulcers with oral potassium tablets.
Quinidine	Increased dicyclomine effect.
Sedatives* or central nervous system (CNS) depressants*	Increased sedative effect of both drugs.
Vitamin C	Decreased dicyclomine effect. Avoid large doses of vitamin C.

POSSIBLE INTERACTION WITH OTHER SUBSTANCES

INTERACTS WITH	COMBINED EFFECT
Alcohol:	None expected.
Beverages:	None expected.
Cocaine:	Excessively rapid heartbeat. Avoid.
Foods:	None expected.
Marijuana:	Drowsiness and dry mouth.
Tobacco:	None expected.

*See Glossary

DIFENOXIN & ATROPINE

Motofen

BASIC INFORMATION

Habit forming? Yes
Prescription needed? Yes
Available as generic? No
Drug class: Antidiarrheal

USES

- Reduces spasms of digestive system.
- Treats severe diarrhea.

DOSAGE & USAGE INFORMATION

How to take:
Tablet—Swallow with liquid or food to lessen stomach irritation.

When to take:
After each loose stool or every 3 to 4 hours. No more than 5 tablets in 12 hours.

If you forget a dose:
Take as soon as you remember. Don't double this dose.

What drug does:
- Blocks nerve impulses at parasympathetic nerve endings, preventing muscle contractions and gland secretions of organs involved.
- Acts on brain to decrease spasm of smooth muscle.

Time lapse before drug works:
40 to 60 minutes.

Continued next column

OVERDOSE

SYMPTOMS:
Dilated pupils, rapid pulse and breathing, dizziness, fever, hallucinations, confusion, slurred speech, agitation, flushed face, convulsions, coma.
WHAT TO DO:
- **Dial 911 (emergency) for an ambulance or medical help or poison center 1-800-222-1222. Then give first aid immediately.**
- **See emergency information on inside covers.**

Don't take with:
Any medicine that will decrease mentalalertness or reflexes, such as alcohol, other mind-altering drugs, cough/cold medicines, antihistamines, allergy medicine, sedatives, tranquilizers (sleeping pills or "downers") barbiturates, seizure medicine, narcotics, other prescription medicines for pain, muscle relaxants, anesthetics.

POSSIBLE ADVERSE REACTIONS OR SIDE EFFECTS

SYMPTOMS	WHAT TO DO
Life-threatening:	
Shortness of breath, agitation, nervousness.	Discontinue. Seek emergency treatment.
Common:	
Dizziness, drowsiness.	Continue. Call doctor when convenient.
Infrequent:	
• Bloating; constipation; appetite loss; abdominal pain; blurred vision; warm, flushed skin; fast heartbeat; dry mouth.	Discontinue. Call doctor right away.
• Frequent urination, lightheadedness, dry skin, headache, insomnia.	Continue. Call doctor when convenient.
Rare:	
Weakness, confusion, fever.	Continue. Call doctor when convenient.

WARNINGS & PRECAUTIONS

Don't take if:
- You are allergic to any anticholinergic.
- You have trouble with stomach bloating, difficulty emptying your bladder completely, narrow-angle glaucoma, severe ulcerative colitis.
- You are dehydrated.

Before you start, consult your doctor:
- If you have open-angle glaucoma, angina, chronic bronchitis, asthma, liver disease, hiatal hernia, enlarged prostate, myasthenia gravis, peptic ulcer.
- If you will have surgery within 2 months, including dental surgery, requiring general or spinal anesthesia.

Over age 60:
Adverse reactions and side effects may be more frequent and severe than in younger persons.

Pregnancy:
Decide with your doctor whether drug benefits justify risk to unborn child. Risk category C (see page xviii).

Breast-feeding:
Drug passes into milk. Avoid drug or discontinue nursing until you finish medicine. Consult doctor for advice on maintaining milk supply.

Infants & children:
Use only under medical supervision.

Prolonged use:
- Chronic constipation, possible fecal impaction. Consult doctor immediately.
- Talk to your doctor about the need for follow-up medical examinations or laboratory studies to check liver function.

Skin & sunlight:
No problems expected.

Driving, piloting or hazardous work:
Use disqualifies you for piloting aircraft. Don't drive until you learn how medicine affects you. Don't work around dangerous machinery. Don't climb ladders or work in high places. Danger increases if you drink alcohol or take medicine affecting alertness and reflexes, such as antihis-tamines, tranquilizers, sedatives, pain medicine, narcotics and mind-altering drugs.

Discontinuing:
May be unnecessary to finish medicine. Follow doctor's instructions.

Others:
Atropine included at doses below therapeutic level to prevent abuse.

POSSIBLE INTERACTION WITH OTHER DRUGS

GENERIC NAME OR DRUG CLASS	COMBINED EFFECT
Addictive substances (narcotics,* others)	Increased chance of abuse.
Amantadine	Increased atropine effect.
Anticholinergics, other*	Increased atropine effect.
Antidepressants, tricyclic (TCA)*	Increased atropine effect. Increased sedation.
Antihistamines*	Increased atropine effect.
Antihypertensives*	Increased sedation.
Clozapine	Toxic effect on the central nervous system.
Cortisone drugs*	Increased internal eye pressure.
Ethinamate	Dangerous increased effects of ethinamate. Avoid combining.
Fluoxetine	Increased depressant effects of both drugs.
Guanfacine	May increase depressant effects of either drug.
Haloperidol	Increased internal eye pressure.
Leucovorin	High alcohol content of leucovorin may cause adverse effects.
Meperidine	Increased atropine effect.
Methylphenidate	Increased atropine effect.
Methyprylon	Increased sedative effect, perhaps to dangerous level. Avoid.
Monozmine oxidase (MAO) inhibitors*	Increased atropine effect.
Nabilone	Greater depression of central nervous system.
Naltrexone	Triggers withdrawal symptoms.
Narcotics*	Increased sedation. Avoid.

Continued on page 910

POSSIBLE INTERACTION WITH OTHER SUBSTANCES

INTERACTS WITH	COMBINED EFFECT
Alcohol:	Increased sedation. Avoid.
Beverages:	None expected.
Cocaine:	Excessively rapid heartbeat. Avoid.
Foods:	None expected.
Marijuana:	Drowsiness and dry mouth.
Tobacco:	May increase diarrhea. Avoid.

DIGITALIS PREPARATIONS (Digitalis Glycosides)

GENERIC AND BRAND NAMES

DIGITOXIN
Crystodigin

DIGOXIN
Lanoxicaps
Lanoxin
Novodigoxin

BASIC INFORMATION

Habit forming? No
Prescription needed? Yes
Available as generic? Yes
Drug class: Digitalis preparation

USES

- Strengthens weak heart muscle contractions to prevent congestive heart failure.
- Corrects irregular heartbeat.

DOSAGE & USAGE INFORMATION

How to take:
- Tablet or capsule—Swallow with liquid. If you can't swallow whole, crumble tablet or open capsule and take with liquid or food.
- Liquid—Dilute dose in beverage before swallowing.

When to take:
At the same time each day.

If you forget a dose:
Take as soon as you remember up to 12 hours late. If more than 12 hours, wait for next scheduled dose (don't double this dose).

What drug does:
- Strengthens heart muscle contraction.
- Delays nerve impulses to heart.

Time lapse before drug works:
May require regular use for a week or more.

Continued next column

OVERDOSE

SYMPTOMS:
Nausea, vomiting, diarrhea, vision disturbances, halos around lights, fatigue, irregular heartbeat, confusion, hallucinations, convulsions.
WHAT TO DO:
- **Dial 911 (emergency) for an ambulance or medical help or poison center 1-800-222-1222. Then give first aid immediately.**
- **See emergency information on inside covers.**

Don't take with:
Nonprescription drugs without consulting doctor.

POSSIBLE ADVERSE REACTIONS OR SIDE EFFECTS

SYMPTOMS	WHAT TO DO
Life-threatening: In case of overdose, see previous column.	
Common:	
Appetite loss, diarrhea.	Continue. Call doctor when convenient.
Infrequent:	
Extreme drowsiness, lethargy, disorientation, headache, fainting.	Discontinue. Call doctor right away.
Rare:	
• Rash, hives, cardiac arrhythmias, hallucinations, psychosis.	Discontinue. Call doctor right away.
• Double or yellow-green vision; enlarged, sensitive male breasts; tiredness; weakness; depression; decreased sex drive.	Continue. Call doctor when convenient.

WARNINGS & PRECAUTIONS

Don't take if:
- You are allergic to any digitalis preparation.
- Your heartbeat is slower than 50 beats per minute.

Before you start, consult your doctor:
- If you have taken another digitalis preparation in past 2 weeks.
- If you have taken a diuretic within 2 weeks.
- If you have liver or kidney disease.
- If you have a thyroid disorder.
- If you will have surgery within 2 months, including dental surgery, requiring general or spinal anesthesia.

Over age 60:
Adverse reactions and side effects may be more frequent and severe than in younger persons.

Pregnancy:
Decide with you doctor if drug benefits justify risk to unborn child. Risk category C (see page xviii).

Breast-feeding:
Drug filters into milk. May harm child. Avoid.

Infants & children:
Use only under medical supervision.

DIGITALIS PREPARATIONS (Digitalis Glycosides)

Prolonged use:
Talk to your doctor about the need for follow-up medical examinations or laboratory studies to check ECG*, liver function, kidney function, serum electrolytes.

Skin & sunlight:
No problems expected.

Driving, piloting or hazardous work:
Possible vision disturbances. Otherwise, no problems expected.

Discontinuing:
Don't stop without doctor's advice.

Others:
Some digitalis products contain tartrazine dye. Avoid, especially if you are allergic to aspirin.

POSSIBLE INTERACTION WITH OTHER DRUGS

GENERIC NAME OR DRUG CLASS	COMBINED EFFECT
Adrenocorticoids, systemic	Dangerous potassium depletion. Possible digitalis toxicity.
Amiodarone	Increased digitalis effect.
Amphotericin B	Decreased potassium. Increased toxicity of amphotericin B.
Antacids*	Decreased digitalis effect.
Anticonvulsants, hydantoin*	Increased digitalis effect at first, then decreased.
Anticholinergics*	Possible increased digitalis effect.
Attapulgite	May decrease effectiveness of digitalis.
Beta-adrenergic blocking agents*	Increased digitalis effect.
Beta-agonists*	Increased risk of heartbeat irregularity.
Calcium supplements*	Decreased digitalis effects.
Carteolol	Can either increase or decrease heart rate. Improves irregular heartbeat.
Cholestyramine	Decreased digitalis effect.
Colestipol	Decreased digitalis effect.
Dextrothyroxine	Decreased digitalis effect.
Disopyramide	Possible decreased digitalis effect.
Diuretics*	Possible digitalis toxicity. Excessive potassium loss that may cause irregular heartbeat.
Ephedrine	Disturbed heart rhythm. Avoid.
Epinephrine	Disturbed heart rhythm. Avoid.
Erythromycins*	May increase digitalis absorption.
Flecainide	May increase digitalis blood level.
Fluoxetine	May cause confusion, agitation, convulsions and high blood pressure. Avoid combining.
Hydroxychloroquine	Possible increased digitalis toxicity.
Itraconazole	Possible toxic levels of digitalis.
Laxatives*	Decreased digitalis effect.
Metformin	Increased metformin effect.

Continued on page 910

POSSIBLE INTERACTION WITH OTHER SUBSTANCES

INTERACTS WITH	COMBINED EFFECT
Alcohol:	None expected.
Beverages: Caffeine drinks.	Irregular heartbeat. Avoid.
Cocaine:	Irregular heartbeat. Avoid.
Foods: Prune juice, bran cereals, foods high in fiber.	Decreased digitalis effect.
Marijuana:	Decreased digitalis effect.
Tobacco:	Irregular heartbeat. Avoid.

***See Glossary**

DIMETHYL SULFOXIDE (DMSO)

BRAND NAMES

Rimso-50

BASIC INFORMATION

Habit forming? No
Prescription needed? Yes
Available as generic? Yes
Drug class: Anti-inflammatory (local)

USES

When applied directly to the bladder's membrane lining, DMSO relieves symptoms of bladder inflammation.

DOSAGE & USAGE INFORMATION

How to use:
Under doctor's guidance, directly instill into urinary bladder using a catheter or aseptic syringe. Allow to remain in bladder about 15 minutes, then void. *Note:* Follow doctor's instructions.

When to use:
Follow doctor's instructions.

If you forget a dose:
Take as soon as you remember up to 2 hours late. If more than 2 hours, wait for next scheduled dose (don't double this dose).

What drug does:
Reduces inflammation by unknown mechanism.

Time lapse before drug works:
Works quickly (within minutes).

Don't take with:
Any other medicines (including over-the-counter drugs such as cough and cold medicines, laxatives, antacids, diet pills, caffeine, nose drops or vitamins) without consulting your doctor.

OVERDOSE

SYMPTOMS:
None expected.
WHAT TO DO:
Overdose unlikely to threaten life. If person takes much larger amount than prescribed, call doctor, poison center 1-800-222-1222 or hospital emergency room for instructions.

POSSIBLE ADVERSE REACTIONS OR SIDE EFFECTS

SYMPTOMS	WHAT TO DO
Life-threatening:	
Breathing difficulty.	Seek emergency treatment immediately.
Common:	
Garlic-like taste for up to 72 hours.	No action necessary.
Infrequent:	
Vision problems (not documented in humans, but well documented in animals).	Continue. Call doctor when convenient.
Rare:	
Nasal congestion, itching, hives, facial swelling.	Discontinue. Seek emergency treatment.

DIMETHYL SULFOXIDE (DMSO)

WARNINGS & PRECAUTIONS

Don't use if:
- You have a bladder malignancy.
- You are allergic to DMSO.

Before you start, consult your doctor:
If you have visual problems.

Over age 60:
No special problems expected.

Pregnancy:
Decide with you doctor if drug benefits justify risk to unborn child. Risk category C (see page xviii).

Breast-feeding:
Effect not documented. Consult your doctor.

Infants & children:
Not recommended.

Prolonged use:
Talk to your doctor about the need for follow-up medical examinations or laboratory studies to check liver and kidney function, complete blood counts (white blood cell count, platelet count, red blood cell count, hemoglobin, hematocrit) and vision.

Skin & sunlight:
No special problems expected.

Driving, piloting or hazardous work:
No special problems expected.

Discontinuing:
No special problems expected.

Others:
Although readily available in impure forms, DMSO has not proven effective or safe for sprains, strains, arthritis, scleroderma, gout, skin infections, burns or other uses. Many studies are underway for safety and efficacy for conditions other than bladder inflammation.

POSSIBLE INTERACTION WITH OTHER DRUGS

GENERIC NAME OR DRUG CLASS	COMBINED EFFECT
Any other drug used inside the bladder	Increased effect of both medicines.

POSSIBLE INTERACTION WITH OTHER SUBSTANCES

INTERACTS WITH	COMBINED EFFECT
Alcohol:	No special problems expected.
Beverages:	No special problems expected.
Cocaine:	No special problems expected.
Foods:	No special problems expected.
Marijuana:	No special problems expected.
Tobacco:	No special problems expected.

***See Glossary**

DIPHENIDOL

BRAND NAMES

Vontrol

BASIC INFORMATION

Habit forming? No
Prescription needed? Yes
Available as generic? No
Drug class: Antiemetic, antivertigo

USES

- Prevents motion sickness.
- Controls nausea and vomiting (do not use during pregnancy).

DOSAGE & USAGE INFORMATION

How to take:
Tablet—Swallow with liquid or food to lessen stomach irritation. If you can't swallow whole, crumble tablet and chew or take with liquid or food.

When to take:
30 to 60 minutes before traveling.

If you forget a dose:
Take as soon as you remember. Wait 4 hours for next dose.

What drug does:
Reduces sensitivity of nerve endings in inner ear, blocking messages to brain's vomiting center.

Time lapse before drug works:
30 to 60 minutes.

Don't take with:
Any other medicine without consulting your doctor or pharmacist.

OVERDOSE

SYMPTOMS:
Drowsiness, confusion, incoordination, weak pulse, shallow breathing, stupor, coma.
WHAT TO DO:
- **Dial 911 (emergency) for an ambulance or medical help or poison center 1-800-222-1222. Then give first aid immediately.**
- **See emergency information on inside covers.**

POSSIBLE ADVERSE REACTIONS OR SIDE EFFECTS

SYMPTOMS	WHAT TO DO
Life-threatening: In case of overdose, see previous column.	
Common:	
Drowsiness.	Continue. Tell doctor at next visit.
Infrequent:	
• Headache, diarrhea or constipation, heartburn.	Continue. Call doctor when convenient.
• Dry mouth, nose or throat; dizziness.	Continue. Tell doctor at next visit.
Rare:	
• Hallucinations, confusion.	Discontinue. Seek emergency treatment.
• Rash or hives, depression, jaundice.	Discontinue. Call doctor right away.
• Restlessness; excitement; insomnia; blurred vision; urgent, painful or difficult urination.	Continue. Call doctor when convenient.
• Appetite loss, nausea, weakness.	Continue. Tell doctor at next visit.

WARNINGS & PRECAUTIONS

Don't take if:
- You have severe kidney disease.
- You are allergic to diphenidol or meclizine.

Before you start, consult your doctor:
- If you have prostate enlargement.
- If you have glaucoma.
- If you have heart disease.
- If you have intestinal obstruction or ulcers in the gastrointestinal tract.
- If you have kidney disease.
- If you have low blood pressure.
- If you will have surgery within 2 months, including dental surgery, requiring general or spinal anesthesia.

Over age 60:
Adverse reactions and side effects may be more frequent and severe than in younger persons.

Pregnancy:
Decide with your doctor whether drug benefits justify risk to unborn child. Risk category C (see page xviii).

Breast-feeding:
Drug passes into milk. Avoid drug or discontinue nursing until you finish medicine. Consult doctor for advice on maintaining milk supply.

Infants & children:
No problems expected.

Prolonged use:
No problems expected.

Skin & sunlight:
No problems expected.

Driving, piloting or hazardous work:
Don't fly aircraft. Don't drive until you learn how medicine affects you. Don't work around dangerous machinery. Don't climb ladders or work in high places. Danger increases if you drink alcohol or take medicine affecting alertness and reflexes, such as antihistamines, tranquilizers, sedatives, pain medicine, narcotics and mind-altering drugs.

Discontinuing:
No problems expected.

Others:
No problems expected.

POSSIBLE INTERACTION WITH OTHER DRUGS

GENERIC NAME OR DRUG CLASS	COMBINED EFFECT
Anticonvulsants*	Increased effect of both drugs.
Antidepressants, tricyclic*	Increased sedative effect of both drugs.
Antihistamines*	Increased sedative effect of both drugs.
Atropine	Increased chance of toxic effect of atropine and atropine-like medicines.
Narcotics*	Increased sedative effect of both drugs.
Sedatives*	Increased sedative effect of both drugs.
Tranquilizers*	Increased sedative effect of both drugs.

POSSIBLE INTERACTION WITH OTHER SUBSTANCES

INTERACTS WITH	COMBINED EFFECT
Alcohol:	Increased sedation. Avoid.
Beverages: Caffeine.	May decrease drowsiness.
Cocaine:	Increased chance of toxic effects of cocaine. Avoid.
Foods:	None expected.
Marijuana:	Increased drowsiness, dry mouth.
Tobacco:	None expected.

*See Glossary

DIPHENOXYLATE & ATROPINE

BRAND NAMES

Diphenatol
Lofene
Logen
Lomanate
Lomotil
Lonox
Lo-Trol
Nor-Mil

BASIC INFORMATION

Habit forming? Yes
Prescription needed? Yes
Available as generic? Yes
Drug class: Antidiarrheal

USES

Relieves diarrhea and intestinal cramps.

DOSAGE & USAGE INFORMATION

How to take:

- Tablet—Swallow with liquid or food to lessen stomach irritation.
- Drops or liquid—Follow label instructions and use marked dropper.

When to take:
No more often than directed on label.

If you forget a dose:
Take as soon as you remember up to 2 hours late. If more than 2 hours, wait for next scheduled dose (don't double this dose).

What drug does:
Blocks digestive tract's nerve supply, which reduces propelling movements.

Continued next column

Time lapse before drug works:
May require 12 to 24 hours of regular doses to control diarrhea.

Don't take with:
Any other medicine without consulting your doctor or pharmacist.

OVERDOSE

SYMPTOMS:
Excitement, constricted pupils, shallow breathing, coma.
WHAT TO DO:

- **Dial 911 (emergency) for an ambulance or medical help or poison center 1-800-222-1222. Then give first aid immediately.**
- **If patient is unconscious and not breathing, give mouth-to-mouth breathing. If there is no heartbeat, use cardiac massage and mouth-to-mouth breathing (CPR). Don't try to make patient vomit. If you can't get help quickly, take patient to nearest emergency facility.**
- **See emergency information on inside covers.**

POSSIBLE ADVERSE REACTIONS OR SIDE EFFECTS

SYMPTOMS	WHAT TO DO
Life-threatening:	
Hives, rash, intense itching, faintness soon after a dose (anaphylaxis).	Seek emergency treatment immediately.
Common:	
None expected.	
Infrequent:	
Dry mouth or skin, numbness of hands or feet, dizziness, depression, rash or itch, blurred vision, decreased urination, drowsiness, headache, swollen gums (these symptoms usually mean too much of the drug has been taken).	Discontinue. Call doctor right away.
Rare:	
Severe stomach pain, nausea, vomiting, constipation, bloating, loss of appetite.	Discontinue. Call doctor right away.

WARNINGS & PRECAUTIONS

Don't take if:

- You are allergic to diphenoxylate and atropine or any narcotic or anticholinergic.
- You have jaundice.
- You have infectious diarrhea or antibiotic-associated diarrhea.
- Patient is younger than 2.

Before you start, consult your doctor:

- If you have had liver problems.
- If you have ulcerative colitis.
- If you plan to become pregnant within medication period.
- If you have any medical disorder.
- If you take any medication, including nonprescription drugs.

Over age 60:
Adverse reactions and side effects may be more frequent and severe than in younger persons.

Pregnancy:
Decide with your doctor if drug benefits justify risk to unborn child. Risk category C (see page xviii).

Breast-feeding:
Drug passes into milk. Avoid drug or discontinue nursing until you finish medicine. Consult doctor for advice on maintaining milk supply.

Infants & children:
Don't give to children under 2 years of age. Use only under doctor's supervision for children older than 2.

Prolonged use:
- May be habit forming if larger doses than recommended are taken for a long period of time.
- Talk to your doctor about the need for follow-up medical examinations or laboratory studies to check liver function.

Skin & sunlight:
No problems expected.

Driving, piloting or hazardous work:
Don't drive or pilot aircraft until you learn how medicine affects you. Don't work around dangerous machinery. Don't climb ladders or work in high places. Danger increases if you drink alcohol or take medicine affecting alertness and reflexes.

Discontinuing:
- May be unnecessary to finish medicine. Follow doctor's instructions.
- After discontinuing, consult doctor if you experience muscle cramps, nausea, vomiting, trembling, stomach cramps or unusual sweating.

Others:
If diarrhea lasts longer than 2 days, discontinue and call doctor.

POSSIBLE INTERACTION WITH OTHER DRUGS

GENERIC NAME OR DRUG CLASS	COMBINED EFFECT
Barbiturates*	Increased effect of both drugs.
Clozapine	Toxic effect on the central nervous system.
Ethinamate	Dangerous increased effects of ethinamate. Avoid combining.
Fluoxetine	Increased depressant effects of both drugs.
Guanfacine	May increase depressant effects of either drug.
Leucovorin	High alcohol content of leucovorin may cause adverse effects.
Methyprylon	Increased sedative effect, perhaps to dangerous level. Avoid.
Monozmine oxidase (MAO) inhibitors*	May increase blood pressure excessively.
Naltrexone	Triggers withdrawal symptoms.
Narcotics*	Increased sedation. Avoid.
Sedatives*	Increased effect of both drugs.
Sertraline	Increased depressive effects of both drugs.
Tranquilizers*	Increased effect of both drugs.

POSSIBLE INTERACTION WITH OTHER SUBSTANCES

INTERACTS WITH	COMBINED EFFECT
Alcohol:	Depressed brain function. Avoid.
Beverages:	None expected.
Cocaine:	Decreased effect of diphenoxylate and atropine.
Foods:	None expected.
Marijuana:	None expected.
Tobacco:	None expected.

DIPYRIDAMOLE

BRAND NAMES

Aggrenox
Apo-Dipyridamole
Dipimol
Dipridacot
Novodipiradol
Persantine
Pyridamole

BASIC INFORMATION

Habit forming? No
Prescription needed?
U.S.: Yes
Canada: No
Available as generic? Yes
Drug class: Platelet aggregation inhibitor

USES

- May reduce frequency and intensity of angina attacks.
- May reduce the risk of blood clots after heart surgery.

DOSAGE & USAGE INFORMATION

How to take:
Tablet—Swallow with a full glass of water. If you can't swallow whole, crumble tablet and take with liquid.

When to take:
1 hour before or 2 hours after meals.

If you forget a dose:
Take as soon as you remember up to 2 hours late. If more than 2 hours, wait for next scheduled dose (don't double this dose).

Continued next column

OVERDOSE

SYMPTOMS:
Decreased blood pressure; weak, rapid pulse; cold, clammy skin; collapse.
WHAT TO DO:

- **Dial 911 (emergency) for an ambulance or medical help or poison center 1-800-222-1222. Then give first aid immediately.**
- **If patient is unconscious and not breathing, give mouth-to-mouth breathing. If there is no heartbeat, use cardiac massage and mouth-to-mouth breathing (CPR). Don't try to make patient vomit. If you can't get help quickly, take patient to nearest emergency facility.**
- **See emergency information on inside covers.**

What drug does:

- Probably dilates blood vessels to increase oxygen to heart.
- May reduce platelet clumping, which causes blood clots.

Time lapse before drug works:
3 months of continual use.

Don't take with:
Any other medicine without consulting your doctor or pharmacist.

POSSIBLE ADVERSE REACTIONS OR SIDE EFFECTS

SYMPTOMS	WHAT TO DO
Life-threatening:	
In case of overdose, see previous column.	
Common:	
Dizziness.	Continue. Call doctor when convenient.
Infrequent:	
• Fainting, headache.	Discontinue. Call doctor right away.
• Red flush, rash, nausea, vomiting, cramps, weakness.	Continue. Call doctor when convenient.
Rare:	
Chest pain.	Discontinue. Call doctor right away.

WARNINGS & PRECAUTIONS

Don't take if:

- You are allergic to dipyridamole.
- You are recovering from a heart attack.

Before you start, consult your doctor:

- If you have low blood pressure.
- If you have liver disease.

Over age 60:
Begin treatment with small doses.

Pregnancy:
No proven harm to unborn child. Avoid if possible. Consult doctor. Risk category B (see page xviii).

Breast-feeding:
No proven problems. Consult doctor.

Infants & children:
Not recommended.

Prolonged use:
Talk to your doctor about the need for follow-up medical examinations or laboratory studies.

Skin & sunlight:
No problems expected.

Driving, piloting or hazardous work:
Avoid if you feel dizzy. Otherwise, no problems expected.

Discontinuing:
Don't discontinue without doctor's advice until you complete prescribed dose, even though symptoms diminish or disappear.

Others:

- Drug increases your ability to be active without angina pain. Avoid excessive physical exertion that might injure heart.
- Advise any doctor or dentist whom you consult that you take this medicine.

POSSIBLE INTERACTION WITH OTHER DRUGS

GENERIC NAME OR DRUG CLASS	COMBINED EFFECT
Anticoagulants, oral*	Increased anticoagulant effect. Bleeding tendency.
Aspirin and combination drugs containing aspirin	Increased dipyridamole effect. Dose may need adjustment.

POSSIBLE INTERACTION WITH OTHER SUBSTANCES

INTERACTS WITH	COMBINED EFFECT
Alcohol:	May lower blood pressure excessively.
Beverages:	None expected.
Cocaine:	No proven problems.
Foods:	Decreased dipyridamole absorption unless taken 1 hour before eating.
Marijuana:	Daily use—Decreased dipyridamole effect.
Tobacco: Nicotine.	May decrease dipyridamole effect.

*See Glossary

DISOPYRAMIDE

BRAND NAMES

Norpace
Norpace CR
Rythmodan
Rythmodan-LA

BASIC INFORMATION

Habit forming? No
Prescription needed? Yes
Available as generic? Yes
Drug class: Antiarrhythmic

USES

Corrects heart rhythm disorders.

DOSAGE & USAGE INFORMATION

How to take:

- Extended-release tablet or capsule—Swallow with liquid. Do not crush tablet or open capsule.
- Capsule—Swallow with liquid. If you can't swallow whole, ask your pharmacist to prepare a liquid suspension for your use.

When to take:
At the same times each day.

If you forget a dose:
Take as soon as you remember up to 2 hours late. If more than 2 hours, wait for next scheduled dose (don't double this dose).

What drug does:
Delays nerve impulses to heart to regulate heartbeat.

Continued next column

Time lapse before drug works:
Begins in 30 to 60 minutes. Must use for 5 to 7 days to determine effectiveness.

Don't take with:
Any other medicine without consulting your doctor or pharmacist.

OVERDOSE

SYMPTOMS:
Blood-pressure drop, irregular heartbeat, apnea, loss of consciousness.
WHAT TO DO:

- **Dial 911 (emergency) for an ambulance or medical help or poison center 1-800-222-1222. Then give first aid immediately.**
- **If patient is unconscious and not breathing, give mouth-to-mouth breathing. If there is no heartbeat, use cardiac massage and mouth-to-mouth breathing (CPR). Don't try to make patient vomit. If you can't get help quickly, take patient to nearest emergency facility.**
- **See emergency information on inside covers.**

POSSIBLE ADVERSE REACTIONS OR SIDE EFFECTS

SYMPTOMS	WHAT TO DO
Life-threatening:	
Hives, rash, intense itching, faintness soon after a dose (anaphylaxis).	Seek emergency treatment immediately.
Common:	
• Hypoglycemia (cold sweats, fast heartbeat, extreme hunger, shakiness and nervousness, anxiety, cool and pale skin, drowsiness, headache).	Discontinue. Call doctor right away.
• Dry mouth, constipation, painful or difficult urination, rapid weight gain, blurred vision.	Continue. Call doctor when convenient.
Infrequent:	
• Dizziness, fainting, confusion, chest pain, nervousness, depression, slow or fast heartbeat.	Discontinue. Call doctor right away.
• Swollen feet.	Continue. Call doctor when convenient.
Rare:	
• Shortness of breath, psychosis.	Discontinue. Seek emergency treatment.
• Rash, sore throat, fever, headache, jaundice, muscle weakness.	Discontinue. Call doctor right away.
• Eye pain, diminished sex drive, numbness or tingling of hands and feet, bleeding tendency.	Continue. Call doctor when convenient.

WARNINGS & PRECAUTIONS

Don't take if:

- You are allergic to disopyramide or any antiarrhythmic.
- You have second- or third-degree heart block.
- You have heart failure.

Before you start, consult your doctor:
- If you react unfavorably to other antiarrhythmic drugs.
- If you have had heart disease.
- If you have low blood pressure.
- If you have liver disease.
- If you have glaucoma.
- If you have enlarged prostate.
- If you have myasthenia gravis.
- If you take digitalis preparations or diuretics.

Over age 60:
- May require reduced dose.
- More likely to have difficulty urinating or be constipated.
- More likely to have blood pressure drop.

Pregnancy:
Decide with your doctor if drug benefits justify risk to unborn child. Risk category C (see page xviii).

Breast-feeding:
Drug passes into milk. Avoid drug or discontinue nursing until you finish medicine. Consult doctor for advice on maintaining milk supply.

Infants & children:
Safety not established. Don't use.

Prolonged use:
Talk to your doctor about the need for follow-up medical examinations or laboratory studies to check liver function, kidney function, ECG*, blood pressure, serum potassium.

Skin & sunlight:
May cause rash or intensify sunburn in areas exposed to sun or ultraviolet light photosensitivity reaction). Avoid overexposure. Notify doctor if reaction occurs.

Driving, piloting or hazardous work:
Don't drive or pilot aircraft until you learn how medicine affects you. Don't work around dangerous machinery. Don't climb ladders or work in high places. Danger increases if you drink alcohol or take medicine affecting alertness and reflexes, such as antihistamines, tranquilizers, sedatives, pain medicine, narcotics, or mind-altering drugs.

Discontinuing:
Don't discontinue without doctor's advice until you complete prescribed dose, even though symptoms diminish or disappear.

Others:
If new illness, injury or surgery occurs, tell doctors of disopyramide use.

POSSIBLE INTERACTION WITH OTHER DRUGS

GENERIC NAME OR DRUG CLASS	COMBINED EFFECT
Antiarrhythmics*	May increase effect and toxicity of each drug.
Anticholinergics*	Increased anticholinergic effect.
Anticoagulants, oral*	Possible increased anticoagulant effect.
Antihypertensives*	Increased anti-hypertensive effect.
Cisapride	Decreased disopyramide effect.
Encainide	Increased effect of toxicity on the heart muscle.
Flecainide	Possible irregular heartbeat.
Nicardipine	May cause dangerously slow, fast or irregular heartbeat.
Nimodipine	May cause dangerous irregular, slow or fast heartbeat.
Phenobarbital	Increased metabolism, decreased disopyramide effect.
Phenytoin	Increased metabolism, decreased disopyramide effect.
Propafenone	Increased effect of both drugs and increased risk of toxicity.
Rifampin	Increased metabolism, decreased disopyramide effect.
Tocainide	Increased likelihood of adverse reactions with either drug.

POSSIBLE INTERACTION WITH OTHER SUBSTANCES

INTERACTS WITH	COMBINED EFFECT
Alcohol:	Decreased blood pressure and blood sugar. Use caution.
Beverages:	None expected.
Cocaine:	Irregular heartbeat.
Foods:	None expected.
Marijuana:	Unpredictable. May decrease disopyramide effect.
Tobacco:	May decrease disopyramide effect.

*See Glossary

DISULFIRAM

BRAND NAMES

Antabuse

BASIC INFORMATION

Habit forming? No
Prescription needed? Yes
Available as generic? Yes
Drug class: None

USES

Treatment for alcoholism. Will not cure alcoholism, but is a powerful deterrent to drinking.

DOSAGE & USAGE INFORMATION

How to take:
Tablet—Swallow with liquid.

When to take:
Morning or bedtime. Avoid if you have used *any* alcohol, tonics, cough syrups, fermented vinegar, after-shave lotion or backrub solutions within 12 hours.

If you forget a dose:
Take as soon as you remember up to 12 hours late. If more than 12 hours, wait for next scheduled dose (don't double this dose).

What drug does:
In combination with alcohol, produces a metabolic change that causes severe, temporary toxicity.

Time lapse before drug works:
3 to 12 hours.

Continued next column

OVERDOSE

SYMPTOMS:
Memory loss, behavior disturbances, lethargy, confusion and headaches; nausea, vomiting, stomach pain and diarrhea; weakness and unsteady walk; temporary paralysis.
WHAT TO DO:
- **Dial 911 (emergency) for an ambulance or medical help or poison center 1-800-222-1222. Then give first aid immediately.**
- **See emergency information at end of book.**

Don't take with:
- Nonprescription drugs that contain *any* alcohol.
- Any other central nervous system (CNS) depressant drugs*.

POSSIBLE ADVERSE REACTIONS OR SIDE EFFECTS

SYMPTOMS	WHAT TO DO
Life-threatening:	
In case of overdose, see previous column.	
Common:	
Drowsiness.	Continue. Tell doctor at next visit.
Infrequent:	
• Eye pain, vision changes, abdominal discomfort, throbbing headache, numbness in hands and feet.	Continue. Call doctor when convenient.
• Mood change, decreased sexual ability in men, tiredness.	Continue. Tell doctor at next visit.
• Bad taste in mouth (metal or garlic).	No action necessary.
Rare:	
Rash, jaundice.	Discontinue. Call doctor right away.

WARNINGS & PRECAUTIONS

Don't take if:
- You are allergic to disulfiram (alcohol-disulfiram combination is not an allergic reaction).
- You have used alcohol in any form or amount within 12 hours.
- You have taken paraldehyde within 1 week.
- You have heart disease.

Before you start, consult your doctor:
- If you have allergies.
- If you plan to become pregnant within medication period.
- If no one has explained to you how disulfiram reacts with alcohol.
- If you think you cannot avoid drinking.
- If you have diabetes, epilepsy, liver or kidney disease.
- If you take other drugs.

Over age 60:
Adverse reactions and side effects may be more frequent and severe than in younger persons.

Pregnancy:
Decide with your doctor if drug benefits justify risk to unborn child. Risk category C (see page xviii).

Breast-feeding:
Studies inconclusive. Consult your doctor.

Infants & children:
Not recommended.

Prolonged use:
Periodic blood cell counts and liver function tests recommended if you take this drug a long time.

Skin & sunlight:
No problems expected.

Driving, piloting or hazardous work:
Avoid if you feel drowsy or have vision side effects. Otherwise, no restrictions.

Discontinuing:
Don't discontinue without consulting doctor. Dose may require gradual reduction if you have taken drug for a long time. Doses of other drugs may also require adjustment. Avoid alcohol at least 14 days following last dose.

Others:
- Check all liquids that you take or rub on for presence of alcohol.
- Advise any doctor or dentist whom you consult that you take this medicine.

POSSIBLE INTERACTION WITH OTHER DRUGS

GENERIC NAME OR DRUG CLASS	COMBINED EFFECT
Anticoagulants*	Possible unexplained bleeding.
Anticonvulsants*	Excessive sedation.
Barbiturates*	Excessive sedation.
Central nervous system (CNS) depressants*	Increased depressive effect.
Clozapine	Toxic effect on the central nervous system.
Guanfacine	May increase depressant effects of either drug.
Isoniazid	Unsteady walk and disturbed behavior.
Leucovorin	High alcohol content of leucovorin may cause disulfiram reaction*.
Methyprylon	Increased sedative effect, perhaps to dangerous level. Avoid.
Metronidazole	Disulfiram reaction*.
Nabilone	Greater depression of central nervous system.
Sedatives*	Excessive sedation.
Theophylline	Increased theophylline effect; possibly toxic levels.

POSSIBLE INTERACTION WITH OTHER SUBSTANCES

INTERACTS WITH	COMBINED EFFECT
Alcohol: *Any* form or amount.	Possible life-threatening toxicity. See disulfiram reaction*.
Beverages: Punch or fruit drink that may contain alcohol.	Disulfiram reaction*.
Cocaine:	Increased disulfiram effect.
Foods: Sauces, fermented vinegar, marinades, desserts or other foods prepared with *any* alcohol.	Disulfiram reaction*.
Marijuana:	None expected.
Tobacco:	None expected.

***See Glossary**

DIURETICS, LOOP

GENERIC AND BRAND NAMES

BUMETADINE
Bumex
ETHACRYNIC ACID
Edecrin
FUROSEMIDE
Apo-Furosemide
Furoside
Lasix
Lasix Special
Myrosemide
Novosemide
Uritol
TORSEMIDE
Demadex

BASIC INFORMATION

Habit forming? No
Prescription needed? Yes
Available as generic? Yes
Drug class: Diuretic (loop), antihypertensive

USES

- Lowers high blood pressure.
- Decreases fluid retention.

DOSAGE & USAGE INFORMATION

How to take:
Tablet or liquid—Swallow with liquid. If you can't swallow whole, crumble tablet and take with liquid or food.

When to take:
- 1 dose a day—Take after breakfast.
- More than 1 dose a day—Take last dose no later than 6 p.m. unless otherwise directed.

If you forget a dose:
- 1 dose a day—Take as soon as you remember up to 12 hours late. If more than 12 hours, wait for next scheduled dose (don't double this dose).

Continued next column

OVERDOSE

SYMPTOMS:
Weakness, lethargy, dizziness, confusion, nausea, vomiting, leg muscle cramps, thirst, stupor, deep sleep, weak and rapid pulse, cardiac arrest.
WHAT TO DO:
- **Dial 911 (emergency) for an ambulance or medical help or poison center 1-800-222-1222. Then give first aid immediately.**
- **See emergency information on inside covers.**

- More than 1 dose a day—Take as soon as you remember up to 2 hours late. If more than 2 hours, wait for next scheduled dose (don't double this dose).

What drug does:
Increases elimination of sodium, potassium and water from body. Decreased body fluid reduces blood pressure.

Time lapse before drug works:
1 hour to increase water loss. Requires 2 to 3 weeks to lower blood pressure.

Don't take with:
- Nonprescription drugs with aspirin.
- Any other medicine without consulting your doctor.

POSSIBLE ADVERSE REACTIONS OR SIDE EFFECTS

SYMPTOMS	WHAT TO DO
Life-threatening:	
In case of overdose, see previous column.	
Common:	
Dizziness.	Continue. Call doctor when convenient.
Infrequent:	
Mood change, fatigue, appetite loss, diarrhea, irregular heartbeat, muscle cramps, low blood pressure, abdominal pain, weakness.	Discontinue. Call doctor right away.
Rare:	
Rash or hives, yellow vision, ringing in ears, hearing loss, sore throat, fever, dry mouth, thirst, side or stomach pain, nausea, vomiting, unusual bleeding or bruising, joint pain, jaundice, numbness or tingling in hands or feet.	Discontinue. Call doctor right away.

WARNINGS & PRECAUTIONS

Don't take if:
You are allergic to loop diuretics.

Before you start, consult your doctor:
- If you are taking any other prescription or nonprescription medicine.
- If you are allergic to any sulfa drug.
- If you have liver or kidney disease.
- If you have gout, diabetes or impaired hearing.
- If you will have surgery within 2 months, including dental surgery, requiring general or spinal anesthesia.

Over age 60:
Adverse reactions and side effects may be more frequent and severe than in younger persons.

Pregnancy:
Risk factors vary for drugs in this group. See category list on page xviii and consult doctor.

Breast-feeding:
Drug filters into milk. May harm child. Avoid.

Infants & children:
Use only under medical supervision.

Prolonged use:
- Impaired balance of water and salt, with low potassium level in blood and body tissues.
- Possible diabetes.

Skin & sunlight:
One or more drugs in this group may cause rash or intensify sunburn in areas exposed to sun or ultraviolet light (photosensitivity reaction). Avoid overexposure. Notify doctor if reaction occurs.

Driving, piloting or hazardous work:
Avoid if you feel dizzy; otherwise no problems expected.

Discontinuing:
Don't discontinue without doctor's advice until you complete prescribed dose, even though symptoms diminish or disappear.

Others:
Frequent laboratory studies to monitor potassium level in blood recommended. Eat foods rich in potassium or take potassium supplements. Consult doctor.

POSSIBLE INTERACTION WITH OTHER DRUGS

GENERIC NAME OR DRUG CLASS	COMBINED EFFECT
Adrenocorticoids, systemic	Potassium depletion.
Allopurinol	Decreased allopurinol effect.
Amiodarone	Increased risk of heartbeat irregularity due to low potassium.
Angiotensin-converting enzyme (ACE) inhibitors*	Possible excessive potassium in blood.
Anticoagulants*	Abnormal clotting.
Antidepressants, tricyclic*	Excessive blood pressure drop.
Antidiabetics, oral*	Decreased anti-diabetic effect.
Antihypertensives*	Increased anti-hypertensive effect. Dosages may require adjustment.
Anti-inflammatory drugs, nonsteroidal (NSAIDs)*	Decreased diuretic effect.
Antivirals, HIV/AIDS*	Increased risk of pancreatitis with furosemide.
Barbiturates*	Low blood pressure.
Beta-adrenergic blocking agents*	Increased anti-hypertensive effect. Dosages may require adjustment.
Corticosteroids*	Decreased potassium.
Digitalis preparations*	Excessive potassium loss could lead to serious heart rhythm disorders.
Diuretics, other*	Increased diuretic effect.
Hypokalemia-causing medicines*	Increased risk of excessive potassium loss.
Insulin	Decreased insulin effect.
Lithium	Increased lithium toxicity.
Metformin	Increased metformin effect with furosemide.
Narcotics*	Dangerous low blood pressure. Avoid.

Continued on page 911

POSSIBLE INTERACTION WITH OTHER SUBSTANCES

INTERACTS WITH	COMBINED EFFECT
Alcohol:	Blood pressure drop. Avoid.
Beverages:	None expected.
Cocaine:	Dangerous blood pressure drop. Avoid.
Foods:	None expected.
Marijuana:	Increased thirst and urinary frequency, fainting.
Tobacco:	Decreased furosemide effect.

DIURETICS, POTASSIUM-SPARING

GENERIC AND BRAND NAMES

AMILORIDE
Midamor
SPIRONOLACTONE
Aldactone
Novospiroton
TRIAMTERENE
Dyrenium

BASIC INFORMATION

Habit forming? No
Prescription needed? Yes
Available as generic? Yes
Drug class: Diuretic, antihypertensive, antihypokalemic

USES

- Treatment for high blood pressure (hypertension) and congestive heart failure. Decreases fluid retention and prevents potassium loss.
- Treatment for hypokalemia (low potassium), polycystic ovary syndrome and hirsutism in women.

DOSAGE & USAGE INFORMATION

How to take:
Capsule or tablet—Swallow with liquid. If you can't swallow whole, open capsule or crush tablet and take with liquid or food. May take with meal to lessen stomach irritation.

When to take:
At the same times each day. May interfere with sleep if taken after 6 p.m.

Continued next column

OVERDOSE

SYMPTOMS:
Rapid, irregular heartbeat; confusion; shortness of breath; nervousness; extreme weakness; stupor; coma.
WHAT TO DO:
- **Dial 911 (emergency) for an ambulance or medical help or poison center 1-800-222-1222. Then give first aid immediately.**
- **If patient is unconscious and not breathing, give mouth-to-mouth breathing. If there is no heartbeat, use cardiac massage and mouth-to-mouth breathing (CPR). Don't try to make patient vomit. If you can't get help quickly, take patient to nearest emergency facility.**
- **See emergency information on inside covers.**

If you forget a dose:
Take as soon as you remember. If it is almost time for the next dose, wait for next scheduled dose (don't double this dose).

What drug does:
- Blocks exchange of certain chemicals in the kidneys so sodium and water are excreted. Conserves potassium.
- In polycystic ovary syndrome and hirsutism, blocks androgen hormones.

Time lapse before drug works:
2 to 4 hours.

Don't take with:
Any other medicine without consulting your doctor or pharmacist.

POSSIBLE ADVERSE REACTIONS OR SIDE EFFECTS

SYMPTOMS	WHAT TO DO
Life-threatening: In case of overdose, see previous column.	
Common: Headache, nausea, appetite loss, vomiting, mild diarrhea.	Continue. Call doctor when convenient.
Infrequent: Dizziness, headache, muscle cramps, dry mouth, decreased sexual drive, muscle cramps, constipation.	Continue. Call doctor when convenient.
Rare: Shortness of breath, skin rash or itch (with amiloride); cough or hoarseness, painful urination, back or side pain (with triamterene and spironolactone); potassium changes (confusion, dry mouth, breathing difficulty, irregular heartbeat, unusual tiredness or weakness, mood or mental changes, muscle cramps, tingling in body); red, burning, inflamed feeling of tongue (with triamterene).	Discontinue. Call doctor right away.

WARNINGS & PRECAUTIONS

Don't take if:
- You are allergic to potassium-sparing diuretics.
- Your serum potassium level is high.

Before you start, consult your doctor:
- If you have diabetes.
- If you have heart disease, kidney or liver disease or gout.

Over age 60:
Adverse reactions and side effects may be more frequent and severe than in younger persons. More likely to exceed safe potassium blood levels.

Pregnancy:
Avoid if possible. Consult doctor. Risk category B (see page xviii).

Breast-feeding:
Drug may pass into milk. Avoid drug or discontinue nursing until you finish medicine. Consult doctor for advice on maintaining milk supply.

Infants & children:
No special problems expected.

Prolonged use:
Talk to your doctor about the need for follow-up medical examinations or laboratory studies to check blood pressure, kidney function, ECG* and serum electrolytes.

Skin & sunlight:
One or more of these drugs may cause increased sensitivity to sunlight (photosensitivity reaction). Avoid overexposure. If reaction occurs, notify doctor.

Driving, piloting or hazardous work:
Don't drive or pilot aircraft until you learn how medicine affects you. Don't work around dangerous machinery. Don't climb ladders or work in high places. Danger increases if you drink alcohol or take medicine affecting alertness and reflexes.

Discontinuing:
Don't discontinue without doctor's advice until you complete prescribed dose, even though symptoms diminish or disappear.

Others:
- Periodic physical checkups and potassium-level tests recommended.
- Advise any doctor or dentist whom you consult that you take this medicine.
- If you experience an illness with severe vomiting and diarrhea, consult doctor.
- A special diet may be recommended in addition to this medicine. Follow doctor's advice.

POSSIBLE INTERACTION WITH OTHER DRUGS

GENERIC NAME OR DRUG CLASS	COMBINED EFFECT
Amantadine	Increased effect of amantadine (with triamterene).
Angiotensin-converting enzyme (ACE) inhibitors*	Possible excessive potassium in blood.
Anticoagulants*, oral	Decreased anticoagulant effect.
Antigout drugs*	Decreased antigout effect.
Antihypertensives*	Increased effect of both drugs.
Anti-inflammatory drugs, nonsteroidal (NSAIDs)*	Increased potassium levels.
Cyclosporine	Increased potassium levels.
Digoxin	Increased digoxin effect (with spironolactone).
Diuretics*, other	Increased effect of both drugs.
Dofetilide	Increased risk of heart problems.
Folic acid	Decreased effect of folic acid.
Lithium	Possible lithium toxicity.
Metformin	Increased metformin effect.
Potassium supplements*	Increased potassium levels.

POSSIBLE INTERACTION WITH OTHER SUBSTANCES

INTERACTS WITH	COMBINED EFFECT
Alcohol:	Increased blood pressure drop. Avoid.
Beverages: Low-salt milk.	Possible excess potassium levels. Low-salt milk has extra potassium.
Cocaine:	Blood pressure rise. Avoid.
Foods: Salt substitutes.	Possible excess potassium levels.
Marijuana:	None expected.
Tobacco:	None expected.

DIURETICS, POTASSIUM-SPARING & HYDROCHLOROTHIAZIDE

GENERIC AND BRAND NAMES

AMILODINE & HYDROCHLOROTHIAZIDE
- **Moduret**
- **Moduretic**

SPIRONOLACTONE & HYDROCHLOROTHIAZIDE
- **Aldactazide**
- **Spirozide**

TRIAMTERENE & HYDROCHLOROTHIAZIDE
- **Apo-Triazide**
- **Diazide**
- **Maxzide**
- **Novo-Triamzide**

BASIC INFORMATION

Habit forming? No
Prescription needed? Yes
Available as generic? Yes
Drug class: Diuretic, antihypertensive, antihypokalemic

USES

- Treats, but does not cure, high blood pressure (hypertension) and congestive heart failure. Decreases fluid retention and prevents potassium loss.
- Treatment for hypokalemia (low potassium).

DOSAGE & USAGE INFORMATION

How to take:
Capsule or tablet—Swallow with liquid. Take with meals or milk if stomach irritation occurs.

When to take:
At the same time or times each day. May interfere with sleep if taken after 6 p.m.

Continued next column

OVERDOSE

SYMPTOMS: Rapid, irregular heartbeat; confusion; shortness of breath; nervousness; extreme weakness.
WHAT TO DO:
- **Dial 911 (emergency) for ambulance or medical help or poison center 1-800-222-1222. Give first aid immediately.**
- **If patient is unconscious and not breathing, give mouth-to-mouth breathing. If no heartbeat, use cardiac massage and mouth-to-mouth breathing (CPR). Don't make patient vomit. If you can't get help quickly, take patient to nearest emergency facility.**
- **See emergency information on inside covers.**

If you forget a dose:
Take as soon as you remember. If it is almost time for the next dose, wait for next scheduled dose (don't double this dose).

What drug does:
This is a combination of 2 diuretics that blocks exchange of certain chemicals in the kidneys so sodium and water are excreted. Conserves potassium.

Time lapse before drug works:
Starts in 2 to 4 hours; several days for full effect.

Don't take with:
Any other medicine without consulting your doctor or pharmacist. This includes any nonprescription medicines for colds, coughs, hay fever, sinus problems, appetite control or asthma.

POSSIBLE ADVERSE REACTIONS OR SIDE EFFECTS

SYMPTOMS	WHAT TO DO
Life-threatening: In case of overdose, see previous column.	
Common:	
Nausea or mild vomiting, appetite loss, stomach cramps, mild diarrhea, constipation (with amiloride).	Continue. Call doctor when convenient.
Infrequent:	
Dizziness, muscle cramps, headache, skin sensitive to sun, dry mouth, decreased interest in sex. With spironolactone—tender breasts, deepening of voice, menstrual changes, and increased hair growth in females; breast enlargement in males; increased sweating in both sexes.	Continue. Call doctor when convenient.
Rare:	
Black, tarry or bloody stools; blood in urine; pain or difficulty in urinating; fever or chills; pain in back, side or joints; spots, rash or hives on skin; severe stomach pain; unusual bleeding or bruising, yellow skin or eyes; potassium changes (confusion, dry mouth, breathing difficulty, irregular heartbeat,	Discontinue. Call doctor right away.

unusual tiredness or weakness, mood or mental changes, muscle cramps, tingling in body); red, burning, inflamed feeling of tongue (with triamterene).

WARNINGS & PRECAUTIONS

Don't take if:
- You are allergic to potassium-sparing or thiazide diuretics* or sulfa drugs*.
- Your serum potassium level is high.

Before you start, consult your doctor:
- If you have diabetes or lupus erythematosus.
- If you have menstrual problems (in females) or enlarged breast (in males).
- If you have heart or blood vessel disease, kidney or liver disease, pancreatitis or gout.

Over age 60:
Adverse reactions and side effects may be more frequent and severe than in younger persons. More likely to exceed safe potassium blood levels.

Pregnancy:
Does not control pregnancy symptoms of swollen hands and feet. Avoid if possible. Consult doctor. Risk category B (see page xviii).

Breast-feeding:
Drug passes into milk. Avoid drug or discontinue nursing until you finish medicine. Consult doctor for advice on maintaining milk supply.

Infants & children:
Unknown effect. Use only with doctor's approval.

Prolonged use:
Talk to your doctor about the need for follow-up medical examinations or laboratory studies to check blood pressure, kidney function, ECG* and serum electrolytes.

Skin & sunlight:
One or more of these drugs may cause increased sensitivity to sunlight (photosensitivity reaction). Avoid overexposure. If reaction occurs, notify doctor.

Driving, piloting or hazardous work:
Don't drive or pilot aircraft until you learn how medicine affects you. Don't work around dangerous machinery. Don't climb ladders or work in high places. Danger increases if you drink alcohol or take medicine affecting alertness and reflexes, such as antihistamines, tranquilizers, sedatives, pain medicine, narcotics and mind-altering drugs.

Discontinuing:
Don't discontinue without doctor's approval, even though symptoms diminish or disappear.

Others:
- Your doctor may prescribe a special diet.
- Advise any doctor or dentist whom you consult that you take this medicine.
- If you experience an illness with severe vomiting or diarrhea, consult doctor.

POSSIBLE INTERACTION WITH OTHER DRUGS

GENERIC NAME OR DRUG CLASS	COMBINED EFFECT
Amantadine	Increased effect of amantadine (with triamterene).
Angiotensin-converting enzyme (ACE) inhibitors*	Possible excessive potassium in blood.
Anticoagulants*, oral	Decreased anticoagulant effect.
Antigout drugs*	Decreased antigout effect.
Antihypertensives*	Increased effect of both drugs.
Anti-inflammatory drugs, nonsteroidal (NSAIDs)*	Increased potassium levels.
Cholestyramine	Decreased diuretic effect. Take 1 hour before diuretic.

Continued on page 911

POSSIBLE INTERACTION WITH OTHER SUBSTANCES

INTERACTS WITH	COMBINED EFFECT
Alcohol:	Increased blood pressure drop. Avoid.
Beverages: Low-salt milk.	Possible excess potassium levels. Low-salt milk has extra potassium.
Cocaine:	Blood pressure rise. Avoid.
Foods: Salt substitutes.	Possible excess potassium levels.
Marijuana:	None expected.
Tobacco:	None expected.

DIURETICS, THIAZIDE

GENERIC AND BRAND NAMES

See complete list of generic and brand names in the *Generic and Brand Name Directory*, page 862.

BASIC INFORMATION

Habit forming? No
Prescription needed? Yes
Available as generic? Yes, for some.
Drug class: Antihypertensive, diuretic (thiazide)

USES

- Controls, but doesn't cure, high blood pressure.
- Reduces fluid retention (edema) caused by conditions such as heart disorders and liver disease.

DOSAGE & USAGE INFORMATION

How to take:
Tablet, capsule or liquid—Swallow with liquid. If you can't swallow whole, crumble tablet or open capsule and take with liquid or food. Don't exceed dose.

When to take:
At the same time each day.

If you forget a dose:
Take as soon as you remember up to 2 hours late. If more than 2 hours, wait for next scheduled dose (don't double this dose).

What drug does:
- Forces sodium and water excretion, reducing body fluid.
- Relaxes muscle cells of small arteries.
- Reduced body fluid and relaxed arteries lower blood pressure.

Continued next column

OVERDOSE

SYMPTOMS:
Cramps, weakness, drowsiness, weak pulse, coma.
WHAT TO DO:
- **Dial 911 (emergency) for an ambulance or medical help or poison center 1-800-222-1222. Then give first aid immediately.**
- **See emergency information on inside covers.**

Time lapse before drug works:
4 to 6 hours. May require several weeks to lower blood pressure.

Don't take with:
Nonprescription drugs without consulting doctor.

POSSIBLE ADVERSE REACTIONS OR SIDE EFFECTS

SYMPTOMS	WHAT TO DO
Life-threatening:	
In case of overdose, see previous column.	
Common:	
Muscle cramps.	Discontinue. Call doctor right away.
Infrequent:	
• Blurred vision, severe abdominal pain, nausea, vomiting, irregular heartbeat, weak pulse.	Discontinue. Call doctor right away.
• Dizziness, mood changes, headaches, weakness, tiredness, weight changes, decreased sex drive, diarrhea.	Continue. Call doctor when convenient.
• Dry mouth, thirst.	Continue. Tell doctor at next visit.
Rare:	
• Rash or hives.	Discontinue. Seek emergency treatment.
• Jaundice, joint pain, black stools.	Discontinue. Call doctor right away.
• Sore throat, fever.	Continue. Tell doctor at next visit.

WARNINGS & PRECAUTIONS

Don't take if:
You are allergic to any thiazide diuretic drug.

Before you start, consult your doctor:
- If you are allergic to any sulfa drug or tartrazine dye.
- If you have gout, systemic lupus erythematosis.
- If you have liver, pancreas, diabetes or kidney disorder.

Over age 60:
Adverse reactions and side effects may be more frequent and severe than in younger persons, especially dizziness and excessive potassium loss.

Pregnancy:
Risk factors vary for drugs in this group. See category list on page xviii and consult doctor.

Breast-feeding:
Drug passes into milk. Avoid drug or discontinue nursing.

Infants & children:
No problems expected.

Prolonged use:
- You may need medicine to treat high blood pressure for the rest of your life.
- Talk to your doctor about the need for follow-up medical examinations or laboratory studies to check blood sugar, kidney function, blood pressure, serum electrolytes.

Skin & sunlight:
One or more drugs in this group may cause rash or intensify sunburn in areas exposed to sun or ultraviolet light (photosensitivity reaction). Avoid overexposure. Notify doctor if reaction occurs.

Driving, piloting or hazardous work:
Don't drive or pilot aircraft until you learn how medicine affects you. Don't work around dangerous machinery. Don't climb ladders or work in high places. Danger increases if you drink alcohol or take medicine affecting alertness and reflexes, such as antihistamines, tranquilizers, sedatives, pain medicine, narcotics and mind-altering drugs.

Discontinuing:
Don't discontinue without medical advice.

Others:
- Hot weather and fever may cause dehydration and drop in blood pressure. Dose may require temporary adjustment. Weigh daily and report any unexpected weight decreases to your doctor.
- May cause rise in uric acid, leading to gout.
- May cause blood-sugar rise in diabetics.
- May affect results in some medical tests.
- Advise any doctor or dentist whom you consult that you take this medicine.

POSSIBLE INTERACTION WITH OTHER DRUGS

GENERIC NAME OR DRUG CLASS	COMBINED EFFECT
Adrenocorticoids, systemic	Potassium depletion.
Allopurinol	Decreased allopurinol effect.
Amiodarone	Increased risk of heartbeat irregularity due to low potassium.
Amphotericin B	Increased potassium.
Angiotensin-converting enzyme (ACE) inhibitors*	Decreased blood pressure.
Antidepressants, tricyclic*	Dangerous drop in blood pressure. Avoid combination unless under medical supervision.
Antidiabetic agents, oral*	Increased blood sugar.
Antihypertensives*	Increased hypertensive effect.
Antivirals, HIV/AIDS*	Increased risk of pancreatitis.
Barbiturates*	Increased anti-hypertensive effect.
Beta-adrenergic blocking agents*	Increased anti-hypertensive effect. Dosages of both drugs may require adjustments.
Calcium supplements*	Increased calcium in blood.
Carteolol	Increased anti-hypertensive effect.
Cholestyramine	Decreased anti-hypertensive effect.
Colestipol	Decreased anti-hypertensive effect.
Digitalis preparations*	Excessive potassium loss that causes dangerous heart rhythms.
Diuretics, thiazide*, other	Increased effect of other thiazide diuretics.

Continued on page 912

POSSIBLE INTERACTION WITH OTHER SUBSTANCES

INTERACTS WITH	COMBINED EFFECT
Alcohol:	Dangerous blood pressure drop.
Beverages:	None expected.
Cocaine	Increased risk of heart block and high blood pressure.
Foods: Licorice.	Excessive potassium loss that causes dangerous heart rhythms.
Marijuana:	May increase blood pressure.
Tobacco:	None expected.

*See Glossary

DIVALPROEX

BRAND NAMES

Depakote
Depakote Sprinkle
Epival

BASIC INFORMATION

Habit forming? No
Prescription needed? Yes
Available as generic? No
Drug class: Anticonvulsant

USES

- Controls petit mal (absence) seizures in treatment of epilepsy.
- Treats the manic episodes associated with bipolar disorder.
- Treats migraine headaches.

DOSAGE & USAGE INFORMATION

How to take:
Delayed-release capsule or delayed-release tablet—Swallow with liquid or food to lessen stomach irritation. Do not crumble capsule or crush tablet.

When to take:
One to three times a day as directed by your doctor.

If you forget a dose:
Take as soon as you remember. Don't ever double dose.

What drug does:
Increases concentration of gamma aminobutyric acid, which inhibits nerve transmission in parts of brain.

Continued next column

OVERDOSE

SYMPTOMS:
Coma.
WHAT TO DO:
- **Dial 911 (emergency) for an ambulance or medical help or poison center 1-800-222-1222. Then give first aid immediately.**
- **If patient is unconscious and not breathing, give mouth-to-mouth breathing. If there is no heartbeat, use cardiac massage and mouth-to-mouth breathing (CPR). Don't try to make patient vomit. If you can't get help quickly, take patient to nearest emergency facility.**
- **See emergency information on inside covers.**

Time lapse before drug works:
1 to 4 hours.

Don't take with:
Any other medicine without consulting your doctor or pharmacist.

POSSIBLE ADVERSE REACTIONS OR SIDE EFFECTS

SYMPTOMS	WHAT TO DO
Life-threatening: In case of overdose, see previous column.	
Common: Loss of appetite, indigestion, nausea, vomiting, stomach cramps, diarrhea, tremor, unusual weight gain or loss, menstrual changes.	Continue. Call doctor when convenient.
Infrequent: Clumsiness or unsteadiness, constipation, skin rash, dizziness, drowsiness, unusual excitement or irritability.	Continue. Call doctor when convenient.
Rare: Mood or behavior changes; continued nausea, vomiting and appetite loss; increase in number of seizures; swelling of face, feet or legs; yellow skin or eyes; tiredness or weakness; back-and-forth eye movements (nystagmus); seeing double or seeing spots; severe stomach cramps; unusual bleeding or bruising.	Continue, but call doctor right away.

WARNINGS & PRECAUTIONS

Don't take if:
You are allergic to divalproex or valproic acid.

Before you start, consult your doctor:
- If you have blood, kidney or liver disease.
- If you will have surgery within 2 months, including dental surgery, requiring general or spinal anesthesia.

Over age 60:
Adverse reactions and side effects may be more frequent and severe than in younger persons.

Pregnancy:
Risk to unborn child outweighs drug benefits. Don't use. Risk category D (see page xviii).

Breast-feeding:
Unknown effect. Consult doctor.

Infants & children:
Under close medical supervision only.

Prolonged use:
Request periodic blood tests, liver and kidney function tests.

Skin & sunlight:
No problems expected.

Driving, piloting or hazardous work:
Don't drive or pilot aircraft until you learn how medicine affects you. Don't work around dangerous machinery. Don't climb ladders or work in high places. Danger increases if you drink alcohol or take medicine affecting alertness and reflexes, such as antihistamines, tranquilizers, sedatives, pain medicine, narcotics and mind-altering drugs.

Discontinuing:
Don't discontinue without consulting doctor. Dose may require gradual reduction if you have taken drug for a long time. Doses of other drugs may also require adjustment.

Others:
- Advise any doctor or dentist whom you consult that you take this medicine.
- Be sure you and the doctor discuss benefits and risks of this drug before starting.
- Wear a medical identification that indicates the use of this medicine.
- Use as directed. Don't increase or decrease dosage without doctor's approval.

POSSIBLE INTERACTION WITH OTHER DRUGS

GENERIC NAME OR DRUG CLASS	COMBINED EFFECT
Anticoagulants*	Increases chance of bleeding.
Aspirin	Increases chance of bleeding.
Central nervous system (CNS) depressants*	Increases sedative effect.
Clonazepam	May cause or prolong seizure.
Dipyridamole	Increases chance of bleeding.
Monoamine oxidase (MAO) inhibitors*	Increases sedative effect.
Nabilone	Greater depression of central nervous system.
Phenobarbital	Increases chance of toxicity.
Phenytoin	Unpredictable. May require increased or decreased dosage.
Primidone	Increases chance of toxicity.
Sertraline	Increased depressive effect of both drugs.
Sulfinpyrazone	Increases chance of bleeding.

POSSIBLE INTERACTION WITH OTHER SUBSTANCES

INTERACTS WITH	COMBINED EFFECT
Alcohol:	Deep sedation. Avoid.
Beverages:	None expected.
Cocaine:	Increased brain sensitivity. Avoid.
Foods:	None expected.
Marijuana:	Increased brain sensitivity. Avoid.
Tobacco:	Increased brain sensitivity. Avoid.

***See Glossary**

DOFETILIDE

BRAND NAMES

Tikosyn

BASIC INFORMATION

Habit forming? No
Prescription needed? Yes
Available as generic? No
Drug class: Antiarrhythmic

USES

Corrects irregular heartbeats to a normal rhythm.

DOSAGE & USAGE INFORMATION

How to take:
Capsules—Take with full glass of water.

When to take:
At the same times each day.

If you forget a dose:
Skip the missed dose and go back to your regular dosing schedule (don't double this dose).

What drug does:
Slows the nerve impulses in the heart.

Time lapse before drug works:
2 to 3 hours.

Don't take with:
Any other medicine without consulting your doctor or pharmacist.doctor or pharmacist.

OVERDOSE

SYMPTOMS:
Cardiac arrest, irregular heartbeat, fainting, shortness of breath, unusual tiredness or weakness.
WHAT TO DO:
Dial 911 (emergency) for an ambulance or medical help or poison center 1-800-222-1222. Then give first aid immediately.

POSSIBLE ADVERSE REACTIONS OR SIDE EFFECTS

SYMPTOMS	WHAT TO DO
Life-threatening: In case of overdose, see previous column.	
Common:	
Dizziness, fainting, fast or irregular heartbeat.	Discontinue. Seek emergency evaluation right away.
Infrequent:	
• Unusual swelling of, the extremities, chest pain, slow heartbeat, sudden numbness or tingling (hands, feet or face), paralysis, confusion, weakness, slurred speech, shortness of breath, yellow eyes or skin.	Discontinue. Call doctor right away.
• Abdominal pain, back pain, diarrhea, chills, cough, fever, general feeling of illness, joint pain, headache, nausea, runny nose, sore throat, vomiting, sleeplessness, rash.	Continue. Call doctor if symptoms persist.
Rare:	
Slow heart beat.	Discontinue. Call doctor right away.

WARNINGS & PRECAUTIONS

Don't take if:
You are allergic to dofetilide.

Before you start, consult your doctor:
- If you are using any other medication.
- You have electrolyte disorders, such as low potassium or magnesium levels.
- You have been diagnosed with kidney or liver disease.

Over age 60:
Side effects or problems experienced with this medication appear to be the same in older people as in younger adults, however, older patients are more likely to have kidney problems and should be monitored regularly for possible dosage adjustment.

Pregnancy:
Decide with your doctor if drug benefits justify risk to unborn child. Risk category C (see page xviii).

Breast-feeding:
Drug may pass into milk. Avoid drug or discontinue nursing until you finish medicine. Consult doctor for advice on maintaining milk supply.

Infants & children:
Studies on this medicine have been done only in adult patients. Consult doctor before giving this medicine to persons under age 18.

Prolonged use:
Talk to your doctor about the need for follow up laboratory studies to determine the effect of the medicine on your body.

Skin & sunlight:
None expected.

Driving, piloting or hazardous work:
Don't drive or pilot aircraft until you learn how medicine affects you. Don't work around dangerous machinery. Don't climb ladders or work in high places. Danger increases if you drink alcohol or take medicine affecting alertness and reflexes.

Discontinuing:
Don't discontinue without consulting doctor.

Others:
Advise any doctor or dentist whom you consult that you take this medicine.

POSSIBLE INTERACTION WITH OTHER DRUGS

GENERIC NAME OR DRUG CLASS	COMBINED EFFECT
Antiarrhythmics, other*	Increased dofetilide effect.
Antidepressants, tricyclic*	Increased risk of heart problems.
Calcium channel blockers*	Increased risk of heart problems.
Cimetidine	Increased risk of heart problems.
Diuretics*	Increased risk of heart problems.
Enzyme inhibitors*	Increased dofetilide effect.
Ketoconazole	Increased risk of heart problems.
Macrolides, oral*	Increased risk of heart problems.
Megestrol	Increased dofetilide effect.
Metformin	Increased dofetilide effect.
Norfloxacin	Increased dofetilide effect.
Phenothiazines*	Increased risk of heart problems.
Progestins*	Increased risk of heart problems.
Selective serotonin reuptake inhibitors*	Increased dofetilide effect.
Trimethoprim	Increased dofetilide effect.
Zafirlukast	Increased dofetilide effect.

POSSIBLE INTERACTION WITH OTHER SUBSTANCES

INTERACTS WITH	COMBINED EFFECT
Alcohol:	Increases the chance of liver problems.
Beverages: Grapefruit juice	May increase effect of dofetilide.
Cocaine:	Effect unknown. Avoid.
Foods:	None expected.
Marijuana:	Effect unknown. Avoid
Tobacco:	None expected.

*See Glossary

DOXEPIN (Topical)

BRAND NAMES

Prudoxin
Zonalon

BASIC INFORMATION

Habit forming? No
Prescription needed? Yes
Available as generic? No
Drug class: Antipruritic (topical)

USES

- Treats itching of the skin caused by certain types of eczema (an inflammation of the skin).
- Treatment of moderate itching of atopic dermatitis and lichensimplex chronicus in adult patients.

DOSAGE & USAGE INFORMATION

How to use:
Cream—Apply a thin layer to the affected area of skin and gently rub it in. Do not cover the treated area with a bandage or other dressing.

When to use:
Up to 4 times a day. Allow 3 to 4 hours between applications. Not to be used longer than 8 days.

If you forget a dose:
Use as soon as you remember. If it is almost time for the next dose, wait for the next scheduled dose (don't double this dose).

Continued next column

OVERDOSE

SYMPTOMS:
An overdose of topical medicine is unlikely to occur, but if too much is applied, it can be absorbed into the system.

- **Mild effects include blurred vision, drowsiness, very dry mouth, decreased awareness or responsiveness.**
- **More severe effects include irregular or fast heartbeat, enlarged pupils, jerking movements, dizziness, fainting, abdominal pain or swelling, weak or feeble pulse, high fever or low temperature, vomiting, incurable constipation, seizures, breathing difficulty, unconsciousness.**

WHAT TO DO:

- **Dial 911 (emergency) for an ambulance or medical help or poison center 1-800-222-1222. Then give first aid immediately.**
- **See emergency information on inside covers.**

What drug does:
The exact mechanism is unknown. It appears to block histamine* reactions, which can cause the itching. The drug also has a sedating effect on some people, which can help to relieve the itching symptoms. Variable and sometimes significant amounts of the drug are absorbed through the skin.

Time lapse before drug works:
May take up to 8 days for maximum benefit.

Don't take with:
Any other oral or topical medication without consulting your doctor or pharmacist. This includes nonprescription drugs such as cold or allergy remedies that may contain alcohol or antihistamines. They increase the risk of drowsiness.

POSSIBLE ADVERSE REACTIONS OR SIDE EFFECTS

SYMPTOMS	WHAT TO DO
Life-threatening:	
In case of overdose, see previous column.	
Common:	
• Swelling of the skin where drug is applied; worsening of the itching; burning, tingling or crawling feeling in the skin.	Discontinue. Call doctor right away.
• Stinging of skin where drug is applied, dryness or tightness of skin, taste changes, dizziness, drowsiness, dry mouth or lips, thirst, emotional changes, fatigue, headache, drowsiness.	Continue. Call doctor when convenient.
Infrequent:	
Scaling or cracking of the skin, nausea, anxiety, irritation.	Continue. Call doctor when convenient.
Rare:	
Fever.	Discontinue. Call doctor right away.

Note: **Though the drug is applied topically, it is absorbed into the bloodstream and can cause systemic reactions. Adverse reactions are more likely in patients who use the drug on more than 10% of their body surface.**

WARNINGS & PRECAUTIONS

Don't use if:
You are allergic to doxepin.

Before you start, consult your doctor:
- If you have narrow-angle glaucoma.
- If you are allergic to any other medications.
- If you have a problem with urinary retention.

Over age 60:
No special problems expected.

Pregnancy:
Consult doctor. Risk category B (page xviii).

Breast-feeding:
Drug passes into milk. Avoid drug or discontinue nursing until you finish medicine. Consult doctor for advice on maintaining milk supply.

Infants & children:
Safety in children has not been established. Use only under close medical supervision.

Prolonged use:
Don't use for more than 8 days unless directed by doctor. Longer use can increase the risk of side effects or adverse reactions.

Skin & sunlight:
No special problems expected.

Driving, piloting or hazardous work:
Don't drive or pilot aircraft until you learn how medicine affects you. Don't work around dangerous machinery. Don't climb ladders or work in high places. Danger increases if you drink alcohol or take medicine affecting alertness and reflexes.

Discontinuing:
To be sure of maximum benefit, don't discontinue this medicine before the treatment has been completed unless advised to do so by your doctor.

Others:
- Use medicine only on affected area. It is not to be used in the mouth, the eyes or the vagina.
- Advise any doctor or dentist whom you consult that you are using this medicine.
- If your skin condition doesn't improve within 8 days, consult doctor.
- Use medicine only as directed. Do not increase or reduce dosage without doctor's approval.

POSSIBLE INTERACTION WITH OTHER DRUGS

GENERIC NAME OR DRUG CLASS	COMBINED EFFECT
Antidepressants*	Increased risk of toxicity of both drugs.
Carbamazepine	Increased risk of toxicity of both drugs.
Central nervous system (CNS) depressants*	Increased sedation. May need dosage adjustment.
Cimetidine	Increased risk of doxepin toxicity.
Dextromethorphan	Increased risk of toxicity of both drugs.
Flecainide	Increased risk of toxicity of both drugs.
Monoamine oxidase (MAO) inhibitors*	Potentially life-threatening. Allow 14 days between use of the 2 drugs.
Phenothiazines*	Increased risk of toxicity of both drugs.
Propafenone	Increased risk of toxicity of both drugs.
Quinidine	Increased risk of toxicity of both drugs.

POSSIBLE INTERACTION WITH OTHER SUBSTANCES

INTERACTS WITH	COMBINED EFFECT
Alcohol:	Increased sedative effect. Avoid.
Beverages:	None expected.
Cocaine:	Problems not known. Best to avoid.
Foods:	None expected.
Marijuana:	Problems not known. Best to avoid.
Tobacco:	None expected.

*See Glossary

DRONABINOL (THC, Marijuana)

BRAND NAMES

Marinol

BASIC INFORMATION

Habit forming? Yes
Prescription needed? Yes
Available as generic? No
Drug class: Antiemetic

USES

- Prevents nausea and vomiting that may accompany taking anticancer medication (cancer chemotherapy). Should not be used unless other antinausea medicines fail.
- Appetite stimulant. Used to treat appetite loss in AIDS patients.

DOSAGE & USAGE INFORMATION

How to take:
Capsule—Swallow with liquid.

When to take:
Under supervision, a total of no more than 4 to 6 doses per day, every 2 to 4 hours after cancer chemotherapy for prescribed number of days.

If you forget a dose:
Take as soon as you remember up to 2 hours late. If more than 2 hours, wait for next scheduled dose (don't double this dose).

What drug does:
Affects nausea and vomiting center in brain to make it less irritable following cancer chemotherapy. Exact mechanism is unknown.

Time lapse before drug works:
2 to 4 hours.

Don't take with:
Nonprescription drugs without consulting doctor.

OVERDOSE

SYMPTOMS:
Pounding, rapid heart rate; high or low blood pressure; confusion; hallucinations; drastic mood changes; nervousness or anxiety.
WHAT TO DO:
Overdose unlikely to threaten life. If person takes much larger amount than prescribed, call doctor, poison center 1-800-222-1222 or hospital emergency room for instructions.

POSSIBLE ADVERSE REACTIONS OR SIDE EFFECTS

SYMPTOMS	WHAT TO DO
Life-threatening:	
In case of overdose, see previous column.	
Common:	
• Rapid, pounding heartbeat.	Discontinue. Call doctor right away.
• Dizziness, irritability, drowsiness, euphoria, decreased coordination.	Continue. Call doctor when convenient.
• Red eyes, dry mouth.	No action necessary.
Infrequent:	
• Depression, anxiety, nervousness, headache, hallucinations, dramatic mood changes.	Discontinue. Call doctor right away.
• Blurred or changed vision.	Continue. Call doctor when convenient.
Rare:	
• Rapid heartbeat, fainting, frequent or difficult urination, convulsions, shortness of breath.	Discontinue. Call doctor right away.
• Paranoia, nausea, loss of appetite, dizziness when standing after sitting or lying down, diarrhea.	Continue. Call doctor when convenient.

WARNINGS & PRECAUTIONS

Don't take if:

- Your nausea and vomiting is caused by anything other than cancer chemotherapy.
- You are sensitive or allergic to any form of marijuana or sesame oil.
- Your cycle of chemotherapy is longer than 7 consecutive days. Harmful side effects may occur.

Before you start, consult your doctor:

- If you have heart disease or high blood pressure.
- If you are an alcoholic or drug addict.
- If you are pregnant or intend to become pregnant.
- If you are nursing an infant.
- If you have schizophrenia or a manic-depressive disorder.

Over age 60:
Adverse reactions and side effects may be more frequent and severe than in younger persons.

Pregnancy:
Decide with your doctor if drug benefits justify risk to unborn child. Risk category C (see page xviii).

Breast-feeding:
Drug passes into milk. Avoid drug or discontinue nursing until you finish medicine. Consult doctor about maintaining milk supply.

Infants & children:
Not recommended.

Prolonged use:
- Avoid. Habit forming.
- Talk to your doctor about the need for follow-up medical examinations or laboratory studies to check heart function.

Skin & sunlight:
No problems expected.

Driving, piloting or hazardous work:
Don't drive or pilot aircraft until you learn how medicine affects you. Don't work around dangerous machinery. Don't climb ladders or work in high places. Danger increases if you drink alcohol or take medicine affecting alertness and reflexes, such as antihistamines, tranquilizers, sedatives, pain medicine, narcotics and mind-altering drugs.

Discontinuing:
Withdrawal effects such as irritability, insomnia, restlessness, sweating, diarrhea, hiccups, loss of appetite and hot flashes may follow abrupt withdrawal within 12 hours. Should they occur, these symptoms will probably subside within 96 hours.

Others:
Store in refrigerator.

POSSIBLE INTERACTION WITH OTHER DRUGS

GENERIC NAME OR DRUG CLASS	COMBINED EFFECT
Anesthetics*	Oversedation.
Anticonvulsants*	Oversedation.
Antidepressants, tricyclic*	Oversedation.
Antihistamines*	Oversedation.
Barbiturates*	Oversedation.
Clozapine	Toxic effect on the central nervous system.
Ethinamate	Dangerous increased effects of ethinamate. Avoid combining.
Fluoxetine	Increased depressant effects of both drugs.
Guanfacine	May increase depressant effects of either drug.
Leucovorin	High alcohol content of leucovorin may cause adverse effects.
Methyprylon	Increased sedative effect, perhaps to dangerous level. Avoid.
Molindone	Increased effects of both drugs. Avoid.
Muscle relaxants*	Oversedation.
Nabilone	Greater depression of central nervous system.
Narcotics*	Oversedation.
Sedatives*	Oversedation.
Sertraline	Increased depressive effects of both drugs.
Tranquilizers*	Oversedation.

POSSIBLE INTERACTION WITH OTHER SUBSTANCES

INTERACTS WITH	COMBINED EFFECT
Alcohol:	Oversedation.
Beverages:	None expected.
Cocaine:	None expected.
Foods:	None expected.
Marijuana:	Oversedation.
Tobacco:	None expected.

EFLORNITHINE (Topical)

BRAND NAMES

Vaniqa

BASIC INFORMATION

Habit forming? No
Prescription needed? Yes
Available as generic? No
Drug class: Enzyme Inhibitor (topical)

USES

Treatment for unwanted facial hair on women.

DOSAGE & USAGE INFORMATION

How to take:
Cream—Follow directions on package label. Usually requires twice-daily application. Limit application to facial area and avoid getting medication in eyes, nose or mouth. Apply at least five minutes after hair removal technique (shaving). Do not apply cosmetics until the medication dries. Do not wash face for at least four hours after applying medication.

When to take:
At the same times each day at least 8 hours apart.

If you forget a dose:
Use as soon as possible. Do not use if it is almost time for your next application. Do not double dose.

What drug does:
Inhibits the enzyme that encourages hair growth.

Time lapse before drug works:
4 -8 weeks for improvement to be seen.

Don't take with:
Any other medicine without consulting your doctor or pharmacist.

OVERDOSE

SYMPTOMS:
None expected.
WHAT TO DO:
Not intended for internal use. If child accidentally swallows, call poison center 1-800-222-1222.

POSSIBLE ADVERSE REACTIONS OR SIDE EFFECTS

SYMPTOMS	WHAT TO DO
Life-threatening: None expected.	
Common: Stinging skin, acne breakout.	Continue. Call doctor if condition persists.
Infrequent: Skin symptoms (tingling, redness, chapped, swollen, burning, bleeding, rash, hair bumps, continued acne).	Continue. Call doctor when convenient.
Rare: None expected.	

WARNINGS & PRECAUTIONS

Don't take if:
You are allergic to eflornithine.

Before you start, consult your doctor:
If you have facial abrasions, cuts or scrapes.

Over age 60:
No problems expected.

Pregnancy:
Consult doctor. Risk category C (see page xviii).

Breast-feeding:
It is unknown if eflornithine passes into breast milk. Avoid drug or discontinue nursing until you finish medicine. Consult doctor for advice on maintaining milk supply.

Infants & children:
Safety and efficacy has not been established in children under 12 years of age.

Prolonged use:
If no improvement is seen after six months of using this medicine, consult doctor.

Skin & sunlight:
No problems expected. However, if skin irritation occurs after prolonged exposure to sun, consult doctor.

Driving, piloting or hazardous work:
No problems expected.

Discontinuing:
Consult doctor before discontinuing.

Others:
Advise any doctor or dentist whom you consult that you use this drug.

POSSIBLE INTERACTION WITH OTHER DRUGS

GENERIC NAME OR DRUG CLASS	COMBINED EFFECT
None significant.	

POSSIBLE INTERACTION WITH OTHER SUBSTANCES

INTERACTS WITH	COMBINED EFFECT
Alcohol:	None expected.
Beverages:	None expected.
Cocaine:	None expected.
Foods:	None expected.
Marijuana:	None expected.
Tobacco:	None expected.

EPHEDRINE

BRAND NAMES

See complete list of brand names in the *Generic and Brand Name Directory*, page 862.

BASIC INFORMATION

Habit forming? No
Prescription needed?
Low Strength: No
High Strength: Yes
Available as generic? Yes, for some.
Drug class: Sympathomimetic

USES

- Relieves bronchial asthma.
- Decreases congestion of breathing passages.
- Suppresses allergic reactions.

DOSAGE & USAGE INFORMATION

How to take:
- Tablet or capsule—Swallow with liquid. You may chew or crush tablet.
- Extended-release tablets or capsules—Swallow each dose whole.
- Syrup—Take as directed on bottle.
- Drops—Dilute dose in beverage.

When to take:
As needed, no more often than every 4 hours. To prevent insomnia, take last dose at least 2 hours before bedtime.

If you forget a dose:
Take up to 2 hours late. If more than 2 hours, wait for next dose (don't double this dose).

What drug does:
- Prevents cells from releasing allergy-causing chemicals (histamines).
- Relaxes muscles of bronchial tubes.
- Decreases blood vessel size and blood flow, thus causing decongestion.

Continued next column

OVERDOSE

SYMPTOMS:
Severe anxiety, confusion, delirium, muscle tremors, rapid and irregular pulse.
WHAT TO DO:
- **Dial 911 (emergency) for an ambulance or medical help or poison center 1-800-222-1222. Then give first aid immediately.**
- **See emergency information on inside covers.**

Time lapse before drug works:
30 to 60 minutes.

Don't take with:
- Nonprescription drugs with ephedrine, pseudoephedrine or epinephrine.
- Nonprescription drugs for cough, cold, allergy or asthma without consulting doctor.

POSSIBLE ADVERSE REACTIONS OR SIDE EFFECTS

SYMPTOMS	WHAT TO DO
Life-threatening:	
In case of overdose, see previous column.	
Common:	
• Nervousness, headache, paleness, rapid heartbeat.	Continue. Call doctor when convenient.
• Insomnia.	Continue. Tell doctor at next visit.
Infrequent:	
• Irregular heartbeat.	Discontinue. Call doctor right away.
• Dizziness, appetite loss, nausea, vomiting, painful or difficult urination.	Continue. Call doctor when convenient.
Rare:	
None expected.	

WARNINGS & PRECAUTIONS

Don't take if:
You are allergic to ephedrine or any sympathomimetic* drug.

Before you start, consult your doctor:
- If you have high blood pressure.
- If you have diabetes.
- If you have overactive thyroid gland.
- If you have difficulty urinating.
- If you have taken any MAO inhibitor in past 2 weeks.
- If you have taken digitalis preparations in the last 7 days.
- If you will have surgery within 2 months, including dental surgery, requiring general or spinal anesthesia.

Over age 60:
More likely to develop high blood pressure, heart-rhythm disturbances, angina and to feel drug's stimulant effects.

Pregnancy:
Decide with your doctor if drug benefits justify risk to unborn child. Risk category C (see page xviii).

Breast-feeding:
Drug passes into milk. Avoid drug or discontinue nursing until you finish medicine. Consult doctor for advice on maintaining milk supply.

Infants & children:
No problems expected.

Prolonged use:
- Excessive doses—Rare toxic psychosis.
- Men with enlarged prostate gland may have more urination difficulty.

Skin & sunlight:
No problems expected.

Driving, piloting or hazardous work:
Avoid if you feel dizzy. Otherwise, no problems expected.

Discontinuing:
May be unnecessary to finish medicine. Follow doctor's instructions.

Others:
No problems expected.

POSSIBLE INTERACTION WITH OTHER DRUGS

GENERIC NAME OR DRUG CLASS	COMBINED EFFECT
Adrenocorticoids, systemic	Decreased adrenocorticoid effect.
Antidepressants, tricyclic*	Increased effect of ephedrine. Excessive stimulation of heart and blood pressure.
Antihypertensives*	Decreased antihypertensive effect.
Beta-adrenergic blocking agents*	Decreased effects of both drugs.
Dextrothyroxine	Increased ephedrine effect.
Digitalis preparations*	Serious heart rhythm disturbances.
Epinephrine	Increased epinephrine effect.
Ergot preparations*	Serious blood pressure rise.
Furazolidine	Sudden, severe increase in blood pressure.
Guanadrel	Decreased effect of both drugs.
Guanethidine	Decreased effect of both drugs.
Methyldopa	Possible increased blood pressure.
Monoamine oxidase (MAO) inhibitors*	Increased ephedrine effect. Dangerous blood pressure rise.
Nitrates*	Possible decreased effects of both drugs.
Phenothiazines*	Possible increased ephedrine toxicity. Possible decreased ephedrine effect.
Pseudoephedrine	Increased pseudoephedrine effect.
Rauwolfia	Decreased rauwolfia effect.
Sympathomimetics*	Increased ephedrine effect.
Terazosin	Decreases effectiveness of terazosin.
Theophylline	Increased gastrointestinal intolerance.

POSSIBLE INTERACTION WITH OTHER SUBSTANCES

INTERACTS WITH	COMBINED EFFECT
Alcohol:	None expected.
Beverages: Caffeine drinks.	Nervousness or insomnia.
Cocaine:	High risk of heartbeat irregularities and high blood pressure.
Foods:	None expected.
Marijuana:	Rapid heartbeat, possible heart rhythm disturbance.
Tobacco:	None expected.

*See Glossary

ERGOLOID MESYLATES

BRAND NAMES

Gerimal
Hydergine
Hydergine LC
Niloric

BASIC INFORMATION

Habit forming? No
Prescription needed? Yes
Available as generic? Yes
Drug class: Ergot preparation

USES

Treatment for reduced alertness, poor memory, confusion, depression or lack of motivation in the elderly.

DOSAGE & USAGE INFORMATION

How to take:

- Tablet or capsule—Swallow with liquid. If you can't swallow whole, crumble tablet or open capsule and take with liquid or food.
- Liquid—Take as directed on label.
- Sublingual tablets—Dissolve tablet under tongue.

When to take:
At the same times each day.

If you forget a dose:
Take as soon as you remember up to 2 hours late. If more than 2 hours, wait for next scheduled dose (don't double this dose).

What drug does:
Stimulates brain-cell metabolism to increase use of oxygen and nutrients.

Time lapse before drug works:
Gradual improvements over 3 to 4 months.

Continued next column

OVERDOSE

SYMPTOMS:
Headache, flushed face, nasal congestion, nausea, vomiting, blood pressure drop, blurred vision, weakness, collapse, coma.
WHAT TO DO:

- **Dial 911 (emergency) for an ambulance or medical help or poison center 1-800-222-1222. Then give first aid immediately.**
- **See emergency information on inside covers.**

Don't take with:

- Nonprescription drugs containing alcohol without consulting doctor.
- Any other medication without consulting your doctor or pharmacist.

POSSIBLE ADVERSE REACTIONS OR SIDE EFFECTS

SYMPTOMS	WHAT TO DO
Life-threatening:	
In case of overdose, see previous column.	
Common:	
Runny nose, skin flushing, headache.	Continue. Tell doctor at next visit.
Infrequent:	
• Slow heartbeat, tingling fingers.	Discontinue. Call doctor right away.
• Blurred vision.	Continue. Call doctor when convenient.
Rare:	
• Fainting.	Discontinue. Seek emergency treatment.
• Rash, nausea, vomiting, stomach cramps, dizziness when getting up, drowsiness, soreness under tongue, appetite loss.	Continue. Call doctor when convenient.

WARNINGS & PRECAUTIONS

Don't use if:

- If you are allergic to any ergot preparation.
- Your heartbeat is less than 60 beats per minute.
- Your systolic blood pressure is consistently below 100.

Before you start, consult your doctor:

- If you have had low blood pressure.
- If you have liver disease.
- If you have severe mental illness.

Over age 60:
Primarily used in persons older than 60. Results unpredictable, but many patients show improved brain function.

Pregnancy:
Decide with your doctor if drug benefits justify risk to unborn child. Risk category C (see page xviii).

Breast-feeding:
Risk to nursing child outweighs drug benefits. Don't use.

Infants & children:
Not recommended.

Prolonged use:
Talk to your doctor about the need for follow-up medical examinations or laboratory studies.

Skin & sunlight:
No problems expected.

Driving, piloting or hazardous work:
Avoid if you feel dizzy, faint or have blurred vision. Otherwise, no problems expected.

Discontinuing:
No problems expected.

Others:
May lessen your body's ability to adjust to cold temperatures.

POSSIBLE INTERACTION WITH OTHER DRUGS

GENERIC NAME OR DRUG CLASS	COMBINED EFFECT
Ergot preparations, other	May cause decreased circulation to arms, legs, feet and hands. Avoid.
Sympathomimetics*	May cause decreased circulation to arms, legs, feet and hands. Avoid.

POSSIBLE INTERACTION WITH OTHER SUBSTANCES

INTERACTS WITH	COMBINED EFFECT
Alcohol:	Use caution. May drop blood pressure excessively.
Beverages:	None expected.
Cocaine:	Overstimulation. Avoid.
Foods:	None expected.
Marijuana:	Decreased effect of ergot alkaloids.
Tobacco:	Decreased ergoloid effect. Don't smoke.

*See Glossary

ERGONOVINE

BRAND NAMES

Ergometrine
Ergotrate
Ergotrate Maleate

BASIC INFORMATION

Habit forming? No
Prescription needed? Yes
Available as generic? Yes
Drug class: Ergot preparation (uterine stimulant)

USES

Retards excessive post-delivery bleeding.

DOSAGE & USAGE INFORMATION

How to take:
Tablet—Swallow with liquid or food to lessen stomach irritation.

When to take:
At the same times each day.

If you forget a dose:
Don't take missed dose and don't double next one. Wait for next scheduled dose.

What drug does:
Causes smooth muscle cells of uterine wall to contract and surround bleeding blood vessels of relaxed uterus.

Time lapse before drug works:
Tablets—20 to 30 minutes.

Don't take with:
Any other medicine without consulting your doctor or pharmacist.

OVERDOSE

SYMPTOMS:
Vomiting, diarrhea, weak pulse, low blood pressure, difficult breathing, angina, convulsions.

WHAT TO DO:
- **Dial 911 (emergency) for an ambulance or medical help or poison center 1-800-222-1222. Then give first aid immediately.**
- **If patient is unconscious and not breathing, give mouth-to-mouth breathing. If there is no heartbeat, use cardiac massage and mouth-to-mouth breathing (CPR). Don't try to make patient vomit. If you can't get help quickly, take patient to nearest emergency facility.**
- **See emergency information on inside covers.**

POSSIBLE ADVERSE REACTIONS OR SIDE EFFECTS

SYMPTOMS	WHAT TO DO
Life-threatening:	
In case of overdose, see previous column.	
Common:	
Nausea, vomiting, severe lower abdominal menstrual-like cramps.	Discontinue. Call doctor right away.
Infrequent:	
• Confusion, ringing in ears, diarrhea, muscle cramps.	Discontinue. Call doctor right away.
• Unusual sweating.	Continue. Call doctor when convenient.
Rare:	
Sudden, severe headache; shortness of breath; chest pain; numb, cold hands and feet.	Discontinue. Seek emergency treatment.

WARNINGS & PRECAUTIONS

Don't take if:
You are allergic to any ergot preparation.

Before you start, consult your doctor:
- If you have coronary artery or blood vessel disease.
- If you have liver or kidney disease.
- If you have high blood pressure.
- If you have postpartum infection.

Over age 60:
Not recommended.

Pregnancy:
Risk to unborn child outweighs drug benefits. Don't use. Risk category X (see page xviii).

Breast-feeding:
Drug passes into milk. Avoid drug or discontinue nursing until you finish medicine. Consult doctor for advice on maintaining milk supply.

Infants & children:
Not recommended.

Prolonged use:
Talk to your doctor about the need for follow-up medical examinations or laboratory studies to check blood pressure, ECG*.

Skin & sunlight:
No problems expected.

Driving, piloting or hazardous work:
No problems expected.

Discontinuing:
May be unnecessary to finish medicine. Follow doctor's instructions.

Others:
Drug should be used for short time only following childbirth or miscarriage.

POSSIBLE INTERACTION WITH OTHER DRUGS

GENERIC NAME OR DRUG CLASS	COMBINED EFFECT
Beta-adrenergic blocking agents*	Possible vasospasm (peripheral and cardiac).
Ergot preparations, other	May cause decreased circulation to arms, legs, feet and hands. Avoid.
Sympathomimetics*	May cause decreased circulation to arms, legs, feet and hands. Avoid.

POSSIBLE INTERACTION WITH OTHER SUBSTANCES

INTERACTS WITH	COMBINED EFFECT
Alcohol:	None expected.
Beverages:	None expected.
Cocaine:	None expected.
Foods:	None expected.
Marijuana:	None expected.
Tobacco:	Decreased ergonovine effect. Don't smoke.

*See Glossary

ERGOTAMINE

BRAND NAMES

Cafergot
Cafergot-PB
Cafertine
Cafetrate
Ercaf
Ergo-Caff
Ergomar
Ergostat
Gotamine
Gynergen
Medihaler
Ergotamine
Migergot
Wigraine

BASIC INFORMATION

Habit forming? No
Prescription needed? Yes
Available as generic? No
Drug class: Vasoconstrictor, ergot preparation

USES

Relieves pain of migraines and other headaches caused by dilated blood vessels. Will not prevent headaches.

DOSAGE & USAGE INFORMATION

How to take:
- Tablet—Swallow with liquid. If you can't swallow whole, crumble tablet and take with liquid or food.
- Sublingual tablet—Don't swallow whole. Let dissolve under tongue. Don't eat or drink while tablet is dissolving.
- Suppositories—Remove wrapper and moisten suppository with water. Gently insert larger end into rectum. Push well into rectum with finger.
- Aerosol inhaler—Use only as directed on prescription label.
- Lie down in quiet, dark room after taking.

Continued next column

OVERDOSE

SYMPTOMS:
Tingling, cold extremities and muscle pain. Progresses to nausea, vomiting, diarrhea, cold skin, rapid and weak pulse, severe numbness of extremities, confusion, convulsions, coma.
WHAT TO DO:
- **Dial 911 (emergency) for an ambulance or medical help or poison center 1-800-222-1222. Then give first aid immediately.**
- **See emergency information on inside covers.**

When to take:
At first sign of vascular or migraine headache.

If you forget a dose:
Take as soon as you remember. Wait 4 hours for next dose.

What drug does:
Constricts blood vessels in the head.

Time lapse before drug works:
30 to 60 minutes.

Don't take with:
Any other medicine without consulting your doctor or pharmacist.

POSSIBLE ADVERSE REACTIONS OR SIDE EFFECTS

SYMPTOMS	WHAT TO DO
Life-threatening: In case of overdose, see previous column.	
Common:	
• Dizziness, nausea, diarrhea, vomiting, increased frequency or severity of headaches.	Continue. Call doctor when convenient.
• Feet and ankle swelling.	Discontinue. Call doctor right away.
Infrequent: Itchy or swollen skin; cold, pale hands or feet; pain or weakness in arms, legs, back.	Discontinue. Call doctor right away.
Rare: Anxiety or confusion; red or purple blisters, especially on hands, feet; change in vision; extreme thirst; stomach pain or bloating; unusually fast or slow heartbeat; chest pain; numbness or tingling in face, fingers, toes.	Discontinue. Call doctor right away.

WARNINGS & PRECAUTIONS

Don't take if:
You are allergic to any ergot preparation.

Before you start, consult your doctor:
- If you plan to become pregnant within medication period.
- If you have an infection.
- If you have angina, heart problems, high blood pressure, hardening of the arteries or vein problems.
- If you have kidney or liver disease.
- If you are allergic to other spray inhalants.

Over age 60:
Adverse reactions and side effects may be more frequent and severe than in younger persons.

Pregnancy:
Risk to unborn child outweighs drug benefits. Don't use. Risk category X (see page xviii).

Breast-feeding:
Drug filters into milk. May harm child. Avoid.

Infants & children:
Studies inconclusive on harm to children. Consult your doctor.

Prolonged use:
Cold skin, muscle pain, gangrene of hands and feet. This medicine not intended for uninterrupted use.

Skin & sunlight:
No problems expected.

Driving, piloting or hazardous work:
Don't drive or pilot aircraft until you learn how medicine affects you. Don't work around dangerous machinery. Don't climb ladders or work in high places. Danger increases if you drink alcohol or take medicine affecting alertness and reflexes, such as antihistamines, tranquilizers, sedatives, pain medicine, narcotics and mind-altering drugs.

Discontinuing:
May be unnecessary to finish medicine. Follow doctor's instructions.

Others:
- Impaired blood circulation can lead to gangrene in intestines or extremities. Never exceed recommended dose.
- May affect results in some medical tests.

POSSIBLE INTERACTION WITH OTHER DRUGS

GENERIC NAME OR DRUG CLASS	COMBINED EFFECT
Amphetamines*	Dangerous blood pressure rise.
Beta-adrenergic blocking agents*	Narrowed arteries in heart if ergotamine is taken in high doses.
Ephedrine	Dangerous blood pressure rise.
Epinephrine	Dangerous blood pressure rise.
Ergot preparations, other	May cause decreased circulation to arms, legs, feet and hands. Avoid.
Erythromycin	Decreased ergotamine effect.
Nitroglycerin	Decreased nitroglycerin effect.
Pseudoephedrine	Dangerous blood pressure rise.
Sumatriptan	Increased vasoconstriction. Delay 24 hours between drugs.
Sympathomimetics*	May cause decreased circulation to arms, legs, feet and hands. Avoid.
Troleandomycin	Decreased ergotamine effect.

POSSIBLE INTERACTION WITH OTHER SUBSTANCES

INTERACTS WITH	COMBINED EFFECT
Alcohol:	Dilates blood vessels. Makes headache worse.
Beverages: Caffeine drinks.	May help relieve headache.
Cocaine:	Decreased ergotamine effect.
Foods: Any to which you are allergic.	May make headache worse. Avoid.
Marijuana:	Occasional use—Cool extremities. Regular use—Persistent chill.
Tobacco:	Decreased effect of ergotamine. Makes headache worse.

*See Glossary

ERGOTAMINE, BELLADONNA & PHENOBARBITAL

BRAND NAMES

Bellergal
Bellergal-S
Bellergal Spacetabs

BASIC INFORMATION

Habit forming? Yes
Prescription needed? Yes
Available as generic? No
Drug class: Analgesic, antispasmodic, vasoconstrictor

USES

- Reduces anxiety or nervous tension (low dose).
- Prevents vascular headaches.

DOSAGE & USAGE INFORMATION

How to take:
- Tablet or extended-release tablet—Swallow with liquid, or let dissolve under tongue.
- Lie down in quiet, dark room after taking.

When to take:
At first sign of vascular or migraine headache.

If you forget a dose:
Take as soon as you remember. Wait 4 hours for next dose.

What drug does:
- Constricts blood vessels in the head.
- Blocks nerve impulses at parasympathetic nerve endings, preventing muscle contractions and gland secretions of organs involved.

Continued next column

OVERDOSE

SYMPTOMS:
Tingling, cold extremities; muscle pain; nausea; vomiting; diarrhea; cold skin; rapid and weak pulse; severe numbness of extremities; confusion; dilated pupils; rapid pulse and breathing; dizziness; fever; hallucinations; slurred speech; agitation; flushed face; convulsions; coma.

WHAT TO DO:
- **Dial 911 (emergency) for an ambulance or medical help or poison center 1-800-222-1222. Then give first aid immediately.**
- **See emergency information on inside covers.**

Time lapse before drug works:
15 to 30 minutes.

Don't take with:
Nonprescription drugs without consulting doctor.

POSSIBLE ADVERSE REACTIONS OR SIDE EFFECTS

SYMPTOMS	WHAT TO DO
Life-threatening:	
In case of overdose, see previous column.	
Common:	
• Flushed skin, fever, drowsiness, bloating, depression, frequent urination.	Discontinue. Call doctor right away.
• Constipation, dizziness, drowsiness, "hangover" effect, increased frequency or severity of headaches.	Continue. Call doctor when convenient.
Infrequent:	
• Swollen feet and ankles, numbness or tingling in hands or feet, cold hands and feet, rash.	Discontinue. Call doctor right away.
• Nasal congestion, altered taste.	Continue. Call doctor when convenient.
Rare:	
Jaundice, weak legs, swallowing difficulty, dry mouth, increased sensitivity to sunlight, nausea, vomiting, decreased sweating.	Discontinue. Call doctor right away.

WARNINGS & PRECAUTIONS

Don't take if:
- You are allergic to any barbiturate, tartrazine dye, anticholinergic or ergot preparation.
- You have porphyria, trouble with stomach bloating, difficulty emptying your bladder completely, narrow-angle glaucoma, severe ulcerative colitis, enlarged prostate.

Before you start, consult your doctor:
- If you have epilepsy; kidney, thyroid or liver damage; anemia; chronic pain; open-angle glaucoma; angina; fast heartbeat; heart problems; high blood pressure; hardening of the arteries; vein problems; chronic bronchitis; asthma; hiatal hernia; enlarged prostate; myasthenia gravis; peptic ulcer; an infection.
- If you plan to become pregnant within medication period.

- If you will have surgery within 2 months, including dental surgery, requiring general or spinal anesthesia.

Over age 60:
Adverse reactions and side effects may be more frequent and severe than in younger persons.

Pregnancy:
Risk to unborn child outweighs drug benefits. Don't use. Risk category X (see page xviii).

Breast-feeding:
Drug passes into milk. Avoid drug or discontinue nursing until you finish medicine. Consult doctor for advice on maintaining milk supply.

Infants & children:
Not recommended.

Prolonged use:
- May cause addiction, anemia, chronic intoxication.
- May lower body temperature, making exposure to cold temperatures hazardous.
- Chronic constipation, possible fecal impaction.
- Cold skin, muscle pain, gangrene of hands and feet. This medicine not intended for uninterrupted use.

Skin & sunlight:
One or more drugs in this group may cause rash or intensify sunburn in areas exposed to sun or ultraviolet light (photosensitivity reaction). Avoid overexposure. Notify doctor if reaction occurs.

Driving, piloting or hazardous work:
Don't drive or pilot aircraft until you learn how medicine affects you. Don't work around dangerous machinery. Don't climb ladders or work in high places. Danger increases if you drink alcohol or take medicine affecting alertness and reflexes, such as antihistamines, tranquilizers, sedatives, pain medicine, narcotics and mind-altering drugs.

Discontinuing:
May be unnecessary to finish medicine. Follow doctor's instructions. If you develop withdrawal symptoms of hallucinations, agitation or sleeplessness after discontinuing, call doctor right away.

Others:
- Impaired blood circulation can lead to gangrene in intestines or extremities. Never exceed recommended dose.
- May affect results in some medical tests.

POSSIBLE INTERACTION WITH OTHER DRUGS

GENERIC NAME OR DRUG CLASS	COMBINED EFFECT
Amantadine	Increased belladonna effect.
Amphetamines*	Dangerous blood pressure rise.
Anticholinergics, other*	Increased belladonna effect.
Anticoagulants, oral*	Decreased anticoagulant effect.
Anticonvulsants*	Changed seizure patterns.
Antidepressants, tricyclic*	Decreased anti-depressant effect. Possible dangerous oversedation.
Antidiabetics, oral*	Increased phenobarbital effect.
Antihistamines*	Dangerous sedation. Avoid.
Aspirin	Decreased aspirin effect.
Beta-adrenergic blocking agents*	Narrowed arteries in heart if taken in large doses.
Contraceptives, oral*	Decreased contraceptive effect.
Cortisone drugs*	Decreased cortisone effect. Increased internal eye pressure.
Digitoxin	Decreased digitoxin effect.
Doxycycline	Decreased doxycycline effect.
Dronabinol	Increased effect of drugs.

Continued on page 912

POSSIBLE INTERACTION WITH OTHER SUBSTANCES

INTERACTS WITH	COMBINED EFFECT
Alcohol:	Possible fatal oversedation. Avoid.
Beverages:	None expected.
Cocaine:	Excessively rapid heartbeat. Avoid.
Foods:	None expected.
Marijuana:	Drowsiness and dry mouth, excessive sedation. Avoid.
Tobacco:	None expected.

***See Glossary**

ERYTHROMYCINS

GENERIC AND BRAND NAMES

See complete list of generic and brand names in the *Generic and Brand Name Directory*, page 862.

BASIC INFORMATION

Habit forming? No
Prescription needed? Yes
Available as generic? Yes
Drug class: Antibacterial; antiacne agent

USES

- Treatment of infections responsive to erythromycin.
- Treatment for acne.

DOSAGE & USAGE INFORMATION

How to take:

- Tablet or capsule—Swallow with liquid. You may chew or crush.
- Extended-release tablets or capsules—Swallow each dose whole.
- Oral suspension—Shake well before using. Use dropper supplied with prescription or use a specially marked measuring spoon to measure dose.

When to take:
At the same times each day, 1 hour before or 2 hours after eating. May be taken with food if stomach upset occurs. Enteric-coated tablets may be taken with or without food.

If you forget a dose:

- If you take 3 or more doses daily—Take as soon as you remember. Return to regular schedule.
- If you take 2 doses daily—Take as soon as you remember. Wait 5 to 6 hours for next dose. Return to regular schedule.

Continued next column

What drug does:
Prevents growth and reproduction of susceptible bacteria.

Time lapse before drug works:
2 to 5 days.

Don't take with:
Any other medicine without consulting your doctor or pharmacist.

OVERDOSE

SYMPTOMS:
Nausea, vomiting, abdominal discomfort, diarrhea.
WHAT TO DO:
Overdose unlikely to threaten life. If person takes much larger amount than prescribed, call doctor, poison center 1-800-222-1222 or hospital emergency room for instructions.

POSSIBLE ADVERSE REACTIONS OR SIDE EFFECTS

SYMPTOMS	WHAT TO DO
Life-threatening: None expected.	
Common: Mild nausea.	Continue. Call doctor when convenient.
Infrequent:	
• Mild diarrhea, stomach cramps or vomiting, sore mouth or tongue, skin dryness, irritation or stinging (with use of skin solution).	Continue. Call doctor when convenient.
• Fever with severe nausea and vomiting, severe stomach pain, unusual tiredness or weakness, yellow eyes or skin, allergic skin reaction (skin rash, redness or itch).	Discontinue. Call doctor right away.
Rare: Irregular or slow heartbeat, any hearing loss, fainting.	Discontinue. Call doctor right away.

WARNINGS & PRECAUTIONS

Don't take if:
You are allergic to any erythromycin or macrolides*.

Before you start, consult your doctor:

- You have had liver disease or impaired liver function.
- If you have taken erythromycin estolate in the past.
- If you have a hearing loss.
- If you have a history of heart rhythm problems.

Over age 60:
Adverse reactions and side effects may be more frequent and severe than in younger persons, especially skin reactions around genitals and anus.

Pregnancy:
Decide with your doctor if drug benefits justify risk to unborn child. Risk category B (see page xviii).

Breast-feeding:
Drug passes into milk. Avoid drug or discontinue nursing until you finish medicine. Consult doctor for advice on maintaining milk supply.

Infants & children:
Use only under medical supervision.

Prolonged use:
- You may become more susceptible to infections caused by germs not responsive to erythromycin.
- Talk to your doctor about the need for follow-up medical examinations or laboratory studies to check liver function.

Skin & sunlight:
No problems expected.

Driving, piloting or hazardous work:
No problems expected.

Discontinuing:
You must take full dose at least 10 consecutive days for streptococcal or staphylococcal infections.

Others:
Advise any doctor or dentist whom you consult that you take this medicine.

POSSIBLE INTERACTION WITH OTHER DRUGS

GENERIC NAME OR DRUG CLASS	COMBINED EFFECT
Aminophylline	Increased effect of aminophylline in blood.
Astemizole	Serious heart rhythm problems. Avoid.
Caffeine	Increased effect of caffeine.
Carbamazepine	Increased risk of carbamazepine toxicity.
Cefixime	Decreased antibiotic effect of cefixime.
Chloramphenicol	Decreased chloramphenicol effect.
Cyclosporins	May increase cyclosporin toxicity.
Digoxins*	Increased risk of digoxin toxicity.
Hepatotoxics*	Increased risk of liver toxicity.
HMG-CoA reductase inhibitors	Increased risk of muscle and kidney problems.
Leukotriene modifiers	Decreased effect of zafirlukast.
Lincomycins*	Decreased lincomycin effect.
Mifepristone	Decreased effect of mifepristone.
Oxtriphylline	Increased level of oxtriphylline in blood.
Penicillins*	Decreased penicillin effect.
Sibutramine	Increased sibutramine effect.
Sildenafil	Increased effect of sildenafil.
Theophylline	Increased level of theophylline in blood.
Valproic acid	Increased risk of valproic acid toxicity.
Warfarin	Increased risk of bleeding.

POSSIBLE INTERACTION WITH OTHER SUBSTANCES

INTERACTS WITH	COMBINED EFFECT
Alcohol:	Possible liver damage.
Beverages:	None expected.
Cocaine:	None expected.
Foods:	None expected.
Marijuana:	None expected.
Tobacco:	None expected.

*See Glossary

ESTRAMUSTINE

BRAND NAMES

Emcyt

BASIC INFORMATION

Habit forming? No
Prescription needed? Yes
Available as generic? No
Drug class: Antineoplastic

USES

Treats prostate cancer.

DOSAGE & USAGE INFORMATION

How to take:
Capsule—Swallow with liquid. If you can't swallow whole, open capsule and take with liquid or food. Instructions to take on empty stomach mean 1 hour before or 2 hours after eating.

When to take:
According to doctor's instructions. Try to take 1 hour before or 2 hours after eating or drinking any milk products.

If you forget a dose:
Skip dose. Never double dose.

What drug does:
Suppresses growth of cancer cells.

Time lapse before drug works:
Within 20 hours.

Don't take with:
Any other medicines (including over-the-counter drugs such as cough and cold medicines, laxatives, antacids, diet pills, caffeine, nose drops or vitamins) without consulting your doctor.

OVERDOSE

SYMPTOMS:
None expected.
WHAT TO DO:
Overdose unlikely to threaten life. If person takes much larger amount than prescribed, call doctor, poison center 1-800-222-1222 or hospital emergency room for instructions.

POSSIBLE ADVERSE REACTIONS OR SIDE EFFECTS

SYMPTOMS	WHAT TO DO
Life-threatening:	
Sudden headaches, chest pain, shortness of breath, leg pain, vision changes, slurred speech.	Seek emergency treatment immediately.
Common:	
• Skin rash, itching.	Discontinue. Call doctor right away.
• Increased sun sensitivity.	Decrease sun exposure. Call doctor when convenient.
• Diarrhea, dizziness, nausea, vomiting, headache, swelling in hands or feet.	Continue. Call doctor when convenient.
Infrequent:	
• Joint or muscle pain, difficulty swallowing, sore throat and fever, peeling skin, jaundice.	Discontinue. Call doctor right away.
• Mouth or tongue irritation, breast tenderness or enlargement, decreased interest in sex.	Continue. Call doctor when convenient.
Rare:	
Bloody urine, hearing loss, back pain, abdominal pain.	Discontinue. Call doctor right away.

WARNINGS & PRECAUTIONS

Don't take if:
You have active thrombophlebitis.

Before you start, consult your doctor:
- If you have jaundice.
- If you have history of thrombophlebitis.
- If you have peptic ulcer.
- If you have mental depression.
- If you have migraine headaches.
- If you have or recently had chicken pox.
- If you have shingles (herpes zoster).
- If you have had a recent heart attack.

Over age 60:
Adverse reactions and side effects may be more frequent and severe than in younger persons. You may need smaller doses for shorter periods of time.

Pregnancy:
Used in men only.

Breast-feeding:
Used in men only.

Infants & children:
Not used.

Prolonged use:
Talk to your doctor about the need for follow-up medical examinations or laboratory studies to check complete blood counts (white blood cell count, platelet count, red blood cell count, hemoglobin, hematocrit), blood pressure, liver function, serum acid, serum calcium and alkaline phosphatase.

Skin & sunlight:
No problems expected.

Driving, piloting or hazardous work:
No special problems expected.

Discontinuing:
No special problems expected.

Others:
- Advise any doctor or dentist whom you consult that you take this medicine.
- May affect results in some medical tests.
- May decrease sperm count in males.

POSSIBLE INTERACTION WITH OTHER DRUGS

GENERIC NAME OR DRUG CLASS	COMBINED EFFECT
Calcium supplements*	Decreased absorption of estramustine.
Hepatotoxic medications*	Increased risk of liver toxicity.

POSSIBLE INTERACTION WITH OTHER SUBSTANCES

INTERACTS WITH	COMBINED EFFECT
Alcohol:	Increased "hangover effect" and other gastrointestinal symptoms.
Beverages: Milk and milk products.	Decreased absorption of estramustine.
Cocaine:	None expected.
Foods: Foods high in calcium.	Decreased absorption of estramustine.
Marijuana:	None expected.
Tobacco:	Increased risk of heart attack and blood clots.

***See Glossary**

ESTROGENS

GENERIC AND BRAND NAMES

See complete list of generic and brand names in *Generic and Brand Name Directory*, page 862.

BASIC INFORMATION

Habit forming? No
Prescription needed? Yes
Available as generic? Yes
Drug class: Female sex hormone (estrogen)

USES

- Treatment for estrogen deficiency.
- Treatment for symptoms of menopause and menstrual cycle irregularity.
- Treatment for estrogen-deficiency osteoporosis (bone softening from calcium loss).
- Treatment for vulvar squamous hyperplasia.
- Treatment for atrophic vaginitis.
- Treatment for prostate cancer.
- Reduces the risk of heart attack.

DOSAGE & USAGE INFORMATION

How to take:

- Tablet or capsule—Take with or after food to reduce nausea. Swallow with liquid. If you can't swallow whole, crumble tablet or open capsule and take with liquid or food.
- Vaginal cream or suppositories—Use as directed on label.
- By injection under medical supervision.
- Transdermal patches—Follow package instructions.
- Vaginal insert—Follow package instructions.

When to take:

- Oral estrogen—Take at the same time each day.
- Creams, suppositories, injections or patches—Follow label instructions.

Continued next column

OVERDOSE

SYMPTOMS:
Nausea, vomiting, fluid retention, breast enlargement and discomfort, abnormal vaginal bleeding.
WHAT TO DO:
Overdose unlikely to threaten life. If person takes much larger amount than prescribed, call doctor, poison center 1-800-222-1222 or hospital emergency room for instructions.

If you forget a dose:
Take as soon as you remember up to 12 hours late. If more than 12 hours, wait for next scheduled dose (don't double this dose).

What drug does:

- Restores normal estrogen level in tissues.
- Combined with progestins for contraception.

Time lapse before drug works:
10 to 20 days.

Don't take with:
Any other medicine without consulting your doctor or pharmacist.

POSSIBLE ADVERSE REACTIONS OR SIDE EFFECTS

SYMPTOMS	WHAT TO DO
Life-threatening:	
Profuse bleeding.	Seek emergency treatment.
Common:	
• Stomach cramps.	Discontinue. Call doctor right away.
• Appetite loss.	Continue. Call doctor when convenient.
• Nausea; diarrhea; swollen feet and ankles; tender, swollen breasts; acne; intolerance of contact lenses; change in menstruation.	Continue. Tell doctor at next visit.
Infrequent:	
• Rash, stomach or side pain, joint or muscle pain, bloody skin blisters, breast lumps.	Discontinue. Call doctor right away.
• Depression, dizziness, migraine headache, irritability, vomiting.	Continue. Call doctor when convenient.
• Brown blotches, hair loss, vaginal discharge or bleeding, changes in sex drive.	Continue. Tell doctor at next visit.
Rare:	
Jaundice, hypercalcemia in breast cancer. Involuntary movements.	Discontinue. Call doctor right away.

WARNINGS & PRECAUTIONS

Don't take if:

- You are allergic to any estrogen-containing drugs.
- You have impaired liver function.
- You have had blood clots, stroke or heart attack.
- You have unexplained vaginal bleeding.

Before you start, consult your doctor:

- If you have had cancer of the breast or reproductive organs, fibrocystic breast disease, fibroid tumors of the uterus or endometriosis.
- If you have had migraine headaches, epilepsy or porphyria.
- If you have diabetes, high blood pressure, asthma, congestive heart failure, kidney disease or gallstones.
- If you plan to become pregnant within 3 months.

Over age 60:
Controversial. You and your doctor must decide if risks of drug outweigh benefits.

Pregnancy:
Risk to unborn child outweighs benefits of drug. Don't use. Risk category X (see page xviii).

Breast-feeding:
Drug filters into milk. May harm child. Avoid.

Infants & children:
Not recommended.

Prolonged use:

- Increased growth of fibroid tumors of uterus. Possible association with cancer of uterus.
- Talk to your doctor about the need for follow-up medical examinations or laboratory studies to check pap smear, liver function, mammogram.

Skin & sunlight:
One or more drugs in this group may cause rash or intensify sunburn in areas exposed to sun or ultraviolet light (photosensitivity reaction). Avoid overexposure. Notify doctor if reaction occurs.

Driving, piloting or hazardous work:
No problems expected.

Discontinuing:
You may need to discontinue estrogens periodically. Consult your doctor.

Others:

- In rare instances, may cause blood clot in lung, brain or leg. Symptoms are sudden severe headache, coordination loss, vision change, chest pain, breathing difficulty, slurred speech, pain in legs or groin. Seek emergency treatment immediately.
- Carefully read the paper called "Information for the Patient" that was given to you with your prescription. If you lose it, ask your pharmacist for a copy.

POSSIBLE INTERACTION WITH OTHER DRUGS

GENERIC NAME OR DRUG CLASS	COMBINED EFFECT
Adrenocorticoids, systemic	Increased adreno-corticoid effect.
Alpha adrenergic receptor blockers	Decreased effect of alpha adrenergic blocker.
Anticoagulants, oral*	Decreased anti-coagulant effect.
Anticonvulsants, hydantoin*	Decreased estrogen effect.
Antidepressants, tricyclic*	Increased toxicity of antidepressants.
Antidiabetics, oral*	Unpredictable increase or decrease in blood sugar.
Antifibrinolytic agents*	Increased possibility of blood clotting.
Antivirals, HIV/AIDS*	Increased risk of pancreatitis.
Carbamazepine	Decreased estrogen effect.
Clofibrate	Decreased clofibrate effect.
Dextrothyroxine	Decreased dextrothyroxine effect.
Guanfacine	May decrease antihypertensive effects of guanfacine.
Insulin	Possible decreased insulin effect. May require dosage adjustment.

Continued on page 913

POSSIBLE INTERACTION WITH OTHER SUBSTANCES

INTERACTS WITH	COMBINED EFFECT
Alcohol:	None expected.
Beverages:	
Grapefruit juice.	Possible increased estrogen effect.
Cocaine:	None expected.
Foods:	None expected.
Marijuana:	Possible menstrual irregularities and bleeding between periods.
Tobacco:	Increased risk of blood clots leading to stroke or heart attack.

*See Glossary

ETHCHLORVYNOL

BRAND NAMES

Placidyl

BASIC INFORMATION

Habit forming? Yes
Prescription needed? Yes
Available as generic? No
Drug class: Sleep inducer (hypnotic)

USES

Treatment of insomnia for short periods. Prolonged use is not recommended.

DOSAGE & USAGE INFORMATION

How to take:
Capsules—Take with food or milk to lessen side effects.

When to take:
At or near bedtime.

If you forget a dose:
Bedtime dose—If you forget your once-a-day bedtime dose, don't take it more than 3 hours late.

What drug does:
Affects brain centers that control waking and sleeping.

Time lapse before drug works:
30 to 60 minutes.

Don't take with:
Any other medicine without consulting your doctor or pharmacist.

OVERDOSE

SYMPTOMS:
Excitement, delirium, incoordination, shortness of breath, slow heartbeat, excessive drowsiness, deep coma.
WHAT TO DO:
- **Dial 911 (emergency) for an ambulance or medical help or poison center 1-800-222-1222. Then give first aid immediately.**
- **If patient is unconscious and not breathing, give mouth-to-mouth breathing. If there is no heartbeat, use cardiac massage and mouth-to-mouth breathing (CPR). Don't try to make patient vomit. If you can't get help quickly, take patient to nearest emergency facility.**
- **See emergency information on inside covers.**

POSSIBLE ADVERSE REACTIONS OR SIDE EFFECTS

SYMPTOMS	WHAT TO DO
Life-threatening:	
In case of overdose, see previous column.	
Common:	
• Indigestion, nausea, vomiting, stomach pain.	Discontinue. Call doctor right away.
• Blurred vision, dizziness.	Continue. Call doctor when convenient.
• Unpleasant taste in mouth, fatigue, weakness.	Continue. Tell doctor at next visit.
Infrequent:	
Jitters, clumsiness, unsteadiness, drowsiness, confusion, rash, hives, unusual bleeding or bruising, facial numbness.	Discontinue. Call doctor right away.
Rare:	
Slow heartbeat, difficult breathing, fainting, jaundice, slurred speech, trembling, uncontrolled eye movements.	Discontinue. Call doctor right away.

WARNINGS & PRECAUTIONS

Don't take if:
- You are allergic to any hypnotic.
- You have porphyria.
- Patient is younger than 12.

Before you start, consult your doctor:
- If you plan to become pregnant within medication period.
- If you have kidney or liver disease.

Over age 60:
Adverse reactions and side effects, especially a "hangover" effect, may be more frequent and severe than in younger persons.

Pregnancy:
Decide with your doctor if drug benefits justify risk to unborn child. Risk category C (see page xviii).

Breast-feeding:
No problems expected, but observe child and ask doctor for guidance.

Infants & children:
Not recommended.

Prolonged use:
Impaired vision.

Skin & sunlight:
No problems expected.

Driving, piloting or hazardous work:
Don't drive or pilot aircraft until you learn how medicine affects you. Don't work around dangerous machinery. Don't climb ladders or work in high places. Danger increases if you drink alcohol or take medicine affecting alertness and reflexes.

Discontinuing:
- Don't discontinue without consulting doctor. Dose may require gradual reduction if you have taken drug for a long time. Doses of other drugs may also require adjustment.
- Many side effects may occur when you stop taking this drug, including irritability, muscle twitching, hallucinations or seizures. Consult your doctor.

Others:
No problems expected.

POSSIBLE INTERACTION WITH OTHER DRUGS

GENERIC NAME OR DRUG CLASS	COMBINED EFFECT
Anticoagulants, oral*	Decreased anticoagulant effect.
Antidepressants, tricyclic* (especially amitriptyline)	Delirium and deep sedation.
Antihistamines*	Increased antihistamine effect.
Clozapine	Toxic effect on the central nervous system.
Ethinamate	Dangerous increased effects of ethinamate. Avoid combining.
Fluoxetine	Increased depressant effects of both drugs.
Guanfacine	May increase depressant effects of either drug.
Leucovorin	High alcohol content of leucovorin may cause adverse effects.
Methyprylon	Increased sedative effect, perhaps to dangerous level. Avoid.
Molindone	Increased sedative effect.
Monoamine oxidase (MAO) inhibitors*	Increased sedation.
Nabilone	Greater depression of central nervous system.
Narcotics*	Increased narcotic effect.
Pain relievers*	Increased effect of pain reliever.
Sedatives*	Increased sedative effect.
Sertraline	Increased depressive effects of both drugs.
Tranquilizers*	Increased tranquilizer effect.

POSSIBLE INTERACTION WITH OTHER SUBSTANCES

INTERACTS WITH	COMBINED EFFECT
Alcohol:	Excessive depressant and sedative effect. Avoid.
Beverages:	None expected.
Cocaine:	Decreased ethchlorvynol effect.
Foods:	None expected.
Marijuana:	Occasional use—Drowsiness, unsteadiness, depressed function. Frequent use—Severe drowsiness, impaired physical and mental function.
Tobacco:	None expected.

ETHIONAMIDE

BRAND NAMES

Trecator-SC

BASIC INFORMATION

Habit forming? No
Prescription needed? Yes
Available as generic? No
Drug class: Antimycobacterial (antituberculosis)

USES

Treats tuberculosis. Used in combination with other antituberculosis drugs such as isoniazid, streptomycin, rifampin, ethambutol.

DOSAGE & USAGE INFORMATION

How to take:
Tablets—Swallow with liquid or food to lessen stomach irritation. If you can't swallow whole, crumble tablet and take with liquid or food.

When to take:
Usually every 8 to 12 hours, with or after meals.

If you forget a dose:
Take as soon as you remember up to 2 hours late. If more than 2 hours, wait for next scheduled dose. Don't double this dose.

What drug does:
Kills germs that cause tuberculosis.

Time lapse before drug works:
Within 3 hours.

Don't take with:
Any other medicine without consulting your doctor or pharmacist.

OVERDOSE

SYMPTOMS:
None expected.
WHAT TO DO:
Overdose unlikely to threaten life. If person takes much larger amount than prescribed, call doctor, poison center 1-800-222-1222 or hospital emergency room for instructions.

POSSIBLE ADVERSE REACTIONS OR SIDE EFFECTS

SYMPTOMS	WHAT TO DO
Life-threatening: None expected.	
Common:	
• Vomiting.	Discontinue. Call doctor right away.
• Dizziness, sore mouth, nausea, metallic taste.	Continue. Call doctor when convenient.
Infrequent: Jaundice (yellow eyes and skin); numbness, tingling, pain in hands or feet; depression; confusion.	Discontinue. Call doctor right away.
Rare:	
• Hunger, shakiness, rapid heartbeat; blurred vision; vision changes; skin rash.	Discontinue. Call doctor right away.
• Gradual swelling in the neck (thyroid gland).	Continue. Call doctor when convenient.
• Enlargement of breasts (male).	No action necessary.

WARNINGS & PRECAUTIONS

Don't take if:
You know you are hypersensitive to ethionamide.

Before you start, consult your doctor:
- If you have diabetes mellitus.
- If you have liver disease.

Over age 60:
No information available.

Pregnancy:
Decide with your doctor if drug benefits justify risk to unborn child. Risk category C (see page xviii).

Breast-feeding:
Effect not documented. Consult your family doctor or pediatrician.

Infants & children:
Effect not documented. Consult your family doctor or pediatrician.

Prolonged use:
No special problems expected.

Skin & sunlight:
No special problems expected.

Driving, piloting or hazardous work:
Don't drive or pilot aircraft until you learn how medicine affects you. Don't work around dangerous machinery. Don't climb ladders or work in high places. Danger increases if you drink alcohol or take medicine affecting alertness and reflexes.

Discontinuing:
Don't discontinue without consulting doctor.

Others:
- Advise any doctor or dentist whom you consult that you take this medicine.
- Request occasional laboratory studies for liver function.
- Request occasional eye examinations.
- Treatment may take months or years.
- You should take pyridoxine (vitamin B-6) supplements while taking ethionamide.

POSSIBLE INTERACTION WITH OTHER DRUGS

GENERIC NAME OR DRUG CLASS	COMBINED EFFECT
Antivirals, HIV/AIDS*	Increased risk of peripheral neuropathy.
Cycloserine	Increased risk of seizures.
Pyridoxine	Increased excretion by kidney. (Should take pyridoxine supplements while on ethionamide to prevent development of neuritis in feet and hands).

POSSIBLE INTERACTION WITH OTHER SUBSTANCES

INTERACTS WITH	COMBINED EFFECT
Alcohol:	Increased incidence of liver diseases.
Beverages: Any alcoholic beverage.	Increased incidence of liver diseases.
Cocaine:	None expected.
Foods:	None expected.
Marijuana:	No interaction expected, but may slow body's recovery.
Tobacco:	No interaction expected, but may slow body's recovery.

**See Glossary*

ETIDRONATE

BRAND NAMES

Didronel
EHDP

BASIC INFORMATION

Habit forming? No
Prescription needed? Yes
Available as generic? No
Drug class: Antihypercalcemic

USES

- Treats Paget's disease of the bone.
- Aids healing following hip replacement or spinal cord injury.

DOSAGE & USAGE INFORMATION

How to take:
Tablet—Swallow with water. Do not take with milk.

When to take:
According to doctor's instructions. Take 1 hour before or 2 hours after eating.

If you forget a dose:
Take as soon as you remember up to 6 hours late. If more than 6 hours, wait for next dose (don't double this dose).

What drug does:
Unknown. Appears to retard bone loss and stimulates bone formation.

Time lapse before drug works:
- Paget's disease—1 month.
- Other uses—1 day to several months.

Don't take with:
Any other medicine without consulting your doctor or pharmacist.

OVERDOSE

SYMPTOMS:
None expected.
WHAT TO DO:
Overdose unlikely to threaten life. If person takes much larger amount than prescribed, call doctor, poison center 1-800-222-1222 or hospital emergency room for instructions.

POSSIBLE ADVERSE REACTIONS OR SIDE EFFECTS

SYMPTOMS	WHAT TO DO
Life-threatening:	
None expected.	
Common:	
Tenderness or pain in bones, diarrhea, nausea.	Continue. Call doctor when convenient.
Infrequent:	
None expected.	
Rare:	
Rash; hives; swelling of hands, feet, lips, throat.	Discontinue. Call doctor right away.

WARNINGS & PRECAUTIONS

Don't take if:
You are allergic to etidronate or alendronate.

Before you start, consult your doctor:
If you have kidney disease, heart failure, bone fractures or colitis.

Over age 60:
No special problems expected.

Pregnancy:
Consult doctor. Risk category B (see page xviii).

Breast-feeding:
Safety not established. Consult doctor.

Infants & children:
Use only under supervision of a medical professional.

Prolonged use:
No special problems expected.

Skin & sunlight:
No special problems expected.

Driving, piloting or hazardous work:
No special problems expected.

Discontinuing:
Don't discontinue without doctor's advice, even though symptoms diminish or disappear.

Others:
- Medicine may be prescribed for 2 weeks, stopped for 2 to 3 months, then started again.
- Have regular check-ups with your doctor even if you currently are not undergoing treatment.

POSSIBLE INTERACTION WITH OTHER DRUGS

GENERIC NAME OR DRUG CLASS	COMBINED EFFECT
Antacids*	Decreased effect of etidronate.
Mineral supplements*	Decreased effect of etidronate.

POSSIBLE INTERACTION WITH OTHER SUBSTANCES

INTERACTS WITH	COMBINED EFFECT
Alcohol:	None expected.
Beverages: Milk.	Decreased effect of etidronate.
Cocaine:	None expected.
Foods: Dairy products or foods containing high levels of calcium.	Decreased effect of etidronate.
Marijuana:	None expected.
Tobacco:	None expected.

***See Glossary**

ETOPOSIDE

BRAND NAMES

VePesid   VP-16

BASIC INFORMATION

Habit forming? No
Prescription needed? Yes
Available as generic? No
Drug class: Antineoplastic

USES

- Treats testicle, lung and bladder cancer.
- Treats Hodgkin's disease and some other forms of cancer.

DOSAGE & USAGE INFORMATION

How to take:

- Capsules—Swallow with liquid. If you can't swallow whole, open capsule and take with liquid or food. Instructions to take on empty stomach mean 1 hour before or 2 hours after eating.
- Injection—Given under doctor's supervision.

When to take:
According to your doctor's instructions.

If you forget a dose:
Skip this dose. Never double dose. Resume regular schedule.

What drug does:
Inhibits DNA in cancer cells.

Time lapse before drug works:
Unpredictable.

Don't take with:
Any other medicines (including over-the-counter drugs such as cough and cold medicines, laxatives, antacids, diet pills, caffeine, nose drops or vitamins) without consulting your doctor.

OVERDOSE

SYMPTOMS:
Rapid pulse, shortness of breath, wheezing, fainting, coma.
WHAT TO DO:

- **Dial 911 (emergency) for an ambulance or medical help or poison center 1-800-222-1222. Then give first aid immediately.**
- **See emergency information on inside covers.**

POSSIBLE ADVERSE REACTIONS OR SIDE EFFECTS

SYMPTOMS	WHAT TO DO
Life-threatening: In case of overdose, see previous column.	
Common:	
• Appetite loss, nausea, vomiting.	Continue. Call doctor when convenient.
• Loss of hair	No action necessary.
Infrequent:	
Symptoms of low white blood cell count and low platelet count: black, tarry stools; bloody urine; cough; chills or fever; low back pain; bruising.	Discontinue. Call doctor right away.
Rare:	
Mouth sores.	Continue. Call doctor when convenient.

WARNINGS & PRECAUTIONS

Don't take if:
- You have chicken pox.
- You have shingles (herpes zoster).

Before you start, consult your doctor:
If you have liver or kidney disease.

Over age 60:
No special problems expected.

Pregnancy:
Risk to unborn child outweighs drug benefits. Don't use. Risk category D (see page xviii).

Breast-feeding:
Drug passes into milk. Avoid drug or discontinue nursing until you finish medicine. Consult doctor for advice on maintaining milk supply.

Infants & children:
Effect not documented. Consult your doctor.

Prolonged use:
- Talk to your doctor about the need for follow-up medical examinations or laboratory studies to check complete blood counts (white blood cell count, platelet count, red blood cell count, hemoglobin, hematocrit).
- Check mouth frequently for ulcers.

Skin & sunlight:
No problems expected.

Driving, piloting or hazardous work:
Avoid if you feel confused, drowsy or dizzy.

Discontinuing:
May still experience symptoms of bone marrow depression, such as: blood in stools, fever or chills, blood spots under the skin, back pain, hoarseness, bloody urine. If any of these occur, call your doctor right away.

Others:
- Advise any doctor or dentist whom you consult that you take this medicine.
- May affect results in some medical tests.
- Etoposide may be used in combinations with other antineoplastic treatment plans. The incidence and severity of side effects may be different when used in combinations such as doxorubicin, procarbazine and etoposide (APE); etoposide, cyclophosphamide, doxorubicin and vincristine (CAVE, ECHO, CAPO, EVAC or VOCA); cyclophosphamide, doxorubicin and etoposide (CAE or ACE); cisplatin, bleomycin, doxorubicin and etoposide; cisplatin, bleomycin and etoposide; cisplatin and etoposide. For further information regarding these combinations, consult your doctor.

POSSIBLE INTERACTION WITH OTHER DRUGS

GENERIC NAME OR DRUG CLASS	COMBINED EFFECT
Angiotensin-converting enzyme (ACE) inhibitors*	May increase bone marrow depression or make kidney damage more likely.
Antineoplastic (cancer-treating) drugs*	May increase bone marrow depression or make kidney damage more likely.
Clozapine	Toxic effect on bone marrow.
Tiopronin	Increased risk of toxicity to bone marrow.
Vaccines, live or killed virus	Increased likelihood of toxicity or reduced effectiveness of vaccine. Wait 3 months to 1 year after etoposide treatment before getting vaccine.

POSSIBLE INTERACTION WITH OTHER SUBSTANCES

INTERACTS WITH	COMBINED EFFECT
Alcohol:	Increased likelihood of adverse reactions. Avoid.
Beverages:	None expected.
Cocaine:	Increased likelihood of adverse reactions. Avoid.
Foods:	None expected.
Marijuana:	Increased likelihood of adverse reactions. Avoid.
Tobacco:	None expected.

***See Glossary**

FELBAMATE

BRAND AND GENERIC NAMES

FBM Felbatol

BASIC INFORMATION

Habit forming? No
Prescription needed? Yes
Available as generic? No
Drug class: Anticonvulsant

USES

- Treatment for partial epileptic seizures.
- Treatment for Lennox-Gastaut syndrome (a severe form of epilepsy in children).

DOSAGE & USAGE INFORMATION

How to take:
- Tablet—Swallow with liquid. May be taken with food to lessen stomach upset unless the doctor has directed taking on an empty stomach.
- Oral suspension—Shake bottle well before measuring. Use specially marked measuring device to measure each dose accurately. Don't measure with a regular household teaspoon.

When to take:
At the same times each day. Your doctor will determine the best schedule. Dosages will gradually be increased over the first 3 weeks.

If you forget a dose:
Take as soon as you remember up to 2 hours late. If more than 2 hours, wait for next scheduled dose (don't double this dose).

What drug does:
- Decreases the frequency of partial seizures that start in a localized part of the brain, including those that progress into more generalized grand mal seizures.
- Decreases seizure activity and improves quality of life in children with Lennox-Gastaut syndrome.

Continued next column

OVERDOSE

SYMPTOMS:
Gastric distress, increased heart rate.
WHAT TO DO:
Overdose unlikely to threaten life. If person takes much larger amount than prescribed, call doctor, poison center 1-800-222-1222 or hospital emergency room for instructions.

Time lapse before drug works:
May take several weeks for maximum effectiveness.

Don't take with:
Any other prescription or nonprescription drug without consulting your doctor.

POSSIBLE ADVERSE REACTIONS OR SIDE EFFECTS

SYMPTOMS	WHAT TO DO
Life-threatening: None expected.	
Common:	
• Fever, red or purple spots on skin, walking in unusual manner.	Continue, but call doctor right away.
• Abdominal pain, taste changes, constipation, sleeping difficulty, dizziness, headache, nausea or vomiting, indigestion, appetite loss.	Continue. Call doctor when convenient.
Infrequent:	
• Mood or mental changes, clumsiness, skin rash, tremor.	Continue, but call doctor right away.
• Vision changes, diarrhea, drowsiness, coughing or sneezing, ear pain or fullness, runny nose, weight loss.	Continue. Call doctor when convenient.
Rare:	
Black or tarry stools, bloody or dark-colored urine, unusual bruising or bleeding, breathing difficulty, wheezing, pain or tightness in chest, sore throat, mouth or lip sores, swollen face, swollen or painful glands or lymph nodes, yellow skin or eyes, chills, general tired feeling, continuing headache or abdominal pain, hives, itching, muscle cramps, stuffy nose, skin reaction to sunlight.	Continue, but call doctor right away.

WARNINGS & PRECAUTIONS

Don't take if:
You are allergic to felbamate.

Before you start, consult your doctor:
- If you have a sensitivity to other carbamate drugs*, other medications or other substances.
- If you have any blood disorder.
- If you have a history of bone marrow depression.
- If you have or have had any liver disease.

Over age 60:
Adverse reactions and side effects may be more frequent and severe than in younger persons.

Pregnancy:
Decide with your doctor if drug benefits justify risks to unborn child. Risk category B (see page xviii).

Breast-feeding:
Drug passes into milk. Unknown effect. Consult your doctor.

Infants & children:
Give only under close medical supervision.

Prolonged use:
Talk to your doctor about the need for follow-up medical examinations or laboratory studies to check complete blood counts (white blood cell count, platelet count, red blood cell count, hemoglobin, hematocrit), iron concentrations and liver function studies.

Skin & sunlight:
No problems expected.

Driving, piloting or hazardous work:
Don't drive or pilot aircraft until you learn how medicine affects you. Don't work around dangerous machinery. Don't climb ladders or work in high places. Danger increases if you drink alcohol or take other medicines affecting alertness and reflexes such as antihistamines, tranquilizers, sedatives, pain medicine, narcotics and mind-altering drugs.

Discontinuing:
Don't discontinue without doctor's approval due to risk of increased seizure activity.

Others:
- Felbamate may cause serious side effects including blood problems and liver problems (rarely fatal). Decide with your doctor if drug benefits justify risks.
- Advise any doctor or dentist whom you consult that you take this medicine.
- Felbamate may be used alone or combined with other antiepileptic drugs. The dosages of other antiepileptic drugs you currently use will be reduced to minimize side effects and adverse reactions due to interactions.
- Wear medical identification that indicates the use of this medicine.

POSSIBLE INTERACTION WITH OTHER DRUGS

GENERIC NAME OR DRUG CLASS	COMBINED EFFECT
Carbamazepine	Increased side effects and adverse reactions.
Phenytoin	Increased side effects and adverse reactions.
Valproic acid	Increased side effects and adverse reactions.

POSSIBLE INTERACTION WITH OTHER SUBSTANCES

INTERACTS WITH	COMBINED EFFECT
Alcohol:	None expected.
Beverages:	None expected.
Cocaine:	None expected.
Foods:	None expected.
Marijuana:	None expected.
Tobacco:	None expected.

***See Glossary**

FIBRATES

GENERIC AND BRAND NAMES

CLOFIBRATE
- **Abitrate**
- **Atromid-S**
- **Claripex**
- **Novofibrate**

FENOFIBRATE
- **Lipidil**
- **Tricor**

BASIC INFORMATION

Habit forming? No
Prescription needed? Yes
Available as generic? Yes
Drug class: Antihyperlipidemic

USES

Reduces fatty substances in the blood (triglycerides).

DOSAGE & USAGE INFORMATION

How to take:
Capsule—Swallow with liquid or food to lessen stomach irritation.

When to take:
At the same times each day.

If you forget a dose:
Take as soon as you remember up to 2 hours late. If more than 2 hours, wait for next scheduled dose (don't double this dose).

What drug does:
Inhibits formation of fatty substances.

Time lapse before drug works:
3 months or more.

Don't take with:
Any other medicine without consulting your doctor or pharmacist.

OVERDOSE

SYMPTOMS:
Diarrhea, headache, muscle pain.
WHAT TO DO:
Overdose unlikely to threaten life. If person takes much larger amount than prescribed, call doctor, poison center 1-800-222-1222 or hospital emergency room for instructions.

POSSIBLE ADVERSE REACTIONS OR SIDE EFFECTS

SYMPTOMS	WHAT TO DO
Life-threatening: None expected.	
Common: None expected.	
Infrequent:	
• Chest pain, shortness of breath, irregular heartbeat.	Discontinue. Seek emergency treatment.
• Nausea, flu-like illness, vomiting.	Discontinue. Call doctor right away.
• Diarrhea, abdominal pain, belching, constipation, muscle aches and pains.	Continue. Call doctor when convenient.
Rare:	
• Cardiac arrhythmias, angina.	Discontinue. Seek emergency treatment.
• Rash, itch; mouth or lip sores; sore throat; swollen feet, legs; blood in urine; painful urination; fever; chills; anemia.	Discontinue. Call doctor right away.
• Dizziness, weakness, drowsiness, muscle cramps, headache, diminished sex drive, hair loss, dry mouth, bloating or stomach pain, chronic indigestion, loss of appetite, nausea, unusual bleeding or bruising, unusual tiredness, vomiting, yellow eyes or skin.	Continue. Call doctor when convenient.

WARNINGS & PRECAUTIONS

Don't take if:
- You are allergic to any fibrates.
- You have had serious liver disease.

Before you start, consult your doctor:
- If you have had liver or kidney disease.
- If you have had peptic ulcer disease.
- If you have had gallbladder disease or gallstones.
- If you have diabetes.

Over age 60:
Adverse reactions and side effects may be more frequent and severe than in younger persons. May develop flu-like symptoms.

Pregnancy:
Decide with your doctor if drug benefits justify risk to unborn child. Risk category C (see page xviii).

Breast-feeding:
May harm child. Avoid. Consult doctor.

Infants & children:
Not recommended.

Prolonged use:
- May cause gallbladder infection.
- Possible cause of stomach cancer.
- Talk to your doctor about the need for follow-up medical examinations or laboratory studies to check complete blood counts (white blood cell count, platelet count, red blood cell count, hemoglobin, hematocrit) and serum low-density lipoprotein.

Skin & sunlight:
May cause rash or intensify sunburn in areas exposed to sun or ultraviolet light (photosensitivity reaction). Avoid overexposure. Notify doctor if reaction occurs.

Driving, piloting or hazardous work:
Avoid if you feel drowsy or dizzy. Otherwise, no problems expected.

Discontinuing:
Don't discontinue without doctor's advice until you complete prescribed dose, even though symptoms diminish or disappear.

Others:
- Periodic blood cell counts and liver-function studies recommended if you take clofibrate for a long time.
- Some studies question effectiveness. Many studies warn of toxicity.

POSSIBLE INTERACTION WITH OTHER DRUGS

GENERIC NAME OR DRUG CLASS	COMBINED EFFECT
Anticoagulants, oral*	Increased anticoagulant effect. Dose reduction of anticoagulant necessary.
Antidiabetics, oral*	Increased antidiabetic effect.
Contraceptives, oral*	Decreased fibrate effect.
Cyclosporine	May cause kidney problems, or worsen them.
Desmopressin	May decrease desmopressin effect.
Dexfenfluramine	May require dosage change as weight loss occurs.
Estrogens*	Decreased fibrate effect.
Furosemide	Possible toxicity of both drugs.
HMG-CoA reductase inhibitors	May cause muscle or kidney problems or make them worse.
Insulin	Increased insulin effect.
Insulin lispro	May need decreased dosage of insulin.
Probenecid	Increased effect and toxicity of fibrate.
Thyroid hormones*	Increased fibrate effect.
Ursodiol	Decreased effect of ursodiol.

POSSIBLE INTERACTION WITH OTHER SUBSTANCES

INTERACTS WITH	COMBINED EFFECT
Alcohol:	None expected.
Beverages:	None expected.
Cocaine:	None expected.
Foods: Fatty foods.	Decreased fibrate effect.
Marijuana:	None expected.

***See Glossary**

FLAVOXATE

BRAND NAMES

Urispas

BASIC INFORMATION

Habit forming? No
Prescription needed? Yes
Available as generic? No
Drug class: Antispasmodic (urinary tract)

USES

Relieves urinary pain, urgency, nighttime urination, unusual frequency of urination associated with urinary system disorders.

DOSAGE & USAGE INFORMATION

How to take:
Tablet—Swallow with liquid or food to lessen stomach irritation.

When to take:
30 minutes before meals (unless directed otherwise by doctor).

If you forget a dose:
Take as soon as you remember up to 2 hours late. If more than 2 hours, wait for next scheduled dose (don't double this dose).

What drug does:
Blocks nerve impulses at smooth muscle nerve endings, preventing muscle contractions and gland secretions of organs involved.

Time lapse before drug works:
15 to 30 minutes.

Don't take with:
Any other medicine without consulting your doctor or pharmacist.

OVERDOSE

SYMPTOMS:
Dilated pupils, rapid pulse and breathing, dizziness, fever, hallucinations, confusion, slurred speech, agitation, flushed face, convulsions, coma.
WHAT TO DO:
- **Dial 911 (emergency) for an ambulance or medical help or poison center 1-800-222-1222. Then give first aid immediately.**
- **See emergency information on inside covers.**

POSSIBLE ADVERSE REACTIONS OR SIDE EFFECTS

SYMPTOMS	WHAT TO DO
Life-threatening: In case of overdose, see previous column.	
Common:	
• Confusion, delirium, rapid heartbeat.	Discontinue. Call doctor right away.
• Nausea, vomiting, less perspiration, drowsiness.	Continue. Call doctor when convenient.
• Constipation.	Continue. Tell doctor at next visit.
• Dry ears, nose, throat.	No action necessary.
Infrequent:	
• Unusual excitement, irritability, restlessness, clumsiness, hallucinations.	Discontinue. Call doctor right away.
• Headache, increased sensitivity to light, painful or difficult urination.	Continue. Call doctor when convenient.
Rare:	
• Shortness of breath.	Discontinue. Seek emergency treatment.
• Rash or hives; eye pain; blurred vision; sore throat, fever, mouth sores; abdominal pain.	Discontinue. Call doctor right away.
• Dizziness.	Continue. Call doctor when convenient.

WARNINGS & PRECAUTIONS

Don't take if:
- You are allergic to any anticholinergic.
- You have trouble with stomach bloating.
- You have difficulty emptying your bladder completely.
- You have narrow-angle glaucoma.
- You have severe ulcerative colitis.

Before you start, consult your doctor:
- If you have open-angle glaucoma.
- If you have angina.
- If you have chronic bronchitis or asthma.
- If you have liver disease.
- If you have hiatal hernia.
- If you have enlarged prostate.
- If you have myasthenia gravis.
- If you have peptic ulcer.
- If you will have surgery within 2 months, including dental surgery, requiring general or spinal anesthesia.

Over age 60:
Adverse reactions and side effects, particularly mental confusion, may be more frequent and severe than in younger persons.

Pregnancy:
Consult doctor. Risk category B (see page xviii).

Breast-feeding:
Drug passes into milk. Avoid drug or discontinue nursing until you finish medicine. Consult doctor for advice on maintaining milk supply.

Infants & children:
Use only under medical supervision.

Prolonged use:
Chronic constipation, possible fecal impaction. Consult doctor immediately.

Skin & sunlight:
No problems expected.

Driving, piloting or hazardous work:
Use disqualifies you for piloting aircraft. Don't drive until you learn how medicine affects you. Don't work around dangerous machinery. Don't climb ladders or work in high places. Danger increases if you drink alcohol or take medicine affecting alertness and reflexes, such as antihistamines, tranquilizers, sedatives, pain medicine, narcotics and mind-altering drugs.

Discontinuing:
May be unnecessary to finish medicine. Follow doctor's instructions.

Others:
No problems expected.

POSSIBLE INTERACTION WITH OTHER DRUGS

GENERIC NAME OR DRUG CLASS	COMBINED EFFECT
Antimuscarinics*	Increased effect of flavoxate.
Central nervous system (CNS) depressants, other*	Increased effect of both drugs.
Clozapine	Toxic effect on the central nervous system.
Ethinamate	Dangerous increased effects of ethinamate. Avoid combining.
Fluoxetine	Increased depressant effects of both drugs.
Guanfacine	May increase depressant effects of either drug.
Leucovorin	High alcohol content of leucovorin may cause adverse effects.
Methyprylon	Increased sedative effect, perhaps to dangerous level. Avoid.
Nabilone	Greater depression of central nervous system.
Nizatidine	Increased nizatidine effect.
Sertraline	Increased depressive effects of both drugs.

POSSIBLE INTERACTION WITH OTHER SUBSTANCES

INTERACTS WITH	COMBINED EFFECT
Alcohol:	None expected.
Beverages:	None expected.
Cocaine:	Excessively rapid heartbeat. Avoid.
Foods:	None expected.
Marijuana:	Drowsiness, dry mouth.
Tobacco:	None expected.

*See Glossary

FLECAINIDE ACETATE

BRAND NAMES

Tambocor

BASIC INFORMATION

Habit forming? No
Prescription needed? Yes
Available as generic? No
Drug class: Antiarrhythmic

USES

Stabilizes irregular heartbeat.

DOSAGE & USAGE INFORMATION

How to take:
Tablet—Swallow with liquid. If you can't swallow whole, crumble tablet and take with liquid or food.

When to take:
At the same time each day, according to instructions on prescription label. Take tablets approximately 12 hours apart.

If you forget a dose:
Take as soon as you remember up to 4 hours late. If more than 4 hours, wait for next scheduled dose (don't double this dose).

What drug does:
Decreases conduction of abnormal electrical activity in the heart muscle or its regulating systems.

Continued next column

OVERDOSE

SYMPTOMS:
Low blood pressure or unconsciousness, irregular or rapid heartbeat, sleepiness, tremor, sweating.

WHAT TO DO:
- **Dial 911 (emergency) for an ambulance or medical help or poison center 1-800-222-1222. Then give first aid immediately.**
- **If patient is unconscious and not breathing, give mouth-to-mouth breathing. If there is no heartbeat, use cardiac massage and mouth-to-mouth breathing (CPR). Don't try to make patient vomit. If you can't get help quickly, take patient to nearest emergency facility.**
- **See emergency information on inside covers.**

Time lapse before drug works:
1 to 6 hours. May need doses daily for 2 to 3 days for maximum effect.

Don't take with:
Any other medicine without consulting your doctor or pharmacist.

POSSIBLE ADVERSE REACTIONS OR SIDE EFFECTS

SYMPTOMS	WHAT TO DO
Life-threatening:	
In case of overdose, see previous column.	
Common:	
Blurred vision, dizziness.	Continue. Call doctor when convenient.
Infrequent:	
• Chest pain, irregular heartbeat.	Discontinue. Seek emergency treatment.
• Shakiness, rash, nausea, vomiting.	Continue, but call doctor right away.
• Anxiety; depression; weakness; headache; appetite loss; weakness in muscles, bones, joints; swollen feet, ankles or legs; loss of taste; numbness or tingling in hands or feet, abdominal pain.	Continue. Call doctor when convenient.
• Constipation.	Continue. Tell doctor at next visit.
Rare:	
• Shortness of breath.	Discontinue. Seek emergency treatment.
• Sore throat, jaundice, fever.	Continue, but call doctor right away.

WARNINGS & PRECAUTIONS

Don't take if:
You are allergic to flecainide or a local anesthetic such as novocaine, xylocaine or other drug whose generic name ends with "caine."

Before you start, consult your doctor:
- If you have kidney disease.
- If you have liver disease.
- If you have had a heart attack in past 3 weeks.
- If you have a pacemaker.

Over age 60:
Adverse reactions and side effects may be more frequent and severe than in younger persons.

Pregnancy:
Decide with your doctor whether drug benefits justify risk to unborn child. Risk category C (see page xviii).

Breast-feeding:
Drug passes into milk. Avoid drug or discontinue nursing until you finish medicine. Consult doctor for advice on maintaining milk supply.

Infants & children:
Not recommended. Safety and dosage have not been established.

Prolonged use:
Talk to your doctor about the need for follow-up medical examinations or laboratory studies to check complete blood counts (white blood cell count, platelet count, red blood cell count, hemoglobin, hematocrit), ECG*.

Skin & sunlight:
No problems expected.

Driving, piloting or hazardous work:
Don't drive or pilot aircraft until you learn how medicine affects you. Don't work around dangerous machinery. Don't climb ladders or work in high places. Danger increases if you drink alcohol or take medicine affecting alertness and reflexes, such as antihistamines, tranquilizers, sedatives, pain medicine, narcotics and mind-altering drugs.

Discontinuing:
Don't discontinue without consulting doctor. Dose may require gradual reduction if you have taken drug for a long time. Doses of other drugs may also require adjustment.

Others:
Wear identification bracelet or carry an identification card with inscription of medicine you take.

POSSIBLE INTERACTION WITH OTHER DRUGS

GENERIC NAME OR DRUG CLASS	COMBINED EFFECT
Antacids* (high dose)	Possible increased flecainide acetate effect.
Antiarrhythmics, other*	Possible irregular heartbeat.
Beta-adrenergic blocking agents*	Possible decreased efficiency of heart muscle contraction, leading to congestive heart failure.
Bone marrow depressants*	Possible decreased production of blood cells in bone marrow.
Carbonic anhydrase inhibitors*	Possible increased flecainide acetate effect.
Cimetidine	Increased effect of flecainide.
Digitalis preparations*	Possible increased digitalis effect. Possible irregular heartbeat.
Disopyramide	Possible decreased efficiency of heart muscle contraction, leading to congestive heart failure.
Doxepin (topical)	Increased risk of toxicity of both drugs.
Nicardipine	Possible increased effect and toxicity of each drug.
Paroxetine	Increased effect of both drugs.
Propafenone	Increased effect of both drugs and increased risk of toxicity.
Sodium bicarbonate	Possible increased flecainide acetate effect.
Verapamil	Possible decreased efficiency of heart muscle contraction, leading to congestive heart failure.

POSSIBLE INTERACTION WITH OTHER SUBSTANCES

INTERACTS WITH	COMBINED EFFECT
Alcohol:	May further depress normal heart function.
Beverages: Caffeine-containing beverages.	Possible decreased flecainide effect.
Cocaine:	Possible decreased flecainide effect.
Foods:	None expected.
Marijuana:	Possible decreased flecainide effect.
Tobacco:	Possible decreased flecainide effect.

FLUOROQUINOLONES

GENERIC AND BRAND NAMES

CIPROFLOXACIN
Cipro
ENOXACIN
Penetrex
GATIFLOXACIN
Tequin
LEVOFLOXACIN
Levaquin
LOMEFLOXACIN
Maxaquin
MOXIFLOXACIN
Avelox
Noroxin
OFLOXACIN
Floxin
SPARFLOXACIN
Zagam
TROVAFLOXACIN
Trovan

BASIC INFORMATION

Habit forming? No
Prescription needed? Yes
Available as generic? No
Drug class: Antibacterial

USES

- Treats a wide range of bacteria that may cause diarrhea, pneumonia, skin and soft tissue infections, urinary tract infections, conjunctivitis, bone infections.
- Treatment for specific agents that could be used in biologic warfare.

DOSAGE & USAGE INFORMATION

How to take:
- Tablets—Take with full glass of water. Take enoxacin and ofloxacin on an empty stomach. Other fluoroquinolones may be taken with or without meals.
- Oral suspension—Take as directed on label.

Continued next column

OVERDOSE

SYMPTOMS:
Confusion and hallucinations, headache, abdominal pain, convulsions.
WHAT TO DO:
- **Dial 911 (emergency) for an ambulance or medical help or poison center 1-800-222-1222. Then give first aid immediately.**
- **If patient is unconscious and not breathing, give mouth-to-mouth breathing. If there is no heartbeat, use cardiac massage and mouth-to-mouth breathing (CPR). Don't try to make patient vomit. If you can't get help quickly, take patient to nearest emergency facility.**
- **See emergency information on inside covers.**

When to take:
As directed by your doctor.

If you forget a dose:
Take as soon as you remember up to 2 hours late. If more than 2 hours, wait for next scheduled dose (don't double this dose).

What drug does:
Destroys bacteria in the body, probably by promoting DNA breakage in germs.

Time lapse before drug works:
1 to 2 weeks for most infections, but some infections may take 6 weeks or more for cure.

Don't take with:
Any other medicine without consulting your doctor or pharmacist.

POSSIBLE ADVERSE REACTIONS OR SIDE EFFECTS

SYMPTOMS	WHAT TO DO
Life-threatening:	
Hives, rash, intense itching, faintness soon after a dose (anaphylaxis).	Seek emergency treatment immediately.
Common:	
• Sparfloxacin may cause fainting, slow irregular heart rate.	Discontinue. Call doctor right away.
• Mild stomach discomfort, nausea, dizziness, drowsiness, nervousness, insomnia, headache, vaginal discharge or pain, lightheadedness, mild diarrhea.	Continue. Call doctor when convenient.
Infrequent:	
Skin (itching, red, blisters, burning, rash, swelling, peeling).	Discontinue. Call doctor right away.
Rare:	
• Abdominal pain or cramps or tenderness, agitation, confusion, hallucinations, tremors, shortness of breath, sweating, swelling (neck, face, calves or legs), pale stools, bloody or dark or cloudy urine, joint or calf pain, diarrhea, tired or weak feeling, tendon problems (inflammation, pain, rupture), yellow eyes or skin, seizures, fast or irregular heartbeat, vomiting, fever.	Discontinue. Call doctor right away.

• Appetite loss, dreams abnormal, muscle or back pain, skin sensitive to sun, sore mouth or tongue, vision problems, vaginal infection, taste changes, flushing.	Continue. Call doctor when convenient.

WARNINGS & PRECAUTIONS

Don't take if:
You are allergic to fluoroquinolones or quinolone derivatives.

Before you start, consult your doctor:
- If you have any disorder of the central nervous system such as epilepsy or stroke.
- If you have had sun sensitivity or tendinitis.
- If you have diabetes or liver, kidney or heart disease.

Over age 60:
No special problems expected.

Pregnancy:
Decide with your doctor if drug benefits justify risk to unborn child. Risk category C (see page xviii).

Breast-feeding:
Drug passes into milk. Avoid drug or discontinue nursing until you finish medicine. Consult doctor for advice on maintaining milk supply.

Infants & children:
Normally not recommended for ages under 18.

Prolonged use:
Usually not prescribed for long-term use.

Skin & sunlight:
One or more drugs in this group may cause rash or intensify sunburn in areas exposed to sun or ultraviolet light (photosensitivity reaction). Avoid overexposure. Notify doctor if reaction occurs.

Driving, piloting or hazardous work:
Don't drive or pilot aircraft until you learn how medicine affects you. Don't work around dangerous machinery. Don't climb ladders or work in high places. Danger increases if you drink alcohol or take medicine affecting alertness and reflexes.

Discontinuing:
Don't discontinue without consulting doctor or completing prescribed dosage. Call doctor if symptoms occur after you stop drug (such as stomach cramps, fever, swelling, calf pain, diarrhea that is watery or bloody).

Others:
- Serious liver problems associated with use of trovafloxacin; can lead to liver transplantation and/or death. Close medical supervision a must.
- May affect accuracy of laboratory test.
- Avoid strenuous exercise. If tendon problems develop, rest and refrain from exercise.
- Drink plenty of fluids while taking drug.
- Advise any doctor or dentist whom you consult that you take this medicine.

POSSIBLE INTERACTION WITH OTHER DRUGS

GENERIC NAME OR DRUG CLASS	COMBINED EFFECT
Aminophylline	Increased effect of aminophylline.
Antacids*	Decreased fluoroquinolone effect.
Antidiabetic agents*	Adverse diabetic reactions.
Anti-inflammatory drugs, nonsteroidal (NSAID's)*	Increased risk of central nervous system problems.
Caffeine	Increased risk of central nervous system problems.
Calcium supplements	Decreased fluoroquinolone effect.
Citrates	Decreased trovafloxacin effect.

Continued on page 913

POSSIBLE INTERACTION WITH OTHER SUBSTANCES

INTERACTS WITH	COMBINED EFFECT
Alcohol:	Increased possibility of central nervous system side effects.
Beverages: Caffeine drinks.	Increased effect of caffeine. Don't use with enoxacin.
Cocaine:	Increased possibility of central nervous system side effects.
Foods: Dairy foods.	Decreased effect of fluoroquinolone.
Marijuana:	Increased possibility of central nervous system side effects.
Tobacco:	Increased possibility of central nervous system side effects.

***See Glossary**

FLUOROURACIL (Topical)

BRAND NAMES

5-FU
Efudex
Fluoroplex

BASIC INFORMATION

Habit forming? No
Prescription needed? Yes
Available as generic? No
Drug class: Antineoplastic (topical)

USES

- Treats precancerous actinic keratoses on skin.
- Treats superficial basal cell carcinomas (skin cancers that don't spread to distant organs and, therefore, do not threaten life).

DOSAGE & USAGE INFORMATION

How to use:
- Apply with cotton-tipped applicator.
- Cream, lotion, ointment—Bathe and dry area before use. Apply small amount and rub gently.
- Wash hands (if fingertips are used to apply) after applying medicine to other parts of body.

When to use:
Once or twice a day or as directed by doctor.

If you forget a dose:
Apply as soon as you remember. Resume basic schedule.

What drug does:
Selectively destroys actively proliferating cells.

Time lapse before drug works:
2 to 3 days.

Don't use with:
Other topical medications unless prescribed by your doctor.

OVERDOSE

SYMPTOMS:
None expected.
WHAT TO DO:
Not for internal use. If child accidentally swallows, call poison center 1-800-222-1222.

POSSIBLE ADVERSE REACTIONS OR SIDE EFFECTS

SYMPTOMS	WHAT TO DO
Life-threatening	
None expected.	
Common	
• Skin redness or swelling.	Discontinue. Call doctor right away.
• After 1 or 2 weeks of use—Skin itching or oozing; rash, tenderness, soreness.	Continue. Call doctor when convenient.
Infrequent	
Skin darkening or scaling.	Continue. Call doctor when convenient.
Rare	
Watery eyes.	Discontinue. Call doctor right away.

WARNINGS & PRECAUTIONS

Don't use if:
You are allergic to fluorouracil.

Before you start, consult your doctor:
- If you have cloasma or acne rosacea.
- If you have any other skin problems.

Over age 60:
No problems expected.

Pregnancy:
Consult doctor. Risk category X (see page xviii).

Breast-feeding:
Avoid drug or discontinue nursing until you finish medicine. Consult doctor for advice on maintaining milk supply.

Infants & children:
No problems expected, but check with doctor.

Prolonged use:
No problems expected, but check with doctor.

Skin & sunlight:
May cause rash or intensify sunburn in areas exposed to sun or ultraviolet light (photosensitivity reaction). Avoid overexposure. Notify doctor if reaction occurs.

Driving, piloting or hazardous work:
No problems expected, but check with doctor.

Discontinuing:
Pink, smooth area remains after treatment (usually fades in 1 to 2 months).

Others:
- Skin lesions may need biopsy before treatment.
- Keep medicine out of eyes or mouth.
- Heat and moisture in bathroom medicine cabinet can cause breakdown of medicine. Store someplace else.

POSSIBLE INTERACTION WITH OTHER DRUGS

GENERIC NAME OR DRUG CLASS	COMBINED EFFECT
None significant.	

POSSIBLE INTERACTION WITH OTHER SUBSTANCES

INTERACTS WITH	COMBINED EFFECT
Alcohol:	None expected.
Beverages:	None expected.
Cocaine:	None expected.
Foods:	None expected.
Marijuana:	None expected.
Tobacco:	None expected.

FOLIC ACID (Vitamin B-9)

BRAND NAMES

Apo-Folic
Folvite
Novo-Folacid
Numerous other multiple vitamin-mineral supplements. Check labels.

BASIC INFORMATION

Habit forming? No
Prescription needed?
High strength: Yes
Vitamin mixtures: No
Available as generic? Yes
Drug class: Vitamin supplement

USES

- Dietary supplement to promote normal growth, development and good health.
- Dietary supplement during pregnancy to prevent spinal defects.
- Treatment for anemias due to folic acid deficiency occurring from alcoholism, liver disease, hemolytic anemia, sprue, infants on artificial formula, pregnancy, breast feeding and use of oral contraceptives.
- Some studies have found that folic acid supplementation alone or in combination with other vitamins taken before conception and during early pregnancy may reduce the incidence of neural tube defects in infants.

DOSAGE & USAGE INFORMATION

How to take:
Tablet—Swallow with liquid or food to lessen stomach irritation. If you can't swallow whole, crumble tablet and take with liquid or food.

When to take:
At the same time each day.

If you forget a dose:
Take when you remember. Don't double next dose. Resume regular schedule.

What drug does:
Essential to normal red blood cell formation.

Continued next column

OVERDOSE

SYMPTOMS:
None expected.
WHAT TO DO:
Overdose unlikely to threaten life. If child accidentally swallows, call poison center 1-800-222-1222.

Time lapse before drug works:
Not determined.

Don't take with:
Any other medicine without consulting your doctor or pharmacist.

POSSIBLE ADVERSE REACTIONS OR SIDE EFFECTS

SYMPTOMS	WHAT TO DO
Life-threatening:	
None expected.	
Common:	
Large dose may produce yellow urine.	Continue. Tell doctor at next visit.
Infrequent:	
None expected.	
Rare:	
Rash, itching, bronchospasm.	Discontinue. Call doctor right away.

FOLIC ACID (Vitamin B-9)

WARNINGS & PRECAUTIONS

Don't take if:
You are allergic to any B vitamin.

Before you start, consult your doctor:
- If you have liver disease.
- If you have pernicious anemia. (Folic acid corrects anemia, but nerve damage of pernicious anemia continues.)

Over age 60:
No problems expected.

Pregnancy:
No problems expected. Consult doctor. Risk category A (see page xviii).

Breast-feeding:
No problems expected. Consult doctor.

Infants & children:
No problems expected.

Prolonged use:
No problems expected.

Skin & sunlight:
No problems expected.

Driving, piloting or hazardous work:
No problems expected.

Discontinuing:
Don't discontinue without doctor's advice until you complete prescribed dose, even though symptoms diminish or disappear.

Others:
- Folic acid removed by kidney dialysis. Dialysis patients should increase intake to 300% of RDA or take as directed.
- A balanced diet should provide all the folic acid a healthy person needs and make supplements unnecessary. Best sources are green, leafy vegetables; fruits; liver and kidney.

POSSIBLE INTERACTION WITH OTHER DRUGS

GENERIC NAME OR DRUG CLASS	COMBINED EFFECT
Analgesics*	Decreased effect of folic acid.
Anticonvulsants, hydantoin*	Decreased effect of folic acid. Possible increased seizure frequency.
Chloramphenicol	Possible decreased folic acid effect.
Contraceptives, oral*	Decreased effect of folic acid.
Cortisone drugs*	Decreased effect of folic acid.
Methotrexate	Decreased effect of folic acid.
Para-aminosalicylic acid (PAS)	Decreased effect of folic acid.
Pyrimethamine	Decreased effect of folic acid.
Sulfasalazine	Decreased dietary absorption of folic acid.
Triamterene	Decreased effect of folic acid.
Trimethoprim	Decreased effect of folic acid.
Zinc supplements	Increased need for zinc.

POSSIBLE INTERACTION WITH OTHER SUBSTANCES

INTERACTS WITH	COMBINED EFFECT
Alcohol:	None expected.
Beverages:	None expected.
Cocaine:	None expected.
Foods:	None expected.
Marijuana:	None expected.
Tobacco:	None expected.

***See Glossary**

FURAZOLIDONE

BRAND NAMES

Furoxone
Furoxone Liquid

BASIC INFORMATION

Habit forming? No
Prescription needed? Yes
Available as generic? No
Drug class: Antiprotozoal, antibacterial (antibiotic)

USES

- As an adjunct in treating most germs that infect the gastrointestinal tract such as cholera, salmonellosis, E. coli, proteus infections, and other bacterial causes of diarrhea.
- Treats giardiasis.

DOSAGE & USAGE INFORMATION

How to take:
- Liquid—Use a measuring spoon to ensure correct dose.
- Tablet—Swallow with liquid or food to lessen stomach irritation. If you can't swallow whole, crumble tablet and take with liquid or food.

When to take:
At the same time each day, according to instructions on prescription label.

If you forget a dose:
Take as soon as you remember up to 2 hours late. If more than 2 hours, wait for next scheduled dose. Don't double this dose.

What drug does:
Kills microscopic germs.

Time lapse before drug works:
Immediate.

Don't take with:
Any other medicine without consulting your doctor or pharmacist.

OVERDOSE

SYMPTOMS:
None expected.
WHAT TO DO:
Overdose unlikely to threaten life. If person takes much larger amount than prescribed, call doctor, poison center 1-800-222-1222 or hospital emergency room for instructions.

POSSIBLE ADVERSE REACTIONS OR SIDE EFFECTS

SYMPTOMS	WHAT TO DO
Life-threatening: None expected except when taken with forbidden foods (see Possible Interaction with Other Substances).	
Common:	
• Nausea, vomiting.	Continue. Call doctor when convenient.
• Dark yellow or brown urine.	No action necessary.
Infrequent:	
• Abdominal pain.	Discontinue. Call doctor right away.
• Headache.	Continue. Call doctor when convenient.
Rare:	
Sore throat, fever, skin rash, itching, joint pain.	Discontinue. Call doctor right away.

WARNINGS & PRECAUTIONS

Don't take if:
- You have G6PD* deficiency.
- You have hypersensitivity to furazolidone, nitrofurantoin (Furadantin), or nitrofurazone (Furacin).

Before you start, consult your doctor:
If you are taking any other prescription or nonprescription medicine.

Over age 60:
No special problems expected.

Pregnancy:
Decide with your doctor if drug benefits justify risk to unborn child. Risk category C (see page xviii).

Breast-feeding:
Drug may pass into milk. Avoid drug or discontinue nursing until you finish medicine. Consult doctor for advice on maintaining milk supply.

Infants & children:
Don't use for infants without specific instructions from your doctor.

Prolonged use:
No special problems expected.

Skin & sunlight:
No special problems expected.

Driving, piloting or hazardous work:
No special problems expected.

Discontinuing:
Food restrictions outlined in Possible Interaction with Other Substances must be continued for at least 2 weeks after furazolidone is discontinued.

Others:
- Should not be taken with foods or drinks high in tyramine (see Possible Interaction with Other Substances).
- Advise any doctor or dentist whom you consult that you take this medicine.

POSSIBLE INTERACTION WITH OTHER DRUGS

GENERIC NAME OR DRUG CLASS	COMBINED EFFECT
Antidepressants, tricyclic*	Sudden, severe increase in blood pressure.
Monoamine oxidase (MAO) inhibitors*	Sudden, severe increase in blood pressure.
Sumatriptan	Adverse effects unknown. Avoid.
Sympathomimetics*	Sudden, severe increase in blood pressure.

POSSIBLE INTERACTION WITH OTHER SUBSTANCES

INTERACTS WITH	COMBINED EFFECT
Alcohol:	Flushed face, shortness of breath, fever, tightness in chest. Avoid.
Beverages: Any alcoholic beverage.	Flushed face, shortness of breath, fever, tightness in chest. Avoid.
Cocaine:	High blood pressure. Avoid.
Foods: Aged cheese; dark beer; red wine (especially Chianti); sherry; liqueurs; caviar; yeast or protein extracts; fava beans; smoked or pickled meat, poultry, fish; pepperoni, salami, summer sausage; over-ripe fruit.	Sudden, severe high blood pressure that may be life-threatening. Avoid.
Marijuana:	High blood pressure. Avoid.
Tobacco:	No special problems expected.

***See Glossary**

GABAPENTIN

BRAND NAMES

Neurontin

BASIC INFORMATION

Habit forming? No
Prescription needed? Yes
Available as generic? No
Drug class: Anticonvulsant, antiepileptic

USES

Treatment for partial (focal) epileptic seizures. Used in combination with other antiepileptic drugs.

DOSAGE & USAGE INFORMATION

How to take:
Capsule–Swallow with liquid. May be taken with or without food.

When to take:
Your doctor will determine the best schedule. Dosages will be increased rapidly over the first 3 days of use. Further increases may be necessary to achieve maximum benefits.

If you forget a dose:
Take as soon as you remember. If it is almost time for the next dose, skip the missed dose and wait for your next scheduled dose (don't double this dose).

What drug does:
The exact mechanism is unknown. The anticonvulsant action may result from an altered transport of brain amino acids. Amino acids play an important part in chemical reactions within the cells.

Time lapse before drug works:
May take several weeks for effectiveness.

Don't take with:
Any other prescription or nonprescription drug without consulting your doctor.

OVERDOSE

SYMPTOMS:
Double vision, slurred speech, drowsiness, tiredness, diarrhea.
WHAT TO DO:
Overdose unlikely to threaten life. If person takes much larger amount than prescribed, call doctor, poison center 1-800-222-1222 or hospital emergency room for instructions.

POSSIBLE ADVERSE REACTIONS OR SIDE EFFECTS

SYMPTOMS	WHAT TO DO
Life-threatening: None expected.	
Common: Sleepiness, dizziness, fatigue, clumsiness, lack of coordination.	Continue. Call doctor when convenient.
Infrequent: Rapid eye movement (nystagmus), double or blurred vision.	Continue. Call doctor when convenient.
Rare: Rash; nervousness; depression; twitching or swelling in hands, feet or legs; runny nose; dry or sore throat; nausea; vomiting, coughing; dry mouth; constipation; impotence; increased appetite, weight gain; muscle or back ache; forgetfulness; indigestion.	Continue. Call doctor when convenient.

WARNINGS & PRECAUTIONS

Don't take if:
You are allergic to gabapentin.

Before you start, consult your doctor:
If you have kidney disease.

Over age 60:
No special problems expected.

Pregnancy:
Decide with your doctor if drug benefits justify risks to unborn child. Risk category C (see page xviii).

Breast-feeding:
It is unknown if drug passes into milk. Consult your doctor.

Infants & children:
Not recommended for children under age 12.

Prolonged use:
No special problems expected. Follow-up laboratory blood studies may be recommended by your doctor.

Skin & sunlight:
No problems expected.

Driving, piloting or hazardous work:
Don't drive or pilot aircraft until you learn how medicine affects you. Don't work around dangerous machinery. Don't climb ladders or work in high places. Danger increases if you drink alcohol or take other medicines affecting alertness and reflexes such as antihistamines, tranquilizers, sedatives, pain medicine, narcotics and mind-altering drugs.

Discontinuing:
Don't discontinue without doctor's approval due to risk of increased seizure activity.

Others:
- Advise any doctor or dentist whom you consult that you take this medicine.
- Side effects of gabapentin are usually mild to moderate. Because it is normally used with other anticonvulsant drugs, additional side effects may also occur. If they do, discuss them with your doctor.

POSSIBLE INTERACTION WITH OTHER DRUGS

GENERIC NAME OR DRUG CLASS	COMBINED EFFECT
Antacids*	Allow at least 2 hours between the 2 drugs.

POSSIBLE INTERACTION WITH OTHER SUBSTANCES

INTERACTS WITH	COMBINED EFFECT
Alcohol:	None expected.
Beverages:	None expected.
Cocaine:	None expected.
Foods:	None expected.
Marijuana:	None expected.
Tobacco:	None expected.

***See Glossary**

GEMFIBROZIL

BRAND NAMES

Lopid

BASIC INFORMATION

Habit forming? No
Prescription needed? Yes
Available as generic? Yes
Drug class: Antihyperlipidemic

USES

Reduces fatty substances in the blood (triglycerides) and raises high-density lipoprotein (HDL) cholesterol levels.

DOSAGE & USAGE INFORMATION

How to take:
Tablet or capsule—Swallow with liquid or food to lessen stomach irritation.

When to take:
Take 30 minutes before morning and evening meals.

If you forget a dose:
Take as soon as you remember up to 2 hours late. If more than 2 hours, wait for next scheduled dose (don't double this dose).

What drug does:
Inhibits formation of fatty substances.

Time lapse before drug works:
3 months or more.

Don't take with:
Any other medicine without consulting your doctor or pharmacist.

OVERDOSE

SYMPTOMS:
Diarrhea, headache, muscle pain.
WHAT TO DO:
Overdose unlikely to threaten life. If person takes much larger amount than prescribed, call doctor, poison center 1-800-222-1222 or hospital emergency room for instructions.

POSSIBLE ADVERSE REACTIONS OR SIDE EFFECTS

SYMPTOMS	WHAT TO DO
Life-threatening:	
None expected.	
Common:	
Indigestion.	Continue. Call doctor when convenient.
Infrequent:	
Chest pain, shortness of breath, irregular heartbeat, nausea, vomiting, diarrhea, stomach pain.	Discontinue. Call doctor right away.
Rare:	
• Rash, itch; sores in mouth, on lips; sore throat; swollen feet, legs; blood in urine; painful urination; fever; chills.	Discontinue. Call doctor right away.
• Dizziness, headache, drowsiness, muscle cramps, dry skin, backache, unusual tiredness, decreased sex drive.	Continue. Call doctor when convenient.

WARNINGS & PRECAUTIONS

Don't take if:
You are allergic to any antihyperlipidemic.

Before you start, consult your doctor:
- If you have had liver or kidney disease.
- If you have gallstones or gallbladder disease.
- If you have had peptic-ulcer disease.
- If you have diabetes.

Over age 60:
Adverse reactions and side effects may be more frequent and severe than in younger persons.

Pregnancy:
Decide with your doctor if drug benefits justify risks to unborn child. Risk category C (see page xviii).

Breast-feeding:
It is not known if drug passes into milk. Avoid drug or discontinue nursing until you finish medicine. Consult doctor for advice on maintaining milk supply.

Infants & children:
Not recommended.

Prolonged use:
Periodic blood cell counts and liver function studies recommended if you take gemfibrozil for a long time.

Skin & sunlight:
No problems expected.

Driving, piloting or hazardous work:
Avoid if you feel drowsy or dizzy. Otherwise, no problems expected.

Discontinuing:
Don't discontinue without doctor's advice until you complete prescribed dose.

Others:
- Some studies question effectiveness. Many studies warn against toxicity.
- May affect results in some medical tests.

POSSIBLE INTERACTION WITH OTHER DRUGS

GENERIC NAME OR DRUG CLASS	COMBINED EFFECT
Anticoagulants, oral*	Increased anti-coagulant effect. Dose reduction of anticoagulant necessary.
Antidiabetics, oral*	Increased antidiabetic effect.
Contraceptives, oral*	Decreased gemfibrozil effect.
Dexfenfluramine	May require dosage change as weight loss occurs.
Estrogens*	Decreased gemfibrozil effect.
Furosemide	Possible toxicity of both drugs.
HMG-CoA reductase inhibitors	Increased risk of muscle inflammation and kidney failure.
Insulin	Increased insulin effect.
Lovastatin	Increased risk of kidney problems.
Thyroid hormones*	Increased gemfibrozil effect.

POSSIBLE INTERACTION WITH OTHER SUBSTANCES

INTERACTS WITH	COMBINED EFFECT
Alcohol:	None expected.
Beverages:	None expected.
Cocaine:	Decreased effect of gemfibrozil. Avoid.
Foods: Fatty foods.	Decreased gemfibrozil effect.
Marijuana:	None expected.
Tobacco:	Decreased gemfibrozil absorption. Avoid.

*See Glossary

GLUCAGON

BRAND NAMES

Glucagon for Injection

BASIC INFORMATION

Habit forming? No
Prescription needed? Yes
Available as generic? Yes
Drug class: Antihypoglycemic, diagnostic aid

USES

- Treats low blood sugar (hypoglycemia) in diabetics.
- Used as antidote for overdose of beta-adrenergic blockers, quinidine and tricyclic antidepressants.

DOSAGE & USAGE INFORMATION

How to take:
Injection—As directed by your doctor.

When to take:
When there are signs of low blood sugar (anxiety; chills; cool, pale skin; hunger; nausea; tremors; sweating; weakness; stomach pain; confusion; drowsiness; fast heartbeat; continuing headache; unsteady walk; unusual tiredness or weakness; vision changes; unconsciousness) in diabetics who don't respond to eating some form of sugar.

If you forget a dose:
Single dose only.

What drug does:
Forces liver to make more sugar and release it into the bloodstream.

Continued next column

OVERDOSE

SYMPTOMS:
Nausea, vomiting, severe weakness, irregular heartbeat, hoarseness, cramps.
WHAT TO DO:
- **Dial 911 (emergency) for an ambulance or medical help or poison center 1-800-222-1222. Then give first aid immediately.**
- **See emergency information on inside covers.**

Time lapse before drug works:
- For hypoglycemic condition—5 to 20 minutes.
- For muscle relaxant—1 to 10 minutes.

Don't take with:
Any other medicines (including over-the-counter drugs such as cough and cold medicines, laxatives, antacids, diet pills, caffeine, nose drops or vitamins) without consulting your doctor.

POSSIBLE ADVERSE REACTIONS OR SIDE EFFECTS

SYMPTOMS	WHAT TO DO
Life-threatening:	
Unconsciousness.	Seek emergency treatment immediately.
Common:	
Nausea.	Continue. Call doctor when convenient.
Infrequent:	
Lightheadedness, breathing difficulty, skin rash.	Discontinue. Call doctor right away.
Rare:	
None expected.	

WARNINGS & PRECAUTIONS

Don't take if:
You can't tolerate glucagon.

Before you start, consult your doctor:
- If you are allergic to beef or pork.
- If you have pheochromocytoma.*

Over age 60:
No special problems expected.

Pregnancy:
No proven harm to unborn child, but avoid if possible. Consult doctor. Risk category B (see page xviii).

Breast-feeding:
No special problems expected. Consult doctor.

Infants & children:
No special problems expected.

Prolonged use:
To be used intermittently and not for prolonged periods.

Skin & sunlight:
No problems expected.

Driving, piloting or hazardous work:
Don't drive or pilot aircraft until you learn how medicine affects you. Don't work around dangerous machinery. Don't climb ladders or work in high places. Danger increases if you drink alcohol or take medicine affecting alertness and reflexes.

Discontinuing:
No special problems expected.

Others:
- May affect results in some medical tests.
- Explain to other family members how to inject glucagon.
- Before injecting, try to eat some form of sugar, such as glucose tablets, corn syrup, honey, orange juice, hard candy or sugar cubes.
- Store unmixed glucagon at room temperature. Store mixed glucagon in refrigerator, but don't freeze. Mixed solution is only good for 48 hours.
- Check expiration date regularly and replace drug before it expires.

POSSIBLE INTERACTION WITH OTHER DRUGS

GENERIC NAME OR DRUG CLASS	COMBINED EFFECT
Anticoagulants*	Increased anticoagulant effect.

POSSIBLE INTERACTION WITH OTHER SUBSTANCES

INTERACTS WITH	COMBINED EFFECT
Alcohol:	Decreased glucagon effect.
Beverages:	None expected.
Cocaine:	Increased adverse reactions.
Foods: Sugar, fruit juice, candy.	Enhances glucagon effect.
Marijuana:	Increased adverse reactions.
Tobacco:	None expected.

***See Glossary**

GLYCOPYRROLATE

BRAND NAMES

Robinul
Robinul Forte

BASIC INFORMATION

Habit forming? No
Prescription needed? Yes
Available as generic? Yes
Drug class: Antispasmodic, anticholinergic

USES

- Reduces spasms of digestive system.
- Reduces production of saliva during dental procedures.
- Treats peptic ulcer by reducing gastric acid secretion.

DOSAGE & USAGE INFORMATION

How to take:
Tablet—Swallow with liquid. If you can't swallow whole, crumble tablet and take with small amount of liquid or food.

When to take:
30 minutes before meals (unless directed otherwise by doctor).

If you forget a dose:
Wait for next scheduled dose (don't double this dose).

What drug does:
Blocks nerve impulses at parasympathetic nerve endings, preventing smooth (involuntary) muscle contractions and gland secretions of organs involved.

Time lapse before drug works:
15 to 30 minutes.

Don't take with:
Any other medicine without consulting your doctor or pharmacist.

OVERDOSE

SYMPTOMS:
Dry mouth, blurred vision, low blood pressure, decreased breathing rate, rapid heartbeat, flushed skin, drowsiness.
WHAT TO DO:
- **Dial 911 (emergency) for an ambulance or medical help or poison center 1-800-222-1222. Then give first aid immediately.**
- **See emergency information on inside covers.**

POSSIBLE ADVERSE REACTIONS OR SIDE EFFECTS

SYMPTOMS	WHAT TO DO
Life-threatening:	
Hives, rash, intense itching, faintness soon after a dose (anaphylaxis).	Seek emergency treatment immediately.
Common:	
Dry mouth, loss of taste, constipation, difficult urination.	Continue. Call doctor when convenient.
Infrequent:	
• Confusion; dizziness; drowsiness; eye pain; headache; rash; sleep disturbance such as nightmares, frequent waking; nausea; vomiting; rapid heartbeat; lightheadedness.	Discontinue. Call doctor right away.
• Insomnia, blurred vision, diminished sex drive, decreased sweating, nasal congestion, altered taste.	Continue. Call doctor when convenient.
Rare:	
Rash, hives.	Discontinue. Call doctor right away.

WARNINGS & PRECAUTIONS

Don't take if:
- You are allergic to any anticholinergic.
- You have trouble with stomach bloating.
- You have difficulty emptying your bladder completely.
- You have narrow-angle glaucoma.
- You have severe ulcerative colitis.

Before you start, consult your doctor:
- If you have open-angle glaucoma.
- If you have angina, chronic bronchitis or asthma, liver disease, hiatal hernia, enlarged prostate, myasthenia gravis, peptic ulcer, kidney or thyroid disease.
- If you will have surgery within 2 months, including dental surgery, requiring general or spinal anesthesia.

Over age 60:
Adverse reactions and side effects may be more frequent and severe than in younger persons.

Pregnancy:
Consult doctor. Risk category B (see page xviii).

Breast-feeding:
Drug passes into milk and decreases milk flow. Avoid drug or discontinue nursing until you finish medicine. Consult doctor for advice on maintaining milk supply.

Infants & children:
Use only under medical supervision.

Prolonged use:
Chronic constipation, possible fecal impaction. Consult doctor immediately.

Skin & sunlight:
No problems expected.

Driving, piloting or hazardous work:
Use disqualifies you for piloting aircraft. Otherwise, no problems expected.

Discontinuing:
May be unnecessary to finish medicine. Follow doctor's instructions.

Others:
- Heatstroke more likely if you become overheated during exertion.
- Advise any doctor or dentist whom you consult that you take this medicine.

POSSIBLE INTERACTION WITH OTHER DRUGS

GENERIC NAME OR DRUG CLASS	COMBINED EFFECT
Adrenocorticoids, systemic	Possible glaucoma.
Antacids*	Decreased glycopyrrolate absorption effect.
Amantadine	Increased glycopyrrolate effect.
Anticholinergics, other*	Increased glycopyrrolate effect.
Antidepressants, tricyclic*	Increased glycopyrrolate effect.
Antidiarrheals*	Decreased glycopyrrolate absorption effect.
Attapulgite	Decreased effect of anticholinergic.
Buclizine	Increased glycopyrrolate effect.
Digitalis	Possible decreased absorption of digitalis.
Haloperidol	Increased internal eye pressure.
Ketoconazole	Decreased ketoconazole effect.
Meperidine	Increased glycopyrrolate effect.
Methylphenidate	Increased anticholinergic effect.
Molindone	Increased nizatidine effect.
Monoamine oxidase (MAO) inhibitors*	Increased glycopyrrolate effect.
Orphenadrine	Increased glycopyrrolate effect
Phenothiazines	Increased glycopyrrolate effect.
Pilocarpine	Increased glycopyrrolate effect. Loss of pilocarpine effect in glaucoma treatment.
Potassium chloride tabs	Increased side effects of potassium tablets.
Quinidine	Increased glycopyrrolate effect.
Retocunazole	Decreased absorption of both.
Sedatives* or central nervous system (CNS) depressants*	Increased sedative effect of both drugs.
Vitamin C	Increased glycopyrrolate effect. Avoid large vitamin C doses.

POSSIBLE INTERACTION WITH OTHER SUBSTANCES

INTERACTS WITH	COMBINED EFFECT
Alcohol:	None expected.
Beverages:	None expected.
Cocaine:	Excessively rapid heartbeat.
Foods:	None exected.
Marijuana:	Drowsiness and dry mouth.
Tobacco:	None expected.

*See Glossary

GOLD COMPOUNDS

GENERIC AND BRAND NAMES

AURANOFIN
Ridaura-Oral

GOLD SODIUM THIOMOLATE
Myocrisin

BASIC INFORMATION

Habit forming? No
Prescription needed? Yes
Available as generic? No
Drug class: Gold compounds

USES

Treatment for rheumatoid arthritis and juvenile arthritis.

DOSAGE & USAGE INFORMATION

How to take:
- Capsules—Swallow with full glass of fluid. Follow prescription directions. Taking too much can cause serious adverse reactions.
- Injections—Under medical supervision.

When to take:
Once or twice daily, morning and night.

If you forget a dose:
Take as soon as you remember up to 6 hours late, then go back to usual schedule.

What drug does:
Modifies disease activity of rheumatoid arthritis by mechanisms not yet understood.

Time lapse before drug works:
3 to 6 months.

Don't take with:
Any other medicine without consulting your doctor or pharmacist.

OVERDOSE

SYMPTOMS:
Confusion, delirium, numbness and tingling in feet and hands.
WHAT TO DO:
- **Induce vomiting with syrup of ipecac if available.**
- **Dial 911 (emergency) for an ambulance or medical help or poison center 1-800-222-1222. Then give first aid immediately.**
- **See emergency information on inside covers.**

POSSIBLE ADVERSE REACTIONS OR SIDE EFFECTS

SYMPTOMS	WHAT TO DO
Life-threatening:	
Hives, rash, intense itching, faintness soon after a dose (anaphylaxis).	Seek emergency treatment immediately.
Common:	
• Itch; hives; sores or white spots in mouth, throat; appetite loss; diarrhea; vomiting; skin rashes; fever.	Discontinue. Call doctor right away.
• Indigestion, constipation.	Continue. Call doctor when convenient.
Infrequent:	
• Excessive fatigue; sore tongue, mouth or gums; metallic or odd taste; unusual bleeding or bruising; blood in urine; vaginal discharge; flushing; fainting; dizziness; sweating after injection.	Discontinue. Call doctor right away.
• Hair loss; pain in muscles, bones and joints (with injections).	Continue. Call doctor when convenient.
Rare:	
• Blood in stool, difficult breathing, coughing, seizures.	Discontinue. Seek emergency treatment.
• Abdominal pain, jaundice, numbness or tingling in hands or feet, muscle weakness.	Discontinue. Call doctor right away.
• "Pink eye."	Continue. Call doctor when convenient.

WARNINGS & PRECAUTIONS

Don't take if:
- You have history of allergy to gold or other metals.
- You have any blood disorder.
- You have kidney disease.

Before you start, consult your doctor:
- If you are pregnant or may become pregnant.
- If you have lupus erythematosus.
- If you have Sjögren's syndrome.
- If you have chronic skin disease.
- If you are debilitated.
- If you have blood dyscrasias.

Over age 60:
Adverse reactions and side effects may be more frequent and severe than in younger persons.

Pregnancy:
Decide with your doctor if drug benefits justify risks to unborn child. Risk category C (see page xviii).

Breast-feeding:
Drug may filter into milk, causing side effects in infants. Avoid. Consult doctor.

Infants & children:
Not recommended. Safety and dosage have not been established.

Prolonged use:
Request periodic laboratory studies of blood counts, urine and liver function. These should be done before use and at least once a month during treatment.

Skin & sunlight:
- One or more drugs in this group may cause rash or intensify sunburn in areas exposed to sun or ultraviolet light (photosensitivity reaction). Avoid overexposure. Notify doctor if reaction occurs.
- Blue-gray pigmentation in skin exposed to sunlight.

Driving, piloting or hazardous work:
Avoid if you have serious adverse reactions or side effects. Otherwise, no problems expected.

Discontinuing:
Don't discontinue without doctor's advice until you complete prescribed dose.

Others:
- Side effects and adverse reactions may appear during treatment or for many months after discontinuing.
- Gold has been shown to cause kidney tumors and kidney cancer in animals given excessive doses.
- May interfere with the accuracy of some medical tests.

POSSIBLE INTERACTION WITH OTHER DRUGS

GENERIC NAME OR DRUG CLASS	COMBINED EFFECT
Bone marrow depressants*	Increased risk of toxicity of both drugs.
Hepatotoxics*	Increased risk of toxicity of both drugs.
Nephrotoxics*	Increased risk of toxicity of both drugs.
Penicillamine	Increased likelihood of kidney damage.
Phenytoin	Increased phenytoin blood levels. Phenytoin dosage may require adjustment.

POSSIBLE INTERACTION WITH OTHER SUBSTANCES

INTERACTS WITH	COMBINED EFFECT
Alcohol:	None expected.
Beverages:	None expected.
Cocaine:	None expected.
Foods:	None expected.
Marijuana:	None expected.
Tobacco:	None expected.

***See Glossary**

GRISEOFULVIN

BRAND NAMES

Fulvicin P/G
Fulvicin U/F
Grifulvin V
Grisactin
Grisactin Ultra
Grisovin-FP
Gris-PEG

BASIC INFORMATION

Habit forming? No
Prescription needed? Yes
Available as generic? Yes
Drug class: Antifungal

USES

Treatment for fungal infections susceptible to griseofulvin.

DOSAGE & USAGE INFORMATION

How to take:

- Tablet or capsule—Swallow with liquid or food to lessen stomach irritation. If you can't swallow whole, crumble tablet or open capsule and take with liquid or food.
- Liquid—Follow label instructions.

When to take:
With or immediately after meals.

If you forget a dose:
Take as soon as you remember up to 2 hours late. If more than 2 hours, wait for next scheduled dose (don't double this dose).

What drug does:
Prevents fungi from growing and reproducing.

Time lapse before drug works:
2 to 10 days for skin infections. 2 to 4 weeks for infections of fingernails or toenails. Complete cure of either may require several months.

Don't take with:
Any other medicine without consulting your doctor or pharmacist.

OVERDOSE

SYMPTOMS:
Nausea, vomiting, diarrhea. In sensitive individuals, severe diarrhea may occur without overdosing.
WHAT TO DO:
Overdose unlikely to threaten life. If person takes much larger amount than prescribed, call doctor, poison center 1-800-222-1222 or hospital emergency room for instructions.

POSSIBLE ADVERSE REACTIONS OR SIDE EFFECTS

SYMPTOMS	WHAT TO DO
Life-threatening: In case of overdose, see previous column.	
Common: Headache.	Continue. Tell doctor at next visit.
Infrequent:	
• Confusion; rash, hives, itch; mouth or tongue irritation; soreness; nausea; vomiting; diarrhea; stomach pain.	Discontinue. Call doctor right away.
• Insomnia, tiredness.	Continue. Call doctor when convenient.
Rare: Sore throat, fever, numbness or tingling in hands or feet, cloudy urine, sensitivity to sunlight, yellow skin or eyes, sensitivity of skin to sunlight (these symptoms are more likely to occur with high doses taken for long periods).	Discontinue. Call doctor right away.

WARNINGS & PRECAUTIONS

Don't take if:
- You are allergic to any antifungal medicine.
- You are allergic to penicillin.
- You have liver disease.
- You have porphyria.
- The infection is minor and will respond to less potent drugs.

Before you start, consult your doctor:
- If you plan to become pregnant within medication period.
- If you have liver disease.
- If you have lupus.

Over age 60:
Adverse reactions and side effects may be more frequent and severe than in younger persons.

Pregnancy:
Risk to unborn child outweighs drug benefits. Don't use. Risk category X (see page xviii).

Breast-feeding:
No problems expected, but consult your doctor.

Infants & children:
Not recommended for children younger than 2.

Prolonged use:
- You may become susceptible to infections caused by germs not responsive to griseofulvin.
- Talk to your doctor about the need for follow-up medical examinations or laboratory studies to check complete blood counts (white blood cell count, platelet count, red blood cell count, hemoglobin, hematocrit), liver function, kidney function.

Skin & sunlight:
May cause rash or intensify sunburn in areas exposed to sun or ultraviolet light (photosensitivity reaction). Avoid overexposure. Notify doctor if reaction occurs.

Driving, piloting or hazardous work:
Don't drive or pilot aircraft until you learn how medicine affects you. Don't work around dangerous machinery. Don't climb ladders or work in high places. Danger increases if you drink alcohol or take medicine affecting alertness and reflexes.

Discontinuing:
Don't discontinue without doctor's advice until you complete prescribed dose, even though symptoms diminish or disappear.

Others:
- Periodic laboratory blood studies and liver and kidney function tests recommended.
- Advise any doctor or dentist whom you consult that you take this medicine.

POSSIBLE INTERACTION WITH OTHER DRUGS

GENERIC NAME OR DRUG CLASS	COMBINED EFFECT
Anticoagulants, oral*	Decreased anti-anticoagulant effect.
Barbiturates*	Decreased griseofulvin effect.
Contraceptives, oral*	Decreased contraceptive effect.
Photosensitizing medications*	Increased sun hazard.

POSSIBLE INTERACTION WITH OTHER SUBSTANCES

INTERACTS WITH	COMBINED EFFECT
Alcohol:	Increased intoxication. Possible disulfiram reaction.*
Beverages:	None expected.
Cocaine:	None expected.
Foods:	None expected, but foods high in fat will improve drug absorption.
Marijuana:	None expected.
Tobacco:	None expected.

*See Glossary

GUAIFENESIN

BRAND NAMES

See complete list of brand names in the *Generic and Brand Name Directory*, page 862.

BASIC INFORMATION

Habit forming? No
Prescription needed? No
Available as generic? Yes
Drug class: Expectorant

USES

Loosens mucus in respiratory passages from allergies and infections (hay fever, cough, cold).

DOSAGE & USAGE INFORMATION

How to take:

- Tablet or capsule—Swallow with liquid. If you can't swallow whole, crumble tablet or open capsule and take with liquid or food.
- Extended-release tablet or extended-release capsule—Swallow with liquid.
- Syrup, oral solution or lozenge—Take as directed on label. Follow with 8 oz. water.

When to take:
As needed, no more often than every 4 hours.

If you forget a dose:
Take as soon as you remember. Wait 4 hours for next dose.

What drug does:
Increases production of watery fluids to thin mucus so it can be coughed out or absorbed.

Time lapse before drug works:
15 to 30 minutes. Regular use for 5 to 7 days necessary for maximum benefit.

Don't take with:
Any other medicine without consulting your doctor or pharmacist.

OVERDOSE

SYMPTOMS:
Drowsiness, mild weakness, nausea, vomiting.
WHAT TO DO:
Overdose unlikely to threaten life. If person takes much larger amount than prescribed, call doctor, poison center 1-800-222-1222 or hospital emergency room for instructions.

POSSIBLE ADVERSE REACTIONS OR SIDE EFFECTS

SYMPTOMS	WHAT TO DO
Life-threatening: None expected.	
Common: None expected.	
Infrequent: Drowsiness, rash, stomach pain, diarrhea, nausea.	Continue. Call doctor when convenient.
Rare: None expected.	

WARNINGS & PRECAUTIONS

Don't take if:
You are allergic to any cough or cold preparation containing guaifenesin.

Before you start, consult your doctor:
If you are allergic to any medicine, food or other substance.

Over age 60:
Adverse reactions and side effects may be more frequent and severe than in younger persons. For drug to work, you must drink 8 to 10 glasses of fluid per day.

Pregnancy:
Decide with your doctor if drug benefits justify risks to unborn child. Risk category C (see page xviii).

Breast-feeding:
No proven problems. Consult your doctor.

Infants & children:
No problems expected.

Prolonged use:
No problems expected.

Skin & sunlight:
No problems expected.

Driving, piloting or hazardous work:
Avoid if you feel drowsy. Otherwise, no problems expected.

Discontinuing:
May be unnecessary to finish medicine. Discontinue when symptoms disappear. If symptoms persist more than 1 week, consult doctor.

Others:
Some guaifenesin syrup products contain alcohol. Read labels for alcohol content if you want to avoid these products.

POSSIBLE INTERACTION WITH OTHER DRUGS

GENERIC NAME OR DRUG CLASS	COMBINED EFFECT
Anticoagulants*	Possible risk of bleeding.

POSSIBLE INTERACTION WITH OTHER SUBSTANCES

INTERACTS WITH	COMBINED EFFECT
Alcohol:	None expected.
Beverages:	You must drink 8 to 10 glasses of fluid per day for drug to work.
Cocaine:	None expected.
Foods:	None expected.
Marijuana:	None expected.
Tobacco:	None expected.

***See Glossary**

GUANABENZ

BRAND NAMES

Wytensin

BASIC INFORMATION

Habit forming? No
Prescription needed? Yes
Available as generic? No
Drug class: Antihypertensive

USES

Controls, but doesn't cure, high blood pressure.

DOSAGE & USAGE INFORMATION

How to take:
Tablet—Swallow with liquid or food to lessen stomach irritation. If you can't swallow whole, crumble tablet and take with liquid or food.

When to take:
At the same times each day.

If you forget a dose:
Take as soon as you remember up to 2 hours late. If more than 2 hours, wait for next scheduled dose (don't double this dose).

What drug does:
- Relaxes muscle cells of small arteries.
- Slows heartbeat.

Time lapse before drug works:
1 hour.

Don't take with:
Any other medicine without consulting your doctor or pharmacist.

OVERDOSE

SYMPTOMS:
Severe dizziness, slow heartbeat, unusual tiredness or weakness, pinpoint pupils, fainting, coma.
WHAT TO DO:
- **Dial 911 (emergency) for an ambulance or medical help or poison center 1-800-222-1222. Then give first aid immediately.**
- **If patient is unconscious and not breathing, give mouth-to-mouth breathing. If there is no heartbeat, use cardiac massage and mouth-to-mouth breathing (CPR). Don't try to make patient vomit. If you can't get help quickly, take patient to nearest emergency facility.**
- **See emergency information on inside covers.**

POSSIBLE ADVERSE REACTIONS OR SIDE EFFECTS

SYMPTOMS	WHAT TO DO
Life-threatening: In case of overdose, see previous column.	
Common:	
• Dry mouth, drowsiness.	Continue. Call doctor when convenient.
• Insomnia, weakness.	Continue. Tell doctor at next visit.
Infrequent:	
• Irregular heartbeat, shakiness in hands.	Discontinue. Call doctor right away.
• Dizziness, appetite loss, nausea, vomiting, painful or difficult urination, headache.	Continue. Call doctor when convenient.
Rare:	
Decreased sex drive.	Continue. Call doctor when convenient.

WARNINGS & PRECAUTIONS

Don't take if:
You are allergic to any sympathomimetic drug.

Before you start, consult your doctor:
- If you have blood disease.
- If you have heart disease.
- If you have liver disease.
- If you have diabetes or overactive thyroid.
- If you will have surgery within 2 months, including dental surgery, requiring general or spinal anesthesia.

Over age 60:
Adverse reactions and side effects may be more frequent and severe than in younger persons. Hot weather may cause need to reduce dosage.

Pregnancy:
Decide with your doctor if drug benefits justify risks to unborn child. Risk category C (see page xviii).

Breast-feeding:
Unknown effect. Consult doctor.

Infants & children:
Not recommended.

Prolonged use:
Side effects tend to diminish. Request uric acid and kidney function studies periodically.

Skin & sunlight:
No problems expected.

Driving, piloting or hazardous work:
Avoid if you feel dizzy; otherwise, no problems expected.

Discontinuing:
Don't discontinue without consulting doctor. Dose may require gradual reduction if you have taken drug for a long time. Doses of other drugs may also require adjustment. Abruptly discontinuing may cause anxiety, chest pain, salivation, headache, abdominal cramps, fast heartbeat, increased sweating, tremors, insomnia.

Others:
- Stay away from high-sodium foods. Lose weight if you are overweight.
- May interfere with the accuracy of some medical tests.

POSSIBLE INTERACTION WITH OTHER DRUGS

GENERIC NAME OR DRUG CLASS	COMBINED EFFECT
Angiotensin-converting enzyme (ACE) inhibitors*	Possible excessive potassium in blood.
Antihypertensives, other*	Decreases blood pressure more than either alone. May be beneficial, but requires dosage adjustment.
Beta-adrenergic blocking agents*	Blood pressure control more difficult.
Central nervous system (CNS) depressants* (sedatives,* sleeping pills,* tranquilizers,* antidepressants,* narcotics*)	Increased brain depression. Avoid.
Clozapine	Toxic effect on the central nervous system.
Diuretics*	Decreases blood pressure more than either alone. May be beneficial, but requires dosage adjustment.
Ethinamate	Dangerous increased effects of ethinamate. Avoid combining.
Fluoxetine	Increased depressant effects of both drugs.
Guanfacine	May increase depressant effects of either drug.
Leucovorin	High alcohol content of leucovorin may cause adverse effects.
Methyprylon	Increased sedative effect, perhaps to dangerous level. Avoid.
Nabilone	Greater depression of central nervous system.
Nicardipine	Blood pressure drop. Dosages may require adjustment.
Nimodipine	Dangerous blood pressure drop.
Sertraline	Increased depressive effects of both drugs.

POSSIBLE INTERACTION WITH OTHER SUBSTANCES

INTERACTS WITH	COMBINED EFFECT
Alcohol:	Oversedation. Avoid.
Beverages: Caffeine.	Overstimulation. Avoid.
Cocaine:	Overstimulation. Avoid.
Foods: Salt.	Decrease salt intake to increase beneficial effects of guanabenz.
Marijuana:	Overstimulation. Avoid.
Tobacco:	Decreased guanabenz effect.

*See Glossary

GUANADREL

BRAND NAMES

Hylorel

BASIC INFORMATION

Habit forming? No
Prescription needed? Yes
Available as generic? No
Drug class: Antihypertensive

USES

Controls, but doesn't cure, high blood pressure.

DOSAGE & USAGE INFORMATION

How to take:
Tablet—Swallow with liquid or food to lessen stomach irritation. If you can't swallow whole, crumble tablet and take with liquid or food.

When to take:
At the same time each day.

If you forget a dose:
Take as soon as you remember up to 2 hours late. If more than 2 hours, wait for next scheduled dose (don't double this dose).

What drug does:
Relaxes muscle cells of small arteries.

Time lapse before drug works:
4 to 6 hours. May need to take for lifetime.

Don't take with:
Any other medicine without consulting your doctor or pharmacist.

OVERDOSE

SYMPTOMS:
Severe blood pressure drop; fainting; blurred vision; slow, weak pulse; cold, sweaty skin; loss of consciousness.
WHAT TO DO:
- **Dial 911 (emergency) for an ambulance or medical help or poison center 1-800-222-1222. Then give first aid immediately.**
- **See emergency information on inside covers.**

POSSIBLE ADVERSE REACTIONS OR SIDE EFFECTS

SYMPTOMS	WHAT TO DO
Life-threatening: In case of overdose, see previous column.	
Common:	
• Diarrhea, more bowel movements, fatigue, weakness.	Continue. Call doctor when convenient.
• Dizziness, lower sex drive, feet and ankle swelling, drowsiness.	Continue. Tell doctor at next visit.
• Stuffy nose, dry mouth.	No action necessary.
Infrequent:	
• Rash, blurred vision, drooping eyelids, chest pain or shortness of breath, muscle pain or tremor.	Discontinue. Call doctor right away.
• Nausea or vomiting, headache.	Continue. Call doctor when convenient.
• Impotence, nighttime urination.	Continue. Tell doctor at next visit.
Rare:	
Decreased white blood cells causing sore throat, fever.	Discontinue. Call doctor right away.

WARNINGS & PRECAUTIONS

Don't take if:
- You are allergic to guanadrel.
- You have taken MAO inhibitors* within 2 weeks.

Before you start, consult your doctor:
- If you have stroke or heart disease.
- If you have asthma.
- If you have had kidney disease.
- If you have peptic ulcer or chronic acid indigestion.
- If you will have surgery within 2 months, including dental surgery, requiring general or spinal anesthesia.

Over age 60:
Adverse reactions and side effects may be more frequent and severe than in younger persons. Start with small doses and monitor blood pressure frequently.

Pregnancy:
No proven harm to unborn child. Avoid if possible. Consult doctor. Risk category B (see page xviii).

Breast-feeding:
No proven harm to nursing infant. Avoid if possible. Consult doctor.

Infants & children:
Not recommended.

Prolonged use:
- Due to drug's cumulative effect, dose will require adjustment to prevent wide fluctuations in blood pressure.
- Talk to your doctor about the need for follow-up medical examinations or laboratory studies.

Skin & sunlight:
No problems expected.

Driving, piloting or hazardous work:
Don't drive or pilot aircraft until you learn how medicine affects you. Don't work around dangerous machinery. Don't climb ladders or work in high places. Danger increases if you drink alcohol or take medicine affecting alertness and reflexes, such as antihistamines, tranquilizers, sedatives, pain medicine, narcotics and mind-altering drugs.

Discontinuing:
Don't discontinue without consulting doctor. Dose may require gradual reduction if you have taken drug for a long time. Doses of other drugs may also require adjustment.

Others:
- Hot weather further lowers blood pressure, particularly in patients over 60.
- Advise any doctor or dentist whom you consult that you take this medicine.

POSSIBLE INTERACTION WITH OTHER DRUGS

GENERIC NAME OR DRUG CLASS	COMBINED EFFECT
Angiotensin-converting enzyme (ACE) inhibitors*	Possible excessive potassium in blood.
Antidepressants, tricyclic*	Decreased effect of guanadrel.
Antihypertensives, other*	Increased effect of guanadrel.
Beta-adrenergic blocking agents*	Increased likelihood of dizziness and fainting.
Carteolol	Increased anti-hypertensive effect.
Contraceptives, oral*	Increased side effects of oral contraceptives.
Central nervous system (CNS) depressants* (anticonvulsants,* antihistamines,* muscle relaxants,* narcotics,* sedatives,* tranquilizers*)	Decreased effect of guanadrel.
Diuretics*	Increased likelihood of dizziness and fainting.
Haloperidol	Decreased effect of guanadrel.
Insulin	Increased insulin effect.
Loxapine	Decreased effect of guanadrel.
Monoamine oxidase (MAO) inhibitors*	Severe high blood pressure. Avoid.
Nicardipine	Blood pressure drop. Dosages may require adjustment.
Nimodipine	Dangerous blood pressure drop.
Phenothiazines*	Decreased effect of guanadrel.
Rauwolfia alkaloids*	Increased likelihood of dizziness and fainting.
Sotalol	Increased anti-hypertensive effect.
Sympathomimetics*	Decreased effect of guanadrel.
Terazosin	Decreases effective-ness of terazosin.
Thioxanthenes*	Decreased effect of guanadrel.
Trimeprazine	Decreased effect of guanadrel.

POSSIBLE INTERACTION WITH OTHER SUBSTANCES

INTERACTS WITH	COMBINED EFFECT
Alcohol:	Decreased effect of guanadrel. Avoid.
Beverages: Caffeine.	Decreased effect of guanadrel.
Cocaine:	Increased risk of heart block and high blood pressure.
Foods:	None expected.
Marijuana:	Higher blood pressure. Avoid.
Tobacco:	Higher blood pressure. Avoid.

GUANETHIDINE

BRAND NAMES

Apo-Guanethidine
Ismelin

BASIC INFORMATION

Habit forming? No
Prescription needed? Yes
Available as generic? Yes
Drug class: Antihypertensive

USES

Reduces high blood pressure.

DOSAGE & USAGE INFORMATION

How to take:
Tablet—Swallow with liquid. If you can't swallow tablet whole, crumble and take with liquid or food.

When to take:
At the same time each day.

If you forget a dose:
Take as soon as you remember up to 2 hours late. If more than 2 hours, wait for next scheduled dose (don't double this dose).

What drug does:
Displaces norepinephrine—hormone necessary to maintain small blood vessel tone. Blood vessels relax and high blood pressure drops.

Time lapse before drug works:
Regular use for several weeks may be necessary to determine effectiveness.

Don't take with:
- Nonprescription drugs containing alcohol without consulting doctor.
- Any other medicine without consulting your doctor or pharmacist.

OVERDOSE

SYMPTOMS:
Severe blood pressure drop; fainting; blurred vision; slow, weak pulse; cold, sweaty skin; loss of consciousness.
WHAT TO DO:
- **Dial 911 (emergency) for an ambulance or medical help or poison center 1-800-222-1222. Then give first aid immediately.**
- **See emergency information on inside covers.**

POSSIBLE ADVERSE REACTIONS OR SIDE EFFECTS

SYMPTOMS	WHAT TO DO
Life-threatening:	
In case of overdose, see previous column.	
Common:	
• Unusually slow heartbeat.	Discontinue. Call doctor right away.
• Diarrhea; more bowel movements; swollen feet, legs; fatigue, weakness.	Continue. Call doctor when convenient.
• Dizziness, lower sex drive.	Continue. Tell doctor at next visit.
• Stuffy nose, dry mouth.	No action necessary.
Infrequent:	
• Rash, blurred vision, drooping eyelids, chest pain or shortness of breath, muscle pain or tremor.	Discontinue. Call doctor right away.
• Nausea or vomiting, headache.	Continue. Call doctor when convenient.
• Impotence, nighttime urination, hair loss.	Continue. Tell doctor at next visit.
Rare:	
Decreased white blood cells causing sore throat, fever.	Discontinue. Call doctor right away.

WARNINGS & PRECAUTIONS

Don't take if:
- You are allergic to guanethidine.
- You have taken MAO inhibitors within 2 weeks.

Before you start, consult your doctor:
- If you have had stroke or heart disease.
- If you have asthma.
- If you have had kidney disease.
- If you have peptic ulcer or chronic acid indigestion.
- If you will have surgery within 2 months, including dental surgery, requiring general or spinal anesthesia.

Over age 60:
Adverse reactions and side effects may be more frequent and severe than in younger persons. Start with small doses and monitor blood pressure frequently.

Pregnancy:
Decide with your doctor if drug benefits justify risk to unborn child. Risk category C (see page xviii).

Breast-feeding:
Unknown effect. Consult doctor.

Infants & children:
Not recommended.

Prolonged use:
- Due to drug's cumulative effect, dose will require adjustment to prevent wide fluctuations in blood pressure.
- Talk to your doctor about the need for follow-up medical examinations or laboratory studies.

Skin & sunlight:
No problems expected.

Driving, piloting or hazardous work:
Don't drive or pilot aircraft until you learn how medicine affects you. Don't work around dangerous machinery. Don't climb ladders or work in high places. Danger increases if you drink alcohol or take medicine affecting alertness and reflexes, such as antihistamines, tranquilizers, sedatives,pain medicine, narcotics and mind-altering drugs.

Discontinuing:
Don't discontinue without consulting doctor. Dose may require gradual reduction if you have taken drug for a long time. Doses of other drugs may also require adjustment.

Others:
Hot weather further lowers blood pressure.

POSSIBLE INTERACTION WITH OTHER DRUGS

GENERIC NAME OR DRUG CLASS	COMBINED EFFECT
Amphetamines*	Decreased guanethidine effect.
Angiotensin-converting enzyme (ACE) inhibitors*	Possible excessive potassium in blood.
Antidepressants, tricyclic*	Decreased guanethidine effect.
Antidiabetics, oral*	Increased guanethidine effect.
Antihistamines*	Decreased guanethidine effect.
Carteolol	Increased anti-hypertensive effect.
Contraceptives, oral*	Decreased guanethidine effect. Increased side effects of oral contraceptives.
Digitalis preparations*	Slower heartbeat.
Diuretics, thiazide*	Increased guanethidine effect.
Haloperidol	Decreased guanethidine effect.
Indapamide	Possible increased effects of both drugs. When monitored carefully, combination may be beneficial in controlling hypertension.
Insulin	Increased insulin effect.
Loxapine	Decreased effect of guanethidine.
Minoxidil	Dosage adjustments may be necessary to keep blood pressure at proper level.
Monoamine oxidase (MAO) inhibitors*	Increased blood pressure.
Nicardipine	Blood pressure drop. Dosages may require adjustment.
Nimodipine	Dangerous blood pressure drop.
Phenothiazines*	Decreased guanethidine effect.

Continued on page 913

POSSIBLE INTERACTION WITH OTHER SUBSTANCES

INTERACTS WITH	COMBINED EFFECT
Alcohol:	Use caution. Decreases blood pressure.
Beverages: Carbonated drinks.	Use sparingly. Sodium content increases blood pressure.
Cocaine:	Increased risk of heart block and high blood pressure.
Foods: Spicy or acid foods.	Avoid if subject to indigestion or peptic ulcer.
Marijuana:	Excessively low blood pressure. Avoid.
Tobacco:	Possible blood pressure rise. Avoid.

GUANETHIDINE & HYDROCHLOROTHIAZIDE

BRAND NAMES

Esimil
Ismelin-Esidrix

BASIC INFORMATION

Habit forming? No
Prescription needed? Yes
Available as generic? No
Drug class: Antihypertensive, diuretic

USES

- Controls, but doesn't cure, high blood pressure.
- Reduces fluid retention (edema).

DOSAGE & USAGE INFORMATION

How to take:
Tablet—Swallow with liquid. If you can't swallow whole, crumble tablet and take with liquid or food.

When to take:
At the same time each day.

If you forget a dose:
Take as soon as you remember up to 2 hours late. If more than 2 hours, wait for next scheduled dose (don't double this dose).

What drug does:
- Forces sodium and water secretion, reducing body fluid.
- Displaces norepinephrine—hormone necessary to maintain small blood vessel tone. Blood vessels relax and high blood pressure drops.

Time lapse before drug works:
Regular use for several weeks may be necessary to determine effectiveness.

Don't take with:
- Nonprescription drugs containing alcohol without consulting doctor.
- Any other medicine without consulting your doctor or pharmacist.

OVERDOSE

SYMPTOMS:
Cramps, weakness, drowsiness, blurred vision, weak pulse, severe blood pressure drop, fainting, cold and sweaty skin, loss of consciousness, coma.
WHAT TO DO:
- **Dial 911 (emergency) for an ambulance or medical help or poison center 1-800-222-1222. Then give first aid immediately.**
- **See emergency information on inside covers.**

POSSIBLE ADVERSE REACTIONS OR SIDE EFFECTS

SYMPTOMS	WHAT TO DO
Life-threatening:	
Chest pain, shortness of breath, irregular heartbeat.	Discontinue. Seek emergency treatment.
Common:	
• Slow heartbeat, swollen feet and ankles, fatigue, weakness.	Discontinue. Call doctor right away.
• Dizziness, stuffy nose, dry mouth, diarrhea, diminished sex drive.	Continue. Call doctor when convenient.
Infrequent:	
• Mood change, rash or hives, blurred vision, drooping eyelids, muscle pain or tremors.	Discontinue. Call doctor right away.
• Increased nighttime urination, abdominal pain, vomiting, nausea, headache, weakness.	Continue. Call doctor when convenient.
• Impotence, nighttime urination, hair loss.	Continue. Tell doctor at next visit.
Rare:	
• Decreased white blood cells causing sore throat, fever; jaundice.	Discontinue. Call doctor right away.
• Weight gain or loss.	Continue. Call doctor when convenient.

WARNINGS & PRECAUTIONS

Don't take if:
- You are allergic to any thiazide diuretic drug or guanethidine.
- You have taken MAO inhibitors within 2 weeks.

Before you start, consult your doctor:
- If you are allergic to any sulfa drug.
- If you have gout, asthma, liver, pancreas or kidney disorder, peptic ulcer or chronic acid indigestion.
- If you have had stroke or heart disease.
- If you will have surgery within 2 months, including dental surgery, requiring general or spinal anesthesia.

Continued next column

Over age 60:
Adverse reactions and side effects may be more frequent and severe than in younger persons, especially dizziness and excessive potassium loss.

Pregnancy:
Decide with your doctor if drug benefits justify risk to unborn child. Risk category C (see page xviii).

Breast-feeding:
Drug passes into milk. Avoid drug or discontinue nursing until you finish medicine. Consult doctor for advice on maintaining milk supply.

Infants & children:
Not recommended.

Prolonged use:
- Due to drug's cumulative effect, dose will require adjustment to prevent wide fluctuations in blood pressure.
- Talk to your doctor about the need for follow-up medical examinations or laboratory studies.

Skin & sunlight:
One or more drugs in this group may cause rash or intensify sunburn in areas exposed to sun or ultraviolet light (photosensitivity reaction). Avoid overexposure. Notify doctor if reaction occurs.

Driving, piloting or hazardous work:
Don't drive or pilot aircraft until you learn how medicine affects you. Don't work around dangerous machinery. Don't climb ladders or work in high places. Danger increases if you drink alcohol or take medicine affecting alertness and reflexes, such as antihistamines, tranquilizers, sedatives, pain medicine, narcotics and mind-altering drugs.

Discontinuing:
Don't discontinue without consulting doctor. Dose may require gradual reduction if you have taken drug for a long time. Doses of other drugs may also require adjustment.

Others:
- Hot weather and fever may cause dehydration and drop in blood pressure. Dose may require temporary adjustment. Weigh daily and report any unexpected weight decreases to your doctor.
- May cause rise in uric acid, leading to gout.
- May cause blood sugar rise in diabetics.

POSSIBLE INTERACTION WITH OTHER DRUGS

GENERIC NAME OR DRUG CLASS	COMBINED EFFECT
Allopurinol	Decreased allopurinol effect.
Amphetamines*	Decreased guanethidine effect.
Antidepressants, tricyclic*	Dangerous drop in blood pressure. Avoid combination unless under medical supervision.
Antihistamines*	Decreased guanethidine effect.
Barbiturates*	Increased hydrochlorothiazide effect.
Beta-adrenergic blocking agents*	Increased anti-hypertensive effect. Dosages of both drugs may require adjustments.
Carteolol	Increased anti-hypertensive effect.
Cholestyramine	Decreased hydrochlorothiazide effect.
Contraceptives, oral*	Decreased guanethidine effect.

Continued on page 914

POSSIBLE INTERACTION WITH OTHER SUBSTANCES

INTERACTS WITH	COMBINED EFFECT
Alcohol:	Use caution Decreases blood pressure.
Beverages: Carbonated drinks.	Use sparingly. Sodium content increases blood pressure.
Cocaine:	Raises blood pressure. Avoid.
Foods: Spicy or acid foods.	Avoid if subject to indigestion or peptic ulcer.
Licorice.	Excessive potassium loss that causes dangerous heart rhythms.
Marijuana:	Effect on blood pressure unpredictable.
Tobacco:	Possible blood pressure rise. Avoid.

***See Glossary**

GUANFACINE

BRAND NAMES

Tenex

BASIC INFORMATION

Habit forming? No
Prescription needed? Yes
Available as generic? No
Drug class: Antihypertensive

USES

Treats high blood pressure, usually in combination with a diuretic drug.

DOSAGE & USAGE INFORMATION

How to take:
Tablets—Swallow with liquid or food to lessen stomach irritation. If you can't swallow whole, crumble tablet and take with liquid or food.

When to take:
Usually at bedtime to minimize daytime drowsiness.

If you forget a dose:
Take as soon as you remember up to 2 hours late. If more than 2 hours, wait for next scheduled dose (don't double this dose).

What drug does:
- Decreases stimulating effects of the sympathetic nervous system on the heart, kidneys and arteries throughout the body.
- Decreases both systolic and diastolic blood pressure.

Time lapse before drug works:
Within 1 week.

Don't take with:
Any other medicine without consulting your doctor or pharmacist.

OVERDOSE

SYMPTOMS:
Difficulty breathing, loss of consciousness, dizziness, very slow heartbeat.
WHAT TO DO:
- **Dial 911 (emergency) for an ambulance or medical help or poison center 1-800-222-1222. Then give first aid immediately.**
- **See emergency information on inside covers.**

POSSIBLE ADVERSE REACTIONS OR SIDE EFFECTS

SYMPTOMS	WHAT TO DO
Life-threatening:	
Shortness of breath.	Seek emergency treatment immediately.
Common:	
• Decreased sexual function, drowsiness, constipation.	Continue. Call doctor when convenient.
• Increased dental problems because of dry mouth and less salivation.	Consult your dentist about a prevention program.
Infrequent:	
• Confusion, dizziness or fainting, slow heartbeat.	Continue, but call doctor right away.
• Mental depression, eye irritation, insomnia, tiredness or weakness, headache, nausea and/or vomiting.	Continue. Call doctor when convenient.
Rare:	
May occur if medicine is abruptly discontinued—Anxiety, chest pain, heartbeat irregularities, excess salivation, sleep problems, nervousness, sweating.	Seek emergency treatment.

WARNINGS & PRECAUTIONS

Don't take if:
You have had a recent heart attack.

Before you start, consult your doctor:
- If you have heart disease or liver disease.
- If you have coronary insufficiency.
- If you have mental depression.

Over age 60:
None significant.

Pregnancy:
No proven harm to unborn child, but avoid if possible. Consult doctor. Risk category B (see page xviii).

Breast-feeding:
Effect not documented. Consult your doctor.

Infants & children:
Effect not documented. Consult your pediatrician.

Prolonged use:
Talk to your doctor about the need for follow-up medical examinations or laboratory studies to check blood pressure.

Skin & sunlight:
No problems expected.

Driving, piloting or hazardous work:
Don't drive or pilot aircraft until you learn how medicine affects you. Don't work around dangerous machinery. Don't climb ladders or work in high places. Danger increases if you drink alcohol or take medicine affecting alertness and reflexes.

Discontinuing:
- Don't discontinue without consulting doctor. Dose may require gradual reduction if you have taken drug for a long time. Doses of other drugs may also require adjustment.
- May occur if medicine is discontinued abruptly: anxiety, chest pain, heartbeat irregularities, excess salivation, sleep problems, nervousness, sweating.

Others:
- This medication works better if you attempt to reduce your weight to normal, exercise regularly, restrict salt in your diet and reduce stress wherever possible. Continue taking medicine even when you feel good.
- Adverse reactions are usually dose-related and diminish when dosage is reduced.

POSSIBLE INTERACTION WITH OTHER DRUGS

GENERIC NAME OR DRUG CLASS	COMBINED EFFECT
Antihypertensives, other*	May increase effects of guanfacine and other medicines.
Anti-inflammatory drugs, nonsteroidal (NSAIDs)*	May decrease anti-hypertensive effects of guanfacine.
Carteolol	Increased anti-hypertensive effect.
Central nervous system (CNS) depressants*	Increases depressant effect of both drugs.
Clozapine	Toxic effect on the central nervous system.
Estrogens*	May decrease anti-hypertensive effects of guanfacine.
Ethinamate	Dangerous increased effects of ethinamate. Avoid combining.
Fluoxetine	Increased depressant effects of both drugs.
Leucovorin	High alcohol content of leucovorin may cause adverse effects.
Lisinopril	Increased anti-hypertensive effect. Dosage of each may require adjustment.
Methyprylon	Increased sedative effect, perhaps to dangerous level. Avoid.
Nabilone	Greater depression of central nervous system.
Nicardipine	Blood pressure drop. Dosages may require adjustment.
Nimodipine	Dangerous blood pressure drop.
Propafenone	Increased effect of both drugs and increased risk of toxicity.
Sertraline	Increased depressive effects of both drugs.
Sotalol	Increased anti-hypertensive effect.

Continued on page 914

POSSIBLE INTERACTION WITH OTHER SUBSTANCES

INTERACTS WITH	COMBINED EFFECT
Alcohol:	Excess use may lead to dangerous drop in blood pressure.
Beverages: Any containing caffeine, such as coffee, tea or cocoa.	May decrease anti-hypertensive effect of guanfacine.
Cocaine:	Increased risk of heart block and high blood pressure.
Foods:	None expected.
Marijuana:	May decrease anti-hypertensive effect of guanfacine.
Tobacco:	May decrease anti-hypertensive effect of guanfacine.

***See Glossary**

HALOPERIDOL

BRAND NAMES

Apo-Haloperidol
Haldol
Haldol Decanoate
Haldol LA
Halperon
Novo-Peridol
Peridol
PMS Haloperidol

BASIC INFORMATION

Habit forming? No
Prescription needed? Yes
Available as generic? Yes
Drug class: Antipsychotic

USES

- Reduces severe anxiety, agitation and psychotic behavior.
- Treatment for Tourette's syndrome
- Treatment for infantile autism.
- Treatment for Huntington's chorea.

DOSAGE & USAGE INFORMATION

How to take:
- Tablet—Swallow with liquid. If you can't swallow whole, crumble tablet and take with liquid or food.
- Drops—Dilute dose in beverage before swallowing.

When to take:
At the same times each day.

Continued next column

If you forget a dose:
Take as soon as you remember up to 2 hours late. If more than 2 hours, wait for next scheduled dose (don't double this dose).

What drug does:
Corrects an imbalance in nerve impulses from brain; blocks effect of dopamine*.

Time lapse before drug works:
Up to 4 weeks.

Don't take with:
- Nonprescription drugs without consulting doctor.
- Any other medicine without consulting your doctor or pharmacist.

OVERDOSE

SYMPTOMS:
Weak, rapid pulse; shallow, slow breathing; tremor or muscle weakness; very low blood pressure; convulsions; deep sleep ending in coma.
WHAT TO DO:
- **Dial 911 (emergency) for an ambulance or medical help or poison center 1-800-222-1222. Then give first aid immediately.**
- **If patient is unconscious and not breathing, give mouth-to-mouth breathing. If there is no heartbeat, use cardiac massage and mouth-to-mouth breathing (CPR). Don't try to make patient vomit. If you can't get help quickly, take patient to nearest emergency facility.**
- **See emergency information at end of book.**

POSSIBLE ADVERSE REACTIONS OR SIDE EFFECTS

SYMPTOMS	WHAT TO DO
Life-threatening:	
High fever, rapid pulse, profuse sweating, muscle rigidity, confusion and irritability, seizures.	Discontinue. Seek emergency treatment.
Common:	
• Jerky or involuntary movements, especially of the face, lips, jaw, tongue; slow-frequency tremor of head or limbs, especially while moving; muscle rigidity, lack of facial expression and slow inflexible movements.	Discontinue. Call doctor right away.
• Pacing or restlessness; intermittent spasms of muscles of face, eyes, tongue, jaw, neck, body or limbs.	Continue. Call doctor when convenient.
Infrequent:	
Dry mouth, blurred vision, constipation, difficulty urinating; sedation, low blood pressure, dizziness.	Continue. Call doctor when convenient.
Rare:	
Other symptoms not listed above.	Continue. Call doctor when convenient.

WARNINGS & PRECAUTIONS

Don't take if:
- You have ever been allergic to haloperidol.
- You are depressed.
- You have Parkinson's disease.
- Patient is younger than 3 years old.

Before you start, consult your doctor:
- If you take sedatives, sleeping pills, tranquilizers, antidepressants, antihistamines, narcotics or mind-altering drugs.
- If you have a history of mental depression.
- If you have had kidney or liver problems.
- If you have diabetes, epilepsy, glaucoma, high blood pressure or heart disease, prostate trouble, overactive thyroid or asthma.
- If you drink alcoholic beverages frequently.

Over age 60:
Adverse reactions and side effects may be more frequent and severe than in younger persons.

Pregnancy:
Decide with your doctor if drug benefits justify risk to unborn child. Risk category C (see page xviii).

Breast-feeding:
Drug passes into milk. Avoid drug or discontinue nursing until you finish medicine. Consult doctor about maintaining milk supply.

Infants & children:
Not recommended. Side effects may be more common.

Prolonged use:
- May develop tardive dyskinesia (involuntary movements of jaws, lips and tongue).
- Talk to your doctor about the need for follow-up medical examinations or laboratory studies to check blood pressure, liver function.

Skin & sunlight:
- May cause rash or intensify sunburn in areas exposed to sun or ultraviolet light (photosensitivity). Avoid overexposure and use sunscreen. Consult doctor if reaction occurs.
- Avoid getting overheated. The drug affects body temperature and sweating.

Driving, piloting or hazardous work:
Don't drive or pilot aircraft until you learn how medicine affects you. Don't work around dangerous machinery. Don't climb ladders or work in high places. Danger increases if you drink alcohol or take medicine affecting alertness and reflexes.

Discontinuing:
Don't discontinue without consulting doctor. Dose may require gradual reduction if you have taken drug for a long time. Doses of other drugs may also require adjustment.

Others:
- For dry mouth, suck on sugarless hard candy or chew sugarless gum. If dry mouth persists, consult your dentist
- Advise any doctor or dentist whom you consult that you take this medicine.

POSSIBLE INTERACTION WITH OTHER DRUGS

GENERIC NAME OR DRUG CLASS	COMBINED EFFECT
Anticholinergics*	Increased anti-cholinergic effect. May cause elevated pressure within the eye.
Anticonvulsants*	Changed seizure pattern.
Antidepressants*	Excessive sedation.
Antihistamines*	Excessive sedation.
Antihypertensives*	May cause severe blood pressure drop.
Barbiturates*	Excessive sedation.
Bupropion	Increased risk of seizures.
Central nervous system (CNS) depressants*	Increased CNS depression; increased blood pressure drop.
Clozapine	Toxic effect on the nervous system.

Continued on page 914

POSSIBLE INTERACTION WITH OTHER SUBSTANCES

INTERACTS WITH	COMBINED EFFECT
Alcohol:	Excessive sedation and depressed brain function. Avoid.
Beverages:	None expected.
Cocaine:	Decreased effect of haloperidol. Avoid.
Foods:	None expected.
Marijuana:	Occasional use—Increased sedation. Frequent use—Possible toxic psychosis.
Tobacco:	None expected.

***See Glossary**

HISTAMINE H_2 RECEPTOR ANTAGONISTS

GENERIC AND BRAND NAMES

CIMETIDINE
- **Apo-Cimetidine**
- **Liquid Tagamet**
- **Novocimetine**
- **Peptol**
- **Tagamet**
- **Tagamet HB**

FAMOTIDINE
- **Mylanta-AR**
- **Pepcid**
- **Pepcid AC**
- **Ulcidine**

NIZATIDINE
- **Axid**

RANITIDINE
- **Apo-Ranitidine**
- **Zantac**
- **Zantac 75**
- **Zantac-C**
- **Zantac Efferdose**
- **Zantac Geldose**

BASIC INFORMATION

Habit forming? No
Prescription needed? Yes, for some
Available as generic? No
Drug class: Histamine H_2 antagonist

USES

- Treatment for duodenal and gastric ulcers and other conditions in which stomach produces excess hydrochloric acid.
- Treatment for and prevention of heartburn.
- Maintenance of healing of erosive esophagitis.

DOSAGE & USAGE INFORMATION

How to take:
- Chewable tablet (Pepcid AC)—Chew thoroughly and swallow with water.
- Tablet, capsule or liquid—Swallow with liquid.
- Oral suspension or effervescent tablets for oral solution—Follow instructions on label.

When to take:
- 1 dose per day—Take at bedtime.
- 2 or more doses per day—Take at the same times each day.

Continued next column

If you forget a dose:
Take as soon as you remember up to 2 hours late. If more than 2 hours, wait for next scheduled dose (don't double this dose).

What drug does:
Blocks histamine release so stomach secretes less acid.

Time lapse before drug works:
- Begins in 30 minutes. May require several days to relieve pain.
- Lower dosages in nonprescription medicines may take 45 minutes ro relieve heartburn.

Don't take with:
Any other medicine without consulting your doctor or pharmacist.

OVERDOSE

SYMPTOMS:
Confusion, slurred speech, breathing difficulty, rapid heartbeat, delirium.
WHAT TO DO:
Overdose unlikely to threaten life. If person takes much larger amount than prescribed, call doctor, poison center 1-800-222-1222 or hospital emergency room for instructions.

POSSIBLE ADVERSE REACTIONS OR SIDE EFFECTS

SYMPTOMS	WHAT TO DO
Life-threatening: In case of overdose, see previous column.	
Common: None expected.	
Infrequent:	
• Dizziness or headache, diarrhea.	Continue. Call doctor when convenient.
• Diminished sex drive, unusual milk flow in females, hair loss.	Continue. Tell doctor at next visit.
Rare:	
• Confusion; rash, hives; sore throat, fever; slow, fast or irregular heartbeat; unusual bleeding or bruising; muscle cramps or pain; fatigue; weakness.	Discontinue. Call doctor right away.
• Constipation.	Continue. Call doctor when convenient.

WARNINGS & PRECAUTIONS

Don't take if:
You are allergic to any histamine H_2 antagonist.

Before you start, consult your doctor:
- If you plan to become pregnant while on medication.
- If you take aspirin. Aspirin may irritate stomach.

Over age 60:
Adverse reactions and side effects may be more frequent and severe than in younger persons.

Pregnancy:
Risk factors vary for drugs in this group. See category list on page xviii and consult doctor.

Breast-feeding:
Drug passes into milk. Avoid drug or discontinue nursing until you finish medicine. Consult doctor about maintaining milk supply.

Infants & children:
Not recommended.

Prolonged use:
- Possible liver damage.
- Talk to your doctor about the need for follow-up medical examinations or laboratory studies to check blood levels of vitamin B-12.

Skin & sunlight:
No problems expected.

Driving, piloting or hazardous work:
Don't drive or pilot aircraft until you learn how medicine affects you. Don't work around dangerous machinery. Don't climb ladders or work in high places. Danger increases if you drink alcohol or take medicine affecting alertness and reflexes, such as antihistamines, tranquilizers, sedatives, pain medicine, narcotics and mind-altering drugs.

Discontinuing:
Don't discontinue without consulting a doctor. Dose may require gradual reduction if you have taken drug for a long time. Doses of other drugs may also require adjustment.

Others:
- Patients on kidney dialysis—Take at end of dialysis treatment.
- May interfere with the accuracy of some medical tests.

POSSIBLE INTERACTION WITH OTHER DRUGS

GENERIC NAME OR DRUG CLASS	COMBINED EFFECT
Alprazolam	Increased effect and toxicity of alprazolam.
Antacids*	Decreased absorption of histamine H_2 receptor antagonist.
Anticoagulants, oral*	Increased anticoagulant effect.
Anticholinergics*	Increased histamine H_2 receptor antagonist effect.
Antivirals, HIV/AIDS*	Increased antiviral effect with cimetidine.
Azelastine	Increased azelastine effect.
Bupropion	Increased bupropion effect.
Carbamazepine	Increased effect and toxicity of carbamazepine.
Carmustine (BCNU)	Severe impairment of red blood cell production; some interference with white blood cell formation.
Chlordiazepoxide	Increased effect and toxicity of chlordiazepoxide.
Cisapride	Decreased histamine H_2 receptor effect.
Citalopram	Increased effect of citalopram.
Diazepam	Increased effect and toxicity of diazepam.

Continued on page 915

POSSIBLE INTERACTION WITH OTHER SUBSTANCES

INTERACTS WITH	COMBINED EFFECT
Alcohol:	No interactions expected, but alcohol may slow body's recovery. Avoid.
Beverages:	
Milk.	Enhanced effectiveness. Small amounts useful for taking medication.
Caffeine drinks.	May increase acid secretion and delay healing.
Cocaine:	Decreased effect of histamine H_2 receptor antagonist.
Foods:	Enhanced effectiveness. Protein-rich foods should be eaten in moderation to minimize secretion of stomach acid.
Marijuana:	Increased chance of low sperm count. Marijuana may slow body's recovery. Avoid.
Tobacco:	Reversed effect of histamine H_2 receptor antagonist. Tobacco may slow body's recovery. Avoid.

***See Glossary**

HMG-CoA REDUCTASE INHIBITORS

GENERIC AND BRAND NAMES

ATORVASTATIN
Lipitor
CERIVASTATIN
Baycol
FLUVASTATIN
Lescol
Lescol XL
LOVASTATIN
Advicor
Mevacor
Mevinolin
PRAVASTATIN
Eptastatin
Pravachol
SIMVASTATIN
Epistatin
Synvinolin
Zocor

BASIC INFORMATION

Habit forming? No
Prescription needed? Yes
Available as generic? No
Drug class: Antihyperlipidemic

USES

- Lowers blood cholesterol levels caused by low-density lipoproteins (LDL) in persons who haven't improved by exercising, dieting or using other measures and raises high density lipoproteins (HDL-C).
- Used in combination with a low-fat diet to slow the progression of atherosclerosis in patients with coronary heart disease and high cholesterol levels.
- Lowers triglyceride levels.

DOSAGE & USAGE INFORMATION

How to take:
Tablet or capsule—Swallow with liquid. If you can't swallow whole, crumble tablet and take with liquid or food.

When to take:
According to directions on prescription.

Continued next column

OVERDOSE

SYMPTOMS:
None expected.
WHAT TO DO:
Overdose not expected to threaten life. If person takes much larger amount than prescribed, call doctor, poison center 1-800-222-1222 or hospital emergency room for instructions.

If you forget a dose:
Take as soon as you remember up to 2 hours late. If more than 2 hours, wait for next scheduled dose (don't double this dose).

What drug does:
Inhibits an enzyme in the liver.

Time lapse before drug works:
2 to 4 weeks.

Don't take with:
- A high-fat diet.
- Any other medicine without consulting your doctor or pharmacist.

POSSIBLE ADVERSE REACTIONS OR SIDE EFFECTS

SYMPTOMS	WHAT TO DO
Life-threatening: None expected.	
Common: None expected.	
Infrequent:	
• Aching muscles, fever, blurred vision.	Discontinue. Call doctor right away.
• Constipation, nausea, tiredness, weakness, dizziness, skin rash, headache, diarrhea, heartburn.	Continue. Call doctor when convenient.
Rare:	
• Muscle or stomach pain, unusual tiredness or weakness.	Discontinue. Call doctor right away.
• Impotence, insomnia.	Continue. Call doctor when convenient.

WARNINGS & PRECAUTIONS

Don't take if:
You are allergic to any HMG-CoA reductase inhibitor.

Before you start, consult your doctor:
- If you take immunosuppressive drugs, particularly following an organ transplant.
- If you have low blood pressure.
- If you have hormone abnormalities.
- If you have an active infection.
- If you have active liver disease.
- If you have a seizure disorder.
- If you have a history of alcohol abuse.
- If you have had recent surgery.

Over age 60:
Likely to be more sensitive to drug.

Pregnancy:
Consult doctor. Risk category X (see page xviii).

Breast-feeding:
Discontinue nursing until you finish medicine. Consult doctor for advice on maintaining milk supply.

Infants & children:
Not recommended for children.

Prolonged use:
Talk to your doctor about the need for follow-up medical examinations or laboratory studies to check liver function, serum cholesterol, eyes.

Skin & sunlight:
No problems expected.

Driving, piloting or hazardous work:
No special problems expected.

Discontinuing:
Don't discontinue without consulting doctor. Dose may require gradual reduction if you have taken drug for a long time. Doses of other drugs may also require adjustment.

Others:
- Request liver function tests and eye examinations before beginning this medicine and repeat every 2 to 6 months.
- Advise any doctor or dentist whom you consult that you take this medicine.
- Use an effective form of birth control while taking this drug. Notify your doctor immediately if you become pregnant.

POSSIBLE INTERACTION WITH OTHER DRUGS

GENERIC NAME OR DRUG CLASS	COMBINED EFFECT
Antifungals, azole*	Increased effect of HMG-CoA reductase inhibitor.
Cholestyramine	Decreased effect of HMG-CoA reductase inhibitor if taken at same time.
Colestipol	Decreased effect of HMG-CoA reductase inhibitor if taken at same time.
Cyclosporine	Increased risk of muscle and kidney problems.
Digoxin	Increased digoxin effect.
Diltiazem	Increased effect of HMG-CoA inhibitor.
Erythromycins*	Increased risk of muscle and kidney problems.
Gemfibrozil	Increased risk of muscle and kidney problems and muscle inflammation.
Immunosuppressants*	Increased risk of muscle or kidney problems.
Niacin	Increased risk of muscle and kidney problems.
Orlistat	Increased effect of HMG-CoA reductase inhibitor.

POSSIBLE INTERACTION WITH OTHER SUBSTANCES

INTERACTS WITH	COMBINED EFFECT
Alcohol:	Best to avoid alcohol while taking this drug.
Beverages:	None expected.
Cocaine:	None expected.
Foods:	None expected.
Marijuana:	None expected.
Tobacco:	None expected.

*See Glossary

HYDRALAZINE

BRAND NAMES

Apresoline
Novo-Hylazin

BASIC INFORMATION

Habit forming? No
Prescription needed? Yes
Available as generic? Yes
Drug class: Antihypertensive

USES

Treatment for high blood pressure and congestive heart failure.

DOSAGE & USAGE INFORMATION

How to take:
Tablet—Swallow with liquid. If you can't swallow whole, crumble tablet and take with liquid or food.

When to take:
At the same time each day. Should be taken with food.

If you forget a dose:
Take as soon as you remember up to 2 hours late. If more than 2 hours, wait for next scheduled dose (don't double this dose).

What drug does:
Relaxes and expands blood vessel walls, lowering blood pressure.

Time lapse before drug works:
Regular use for several weeks may be necessary to determine drug's effectiveness.

Continued next column

OVERDOSE

SYMPTOMS:
Rapid and weak heartbeat, fainting, extreme weakness, cold and sweaty skin, flushing.
WHAT TO DO:

- **Dial 911 (emergency) for an ambulance or medical help or poison center 1-800-222-1222. Then give first aid immediately.**
- **If patient is unconscious and not breathing, give mouth-to-mouth breathing. If there is no heartbeat, use cardiac massage and mouth-to-mouth breathing (CPR). Don't try to make patient vomit. If you can't get help quickly, take patient to nearest emergency facility.**
- **See emergency information on inside covers.**

Don't take with:

- Nonprescription drugs containing alcohol without consulting doctor.
- Any other medicine without consulting your doctor or pharmacist.

POSSIBLE ADVERSE REACTIONS OR SIDE EFFECTS

SYMPTOMS	WHAT TO DO
Life-threatening: In case of overdose, see previous column.	
Common:	
• Nausea or vomiting, rapid or irregular heartbeat.	Discontinue. Call doctor right away.
• Headache, diarrhea, appetite loss, painful or difficult urination.	Continue. Tell doctor at next visit.
Infrequent:	
• Hives or rash, flushed face, sore throat, fever, chest pain, swelling of lymph glands, skin blisters, swelling in feet or legs, joint pain.	Discontinue. Call doctor right away.
• Confusion, dizziness, anxiety, depression, joint pain, general discomfort or weakness, fever, muscle pain, chest pain.	Continue. Call doctor when convenient.
• Watery eyes and irritation, constipation.	Continue. Tell doctor at next visit.
Rare:	
• Weakness and faintness when arising from bed or chair, jaundice.	Discontinue. Call doctor right away.
• Numbness or tingling in hands or feet, nasal congestion, impotence.	Continue. Call doctor when convenient.

WARNINGS & PRECAUTIONS

Don't take if:

- You are allergic to hydralazine or tartrazine dye.
- You have history of coronary artery disease or rheumatic heart disease.

Before you start, consult your doctor:

- If you feel pain in chest, neck or arms on physical exertion.
- If you have had lupus.
- If you have had a stroke.

- If you have had kidney disease or impaired kidney function.
- If you will have surgery within 2 months, including dental surgery, requiring general or spinal anesthesia.

Over age 60:
Adverse reactions and side effects may be more frequent and severe than in younger persons.

Pregnancy:
Decide with your doctor if drug benefits justify risk to unborn child. Risk category C (see page xviii).

Breast-feeding:
Drug filters into milk. May harm child. Avoid.

Infants & children:
Not recommended.

Prolonged use:
- May cause lupus (arthritis-like illness).
- Possible psychosis.
- May cause numbness, tingling in hands or feet.
- Talk to your doctor about the need for follow-up medical examinations or laboratory studies to check blood pressure, complete blood counts (white blood cell count, platelet count, red blood cell count, hemoglobin, hematocrit), ANA titers*.

Skin & sunlight:
No problems expected.

Driving, piloting or hazardous work:
Don't drive or pilot aircraft until you learn how medicine affects you. Don't work around dangerous machinery. Don't climb ladders or work in high places. Danger increases if you drink alcohol or take medicine affecting alertness and reflexes, such as antihistamines, tranquilizers, sedatives, pain medicine, narcotics and mind-altering drugs.

Discontinuing:
Don't discontinue without doctor's advice until you complete prescribed dose, even though symptoms diminish or disappear.

Others:
- Vitamin B-6 diet supplement may be advisable. Consult doctor.
- Some products contain tartrazine dye. Avoid, especially if you are allergic to aspirin.
- May interfere with the accuracy of some medical tests.

POSSIBLE INTERACTION WITH OTHER DRUGS

GENERIC NAME OR DRUG CLASS	COMBINED EFFECT
Amphetamines*	Decreased hydralazine effect.
Antihypertensives, other*	Increased anti-hypertensive effect.
Anti-inflammatory drugs, nonsteroidal (NSAIDs)*	Decreased effect of hydralazine.
Antivirals, HIV/AIDS*	Increased risk of peripheral neuropathy.
Carteolol	Increased anti-hypertensive effect.
Diazoxide & other anti-hypertensive drugs	Increased anti-hypertensive effect.
Diuretics, oral*	Increased effects of both drugs. When monitored carefully, combination may be beneficial in controlling hypertension.
Guanfacine	Increased effects of both drugs.
Lisinopril	Increased anti-hypertensive effect. Dosage of each may require adjustment.
Monoamine oxidase (MAO) inhibitors*	Increased hydralazine effect.
Nicardipine	Blood pressure drop. Dosages may require adjustment.
Nimodipine	Dangerous blood pressure drop.

Continued on page 915

POSSIBLE INTERACTION WITH OTHER SUBSTANCES

INTERACTS WITH	COMBINED EFFECT
Alcohol:	May lower blood pressure excessively. Use extreme caution.
Beverages:	None expected.
Cocaine:	Increased risk of heart block and high blood pressure.
Foods:	Increased hydralazine absorption.
Marijuana:	Weakness on standing.
Tobacco:	Possible angina attacks.

***See Glossary**

HYDRALAZINE & HYDROCHLOROTHIAZIDE

BRAND NAMES

Apresazide
Apresoline-Esidrix
Aprozide
Hydra-zide

BASIC INFORMATION

Habit forming? No
Prescription needed? Yes
Available as generic? Yes
Drug class: Antihypertensive, diuretic

USES

- Controls, but doesn't cure, high blood pressure.
- Reduces fluid retention (edema).

DOSAGE & USAGE INFORMATION

How to take:
Tablet or capsule—Swallow with liquid. If you can't swallow whole, crumble tablet or open capsule and take with liquid or food.

When to take:
At the same time each day.

If you forget a dose:
Take as soon as you remember up to 2 hours late. If more than 2 hours, wait for next scheduled dose (don't double this dose).

Continued next column

OVERDOSE

SYMPTOMS:
Cramps, drowsiness, weak pulse, rapid and weak heartbeat, fainting, extreme weakness, cold and sweaty skin, coma.
WHAT TO DO:
- **Dial 911 (emergency) for an ambulance or medical help or poison center 1-800-222-1222. Then give first aid immediately.**
- **If patient is unconscious and not breathing, give mouth-to-mouth breathing. If there is no heartbeat, use cardiac massage and mouth-to-mouth breathing (CPR). Don't try to make patient vomit. If you can't get help quickly, take patient to nearest emergency facility.**
- **See emergency information on inside covers.**

What drug does:
- Forces sodium and water excretion, reducing body fluid.
- Relaxes and expands blood vessel walls, lowering blood pressure.
- Reduced body fluid and relaxed arteries lower blood pressure.

Time lapse before drug works:
Regular use for several weeks may be necessary to determine drug's effectiveness.

Don't take with:
- Nonprescription drugs containing alcohol without consulting doctor.
- Any other medicine without consulting your doctor or pharmacist.

POSSIBLE ADVERSE REACTIONS OR SIDE EFFECTS

SYMPTOMS	WHAT TO DO
Life-threatening:	
Chest pain, irregular and fast heartbeat, weak pulse.	Discontinue. Seek emergency treatment.
Common:	
• Nausea, vomiting.	Discontinue. Call doctor right away.
• Headache, diarrhea, appetite loss, frequent urination, dry mouth, thirst.	Continue. Call doctor when convenient.
Infrequent:	
• Rash; black, bloody or tarry stool; red or flushed face; sore throat, fever, mouth sores; constipation; lymph glands swelling; blurred vision; skin blisters; swelling in feet or legs.	Discontinue. Call doctor right away.
• Dizziness; confusion; watery eyes; weight gain or loss; joint, muscle or chest pain; depression; anxiety; fever.	Continue. Call doctor when convenient.
Rare:	
• Weakness and faintness when arising from bed or chair, jaundice.	Discontinue. Call doctor right away.
• Numbness or tingling in hands or feet, nasal congestion, impotence.	Continue. Call doctor when convenient.

HYDRALAZINE & HYDROCHLOROTHIAZIDE

WARNINGS & PRECAUTIONS

Don't take if:
- You are allergic to hydralazine, any thiazide diuretic drug or tartrazine dye.
- You have history of coronary artery disease or rheumatic heart disease.

Before you start, consult your doctor:
- If you feel pain in chest, neck or arms on physical exertion.
- If you are allergic to any sulfa drug.
- If you have had lupus or a stroke.
- If you have gout, liver, pancreas or kidney disorder.
- If you will have surgery within 2 months, including dental surgery, requiring general or spinal anesthesia.

Over age 60:
Adverse reactions and side effects may be more frequent and severe than in younger persons, especially dizziness and excessive potassium loss.

Pregnancy:
Decide with your doctor if drug benefits justify risk to unborn child. Risk category C (see page xviii).

Breast-feeding:
Drug passes into milk. Avoid drug or discontinue nursing until you finish medicine. Consult doctor for advice on maintaining milk supply.

Infants & children:
Not recommended.

Prolonged use:
- May cause lupus (arthritis-like illness).
- Possible psychosis.
- May cause numbness, tingling in hands or feet.
- Talk to your doctor about the need for follow-up medical examinations or laboratory studies to check blood pressure, complete blood counts (white blood cell count, platelet count, red blood cell count, hemoglobin, hematocrit), ANA titers*.

Skin & sunlight:
One or more drugs in this group may cause rash or intensify sunburn in areas exposed to sun or ultraviolet light (photosensitivity reaction). Avoid overexposure. Notify doctor if reaction occurs.

Driving, piloting or hazardous work:
Don't drive or pilot aircraft until you learn how medicine affects you. Don't work around dangerous machinery. Don't climb ladders or work in high places. Danger increases if you drink alcohol or take medicine affecting alertness and reflexes, such as antihistamines, tranquilizers, sedatives, pain medicine, narcotics and mind-altering drugs.

Discontinuing:
Don't discontinue without consulting doctor's advice until you complete prescribed dose, even though symptoms diminish or disappear.

Others:
- Vitamin B-6 diet supplement may be advisable. Consult doctor.
- Hot weather and fever may cause dehydration and drop in blood pressure. Dose may require temporary adjustment. Weigh daily and report any unexpected weight decreases to your doctor.
- May cause rise in uric acid, leading to gout.
- May cause blood sugar rise in diabetics.

POSSIBLE INTERACTION WITH OTHER DRUGS

GENERIC NAME OR DRUG CLASS	COMBINED EFFECT
Acebutolol	Decreased anti-hypertensive effect of acebutolol.
Allopurinol	Decreased allopurinol effect.
Amphetamines*	Decreased hydralazine effect.
Antidepressants, tricyclic*	Dangerous drop in blood pressure. Avoid combination unless under medical supervision.

Continued on page 916

POSSIBLE INTERACTION WITH OTHER SUBSTANCES

INTERACTS WITH	COMBINED EFFECT
Alcohol:	May lower blood pressure excessively. Use extreme caution.
Beverages:	None expected.
Cocaine:	Dangerous blood pressure rise. Avoid.
Foods: Licorice.	Excessive potassium loss that causes dangerous heart rhythms.
Marijuana:	Weakness on standing. May increase blood pressure.
Tobacco:	Possible angina attacks.

*See Glossary

HYDROCORTISONE (Rectal)

BRAND NAMES

Anucort
Anusol-H.C.
Cort-Dome High Potency
Corticaine
Cortiment-10
Cortiment-40
Dermolate
Hemril-HC
Proctocort
Rectocort

BASIC INFORMATION

Habit forming? No
Prescription needed? Yes
Available as generic? Yes, for some
Drug class: Anti-inflammatory, steroidal (rectal); anesthetic (rectal)

USES

In or around the rectum to relieve swelling, itching and pain for hemorrhoids (piles) and other rectal conditions. Frequently used after hemorrhoid surgery.

DOSAGE & USAGE INFORMATION

How to use:
- Follow instructions in package.
- Rectal cream or ointment—Apply to surface of rectum with fingers. Insert applicator into rectum no farther than halfway and apply inside. Wash applicator with warm soapy water or discard.
- Suppository—Remove wrapper and moisten with water. Lie on side. Push blunt end of suppository into rectum with finger. If suppository is too soft, run cold water over it or put in refrigerator for 15 to 45 minutes before using.
- Aerosol foam—Read patient instructions. Don't insert into rectum. Use the special applicator and wash carefully after using.

When to use:
Follow instructions in package or when needed.

Continued next column

OVERDOSE

SYMPTOMS:
None expected.
WHAT TO DO:
Not intended for internal use. If child accidentally swallows, call poison center 1-800-222-1222.

If you forget a dose:
Use as soon as you remember.

What drug does:
- Reduces inflammation.
- Relieves pain and itching.

Time lapse before drug works:
5 to 15 minutes.

Don't use with:
Other rectal medicines without consulting your doctor.

POSSIBLE ADVERSE REACTIONS OR SIDE EFFECTS

SYMPTOMS	WHAT TO DO
Life-threatening	
None expected.	
Common	
None expected.	
Infrequent	
• Nervousness, trembling, hives, rash, itch, inflammation or tenderness not present before application, slow heartbeat.	Discontinue. Call doctor right away.
• Dizziness, blurred vision, swollen feet.	Continue. Call doctor when convenient.
Rare	
• Blood in urine.	Discontinue. Call doctor right away.
• Increased or painful urination.	Continue. Call doctor when convenient.

WARNINGS & PRECAUTIONS

Don't use if:
You are allergic to any topical anesthetic.

Before you start, consult your doctor:
- If you have skin infection at site of treatment.
- If you have had severe or extensive skin disorders such as eczema or psoriasis.
- If you have bleeding hemorrhoids.

Over age 60:
Adverse reactions and side effects may be more frequent and severe than in younger persons.

Pregnancy:
Decide with your doctor if drug benefits justify risk to unborn child. Risk category C (see page xviii).

Breast-feeding:
No problems expected. Consult doctor.

Infants & children:
Don't use without careful medical supervision. Too much may be absorbed into the blood stream and affect growth.

Prolonged use:
Possible excess absorption. Don't use longer than 3 days for any one problem.

Skin & sunlight:
No problems expected.

Driving, piloting or hazardous work:
No problems expected.

Discontinuing:
May be unnecessary to finish medicine. Follow doctor's instructions.

Others:
- Report any rectal bleeding to your doctor.
- Keep cool, but don't freeze.

POSSIBLE INTERACTION WITH OTHER DRUGS

GENERIC NAME OR DRUG CLASS	COMBINED EFFECT
Sulfa drugs*	Decreased anti-infective effect of sulfa drugs.

POSSIBLE INTERACTION WITH OTHER SUBSTANCES

INTERACTS WITH	COMBINED EFFECT
Alcohol:	None expected.
Beverages:	None expected.
Cocaine:	Possible nervous system toxicity. Avoid.
Foods:	None expected.
Marijuana:	None expected.
Tobacco:	None expected.

***See Glossary**

HYDROXYCHLOROQUINE

BRAND NAMES

Plaquenil

BASIC INFORMATION

Habit forming? No
Prescription needed? Yes
Available as generic? No
Drug class: Antiprotozoal, antirheumatic

USES

- Treatment for protozoal infections, such as malaria and amebiasis.
- Treatment for some forms of arthritis and lupus.

DOSAGE & USAGE INFORMATION

How to take:
Tablet—Swallow with food or milk to lessen stomach irritation.

When to take:
- Depends on condition. Is adjusted during treatment.
- Malaria prevention—Begin taking medicine 2 weeks before entering areas where malaria is present and until 8 weeks after return.

If you forget a dose:
- 1 or more doses a day—Take as soon as you remember up to 2 hours late. If more than 2 hours, wait for next scheduled dose (don't double this dose).
- 1 dose weekly—Take as soon as possible, then return to regular dosing schedule.

What drug does:
- Inhibits parasite multiplication.
- Decreases inflammatory response in diseased joint.

Time lapse before drug works:
1 to 2 hours.

Continued next column

OVERDOSE

SYMPTOMS:
Severe breathing difficulty, drowsiness, faintness, headache, seizures.
WHAT TO DO:
- **Dial 911 (emergency) for an ambulance or medical help or poison center 1-800-222-1222. Then give first aid immediately.**
- **See emergency information on inside covers.**

Don't take with:
Any other medicine without consulting your doctor or pharmacist.

POSSIBLE ADVERSE REACTIONS OR SIDE EFFECTS

SYMPTOMS	WHAT TO DO
Life-threatening: In case of overdose, see previous column.	
Common:	
Headache, appetite loss, abdominal pain.	Continue. Tell doctor at next visit.
Infrequent:	
• Blurred vision, changes in vision.	Discontinue. Call doctor right away.
• Rash or itch, diarrhea, nausea, vomiting, hair loss, blue-black skin or mouth, dizziness, nervousness.	Continue. Call doctor when convenient.
Rare:	
• Mood or mental changes, seizures, sore throat, fever, unusual bleeding or bruising, muscle weakness, convulsions.	Discontinue. Call doctor right away.
• Ringing or buzzing in ears, hearing loss.	Continue. Call doctor when convenient.

WARNINGS & PRECAUTIONS

Don't take if:
You are allergic to chloroquine or hydroxychloroquine.

Before you start, consult your doctor:
- If you plan to become pregnant within the medication period.
- If you have blood disease.
- If you have eye or vision problems.
- If you have a G6PD* deficiency.
- If you have liver disease.
- If you have nerve or brain disease (including seizure disorders).
- If you have porphyria.
- If you have psoriasis.
- If you have stomach or intestinal disease.
- If you drink more than 3 oz. of alcohol daily.

Over age 60:
Adverse reactions and side effects may be more frequent and severe than in younger persons.

Pregnancy:
Decide with your doctor if drug benefits justify risk to unborn child. Risk category C (see page xviii).

Breast-feeding:
Drug passes into milk. Avoid drug or discontinue nursing. Consult doctor for advice on maintaining milk supply.

Infants & children:
Not recommended. Dangerous.

Prolonged use:
- Permanent damage to the retina (back part of the eye) or nerve deafness.
- Talk to your doctor about the need for follow-up medical examinations or laboratory studies to check complete blood counts (white blood cell count, platelet count, red blood cell count, hemoglobin, hematocrit), eyes.

Skin & sunlight:
No special problems expected.

Driving, piloting or hazardous work:
Don't drive or pilot aircraft until you learn how medicine affects you. Don't work around dangerous machinery. Don't climb ladders or work in high places. Danger increases if you drink alcohol or take medicine affecting alertness and reflexes.

Discontinuing:
Don't discontinue without doctor's advice until you complete prescribed dose, even though symptoms diminish or disappear.

Others:
- Periodic physical and blood examinations recommended.
- If you are in a malaria area for a long time, you may need to change to another preventive drug every 2 years.

POSSIBLE INTERACTION WITH OTHER DRUGS

GENERIC NAME OR DRUG CLASS	COMBINED EFFECT
Estrogens*	Possible liver toxicity.
Gold compounds*	Risk of severe rash and itch.
Kaolin	Decreased absorption of hydroxychloroquine.
Magnesium trisilicate	Decreased absorption of hydroxychloroquine.
Penicillamine	Possible blood or kidney toxicity.

POSSIBLE INTERACTION WITH OTHER SUBSTANCES

INTERACTS WITH	COMBINED EFFECT
Alcohol:	Possible liver toxicity. Avoid.
Beverages:	None expected.
Cocaine:	None expected.
Foods:	None expected.
Marijuana:	None expected.
Tobacco:	None expected.

***See Glossary**

HYDROXYUREA

BRAND NAMES

Droxia
Hydrea

BASIC INFORMATION

Habit forming? No
Prescription needed? Yes
Available as generic? Yes
Drug class: Antineoplastic

USES

- Treats head, neck, ovarian and cervical cancer.
- Treats leukemia, melanoma and polycythemia vera.
- Treats sickle cell disease.

DOSAGE & USAGE INFORMATION

How to take:
Capsules—Swallow with liquid. If you can't swallow whole, open capsule and take with liquid or food. Instructions to take on empty stomach mean 1 hour before or 2 hours after eating.

When to take:
According to doctor's instructions.

If you forget a dose:
Skip this dose. Never double dose. Resume regular schedule.

What drug does:
Probably interferes with synthesis of DNA.

Time lapse before drug works:
2 hours.

Don't take with:
Any other medicines (including over-the-counter drugs such as cough and cold medicines, laxatives, antacids, diet pills, caffeine, nose drops or vitamins) without consulting your doctor.

OVERDOSE

SYMPTOMS:
Black, tarry stools; fainting; seizures.
WHAT TO DO:
- **Dial 911 (emergency) for an ambulance or medical help or poison center 1-800-222-1222. Then give first aid immediately.**
- **See emergency information on inside covers.**

POSSIBLE ADVERSE REACTIONS OR SIDE EFFECTS

SYMPTOMS	WHAT TO DO
Life-threatening:	
In case of overdose, see previous column.	
Common:	
• Skin rash, fever, chills, cough, back pain.	Discontinue. Call doctor right away.
• Diarrhea, drowsiness, nausea, vomiting.	Continue. Call doctor when convenient.
Infrequent:	
Mouth sores, bruising, constipation, red skin.	Discontinue. Call doctor right away.
Rare:	
Confusion, hallucinations, headache, swollen feet.	Continue. Call doctor when convenient.

WARNINGS & PRECAUTIONS

Don't take if:

- You have chicken pox.
- You have shingles (herpes zoster).

Before you start, consult your doctor:

- If you have anemia.
- If you have gout.
- If you have an infection.
- If you have kidney disease.

Over age 60:
Adverse reactions and side effects may be more frequent and severe than in younger persons. You may need smaller doses for shorter periods of time.

Pregnancy:
Decide with your doctor if drug benefits justify risk to unborn child. Risk category C (see page xviii).

Breast-feeding:
Drug passes into milk. Avoid drug or discontinue nursing until you finish medicine. Consult doctor for advice on maintaining milk supply.

Infants & children:
Effect not documented. Consult your pediatrician.

Prolonged use:
Talk to your doctor about the need for follow-up medical examinations or laboratory studies to check kidney function, complete blood counts (white blood cell count, platelet count, red blood cell count, hemoglobin, hematocrit) and serum uric acid.

Skin & sunlight:
No problems expected.

Driving, piloting or hazardous work:
Avoid if you feel confused, drowsy or dizzy.

Discontinuing:
May still experience symptoms of bone marrow depression, such as: blood in stools, fever or chills, blood spots under the skin, back pain, hoarseness, bloody urine. If any of these occur, call your doctor right away.

Others:

- Advise any doctor or dentist whom you consult that you take this medicine.
- May affect results in some medical tests.

POSSIBLE INTERACTION WITH OTHER DRUGS

GENERIC NAME OR DRUG CLASS	COMBINED EFFECT
Bone marrow depressants, other*	Dangerous suppression of bone marrow activity.
Clozapine	Toxic effect on bone marrow.
Levamisole	Increased risk of bone marrow depression.
Probenecid	May require increased dosage to treat gout.
Sulfinpyrazone	May require increased dosage to treat gout.
Tiopronin	Increased risk of toxicity to bone marrow.
Vaccines, live or killed virus	Increased risk of side effects.

POSSIBLE INTERACTION WITH OTHER SUBSTANCES

INTERACTS WITH	COMBINED EFFECT
Alcohol:	None expected.
Beverages:	None expected.
Cocaine:	None expected.
Foods:	None expected.
Marijuana:	None expected.
Tobacco:	None expected.

*See Glossary

HYDROXYZINE

BRAND NAMES

Ami Rax
Anxanil
Apo-Hydroxyzine
Atarax
Hydrophed
Marax
Novo-Hydroxyzin
T.E.H.Compound
Theomax
Vistaril

BASIC INFORMATION

Habit forming? No
Prescription needed? Yes
Available as generic? Yes
Drug class: Tranquilizer, antihistamine

USES

- Treatment for anxiety, tension and agitation.
- Relieves itching from allergic reactions.

DOSAGE & USAGE INFORMATION

How to take:
- Tablet, syrup or capsule—Swallow with liquid. If you can't swallow whole, crumble tablet or open capsule and take with liquid or food.
- Liquid—If desired, dilute dose in beverage before swallowing.

When to take:
At the same times each day.

If you forget a dose:
Take as soon as you remember up to 2 hours late. If more than 2 hours, wait for next scheduled dose (don't double this dose).

What drug does:
Blocks action of histamine after an allergic response triggers histamine release. Histamines cause itching, sneezing, runny nose and eyes and other symptoms.

Time lapse before drug works:
15 to 30 minutes.

Don't take with:
Any other medicine without consulting your doctor or pharmacist.

OVERDOSE

SYMPTOMS:
Drowsiness, unsteadiness, agitation, purposeless movements, tremor, convulsions.
WHAT TO DO:
- **Dial 911 (emergency) for an ambulance or medical help or poison center 1-800-222-1222. Then give first aid immediately.**
- **See emergency information at end of book.**

POSSIBLE ADVERSE REACTIONS OR SIDE EFFECTS

SYMPTOMS	WHAT TO DO
Life-threatening: In case of overdose, see previous column.	
Common:	
Drowsiness; dizziness; dryness of mouth, nose or throat; nausea.	Continue. Call doctor when convenient.
Infrequent:	
• Change in vision, clumsiness, rash.	Discontinue. Call doctor right away.
• Less tolerance for contact lenses, painful or difficult urination.	Continue. Call doctor when convenient.
• Appetite loss.	Continue. Tell doctor at next visit.
Rare:	
Nightmares, agitation, irritability, sore throat, fever, rapid heartbeat, unusual bleeding or bruising, fatigue, weakness, confusion, fainting, seizures.	Discontinue. Call doctor right away.

WARNINGS & PRECAUTIONS

Don't take if:
You are allergic to any antihistamine.

Before you start, consult your doctor:
- If you have asthma or kidney disease.
- If you will have surgery within 2 months, including dental surgery, requiring general or spinal anesthesia.

Over age 60:
- Adverse reactions and side effects may be more frequent and severe than in younger persons.
- Drug likely to increase urination difficulty caused by enlarged prostate gland.

Pregnancy:
Decide with your doctor if drug benefits justify risk to unborn child. Risk category C (see page xviii).

Breast-feeding:
Drug passes into milk. Avoid drug or discontinue nursing until you finish medicine. Consult doctor for advice on maintaining milk supply.

Infants & children:
Use only under medical supervision.

Prolonged use:
Tolerance* develops and reduces effectiveness.

Skin & sunlight:
No problems expected.

Driving, piloting or hazardous work:
Don't drive or pilot aircraft until you learn how medicine affects you. Don't work around dangerous machinery. Don't climb ladders or work in high places. Danger increases if you drink alcohol or take medicine affecting alertness and reflexes, such as antihistamines, tranquilizers, sedatives, pain medicine, narcotics and mind-altering drugs.

Discontinuing:
Don't discontinue without consulting doctor. Dose may require gradual reduction if you have taken drug for a long time. Doses of other drugs may also require adjustment.

Others:
Advise any doctor or dentist whom you consult that you take this medicine.

POSSIBLE INTERACTION WITH OTHER DRUGS

GENERIC NAME OR DRUG CLASS	COMBINED EFFECT
Antidepressants, tricyclic*	Increased effects of both drugs.
Antihistamines*	Increased hydroxyzine effect.
Attapulgite	Decreased hydroxyzine effect.
Carteolol	Decreased antihistamine effect.
Central nervous system (CNS) depressants*	Greater depression of central nervous system.
Clozapine	Toxic effect on the central nervous system.
Fluoxetine	Increased depressant effects of both drugs.
Guanfacine	May increase depressant effects of either drug.
Leucovorin	High alcohol content of leucovorin may cause adverse effects.
Narcotics*	Increased effects of both drugs.
Pain relievers*	Increased effects of both drugs.
Sertraline	Increased depressive effects of both drugs.
Sotalol	Increased antihistamine effect.

POSSIBLE INTERACTION WITH OTHER SUBSTANCES

INTERACTS WITH	COMBINED EFFECT
Alcohol:	Increased sedation and intoxication. Use with caution.
Beverages: Caffeine drinks.	Decreased tranquilizer effect of hydroxyzine.
Cocaine:	Decreased hydroxyzine effect. Avoid.
Foods:	None expected.
Marijuana:	None expected.
Tobacco:	None expected.

*See Glossary

HYOSCYAMINE

BRAND NAMES

Anaspaz
Anaspaz PB
Atrohist Plus
Barbidonna
Barbidonna 2
Belladenal
Neoquess
Bellafoline
Cystospaz
Cystospaz-M
Gastrosed
Kinesed
Levbid
Levsin
Levsin S/L
Levsinex
Levsinex Timecaps
Nulev
Phenahist TR
Phenchlor SHA
Ru-Tuss
Stahist

BASIC INFORMATION

Habit forming? No
Prescription needed?
Low strength: No
High strength: Yes
Available as generic? No
Drug class: Antispasmodic, anticholinergic

USES

Reduces spasms of digestive system, bladder and urethra.

DOSAGE & USAGE INFORMATION

How to take:
- Tablet or liquid—Swallow with liquid or food to lessen stomach irritation. You may chew or crush tablets.
- Extended-release capsules or tablets—Swallow each dose whole.
- Drops—Dilute dose in beverage before swallowing.

When to take:
30 minutes before meals (unless directed otherwise by doctor).

Continued next column

OVERDOSE

SYMPTOMS:
Dilated pupils, rapid pulse and breathing, dizziness, fever, hallucinations, confusion, slurred speech, agitation, flushed face, convulsions, coma.
WHAT TO DO:
- **Dial 911 (emergency) for an ambulance or medical help or poison center 1-800-222-1222. Then give first aid immediately.**
- **See emergency information on inside covers.**

If you forget a dose:
Take as soon as you remember up to 2 hours late. If more than 2 hours, wait for next scheduled dose (don't double this dose).

What drug does:
Blocks nerve impulses at parasympathetic nerve endings, preventing muscle contractions and gland secretions of organs involved.

Time lapse before drug works:
15 to 30 minutes.

Don't take with:
- Antacids* or antidiarrheals*.
- Any other medicine without consulting your doctor or pharmacist.

POSSIBLE ADVERSE REACTIONS OR SIDE EFFECTS

SYMPTOMS	WHAT TO DO
Life-threatening:	
In case of overdose, see previous column.	
Common:	
• Confusion, delirium, rapid heartbeat.	Discontinue. Call doctor right away.
• Nausea, vomiting, decreased sweating.	Continue. Call doctor when convenient.
• Constipation.	Continue. Tell doctor at next visit.
• Dryness in ears, nose, throat, mouth.	No action necessary.
Infrequent:	
• Headache, painful or difficult urination, nasal congestion, altered taste.	Continue. Call doctor when convenient.
• Lightheadedness.	Discontinue. Call doctor right away.
Rare:	
Rash or hives, eye pain, blurred vision.	Discontinue. Call doctor right away.

WARNINGS & PRECAUTIONS

Don't take if:
- You are allergic to any anticholinergic.
- You have trouble with stomach bloating.
- You have difficulty emptying your bladder completely.
- You have narrow-angle glaucoma.
- You have severe ulcerative colitis.

Before you start, consult your doctor:
- If you have open-angle glaucoma.
- If you have angina.
- If you have chronic bronchitis or asthma.
- If you have hiatal hernia.
- If you have liver, kidney or thyroid disease.
- If you have enlarged prostate.
- If you have myasthenia gravis.
- If you have peptic ulcer.
- If you will have surgery within 2 months, including dental surgery, requiring general or spinal anesthesia.

Over age 60:
Adverse reactions and side effects may be more frequent and severe than in younger persons.

Pregnancy:
Decide with your doctor if drug benefits justify risk to unborn child. Risk category C (see page xviii).

Breast-feeding:
Drug passes into milk and decreases milk flow. Avoid drug or discontinue nursing until you finish medicine. Consult doctor for advice on maintaining milk supply.

Infants & children:
Use only under medical supervision.

Prolonged use:
Chronic constipation, possible fecal impaction. Consult doctor immediately.

Skin & sunlight:
No problems expected.

Driving, piloting or hazardous work:
Use disqualifies you for piloting aircraft. Otherwise, no problems expected.

Discontinuing:
May be unnecessary to finish medicine. Follow doctor's instructions.

Others:
Advise any doctor or dentist whom you consult that you take this medicine.

POSSIBLE INTERACTION WITH OTHER DRUGS

GENERIC NAME OR DRUG CLASS	COMBINED EFFECT
Amantadine	Increased hyoscyamine effect.
Anticholinergics, other*	Increased hyoscyamine effect.
Antidepressants, tricyclic*	Increased hyoscyamine effect.
Antihistamines*	Increased hyoscyamine effect.
Cortisone drugs*	Increased internal eye pressure.
Haloperidol	Increased internal eye pressure.
Ketoconazole	Decreased ketoconazole effect.
Meperidine	Increased hyoscyamine effect.
Methylphenidate	Increased hyoscyamine effect.
Molindone	Increased anticholinergic effect.
Monoamine oxidase (MAO) inhibitors*	Increased hyoscyamine effect.
Nizatidine	Increased nizatidine effect.
Orphenadrine	Increased hyoscyamine effect.
Phenothiazines*	Increased hyoscyamine effect.
Pilocarpine	Loss of pilocarpine effect in glaucoma treatment.
Sedatives* or central nervous system (CNS) depressants*	Increased sedative effect of both drugs.
Vitamin C	Decreased hyoscyamine effect. Avoid large doses of vitamin C.

POSSIBLE INTERACTION WITH OTHER SUBSTANCES

INTERACTS WITH	COMBINED EFFECT
Alcohol:	None expected.
Beverages:	None expected.
Cocaine:	Excessively rapid heartbeat. Avoid.
Foods:	None expected.
Marijuana:	Drowsiness and dry mouth.
Tobacco:	None expected.

*See Glossary

IMATINIB

BRAND NAMES

Gleevec

BASIC INFORMATION

Habit forming? No
Prescription needed? Yes
Available as generic? No
Drug class: Antineoplastic

USES

- Treatment for chronic myeloid leukemia (CML).
- Treatment for gastrointestinal stomal tumors.

DOSAGE & USAGE INFORMATION

How to take:
Capsule—Swallow with large glass of water to minimize the risk of stomach and gastrointestinal irritation.

When to take:
Usually once a day at mealtime or according to doctor's instructions.

If you forget a dose:
Do not take the missed dose at all. Return to your regular dosing schedule at the prescribed time. Never double a dose to make up for a missed dose. Consult your doctor.

What drug does:
Reduces substantially the level of cancerous cells in the bone marrow and blood of treated patients.

Time lapse before drug works:
Starts working in 2-4 hours, but effectiveness may take 1-3 months.

Don't take with:

Any other medicines (including over-the-counter drugs such as cough and cold medicines, laxatives, antacids, diet pills, caffeine, nose drops or vitamins) without consulting your doctor.

OVERDOSE

SYMPTOMS:
Unknown effect.
WHAT TO DO:
If person takes much larger amount than prescribed, call doctor, poison center 1-800-222-1222 or hospital emergency room for instructions.

POSSIBLE ADVERSE REACTIONS OR SIDE EFFECTS

SYMPTOMS	WHAT TO DO
Life-threatening:	
Some adverse effects from advanced cancer and/or the medicine can be serious or life threatening.	Seek emergency treatment for any symptoms that appear severe or critical.
Common:	
• Chest pain, shortness of breath, swelling (face, hands, legs. feet), black tarry stools, nausea or vomiting, muscle pain or cramps, blood in urine, decreased or painful urination, fever, chills, pale skin, quick weight gain, stomach cramps, sore throat, sores on body, ulcers or white spots on lips or in mouth, swollen glands, unusual bleeding or tiredness or weakness.	Continue. Call doctor right away.
• Joint or bone pain, diarrhea, skin rash. fatigue.	Continue. Call doctor when convenient.
Infrequent:	
• Convulsions, irregular heartbeat, wheezing, tightness in chest, numbness or tingling (in hands, feet, or lips), pinpoint red spots on skin.	Continue. Call doctor right away.
• Bloody nose, mood changes, slow weight gain, weight loss, sneezing, joint pain, constipation, loss of appetite, headache, increased thirst, dry mouth.	Continue. Call doctor when convenient.
Rare:	
Acid indigestion or upset stomach, stuffy nose, itchy skin.	Continue. Call doctor when convenient.

Note: Side effects are often unavoidable with drugs used to treat cancer. Discuss any concerns or questions or other symptoms with your doctor.

PRECAUTIONS

Don't take if:
You are allergic to imatinib.

Before you start, consult your doctor:
- If you have any infection.
- If you have anemia.
- If you have leukopenia, neutropenia. or thrombocytopenia.
- If you have bone marrow depression.
- If you have recent chickenpox or herpes zoster.
- If you have liver problems.

Over age 60:
Other than a higher incidence of edema, studies to date have not shown problems that would limit the usefulness of imatinib.

Pregnancy:
Not recommended. Consult doctor. Risk category D (see page xviii).

Breast-feeding:
It is unknown if drug passes into milk. Avoid drug or discontinue nursing until you finish medicine. Consult doctor for advice on maintaining milk supply.

Infants & children:
Safety and efficacy have not been established in children under 18 years of age.

Prolonged use:
- Talk to your doctor about the need for follow-up medical examinations or laboratory studies to check your response to the drug, blood studies, weight gain and liver function.
- The long term effects of the drug are not yet known.

Skin & sunlight:
No problems expected.

Driving, piloting or hazardous work:
No problems expected.

Discontinuing:
No special problems expected. Don't discontinue drug without doctor's approval.

Others:
- Advise any doctor or dentist whom you consult that you take this medicine.
- Do not have any immunizations without your doctors approval. Imatinib may lower your resistance to the infection that you are getting the immunization for.
- Avoid persons who have recently taken the oral polio virus vaccine, they may pass the virus on to you.
- Avoid people with infections, because you have an increased chance of getting the infection.
- Advise your doctor of any unusual symptoms, infections or injuries.
- Be careful when brushing or flossing teeth, or using a razor or other sharp object to avoid being injured.
- May affect results in some medical tests.
- This is a new drug and additional information should become available as more patients use it for longer periods of time.
- Avoid contact sports or activities that could cause, injury, bruising or bleeding.

POSSIBLE INTERACTION WITH OTHER DRUGS

GENERIC NAME OR DRUG CLASS	COMBINED EFFECT
Anticoagulants*	Blood clotting problems.
Blood dyscrasia-causing medications*	Increased risk of adverse effects of imatinib.
Bone marrow depressants, other*	Increased bone marrow suppression.
Cyclosporine	Increased effect of cyclosporine.
Enzyme inducers*	Decreased effect of imatinib.
Enzyme inhibitors*	Increased effect of imatinib.
HMG-CoA reductase inhibitors	Increased effect of HMG-CoA reductase inhibitor.
Pimozide	Increased effect of pimozide.
Vaccines (live)	Increased risk of getting the disease the vaccine prevents.
Vaccines (killed)	Decreased effective-ness of vaccine.

POSSIBLE INTERACTION WITH OTHER SUBSTANCES

INTERACTS WITH	COMBINED EFFECT
Alcohol:	None expected.
Beverages:	None expected.
Cocaine:	None expected. Best to avoid.
Foods:	None expected.
Marijuana:	None expected. Best to avoid.
Tobacco:	None expected.

*See Glossary

IMMUNOSUPPRESSIVE AGENTS

GENERIC AND BRAND NAMES

MYCOPHENOLATE	TACROLIMUS
CellCept	Prograf

BASIC INFORMATION

Habit forming? No
Prescription needed? Yes
Available as generic? No
Drug class: Immunosuppressant

USES

Helps to suppress the immune system and prevent rejection in patients who have undergone organ transplants.

DOSAGE & USAGE INFORMATION

How to take:

- Oral suspension—Take as directed on label.
- Tablet or capsule—Swallow with liquid. Do not open capsule or crush tablet. Tacrolimus may be taken with or without food. Take mycophenolate on an empty stomach (1 hour before or 2 hours after a meal).

When to take:
At the same times each day, according to instructions on prescription label.

If you forget a dose:
Take as soon as you remember. If it is almost time for the next dose, wait for next scheduled dose (don't double this dose). Consult doctor if you are unsure about dosing schedule.

What drug does:
Tacrolimus and myclophenolate are 2 different types of immunsuppressive drugs. They suppress immune reactions (to transplanted organs) in certain cells by inhibiting their growth.

Time lapse before drug works:
3 to 3-1/2 hours. May take several weeks to evaluate effectiveness against organ rejection.

Continued next column

OVERDOSE

SYMPTOMS:
Increased severity of adverse reactions, coma, delirium.
WHAT TO DO:

- **Dial 911 (emergency) for an ambulance or medical help or poison center 1-800-222-1222. Then give first aid immediately.**
- **See emergency information on inside covers.**

Don't take with:
Any other medicine without consulting your doctor or pharmacist.

POSSIBLE ADVERSE REACTIONS OR SIDE EFFECTS

SYMPTOMS	WHAT TO DO
Life-threatening: In case of overdose, see previous column.	
Common:	
• Infections (fever, chills, hoarseness, cough, trouble urinating, back or side pain); headache; tingling or numbness of hands or feet; chest pain; blood in urine; trouble sleeping; trembling of hands; shortness of breath.	Continue, but call doctor right away.
• Mild back pain, constipation or diarrhea, stomach pain, heartburn.	Continue. Call doctor when convenient.
Infrequent:	
• Bloody vomit; anxiety; nervousness; white patches on mouth, tongue or throat; weakness; seizures.	Continue, but call doctor right away.
• Hair loss or excess hair growth, nausea, mild vomiting, skin rash or itch, muscle or joint pain, dizziness.	Continue. Call doctor when convenient.
Rare:	
• Bloody, black or tarry stools; small red spots on skin; unusual bleeding or bruising; irregular heartbeat.	Continue, but call doctor right away.
• Mood or mental changes, any other side effects not listed.	Continue. Call doctor when convenient

WARNINGS & PRECAUTIONS

Don't take if:
You are allergic to mycophenolate or tacrolimus.

Before you start, consult your doctor:

- If you have liver or kidney disease.
- If you have a digestive system disease.
- If you have an infection.
- If you have chickenpox (or have recently been exposed) or herpes zoster (shingles).

Over age 60:
No special problems expected.

Pregnancy:
Decide with your doctor if drug benefits justify risk to unborn child. Risk category C (see page xviii).

Breast-feeding:
Tacrolimus passes into milk; mycophenolate may pass into milk. Avoid drugs or discontinue nursing until you finish medicine. Consult doctor for advice on maintaining milk supply.

Infants & children:
Safety and effectiveness of mycophenolate are not established. Tacrolimus has been used successfully in liver transplants in pediatric patients.

Prolonged use:
- Can cause reduced function of kidneys.
- Can increase risk of developing lymphoma (cancer of lymph glands).
- Talk to your doctor about the need for follow-up medical examinations or laboratory studies to check blood concentration of drug, kidney function, liver function, potassium levels, drug's effectiveness and adverse reactions.

Skin & sunlight:
No special problems expected.

Driving, piloting or hazardous work:
Don't drive or pilot aircraft until you learn how medicine affects you. Don't work around dangerous machinery. Don't climb ladders or work in high places. Danger increases if you drink alcohol or take medicine affecting alertness and reflexes.

Discontinuing:
Don't discontinue without consulting doctor. You probably will require this medicine for the remainder of your life.

Others:
- Advise any doctor or dentist whom you consult that you take this drug. May interfere with results of some medical tests.
- Wear medical identification stating that you have had a transplant and take this drug.
- Check blood pressure routinely at home. Drug may sometimes cause hypertension.
- Avoid any immunizations except those specifically recommended by your doctor.
- Maintain good dental hygiene. Immunosuppression can cause gum problems.

POSSIBLE INTERACTION WITH OTHER DRUGS

GENERIC NAME OR DRUG CLASS	COMBINED EFFECT
Acyclovir	Increased effect of mycophenolate.
Antacids*	Decreased effect of mycophenolate.
Cholestyramine	Decreased effect of mycophenolate.
Diuretics, potassium-sparing*	Increased risk of potassium toxicity.
Enzyme inducers*	Decreased effect of tacrolimus.
Enzyme inhibitors*	Increased effect of tacrolimus.
Gancyclovir	Increased effect of mycophenolate.
Immunosuppressants*, other	Increased immunosuppressive effect.
Nephrotoxic medications*	Increased risk of kidney problems.
Potassium supplements	Increased risk of potassium toxicity.
Probenecid	Increased effect of mycophenolate.
Troglitazone	Decreased effect of tacrolimus.
Vaccinations	Avoid unless doctor approves.

POSSIBLE INTERACTION WITH OTHER SUBSTANCES

INTERACTS WITH	COMBINED EFFECT
Alcohol:	May increase possibility of toxic effects. Avoid.
Beverages: Grapefruit juice.	Increased effect and toxicity of drug. Avoid.
Cocaine:	May increase possibility of toxic effects. Avoid.
Foods:	No special problems expected.
Marijuana:	May increase possibility of toxic effects. Avoid.
Tobacco:	None expected.

*See Glossary

INDAPAMIDE

BRAND NAMES

Lozide Lozol

BASIC INFORMATION

Habit forming? No
Prescription needed? Yes
Available as generic? Yes
Drug class: Antihypertensive, diuretic

USES

- Controls, but doesn't cure, high blood pressure.
- Reduces fluid retention (edema) caused by conditions such as heart disorders.

DOSAGE & USAGE INFORMATION

How to take:
Tablet—Swallow with liquid or food to lessen stomach irritation.

When to take:
At the same times each day, usually at bedtime.

If you forget a dose:
Bedtime dose—If you forget your once-a-day bedtime dose, don't take it more than 3 hours late. Never double dose.

What drug does:
Forces kidney to excrete more sodium and causes excess salt and fluid to be excreted.

Time lapse before drug works:
2 hours for effect to begin. May require 1 to 4 weeks for full effects.

Continued next column

OVERDOSE

SYMPTOMS:
Nausea, vomiting, diarrhea, very dry mouth, thirst, weakness, excessive fatigue, very rapid heart rate, weak pulse.
WHAT TO DO:
- **Dial 911 (emergency) for an ambulance or medical help or poison center 1-800-222-1222. Then give first aid immediately.**
- **If patient is unconscious and not breathing, give mouth-to-mouth breathing. If there is no heartbeat, use cardiac massage and mouth-to-mouth breathing (CPR). Don't try to make patient vomit. If you can't get help quickly, take patient to nearest emergency facility.**
- **See emergency information on inside covers.**

Don't take with:
Any other medicine without consulting your doctor or pharmacist.

POSSIBLE ADVERSE REACTIONS OR SIDE EFFECTS

SYMPTOMS	WHAT TO DO
Life-threatening: In case of overdose, see previous column.	
Common:	
• Excessive tiredness or weakness, muscle cramps.	Discontinue. Call doctor right away.
• Frequent urination.	Continue. Tell doctor at next visit.
Infrequent:	
Insomnia, mood change, dizziness on changing position, headache, excessive thirst, diarrhea, appetite loss, nausea, dry mouth, decreased sex drive..	Continue. Call doctor when convenient.
Rare:	
• Weak pulse.	Discontinue. Seek emergency treatment.
• Itching, rash, hives, irregular heartbeat.	Discontinue. Call doctor right away.

WARNINGS & PRECAUTIONS

Don't take if:
- You are allergic to indapamide or to any sulfa drug or thiazide diuretic.*
- You have severe kidney disease.

Before you start, consult your doctor:
- If you have severe kidney disease.
- If you have diabetes.
- If you have gout.
- If you have liver disease.
- If you will have surgery within 2 months, including dental surgery, requiring general or spinal anesthesia.
- If you have lupus erythematosus.
- If you are pregnant or plan to become pregnant.

Over age 60:
Adverse reactions and side effects may be more frequent and severe than in younger persons.

Pregnancy:
Consult doctor. Risk category B (see page xviii).

Breast-feeding:
Unknown effect on child. Consult doctor.

Infants & children:
Use only under close medical supervision.

Prolonged use:
Request laboratory studies for blood sugar, BUN*, uric acid and serum electrolytes (potassium and sodium).

Skin & sunlight:
May cause rash or intensify sunburn in areas exposed to sun or ultraviolet light (photosensitivity reaction). Avoid overexposure. Notify doctor if reaction occurs.

Driving, piloting or hazardous work:
Don't drive or pilot aircraft until you learn how medicine affects you. Don't work around dangerous machinery. Don't climb ladders or work in high places. Danger increases if you drink alcohol or take medicine affecting alertness and reflexes, such as antihistamines, tranquilizers, sedatives, pain medicine, narcotics and mind-altering drugs.

Discontinuing:
Don't discontinue without consulting doctor. Dose may require gradual reduction if you have taken drug for a long time. Doses of other drugs may also require adjustment.

Others:
No problems expected.

POSSIBLE INTERACTION WITH OTHER DRUGS

GENERIC NAME OR DRUG CLASS	COMBINED EFFECT
Adrenocorticoids, systemic	Possible excessive potassium loss.
Allopurinol	Decreased allopurinol effect.
Amiodarone	Increased risk of heartbeat irregularity due to low potassium.
Amphotericin B	Increased potassium.
Angiotensin-converting enzyme (ACE) inhibitors*	Decreased blood pressure. Possible excessive potassium in blood.
Antidepressants, tricyclic*	Dangerous drop in blood pressure.
Antidiabetic agents, oral*	Increased blood sugar.
Antihypertensives, other*	Increased anti-hypertensive effect.
Barbiturates*	Increased indapamide effect.
Beta-adrenergic blocking agents*	Increased effect of indapamide.
Calcium supplements*	Increased calcium in blood.
Carteolol	Increased anti-hypertensive effect.
Cholestyramine	Decreased indapamide effect.
Colestipol	Decreased indapamide effect.
Digitalis preparations*	Excessive potassium loss that may cause dangerous heart rhythms.
Diuretics, thiazide*	Increased effect of thiazide diuretics.
Indomethacin	Decreased indapamide effect.
Lithium	High risk of lithium toxicity.
Monoamine oxidase (MAO) inhibitors*	Increased indapamide effect.
Nicardipine	Dangerous blood pressure drop. Dosages may require adjustment.
Nimodipine	Dangerous blood pressure drop.

Continued on page 916

POSSIBLE INTERACTION WITH OTHER SUBSTANCES

INTERACTS WITH	COMBINED EFFECT
Alcohol:	Dangerous blood pressure drop. Avoid.
Beverages:	No problems expected.
Cocaine:	Increased risk of heart block and high blood pressure.
Foods: Licorice.	Excessive potassium loss that may cause dangerous heart rhythms.
Marijuana:	Reduced effectiveness of indapamide. Avoid.
Tobacco:	Reduced effectiveness of indapamide. Avoid.

***See Glossary**

INSULIN

BRAND NAMES

See complete list of brand names in the *Generic and Brand Name Directory*, page 862.

BASIC INFORMATION

Habit forming? No
Prescription needed? No
Available as generic? Yes
Drug class: Antidiabetic

USES

Controls diabetes mellitus, a metabolic disorder, in which the body does not manufacture insulin.

DOSAGE & USAGE INFORMATION

How to take:
Taken by injection under the skin. Use disposable, sterile needles. Rotate injection sites.

When to take:
At the same time each day.

If you forget a dose:
Take as soon as you remember. Wait at least 4 hours for next dose. Resume regular schedule.

What drug does:
Facilitates passage of blood sugar through cell membranes so sugar is usable.

Time lapse before drug works:
30 minutes to 8 hours, depending on type of insulin used.

Continued next column

OVERDOSE

SYMPTOMS:
Low blood sugar (hypoglycemia)—Anxiety; chills, cold sweats, pale skin; drowsiness; excessive hunger; headache; nausea; nervousness; fast heartbeat; shakiness; unusual tiredness or weakness.
WHAT TO DO:

- **Eat some type of sugar immediately, such as glucose product, orange juice (ad some sugar), nondiet sodas, candy (such as 5 Lifesavers), honey.**
- **If patient loses consciousness, give glucagon if you have it and know how to use it.**
- **Otherwise, dial 911 (emergency) for an ambulance or medical help or poison center 1-800-222-1222. Then give first aid immediately.**
- **See emergency information on inside covers.**

Don't take with:
Any other medicine without consulting your doctor or pharmacist.

POSSIBLE ADVERSE REACTIONS OR SIDE EFFECTS

SYMPTOMS	WHAT TO DO
Life-threatening:	
Hives, rash, intense itching, faintness soon after a dose (anaphylaxis).	Seek emergency treatment immediately.
Common:	
None expected.	
Infrequent:	
• Symptoms of low blood sugar—nervousness, hunger (excessive), cold sweats, rapid pulse, anxiety, cold skin, chills, confusion, concentration loss, drowsiness, headache, nausea, weakness, shakiness, vision changes.	Seek treatment (eat some form of quick-acting sugar—glucose tablets, sugar, fruit juice, corn syrup, honey).
• Symptoms of high blood sugar—increased urination, unusual thirst, dry mouth, drowsiness, flushed or dry skin, fruit-like breath odor, appetite loss, stomach pain or vomiting, tiredness, trouble breathing, increased blood sugar level.	Seek emergency treatment immediately.
• Swelling, redness, itch or warmth at injection site.	Continue. Call doctor when convenient.
Rare:	
None expected.	

WARNINGS & PRECAUTIONS

Don't take if:

- Your diagnosis and dose schedule is not established.
- You don't know how to deal with overdose emergencies.

Before you start, consult your doctor:

- If you are allergic to insulin.
- If you take MAO inhibitors.
- If you have liver or kidney disease or low thyroid function.

Over age 60:
Guard against hypoglycemia. Repeated episodes can cause permanent confusion and abnormal behavior.

Pregnancy:
Adhere rigidly to diabetes treatment program. Risk category B (see page xviii).

Breast-feeding:
No problems expected. Consult doctor.

Infants & children:
Use only under medical supervision.

Prolonged use:
Talk to your doctor about the need for follow-up medical examinations or laboratory studies to check blood sugar, serum potassium, urine.

Skin & sunlight:
No problems expected.

Driving, piloting or hazardous work:
No problems expected after dose is established.

Discontinuing:
Don't discontinue without doctor's advice until you complete prescribed dose, even though symptoms diminish or disappear.

Others:
- Diet and exercise affect how much insulin you need. Work with your doctor to determine accurate dose.
- Notify your doctor if you skip a dose, overeat, have fever or infection.
- Notify doctor if you develop symptoms of high blood sugar: drowsiness, dry skin, orange fruit-like odor to breath, increased urination, appetite loss, unusual thirst.
- Never freeze insulin.
- May interfere with the accuracy of some medical tests.

POSSIBLE INTERACTION WITH OTHER DRUGS

GENERIC NAME OR DRUG CLASS	COMBINED EFFECT
Adrenocorticoids, systemic	Decreased insulin effect.
Anticonvulsants, hydantoin*	Decreased insulin effect.
Antidiabetics, oral*	Increased antibiabetic effect.
Beta-adrenergic blocking agents*	Possible increased difficulty in regulating blood sugar levels.
Bismuth subsalicylate	Increased insulin effect. May require dosage adjustment.
Carteolol	Hypoglycemic effects may be prolonged.
Contraceptives, oral*	Decreased insulin effect.
Dexfenfluramine	May require dosage change as weight loss occurs.
Diuretics, thiazide*	Decreased insulin effect.
Furosemide	Decreased insulin effect.
Insulin analogs	May require dosage adjustment.
Monoamine oxidase (MAO) inhibitors*	Increased insulin effect.
Nicotine	Increased insulin effect.
Oxyphenbutazone	Increased insulin effect.
Phenylbutazone	Increased insulin effect.
Salicylates*	Increased insulin effect.
Smoking deterrents	May require insulin dosage adjustment.
Sulfa drugs*	Increased insulin effect.
Tetracyclines*	Increased insulin effect.
Thyroid hormones*	Decreased insulin effect.

POSSIBLE INTERACTION WITH OTHER SUBSTANCES

INTERACTS WITH	COMBINED EFFECT
Alcohol:	Increased insulin effect. Blood sugar problems Avoid.
Beverages:	None expected.
Cocaine:	Unknown effect. Avoid.
Foods:	None expected. Follow your diabetic diet instructions.
Marijuana:	Possible increase in blood sugar. Avoid.
Tobacco:	Decreased insulin absorption. Avoid.

*See Glossary

INSULIN ANALOGS

BENERIC AND BRAND NAMES

INSULIN ASPART
Novolog
INSULIN GLARGINE
Lantus
Glargine
INSULIN LISPRO
Humalog
Humalog Mix 75/25

BASIC INFORMATION

Habit forming? No
Prescription needed? Yes
Available as generic? No
Drug class: Antidiabetic

USES

Controls diabetes mellitus, a metabolic disorder in which the body does not manufacture insulin. These insulins are rapid- or fast-acting; working quickly in the body after injection. Human insulin analogs are variations (analogs) of human insulin. Insulin analogs are being developed to more closely mimic the time action of insulin naturally secreted from the pancreas.

DOSAGE & USAGE INFORMATION

How to take:
Taken by injection under the skin. Use disposable, sterile needles. Rotate injection sites. Follow instructions provided with the product.

Continued next column

OVERDOSE

SYMPTOMS:
Low blood sugar (hypoglycemia)—Anxiety; chills, cold sweats, pale skin; drowsiness; excessive hunger; headache; nausea; nervousness; fast heartbeat; shakiness; unusual tiredness or weakness.
WHAT TO DO:

- **Eat some type of sugar immediately, such as glucose product, orange juice (ad some sugar), nondiet sodas, candy (such as 5 Lifesavers), honey.**
- **If patient loses consciousness, give glucagon if you have it and know how to use it.**
- **Otherwise, dial 911 (emergency) for an ambulance or medical help or poison center 1-800-222-1222. Then give first aid immediately.**
- **See emergency information on inside covers.**

When to take:
At the same times each day. If taken at mealtime, use it within a 15 minute period prior to the meal. May need to be taken in combination with a long-acting insulin to prevent hyperglycemia.

If you forget a dose:
Follow your doctor's instructions. If unsure, call your doctor or pharmacist.

What drug does:
Facilitates passage of blood sugar through cell membranes so sugar is usable. The drug helps keep your blood sugar levels from going too high after you eat.

Time lapse before drug works:
30 minutes to 1 hour, which is faster than regular insulin. Insulin aspart and insulin lispro finish acting in 3-4 hours, insulin glargine in 24 hours.

Don't take with:
Any other medicine without consulting your doctor or pharmacist.

POSSIBLE ADVERSE REACTIONS OR SIDE EFFECTS

SYMPTOMS	WHAT TO DO
Life-threatening:	
Hives, rash, intense itching, faintness, swelling, breathing difficulty soon after a dose (anaphylaxis).	Seek emergency treatment immediately.
Common:	
None expected.	
Infrequent:	
• Symptoms of low blood sugar—nervousness, hunger (excessive), cold sweats, rapid pulse, anxiety, cold skin, chills, confusion, concentration loss, drowsiness, headache, nausea, weakness, shakiness, vision changes.	Seek treatment (eat some form of quick-acting sugar—glucose tablets, sugar, fruit juice, corn syrup, honey).
• Symptoms of high blood sugar—increased urination, unusual thirst, dry mouth, drowsiness, flushed or dry skin, fruit-like breath odor, appetite loss, stomach pain or vomiting, tiredness, trouble breathing, increased blood sugar level.	Seek emergency treatment immediately.

• Swelling, redness, itch or warmth at injection site; other skin changes at injection site (e.g., thinning or thickened skin).	Continue. Call doctor when convenient.
Rare:	
Dry mouth, excessive thirst, weak or fast pulse, heartbeat irregularities, mental or mood changes, nausea or vomiting, unusual tiredness or weakness, muscle cramps (may be symptoms of hypokalemia).	Continue, but call doctor right away.

WARNINGS & PRECAUTIONS

Don't take if:
If you are allergic to insulin.

Before you start, consult your doctor:
- Your diagnosis and dose schedule are not established or you don't know how to deal with overdose emergencies.
- If you take MAO inhibitors*.
- If you have hypoglycemia, liver or kidney disease or low thyroid function.

Over age 60:
Insulin requirements may change. The family should notify the doctor if abnormal behavior or confusion occurs in an older person.

Pregnancy:
Risk category B for lispro and category C for aspart and glargine. See page xviii and consult doctor.

Breast-feeding:
Unknown if drugs pass into milk. May require dosage adjustment. Consult doctor.

Infants & children:
Use only under medical supervision.

Prolonged use:
Talk to your doctor about the need for follow-up medical examinations or laboratory studies to check effectiveness of drug.

Skin & sunlight:
No problems expected.

Driving, piloting or hazardous work:
No problems expected after dose is established. Need to be cautious for signs of hypoglycemia.

Discontinuing:
Don't discontinue without doctor's advice, even though symptoms diminish or disappear.

Others:
- Diet and exercise affect how much insulin you need. Work with your doctor to determine accurate dose. Monitor your glucose levels as directed.
- Notify your doctor if you have a fever, infection, diarrhea, or experience vomiting.
- Advise any doctor or dentist whom you consult that you take this medicine.
- Never freeze insulin.
- Wear medical identification that indicates you have diabetes and take insulin.
- You and your family should educate yourselves about diabetes; learn to recognize hypoglycemia and treat it with sugar or glucagon.
- May interfere with the accuracy of some medical tests.

POSSIBLE INTERACTION WITH OTHER DRUGS

GENERIC NAME OR DRUG CLASS	COMBINED EFFECT
Antidiabetics, oral*	Increased antidiabetic effect.
Hyperglycemia-causing agents*	May need increased dosage of insulin.
Hypoglycemia-causing agents*	May need decreased dosage of insulin.
Insulin	May need dosage adjustment.
Sympatholytics*	Increased insulin effect.
Smoking deterrents	May require insulin dosage adjustment.

POSSIBLE INTERACTION WITH OTHER SUBSTANCES

INTERACTS WITH	COMBINED EFFECT
Alcohol:	Increased insulin effect. Blood sugar problems Avoid.
Beverages:	None expected.
Cocaine:	Unknown effect. Avoid.
Foods:	None expected. Follow your diabetic diet instructions.
Marijuana:	Possible increase in blood sugar. Avoid.
Tobacco:	Decreased insulin absorption. Avoid.

***See Glossary**

INTERMITTENT CLAUDICATION AGENTS

GENERIC AND BRAND NAMES

CILOSTAZOL
Pletal

BASIC INFORMATION

Habit forming? No
Prescription needed?
U.S.: Yes, for some
Canada: No
Available as generic? Yes
Drug class: Vasodilator

USES

- Treats intermittent claudication (leg pain caused by poor circulation).
- May improve poor blood flow to extremities.

DOSAGE & USAGE INFORMATION

How to take:
Tablet or capsule—Swallow with liquid. If you can't swallow whole, crumble tablet or open capsule and take with liquid or food.

When to take:
- For cyclandelate, at the same time each day.
- For cilostazol, take 1 hour before or 2 hours after breakfast and dinner.

If you forget a dose:
Take as soon as you remember up to 2 hours late. If more than 2 hours, wait for next scheduled dose (don't double this dose).

What drug does:
Increases blood flow by relaxing and expanding blood-vessel walls.

Time lapse before drug works:
3-4 weeks.

Don't take with:
Any other medicine, herbal remedy or dietary supplements without consulting your doctor or pharmacist.

OVERDOSE

SYMPTOMS:
Severe headache, diarrhea, dizziness, change in heartbeat, nausea or vomiting; flushed, hot face.
WHAT TO DO:
Overdose unlikely to threaten life. If person takes much larger amount than prescribed, call doctor, poison center 1-800-222-1222 or hospital emergency room for instructions.

POSSIBLE ADVERSE REACTIONS OR SIDE EFFECTS

SYMPTOMS	WHAT TO DO
Life-threatening:	
In case of overdose, see previous column.	
Common:	
• Fever, rapid or irregular heartbeat.	Discontinue. Call doctor right away.
• Abdominal pain, back pain, dizziness, headache, diarrhea, gas, heartburn, cough, muscle stiffness, nausea, swelling of arms and legs.	Continue. Call doctor if symptoms persist.
Infrequent:	
• Irregular heartbeat, tongue swelling, nosebleeds, abnormal bleeding, bloody mucus, bloody stools, stiff neck, runny nose, fainting.	Discontinue. Call doctor right away.
• Dizziness upon arising; headache; weakness; flushed face; tingling in face, fingers or toes; unusual sweating, belching, bone pain, stomach cramping, burning in throat or chest, difficulty in swallowing, ringing in the ears, hives.	Continue. Call doctor when convenient.
Rare:	
None expected.	

INTERMITTENT CLAUDICATION AGENTS

WARNINGS & PRECAUTIONS

Don't take if:
You have had allergic reaction to cilostazol or cyclandelate.

Before you start, consult your doctor:
- If you have glaucoma.
- If you have heart disease, especially chronic heart failure (CHF).
- If you have kidney disease.
- If you smoke.

Over age 60:
Adverse reactions and side effects may be more frequent and severe than in younger persons.

Pregnancy:
Consult doctor. Risk category C (see page xviii).

Breast-feeding:
It is unknown if drug passes into milk. It is not recommended for use in nursing mothers.

Infants & children:
Cyclandelate is not recommended for children. Consult doctor regarding use of cilostazol.

Prolonged use:
No problems expected.

Skin & sunlight:
No problems expected.

Driving, piloting or hazardous work:
Avoid if you feel dizzy or weak. Otherwise, no problems expected.

Discontinuing:
Don't discontinue without doctor's advice until you complete prescribed dose, even though symptoms diminish or disappear.

Others:
- Response to drug varies. If your symptoms don't improve after 3 weeks of use, consult doctor.
- Avoid smoking while taking this medication, as it may worsen your condition.
- Advise any doctor or dentist whom you consult that you take this medicine.

POSSIBLE INTERACTION WITH OTHER DRUGS

GENERIC NAME OR DRUG CLASS	COMBINED EFFECT
Aspirin	Effects unknown.
Enzyme inhibitors*	Increased effect of intermittent claudication agent.
Sertraline	Increased effect of cilostazol.

POSSIBLE INTERACTION WITH OTHER SUBSTANCES

INTERACTS WITH	COMBINED EFFECT
Alcohol:	None expected.
Beverages: Grapefruit juice.	Increased drug effect.
Cocaine:	Decreased drug effect. Avoid.
Foods:	None expected.
Marijuana:	None expected.
Tobacco:	May decrease drug effect. Avoid.

***See Glossary**

IODOQUINOL

BRAND NAMES

Diiodohydroxyquin
Diodoquin
Diquinol
Yodoquinol
Yodoxin

BASIC INFORMATION

Habit forming? No
Prescription needed? Yes
Available as generic? Yes
Drug class: Antiprotozoal, antiparasitic

USES

Treatment for intestinal amebiasis and balantidiasis.

DOSAGE & USAGE INFORMATION

How to take:
Tablets—Mix with applesauce or chocolate syrup if unable to swallow tablets.

When to take:
Three times daily after meals for 20 days. Treatment may be repeated after 2 to 3 weeks.

If you forget a dose:
Take as soon as you remember up to 2 hours late. If more than 2 hours, wait for next scheduled dose (don't double this dose).

What drug does:
Kills amoeba (microscopic parasites) in intestinal tract.

Time lapse before drug works:
May require full course of treatment (20 days) to cure.

Don't take with:
Any other medication without consulting your doctor or pharmacist.

OVERDOSE

SYMPTOMS:

- **Prolonged dosing at high level may produce blurred vision, muscle pain, eye pain, numbness and tingling in hands or feet.**
- **Single overdosage unlikely to threaten life.**

WHAT TO DO:
If person takes much larger amount than prescribed, call doctor, poison center 1-800-222-1222 or hospital emergency room for instructions.

POSSIBLE ADVERSE REACTIONS OR SIDE EFFECTS

SYMPTOMS	WHAT TO DO
Life-threatening: In case of overdose, see previous column.	
Common:	
Diarrhea, nausea, vomiting, abdominal pain.	Continue. Call doctor when convenient.
Infrequent:	
• Clumsiness, rash, hives, itching, blurred vision, muscle pain, numbness or tingling in hands or feet, chills, fever, weakness.	Discontinue. Call doctor right away.
• Swelling of neck. (thyroid gland)	Continue. Call doctor when convenient.
Rare:	
Dizziness, headache, rectal itching.	Continue. Call doctor when convenient.

WARNINGS & PRECAUTIONS

Don't take if:
You have kidney or liver disease.

Before you start, consult your doctor:
If you have optic atrophy or thyroid disease.

Over age 60:
Adverse reactions and side effects may be more frequent and severe than in younger persons.

Pregnancy:
Decide with your doctor if drug benefits justify risk to unborn child. Risk category C (see page xviii).

Breast-feeding:
No proven problems, but avoid if possible. Discontinue nursing until you finish medicine. Consult doctor for advice on maintaining milk supply.

Infants & children:
Not recommended. Safety and dosage has not been established.

Prolonged use:
Not recommended.

Skin & sunlight:
No problems expected.

Driving, piloting or hazardous work:
No problems expected.

Discontinuing:
Don't discontinue without consulting doctor.

Others:
- Thyroid tests may be inaccurate for as long as 6 months after discontinuing iodoquinol treatment.
- May interfere with the accuracy of some medical tests.

POSSIBLE INTERACTION WITH OTHER DRUGS

GENERIC NAME OR DRUG CLASS	COMBINED EFFECT
None expected.	

POSSIBLE INTERACTION WITH OTHER SUBSTANCES

INTERACTS WITH	COMBINED EFFECT
Alcohol:	None expected.
Beverages:	None expected.
Cocaine:	None expected.
Foods:	Taking with food may decrease gastrointestinal side effects.
Marijuana:	None expected.
Tobacco:	None expected.

*See Glossary

IPECAC

BRAND NAMES

Ipecac Syrup
Quelidrine Cough

BASIC INFORMATION

Habit forming? No
Prescription needed? No
Available as generic? Yes
Drug class: Emetic

USES

- Used in emergencies to induce vomiting after medication overdose and in some instances of poisoning.
- Don't use if suspected substance to be vomited is strychnine or a corrosive such as lye, kerosene, gasoline, bleach, strong acid or cleaning fluid.

How to take:
- Call doctor, poison control center or emergency room before giving ipecac to any one.
- Don't give to an unconscious or semiconscious person.
- Syrup, undiluted—Carefully follow instructions on the bottle.
- Drink water immediately after taking ipecac.
- Place person in a head-down position to prevent aspiration of vomitus.

When to take:
- Upon discovery of accidental or intentional poisoning or overdose.
- May repeat in 30 minutes if vomiting doesn't occur with first ipecac dose.
- Don't give more than 2 doses.

If you forget a dose:
One-time use only.

Continued next column

OVERDOSE

SYMPTOMS:
Watery diarrhea, breathing difficulty, stiff muscles.
WHAT TO DO:
- **Dial 911 (emergency) for an ambulance or medical help or poison center 1-800-222-1222. Then give first aid immediately.**
- **See emergency information on inside covers.**

What drug does:
Irritates stomach lining and stimulates the vomiting center in the brain.

Time lapse before drug works:
20 minutes.

Don't take with:
Any other medicines (including over-the-counter drugs such as cough and cold medicines, laxatives, antacids, diet pills, caffeine, nose drops or vitamins) without consulting your doctor.

POSSIBLE ADVERSE REACTIONS OR SIDE EFFECTS

SYMPTOMS	WHAT TO DO
Life-threatening:	
Heartbeat irregularity.	Seek emergency treatment immediately.
Common:	
None expected.	
Infrequent:	
None expected.	
Rare:	
None expected.	

WARNINGS & PRECAUTIONS

Don't take if:
You are intoxicated from any source.

Before you start, consult your doctor:
If you have heart disease (ipecac can be poisonous to a damaged heart).

Over age 60:
No special problems expected.

Pregnancy:
No studies done. Unknown effect. Consult doctor. Risk category C (see page xviii).

Breast-feeding:
Consult your doctor.

Infants & children:
Give only after consulting doctor or poison control center.

Prolonged use:
Not intended for long-term use.

Skin & sunlight:
No problems expected.

Driving, piloting or hazardous work:
Don't drive or pilot aircraft until you learn how medicine affects you. Don't work around dangerous machinery. Don't climb ladders or work in high places. Danger increases if you drink alcohol or take medicine affecting alertness and reflexes.

Discontinuing:
No special problems expected.

Others:
- If you are instructed to also use activated charcoal, don't use until after ipecac has induced vomiting.
- Don't give more than 2 doses to anyone.
- Don't use ipecac as a means of inducing vomiting to lose weight. It can be toxic to the heart and cause death as a result of chronic use.

POSSIBLE INTERACTION WITH OTHER DRUGS

GENERIC NAME OR DRUG CLASS	COMBINED EFFECT
Antiemetics*	Decreased ipecac effect. Possible ipecac toxicity.
Charcoal, activated	Improves treatment. If taken for the same overdose, charcoal should follow vomiting induced by ipecac.
Other medicines or herbs to cause vomiting	Decreased ipecac effect.

POSSIBLE INTERACTION WITH OTHER SUBSTANCES

INTERACTS WITH	COMBINED EFFECT
Alcohol:	Avoid. Vomiting while intoxicated can be dangerous.
Beverages:	
Carbonated.	Stomach distention. Avoid.
Milk.	Decreased ipecac effect.
Cocaine:	Avoid.
Foods:	None expected.
Marijuana:	Avoid. Aspiration of vomitus could be fatal.
Tobacco:	None expected.

*See Glossary

IPRATROPIUM

BRAND NAMES

Apo-Ipravent
Atrovent
Combivent
Duoneb
Kendral-Ipratropium

BASIC INFORMATION

Habit forming? No
Prescription needed? Yes
Available as generic? No
Drug class: Bronchodilator, anticholinergic

USES

- Treats asthma, bronchitis and emphysema.
- Should not be used alone for acute asthma attacks. May be used with inhalation forms of albuterol or fenoterol.
- May be used to treat rhinorrhea (runny nose).

DOSAGE & USAGE INFORMATION

How to use:
- By inhalation. Follow printed instructions on package.
- Avoid contact with eyes.
- Allow 1 minute between inhalations.

When to take:
Follow your doctor's instructions.

If you forget a dose:
Take as soon as you remember up to 2 hours late. If more than 2 hours, wait for next scheduled dose (don't double this dose).

What drug does:
Dilates bronchial tubes or nasal passages by direct effect on them.

Time lapse before drug works:
None. Effect begins right away.

Don't take with:
Any other medicines (including over-the-counter drugs such as cough and cold medicines, laxatives, antacids, diet pills, caffeine, nose drops or vitamins) without consulting your doctor.

OVERDOSE

SYMPTOMS:
None likely.
WHAT TO DO:
Overdose unlikely to threaten life. If person takes much larger amount than prescribed, call doctor, poison center 1-800-222-1222 or hospital emergency room for instructions.

POSSIBLE ADVERSE REACTIONS OR SIDE EFFECTS

SYMPTOMS	WHAT TO DO
Life-threatening:	
Pounding heartbeat.	Discontinue. Call doctor right away.
Common:	
Cough, headache, dizziness, nervousness, nausea.	Continue. Call doctor when convenient.
Infrequent:	
Blurred vision, difficult urination, stuffy nose, insomnia, tremors, weakness.	Continue. Call doctor when convenient.
Rare:	
Skin rash, ulcers on lips or in mouth, hives.	Discontinue. Call doctor right away.

WARNINGS & PRECAUTIONS

Don't take if:
You are sensitive to belladonna or atropine.

Before you start, consult your doctor:
- If you have prostate trouble.
- If you have glaucoma.
- If you have severe dental problems.

Over age 60:
Adverse reactions and side effects may be more frequent and severe than in younger persons. You may need smaller doses for shorter periods of time.

Pregnancy:
Consult doctor. Risk category B (see page xviii).

Breast-feeding:
No special problems expected. Consult doctor.

Infants & children:
Effect not documented. Consult your pediatrician.

Prolonged use:
Decreases saliva flow and may increase cavities, gum disease, thrush and discomfort.

Skin & sunlight:
No problems expected.

Driving, piloting or hazardous work:
Avoid if you feel confused, drowsy or dizzy.

Discontinuing:
No special problems expected.

Others:
- Advise any doctor or dentist whom you consult that you take this medicine.
- Allow 5-minute intervals between ipratropium inhalations and inhalations of cromolyn, cortisone or other inhalant medicines.
- Check with doctor if this medicine doesn't bring relief within 30 minutes.

POSSIBLE INTERACTION WITH OTHER DRUGS

GENERIC NAME OR DRUG CLASS	COMBINED EFFECT
Anticholinergics*	Increased anticholinergic effect.
Cromolyn (inhalation form)	Wait 5 minutes before using cromolyn.

POSSIBLE INTERACTION WITH OTHER SUBSTANCES

INTERACTS WITH	COMBINED EFFECT
Alcohol:	None expected.
Beverages:	None expected.
Cocaine:	Excess central nervous system stimulation. Avoid.
Foods:	None expected.
Marijuana:	Decreased ipratropium effect.
Tobacco:	Decreased ipratropium effect.

***See Glossary**

IRON SUPPLEMENTS

GENERIC AND BRAND NAMES

See complete list of generic and brand names in the *Generic and Brand Name Directory*, page 862.

BASIC INFORMATION

Habit forming? No
Prescription needed?
With folic acid: Yes
Without folic acid: No
Available as generic? Yes
Drug class: Mineral supplement (iron)

USES

Treatment for dietary iron deficiency or iron-deficiency anemia from other causes.

DOSAGE & USAGE INFORMATION

How to take:

- Tablet, capsule or syrup—Swallow with liquid or food to lessen stomach irritation. If you can't swallow whole, crumble tablet or open capsule and take with liquid or food. Place medicine far back on tongue to avoid staining teeth.
- Extended-release capsule—Swallow whole with liquid. Do not crush.
- Chewable tablets—Chew well before swallowing.
- Liquid—Dilute dose in beverage before swallowing and drink through a straw.

When to take:
1 hour before or 2 hours after eating.

If you forget a dose:
Take up to 2 hours late. If more than 2 hours, wait for next dose (don't double this dose).

Continued next column

OVERDOSE

SYMPTOMS:

- **Moderate overdose—Stomach pain, vomiting, diarrhea, black stools, lethargy.**
- **Serious overdose—Weakness and collapse; pallor, weak and rapid heartbeat; shallow breathing; convulsions and coma.**

WHAT TO DO:

- **Dial 911 (emergency) for an ambulance or medical help or poison center 1-800-222-1222. Then give first aid immediately.**
- **See emergency information on inside covers.**

What drug does:
Stimulates bone marrow's production of hemoglobin (red blood cell pigment that carries oxygen to body cells).

Time lapse before drug works:
3 to 7 days. May require 3 weeks for maximum benefit.

Don't take with:

- Multiple vitamin and mineral supplements.
- Any other medicine without consulting your doctor or pharmacist.

POSSIBLE ADVERSE REACTIONS OR SIDE EFFECTS

SYMPTOMS	WHAT TO DO
Life-threatening: In case of overdose, see last column.	
Common:	
• Stomach pain that is continuing.	Discontinue. Call doctor right away.
• Dark green or black stool, teeth stained with liquid iron, constipation, diarrhea, mild nausea or vomiting.	Continue. Call doctor when convenient.
Infrequent: None expected.	
Rare:	
• Throat pain on swallowing, chest pain, cramps, blood in stool or black stool that has sticky constistency.	Discontinue. Call doctor right away.
• Darkened urine, heartburn.	Continue. Call doctor when convenient.

WARNINGS & PRECAUTIONS

Don't take if:

- You are allergic to any iron supplement or tartrazine dye.
- You take iron injections.
- You have acute hepatitis, hemosiderosis or hemochromatosis (conditions involving excess iron in body).
- You have hemolytic anemia.

Before you start, consult your doctor:

- If you plan to become pregnant while on medication.
- If you have had stomach surgery.
- If you have had peptic ulcer, enteritis or colitis.

Over age 60:
May cause hemochromatosis (iron storage disease) with bronze skin, liver damage, diabetes, heart problems and impotence.

Pregnancy:
Take only if your doctor advises. Risk category C (see page xviii).

Breast-feeding:
No problems expected. Take only if your doctor confirms you have a dietary deficiency or an iron-deficiency anemia.

Infants & children:
Use only under medical supervision. Overdose common and dangerous. Keep out of children's reach.

Prolonged use:
- May cause hemochromatosis (iron storage disease) with bronze skin, liver damage, diabetes, heart problems and impotence.
- Talk to your doctor about the need for follow-up medical examinations or laboratory studies to check complete blood counts (white blood cell count, platelet count, red blood cell count, hemoglobin, hematocrit), serum iron, total iron-binding capacity.

Skin & sunlight:
No problems expected.

Driving, piloting or hazardous work:
No problems expected.

Discontinuing:
May be unnecessary to finish medicine. Follow doctor's instructions.

Others:
- Liquid form stains teeth. Mix with water or juice to lessen the effect. Brush with baking soda or hydrogen peroxide to help remove stain.
- Some products contain tartrazine dye. Avoid, especially if you are allergic to aspirin.
- May interfere with the accuracy of some medical tests.
- If using extended-release form or coated tablet and your stools don't turn black, consult doctor. The tablet may not be breaking down, and an underdose may result.

POSSIBLE INTERACTION WITH OTHER DRUGS

GENERIC NAME OR DRUG CLASS	COMBINED EFFECT
Acetohydroxamic acid	Decreased effects of both drugs.
Allopurinol	Possible excess iron storage in liver.
Antacids*	Poor iron absorption.
Chloramphenicol	Decreased effect of iron. Interferes with formation of red blood cells and hemoglobin.
Cholestyramine	Decreased iron effect.
Etidronate	Decreased etidronate effect. Take at least 2 hours after iron supplement.
H_2 antagonists*	Decreased iron effect.
Iron supplements, other*	Possible excess iron storage in liver.
Tetracyclines*	Decreased tetracycline effect. Take iron 3 hours before or 2 hours after taking tetracycline.
Vitamin E	Decreased iron and vitamin E effect.
Zinc supplements	Increased need for zinc.

POSSIBLE INTERACTION WITH OTHER SUBSTANCES

INTERACTS WITH	COMBINED EFFECT
Alcohol:	Increased iron absorption. May cause organ damage. Avoid or use in moderation.
Beverages: Milk, tea.	Decreased iron effect.
Cocaine:	None expected.
Foods: Dairy foods, eggs, whole-grain bread and cereal.	Decreased iron effect.
Marijuana:	None expected.
Tobacco:	None expected.

*See Glossary

ISOMETHEPTENE, DICHLORALPHENAZONE & ACETAMINOPHEN

BRAND NAMES

Amidrine
I.D.A.
Iso-Acetazone
Isocom
Midchlor
Midquin
Midrin
Migquin
Migrapap
Migratine
Migrazone
Migrend
Migrex
Mitride

BASIC INFORMATION

Habit forming? No
Prescription needed? Yes
Available as generic? No
Drug class: Analgesic, sedative, vascular headache suppressant

USES

Treatment of vascular (throbbing or migraine type) and tension headaches.

DOSAGE & USAGE INFORMATION

How to take:
Capsules—Take with fluid. Usual dose—2 capsules at start, then 1 every hour until fully relieved. Don't exceed 5 capsules in 12 hours.

When to take:
At first sign of headache.

If you forget a dose:
Use as soon as you remember.

What drug does:
Causes blood vessels in head to constrict or become narrower. Acetaminophen relieves pain by effects on hypothalamus—the part of the brain that helps regulate body heat and receives body's pain messages.

Time lapse before drug works:
30-60 minutes.

Continued next column

OVERDOSE

SYMPTOMS:
Stomach upsets, irritability, sweating, severe diarrhea, convulsions, coma.
WHAT TO DO:

- **Dial 911 (emergency) for an ambulance or medical help or poison center 1-800-222-1222. Then give first aid immediately.**
- **See emergency information on inside covers.**

Don't take with:
Any medicine that will decrease mental alertness or reflexes, such as alcohol, other mind-altering drugs, cough/cold medicines, antihistamines, allergy medicine, sedatives, tranquilizers (sleeping pills or "downers") barbiturates, seizure medicine, narcotics, other prescription medicine for pain, muscle relaxants, anesthetics.

POSSIBLE ADVERSE REACTIONS OR SIDE EFFECTS

SYMPTOMS	WHAT TO DO
Life-threatening:	
In case of overdose, see previous column.	
Common:	
Dizziness, drowsiness.	Continue. Call doctor when convenient.
Infrequent:	
Diarrhea, vomiting, nausea, abdominal cramps, upper abdominal pain.	Discontinue. Call doctor right away.
Rare:	
Rash; itchy skin; sore throat, fever, mouth sores; unusual bleeding or bruising; weakness; jaundice.	Discontinue. Call doctor right away.

WARNINGS & PRECAUTIONS

Don't take if:

- You are allergic to acetaminophen or any other component of this combination medicine.
- Your symptoms don't improve after 2 days use. Call your doctor.

Before you start, consult your doctor:
If you have kidney disease, liver damage, glaucoma, heart or blood vessel disorder, hypertension, alcoholism (active).

Over age 60:
Don't exceed recommended dose. You can't eliminate drug as efficiently as younger persons.

Pregnancy:
Decide with your doctor if drug benefits justify risk to unborn child. Risk category C (see page xviii).

Breast-feeding:
No proven harm to nursing infant. Consult doctor.

Infants & children:
Give under careful medical supervision only.

Prolonged use:
- May affect blood system and cause anemia. Limit use to 5 days for children 12 and under, and 10 days for adults.
- Talk to your doctor about the need for follow-up medical examinations or laboratory studies to check complete blood counts (white blood cell count, platelet count, red blood cell count, hemoglobin, hematocrit), liver function.

Skin & sunlight:
No problems expected.

Driving, piloting or hazardous work:
Avoid if you feel drowsy. Otherwise, no restrictions.

Discontinuing:
Discontinue in 2 days if symptoms don't improve.

Others:
No problems expected.

POSSIBLE INTERACTION WITH OTHER DRUGS

GENERIC NAME OR DRUG CLASS	COMBINED EFFECT
Anticoagulants, oral*	May increase anticoagulant effect. If combined frequently, prothrombin time should be monitored.
Anti-inflammatory drugs, nonsteroidal (NSAIDs)*	Long-term combined effect (3 years or longer) increases chance of damage to kidney, including malignancy.
Aspirin or other salicylates*	Long-term combined effect (3 years or longer) increases chance of damage to kidney, including malignancy.
Beta-adrenergic blocking agents*	Narrowed arteries in heart if taken in large doses.
Central nervous system (CNS) depressants*	Increased sedative effect.
Monoamine oxidase (MAO) inhibitors*	Sudden increase in blood pressure.
Phenacetin	Long-term combined effect (3 years or longer) increases chance of damage to kidney, including malignancy.
Phenobarbital	Quicker elimination and decreased effect of acetaminophen.
Tetracyclines* (effervescent granules or tablets)	May slow tetracycline absorption. Space doses 2 hours apart.
Zidovudine (AZT)	Increased toxic effect of zidovudine.

POSSIBLE INTERACTION WITH OTHER SUBSTANCES

INTERACTS WITH	COMBINED EFFECT
Alcohol:	Drowsiness. Toxicity to liver. Avoid.
Beverages:	None expected.
Cocaine:	None expected. However, cocaine may slow body's recovery. Avoid.
Foods:	None expected.
Marijuana:	Increased pain relief. However, marijuana may slow body's recovery. Avoid.
Tobacco:	May decrease medicine's effectiveness. Avoid.

*See Glossary

ISONIAZID

BRAND NAMES

INH
Isotamine
Laniazid
Nydrazid
PMS Isoniazid
Rifamate
Tubizid

BASIC INFORMATION

Habit forming? No
Prescription needed? Yes
Available as generic? Yes
Drug class: Antitubercular

USES

Kills tuberculosis germs.

DOSAGE & USAGE INFORMATION

How to take:
- Tablet—Swallow with liquid to lessen stomach irritation.
- Syrup—Follow label directions.

When to take:
At the same time each day.

If you forget a dose:
Take as soon as you remember up to 12 hours late. If more than 12 hours, wait for next scheduled dose (don't double this dose).

What drug does:
Interferes with TB germ metabolism. Eventually destroys the germ.

Continued next column

OVERDOSE

SYMPTOMS:
Difficult breathing, convulsions, coma.
WHAT TO DO:
- **Dial 911 (emergency) for an ambulance or medical help or poison center 1-800-222-1222. Then give first aid immediately.**
- **If patient is unconscious and not breathing, give mouth-to-mouth breathing. If there is no heartbeat, use cardiac massage and mouth-to-mouth breathing (CPR). Don't try to make patient vomit. If you can't get help quickly, take patient to nearest emergency facility.**
- **See emergency information on inside covers.**

Time lapse before drug works:
3 to 6 months. You may need to take drug as long as 2 years.

Don't take with:
Any other medication without consulting your doctor or pharmacist.

POSSIBLE ADVERSE REACTIONS OR SIDE EFFECTS

SYMPTOMS	WHAT TO DO
Life-threatening: In case of overdose, see previous column.	
Common:	
• Muscle pain and pain in joints, tingling or numbness in extremities, jaundice.	Discontinue. Call doctor right away.
• Confusion, unsteady walk.	Continue. Call doctor when convenient.
Infrequent:	
• Swollen glands, nausea, indigestion, diarrhea, vomiting.	Discontinue. Call doctor right away.
• Dizziness, appetite loss.	Continue. Call doctor when convenient.
Rare:	
• Rash, fever, impaired vision, anemia with fatigue, weakness, fever, sore throat, unusual bleeding or bruising.	Discontinue. Call doctor right away.
• Breast enlargement or discomfort.	Continue. Tell doctor at next visit.

WARNINGS & PRECAUTIONS

Don't take if:
You are allergic to isoniazid.

Before you start, consult your doctor:
- If you plan to become pregnant within medication period.
- If you are allergic to athionamide, pyrazinamide or nicotinic acid.
- If you drink alcohol.
- If you have liver or kidney disease.
- If you have epilepsy, diabetes or lupus.

Over age 60:
Adverse reactions and side effects, especially jaundice, may be more frequent and severe than in younger persons. Kidneys may be less efficient.

Pregnancy:
Decide with your doctor if drug benefits justify risk to unborn child. Risk category C (see page xviii).

Breast-feeding:
Drug passes into milk. Avoid drug or discontinue nursing until you finish medicine. Consult doctor for advice on maintaining milk supply.

Infants & children:
Use only under medical supervision.

Prolonged use:
- Numbness and tingling of hands and feet.
- Talk to your doctor about the need for follow-up medical examinations or laboratory studies to check liver function, eyes.

Skin & sunlight:
No problems expected.

Driving, piloting or hazardous work:
Avoid if you feel dizzy. Otherwise, no problems expected.

Discontinuing:
Don't discontinue without doctor's advice until you complete prescribed dose, even though symptoms diminish or disappear.

Others:
- Diabetic patients may have false blood sugar tests.
- Periodic liver function tests and laboratory blood studies recommended.
- Prescription for vitamin B-6 (pyridoxine) recommended to prevent nerve damage.

POSSIBLE INTERACTION WITH OTHER DRUGS

GENERIC NAME OR DRUG CLASS	COMBINED EFFECT
Acetaminophen	Increased risk of liver damage.
Adrenocorticoids, systemic	Decreased isoniazid effect.
Alfentanil	Prolonged duration of alfentanil effect (undesirable).
Antacids* (aluminum-containing)	Decreased absorption of isoniazid.
Anticholinergics*	May increase pressure within eyeball.
Anticoagulants, oral*	Increased anticoagulant effect.
Antidiabetics*	Increased anti-diabetic effect.
Antihypertensives*	Increased anti-hypertensive effect.
Antivirals, HIV/AIDS*	Increased risk of peripheral neuropathy.
Carbamazepine	Increased risk of liver damage.
Cycloserine	Increased risk of central nervous system effects.
Disulfiram	Increased effect of disulfiram.
Laxatives*	Decreased absorption and effect of isoniazid.
Hepatotoxics*	Increased risk of liver damage.
Ketoconazole	Increased risk of liver damage.
Narcotics*	Increased narcotic effect.
Phenytoin	Increased phenytoin effect.
Pyridoxine (Vitamin B-6)	Decreased chance of nerve damage in extremities.
Rifampin	Increased isoniazid toxicity to liver.
Sedatives*	Increased sedative effect.
Stimulants*	Increased stimulant effect.

POSSIBLE INTERACTION WITH OTHER SUBSTANCES

INTERACTS WITH	COMBINED EFFECT
Alcohol:	Increased incidence of liver disease and seizures.
Beverages:	None expected.
Cocaine:	None expected.
Foods: Swiss or Cheshire cheese, fish.	Red or itching skin, fast heartbeat. Seek emergency treatment.
Marijuana:	No interactions expected, but marijuana may slow body's recovery.
Tobacco:	No interactions expected, but tobacco may slow body's recovery.

*See Glossary

ISOTRETINOIN

BRAND NAMES

Accutane
Accutane Roche

BASIC INFORMATION

Habit forming? No
Prescription needed? Yes
Available as generic? No
Drug classification: Antiacne (systemic)

USES

- Decreases cystic acne formation in severe cases.
- Treats certain other skin disorders involving an overabundance of outer skin layer.

DOSAGE & USAGE INFORMATION

How to take:
Capsule—Swallow with liquid or food to lessen stomach irritation. If you can't swallow whole, open capsule and take with liquid or food.

When to take:
Twice a day. Follow prescription directions.

If you forget a dose:
Take as soon as you remember up to 2 hours late. If more than 2 hours, wait for next scheduled dose and double dose.

What drug does:
Reduces sebaceous gland activity and size.

Time lapse before drug works:
May require 15 to 20 weeks to experience full benefit.

Don't take with:
- Vitamin A or supplements containing Vitamin A.
- Any other medication without consulting your doctor or pharmacist.

OVERDOSE

SYMPTOMS:
None reported.
WHAT TO DO:
Overdose unlikely to threaten life. If person takes much larger amount than prescribed, call doctor, poison center 1-800-222-1222 or hospital emergency room for instructions.

POSSIBLE ADVERSE REACTIONS OR SIDE EFFECTS

SYMPTOMS	WHAT TO DO
Life-threatening: None expected.	
Common:	
• Burning, red, itching eyes; lip scaling; burning pain; nosebleeds.	Discontinue. Call doctor right away.
• Itchy skin.	Continue. Call doctor when convenient.
• Dry mouth.	Continue. Tell doctor at next visit. (Suck ice or chew gum).
Infrequent:	
• Rash, infection, nausea, vomiting.	Discontinue. Call doctor right away.
• Pain in muscles, bones, joints; hair thinning; tiredness.	Continue. Call doctor when convenient.
Rare:	
• Severe stomach pain, bleeding gums, blurred vision, severe diarrhea, continuing headache, vomiting, eye pain, rectal bleeding, yellow skin or eyes.	Discontinue. Call doctor right away.
• Mild headache, increased sensitivity to light, stomach upset, peeling of skin on palms or soles of feet, tiredness.	Continue. Call doctor when convenient.

WARNINGS & PRECAUTIONS

Don't take if:
- You are allergic to isotretinoin, etretinate, tretinoin or vitamin A derivatives.
- You are pregnant or plan pregnancy.
- *You are even able to bear children. Read, understand and follow the patient information enclosure with your prescription.*

Before you start, consult your doctor:
- If you have diabetes.
- If you or any member of family have high triglyceride levels in blood.

Over age 60:
Adverse reactions and side effects may be more frequent and severe than in younger persons.

Pregnancy:
Causes birth defects in fetus. Don't use. Risk category X (see page xviii).

Breast-feeding:
Effect unknown. Not recommended. Consult doctor.

Infants & children:
Not recommended.

Prolonged use:
- Possible damage to cornea.
- Talk to your doctor about the need for follow-up medical examinations or laboratory studies to check complete blood counts (white blood cell count, platelet count, red blood cell count, hemoglobin, hematocrit), liver function, blood lipids, blood sugar.

Skin & sunlight:
May cause rash or intensify sunburn in areas exposed to sun or ultraviolet light (photo-sensitivity reaction). Avoid overexposure. Notify doctor if reaction occurs.

Driving, piloting or hazardous work:
Use caution if there is a decrease in your night vision or you are unable to see well. Consult doctor.

Discontinuing:
Single course of treatment is usually all that's needed. If second course required, wait 8 weeks after completing first course.

Others:
- Use only for severe cases of cystic acne that have not responded to less hazardous forms of acne treatment.
- May interfere with the accuracy of some medical tests.
- Don't donate blood for at least 30 days after discontinuing medicine.
- Acne may worsen at the start of treatment.
- Contact lens wearers may experience discomfort during treatment with this drug.
- **If you are planning pregnancy or at risk of pregnancy, don't take this drug.**

POSSIBLE INTERACTION WITH OTHER DRUGS

GENERIC NAME OR DRUG CLASS	COMBINED EFFECT
Antiacne topical preparations* (other), cosmetics (medicated), skin preparations with alcohol, soaps or cleansers (abrasive)	Severe skin irritation.
Etretinate	Increased chance of toxicity of each drug.
Tetracyclines*	Increased risk of developing pseudo-tumor cerebri.*
Topical drugs or cosmetics	May interact with isotretinoin.
Tretinoin	Increased chance of toxicity.
Vitamin A	Additive toxic effect of each. Avoid.

POSSIBLE INTERACTION WITH OTHER SUBSTANCES

INTERACTS WITH	COMBINED EFFECT
Alcohol:	Significant increase in triglycerides in blood. Avoid.
Beverages:	None expected.
Cocaine:	Increased chance of toxicity of isotretinoin. Avoid.
Foods:	None expected.
Marijuana:	Increased chance of toxicity of isotretinoin. Avoid.
Tobacco:	May decrease absorption of medicine. Avoid tobacco while in treatment.

***See Glossary**

ISOXSUPRINE

BRAND NAMES

Vasodilan　　Vasoprine

BASIC INFORMATION

Habit forming? No
Prescription needed? Yes
Available as generic? Yes
Drug class: Vasodilator

USES

- May improve poor blood circulation.
- Management of premature labor.
- Treatment for painful menstruation.

DOSAGE & USAGE INFORMATION

How to take:
Tablet—Swallow with liquid or food to lessen stomach irritation. If you can't swallow whole, crumble tablet and take with liquid or food.

When to take:
At the same times each day.

If you forget a dose:
Take as soon as you remember up to 2 hours late. If more than 2 hours, wait for next scheduled dose (don't double this dose).

What drug does:
Expands blood vessels, increasing flow and permitting distribution of oxygen and nutrients.

Time lapse before drug works:
1 hour.

Continued next column

OVERDOSE

SYMPTOMS:
Headache, dizziness, flush, vomiting, weakness, sweating, fainting, shortness of breath, coma.

WHAT TO DO:

- **Dial 911 (emergency) for an ambulance or medical help or poison center 1-800-222-1222. Then give first aid immediately.**
- **If patient is unconscious and not breathing, give mouth-to-mouth breathing. If there is no heartbeat, use cardiac massage and mouth-to-mouth breathing (CPR). Don't try to make patient vomit. If you can't get help quickly, take patient to nearest emergency facility.**
- **See emergency information on inside covers.**

Don't take with:
Any other medication without consulting your doctor or pharmacist.

POSSIBLE ADVERSE REACTIONS OR SIDE EFFECTS

SYMPTOMS	WHAT TO DO
Life-threatening:	
In case of overdose, see previous column.	
Common:	
None expected.	
Infrequent:	
Nausea, vomiting.	Continue. Call doctor when convenient.
Rare:	
Rapid or irregular heartbeat, rash, chest pain, shortness of breath.	Discontinue. Call doctor right away.

WARNINGS & PRECAUTIONS

Don't take if:
- You are allergic to any vasodilator.
- You have any bleeding disease.

Before you start, consult your doctor:
- If you have high blood pressure, hardening of the arteries or heart disease.
- If you plan to become pregnant within medication period.
- If you have glaucoma.

Over age 60:
Adverse reactions and side effects may be more frequent and severe than in younger persons.

Pregnancy:
Decide with your doctor whether drug benefits justify risk to unborn child. Risk category C (see page xviii).

Breast-feeding:
No problems expected, but consult doctor.

Infants & children:
Not recommended.

Prolonged use:
Talk to your doctor about the need for follow-up medical examinations or laboratory studies.

Skin & sunlight:
No problems expected.

Driving, piloting or hazardous work:
Avoid if you feel dizzy or faint. Otherwise, no problems expected.

Discontinuing:
Don't discontinue without doctor's advice until you complete prescribed dose, even though symptoms diminish or disappear.

Others:
- Be cautious when arising from lying or sitting position, when climbing stairs, or if dizziness occurs.
- May interfere with the accuracy of some medical tests.

POSSIBLE INTERACTION WITH OTHER DRUGS

GENERIC NAME OR DRUG CLASS	COMBINED EFFECT
None significant.	

POSSIBLE INTERACTION WITH OTHER SUBSTANCES

INTERACTS WITH	COMBINED EFFECT
Alcohol:	None expected.
Beverages:	
Milk.	Decreased stomach irritation.
Cocaine:	Decreased blood circulation to extremities. Avoid.
Foods:	None expected.
Marijuana:	Rapid heartbeat.
Tobacco:	Decreased isoxsuprine effect; nicotine constricts blood vessels.

KANAMYCIN

BRAND NAMES

Kantrex

BASIC INFORMATION

Habit forming? No
Prescription needed? Yes
Available as generic? No
Drug class: Bowel preparation

USES

- To cleanse bowel of bacteria prior to intestinal surgery.
- Treats hepatic coma.

DOSAGE & USAGE INFORMATION

How to take:
Capsules—Swallow with liquid. If you can't swallow whole, open capsule and take with liquid or food. Instructions to take on empty stomach mean 1 hour before or 2 hours after eating.

When to take:
At the same time each day, according to instructions on prescription label.

If you forget a dose:
Take as soon as you remember up to 2 hours late. If more than 2 hours, wait for next scheduled dose (don't double this dose).

What drug does:
Kills susceptible bacteria in the intestines.

Time lapse before drug works:
15 to 30 minutes.

Don't take with:
Any other medication without consulting your doctor or pharmacist.

OVERDOSE

SYMPTOMS:
Clumsiness, dizziness, seizures, coma.
WHAT TO DO:

- **Dial 911 (emergency) for an ambulance or medical help or poison center 1-800-222-1222. Then give first aid immediately.**
- **See emergency information on inside covers.**

POSSIBLE ADVERSE REACTIONS OR SIDE EFFECTS

SYMPTOMS	WHAT TO DO
Life-threatening: In case of overdose, see previous column.	
Common: Mouth irritation or soreness, nausea.	Continue. Call doctor when convenient.
Infrequent: Vomiting.	Discontinue. Call doctor right away.
Rare: Decreased urine, hearing loss, ringing in ears, clumsiness, unsteadiness, skin rash.	Discontinue. Call doctor right away.

WARNINGS & PRECAUTIONS

Don't take if:
- You are allergic to kanamycin.
- You can't tolerate any aminoglycoside.

Before you start, consult your doctor:
- If you have hearing difficulty.
- If you have intestinal obstruction.
- If you have severe kidney disease.
- If you have ulcerative colitis.

Over age 60:
Adverse reactions and side effects may be more frequent and severe than in younger persons. You may need smaller doses for shorter periods of time.

Pregnancy:
Consult doctor. Risk category D (see page xviii).

Breast-feeding:
No special problems expected. Consult doctor.

Infants & children:
Not recommended for prolonged use.

Prolonged use:
Not recommended for prolonged use.

Skin & sunlight:
No problems expected.

Driving, piloting or hazardous work:
Avoid if you feel confused, drowsy or dizzy.

Discontinuing:
Not recommended for prolonged use.

Others:
No problems expected.

POSSIBLE INTERACTION WITH OTHER DRUGS

GENERIC NAME OR DRUG CLASS	COMBINED EFFECT
None significant.	

POSSIBLE INTERACTION WITH OTHER SUBSTANCES

INTERACTS WITH	COMBINED EFFECT
Alcohol:	None expected.
Beverages:	None expected.
Cocaine:	None expected.
Foods:	None expected.
Marijuana:	None expected.
Tobacco:	None expected.

KAOLIN & PECTIN

BRAND NAMES

Donnagel-MB
Kao-Con
Kaotin
Kapectolin
Kapectolin with Paregoric
K-C
K-P
K-Pek
Parapectolin

BASIC INFORMATION

Habit forming? No
Prescription needed? No
Available as generic? Yes
Drug class: Antidiarrheal

USES

Treats mild to moderate diarrhea. Used in conjunction with fluids, appropriate diet and rest. Treats symptoms only. Does not cure any disorder that causes diarrhea.

DOSAGE & USAGE INFORMATION

How to take:
Liquid—Swallow prescribed dosage (without diluting) after each loose bowel movement.

When to take:
After each loose bowel movement.

If you forget a dose:
Take when you remember.

What drug does:
Makes loose stools less watery, but may not prevent loss of fluids.

Time lapse before drug works:
15 to 30 minutes.

Don't take with:
Any other medication without consulting your doctor or pharmacist.

OVERDOSE

SYMPTOMS:
Fecal impaction.
WHAT TO DO:
Overdose unlikely to threaten life. If person takes much larger amount than prescribed, call doctor, poison center 1-800-222-1222 or hospital emergency room for instructions.

POSSIBLE ADVERSE REACTIONS OR SIDE EFFECTS

SYMPTOMS	WHAT TO DO
Life-threatening: None expected.	
Common: None expected.	
Infrequent: None expected.	
Rare: Constipation (mild).	Continue. Call doctor when convenient.

WARNINGS & PRECAUTIONS

Don't take if:
You are allergic to kaolin or pectin.

Before you start, consult your doctor:
- If patient is child or infant.
- If you have any chronic medical problem with heart disease, peptic ulcer, asthma or others.
- If you have fever over 101°F.

Over age 60:
Fluid loss caused by diarrhea, especially if taking other medicines, may lead to serious disability. Consult doctor.

Pregnancy:
Consult doctor. Risk category C (see page xviii).

Breast-feeding:
No problems expected.

Infants & children:
Fluid loss caused by diarrhea in infants and children can cause serious dehydration. Consult doctor before giving any medicine for diarrhea.

Prolonged use:
Not recommended.

Skin & sunlight:
No problems expected.

Driving, piloting or hazardous work:
No problems expected.

Discontinuing:
May be unnecessary to finish medicine. Follow doctor's instructions.

Others:
Consult doctor about fluids, diet and rest.

POSSIBLE INTERACTION WITH OTHER DRUGS

GENERIC NAME OR DRUG CLASS	COMBINED EFFECT
Digoxin	Decreases absorption of digoxin. Separate doses by at least 2 hours.
Lincomycins*	Decreases absorption of lincomycin. Separate doses by at least 2 hours.
All other oral medicines	May decrease absorption of other medicines. Separate doses by at least 2 hours.

POSSIBLE INTERACTION WITH OTHER SUBSTANCES

INTERACTS WITH	COMBINED EFFECT
Alcohol:	Increased diarrhea. Prevents action of kaolin and pectin.
Beverages:	None expected.
Cocaine:	Aggravates underlying disease. Avoid.
Foods:	None expected.
Marijuana:	Aggravates underlying disease. Avoid.
Tobacco:	Aggravates underlying disease. Avoid.

***See Glossary**

KAOLIN, PECTIN, BELLADONNA & OPIUM

BRAND NAMES

Amogel PG
Donnagel-PG
Donnapectolin-PG
Kapectolin PG
Quiagel PG

BASIC INFORMATION

Habit forming? Yes
Prescription needed? Yes
Available as generic? No
Drug class: Narcotic, antidiarrheal, antispasmodic

USES

Treats mild to moderate diarrhea. Used in conjunction with fluids, appropriate diet and rest. Treats symptoms only. Does not cure any disorder that causes diarrhea.

DOSAGE & USAGE INFORMATION

How to take:
Liquid—Swallow prescribed dosage (without diluting) after each loose bowel movement.

When to take:
As needed for diarrhea, no more often than every 4 hours.

If you forget a dose:
Take when you remember.

Continued next column

OVERDOSE

SYMPTOMS:
Fecal impaction, rapid pulse, dizziness, fever, hallucinations, confusion, slurred speech, agitation, flushed face, convulsions, deep sleep, slow breathing, slow pulse, warm skin, constricted pupils, coma.

WHAT TO DO:
- **Dial 911 (emergency) for an ambulance or medical help or poison center 1-800-222-1222. Then give first aid immediately.**
- **If patient is unconscious and not breathing, give mouth-to-mouth breathing. If there is no heartbeat, use cardiac massage and mouth-to-mouth breathing (CPR). Don't try to make patient vomit. If you can't get help quickly, take patient to nearest emergency facility.**
- **See emergency information on inside covers.**

What drug does:
- Blocks nerve impulses at parasympathetic nerve endings, preventing muscle contractions and gland secretions of organs involved.
- Makes loose stools less watery, but may not prevent loss of fluids.
- Anesthetizes surface membranes of intestines and blocks nerve impulses.

Time lapse before drug works:
15 to 30 minutes.

Don't take with:
Any other medication without consulting your doctor or pharmacist.

POSSIBLE ADVERSE REACTIONS OR SIDE EFFECTS

SYMPTOMS	WHAT TO DO
Life-threatening:	
Unusually rapid heartbeat (over 100), difficult breathing, slow heartbeat (under 50/minute).	Discontinue. Seek emergency treatment.
Common (with large dosage):	
Weakness, increased sweating, red or flushed face, lightheadedness, headache, dry mouth, dry skin, drowsiness, dizziness, frequent urination, decreased sweating, constipation, confusion, tiredness.	Continue. Call doctor when convenient.
Infrequent:	
• Reduced taste sense, nervousness, eyes, sensitive to sunlight, blurred vision.	Discontinue. Call doctor right away.
• Diminished sex drive, memory loss.	Continue. Call doctor when convenient.
Rare:	
Bloating, abdominal cramps and vomiting, eye pain, hallucinations, shortness of breath, rash, itchy skin, slow heartbeat.	Discontinue. Call doctor right away.

WARNINGS & PRECAUTIONS

Don't take if:
- You are allergic to any anticholinergic, narcotic, kaolin or pectin.
- You have trouble with stomach bloating, difficulty emptying your bladder completely, narrow-angle glaucoma, severe ulcerative colitis.

KAOLIN, PECTIN, BELLADONNA & OPIUM

Before you start, consult your doctor:
- If you have open-angle glaucoma, angina, chronic bronchitis or asthma, hiatal hernia, liver disease, enlarged prostate, myasthenia gravis, peptic ulcer, impaired liver or kidney function, fever over 101F, any chronic medical problem with heart disease, peptic ulcer, asthma or others.
- If patient is child or infant.
- If you will have surgery within 2 months, including dental surgery, requiring general or spinal anesthesia.

Over age 60:
- Adverse reactions and side effects may be more frequent and severe than in younger persons.
- More likely to be drowsy, dizzy, unsteady or constipated.
- Fluid loss caused by diarrhea, especially if taking other medicines, may lead to serious disability. Consult doctor.

Pregnancy:
Decide with your doctor if drug benefits justify risk to unborn child. Risk category C (see page xviii).

Breast-feeding:
Drug passes into milk. Avoid drug or discontinue nursing until you finish medicine. Consult doctor for advice on maintaining milk supply.

Infants & children:
Fluid loss caused by diarrhea in infants and children can cause serious dehydration. Consult doctor before giving any medicine for diarrhea.

Prolonged use:
- Causes psychological and physical dependence. Not recommended.
- Talk to your doctor about the need for follow-up medical examinations or laboratory studies to check liver function, kidney function.

Skin & sunlight:
No special problems expected.

Driving, piloting or hazardous work:
Don't drive or pilot aircraft until you learn how medicine affects you. Don't work around dangerous machinery. Don't climb ladders or work in high places. Danger increases if you drink alcohol or take medicine affecting alertness and reflexes, such as antihistamines, tranquilizers, sedatives, pain medicine, narcotics and mind-altering drugs.

Discontinuing:
May be unnecessary to finish medicine. Follow doctor's instructions.

Others:
- Great potential for abuse.
- Consult doctor about fluids, diet and rest.

POSSIBLE INTERACTION WITH OTHER DRUGS

GENERIC NAME OR DRUG CLASS	COMBINED EFFECT
Amantadine	Increased belladonna effect.
Analgesics*	Increased analgesic effect.
Antidepressants*	Increased sedative effect.
Antihistamines*	Increased sedative effect.
Carteolol	Increased narcotic effect. Dangerous sedation.
Central nervous system (CNS) depressants*	Increased depressant effect of both.
Cortisone drugs*	Increased internal eye pressure.
Digoxin	Decreases absorption of digoxin. Separate doses by at least 2 hours.
Haloperidol	Increased internal eye pressure.

Continued on page 916

POSSIBLE INTERACTION WITH OTHER SUBSTANCES

INTERACTS WITH	COMBINED EFFECT
Alcohol:	Increases alcohol's intoxicating effect, increased diarrhea, prevents action of kaolin and pectin. Avoid.
Beverages:	None expected.
Cocaine:	Aggravates underlying disease. Avoid.
Foods:	None expected.
Marijuana:	Impairs physical and mental performance, aggravates underlying disease. Avoid.
Tobacco:	Aggravates underlying disease. Avoid.

KERATOLYTICS

GENERIC AND BRAND NAMES

See complete list of generic and brand names in the *Generic and Brand Name Directory*, page 862.

BASIC INFORMATION

Habit forming? No
Prescription needed? Yes, on some.
Available as generic? Yes
Drug class: Keratolytic, antiacne (topical), antiseborrheic

USES

Treatment for acne, psoriasis, ichthyosis, keratosis, folliculitis, flat warts, eczema, urticaria, calluses, corns, seborrheic dermatitis, dandruff.

DOSAGE & USAGE INFORMATION

How to use:
Cream, gel, lotion, ointment, pads, plaster, shampoo, soap, topical solution, suspension—Always follow instructions on the label or use as directed by your doctor.

When to use:
At the same time each day or as needed.

If you forget an application:
Use as soon as you remember.

What drug does:
Keratolytics are drugs that soften, loosen and remove keratin (the tough outer layer of the skin).

Time lapse before drug works:
2 to 3 weeks. May require 6 weeks for maximum improvement.

Don't use with:
- Benzoyl peroxide. Apply 12 hours apart.
- Any other medicine without consulting your doctor or pharmacist.

OVERDOSE

SYMPTOMS:
None expected.
WHAT TO DO:
If person swallows drug, call doctor, poison center 1-800-222-1222 or hospital emergency room for instructions.

POSSIBLE ADVERSE REACTIONS OR SIDE EFFECTS

SYMPTOMS	WHAT TO DO
Life-threatening:	
None expected.	
Common:	
• Pigment change in treated area, warmth or stinging, peeling.	Continue. Tell doctor at next visit.
• Sensitivity to wind or cold.	No action necessary.
Infrequent:	
Blistering, crusting, severe burning, swelling, skin irritation that begins after treatment.	Discontinue. Call doctor right away.
Rare:	
Symptoms of systemic toxicity (diarrhea, nausea, dizziness, headache, breathing difficulty, tiredness, weakness).	Discontinue. Call doctor right away.

WARNINGS & PRECAUTIONS

Don't take if:
- You are allergic to resorcinol or salicyclic acid.
- You are sunburned or windburned or have an open skin wound, skin irritation or infection.

Before you start, consult your doctor:
- If you have eczema.
- If you have diabetes mellitus.
- If you have peripheral vascular disease (blood vessel disease).

Over age 60:
No problems expected.

Pregnancy:
Risk factors vary for drugs in this group. See category list on page xviii and consult doctor.

Breast-feeding:
No problems expected. Consult doctor.

Infants & children:
Not recommended. Increased risk of toxicity.

Prolonged use:
No problems expected.

Skin & sunlight:
No special problems expected.

Driving, piloting or hazardous work:
No problems expected.

Discontinuing:
Follow your doctor's instructions or the directions on the label.

Others:
- Acne may get worse before improvement starts in 2 or 3 weeks. Don't wash face more than 2 or 3 times daily.
- Keep medicine away from mouth or eyes. If it accidentally gets into the eyes, flush immediately with clear water.
- Keep medicine away from heat or flame.

POSSIBLE INTERACTION WITH OTHER DRUGS

GENERIC NAME OR DRUG CLASS	COMBINED EFFECT
Antiacne topical preparations (other)	Severe skin irritation.
Cosmetics (medicated)	Severe skin irritation.
Skin preparations with alcohol	Severe skin irritation.
Soaps or cleansers (abrasive)	Severe skin irritation.

POSSIBLE INTERACTION WITH OTHER SUBSTANCES

INTERACTS WITH	COMBINED EFFECT
Alcohol:	None expected.
Beverages:	None expected.
Cocaine:	None expected.
Foods:	None expected.
Marijuana:	None expected.
Tobacco:	None expected.

LAMOTRIGINE

BRAND NAMES

Lamictal

BASIC INFORMATION

Habit forming? No
Prescription needed? Yes
Available as generic? No
Drug class: Anticonvulsant, antiepileptic

USES

Treatment for partial (focal) epileptic seizures. May be used in combination with other antiepileptic drugs.

DOSAGE & USAGE INFORMATION

How to take:
Tablets—Swallow with liquid. May be taken with or without food.

When to take:
Your doctor will determine the best schedule. Dosages may be increased gradually over the first few weeks of use to achieve maximum benefits.

If you forget a dose:
Take as soon as you remember. If it is almost time for the next dose, then skip the missed dose and wait for your next scheduled dose (don't double this dose).

What drug does:
The exact mechanism is unknown. The anticonvulsant action may result from a decrease in the release of stimulatory neurotransmitters (substances that stimulate nerve cells).

Time lapse before drug works:
May take several weeks for effectiveness.

Don't take with:
Any other prescription or nonprescription drug without consulting your doctor.

OVERDOSE

SYMPTOMS:
Severe drowsiness, severe headache, severe dizziness, coma.
WHAT TO DO:
- **Dial 911 (emergency) for an ambulance or medical help or poison center 1-800-222-1222. Then give first aid immediately.**
- **See emergency information on inside covers.**

POSSIBLE ADVERSE REACTIONS OR SIDE EFFECTS

SYMPTOMS	WHAT TO DO
Life-threatening: In case of overdose, see previous column.	
Common:	
• Skin rash, double vision or blurred vision, clumsiness.	Continue, but call doctor right away.
• Dizziness, nausea or vomiting, headache, drowsiness.	Continue. Call doctor when convenient.
Infrequent:	
Anxiety, depression, confusion, irritability, other mood or mental changes, increase in seizure activity, back-and-forth eye movements (nystagmus).	Continue, but call doctor right away.
Rare:	
• Swelling (hands, face, mouth, feet); breathing difficulty; tiredness or weakness; fever; chills; sore throat; unusual bruising or bleeding; skin peeling, blistering or loosening; muscle cramps or pain; sores on mouth or lips; small red or purple dots on skin.	Continue, but call doctor right away.
• Slurred speech, indigestion, runny nose, trembling, trouble sleeping, weakness.	Continue. Call doctor when convenient.

WARNINGS & PRECAUTIONS

Don't take if:
You are allergic to lamotrigine.

Before you start, consult your doctor:
- If you have kidney or liver disease.
- If you have any heart disorder.
- If you are allergic to any medication, food, or other substance.

Over age 60:
No special problems expected.

Pregnancy:
Decide with your doctor if drug benefits justify risks to unborn child. Risk category C (see page xviii).

Breast-feeding:
Drug passes into milk. Avoid drug or discontinue nursing until you finish medicine. Consult doctor for advice on maintaining milk supply.

Infants & children:
Safety not established for children under age 16. Use only under close medical supervision.

Prolonged use:
Schedule regular visits to your doctor to determine if drug is continuing to be effective in controlling seizures. Follow-up laboratory blood studies may be recommended by your doctor.

Skin & sunlight:
No special problems expected.

Driving, piloting or hazardous work:
Don't drive or pilot aircraft until you learn how medicine affects you. Don't work around dangerous machinery. Don't climb ladders or work in high places. Danger increases if you drink alcohol or take other medicines affecting alertness and reflexes, such as antihistamines, tranquilizers, sedatives, pain medicine, narcotics and mind-altering drugs.

Discontinuing:
Don't discontinue without doctor's approval due to risk of increased seizure activity. Dosage may need to be gradually reduced.

Others:
- Advise any doctor or dentist whom you consult that you take this medicine.
- Use as directed. Don't increase or decrease dosage without doctor's approval.
- Wear medical identification stating that you have a seizure disorder and take this medication.
- A skin rash may indicate a serious, and potentially life-threatening, medical problem. If a skin rash develops, it is usually during the first 4 to 6 weeks after treatment with the drug is started. Call your doctor promptly if you develop any skin rash.

POSSIBLE INTERACTION WITH OTHER DRUGS

GENERIC NAME OR DRUG CLASS	COMBINED EFFECT
Carbamazepine	Decreased effect of lamotrigine. Increase in risk of side effects.
Central nervous system (CNS) depressants*	Increased sedation.
Folate antagonists*, other	Folic acid deficiency.
Phenobarbital	Decreased effect of lamotrigine.
Phenytoin	Decreased effect of lamotrigine.
Primidone	Decreased effect of lamotrigine.
Valproic acid	Increased effect of lamotrigine. May increase risk of skin rash.

POSSIBLE INTERACTION WITH OTHER SUBSTANCES

INTERACTS WITH	COMBINED EFFECT
Alcohol:	Increased sedation. Avoid.
Beverages:	None expected.
Cocaine:	Problems not known. Best to avoid.
Foods:	None expected.
Marijuana:	Problems not known. Best to avoid.
Tobacco:	None expected.

LAXATIVES, BULK-FORMING

GENERIC AND BRAND NAMES

See complete list of generic and brand names in the *Generic and Brand Name Directory*, page 862.

BASIC INFORMATION

Habit forming? No
Prescription needed? No
Available as generic? Yes
Drug class: Laxative, bulk-forming

USES

For short-term relief of simple constipation (bowel movements that are abnormally difficult or infrequent). Normal frequency of bowel movements may vary from 2 to 3 times a day to 2 to 3 times a week. Laxatives treat the symptoms of constipation, not the cause.

DOSAGE & USAGE INFORMATION

How to take:
Powder, oral solution, tablets, capsules, granules, chewable tablets, caramels, effervescent powder, wafers—Follow package instructions. Swallow with full glass of water or fruit juice. Drink 6 to 8 glasses of water each day in addition to one taken with each dose. Mix all powders thoroughly to avoid any risk of unmixed powder causing intestinal blockage.

When to take:
As directed on the label or according to doctor's instructions.

If you forget a dose:
Take as soon as you remember.

What drug does:
Adds dietary fiber that is not digested. Once in the intestine, it helps to increase fecal bulk, lubricate and soften the intestinal contents and facilitate the passage of stools.

Continued next column

OVERDOSE

SYMPTOMS:
Weakness, increased sweating, confusion, irregular heartbeat, muscle cramps.
WHAT TO DO:
Overdose unlikely to threaten life. If person takes much larger amount than prescribed, call doctor, poison center 1-800-222-1222 or hospital emergency room for instructions.

Time lapse before drug works:
May work in 12 to 24 hours. Sometimes does not work for 2 to 3 days.

Don't take with:
- Any other medicine without consulting your doctor or pharmacist.
- Don't take within 2 hours of taking another medicine. Laxative interferes with absorption of medicine.

POSSIBLE ADVERSE REACTIONS OR SIDE EFFECTS

SYMPTOMS	WHAT TO DO
Life-threatening:	
None expected.	
Common:	
None expected.	
Infrequent:	
Mild stomach cramps, throat irritation with liquid form.	Continue. Call doctor when convenient.
Rare:	
Allergic skin rash or itching, trouble breathing, swallowing difficulty.	Discontinue. Call doctor right away.

WARNINGS & PRECAUTIONS

Don't take if:
- You have symptoms of appendicitis (abdominal pain, cramping, soreness, bloating, nausea and vomiting). Consult doctor.
- You have dysphagia (swallowing difficulty).
- You are allergic to bulk-forming laxatives.
- You have missed a bowel movement for just 1 or 2 days.

Before you start, consult your doctor:
- If you are allergic to any medicine, food, or other substance or have a family history of allergies.
- If you have diabetes or heart or kidney disease.
- If you have hypertension (high blood pressure) and the laxative contains sodium.
- If you have an intestinal obstruction or undiagnosed rectal bleeding.
- If you are taking other laxatives.

Over age 60:
No special problems expected.

Pregnancy:
Most bulk-forming laxatives contain sodium or sugars, which may cause fluid retention. Risk factors vary or may not be designated for these laxatives. Read categories on page xviii and consult doctor.

Breast-Feeding:
No special problems expected. Consult doctor.

Infants & children:
- Don't give to children under age 6 without doctor's approval. Young children are not able to describe their symptoms accurately, and a proper diagnosis needs to be made before starting any treatment.
- Don't give to a child who refuses to have a bowel movement (toileting refusal). May force a painful bowel movement and cause the child to hold back even more. Consult doctor.
- For children over age 6, follow package instructions or doctor's directions for correct dosage amount.

Prolonged use:
Don't take for more than 1 week unless under doctor's supervision. Bulk-form laxatives are sometimes used for long-term therapy.

Skin & sunlight:
No special problems expected.

Driving, piloting or hazardous work:
No special problems expected.

Discontinuing:
May be unnecessary to finish medicine. Follow doctor's instructions or instructions on label.

Others:
- Don't give to "flush out" the system or as a "tonic."
- Use as directed. Don't increase or decrease dosage without doctor's approval.
- Excessive use of laxatives in a teenager may indicate an eating disorder such as anorexia nervosa or bulimia nervosa. Consult doctor.
- If there is a sudden change in bowel habits or bowel function that lasts longer than 2 weeks, consult doctor.

POSSIBLE INTERACTION WITH OTHER DRUGS

GENERIC NAME OR DRUG CLASS	COMBINED EFFECT
Antacids*	Irritation of stomach or small intestine.
Anticoagulants*	Decreased anti-coagulant effect. Take 2 hours apart.
Digitalis preparations*	Decreased digitalis effect. Take 2 hours apart.
Diuretics, potassium-sparing*	Decreased potassium effect.
Potassium supplements*	Decreased potassium effect.
Salicylates*	Decreased salicylate effect. Take 2 hours apart.
Tetracyclines*	Decreased tetracycline effect. Take 2 hours apart.

POSSIBLE INTERACTION WITH OTHER SUBSTANCES

INTERACTS WITH	COMBINED EFFECT
Alcohol:	None expected.
Beverages:	None expected.
Cocaine:	None expected.
Foods:	None expected.
Marijuana:	None expected.
Tobacco:	None expected.

*See Glossary

LAXATIVES, OSMOTIC

GENERIC AND BRAND NAMES

See complete list of generic and brand names in the *Generic and Brand Name Directory*, page 862.

BASIC INFORMATION

Habit forming? No
Prescription needed? No
Available as generic? Yes
Drug class: Laxative, hyperosmotic

USES

For short-term relief of simple constipation (bowel movements that are abnormally difficult or infrequent). Normal frequency of bowel movements may vary from 2 to 3 times a day to 2 to 3 times a week. Laxatives treat the symptoms of constipation, not the cause.

DOSAGE & USAGE INFORMATION

How to take:

- Oral solution, tablets, crystals, effervescent powder, milk of magnesia—Follow package instructions. Swallow with full glass of water or fruit juice. A second glass of liquid is often recommended for best effect. Drink 6 to 8 glasses of water each day, in addition to one taken with each dose.
- Enema or suppositories—Read and follow package instructions.

When to take:
Since drug produces stool within 30 minutes to 3 hours following a dose, take it at a time that will not interfere with sleep or other scheduled activities. Don't take late in the day on an empty stomach.

If you forget a dose:
Take as soon as you remember.

Continued next column

What drug does:
Draws water into the bowel from surrounding tissue to help loosen and soften the stool and increases bowel action.

Time lapse before drug works:

- Oral forms—30 minutes to 3 hours. May take longer if taken with a meal.
- Rectal forms—2 to 15 minutes.

Don't take with:

- Any other medicine without consulting your doctor or pharmacist.
- Don't take within 2 hours of taking another medicine. Laxative interferes with absorption of medicine.

OVERDOSE

SYMPTOMS:
Weakness, increased sweating, confusion, irregular heartbeat, muscle cramps.
WHAT TO DO:
Overdose unlikely to threaten life. If person takes much larger amount than prescribed, call doctor, poison center 1-800-222-1222 or hospital emergency room for instructions.

POSSIBLE ADVERSE REACTIONS OR SIDE EFFECTS

SYMPTOMS	WHAT TO DO
Life-threatening: None expected.	
Common: None expected.	
Infrequent:	
• Belching, cramps, nausea, diarrhea, increased thirst.	Continue. Call doctor when convenient.
• Rectal bleeding, burning, itching or pain (with rectal forms).	Discontinue. Call doctor right away.
Rare: When used too often or dose is too high—Confusion, irregular heartbeat, muscle cramps, unusual tiredness or weakness, dehydration.	Discontinue. Call doctor right away.

WARNINGS & PRECAUTIONS

Don't take if:

- You are having symptoms of appendicitis (abdominal pain, cramping, soreness, bloating, nausea and vomiting). Consult doctor.
- You are allergic to osmotic laxatives.
- You have missed a bowel movement for just 1 or 2 days.

Before you start, consult your doctor:

- If you are allergic to any medicine, food or other substance or have a family history of allergies.
- If you have hypertension (high blood pressure) and the laxative contains sodium.
- If you have an intestinal obstruction, undiagnosed rectal bleeding or a colostomy or ileostomy.

- If you have diabetes or heart or kidney disease.
- If you are taking other laxatives.

Over age 60:
- Rectal solutions could cause excess fluid in the body. Consult doctor before using.
- No special problems expected with laxatives taken by mouth.

Pregnancy:
Risk factors vary or may not be designated for these laxatives. Read categories on page xviii and consult doctor.

Breast-feeding:
No special problems expected. Consult doctor.

Infants & children:
- Don't give to children under age 6 without doctor's approval. Young children are not able to describe their symptoms accurately, and a proper diagnosis needs to be made before starting any treatment.
- Don't give to a child who refuses to have a bowel movement (toileting refusal). May force a painful bowel movement and cause the child to hold back even more. Consult doctor.
- For children over age 6, follow package instructions or doctor's directions for correct dosage amount.

Prolonged use:
Don't take for more than 1 week unless under doctor's supervision. May cause laxative dependence in which normal bowel function depends on the laxative to produce a bowel movement.

Skin & sunlight:
No special problems expected.

Driving, piloting or hazardous work:
No special problems expected.

Discontinuing:
May be unnecessary to finish medicine. Follow doctor's instructions or instructions on label.

Others:
- Don't give to "flush out" the system or as a "tonic."
- Use as directed. Don't increase or decrease dosage without doctor's approval.
- Excessive use of laxatives in a teenager may indicate an eating disorder such as anorexia nervosa or bulimia nervosa. Consult doctor.
- If there is a sudden change in bowel habits or bowel function that lasts longer than 2 weeks, consult doctor.

POSSIBLE INTERACTION WITH OTHER DRUGS

GENERIC NAME OR DRUG CLASS	COMBINED EFFECT
Antacids*	Irritation of stomach or small intestine.
Anticoagulants*	Decreased anticoagulant effect with aluminum- or magnesium-containing laxatives. Avoid.
Ciprofloxacin	Decreased ciprofloxacin effect with magnesium-containing laxatives. Avoid.
Digitalis preparations*	Decreased digitalis effect with aluminum- or magnesium-containing laxatives. Avoid.
Diuretics, potassium-sparing*	Decreased potassium effect.
Etidronate	Decreased etidronate effect if taken with magnesium-containing laxatives. Take 2 hours apart.
Phenothiazines*	Decreased phenothiazine effect with aluminum- or magnesium-containing laxatives. Avoid.
Potassium supplements*	Decreased potassium effect.
Sodium polystyrene	Fluid imbalance in body with magnesium-containing laxatives. Avoid.
Tetracyclines*	Decreased tetracycline effect. Take 2 hours apart.

POSSIBLE INTERACTION WITH OTHER SUBSTANCES

INTERACTS WITH	COMBINED EFFECT
Alcohol:	None expected.
Beverages:	None expected.
Cocaine:	None expected.
Foods:	None expected.
Marijuana:	None expected.
Tobacco:	None expected.

*See Glossary

LAXATIVES, SOFTENER/LUBRICANT

GENERIC AND BRAND NAMES

See complete list of generic and brand names in the *Generic and Brand Name Directory,* page 862.

BASIC INFORMATION

Habit forming? No
Prescription needed? No
Available as generic? Yes
Drug class: Laxative (stool softener-emollient), lubricant

USES

For short-term relief of simple constipation (bowel movements that are abnormally difficult or infrequent). Normal frequency of bowel movements may vary from 2 to 3 times a day to 2 to 3 times a week. Laxatives treat the symptoms of constipation, not the cause.

DOSAGE & USAGE INFORMATION

How to take:

- Tablets, capsules, syrup, chewable tablets, oral solution—Follow package instructions. Swallow with full glass of water, fruit juice or milk. Drink 6 to 8 glasses of water each day in addition to one taken with each dose.
- Enema or suppositories—Read and follow package instructions.

When to take:
Produces stool within 30 minutes to 3 hours following a dose. Take drug at a time that will not interfere with sleep or scheduled activities. Don't take late in the day on an empty stomach.

If you forget a dose:
Take as soon as you remember.

Continued next column

OVERDOSE

SYMPTOMS:
Weakness, increased sweating, confusion, irregular heartbeat, muscle cramps.
WHAT TO DO:
Overdose unlikely to threaten life. If person takes much larger amount than prescribed, call doctor, poison center 1-800-222-1222 or hospital emergency room for instructions.

What drug does:
Softener laxatives help liquids mix into the stool to help prevent hard stool masses. Lubricant laxatives coat the stool surface with a thin film that helps ease the passage of the stool through the intestines.

Time lapse before drug works:

- When taken by mouth, usually works within 1 to 2 days after first dose, but may take 3 to 5 days for full effectiveness.
- Rectal dosage forms work in 2 to 15 minutes.

Don't take with:

- Any other medicine without consulting your doctor or pharmacist.
- Other stool softener laxatives or mineral oil.
- Don't take within 2 hours of taking another medicine. Laxative interferes with absorption of medicine.

POSSIBLE ADVERSE REACTIONS OR SIDE EFFECTS

SYMPTOMS	WHAT TO DO
Life-threatening:	
None expected.	
Common:	
None expected.	
Infrequent:	
• Mild stomach cramps, throat irritation with liquid forms, diarrhea.	Continue. Call doctor when convenient.
• Rectal bleeding, burning, itching or pain (with rectal forms).	Discontinue. Call doctor right away.
Rare:	
Skin rash.	Discontinue. Call doctor right away.

WARNINGS & PRECAUTIONS

Don't take if:

- You have symptoms of appendicitis (abdominal pain, cramping, soreness, bloating, nausea and vomiting). Consult doctor.
- You are allergic to a softener-emollient or lubricant laxative.
- You have missed a bowel movement for just 1 or 2 days.

Before you start, consult your doctor:
- If you are allergic to any medicine, food or other substance or have a family history of allergies.
- If you have hypertension (high blood pressure) and the laxative contains sodium.
- If you have an intestinal obstruction, undiagnosed rectal bleeding or a colostomy or ileostomy.
- If you are taking other laxatives.
- If you have diabetes or heart or kidney disease.
- If you are taking other laxatives.
- You have dysphagia (swallowing difficulty) and want to take mineral oil.

Over age 60:
Oral mineral oil is not recommended for bedridden elderly patients; otherwise, no special problems expected.

Pregnancy:
Risk factors vary or may not be designated for these laxatives. Read categories on page xviii and consult doctor.

Breast-feeding:
No special problems expected. Consult doctor.

Infants & children:
- Don't give to children under age 6 without doctor's approval. Young children are not able to describe their symptoms accurately, and a proper diagnosis needs to be made before starting any treatment.
- Don't give to a child who refuses to have a bowel movement (toileting refusal). May force a painful bowel movement and cause the child to hold back even more. Consult doctor.
- For children over age 6, follow package instructions or doctor's directions for correct dosage amount.

Prolonged use:
Don't take for more than 1 week unless under doctor's supervision.

Skin & sunlight:
No special problems expected.

Driving, piloting or hazardous work:
No special problems expected.

Discontinuing:
May be unnecessary to finish medicine. Follow doctor's instructions or instructions on label.

Others:
- Don't give to "flush out" the system or as a "tonic."
- Use as directed. Don't increase or decrease dosage without doctor's approval.
- Excessive use of laxatives in a teenager may indicate an eating disorder such as anorexia nervosa or bulimia nervosa. Consult doctor.
- If there is a sudden change in bowel habits or bowel function that lasts longer than 2 weeks, consult doctor.

POSSIBLE INTERACTION WITH OTHER DRUGS

GENERIC NAME OR DRUG CLASS	COMBINED EFFECT
Antacids*	Irritation of stomach or small intestine.
Anticoagulants*	Decreased anti-coagulant effect with mineral oil.
Contraceptives, oral*	Decreased contra-ceptive effect with mineral oil.
Danthron	Increased danthron effect.
Digitalis preparations*	Decreased digitalis effect with mineral oil.
Diuretics, potassium-sparing*	Decreased potassium effect.
Phenophthalein	Increased pheno-phthalein effect.
Potassium supplements*	Decreased potassium effect.
Vitamins A, D, E, K	Decreased vitamin effect with mineral oil.

POSSIBLE INTERACTION WITH OTHER SUBSTANCES

INTERACTS WITH	COMBINED EFFECT
Alcohol:	None expected.
Beverages:	None expected.
Cocaine:	None expected.
Foods:	None expected.
Marijuana:	None expected.
Tobacco:	None expected.

*See Glossary

LAXATIVES, STIMULANT

GENERIC AND BRAND NAMES

See complete list of generic and brand names in the *Generic and Brand Name Directory*, page 862.

BASIC INFORMATION

Habit forming? Potentially
Prescription needed? No
Available as generic? Yes
Drug class: Laxative (stimulant)

USES

For short-term relief of simple constipation (bowel movements that are abnormally difficult or infrequent). Normal frequency of bowel movements may vary from 2 to 3 times a day to 2 to 3 times a week. Laxatives treat the symptoms of constipation, not the cause.

DOSAGE & USAGE INFORMATION

How to take:

- Tablets, chewable tablets, syrup, chewing gum, oral solution, granules, fluidextract, emulsion, wafers—Follow package instructions. Swallow with full glass of water, fruit juice or milk. Give child 6 to 8 glasses of fluid each day in addition to the one taken with each dose to keep stool soft. Give on an empty stomach. Results may be delayed if given with food.
- Enema—Lubricate rectal area with petroleum jelly before inserting enema applicator. Insert carefully to avoid damage to rectal wall. To mix powder for rectal solution, follow instructions on package.
- Suppository—Remove wrapper and moisten suppository with water. Gently insert tapered end into rectum. Push well into rectum with finger. Retain in rectum 20 to 30 minutes.

Continued next column

When to take:
Usually at bedtime on an empty stomach, unless directed otherwise. Castor oil is usually taken late in the day, as it works within 2 to 6 hours.

If you forget a dose:
Take as soon as you remember.

What drug does:
Acts on smooth muscles of intestinal wall to cause vigorous bowel movement.

Time lapse before drug works:
Oral form within 6 to 10 hours (castor oil 2 to 6 hours). Rectal form within15 minutes to 1 hour.

Don't take with:

- Any other medicine without consulting your doctor or pharmacist.
- Don't take within 2 hours of another medicine. Laxative interferes with absorption of medicine.

OVERDOSE

SYMPTOMS:
Weakness, increased sweating, confusion, irregular heartbeat, muscle cramps.
WHAT TO DO:
Overdose unlikely to threaten life. If person takes much larger amount than prescribed, call doctor, poison center 1-800-222-1222 or hospital emergency room for instructions.

POSSIBLE ADVERSE REACTIONS OR SIDE EFFECTS

SYMPTOMS	WHAT TO DO
Life-threatening: None expected.	
Common: None expected.	
Infrequent:	
• Belching, cramps, nausea, diarrhea, throat irritation.	Continue. Call doctor when convenient.
• Rectal bleeding, burning, itching or pain (with rectal forms).	Discontinue. Call doctor right away.
Rare:	
Confusion, irregular heartbeat, muscle cramps, unusual tiredness or weakness; pink to red color of urine and stools (with phenolphthalein); pink, red or violet to brown urine color (with cascara, danthron or senna); yellow to brown color of urine (with cascara, phenolphthalein or senna); skin rash (allergy).	Discontinue. Call doctor right away.

WARNINGS & PRECAUTIONS

Don't take if:
- You have symptoms of appendicitis (abdominal pain, cramping, soreness, bloating, nausea and vomiting). Consult doctor.
- You are allergic to a stimulant laxative.
- You have missed a bowel movement for just 1 or 2 days.

Before you start, consult your doctor:
- If you are a allergic to any medicine, food or other substance or have a family history of allergies.
- If you have hypertension (high blood pressure) and the laxative contains sodium.
- If you have an intestinal obstruction or undiagnosed rectal bleeding.
- If you have diabetes or heart or kidney disease.
- If you are taking other laxatives.

Over age 60:
Excessive use of stimulant laxatives may cause excess loss of body fluid, resulting in weakness and lack of coordination.

Pregnancy:
Risk factors vary or may not be designated for these laxatives. Read categories on page xviii and consult doctor.

Breast-feeding:
Some of the stimulant laxatives may pass into breast milk. Consult doctor.

Infants & children:
- Don't give to children under age 6 without doctor's approval. Young children are not able to describe their symptoms accurately, and a proper diagnosis needs to be made before starting any treatment.
- Don't give to a child who refuses to have a bowel movement (toileting refusal). May force a painful bowel movement and cause the child to hold back even more. Consult doctor.
- For children over age 6, follow package instructions or doctor's directions for correct dosage amount.

Prolonged use:
Don't take for more than 1 week unless under doctor's supervision.

Skin & sunlight:
No special problems expected.

Driving, piloting or hazardous work:
No special problems expected.

Discontinuing:
May be unnecessary to finish medicine. Follow doctor's instructions or instructions on label.

Others:
- Don't give to "flush out" the system or as a "tonic."
- Use as directed. Don't increase or decrease dosage without doctor's approval.
- Excessive use of laxatives in a teenager may indicate an eating disorder such as anorexia nervosa or bulimia nervosa. Consult doctor.
- If there is a sudden change in bowel habits or bowel function that lasts longer than 2 weeks, consult doctor.

POSSIBLE INTERACTION WITH OTHER DRUGS

GENERIC NAME OR DRUG CLASS	COMBINED EFFECT
Antacids*	Irritation of stomach or small intestine.
Diuretics, potassium-sparing*	Decreased potassium effect.
Histamine H_2 receptor antagonists*	Stomach irritation with bisacodyl. Take 1 hour apart.
Potassium supplements*	Decreased potassium effect.

POSSIBLE INTERACTION WITH OTHER SUBSTANCES

INTERACTS WITH	COMBINED EFFECT
Alcohol:	None expected.
Beverages: Milk.	Stomach irritation with bisacodyl. Take 1 hour apart.
Cocaine:	None expected.
Foods:	None expected.
Marijuana:	None expected.
Tobacco:	None expected.

*See Glossary

LEFLUNOMIDE

BRAND NAMES

Arava

BASIC INFORMATION

Habit forming? No
Prescription needed? Yes
Available as generic? No
Drug class: Antirheumatic

USES

Treats symptoms caused by rheumatoid arthritis, such as inflammation, swelling, stiffness and joint pain. Slows joint deterioration.

DOSAGE & USAGE INFORMATION

How to take:
Tablets—Take with full glass of water. If you can't swallow whole, crumble tablet and take with liquid or food.

When to take:
At the same time each day.

If you forget a dose:
Take as soon as you remember. However, if it is almost time for your next dose, skip the missed dose and go back to your regular dosing schedule (don't double this dose).

What drug does:
Stops the body from producing too many of the immune cells that are responsible for the swelling and inflammation (immunosuppressive and antiinflammatory).

Time lapse before drug works:
6 to 12 hours.

Don't take with:
Any other medicine without consulting your doctor or pharmacist.

Continued next column

OVERDOSE

SYMPTOMS:
None expected.
WHAT TO DO:
Overdose unlikely to threaten life. If person takes much larger amount than prescribed, call doctor, poison center 1-800-222-1222 or hospital emergency room for instructions.

POSSIBLE ADVERSE REACTIONS OR SIDE EFFECTS

SYMPTOMS	WHAT TO DO
Life-threatening:	
None expected.	
Common:	
• Chest congestion, cough, difficulty in breathing, loss of appetite, nausea, vomiting, yellow eyes or skin, dizziness, fever, sneezing, sore throat, pain or burning while urinating, frequent urge to urinate.	Continue. Call doctor right away.
• Abdominal pain, hair loss, back pain, diarrhea, heartburn, rash, unexplained weight loss.	Continue. Call doctor if symptoms persist.
Infrequent:	
• Unusual tiredness or weakness, shortness of breath, indigestion, pounding heartbeat, burning or tingling sensation in fingers and toes, joint or muscle pain, rapid heartbeat.	Continue. Call doctor right away.
• Acne, loss of appetite, anxiety, red or irritated eyes, constipation, dry mouth, gas, mouth ulcer, pain or burning in throat, itching, runny nose.	Continue. Call doctor when convenient.
Rare:	
None expected.	

WARNINGS & PRECAUTIONS

Don't take if:
You are allergic to leflunomide.

Before you start, consult your doctor:
- If you are using any other medication.
- You have immune system problems.
- You have severe or uncontrolled infections.
- You have been diagnosed with kidney or liver disease.

Over age 60:
Side effects or problems experienced with this medication appear to be the same in older people as in younger adults.

Pregnancy:
Risk to unborn child outweighs drug benefits. Don't use. Risk category X (see page xviii).

Breast-feeding:
Drug may pass into milk. Avoid drug or discontinue nursing until you finish medicine. Consult doctor for advice on maintaining milk supply.

Infants & children:
Studies on this medicine have been done only in adult patients. Consult doctor before giving this medicine to persons under age 18.

Prolonged use:
Usually not prescribed for long-term use.

Skin & sunlight:
None expected.

Driving, piloting or hazardous work:
None expected.

Discontinuing:
Don't discontinue without consulting doctor or completing prescribed dosage.

Others:
- May affect accuracy of some laboratory test values.
- Women of childbearing age are advised to use reliable contraception before receiving leflunomide. If you become pregnant while taking this drug, notify your doctor immediately.
- Use of leflunomide by men during time of conception may cause birth defects in their children. Therefore, men taking leflunomide should use condoms as a form of birth control.
- Do not have any immunizations during or after treatment with this drug without your doctor's approval.
- Advise any doctor or dentist whom you consult that you take this medicine.

POSSIBLE INTERACTION WITH OTHER DRUGS

GENERIC NAME OR DRUG CLASS	COMBINED EFFECT
Charcoal, activated	Decreased leflunomide effect.
Cholestyramine	Decreased leflunomide effect.
Methotrexate	Increased risk of side effects.
Rifampin	May increase risk of leflunomide toxicity.

POSSIBLE INTERACTION WITH OTHER SUBSTANCES

INTERACTS WITH	COMBINED EFFECT
Alcohol:	Increases the chance of liver problems. Avoid.
Beverages:	None expected.
Cocaine:	Effect unknown. Avoid.
Foods:	None expected.
Marijuana:	Effect unknown. Avoid
Tobacco:	None expected.

LEUCOVORIN

BRAND NAMES

Citrocovorin Calcium
Citrovorum Factor
Folinic Acid
Wellcovorin

BASIC INFORMATION

Habit forming? No
Prescription needed? Yes
Available as generic? Yes
Drug class: Antianemic

USES

- Antidote to folic acid antagonists.
- Treats anemia.

DOSAGE & USAGE INFORMATION

How to take:
Tablets—Swallow with liquid or food to lessen stomach irritation. If you can't swallow whole, crumble tablet and take with liquid or food.

When to take:
At the same time each day, according to instructions on prescription label.

If you forget a dose:
Take as soon as you remember up to 2 hours late. If more than 2 hours, wait for next scheduled dose (don't double this dose).

What drug does:
Favors development of DNA, RNA and protein synthesis.

Time lapse before drug works:
20 to 30 minutes.

Don't take with:
Any other medicine without consulting your doctor or pharmacist.

OVERDOSE

SYMPTOMS:
Unlikely to threaten life. If overdose is suspected, follow instructions below.
WHAT TO DO:
- **Dial 911 (emergency) for an ambulance or medical help or poison center 1-800-222-1222. Then give first aid immediately.**
- **See emergency information on inside covers.**

POSSIBLE ADVERSE REACTIONS OR SIDE EFFECTS

SYMPTOMS	WHAT TO DO
Life-threatening:	
Wheezing.	Seek emergency treatment immediately.
Common:	
None expected.	
Infrequent:	
None expected.	
Rare:	
Skin rash, hives.	Discontinue. Call doctor right away.

WARNINGS & PRECAUTIONS

Don't take if:
- You have pernicious anemia.
- You have vitamin B-12 deficiency.

Before you start, consult your doctor:
- If you have acid urine, acites, dehydration.
- If you have kidney function impairment.

Over age 60:
Adverse reactions and side effects may be more frequent and severe than in younger persons. You may need smaller doses for shorter periods of time.

Pregnancy:
Recommended for the treatment of megaloblastic anemia caused by pregnancy. Decide with your doctor if drug benefits justify risk to unborn child. Risk category C (see page xviii).

Breast-feeding:
No problems expected. Consult doctor.

Infants & children:
May increase frequency of seizures. Avoid if possible.

Prolonged use:
No problems expected.

Skin & sunlight:
No problems expected.

Driving, piloting or hazardous work:
Don't drive or pilot aircraft until you learn how medicine affects you. Don't work around dangerous machinery. Don't climb ladders or work in high places. Danger increases if you drink alcohol or take medicine affecting alertness and reflexes.

Discontinuing:
Don't discontinue without consulting doctor. Dose may require gradual reduction if you have taken drug for a long time. Doses of other drugs may also require adjustment.

Others:
No problems expected.

POSSIBLE INTERACTION WITH OTHER DRUGS

GENERIC NAME OR DRUG CLASS	COMBINED EFFECT
Anticonvulsants, barbiturate and hydantoin*	Large doses of leucovorin may counteract the effects of these medicines.
Central nervous system (CNS) depressants*	High alcohol content of leucovorin may cause adverse effects.
Fluorouracil	Increased levels of fluorouracil.
Primidone	Large doses of leucovorin may counteract the effects of both drugs.

POSSIBLE INTERACTION WITH OTHER SUBSTANCES

INTERACTS WITH	COMBINED EFFECT
Alcohol:	Increased adverse reactions of both.
Beverages:	None expected.
Cocaine:	Increased adverse reactions of both drugs.
Foods:	None expected.
Marijuana:	Increased adverse reactions of both drugs.
Tobacco:	Increased adverse reactions of both.

*See Glossary

LEUKOTRIENE MODIFIERS

GENERIC AND BRAND NAMES

MONTELUKAST
Singulair
ZAFIRLUKAST
Accolate
ZILEUTON
Zyflo

BASIC INFORMATION

Habit forming? No
Prescription needed? Yes
Available as generic? No
Drug class: Antiasthmatic

USES

Treatment of mild to moderate asthma. Not used to treat an active asthma attack. May be used with other asthma medications as directed by your doctor. Montelukast is used for prophylaxis (preventive) and chronic treatment of asthma.

DOSAGE & USAGE INFORMATION

How to take:
- Chewable tablets—(Montelukast) cherry flavor, recommended for children 6 to 15 years old.
- Tablets—Swallow with water, with or without food, except for zafirlukast which must be taken on an empty stomach 1 hour before or 2 hours after a meal.

When to take:
- Montelukast—At the same times each day.
- Zafirlukast—Twice a day at the same times.
- Zileuton—Four times a day at the same times.

If you forget a dose:
Take as soon as you remember, up to 2 hours late. If more than 2 hours, wait for next scheduled dose. Do not double doses.

What drug does:
Inhibits inflammatory cells associated with asthma. Inhibits reflex reactions to irritants, exercise and cold.

Continued next column

OVERDOSE

SYMPTOMS:
It is unknown what symptoms may occur.
WHAT TO DO:
If person uses much larger amount than prescribed, call doctor, poison center 1-800-222-1222 or hospital emergency room for instructions.

Time lapse before drug works:
30 minutes to 4 hours.

Don't take with:
Any other prescription or nonprescription drug without consulting your doctor or pharmacist.

POSSIBLE ADVERSE REACTIONS OR SIDE EFFECTS

SYMPTOMS	WHAT TO DO
Life-threatening: None expected.	
Common: Headache, stomach upset, nausea.	Continue. Call doctor when convenient.
Infrequent: Weak feeling, pain in abdomen, headache, unusual tiredness, cough, dental pain, dizziness, heartburn, fever, nasal congestion, skin rash.	Continue. Call doctor when convenient.
Rare: Liver problems (yellow eyes or skin, fatigue, symptoms of flu, nausea, itching, pain in upper right abdominal area).	Discontinue. Call doctor right away.

WARNINGS & PRECAUTIONS

Don't take if:
You are allergic to this medication.

Before you start, consult your doctor:
- If you have any other medical problem.
- If you have a liver or kidney disease.
- If you have a history of alcoholism.

Over age 60:
In some cases older patients taking zafirlukast experienced more infections; otherwise, no problems expected.

Pregnancy:
Decide with your doctor whether drug benefits justify risk to unborn child. Montelukast and zafirlukast—risk category B; zileuton—risk category C (see page xviii).

Breast-feeding:
- Montelukast and zileuton—It is unknown if drug passes into milk. Avoid drug or discontinue nursing until you finish medicine. Consult doctor for advice on maintaining milk supply.
- Zafirlukast—Drug passes into milk. Avoid drug or discontinue nursing until you finish medicine.

Infants & children:
- Montelukast is approved for children 2 years and older.
- Zafirlukast is approved for children over 6 years.
- Zileuton should only be given under close supervision, especially to children under 12 years old.

Prolonged use:
Schedule regular visits with your doctor to determine if the drug continues its effectiveness in controlling asthma symptoms.

Skin & sunlight:
No problems expected.

Driving, piloting or hazardous work:
No problems expected.

Discontinuing:
Don't discontinue without consulting doctor.

Others:
- In a few rare instances, patients taking zafirlukast while having their oral steroid dosage reduced developed Churg-Strauss syndrome (a rare and sometimes fatal condition). It is not known if the problem is caused by zafirlukast. Symptoms of Churg-Strauss syndrome are similar to those caused by flu. Before starting zafirlukast and reducing oral steroids, discuss the benefits and risk factors with your doctor.
- Advise any doctor or dentist you consult that you take this medicine.
- Talk to your doctor if your asthma attacks are not being controlled by the usual dosage of your fast-acting bronchodilator.
- This drug may affect results in some medical tests.
- This drug should be taken every day, even if you are not having asthma symptoms.

POSSIBLE INTERACTION WITH OTHER DRUGS

GENERIC NAME OR DRUG CLASS	COMBINED EFFECT
Astemizole	Effect unknown. Consult doctor.
Beta adrenergic blocking agents	Increased beta blocker effect.
Calcium channel blockers	Increased effect of calcium channel blocker.
Carbamazepine	Increased effect of carbamazepine.
Cisapride	Increased effect of cisapride.
Cyclosporine	Increased effect of cyclosporine.
Dofetilide	Increased dofetilide effect.
Erythromycin	Decreased effect of zafirlukast.
Phenobarbital	Decreased effect of montelukast.
Phenytoin	Increased effect of phenytoin.
Tolbutamide	Increased effect of tolbutamide.
Warfarin	Increased effect of warfarin.

POSSIBLE INTERACTION WITH OTHER SUBSTANCES

INTERACTS WITH	COMBINED EFFECT
Alcohol:	None expected.
Beverages:	None expected.
Cocaine:	Effects unknown. Avoid.
Foods:	None expected.
Marijuana:	Effects unknown. Avoid.
Tobacco:	None expected.

*See Glossary

LEVAMISOLE

BRAND NAMES

Ergamisol

BASIC INFORMATION

Habit forming? No
Prescription needed? Yes
Available as generic? No
Drug class: Anticancer treatment adjunct

USES

- Treats colorectal cancer when used in combination with fluorouracil.
- Treats malignant melanoma after surgical removal when there is no evidence of spread to organs other than the skin.

DOSAGE & USAGE INFORMATION

How to take:
Tablet—Swallow with liquid or food to lessen stomach irritation. If you can't swallow whole, crumble tablet and take with liquid or food.

When to take:
At the same time each day, according to instructions on prescription label.

If you forget a dose:
Don't take until you notify your doctor.

What drug does:
Acts to help restore the immune system. May activate T-cell lymphocytes and other white cells. Also elevates mood.

Time lapse before drug works:
1-1/2 to 2 hours.

Don't take with:
Any other medicine without consulting your doctor or pharmacist.

OVERDOSE

SYMPTOMS:
None expected.
WHAT TO DO:
Overdose unlikely to threaten life. If person takes much larger amount than prescribed, call doctor, poison center 1-800-222-1222 or hospital emergency room for instructions.

POSSIBLE ADVERSE REACTIONS OR SIDE EFFECTS

SYMPTOMS	WHAT TO DO
Life-threatening:	
Fever, muscle aches, headache, cough, hoarseness, sore throat, painful or difficult urination, low back or side pain.	Seek emergency treatment.
Common:	
• Diarrhea, metallic taste, nausea, joint or muscle pain, skin rash, insomnia, mental depression, nightmares, sleepiness or tiredness, increased dental problems.	Continue. Call doctor when convenient.
• Hair loss.	No action necessary.
Infrequent:	
Mouth, tongue and lip sores.	Call doctor right away.
Rare:	
Unsteady gait while walking; blurred vision; confusion; tremors; tingling or numbness in hands, feet or face; seizures; smacking and puckering of lips; uncontrolled tongue movements.	Call doctor right away.

WARNINGS & PRECAUTIONS

Don't take if:
You are allergic to levamisole.

Before you start, consult your doctor:
- If you take other drugs for cancer.
- If you have an active infection.
- If you have a seizure disorder.
- If you have allergies to other medications.

Over age 60:
No special problems expected.

Pregnancy:
Adequate studies not yet done. Consult your doctor. Risk category C (see page xviii).

Breast-feeding:
Effect unknown. Consult doctor.

Infants & children:
Effect not documented. Consult your doctor.

Prolonged use:
No special problems expected.

Skin & sunlight:
No special problems expected.

Driving, piloting or hazardous work:
No special problems expected.

Discontinuing:
Don't discontinue without consulting doctor. Dose may require gradual reduction if you have taken drug for a long time. Doses of other drugs may also require adjustment.

Others:
- Advise any doctor or dentist whom you consult that you take this medicine.
- Defer dental treatments until your blood count is normal. Pay particular attention to dental hygiene. You may be subject to additional risk of oral infection, delayed healing and bleeding.
- Avoid aspirin. May increase risk of internal bleeding.
- Avoid constipation. May increase risk of internal bleeding.

POSSIBLE INTERACTION WITH OTHER DRUGS

GENERIC NAME OR DRUG CLASS	COMBINED EFFECT
Anticoagulants*	Increased risk of bleeding.
Aspirin	Increased risk of bleeding.
Bone marrow depressants*	Increased risk of bone marrow depression.

POSSIBLE INTERACTION WITH OTHER SUBSTANCES

INTERACTS WITH	COMBINED EFFECT
Alcohol:	Increased risk of gastritis and internal bleeding.
Beverages:	None expected.
Cocaine:	Increased risk of mental disturbances. Avoid.
Foods:	None expected.
Marijuana:	None expected.
Tobacco:	None expected.

***See Glossary**

LEVETIRACETAM

BRAND NAMES

Keppra

BASIC INFORMATION

Habit forming? No
Prescription needed? Yes
Available as generic? No
Drug class: Anticonvulsant, antiepileptic

USES

Used to help control some types of seizures in the treatment of epilepsy. This medicine cannot cure epilepsy and will only work to control seizures for as long as you continue to take it.

DOSAGE & USAGE INFORMATION

How to take:
Tablet–Swallow the tablets with a liquid. May be taken with or without food and on a full or empty stomach.

When to take:
At the same times each day. Your doctor will determine the best schedule. Dosages may be increased every two weeks to achieve maximum benefits.

If you forget a dose:
Take as soon as you remember. If it is almost time for the next dose, skip the missed dose and wait for your next scheduled dose (don't double this dose).

What drug does:
The exact mechanism of the anticonvulsant activity of levetiracetam is unknown.

Time lapse before drug works:
May take several weeks for effectiveness.

Don't take with:
Any other prescription or nonprescription drug without consulting your doctor or pharmacist.

OVERDOSE

SYMPTOMS:
Possibly drowsiness or other symptoms.
WHAT TO DO:
Overdose unlikely to threaten life. If person takes much larger amount than prescribed, call doctor, poison center 1-800-222-1222 or hospital emergency room for instructions.

POSSIBLE ADVERSE REACTIONS OR SIDE EFFECTS

SYMPTOMS	WHAT TO DO
Life-threatening: None expected.	
Common: Cough; dizziness; dry or sore throat; hoarseness; loss of strength or energy; muscle pain or weakness; runny nose; sleepiness tender, swollen glands in neck; trouble in swallowing; unusual tiredness or weakness, voice changes.	Continue. Call doctor when convenient.
Infrequent:	
• Clumsiness or unsteadiness, crying, depression, double vision, fever or chills, headache, loss of memory or problems with memory, lower back or side pain, mood or mental changes, suicidal thoughts or feelings, nervousness, angry outbursts, pain or tenderness around eyes and cheekbones, painful or difficult urination, paranoia, muscle control problems, overreacting, shortness of breath or trouble breathing, stuffy or runny nose, chest tightness, wheezing.	Continue, but call doctor right away.
• Burning, crawling, itching, numbness, prickling, or tingling feelings; feeling of constant movement of self or surroundings; loss of appetite; spinning sensation; weight loss.	Continue. Call doctor when convenient.
Rare: Other symptoms.	Continue. Call doctor when convenient.

WARNINGS & PRECAUTIONS

Don't take if:
You are allergic to levetiracetam.

Before you start, consult your doctor:
- If you have kidney disease.
- If you are allergic to any medication, food or other substance.
- If you have any other medical problems.

Over age 60:
No special problems expected.

Pregnancy:
Decide with your doctor if drug benefits justify risks to unborn child. Risk category C (see page xviii).

Breast-feeding:
It is unknown if drug passes into milk. Avoid drug or discontinue nursing until you finish medicine. Consult doctor for advice on maintaining milk supply.

Infants & children:
Safety and effectiveness in patients below the age of 16 have not been established.

Prolonged use:
No special problems expected. Follow-up laboratory blood studies may be recommended by your doctor.

Skin & sunlight:
No problems expected.

Driving, piloting or hazardous work:
Don't drive or pilot aircraft until you learn how medicine affects you. Don't work around dangerous machinery. Don't climb ladders or work in high places. Danger increases if you drink alcohol or take other medicines affecting alertness and reflexes such as antihistamines, tranquilizers, sedatives, pain medicine, narcotics and mind-altering drugs.

Discontinuing:
Don't discontinue without doctor's approval due to risk of increased seizure activity. The dosage may need to be gradually decreased before stopping the drug completely.

Others:
- Advise any doctor or dentist whom you consult that you take this medicine.
- Levetiracetam may be used with other anticonvulsant drugs and additional side effects may also occur. If they do, discuss them with your doctor.

POSSIBLE INTERACTION WITH OTHER DRUGS

GENERIC NAME OR DRUG CLASS	COMBINED EFFECT
Anticonvulsants*, other	May decrease or increase effect of both drugs.
CNS Depressants*	Increased sedative effect.

POSSIBLE INTERACTION WITH OTHER SUBSTANCES

INTERACTS WITH	COMBINED EFFECT
Alcohol:	Increased sedative. effect. Avoid.
Beverages:	None expected.
Cocaine:	Unknown effect. Avoid.
Foods:	None expected.
Marijuana:	Unknown effect. Avoid.
Tobacco:	None expected.

LEVOCARNITINE

BRAND NAMES

Carnitor
L-Carnitine
VitaCarn

BASIC INFORMATION

Habit forming? No
Prescription needed? Yes
Available as generic? Yes
Drug class: Nutritional supplement

USES

Treats carnitine deficiency, a genetic impairment preventing normal utilization from diet.

DOSAGE & USAGE INFORMATION

How to take:

- Oral solution—Take after meals with liquid to decrease stomach irritation.
- Tablets—Swallow with liquid or food to lessen stomach irritation. If you can't swallow whole, crumble tablet and take with liquid or food.
- Injection—Given by medical professional.

When to take:
Immediately following or during meals to reduce stomach irritation.

If you forget a dose:
Take as soon as you remember up to 2 hours late. If more than 2 hours, wait for next scheduled dose (don't double this dose).

What drug does:
Facilitates normal use of fat to produce energy. Dietary source is meat and milk.

Time lapse before drug works:
Immediate action.

Don't take with:
Any other medicine without consulting your doctor or pharmacist.

OVERDOSE

SYMPTOMS:
Severe muscle weakness.
WHAT TO DO:

- **Dial 911 (emergency) for an ambulance or medical help or poison center 1-800-222-1222. Then give first aid immediately.**
- **See emergency information on inside covers.**

POSSIBLE ADVERSE REACTIONS OR SIDE EFFECTS

SYMPTOMS	WHAT TO DO
Life-threatening: None expected.	
Common: Changed body odor.	Continue. Call doctor when convenient.
Infrequent: Diarrhea, abdominal pain, nausea, vomiting.	Continue, but call doctor right away.
Rare: None expected.	

WARNINGS & PRECAUTIONS

Don't take if:
No contraindications.

Before you start, consult your doctor:
No documented reasons not to take.

Over age 60:
No problems expected.

Pregnancy:
No proven harm to unborn child, but avoid if possible. Consult doctor. Risk category B (see page xviii).

Breast-feeding:
No problems expected. Consult doctor.

Infants & children:
No problems expected. Deficiency can cause impaired growth and development.

Prolonged use:
Talk to your doctor about the need for follow-up medical examinations or laboratory studies to check triglycerides.

Skin & sunlight:
No problems expected.

Driving, piloting or hazardous work:
No problems expected.

Discontinuing:
Don't discontinue without consulting doctor. Dose may require gradual reduction if you have taken drug for a long time. Doses of other drugs may also require adjustment.

Others:
Health food store "vitamin B-T" contains dextro- and levo-carnitine which completely negates the effectiveness of levocarnitine (L-carnitine). Only the L-carnitine form is effective in levocarnitine deficiency.

POSSIBLE INTERACTION WITH OTHER DRUGS

GENERIC NAME OR DRUG CLASS	COMBINED EFFECT
Valproic acid	Decreased levocarnitine effect.

POSSIBLE INTERACTION WITH OTHER SUBSTANCES

INTERACTS WITH	COMBINED EFFECT
Alcohol:	None expected.
Beverages:	None expected.
Cocaine:	None expected.
Foods:	None expected.
Marijuana:	None expected.
Tobacco:	None expected.

LEVODOPA

BRAND NAMES

Dopar
Larodopa

BASIC INFORMATION

Habit forming? No
Prescription needed? Yes
Available as generic? Yes
Drug class: Antiparkinsonism

USES

Controls Parkinson's disease symptoms such as rigidity, tremor and unsteady gait.

DOSAGE & USAGE INFORMATION

How to take:
Tablet or capsule—Swallow with liquid or food to lessen stomach irritation. If you can't swallow whole, crumble tablet or open capsule and take with liquid or food.

When to take:
At the same times each day.

If you forget a dose:
Take as soon as you remember up to 2 hours late. If more than 2 hours, wait for next scheduled dose (don't double this dose).

What drug does:
Restores chemical balance necessary for normal nerve impulses.

Continued next column

OVERDOSE

SYMPTOMS:
Muscle twitch, spastic eyelid closure, nausea, vomiting, diarrhea, irregular and rapid pulse, weakness, fainting, confusion, agitation, hallucination, coma.
WHAT TO DO:
- **Dial 911 (emergency) for an ambulance or medical help or poison center 1-800-222-1222. Then give first aid immediately.**
- **If patient is unconscious and not breathing, give mouth-to-mouth breathing. If there is no heartbeat, use cardiac massage and mouth-to-mouth breathing (CPR). Don't try to make patient vomit. If you can't get help quickly, take patient to nearest emergency facility.**
- **See emergency information on inside covers.**

Time lapse before drug works:
2 to 3 weeks to improve; 6 weeks or longer for maximum benefit.

Don't take with:
Any other medication without consulting your doctor or pharmacist.

POSSIBLE ADVERSE REACTIONS OR SIDE EFFECTS

SYMPTOMS	WHAT TO DO
Life-threatening:	
In case of overdose, see previous column.	
Common:	
• Mood change, diarrhea, depression, anxiety.	Continue. Call doctor when convenient.
• Dry mouth, body odor.	No action necessary.
• Uncontrollable body movements.	Discontinue. Call doctor right away.
Infrequent:	
• Fainting, severe dizziness, headache, insomnia, nightmares, itchy skin, rash, nausea, vomiting, irregular heartbeat, eyelid spasm.	Discontinue. Call doctor right away.
• Flushed face, muscle twitching, discolored or dark urine, difficult urination, blurred vision, appetite loss.	Continue. Call doctor when convenient.
• Constipation, tiredness.	Continue. Tell doctor at next visit.
Rare:	
• High blood pressure.	Discontinue. Call doctor right away.
• Upper abdominal pain, anemia, increased sex drive.	Continue. Call doctor when convenient.

WARNINGS & PRECAUTIONS

Don't take if:
- You are allergic to levodopa or carbidopa.
- You have taken a monoamine oxidase (MAO) inhibitor* in past 2 weeks.
- You have glaucoma (narrow-angle type).

Before you start, consult your doctor:
- If you have diabetes or epilepsy.
- If you have had high blood pressure, heart or lung disease.
- If you have had liver or kidney disease.
- If you have a peptic ulcer.
- If you have malignant melanoma.

- If you will have surgery within 2 months, including dental surgery, requiring general or spinal anesthesia.

Over age 60:
Adverse reactions and side effects may be more frequent and severe than in younger persons.

Pregnancy:
Decide with your doctor if drug benefits justify risk to unborn child. Risk category C (see page xviii).

Breast-feeding:
Drug filters into milk. May harm child. Avoid.

Infants & children:
Not recommended.

Prolonged use:
- May lead to uncontrolled movements of head, face, mouth, tongue, arms or legs.
- Talk to your doctor about the need for follow-up medical examinations or laboratory studies to check complete blood counts (white blood cell count, platelet count, red blood cell count, hemoglobin, hematocrit), kidney function, liver function.

Skin & sunlight:
No problems expected.

Driving, piloting or hazardous work:
Don't drive or pilot aircraft until you learn how medicine affects you. Don't work around dangerous machinery. Don't climb ladders or work in high places. Danger increases if you drink alcohol or take medicine affecting alertness and reflexes, such as antihistamines, tranquilizers, sedatives, pain medicine, narcotics and mind-altering drugs.

Discontinuing:
Don't discontinue without doctor's advice until you complete prescribed dose, even though symptoms diminish or disappear.

Others:
Expect to start with small dose and increase gradually to lessen frequency and severity of adverse reactions.

POSSIBLE INTERACTION WITH OTHER DRUGS

GENERIC NAME OR DRUG CLASS	COMBINED EFFECT
Antidepressants, tricyclic (TCA)*	Decreased blood pressure. Weakness and faintness when arising from bed or chair.
Antiparkinsonism drugs, other*	Increased levodopa effect.
Bupropion	Increased levodopa effect.
Haloperidol	Decreased levodopa effect.
Loxapine	Decreased levodopa effect.
MAO inhibitors*	Dangerous rise in blood pressure.
Methyldopa	Decreased levodopa effect.
Molindone	Decreased levodopa effect.
Olanzapine	May decrease levodopa effect.
Papaverine	Decreased levodopa effect.
Phenothiazines*	Decreased levodopa effect.
Phenytoin	Decreased levodopa effect.
Pyridoxine (Vitamin B-6)	Decreased levodopa effect.
Rauwolfia alkaloids*	Decreased levodopa effect.
Selegiline	May require reduced dosage of levodopa.
Thioxanthenes*	Decreased levodopa effect.
Ziprasidone	Decreased levodopa effect.

POSSIBLE INTERACTION WITH OTHER SUBSTANCES

INTERACTS WITH	COMBINED EFFECT
Alcohol:	None expected.
Beverages:	None expected.
Cocaine:	Increased risk of heartbeat irregularity.
Foods: High-protein diet.	Decreased levodopa effect.
Marijuana:	Increased fatigue, lethargy, fainting.
Tobacco:	None expected.

*See Glossary

LEVONORGESTREL

BRAND NAMES

Norplant

BASIC INFORMATION

Habit forming? No
Prescription needed? Yes
Available as generic? No
Drug class: Female sex hormone (progestin)

USES

Highly effective long-term reversible contraceptive method.

DOSAGE & USAGE INFORMATION

How to take:
Administered by means of implants consisting of six flexible closed capsules (about the size of matchsticks) that are inserted beneath the skin on the inside of the upper arm. Implantation is done by a health-care professional within seven days of the start of the last menstrual period. The drug slowly diffuses into the bloodstream, delivering a nearly constant level of levonorgestrel to the body for up to 5 years.

When to take:
Implanted when long-term (up to 5 years) contraception is desired.

If you forget a dose:
Not a concern.

What drug does:
Inhibits ovulation so that eggs are not produced regularly. Causes the mucus of the cervix to thicken, preventing the sperm from reaching the egg if one is produced.

Time lapse before drug works:
24 hours

Don't take with:
Any other medicine without consulting your doctor or pharmacist.

OVERDOSE

SYMPTOMS:
None expected.

POSSIBLE ADVERSE REACTIONS OR SIDE EFFECTS

SYMPTOMS	WHAT TO DO
Life-threatening: None expected.	
Common: Increased, decreased, irregular or prolonged menstruation; spotting between periods.	Call doctor when convenient.
Infrequent: Headache, acne.	Call doctor when convenient.
Rare:	
• Severe bleeding, infection with pus at implant site, vaginal infection.	Call doctor right away.
• Swelling, numbness, discoloration or tenderness at implant site; breast discharge or tenderness; weight gain or loss; excess hair growth; hair loss from scalp; nausea; dizziness; muscle or abdominal pain; appetite changes; nervousness; depression.	Call doctor when convenient.

WARNINGS & PRECAUTIONS

Don't take if:
- You are allergic to any progestin hormone.
- You are or suspect you might be pregnant.
- You have liver disease or liver tumors.
- You have unexplained vaginal bleeding.
- You have breast cancer.
- You have now, or have a history of, blood clots in the legs, lungs or eyes.

Before you start, consult your doctor:
- If you have a condition that could be aggravated by fluid retention.
- If you have a history of depression or emotional disorders.

Over age 60:
Not recommended.

Pregnancy:
If pregnancy occurs, the capsules should be removed. Risk category X (see page xviii).

Breast-feeding:
Drug passes into milk. Consult your doctor about the advisability of breast-feeding.

Infants & children:
Not recommended.

Prolonged use:
- No problems expected.
- Capsules should be removed at end of five years. New capsules may be implanted if continuing contraception is desired.

Skin & sunlight:
No problems expected.

Driving, piloting or hazardous work:
No problems expected.

Discontinuing:
- Must be removed by a health-care professional.
- May be removed at your request at any time for any reason.
- Removal should be considered if you will be immobile for a long time due to illness or surgery.

Others:
- Review patient information booklet before you have Norplant implanted. You will be given a form to sign indicating you have received information on the risks and benefits of the implants.
- May affect results of some medical tests.
- Does not protect against sexually transmitted diseases. For additional protection, couples may also use condoms and/or spermicidal agents.
- Fertility returns shortly after implants are removed, usually within two weeks.
- Have blood pressure checked by your doctor 3 months after implant.

POSSIBLE INTERACTION WITH OTHER DRUGS

GENERIC NAME OR DRUG CLASS	COMBINED EFFECT
Phenytoin	Decreased contraceptive effect.
Carbamazepine	Decreased contraceptive effect.
Barbiturates*	Decreased contraceptive effect.
Phenylbutazone	Decreased contraceptive effect.
Isoniazid	Decreased contraceptive effect.
Rifampin	Decreased contraceptive effect.

POSSIBLE INTERACTION WITH OTHER SUBSTANCES

INTERACTS WITH	COMBINED EFFECT
Alcohol:	None expected.
Beverages:	None expected.
Cocaine:	None expected.
Foods:	None expected.
Marijuana:	None expected.
Tobacco:	None expected, but consult doctor.

*See Glossary

LINCOMYCIN

BRAND NAMES

Lincocin

BASIC INFORMATION

Habit forming? No
Prescription needed? Yes
Available as generic? Yes
Drug class: Antibacterial

USES

Treatment of bacterial infections that are susceptible to lincomycin.

DOSAGE & USAGE INFORMATION

How to take:
Capsule—Swallow with liquid 1 hour before or 2 hours after eating. Drink 8 ounces of water with each dose.

When to take:
At the same times each day.

If you forget a dose:
Take as soon as you remember up to 2 hours late. If more than 2 hours, wait for next scheduled dose (don't double this dose).

What drug does:
Destroys susceptible bacteria. Does not kill viruses.

Time lapse before drug works:
3 to 5 days.

Don't take with:
Any other medication without consulting your doctor or pharmacist.

OVERDOSE

SYMPTOMS:
Severe nausea, vomiting, diarrhea.
WHAT TO DO:
Overdose unlikely to threaten life. If person takes much larger amount than prescribed, call doctor, poison center 1-800-222-1222 or hospital emergency room for instructions.

POSSIBLE ADVERSE REACTIONS OR SIDE EFFECTS

SYMPTOMS	WHAT TO DO
Life-threatening:	
Hives, wheezing, faintness, itching, coma.	Seek emergency treatment.
Common:	
Bloating	Discontinue. Call doctor right away.
Infrequent:	
• Unusual thirst; vomiting; stomach cramps; severe and watery diarrhea with blood or mucus; painful, swollen joints; jaundice; fever; tiredness; weakness; weight loss.	Discontinue. Call doctor right away.
• Itch around groin, rectum or armpits; white patches in mouth; vaginal discharge, itching.	Continue. Call doctor when convenient.
Rare:	
Skin rash.	Discontinue. Call doctor right away.

WARNINGS & PRECAUTIONS

Don't take if:
- You are allergic to lincomycins.
- You have had ulcerative colitis.
- Prescribed for infant under 1 month old.

Before you start, consult your doctor:
- If you have had yeast infections of mouth, skin or vagina.
- If you will have surgery within 2 months, including dental surgery, requiring general or spinal anesthesia.
- If you have kidney or liver disease.
- If you have allergies of any kind.

Over age 60:
Adverse reactions and side effects may be more frequent and severe than in younger persons.

Pregnancy:
Decide with your doctor if drug benefits justify risk to unborn child. Risk category C (see page xviii).

Breast-feeding:
Drug passes into milk. Avoid drug or discontinue nursing until you finish medicine. Consult doctor for advice on maintaining milk supply.

Infants & children:
Don't give to infants younger than 1 month. Use for children only under medical supervision.

Prolonged use:
- Severe colitis with diarrhea and bleeding.
- You may become more susceptible to infections caused by germs not responsive to lincomycin.
- Talk to your doctor about the need for follow-up medical examinations or laboratory studies to check proctosigmoidoscopy.

Skin & sunlight:
No problems expected.

Driving, piloting or hazardous work:
No problems expected.

Discontinuing:
Don't discontinue without doctor's advice until you complete prescribed dose, even though symptoms diminish or disappear.

Others:
May interfere with the accuracy of some medical tests.

POSSIBLE INTERACTION WITH OTHER DRUGS

GENERIC NAME OR DRUG CLASS	COMBINED EFFECT
Antidiarrheal preparations*	Decreased lincomycin effect.
Attapulgite	May decrease effectiveness of lincomycin.
Chloramphenicol	Decreased lincomycin effect.
Erythromycins*	Decreased lincomycin effect.
Narcotics*	Increased risk of respiratory problems.

POSSIBLE INTERACTION WITH OTHER SUBSTANCES

INTERACTS WITH	COMBINED EFFECT
Alcohol:	None expected.
Beverages:	None expected.
Cocaine:	None expected.
Foods:	None expected.
Marijuana:	None expected.
Tobacco:	None expected.

LINEZOLID

BRAND NAMES

Zyvox

BASIC INFORMATION

Habit forming? No
Prescription needed? Yes
Available as generic? No
Drug class: Antibacterial, antibiotic (oxazolidinone)

USES

Treats bacterial infections of the blood, lungs and skin. It may also be used for other conditions as determined by your doctor.

DOSAGE & USAGE INFORMATION

How to take:

- Tablets—Take with full glass of water. If you can't swallow whole, crumble tablet and take with liquid or food.
- Oral suspension—Take as directed on label. The medicine should be gently mixed by inverting the bottle 3 to 5 times before each dose. Do not shake the bottle.

When to take:
As directed by your doctor. Usually every 12 hours.

If you forget a dose:
Take as soon as you remember. However, if it is almost time for your next dose, skip the missed dose and go back to your regular dosing schedule (don't double this dose).

What drug does:
Destroys bacteria in the body, probably by blocking protein production inside bacteria.

Time lapse before drug works:
10 to 14 days for most infections, but some infections may take longer. Continue taking this medicine for the full time of treatment even if you begin to feel better after a few days.

Don't take with:
Any other medicine without consulting your doctor or pharmacist.

OVERDOSE

SYMPTOMS:
None expected.
WHAT TO DO:
Overdose unlikely to threaten life. If person takes much larger amount than prescribed, call doctor, poison center 1-800-222-1222 or hospital emergency room for instructions.

POSSIBLE ADVERSE REACTIONS OR SIDE EFFECTS

SYMPTOMS	WHAT TO DO
Life-threatening: None expected.	
Common:	
• Diarrhea, headache.	Continue. Call doctor when convenient.
• Nausea.	Continue. Call doctor if symptoms persist.
Infrequent:	
• Fever, sore mouth or tongue, rash, black tarry stools, chest pain, chills, cough, painful or difficult urination, unusual bleeding or bruising, unusual tiredness or weakness, vomiting.	Discontinue. Call doctor right away.
• Constipation, change in taste, sleeplessness, vaginal yeast infection.	Continue. Call doctor when convenient.
Rare: None expected.	

WARNINGS & PRECAUTIONS

Don't take if:
You are allergic to linezolid.

Before you start, consult your doctor:
- If you are using any other medication.
- If you have a history of bleeding problems, diarrhea, high blood pressure or any other medical problems.

Over age 60:
Side effects or problems experienced with this medication appear to be the same in older people as in younger adults.

Pregnancy:
Decide with your doctor if drug benefits justify risk to unborn child. Risk category C (see page xviii).

Breast-feeding:
it is unknown if drug passes into milk. Avoid drug or discontinue nursing until you finish medicine. Consult doctor for advice on maintaining milk supply.

Infants & children:
Studies on this medicine have been done only in adult patients. Consult doctor before giving this medicine to persons under age 18.

Prolonged use:
Usually not prescribed for long-term use.

Skin & sunlight:
None expected.

Driving, piloting or hazardous work:
None expected.

Discontinuing:
Don't discontinue without consulting doctor or completing prescribed dosage.

Others:
- May affect accuracy of some laboratory test values.
- Do not store in the bathroom, near the kitchen sink or in other damp places. Heat or moisture may cause the medicine to break down.
- Advise any doctor or dentist whom you consult that you take this medicine.

POSSIBLE INTERACTION WITH OTHER DRUGS

GENERIC NAME OR DRUG CLASS	COMBINED EFFECT
Phenylpropanolamine	May increase blood pressure.
Pseudoephedrine	May increase blood pressure.

POSSIBLE INTERACTION WITH OTHER SUBSTANCES

INTERACTS WITH	COMBINED EFFECT
Alcohol:	None expected.
Beverages:	None expected.
Cocaine:	Effect unknown. Avoid.
Foods:	None expected.
Marijuana:	Effect unknown. Avoid
Tobacco:	None expected.

LITHIUM

BRAND NAMES

Carbolith
Cibalith-S
Duralith
Eskalith
Eskalith CR
Lithane
Lithizine
Lithobid
Lithonate
Lithotabs

BASIC INFORMATION

Habit forming? No
Prescription needed? Yes
Available as generic? Yes
Drug class: Mood stabilizer

USES

- Normalizes mood and behavior in bipolar (manic-depressive) disorder.
- Treats alcohol toxicity and addiction.
- Treats schizoid personality disorders.

DOSAGE & USAGE INFORMATION

How to take:
- Tablet or capsule—Swallow with liquid or food to lessen stomach irritation. If you can't swallow whole, crumble tablet or open capsule and take with liquid or food. Drink 2 or 3 quarts liquid per day, especially in hot weather.
- Extended-release tablets—Swallow each dose whole. Do not crush.
- Syrup—Take at mealtime. Follow with 8 oz. water.

When to take:
At the same times each day, preferably at mealtime.

If you forget a dose:
Take as soon as you remember up to 2 hours late. If more than 2 hours, wait for next scheduled dose (don't double this dose).

Continued next column

OVERDOSE

SYMPTOMS:
Moderate overdose increases some side effects and may cause diarrhea, nausea. Large overdose may cause vomiting, muscle weakness, convulsions, stupor and coma.
WHAT TO DO:
- **Dial 911 (emergency) for an ambulance or medical help or poison center 1-800-222-1222. Then give first aid immediately.**
- **See emergency information at end of book.**

What drug does:
May correct chemical imbalance in brain's transmission of nerve impulses that influence mood and behavior.

Time lapse before drug works:
1 to 3 weeks. May require 3 months before depressive phase of illness improves.

Don't take with:
Any other medication without consulting your doctor or pharmacist.

POSSIBLE ADVERSE REACTIONS OR SIDE EFFECTS

SYMPTOMS	WHAT TO DO
Life-threatening: In case of overdose, see previous column.	
Common:	
• Dizziness, diarrhea, nausea, vomiting, shakiness, tremor.	Continue. Call doctor when convenient.
• Dry mouth, thirst, decreased sexual ability, increased urination, anorexia.	Continue. Tell doctor at next visit.
Infrequent:	
• Rash, stomach pain, fainting, heartbeat irregularities, shortness of breath, ear noises.	Discontinue. Call doctor right away.
• Swollen hands, feet; slurred speech; thyroid impairment (coldness; dry, puffy skin); muscle aches; headache; weight gain; fatigue; menstrual irregularities, acnelike eruptions.	Continue. Call doctor when convenient.
• Drowsiness, confusion, weakness.	Continue. Tell doctor at next visit.
Rare:	
• Blurred vision, eye pain.	Discontinue. Call doctor right away.
• Jerking of arms and legs, worsening of psoriasis, hair loss.	Continue. Call doctor when convenient.

WARNINGS & PRECAUTIONS

Don't take if:
- You are allergic to lithium or tartrazine dye.
- You have kidney or heart disease.
- Patient is younger than 12.

Before you start, consult your doctor:
- About all medications you take.
- If you plan to become pregnant within medication period.

- If you have diabetes, low thyroid function, epilepsy or any significant medical problem.
- If you are on a low-salt diet or drink more than 4 cups of coffee per day.
- If you plan surgery within 2 months.

Over age 60:
Adverse reactions and side effects may be more frequent and severe than in younger persons.

Pregnancy:
Some fetal risk, but benefits may outweigh risks. Risk category D (see page xviii).

Breast-feeding:
Drug passes into milk. Avoid drug or discontinue nursing until you finish medicine. Consult doctor for advice on maintaining milk supply.

Infants & children:
Don't give to children younger than 12.

Prolonged use:
- Enlarged thyroid with possible impaired function.
- Talk to your doctor about the need for follow-up medical examinations or laboratory studies to check lithium levels, ECG*, kidney function, thyroid, complete blood counts (white blood cell count, platelet count, red blood cell count, hemoglobin, hematocrit).

Skin & sunlight:
No problems expected.

Driving, piloting or hazardous work:
Don't drive or pilot aircraft until you learn how medicine affects you. Don't work around dangerous machinery. Don't climb ladders or work in high places. Danger increases if you drink alcohol or take medicine affecting alertness and reflexes.

Discontinuing:
Don't discontinue without consulting doctor. Dose may require gradual reduction if you have taken drug for a long time. Doses of other drugs may also require adjustment. Quitting this medication when feeling well creates risk of relapse which may not respond to restarting the medication.

Others:
- Regular checkups, periodic blood tests, and tests of lithium levels and thyroid function recommended.
- Avoid exercise in hot weather and other activities that cause heavy sweating. This contributes to lithium poisoning. It is essential to take adequate fluids during hot weather to avoid toxicity.
- Call your doctor if you have an illness that causes heavy sweating, vomiting, or diarrhea. The loss of too much salt and water from your body could cause lithium toxicity.
- Advise any doctor or dentist whom you consult that you take this medicine.
- Some products contain tartrazine dye. Avoid, especially if allergic to aspirin.

POSSIBLE INTERACTION WITH OTHER DRUGS

GENERIC NAME OR DRUG CLASS	COMBINED EFFECT
Acetazolamide	Decreased lithium effect.
Antihistamines*	Possible excessive sedation.
Anti-inflammatory drugs, nonsteroidal (NSAIDs)*	Increased toxic effect of lithium.
Bupropion	Increased risk of seizures.
Carbamazepine	Increased lithium effect.
Desmopressin	Possible decreased desmopressin effect.
Diazepam	Possible hypothermia.
Diclofenac	Possible increase in effect and toxicity.
Didanosine	Increased risk of peripheral neuropathy.
Diuretics*	Increased lithium effect or toxicity.

Continued on page 917

POSSIBLE INTERACTION WITH OTHER SUBSTANCES

INTERACTS WITH	COMBINED EFFECT
Alcohol:	Possible lithium poisoning.
Beverages: Caffeine drinks.	Decreased lithium effect.
Cocaine:	Possible psychosis.
Foods: Salt.	High intake could decrease lithium effect. Low intake could increase lithium effect. *Don't* restrict intake.
Marijuana:	Increased tremor and possible psychosis.
Tobacco:	None expected.

***See Glossary**

LOMUSTINE

BRAND NAMES

CCNU
CeeNU

BASIC INFORMATION

Habit forming? No
Prescription needed? Yes
Available as generic? No
Drug class: Antineoplastic

USES

- Treats brain cancer and Hodgkin's lymphoma.
- Sometimes used to treat breast, lung, skin and gastrointestinal cancer.

DOSAGE & USAGE INFORMATION

How to take:
Capsules—Swallow with liquid. If you can't swallow whole, open capsule and take with liquid or food. Instructions to take on empty stomach mean 1 hour before or 2 hours after eating. Note: There may be two or more different types of capsules in the container. This is not an error.

When to take:
According to doctor's instructions. Usual course of treatment requires single dosage repeated every 6 weeks.

If you forget a dose:
Take as soon as you remember. Don't ever double doses.

What drug does:
Interferes with growth of cancer cells.

Time lapse before drug works:
None. Works immediately.

Don't take with:
Any other medicines (including over-the-counter drugs such as cough and cold medicines, laxatives, antacids, diet pills, caffeine, nose drops or vitamins) without consulting your doctor

OVERDOSE

SYMPTOMS:
Decreased urine (kidney failure); high fever, chills (infection); bloody or black stools (bleeding).
WHAT TO DO:
- **Dial 911 (emergency) for an ambulance or medical help or poison center 1-800-222-1222. Then give first aid immediately.**
- **See emergency information on inside covers.**

POSSIBLE ADVERSE REACTIONS OR SIDE EFFECTS

SYMPTOMS	WHAT TO DO
Life-threatening:	
In case of overdose, see previous column.	
Common:	
• Fever, chills, difficult urination, unusual bleeding.	Continue. Call doctor when convenient.
• Appetite loss, nausea, hair loss.	No action necessary.
Infrequent:	
• Anemia, confusion, slurred speech, mouth sores, skin rash.	Continue. Call doctor when convenient.
• Darkened skin.	No action necessary.
Rare:	
• Jaundice (yellow skin and eyes), cough.	Continue. Call doctor when convenient.
• Shortness of breath.	Discontinue. Call doctor right away.

WARNINGS & PRECAUTIONS

Don't take if:
- You have chicken pox.
- You have shingles (herpes zoster).

Before you start, consult your doctor:
- If you have an infection.
- If you have kidney disease.
- If you have had previous cancer chemotherapy or radiation treatment.

Over age 60:
Adverse reactions and side effects may be more frequent and severe than in younger persons. You may need smaller doses for shorter periods of time.

Pregnancy:
Risk to unborn child outweighs drug benefits. Don't use. Risk category D (see page xviii).

Breast-feeding:
Drug passes into milk. Avoid drug or discontinue nursing until you finish medicine. Consult doctor for advice on maintaining milk supply.

Infants & children:
Effect not documented. Consult your doctor.

Prolonged use:
Talk to your doctor about the need for follow-up medical examinations or laboratory studies to check kidney function, liver function and complete blood counts (white blood cell count, platelet count, red blood cell count, hemoglobin, hematocrit).

Skin & sunlight:
No problems expected.

Driving, piloting or hazardous work:
Don't drive or pilot aircraft until you learn how medicine affects you. Don't work around dangerous machinery. Don't climb ladders or work in high places. Danger increases if you drink alcohol or take medicine affecting alertness and reflexes.

Discontinuing:
Call doctor if any of these occur after discontinuing: black or tarry stools, bloody urine, hoarseness, bleeding or bruising, fever or chills.

Others:
- Advise any doctor or dentist whom you consult that you take this medicine.
- May affect results in some medical tests.
- Most adverse reactions and side effects are unavoidable.
- Avoid immunizations, if possible.
- Avoid persons with infections.
- Check with doctor about brushing or flossing teeth.
- Avoid contact sports.

POSSIBLE INTERACTION WITH OTHER DRUGS

GENERIC NAME OR DRUG CLASS	COMBINED EFFECT
Antineoplastic drugs, other*	Increased chance of drug toxicity.
Blood dyscrasia-causing medicines*	Adverse effect on bone marrow, causing decreased white cells and platelets.
Bone marrow depressants*, other	Increased risk of bone marrow depression.
Clozapine	Toxic effect on bone marrow.
Levamisole	Increased risk of bone marrow depression.
Tiopronin	Increased risk of toxicity to bone marrow.
Vaccines, live or killed virus	Increased chance of toxicity or reduced effectiveness of vaccine. Wait 3 to 12 months after lomustine treatment before getting vaccination.

POSSIBLE INTERACTION WITH OTHER SUBSTANCES

INTERACTS WITH	COMBINED EFFECT
Alcohol:	Increased chance of liver damage.
Beverages:	None expected.
Cocaine:	Increased chance of central nervous system toxicity.
Foods:	None expected.
Marijuana:	None expected.
Tobacco:	None expected.

*See Glossary

LOPERAMIDE

BRAND NAMES

Apo-Loperamide Caplets
Imodium
Imodium A-D
Imodium Advanced
Kaopectate II Caplets
Pepto Diarrhea Control

BASIC INFORMATION

Habit forming? No, unless taken in high doses for long periods.
Prescription needed? Yes, for some
Available as generic? Yes
Drug class: Antidiarrheal

USES

- Treats mild to moderate diarrhea. Used in conjunction with fluids, appropriate diet and rest. Treats symptoms only. Does not cure any disorder that causes diarrhea.
- Treats chronic diarrhea associated with inflammatory bowel disease.

DOSAGE & USAGE INFORMATION

How to take:

- Tablet or capsule—Swallow with food to lessen stomach irritation.
- Liquid—Follow label instructions and use marked dropper.

When to take:
No more often than directed on label.

If you forget a dose:
Take as soon as you remember up to 2 hours late. If more than 2 hours, wait for next scheduled dose (don't double this dose).

What drug does:
Blocks digestive tract's nerve supply, which reduces irritability and contractions in intestinal tract.

Continued next column

OVERDOSE

SYMPTOMS:
Constipation, lethargy, drowsiness or unconsciousness.
WHAT TO DO:
Overdose unlikely to threaten life. If person takes much larger amount than prescribed, call doctor, poison center 1-800-222-1222 or hospital emergency room for instructions.

Time lapse before drug works:
1 to 2 hours.

Don't take with:
Any other medication without consulting your doctor or pharmacist.

POSSIBLE ADVERSE REACTIONS OR SIDE EFFECTS

SYMPTOMS	WHAT TO DO
Life-threatening: None expected.	
Common: None expected.	
Infrequent: None expected.	
Rare:	
• Drowsiness, dizziness, dry mouth.	Continue. Call doctor when convenient.
• Nausea, vomiting, bloating, constipation, appetite loss, rash, abdominal pain.	Discontinue. Call doctor right away.

WARNINGS & PRECAUTIONS

Don't take if:
- You have severe colitis.
- You have colitis resulting from antibiotic treatment or infection.
- You are allergic to loperamide.

Before you start, consult your doctor:
- If you are dehydrated from fluid loss caused by diarrhea.
- If you have liver disease.

Over age 60:
Adverse reactions and side effects may be more frequent and severe than in younger persons.

Pregnancy:
No proven harm. Avoid if possible. Consult doctor. Risk category B (see page xviii).

Breast-feeding:
No proven problems, but avoid if possible or discontinue nursing until you finish medicine. Consult doctor for advice on maintaining milk supply.

Infants & children:
Don't give to infants or toddlers. Use only under doctor's supervision for children older than 2.

Prolonged use:
Habit forming at high dose.

Skin & sunlight:
No problems expected.

Driving, piloting or hazardous work:
Don't drive or pilot aircraft until you learn how medicine affects you. Don't work around dangerous machinery. Don't climb ladders or work in high places. Danger increases if you drink alcohol or take medicine affecting alertness and reflexes.

Discontinuing:
- May be unnecessary to finish medicine. Follow doctor's instructions.
- After discontinuing, consult doctor if you experience muscle cramps, nausea, vomiting, trembling, stomach cramps or unusual sweating.

Others:
If acute diarrhea lasts longer than 48 hours, discontinue and call doctor. In chronic diarrhea, loperamide is unlikely to be effective if diarrhea doesn't improve in 10 days.

POSSIBLE INTERACTION WITH OTHER DRUGS

GENERIC NAME OR DRUG CLASS	COMBINED EFFECT
Antibiotics*	Increased risk of diarrhea.
Narcotic analgesics	Increased risk of severe constipation.

POSSIBLE INTERACTION WITH OTHER SUBSTANCES

INTERACTS WITH	COMBINED EFFECT
Alcohol:	Depressed brain function. Avoid.
Beverages:	None expected.
Cocaine:	Decreased loperamide effect.
Foods:	None expected.
Marijuana:	None expected.
Tobacco:	None expected.

***See Glossary**

LORACARBEF

BRAND NAMES

Lorabid

BASIC INFORMATION

Habit forming? No
Prescription needed? Yes
Available as generic? No
Drug class: Antibacterial

USES

Treatment for bacterial infections of the upper respiratory tract, lower respiratory tract, urinary tract, skin and skin structure.

DOSAGE & USAGE INFORMATION

How to take:

- Capsule—Swallow with liquid. If you can't swallow whole, open capsule and take with liquid. Instructions to take on an empty stomach mean 1 hour before or 2 hours after eating.
- Oral suspension—Follow label instructions for mixing the powder with water. Instructions to take on an empty stomach mean 1 hour before or 2 hours after eating.

When to take:
At the same times each day.

If you forget a dose:
Take as soon as you remember up to 2 hours late. If more than 2 hours, wait for next scheduled dose (don't double this dose).

What drug does:
Kills bacteria susceptible to loracarbef.

Time lapse before drug works:
May require several days to affect infection.

Don't take with:
Any other prescription or nonprescription drug without consulting your doctor.

OVERDOSE

SYMPTOMS:
Nausea, vomiting, diarrhea or abdominal cramps.
WHAT TO DO:
Overdose unlikely to threaten life. If person takes much larger amount than prescribed, call doctor, poison center 1-800-222-1222 or hospital emergency room for instructions.

POSSIBLE ADVERSE REACTIONS OR SIDE EFFECTS

SYMPTOMS	WHAT TO DO
Life-threatening: Hives, rash, intense itching, faintness soon after a dose (anaphylaxis); difficulty in breathing.	Seek emergency treatment immediately.
Common: Abdominal pain, diarrhea, nausea and vomiting, loss of appetite	Continue. Call doctor when convenient.
Infrequent: Itching, skin rash.	Discontinue. Call doctor right away.
Rare: Dizziness, drowsiness, insomnia, nervousness, vaginal itching and discharge.	Continue. Call doctor when convenient.

WARNINGS & PRECAUTIONS

Don't take if:
You are allergic to loracarbef, penicillins* or cephalosporins*.

Before you start, consult your doctor:
- If you have kidney disease.
- If you have a history of colitis.

Over age 60:
Adverse reactions and side effects may be more frequent and severe than in younger persons. You may need smaller doses for shorter periods of time.

Pregnancy:
Consult doctor. Risk category B (see page xviii).

Breast-feeding:
Effect not documented. Consult your doctor.

Infants & children:
Not recommended for patients under 6 months of age.

Prolonged use:
- Kills beneficial bacteria that protect body against other germs. Unchecked germs may cause secondary infections.
- Talk to your doctor about the need for follow-up medical examinations or laboratory studies.

Skin & sunlight:
No problems expected.

Driving, piloting or hazardous work:
Avoid if you feel dizzy or drowsy. Otherwise, no problems expected.

Discontinuing:
Don't discontinue without doctor's advice until you complete prescribed dose, even though symptoms diminish or disappear.

Others:
- Advise any doctor or dentist whom you consult that you take this medicine.
- May affect the results in some medical tests.

POSSIBLE INTERACTION WITH OTHER DRUGS

GENERIC NAME OR DRUG CLASS	COMBINED EFFECT
Probenecid	Increased loracarbef effect.

POSSIBLE INTERACTION WITH OTHER SUBSTANCES

INTERACTS WITH	COMBINED EFFECT
Alcohol:	None expected.
Beverages:	None expected.
Cocaine:	None expected.
Foods:	None expected.
Marijuana:	None expected.
Tobacco:	None expected.

*See Glossary

LOXAPINE

BRAND NAMES

Loxapac
Loxitane
Loxitane C

BASIC INFORMATION

Habit forming? No
Prescription needed? Yes
Available as generic? Yes
Drug class: Tranquilizer, antidepressant

USES

- Treats serious mental illness.
- Treats anxiety and depression.

DOSAGE & USAGE INFORMATION

How to take:
- Oral solution—Take after meals with liquid to decrease stomach irritation.
- Tablets—Swallow with liquid or food to lessen stomach irritation. If you can't swallow whole, crumble tablet and take with liquid or food.
- Capsules—Swallow with liquid or food to lessen stomach irritation. If you can't swallow whole, open capsule and take with liquid or food.

When to take:
At the same times each day, according to instructions on prescription label.

If you forget a dose:
Take as soon as you remember up to 2 hours late. If more than 2 hours, wait for next scheduled dose (don't double this dose).

What drug does:
Probably blocks the effects of dopamine* in the brain.

Time lapse before drug works:
1/2 to 3 hours.

Don't take with:
Any other medicine without consulting your doctor or pharmacist.

OVERDOSE

SYMPTOMS:
Dizziness, drowsiness, severe shortness of breath, muscle spasms, coma.
WHAT TO DO:
- **Dial 911 (emergency) for an ambulance or medical help or poison center 1-800-222-1222. Then give first aid immediately.**
- **See emergency information at end of book.**

POSSIBLE ADVERSE REACTIONS OR SIDE EFFECTS

SYMPTOMS	WHAT TO DO
Life-threatening:	
Severe shortness of breath, skin rash, heartbeat irregularities, profuse sweating, fever, convulsions (rare).	Seek emergency treatment immediately.
Common:	
• Increased dental problems because of dry mouth and less salivation.	Consult your dentist about a prevention program.
• Swallowing difficulty, expressionless face, stiff arms and legs, dizziness.	Discontinue. Call doctor right away.
Infrequent:	
• Chewing movements with lip smacking, loss of balance, shuffling walk, tremor of fingers and hands, uncontrolled tongue movements.	Discontinue. Call doctor right away.
• Constipation, difficult urination, blurred vision, confusion, loss of sex drive, headache, insomnia, menstrual irregularities, weight gain, light sensitivity, nausea.	Continue. Call doctor when convenient.
Rare:	
Rapid heartbeat, fever, sore throat, jaundice, unusual bleeding.	Discontinue. Call doctor right away.

WARNINGS & PRECAUTIONS

Don't take if:
- You are an alcoholic.
- You have liver disease.

Before you start, consult your doctor:
- If you have a seizure disorder.
- If you have an enlarged prostate, glaucoma, Parkinson's disease, heart disease.

Over age 60:
Adverse reactions and side effects may be more frequent and severe than in younger persons. You may need smaller doses for shorter periods of time.

Pregnancy:
Decide with your doctor if drug benefits justify risk to unborn child. Risk category C (see page xviii).

Breast-feeding:
Drug may pass into milk. Avoid drug or discontinue nursing until you finish medicine. Consult doctor for advice on maintaining milk supply.

Infants & children:
Not recommended.

Prolonged use:
Talk to your doctor about the need for follow-up medical examinations or laboratory studies to check complete blood counts (white blood cell count, platelet count, red blood cell count, hemoglobin, hematocrit), liver function, eyes.

Skin & sunlight:
May cause rash or intensify sunburn in areas exposed to sun or ultraviolet light (photosensitivity reaction). Avoid overexposure and use sunscreen. Notify doctor if reaction occurs.

Driving, piloting or hazardous work:
Don't drive or pilot aircraft until you learn how medicine affects you. Don't work around dangerous machinery. Don't climb ladders or work in high places. Danger increases if you drink alcohol or take medicine affecting alertness and reflexes.

Discontinuing:
- Don't discontinue without consulting doctor. Dose may require gradual reduction if you have taken drug for a long time. Doses of other drugs may also require adjustment.
- These symptoms may occur after medicine has been discontinued: dizziness; nausea; abdominal pain; uncontrolled movements of mouth, tongue and jaw.

Others:
Use careful oral hygiene.

POSSIBLE INTERACTION WITH OTHER DRUGS

GENERIC NAME OR DRUG CLASS	COMBINED EFFECT
Anticonvulsants*	Decreased effect of anticonvulsant.
Antidepressants, tricyclic*	May increase toxic effects of both drugs.
Bupropion	Increased risk of seizures.
Central nervous system (CNS) depressants*	Increased sedative effects of both drugs.
Clozapine	Toxic effect on the central nervous system.
Epinephrine	Rapid heart rate and severe drop in blood pressure.
Extrapyramidal reaction*-causing drugs	Increased risk of side effects.
Fluoxetine	Increased depressant effects of both drugs.
Guanadrel	Decreased effect of guanadrel.
Guanethidine	Decreased effect of guanethidine.
Guanfacine	Increased effects of both drugs.
Haloperidol	May increase toxic effects of both drugs.
Leucovorin	High alcohol content of leucovorin may cause adverse effects.
Methyldopa	May increase toxic effects of both drugs.
Metoclopramide	May increase toxic effects of both drugs.
Molindone	May increase toxic effects of both drugs.
Pemoline	Increased central nervous stimulation.
Pergolide	Decreased pergolide effect.
Phenothiazines*	May increase toxic effects of both drugs.
Pimozide	May increase toxic effects of both drugs.

Continued on page 917

POSSIBLE INTERACTION WITH OTHER SUBSTANCES

INTERACTS WITH	COMBINED EFFECT
Alcohol:	May decrease effect of loxapine. Avoid.
Beverages:	None expected.
Cocaine:	May increase toxicity of both drugs. Avoid.
Foods:	None expected.
Marijuana:	May increase toxicity of both drugs. Avoid.
Tobacco:	May increase toxicity.

***See Glossary**

MACROLIDE ANTIBIOTICS

GENERIC AND BRAND NAMES

AZITHROMYCIN
Zithromax
CLARITHROMYCIN
Biaxin
DIRITHROMYCIN
Dynabac

BASIC INFORMATION

Habit forming? No
Prescription needed? Yes
Available as generic? No
Drug class: Antibiotic (macrolide), antibiotic (erythromycin)

USES

Treatment for mild to moderate bacterial infections responsive to macrolide antibiotics. These include bronchitis, tonsillitis, some pneumonias, ear infections, skin infections (e.g., acne), sinusitis, streptococcal sore throat, urethritis and others. Note: Erythromycin is also a macrolide antibiotic. See individual chart for information.

DOSAGE & USAGE INFORMATION

How to take:
- Enteric-coated tablet or delayed release tablet—Swallow with liquid. Do not crush or chew tablet.
- Tablet or capsule—Swallow with liquid. If you can't swallow whole, crumble tablet or open capsule and take with food or water.
- Oral suspension—Swallow with liquid.

When to take:
At the same time each day. Take azithromycin on an empty stomach, 1 hour before or 2 hours after a meal. Clarithromycin may be taken with or without food. Take dirithromycin with food or within 1 hour after eating.

Continued next column

OVERDOSE

SYMPTOMS:
Possibly diarrhea, nausea, vomiting, abdominal pain.
WHAT TO DO:
Overdose unlikely to threaten life. If person takes much larger amount than prescribed, call doctor, poison center 1-800-222-1222 or hospital emergency room for instructions.

If you forget a dose:
Take as soon as you remember. If it is almost time for the next dose, wait for that dose (don't double this dose) and resume regular schedule.

What drug does:
Prevents growth and reproduction of susceptible bacteria.

Time lapse before drug works:
Usually 2 to 5 days. Some infections may require 10 days or longer of therapy to resolve.

Don't take with:
Any other prescription or nonprescription drug without consulting your doctor or pharmacist.

POSSIBLE ADVERSE REACTIONS OR SIDE EFFECTS

SYMPTOMS	WHAT TO DO
Life-threatening:	
Rare allergic reaction—Breathing difficulty; swelling of hands, feet, face, mouth, neck; skin rash; temporary deafness.	Discontinue. Seek emergency treatment.
Common:	
None expected.	
Infrequent:	
Nausea, vomiting, abdominal discomfort, diarrhea.	Continue. Call doctor when convenient.
Rare:	
• Headache, dizziness.	Continue. Call doctor when convenient.
• Allergic reaction (skin rash, itching).	Discontinue. Call right away.

WARNINGS & PRECAUTIONS

Don't take if:
You are allergic to macrolide antibiotics.

Before you start, consult your doctor:
- If you have impaired liver or kidney function.
- If you are allergic to any medication, food or other substance.

Over age 60:
No special problems expected.

Pregnancy:
Risk factors vary for drugs in this group. See page xviii and consult doctor.

Breast-feeding:
One or more of these drugs may pass into milk. Avoid drug or discontinue nursing until you finish medicine. Consult doctor for advice on maintaining milk supply.

Infants & children:
Give only under close medical supervision to those under age 12. Young children may not complain or recognize adverse effects of drug. Observe child closely for any reactions

Prolonged use:
Not recommended. Medicine is discontinued once the infection is cured.

Skin & sunlight:
No special problems expected.

Driving, piloting or hazardous work:
Avoid if you experience dizziness. Otherwise, no problems expected.

Discontinuing:
Don't discontinue without doctor's advice until you complete prescribed dose, even though symptoms diminish or disappear.

Others:
- Advise any doctor or dentist whom you consult that you take this medicine.
- May affect the results of some medical tests.

POSSIBLE INTERACTION WITH OTHER DRUGS

GENERIC NAME OR DRUG CLASS	COMBINED EFFECT
Antacids*, aluminum- or magnesium-containing	Take one hour apart.
Astemizole	May increase risk of heart rhythm problems.
Benzodiazepines	Increased effect of benzodiazepine.
Bromocriptine	Increased effect of bromocriptine.
Carbamazepine	Increased effect of carbamazepine.
Cyclosporine	Increased effect of cyclosporine.
Digoxin	Increased effect of digoxin.
Disopyramide	Unknown effect. Use with caution.
Dofetilide	Increased risk of heart problems.
Histamine H_2 receptor antagonists*	Increased effect of antibiotic.
Lovastatin	Unknown effect. Use with caution.
Rifabutin	Decreased effect of antibiotic.
Rifampin	Decreased effect of antibiotic.
Tacrolimus	Increased effect of tacrolimus.
Theophylline	Increased effect of theophylline.
Triazolam	Increased risk of toxicity.
Warfarin	Increased risk of bleeding.
Zidovudine	Decreased effect of zidovudine.

POSSIBLE INTERACTION WITH OTHER SUBSTANCES

INTERACTS WITH	COMBINED EFFECT
Alcohol:	None expected.
Beverages:	None expected.
Cocaine:	None expected.
Foods:	None expected
Marijuana:	None expected.
Tobacco:	None expected.

*See Glossary

MAPROTILINE

BRAND NAMES

Ludiomil

BASIC INFORMATION

Habit forming? No
Prescription needed? Yes
Available as generic? Yes
Drug class: Antidepressant

USES

Treatment for depression or anxiety associated with depression.

DOSAGE & USAGE INFORMATION

How to take:
Tablet—Swallow with liquid.

When to take:
At the same time each day, usually bedtime.

If you forget a dose:
Bedtime dose—If you forget your once-a-day bedtime dose, don't take it more than 3 hours late. If more than 3 hours, wait for next scheduled dose. Don't double this dose.

What drug does:
Probably affects part of brain that controls messages between nerve cells.

Time lapse before drug works:
Begins in 1 to 2 weeks. May require 4 to 6 weeks for maximum benefit.

Continued next column

OVERDOSE

SYMPTOMS:
Respiratory failure, fever, cardiac arrhythmia, muscle stiffness, drowsiness, hallucinations, convulsions, coma.
WHAT TO DO:
- **Dial 911 (emergency) for an ambulance or medical help or poison center 1-800-222-1222. Then give first aid immediately.**
- **If patient is unconscious and not breathing, give mouth-to-mouth breathing. If there is no heartbeat, use cardiac massage and mouth-to-mouth breathing (CPR). Don't try to make patient vomit. If you can't get help quickly, take patient to nearest emergency facility.**
- **See emergency information at end of book.**

Don't take with:
Nonprescription drugs without consulting your doctor or pharmacist.

POSSIBLE ADVERSE REACTIONS OR SIDE EFFECTS

SYMPTOMS	WHAT TO DO
Life-threatening:	
Seizures.	Seek emergency treatment immediately.
Common:	
• Tremor.	Discontinue. Call doctor right away.
• Headache, dry mouth or unpleasant taste, constipation or diarrhea, nausea, indigestion, fatigue, weakness, drowsiness, nervousness, anxiety, excessive sweating.	Continue. Call doctor when convenient.
• Insomnia, craving sweets.	Continue. Tell doctor at next visit.
Infrequent:	
• Hallucinations, shakiness, dizziness, fainting, blurred vision, eye pain, vomiting, irregular heartbeat or slow pulse, inflamed tongue, abdominal pain, jaundice, hair loss, rash, chills, joint pain, palpitations, hiccups, vision changes.	Discontinue. Call doctor right away.
• Painful or difficult urination; fatigue; decreased sex drive; abnormal dreams; nasal congestion; back pain; muscle aches; frequent urination; painful, absent or irregular menstruation.	Continue. Call doctor when convenient.
Rare:	
Itchy skin; sore throat; jaundice; fever; involuntary movements of jaw, lips and tongue; nightmares; confusion; swollen breasts in men.	Discontinue. Call doctor right away.

WARNINGS & PRECAUTIONS

Don't take if:
- You are allergic to tricyclic antidepressants.
- You drink alcohol.
- You have had a heart attack within 6 weeks.
- You have glaucoma.
- You have taken a monoamine oxidase (MAO) inhibitor* within 2 weeks.

Before you start, consult your doctor:
- If you will have surgery within 2 months, including dental surgery, requiring general or spinal anesthesia.
- If you have an enlarged prostate, heart disease or high blood pressure, stomach or intestinal problems, overactive thyroid, asthma, liver disease, schizophrenia, urinary retention, respiratory disorders, seizure disorders, diabetes, kidney disease.

Over age 60:
More likely to develop urination difficulty and side effects such as hallucinations, shakiness, dizziness, fainting, headache or insomnia.

Pregnancy:
Consult doctor. Risk category B (see page xviii).

Breast-feeding:
Drug passes into milk. Avoid drug or discontinue nursing until you finish medicine. Consult doctor for advice on maintaining milk supply.

Infants & children:
Don't give to children younger than 12.

Prolonged use:
Request blood cell counts, liver function studies; monitor blood pressure closely.

Skin & sunlight:
May cause rash or intensify sunburn in areas exposed to sun or ultraviolet light (photosensitivity reaction). Avoid overexposure and use sunscreen. Notify doctor if reaction occurs.

Driving, piloting or hazardous work:
Don't drive or pilot aircraft until you learn how medicine affects you. Don't work around dangerous machinery. Don't climb ladders or work in high places. Danger increases if you drink alcohol or take medicine affecting alertness and reflexes.

Discontinuing:
Don't discontinue without consulting doctor. Dose may require gradual reduction if you have taken drug for a long time. Doses of other drugs may also require adjustment.

Others:
- Advise any doctor or dentist whom you consult that you take this drug.
- For dry mouth, suck sugarless hard candy or chew sugarless gum. If dry mouth persists, consult your dentist.

POSSIBLE INTERACTION WITH OTHER DRUGS

GENERIC NAME OR DRUG CLASS	COMBINED EFFECT
Anticholinergics*	Increased sedation.
Antiglaucoma agents	Heart rhythm problems, high blood pressure.
Antihistamines*	Increased antihistamine effect.
Barbiturates*	Decreased anti-depressant effect.
Benzodiazepines*	Increased sedation.
Bupropion	Increased risk of seizures.
Central nervous system (CNS) depressants*	Increased sedation.
Cimetidine	Possible increased antidepressant effect and toxicity.
Clonidine	Decreased clonidine effect.
Clozapine	Toxic effect on the central nervous system.
Disulfiram	Delirium.
Diuretics, thiazide*	Increased maprotiline effect.
Ethchlorvynol	Delirium.

Continued on page 917

POSSIBLE INTERACTION WITH OTHER SUBSTANCES

INTERACTS WITH	COMBINED EFFECT
Alcohol: Beverages or medicines with alcohol.	Excessive intoxication. Avoid.
Beverages:	None expected.
Cocaine:	Excessive intoxication. Avoid.
Foods:	None expected.
Marijuana:	Excessive drowsiness. Avoid.
Tobacco:	May decrease absorption of maprotiline. Avoid.

*See Glossary

MASOPROCOL

BRAND NAMES

Actinex

BASIC INFORMATION

Habit forming? No
Prescription needed? Yes
Available as generic? No
Drug class: Antineoplastic (topical)

USES

Treats actinic keratoses (scaly, flat or slightly raised skin lesions).

DOSAGE & USAGE INFORMATION

How to take:
Cream–Wash and dry the skin where lesions are located. Massage cream into affected area. Wash hands immediately after use.

When to take:
Use at the same times each day.

If you forget a dose:
Apply as soon as you remember, then resume regular schedule.

What drug does:
Selectively destroys actively proliferating cells.

Time lapse before drug works:
1 to 2 months.

Don't take with:
Other topical prescription or nonprescription drugs without consulting your doctor.

OVERDOSE

SYMPTOMS:
None reported.
WHAT TO DO:
Not for internal use. If child accidently swallows, call poison center 1-800-222-1222.

POSSIBLE ADVERSE REACTIONS OR SIDE EFFECTS

SYMPTOMS	WHAT TO DO
Life-threatening: None expected.	
Common:	
• Redness and swelling of otherwise normal skin.	Discontinue. Call doctor right away.
• Skin reactions including itching, redness, dryness, flaking where medicine applied.	Continue. Call doctor when convenient.
• Temporary burning sensation right after application.	No action necessary.
Infrequent:	
• Allergic reaction to sulfites—bluish skin, severe dizziness, faintness, wheezing, breathing difficulty.	Discontinue. Seek emergency help.
• Swelling, soreness, persistent burning in treated area.	Continue. Call doctor when convenient.
Rare:	
Bleeding, oozing, blistering skin.	Discontinue. Call doctor right away.

WARNINGS & PRECAUTIONS

Don't take if:
You are allergic to masoprocol.

Before you start, consult your doctor:
If you have a sulfite sensitivity.

Over age 60:
No problems expected.

Pregnancy:
Consult doctor. Risk category B (see page xviii).

Breast-feeding:
Effect not documented. Consult your doctor.

Infants & children:
Not used in this age group.

Prolonged use:
Effects of long-term use unknown. Visit doctor on a regular basis to determine effectiveness of treatment.

Skin & sunlight:
Drug does not cause sensitivity to sunlight. However, keratoses are related to sun exposure, so avoid sunlight when possible.

Driving, piloting or hazardous work:
No problems expected.

Discontinuing:
No problems expected.

Others:
- If you accidently get masoprocol in your eye, promptly wash the eye with water.
- The cream may stain your clothing.
- Get doctor's approval before using cosmetics or make-up on the skin area you are treating.
- Leave the treated skin areas exposed. Don't cover them with a bandage or a dressing.

POSSIBLE INTERACTION WITH OTHER DRUGS

GENERIC NAME OR DRUG CLASS	COMBINED EFFECT
None significant.	

POSSIBLE INTERACTION WITH OTHER SUBSTANCES

INTERACTS WITH	COMBINED EFFECT
Alcohol:	None expected.
Beverages:	None expected.
Cocaine:	None expected.
Foods:	None expected.
Marijuana:	None expected.
Tobacco:	None expected.

MECAMYLAMINE

BRAND NAMES

Inversine

BASIC INFORMATION

Habit forming? No
Prescription needed? Yes
Available as generic? No
Drug class: Antihypertensive

USES

Helps control, but doesn't cure, high blood pressure.

DOSAGE & USAGE INFORMATION

How to take:
Tablets—Swallow with liquid. If you can't swallow whole, crumble tablet and take with liquid or food. Instructions to take on empty stomach mean 1 hour before or 2 hours after eating.

When to take:
- At the same time each day, according to instructions on prescription label.
- Usually twice a day, every 8 or 12 hours apart. Follow label directions.

If you forget a dose:
Take as soon as you remember up to 2 hours late. If more than 2 hours, wait for next scheduled dose (don't double this dose).

What drug does:
Blocks transmission of electrical impulse where two nerve cells connect. Causes constricted blood vessels to relax.

Time lapse before drug works:
30 minutes to 2 hours.

Don't take with:
Any other medicines (including over-the-counter drugs such as cough and cold medicines, laxatives, antacids, diet pills, caffeine, nose drops or vitamins) without consulting your doctor.

OVERDOSE

SYMPTOMS:
Confusion, excitement, seizures, coma.
WHAT TO DO:
- **Dial 911 (emergency) for an ambulance or medical help or poison center 1-800-222-1222. Then give first aid immediately.**
- **See emergency information on inside covers.**

POSSIBLE ADVERSE REACTIONS OR SIDE EFFECTS

SYMPTOMS	WHAT TO DO
Life-threatening:	
In case of overdose, see previous column.	
Common:	
Dizziness upon arising from chair or bed, blurred vision, decreased sex drive, dry mouth, enlarged pupils, constipation.	Continue. Call doctor when convenient.
Infrequent:	
• Confusion, depression, tremors, shortness of breath.	Discontinue. Call doctor right away.
• Difficult urination, tiredness.	Continue. Tell doctor at next visit.
Rare:	
Appetite loss, nausea and vomiting.	Continue. Tell doctor at next visit.

WARNINGS & PRECAUTIONS

Don't take if:
You are allergic to mecamylamine.

Before you start, consult your doctor:
- If you have heart disease.
- If you had a recent heart attack.
- If you have glaucoma or gout.
- If you have kidney disease.

Over age 60:
Adverse reactions and side effects may be more frequent and severe than in younger persons. You may need smaller doses for shorter periods of time.

Pregnancy:
Decide with your doctor if drug benefits justify risk to unborn child. Risk category C (see page xviii).

Breast-feeding:
Effect unknown. Consult doctor.

Infants & children:
Effect not documented. Consult your pediatrician.

Prolonged use:
Talk to your doctor about the need for follow-up medical examinations or laboratory studies to check blood pressure, kidney function and heart function.

Skin & sunlight:
No problems expected.

Driving, piloting or hazardous work:
Avoid if you feel confused, drowsy or dizzy.

Discontinuing:
Don't discontinue without consulting doctor. Dose may require gradual reduction if you have taken drug for a long time. Doses of other drugs may also require adjustment.

Others:
- Advise any doctor or dentist whom you consult that you take this medicine.
- May affect results in some medical tests.
- Get up slowly from chair or bed.
- Dosage may need to be adjusted for hot weather or heavy exercise.

POSSIBLE INTERACTION WITH OTHER DRUGS

GENERIC NAME OR DRUG CLASS	COMBINED EFFECT
Alkalizers, urine*	Prolonged effect of mecamylamine.
Ambenonium	Swallowing difficulty.
Antacids*	Prolonged effect of mecamylamine.
Antibiotics*	Decreased antibiotic effect.
Antiglaucoma, carbonic anhydrase inhibitors	Increased risk of side effects.
Neostigmine	Swallowing difficulty.
Nimodipine	Dangerous blood pressure drop.
Pyridostigmine	Swallowing difficulty.
Sodium bicarbonate	Increased mecamylamine effect.
Sulfa drugs*	Decreased antibiotic effect.

POSSIBLE INTERACTION WITH OTHER SUBSTANCES

INTERACTS WITH	COMBINED EFFECT
Alcohol:	Increased likelihood of fainting.
Beverages:	None expected.
Cocaine:	Increased central nervous system stimulation. Avoid.
Foods: Food with high salt or sodium.	Decreased effectiveness of mecamylamine.
Marijuana:	Increased central nervous system stimulation. Avoid.
Tobacco:	None expected.

MECHLORETHAMINE (Topical)

BRAND NAMES

Mustargen

BASIC INFORMATION

Habit forming? No
Prescription needed? Yes
Available as generic? No
Drug class: Antineoplastic (topical)

USES

- Treats mycosis fungoides.
- Treats other malignancies (by injection).

DOSAGE & USAGE INFORMATION

How to use:

- Solution—Mix according to doctor's instructions. Don't inhale vapors or powder.
- Shower and rinse before treatment.
- Use rubber gloves to apply over entire body.
- Avoid contact with eyes, nose and mouth.
- Ointment—Use according to doctor's instructions.

When to use:
Usually once a day.

If you forget a dose:
Notify your doctor.

What drug does:
Destroys cells that produce mycosis fungoides.

Time lapse before drug works:
None. Works immediately.

Don't use with:
Any other medicines (including over-the-counter drugs such as cough and cold medicines, laxatives, antacids, diet pills, caffeine, nose drops or vitamins) without consulting your doctor.

OVERDOSE

SYMPTOMS:
None expected for topical solutions.
WHAT TO DO:
Not intended for internal use. If child accidentally swallows, call poison center 1-800-222-1222.

POSSIBLE ADVERSE REACTIONS OR SIDE EFFECTS

SYMPTOMS	WHAT TO DO
Life-threatening:	
Immediate hives, shortness of breath.	Seek emergency treatment immediately.
Common:	
Darkening, dry skin.	Continue. Tell doctor at next visit.
Infrequent:	
Allergic reaction with rash, itching, hives.	Seek emergency treatment immediately.
Rare:	
None expected.	

WARNINGS & PRECAUTIONS

Don't use if:
You are allergic to mechlorethamine.

Before you start, consult your doctor:
- If you have chicken pox.
- If you have shingles (herpes zoster).
- If you have skin infection.

Over age 60:
No special problems expected.

Pregnancy:
Risk to unborn child outweighs drug benefits. Don't use. Risk category D (see page xviii).

Breast-feeding:
Drug may be absorbed and pass into milk. Avoid drug or discontinue nursing until you finish medicine. Consult doctor for advice on maintaining milk supply.

Infants & children:
Effect unknown. Consult doctor.

Prolonged use:
- Allergic or hypersensitive reactions more likely.
- Talk to your doctor about the need for follow-up medical examinations or laboratory studies to check liver function, complete blood counts (white blood cell count, platelet count, red blood cell count, hemoglobin, hematocrit) and hearing tests.

Skin & sunlight:
No problems expected.

Driving, piloting or hazardous work:
Don't drive or pilot aircraft until you learn how medicine affects you. Don't work around dangerous machinery. Don't climb ladders or work in high places. Danger increases if you drink alcohol or take medicine affecting alertness and reflexes.

Discontinuing:
No special problems expected.

Others:
- Advise any doctor or dentist whom you consult that you take this medicine.
- May affect results in some medical tests.
- Don't use if solution is discolored.

POSSIBLE INTERACTION WITH OTHER DRUGS

GENERIC NAME OR DRUG CLASS	COMBINED EFFECT
None significant.	

POSSIBLE INTERACTION WITH OTHER SUBSTANCES

INTERACTS WITH	COMBINED EFFECT
Alcohol:	None expected.
Beverages:	None expected.
Cocaine:	None expected.
Foods:	None expected.
Marijuana:	None expected.
Tobacco:	None expected.

MECLIZINE

BRAND NAMES

Antivert
Antivert/25
Antivert/50
Bonamine
Bonine
Dramamine II
D-Vert 15
D-Vert 30
Meni-D
Ru-Vert-M

BASIC INFORMATION

Habit forming? No
Prescription needed?
U.S.: No, for some
Canada: Yes
Available as generic? Yes
Drug class: Antihistamine, antiemetic, anti-motion sickness

USES

- Prevents motion sickness.
- Treatment for vertigo.

DOSAGE & USAGE INFORMATION

How to take:
- Tablet or capsule—Swallow with liquid or food to lessen stomach irritation. If you can't swallow whole, crumble tablet or open capsule and take with liquid or food.
- Chewable tablet—May be chewed, swallowed whole or mixed with food.

When to take:
30 minutes to 1 hour before traveling or as directed by doctor.

If you forget a dose:
Take as soon as you remember. Wait 4 hours for next dose.

What drug does:
Reduces sensitivity of nerve endings in inner ear, blocking messages to brain's vomiting center.

Continued next column

OVERDOSE

SYMPTOMS:
Drowsiness, confusion, incoordination, stupor, coma, weak pulse, shallow breathing, hallucinations.
WHAT TO DO:
- **Dial 911 (emergency) for an ambulance or medical help or poison center 1-800-222-1222. Then give first aid immediately.**
- **See emergency information on inside covers.**

Time lapse before drug works:
30 to 60 minutes.

Don't take with:
Any other medicine without consulting your doctor or pharmacist.

POSSIBLE ADVERSE REACTIONS OR SIDE EFFECTS

SYMPTOMS	WHAT TO DO
Life-threatening:	
In case of overdose, see previous column.	
Common:	
Drowsiness.	Continue. Tell doctor at next visit.
Infrequent:	
• Headache, diarrhea or constipation, fast heartbeat.	Continue. Call doctor when convenient.
• Dry mouth, nose, throat.	Continue. Tell doctor at next visit.
Rare:	
• Rash, hives.	Discontinue. Call doctor right away.
• Restlessness, excitement, insomnia, blurred vision, frequent and difficult urination, hallucinations.	Continue. Call doctor when convenient.
• Appetite loss, nausea.	Continue. Tell doctor at next visit.

WARNINGS & PRECAUTIONS

Don't take if:
- You are allergic to meclizine, buclizine or cyclizine.
- You have taken a monoamine oxidase (MAO) inhibitor* in the past 2 weeks.

Before you start, consult your doctor:
- If you have glaucoma.
- If you have prostate enlargement.
- If you have reacted badly to any antihistamine.

Over age 60:
Adverse reactions and side effects may be more frequent and severe than in younger persons, especially impaired urination from enlarged prostate gland.

Pregnancy:
Consult doctor. Risk category B (see page xviii).

Breast-feeding:
Drug passes into milk. Avoid drug or discontinue nursing until you finish medicine. Consult doctor for advice on maintaining milk supply.

Infants & children:
Safety not established. Avoid if under age 12.

Prolonged use:
No problems expected.

Skin & sunlight:
No problems expected.

Driving, piloting or hazardous work:
Don't fly aircraft. Don't drive until you learn how medicine affects you. Don't work around dangerous machinery. Don't climb ladders or work in high places. Danger increases if you drink alcohol or take medicine affecting alertness and reflexes, such as antihistamines, tranquilizers, sedatives, pain medicine, narcotics and mind-altering drugs.

Discontinuing:
No problems expected.

Others:
Some products contain tartrazine dye. Avoid, especially if you are allergic to aspirin.

POSSIBLE INTERACTION WITH OTHER DRUGS

GENERIC NAME OR DRUG CLASS	COMBINED EFFECT
Amphetamines*	May decrease drowsiness caused by meclizine.
Anticholinergics*	Increased effect of both drugs.
Antidepressants, tricyclic*	Increased effect of both drugs.
Carteolol	Decreased antihistamine effect.
Cisapride	Decreased meclizine effect.
Clozapine	Toxic effect on the central nervous system.
Dronabinol	Increases meclizine effect.
Ethinamate	Dangerous increased effects of ethinamate. Avoid combining.
Fluoxetine	Increased depressant effects of both drugs.
Guanfacine	May increase depressant effects of either drug.
Leucovorin	High alcohol content of leucovorin may cause adverse effects.
Methyprylon	Increased sedative effect, perhaps to dangerous level. Avoid.
Monoamine oxidase (MAO) inhibitors*	Increased meclizine effect.
Nabilone	Greater depression of central nervous system.
Narcotics*	Increased effect of both drugs.
Pain relievers*	Increased effect of both drugs.
Sedatives*	Increased effect of both drugs.
Sertraline	Increased depressive effects of both drugs.
Sleep inducers*	Increased effect of both drugs.
Sotalol	Increased antihistamine effect.
Tranquilizers*	Increased effect of both drugs.

POSSIBLE INTERACTION WITH OTHER SUBSTANCES

INTERACTS WITH	COMBINED EFFECT
Alcohol:	Increased sedation. Avoid.
Beverages: Caffeine drinks.	May decrease drowsiness.
Cocaine:	None expected.
Foods:	None expected.
Marijuana:	Increased drowsiness, dry mouth.
Tobacco:	None expected.

*See Glossary

MEGLITINIDES

GENERIC AND BRAND NAMES

NATEGLINIDE	REPAGLINIDE
Starlix	Prandin

BASIC INFORMATION

Habit forming? No
Prescription needed? Yes
Available as generic? No
Drug class: Antidiabetic

USES

Helps control, but does not cure type 2 (non-insulin dependent) diabetes. Used alone or in combination with other antidiabetic drugs, along with diet and exercise.

DOSAGE & USAGE INFORMATION

Tablets—Take with water between 15-30 minutes before a meal. If you skip the meal, also skip the dose of medicine. If you have an extra meal, take an extra dose.

When to use:
15 - 30 minutes before each meal or as directed by doctor.

If you forget a dose:
If it is almost time for your next dose, take only that dose. Do not double doses.

What drug does:
Increases amount of insulin secreted from the pancreas, which helps to control blood sugar.

Time lapse before drug works:
10-30 minutes, peaks in 1 hour.

Continued next column

OVERDOSE

SYMPTOMS:
Cold sweats, confusion, cool pale skin, difficulty in concentrating, drowsiness, excessive hunger, rapid heartbeat, nausea, nervousness, nightmares, restless sleep, seizures, shakiness, slurred speech, unusual tiredness or weakness, coma.
WHAT TO DO:
- **For mild low blood sugar symptoms, drink or eat something containing sugar right away.**
- **For more severe symptoms, dial 911 (emergency) for an ambulance or medical help or poison center 1-800-222-1222. Then give first aid immediately.**
- **See emergency information on inside covers.**

Don't take with:
Any other medicine without consulting your doctor or pharmacist.

POSSIBLE ADVERSE REACTIONS OR SIDE EFFECTS

SYMPTOMS	WHAT TO DO
Life-threatening:	
In case of overdose or low blood sugar, see previous column.	
Common:	
Symptoms of a cold (sore throat, runny or stuffy nose, cough), back pain, diarrhea, joint pain.	Continue. Call doctor when convenient.
Frequent:	
Low blood sugar symptoms (anxiety, cold sweats, shakiness, rapid heartbeat, blurred vision, pale skin, behavior changes similar to being drunk, confusion or difficulty thinking, drowsiness, excessive hunger, headache, nausea, nightmares, restless sleep, unusual tiredness or weakness.	Treat the low blood sugar. If symptoms are severe, seek emergency treatment.
Infrequent:	
Convulsions (seizures), unconsciousness, bloody or cloudy urine, urination problems (burning, painful, difficult frequent, urge to urinate), wheezing, chills, skin rash or itching or hives, eyes tearing, chest tightness, vomiting.	Discontinue. Call doctor right away.
Rare:	
• Unusual bleeding or bruising, red spots on skin, black tarry stools, hoarseness, lower back or side pain, other side effects not listed occur.	Continue, but call doctor right away.
• Indigestion, feeling of warmth or heat or or burning, stomach pain, constipation, dizziness.	Continue. Call doctor when convenient.

PRECAUTIONS

Don't use if:
You are allergic to either nateglinide or repaglinide.

Before you start, consult your doctor:
- If you have type 1 diabetes or diabetic ketoacidosis (ketones in the blood).
- If you have an infection, fever, an injury or trauma, high stress levels or planning surgery.
- If you have a nervous system disorder.
- If you have kidney or liver disease or underactive adrenal or pituitary gland.
- If you are in a weakened condition or under-nourished.

Over age 60:
Increased risk of developing low blood sugar.

Pregnancy:
Decide with your doctor if drug benefits justify risk to unborn child. Risk category C (see page xviii).

Breast-feeding:
It is not known if drug passes into milk. Avoid drugs or discontinue nursing until you finish medicine. Consult doctor for advice on maintaining milk supply.

Infants & children:
Not recommended. Safety and dosage have not been established.

Prolonged use:
Talk to your doctor about the need for follow up medical examinations or laboratory studies to check blood glucose levels and glycosylated hemoglobin (HbA1c) values.

Skin & sunlight:
No problems expected.

Driving, piloting or hazardous work:
Don't drive or pilot aircraft until you learn how medicine affects you. Don't work around dangerous machinery. Don't climb ladders or work in high places. Danger increases if you drink alcohol or take medicine affecting alertness and reflexes, such as antihistamines, tranquilizers, sedatives, pain medicine, narcotics and mind-altering drugs.

Discontinuing:
Don't discontinue without consulting your doctor even if you feel well. You can have diabetes without feeling any symptoms. Untreated diabetes can cause serious problems.

Others:
- Advise any doctor or dentist whom you consult that you take this medicine. It may interfere with the accuracy of some medical tests.
- Follow any special diet your doctor may prescribe. It can help control diabetes.
- Consult doctor if you become ill with vomiting or diarrhea while taking this drug.
- Use caution when exercising. Ask your doctor about an appropriate exercise program.
- Wear medical identification stating that you have diabetes and take this medication.
- Learn to recognize the symptoms of low and high blood sugar. You and your family need to know what to do if these symptoms occur and when to call the doctor for help.
- Have a glucagon kit and syringe in the event severe low blood sugar occurs.

POSSIBLE INTERACTION WITH OTHER DRUGS

GENERIC NAME OR DRUG CLASS	COMBINED EFFECT
Anti-inflammatory drugs nonsteroidal (NSAID's)	Increased risk of low blood sugar.
Barbiturates	Blood sugar problems.
Beta adrenergic blocking agents	Risk of high or low blood sugar.
Carbamazepine	Blood sugar problems.
Corticosteroids*	Decreased effect of meglitinide.
Diuretics, thiazide	Decreased effect of meglitinide.
Hyperglycemia-causing medications*	Increased risk of loss of glycemic control.
Monoamine oxidase (MAO) inhibitors*	Increased risk of low blood sugar.
Salicylates	Increased risk of low blood sugar.
Sympathomimetics*	Decreased effect of meglitinide.
Thyroid hormones	Decreased effect of meglitinide.

POSSIBLE INTERACTION WITH OTHER SUBSTANCES

INTERACTS WITH	COMBINED EFFECT
Alcohol:	Low blood sugar. Avoid.
Beverages:	None expected.
Cocaine:	None expected.
Foods:	None expected.
Marijuana:	None expected.
Tobacco:	None expected.

*See Glossary

MELATONIN

BRAND NAMES

Numerous brand names are available.

BASIC INFORMATION

Habit forming? No
Prescription needed? No
Available as generic? Yes
Drug class: Hormone

USES

- Melatonin is a hormone produced in the human body by the pineal gland and secreted at night. In most people, the melatonin levels are highest during the normal hours of sleep. The levels increase rapidly in the late evening, peaking after midnight and decreasing toward morning.
- Jet lag: Some research studies have shown that taking melatonin before a flight and continuing for a few days after arrival at the destination helped control jet lag symptoms of fatigue and sleep disturbances. Appears to work best after plane trips that crossed more than six time zones. Timing of doses very important for effectiveness.
- Insomnia and restless leg syndrome: Some research studies have shown that taking melatonin about 2 hours before bedtime decreased the time needed to fall asleep and improved quality of sleep (less wakefulness).
- Other claims that it can slow aging, fight disease, and enhance one's sex life have been less studied and more difficult to prove.

DOSAGE & USAGE INFORMATION

How to take:
For tablet or capsule—Follow instructions on the label or consult your doctor or pharmacist. Different brands supply different doses. Melatonin, as a product, is marketed as a dietary supplement and is not reviewed by the U.S. Food & Drug Administration (FDA) for effectiveness and safety. The melatonin products being sold are made

Continued next column

from animal pineal glands or synthesized. The best dosage amounts are unknown. Use with caution.

When to take:
At the same time each day according to label directions. It is recommended that melatonin be taken at night before bedtime.

If you forget a dose:
Follow label instructions for your particular brand of melatonin. Usually you can take a medication as soon as you remember up to 2 hours late. If more than 2 hours, wait for the next scheduled dose (don't double this dose).

What drug does:

- Glands in the body make chemicals called hormones and release them into the bloodstream. Hormones taken as supplements also end up in the bloodstream. In either case, the blood then carries hormones to different parts of the body. There, hormones influence the way organs and tissues work.
- Hormone supplements may not have the same effects on the body as naturally produced hormones have, because the body processes them differently. Higher doses of supplements may result in higher amounts of hormones in the blood than are healthy.

Time lapse before drug works:
Effectiveness will vary from person to person and will also depend on the reason for taking melatonin.

Don't take with:
Any prescription or nonprescription medicine without consulting your doctor or pharmacist.

OVERDOSE

SYMPTOMS:
It is unknown what symptoms may occur.
WHAT TO DO:
If person takes much larger amount than prescribed, call doctor, poison center 1-800-222-1222 or hospital emergency room for instructions.

POSSIBLE ADVERSE REACTIONS OR SIDE EFFECTS

SYMPTOMS	WHAT TO DO
Life-threatening: None expected.	
Common: Unknown.	
Infrequent: Drowsiness, confusion, headache or grogginess may occur the following morning.	Reduce dosage or discontinue taking.
Rare: Unknown. If symptoms occur that you are concerned about, talk to your doctor or pharmacist. Further research may uncover other side effects.	

WARNINGS & PRECAUTIONS

Don't use if:
You are allergic to melatonin.

Before you start, consult your doctor:
- If you have any chronic health problem.
- If you have high blood pressure (hypertension) or cardiovascular disease. Some studies in animals suggest that melatonin may constrict blood vessels (a condition that could be dangerous for people with these conditions).
- If you are allergic to any medication, food or other substance.

Over age 60:
A lower starting dosage is often recommended until a response is determined.

Pregnancy:
Melatonin is not recommended for pregnant women. Decide with your doctor if drug benefits justify risk to unborn child. Risk category is unknown since melatonin is not regulated by the FDA (see page xviii).

Breast-feeding:
It is unknown if drug passes into milk. Avoid drug or discontinue nursing until you finish medicine. Consult doctor for advice on maintaining milk supply.

Infants & children:
Not recommended for children.

Prolonged use:
Effects are unknown. More research is needed to determine long-term effects of melatonin use.

Skin & sunlight:
No problems expected.

Driving, piloting or hazardous work:
Since it causes drowsiness, don't drive or pilot aircraft until you learn how medicine affects you. Don't work around dangerous machinery. Don't climb ladders or work in high places. Danger increases if you drink alcohol or take medicine affecting alertness and reflexes.

Discontinuing:
No problems expected.

Others:
- Advise any doctor or dentist whom you consult that you take melatonin.
- Melatonin is not researched carefully as yet, but there does not appear to be any particular problems. Some studies are promising as to its effect on health.
- Before starting melatonin, talk to your doctor about your sleep problems or try other things that can help sleep, such as avoidance of caffeine, chocolate, and especially, alcohol in any amount.

POSSIBLE INTERACTION WITH OTHER DRUGS

GENERIC NAME OR DRUG CLASS	COMBINED EFFECT
All medications	Effects are unknown. Talk to your doctor or pharmacist.

POSSIBLE INTERACTION WITH OTHER SUBSTANCES

INTERACTS WITH	COMBINED EFFECT
Alcohol:	Disrupts the night-time melatonin effect. Avoid.
Beverages:	None expected.
Cocaine:	Problems not known. Best to avoid.
Foods:	None expected.
Marijuana:	Problems not known. Best to avoid.
Tobacco:	Smoking can disrupt your normal melatonin cycle. Avoid.

MELOXICAM

BRAND NAMES

Mobic

BASIC INFORMATION

Habit forming? No
Prescription needed? Yes
Available as generic? No
Drug class: Nonsteroidal anti-inflammatory, antirheumatic

USES

Treatment for joint pain, stiffness, inflammation and swelling of rheumatoid arthritis, osteoarthritis and gout.

DOSAGE & USAGE INFORMATION

How to take:
Tablet—Swallow whole with liquid. May be taken with or without food.

When to take:
At the same time each day.

If you forget a dose:
Take as soon as you remember, however, if it is the next day, skip the missed dose and return to your normal schedule (don't double this dose).

What drug does:
Reduces tissue concentration of prostaglandins (hormones which produce inflammation and pain).

Time lapse before drug works:
Begins in 2 to 3 hours. May require 3 weeks of regular use for maximum benefit.

Continued next column

OVERDOSE

SYMPTOMS:
Bloody or black tarry stools; blue lips, fingernails or skin; blurred vision; confusion; changes in urine color or output; difficulty swallowing or breathing; dizziness; fever; chest pain; slow or fast heartbeat; swelling; stomach pain; unusual tiredness or weakness; vomiting of blood or material that looks like coffee grounds; wheezing; yellow eyes or skin.
WHAT TO DO:
- **Dial 911 (emergency) for an ambulance or medical help or poison center 1-800-222-1222.**
- **See emergency information at end of book**

Don't take with:
Any other medicine without consulting your doctor or pharmacist.

POSSIBLE ADVERSE REACTIONS OR SIDE EFFECTS

SYMPTOMS	WHAT TO DO
Life-threatening:	
Hives, rash, intense itching, faintness soon after a dose, breathing difficulties (anaphylaxis).	Seek emergency treatment immediately.
Common:	
Diarrhea, heartburn, indigestion, gas.	Continue. Call doctor when convenient.
Infrequent:	
Abdominal pain, anxiety, confusion, constipation, nausea, nervousness, sleepiness.	Continue. Call doctor when convenient.
Rare:	
Difficulty swallowing, swelling around the face, shortness of breath, tightness in chest, unusual tiredness or weakness, bloody or black tarry stools, vomiting, stomach pain.	Discontinue. Seek emergency treatment.

WARNINGS & PRECAUTIONS

Don't take if:
- You are allergic to aspirin or any other nonsteroidal anti-inflammatory drug (NSAID's).
- You have nasal polyps.

Before you start, consult your doctor:
- If you have a history of alcohol abuse.
- If you have bleeding problems or ulcers.
- If you have any condition that causes fluid retention or dehydration.
- If you have any condition that causes fluid retention (heart problems or high blood pressure).
- If you have used tobacco recently.
- If you have impaired kidney or liver function.
- If you have asthma.

Over age 60:
No problems expected.

Pregnancy:
Decide with your doctor whether drug benefits justify risk to unborn child. Risk category C (see page xviii).

Breast-feeding:
Animal studies show the drug passes into milk. Avoid drug or discontinue nursing until you finish medicine. Consult doctor for advice on maintaining milk supply.

Infants & children:
Not recommended for anyone younger than 18.

Prolonged use:
Talk to your doctor about the need for follow-up medical exams or laboratory studies to check complete blood counts, liver function, stools for blood, and eyes.

Skin & sunlight:
No problems expected.

Driving, piloting or hazardous work:
Don't drive or pilot aircraft until you learn how medicine affects you. Don't work around dangerous machinery. Don't climb ladders or work in high places. Danger increases if you drink alcohol or take medicine affecting alertness and reflexes, such as antihistamines, tranquilizers, sedatives, pain medicine, narcotics and mind-altering drugs.

Discontinuing:
No problems expected. If drug has been taken for a long time, consult doctor before discontinuing.

Others:
- May affect results in some medical tests.
- Advise any doctor or dentist whom you consult that you take this medicine.
- Do not refrigerate.
- Do not store in the bathroom, near the kitchen sink or in other damp places.

POSSIBLE INTERACTION WITH OTHER DRUGS

GENERIC NAME OR DRUG CLASS	COMBINED EFFECT
Angiotensin-converting enzyme (ACE) inhibitors*	May decrease ACE inhibitor effect.
Anti-inflammatory drugs, nonsteroidal (NSAID's)* other	Increased risk of side effects.
Aspirin	Increased risk of stomach ulcer.
Furosemide	Decreased effect of furosemide.
Lithium	Increased lithium effect.
Warfarin	Increased risk of bleeding problems.

POSSIBLE INTERACTION WITH OTHER SUBSTANCES

INTERACTS WITH	COMBINED EFFECT
Alcohol:	Possible stomach ulcer or bleeding. Avoid.
Beverages:	None expected.
Cocaine:	None expected. Best to avoid.
Foods:	None expected.
Marijuana:	Increased pain relief from NSAID's.
Tobacco:	Possible stomach ulcer or bleeding.

*See Glossary

MELPHALAN

BRAND NAMES

Alkeran	Phenylalanine
L-PAM	Mustard

BASIC INFORMATION

Habit forming? No
Prescription needed? Yes
Available as generic? No
Drug class: Antineoplastic

USES

- Treatment for some kinds of cancer.
- Suppresses immune response after organ transplantation and in immune disorders.

DOSAGE & USAGE INFORMATION

How to take:
Tablet—Swallow with liquid after light meal. Don't drink fluids with meals. Drink extra fluids between meals. Avoid sweet or fatty foods.

When to take:
At the same time each day.

If you forget a dose:
Take as soon as you remember. Don't ever double dose.

What drug does:
Inhibits abnormal cell reproduction. May suppress immune system.

Continued next column

OVERDOSE

SYMPTOMS:
Bleeding, chills, fever, collapse, stupor, seizure.
WHAT TO DO:
- **Dial 911 (emergency) for an ambulance or medical help or poison center 1-800-222-1222. Then give first aid immediately.**
- **If patient is unconscious and not breathing, give mouth-to-mouth breathing. If there is no heartbeat, use cardiac massage and mouth-to-mouth breathing (CPR). Don't try to make patient vomit. If you can't get help quickly, take patient to nearest emergency facility.**
- **See emergency information on inside covers.**

Time lapse before drug works:
Up to 6 weeks for full effect.

Don't take with:
Any other medicine without consulting your doctor or pharmacist.

POSSIBLE ADVERSE REACTIONS OR SIDE EFFECTS

SYMPTOMS	WHAT TO DO
Life-threatening: In case of overdose, see previous column.	
Common:	
• Unusual bleeding or bruising, mouth sores with sore throat, chills and fever, black stools, sores in mouth and lips, back pain.	Continue, but call doctor right away.
• Hair loss, joint pain, menstrual. irregularities.	Continue. Call doctor when convenient.
• Nausea, vomiting, diarrhea (unavoidable), tiredness, weakness.	Continue. Tell doctor at next visit.
Infrequent:	
• Skin rash.	Continue, but call doctor right away.
• Mental confusion, shortness of breath.	Continue. Call doctor when convenient.
• Cough.	Continue. Tell doctor at next visit.
Rare:	
Jaundice, swelling in feet or legs.	Continue, but call doctor right away.

WARNINGS & PRECAUTIONS

Don't take if:
- You have had hypersensitivity to alkylating antineoplastic drugs.
- Your physician has not explained serious nature of your medical problem and risks of taking this medicine.

Before you start, consult your doctor:
- If you have gout.
- If you have had kidney stones.
- If you have active infection.
- If you have impaired kidney or liver function.
- If you have taken other antineoplastic drugs or had radiation treatment in last 3 weeks.
- If you have herpes zoster or chicken pox (or been exposed).

Over age 60:
Adverse reactions and side effects may be more frequent and severe than in younger persons.

Pregnancy:
Consult doctor. Risk category D (see page xviii).

Breast-feeding:
Safety not established. Consult doctor.

Infants & children:
Use only under special medical supervision at center experienced in anticancer drugs.

Prolonged use:
- Adverse reactions more likely the longer drug is required.
- Talk to your doctor about the need for follow-up medical examinations or laboratory studies to check complete blood counts (white blood cell count, platelet count, red blood cell count, hemoglobin, hematocrit), kidney function.

Skin & sunlight:
No problems expected.

Driving, piloting or hazardous work:
No problems expected.

Discontinuing:
Don't discontinue without doctor's advice until you complete prescribed dose, even though symptoms diminish or disappear. Some side effects may follow discontinuing. Report to doctor blurred vision, convulsions, confusion, persistent headache, fever or chills, blood in urine, unusual bleeding.

Others:
- May cause sterility.
- May increase chance of developing leukemia.

POSSIBLE INTERACTION WITH OTHER DRUGS

GENERIC NAME OR DRUG CLASS	COMBINED EFFECT
Antigout drugs*	Decreased antigout effect.
Antineoplastic drugs, other*	Increased effect of all drugs (may be beneficial).
Bone marrow depressants*	Increased risk of bone marrow toxicity.
Chloramphenicol	Increased likelihood of toxic effects of both drugs.
Clozapine	Toxic effect on bone marrow.
Lovastatin	Increased heart and kidney damage.
Probenecid	Increased likelihood of bone marrow toxicity.
Sulfinpyrazone	Increased likelihood of bone marrow toxicity.
Tiopronin	Increased risk of toxicity to bone marrow.
Vaccines, live or killed	Increased likelihood of toxicity or reduced effectiveness of vaccine.

POSSIBLE INTERACTION WITH OTHER SUBSTANCES

INTERACTS WITH	COMBINED EFFECT
Alcohol:	May increase chance of intestinal bleeding.
Beverages:	None expected.
Cocaine:	Increases chance of toxicity.
Foods:	Reduces irritation in stomach.
Marijuana:	None expected.
Tobacco:	Increases lung toxicity.

MEPROBAMATE

BRAND NAMES

See complete list of brand names in the *Generic and Brand Name Directory*, page 862.

BASIC INFORMATION

Habit forming? Yes
Prescription needed? Yes
Available as generic? Yes
Drug class: Tranquilizer, antianxiety agent

USES

Reduces mild anxiety, tension and insomnia.

DOSAGE & USAGE INFORMATION

How to take:
- Tablet—Swallow with liquid.
- Extended-release capsules—Swallow each dose whole.

When to take:
At the same times each day.

If you forget a dose:
Take as soon as you remember up to 2 hours late. If more than 2 hours, wait for next scheduled dose (don't double this dose).

What drug does:
Sedates brain centers that control behavior and emotions.

Time lapse before drug works:
1 to 2 hours.

Don't take with:
- Nonprescription drugs containing alcohol or caffeine without consulting doctor.
- Any other medicine without consulting your doctor or pharmacist.

OVERDOSE

SYMPTOMS:
Dizziness, slurred speech, stagger, confusion, depressed breathing and heart function, stupor, coma.
WHAT TO DO:
- **Dial 911 (emergency) for an ambulance or medical help or poison center 1-800-222-1222. Then give first aid immediately.**
- **See emergency information at end of book.**

POSSIBLE ADVERSE REACTIONS OR SIDE EFFECTS

SYMPTOMS	WHAT TO DO
Life-threatening:	
Hives, rash, intense itching, faintness soon after a dose, wheezing (anaphylaxis).	Seek emergency treatment immediately.
Common:	
Dizziness, confusion, agitation, drowsiness, unsteadiness, fatigue, weakness.	Continue. Tell doctor at next visit.
Infrequent:	
• Rash, hives, itchy skin; change in vision; diarrhea, nausea or vomiting.	Discontinue. Call doctor right away.
• False sense of well-being, headache, slurred speech, blurred vision.	Continue. Call doctor when convenient.
Rare:	
Sore throat; fever; rapid, pounding, unusually slow or irregular heartbeat; difficult breathing; unusual bleeding or bruising.	Discontinue. Call doctor right away.

WARNINGS & PRECAUTIONS

Don't take if:
- You are allergic to meprobamate, tybamate, carbromal or carisoprodol.
- You have had porphyria.
- Patient is younger than 6.

Before you start, consult your doctor:
- If you have epilepsy.
- If you have impaired liver or kidney function.
- If you have tartrazine dye allergy.
- If you suffer from drug abuse or alcoholism, active or in remission.
- If you have porphyria.

Over age 60:
Adverse reactions and side effects may be more frequent and severe than in younger persons.

Pregnancy:
Risk to unborn child outweighs drug benefits. Don't use. Risk category D (see page xviii).

Breast-feeding:
Drug passes into milk. May cause sedation in child. Avoid.

Infants & children:
Not recommended.

Prolonged use:
- Habit forming.
- May impair blood cell production.

Skin & sunlight:
No problems expected.

Driving, piloting or hazardous work:
Don't drive or pilot aircraft until you learn how medicine affects you. Don't work around dangerous machinery. Don't climb ladders or work in high places. Danger increases if you drink alcohol or take medicine affecting alertness and reflexes, such as antihistamines, tranquilizers, sedatives, pain medicine, narcotics and mind-altering drugs.

Discontinuing:
Don't discontinue without consulting doctor. Dose may require gradual reduction if you have taken drug for a long time. Doses of other drugs may also require adjustment. Report to your doctor any unusual symptom that begins in the first week you discontinue this medicine. These symptoms may include convulsions, confusion, nightmares, insomnia.

Others:
- Advise any doctor or dentist whom you consult that you take this drug.
- For dry mouth, suck sugarless hard candy or sugarless gum. If dry mouth persists, consult your dentist.

POSSIBLE INTERACTION WITH OTHER DRUGS

GENERIC NAME OR DRUG CLASS	COMBINED EFFECT
Addictive drugs*	Increased risk of addictive effect.
Antidepressants, tricyclic*	Increased anti-depressant effect.
Antihistamines*	Possible excessive sedation.
Central nervous system (CNS) depressants*	Increased depressive effects of both drugs.
Monoamine oxidase (MAO) inhibitors*	Increased meprobamate effect.
Narcotics*	Increased narcotic effect.
Sertraline	Increased depressive effects of both drugs.

POSSIBLE INTERACTION WITH OTHER SUBSTANCES

INTERACTS WITH	COMBINED EFFECT
Alcohol:	Dangerous increased effect of meprobamate.
Beverages: Caffeine drinks.	Decreased calming effect of meprobamate.
Cocaine:	Decreased meprobamate effect.
Foods:	None expected.
Marijuana:	Increased sedative effect of meprobamate.
Tobacco:	None expected.

*See Glossary

MEPROBAMATE & ASPIRIN

BRAND NAMES

Epromate-M
Equagesic
Equazine-M
Heptogesic
Mepro Analgesic
Meprogese
Meprogesic
Meprogesic Q
Micrainin
Q-gesic
Tranquigesic

BASIC INFORMATION

Habit forming? Yes
Prescription needed? Yes
Available as generic? Yes
Drug class: Anti-inflammatory (nonsteroidal), analgesic, tranquilizer

USES

- Reduces mild anxiety, tension and insomnia.
- Reduces pain, fever, inflammation.
- Relieves swelling, stiffness, joint pain.
- Antiplatelet effect.

DOSAGE & USAGE INFORMATION

How to take:
- Tablet—Swallow with liquid.
- Effervescent tablets—Dissolve in water.

When to take:
Pain, fever, inflammation—As needed, no more often than every 4 hours.

If you forget a dose:
Take as soon as you remember up to 2 hours late. If more than 2 hours, wait for next scheduled dose (don't double this dose).

What drug does:
- Sedates brain centers which control behavior and emotions.

Continued next column

- Affects hypothalamus, the part of the brain which regulates temperature by dilating small blood vessels in skin.
- Prevents clumping of platelets (small blood cells) so blood vessels remain open.
- Decreases prostaglandin effect.
- Suppresses body's pain messages.

Time lapse before drug works:
1 to 2 hours.

Don't take with:
- Tetracyclines.
- Nonprescription drugs containing alcohol or caffeine without consulting doctor.
- Any other medicine without consulting your doctor or pharmacist.

OVERDOSE

SYMPTOMS:
Dizziness; slurred speech; stagger; depressed heart function; ringing in ears; nausea; vomiting; fever; deep, rapid breathing; hallucinations; convulsions; stupor; coma.
WHAT TO DO:
- **Dial 911 (emergency) for an ambulance or medical help or poison center 1-800-222-1222. Then give first aid immediately.**
- **See emergency information on inside covers.**

POSSIBLE ADVERSE REACTIONS OR SIDE EFFECTS

SYMPTOMS	WHAT TO DO
Life-threatening:	
Hives, rash, intense itching, faintness soon after a dose (anaphylaxis); difficulty breathing.	Seek emergency treatment immediately.
Common:	
• Nausea, vomiting.	Discontinue. Call doctor right away.
• Dizziness, confusion, agitation, drowsiness, unsteadiness, fatigue, weakness, ears ringing, heartburn, indigestion, abdominal pain.	Continue. Call doctor when convenient.
Infrequent:	
Blurred vision, headache.	Continue. Call doctor when convenient.
Rare:	
• Black, bloody or tarry stool; vomiting blood or black material; blood in urine.	Discontinue. Seek emergency treatment.
• Rash, hives, itchy skin, change in vision, fever, jaundice, mental confusion.	Discontinue. Call doctor right away.

WARNINGS & PRECAUTIONS

Don't take if:
- You are allergic to meprobamate, tybamate, carbromal or carisoprodol.
- You are sensitive to aspirin.
- You have had porphyria.
- You have a peptic ulcer of stomach or duodenum or a bleeding disorder.
- Patient is younger than 6.

Before you start, consult your doctor:
- If you have epilepsy, impaired liver or kidney function, asthma or nasal polyps.
- If you are allergic to tartrazine.
- If you have had gout, stomach or duodenal ulcers.

Over age 60:
Adverse reactions and side effects may be more frequent and severe than in younger persons. More likely to cause hidden bleeding in stomach or intestines. Watch for dark stools.

Pregnancy:
Risk to unborn child outweighs drug benefits. Don't use.

Breast-feeding:
Drug passes into milk. Avoid drug or discontinue nursing until you finish medicine. Consult doctor for advice on maintaining milk supply.

Infants & children:
Not recommended.

Prolonged use:
- Habit forming.
- May impair blood cell production.
- Kidney damage. Periodic kidney function test recommended.

Skin & sunlight:
No special problems expected.

Driving, piloting or hazardous work:
Don't drive or pilot aircraft until you learn how medicine affects you. Don't work around dangerous machinery. Don't climb ladders or work in high places. Danger increases if you drink alcohol or take medicine affecting alertness and reflexes, such as antihistamines, tranquilizers, sedatives, pain medicine, narcotics and mind-altering drugs.

Discontinuing:
Don't discontinue without consulting doctor. Dose may require gradual reduction if you have taken drug for a long time. Doses of other drugs may also require adjustment.

Others:
- Aspirin can complicate surgery; illness; pregnancy, labor and delivery.
- Urine tests for blood sugar may be inaccurate.

POSSIBLE INTERACTION WITH OTHER DRUGS

GENERIC NAME OR DRUG CLASS	COMBINED EFFECT
Acebutolol	Decreased anti-hypertensive effect of acebutolol.
Addictive drugs*	Increased risk of addictive effect.
Adrenocorticoids, systemic	Increased risk of ulcers. Increased adrenocorticoid effect.
Allopurinol	Decreased allopurinol effect.
Angiotensin-converting enzyme (ACE) inhibitors*	Decreased effect of ACE inhibitors.
Antacids*	Decreased aspirin effect.
Anticoagulants*	Increased anticoagulant effect. Abnormal bleeding.
Anticonvulsants*	Change in seizure pattern.
Antidepressants, tricyclic*	Increased anti-depressant effect.
Antidiabetics*, oral	Low blood sugar.
Anti-inflammatory drugs, nonsteroidal (NSAIDs)*	Risk of stomach bleeding and ulcers.
Aspirin, other	Likely aspirin toxicity.
Bumetanide	Possible aspirin toxicity.
Dronabinol	Increased effect of both drugs.

Continued on page 918

POSSIBLE INTERACTION WITH OTHER SUBSTANCES

INTERACTS WITH	COMBINED EFFECT
Alcohol:	Possible stomach irritation and bleeding. Dangerous increased effect of meprobamate. Avoid.
Beverages: Caffeine drinks.	Decreased calming effect of meprobamate.
Cocaine:	Decreased meprobamate effect.
Foods:	None expected.
Marijuana:	Possible increased pain relief, but marijuana may slow body's recovery. Avoid.
Tobacco:	None expected.

*See Glossary

MERCAPTOPURINE

BRAND NAMES

6-MP
Purinethol

BASIC INFORMATION

Habit forming? No
Prescription needed? Yes
Available as generic? No
Drug class: Antineoplastic, immunosuppressant

USES

- Treatment for some kinds of cancer.
- Treatment for regional enteritis and ulcerative colitis and other immune disorders.

DOSAGE & USAGE INFORMATION

How to take:
Tablet—Swallow with liquid.

When to take:
At the same time each day.

If you forget a dose:
Skip the missed dose. Don't double the next dose.

What drug does:
Inhibits abnormal cell reproduction.

Time lapse before drug works:
May require 6 weeks for maximum effect.

Don't take with:
Any other medicine without consulting your doctor or pharmacist.

OVERDOSE

SYMPTOMS:
Headache, stupor, seizures.
WHAT TO DO:

- **Dial 911 (emergency) for an ambulance or medical help or poison center 1-800-222-1222. Then give first aid immediately.**
- **If patient is unconscious and not breathing, give mouth-to-mouth breathing. If there is no heartbeat, use cardiac massage and mouth-to-mouth breathing (CPR). Don't try to make patient vomit. If you can't get help quickly, take patient to nearest emergency facility.**
- **See emergency information on inside covers.**

POSSIBLE ADVERSE REACTIONS OR SIDE EFFECTS

SYMPTOMS	WHAT TO DO
Life-threatening:	
In case of overdose, see previous column.	
Common:	
• Black stools or bloody vomit.	Discontinue. Seek emergency treatment.
• Mouth sores, sore throat, unusual bleeding or bruising.	Discontinue. Call doctor right away.
• Abdominal pain, nausea, vomiting, weakness, tiredness.	Continue. Call doctor when convenient.
Infrequent:	
• Seizures.	Discontinue. Seek emergency treatment.
• Diarrhea, headache, confusion, blurred vision, shortness of breath, joint pain, blood in urine, jaundice, back pain, appetite loss, feet and leg swelling.	Discontinue. Call doctor right away.
• Cough.	Continue. Call doctor when convenient.
• Acne, boils, hair loss, itchy skin.	Continue. Tell doctor at next visit.
Rare:	
Fever and chills.	Discontinue. Call doctor right away.

WARNINGS & PRECAUTIONS

Don't take if:
You are allergic to any antineoplastic.

Before you start, consult your doctor:

- If you are alcoholic.
- If you have blood, liver or kidney disease.
- If you have colitis or peptic ulcer.
- If you have gout.
- If you have an infection.
- If you plan to become pregnant within 3 months.

Over age 60:
Adverse reactions and side effects may be more frequent and severe than in younger persons.

Pregnancy:
Risk to unborn child outweighs drug benefits. Don't use. Risk category D (see page xviii).

Breast-feeding:
Avoid drug or discontinue nursing.

Infants & children:
Use only under special medical supervision.

Prolonged use:
- Adverse reactions more likely the longer drug is required.
- Talk to your doctor about the need for follow-up medical examinations or laboratory studies to check complete blood counts (white blood cell count, platelet count, red blood cell count, hemoglobin, hematocrit), liver function, kidney function, uric acid.

Skin & sunlight:
No problems expected.

Driving, piloting or hazardous work:
Avoid if you feel dizzy, drowsy or confused. Otherwise, no problems expected.

Discontinuing:
Don't discontinue without doctor's advice until you complete prescribed dose, even though symptoms diminish or disappear. Some side effects may follow discontinuing. Report to doctor blurred vision, convulsions, confusion, persistent headache, chills or fever, bloody urine or stools, back pain, jaundice.

Others:
- Drink more water than usual to cause frequent urination.
- Don't give this medicine to anyone else for any purpose. It is a strong drug that requires close medical supervision.
- Report for frequent medical follow-up and laboratory studies.

POSSIBLE INTERACTION WITH OTHER DRUGS

GENERIC NAME OR DRUG CLASS	COMBINED EFFECT
Acetaminophen	Increased likelihood of liver toxicity.
Allopurinol	Increased toxic effect of mercaptopurine.
Anticoagulants,* oral	May increase or decrease anticoagulant effect.
Antineoplastic drugs*, other	Increased effect of both (may be desirable) or increased toxicity of each.
Chloramphenicol	Increased toxicity of each.
Clozapine	Toxic effect on bone marrow.
Cyclosporine	May increase risk of infection.
Hepatotoxic drugs*	Increased risk of liver toxicity.
Immunosuppresants*, other	Increased risk of infections and neoplasms*.
Isoniazid	Increased risk of liver damage.
Levamisole	Increased risk of bone marrow depression.
Lovastatin	Increased heart and kidney damage.
Probenecid	Increased toxic effect of mercaptopurine.
Sulfinpyrazone	Increased toxic effect of mercaptopurine.
Tiopronin	Increased risk of toxicity to bone marrow.
Vaccines, live or killed	Increased risk of toxicity or reduced effectiveness of vaccine.

POSSIBLE INTERACTION WITH OTHER SUBSTANCES

INTERACTS WITH	COMBINED EFFECT
Alcohol:	May increase chance of intestinal bleeding.
Beverages:	None expected.
Cocaine:	Increased chance of toxicity.
Foods:	Reduced irritation in stomach.
Marijuana:	None expected.
Tobacco:	Increased lung toxicity.

*See Glossary

MESALAMINE

BRAND NAMES

5-ASA
Asacol
Canasa
Mesalazine
Pentasa
Rowasa
Salofalk

BASIC INFORMATION

Habit forming? No
Prescription needed? Yes
Available as generic? No
Drug class: Anti-inflammatory (nonsteroidal)

USES

- Treats ulcerative colitis.
- Reduces inflammatory conditions of the lower colon and rectum.

DOSAGE & USAGE INFORMATION

How to use:

- Rectal—Use as an enema. Insert the tip of the pre-packaged medicine container into the rectum. Squeeze container to empty contents. Retain in rectum all night or as long as possible.
- Rectal suppository—Follow instructions on package.
- Delayed-release tablet or extended-release capsule—Swallow with liquid. Do not crush or chew tablet.

When to use:

- Rectal—Each night, preferably after a bowel movement. Continue for 3 to 6 weeks according to your doctor's instructions.
- Rectal suppository—Use 1-3 times a day according to doctor's instructions.
- Tablet—3 to 4 times a day or as directed by doctor.

If you forget a dose:
Take or use as soon as you remember up to 2 hours late. If more than 2 hours, wait for next scheduled dose (don't double this dose).

Continued next column

OVERDOSE

SYMPTOMS:
None expected.
WHAT TO DO:
No action needed.

What drug does:
Decreases production of arachidonic acid forms which are increased in patients with chronic inflammatory bowel disease.

Time lapse before drug works:
3 to 21 days.

Don't take with:

- Oral sulfasalazine concurrently. To do so may increase chances of kidney damage.
- Any other medicine without consulting your doctor or pharmacist.

POSSIBLE ADVERSE REACTIONS OR SIDE EFFECTS

SYMPTOMS	WHAT TO DO
Life-threatening:	
None expected.	
Common:	
None expected.	
Infrequent:	
None expected.	
Rare:	
• Abdominal pain, bloody diarrhea, fever, skin rash, anal irritation, chest pain, short of breath.	Discontinue. Call doctor right away.
• Gaseousness, nausea, headache, mild hair loss, diarrhea.	Continue. Call doctor when convenient.

WARNINGS & PRECAUTIONS

Don't take if:
You are allergic to salicylates* or any medication containing sulfasalazine (such as Azulfidine) or mesalamine.

Before you start, consult your doctor:
- If you have had chronic kidney disease.
- If you have pancreatitis.
- If you have heart inflammation (pericarditis).

Over age 60:
More sensitive to drug. Aggravates symptoms of enlarged prostate. Causes impaired thinking, hallucinations, nightmares. Consult doctor about any of these.

Pregnancy:
Consult doctor. Risk category B (see page xviii).

Breast-feeding:
It is unknown if drug passes into milk. Avoid nursing until you finish medicine. Consult doctor for advice on maintaining milk supply.

Infants & children:
Use for children only under doctor's supervision.

Prolonged use:
Talk to your doctor about the need for follow-up medical examinations or laboratory studies to check urine.

Skin & sunlight:
No problems expected.

Driving, piloting or hazardous work:
Don't drive or pilot aircraft until you learn how medicine affects you. Don't work around dangerous machinery. Don't climb ladders or work in high places. Danger increases if you drink alcohol or take medicine affecting alertness and reflexes.

Discontinuing:
Don't discontinue without consulting doctor. Dose may require gradual reduction if you have taken drug for a long time. Doses of other drugs may also require adjustment.

Others:
- Internal eye pressure should be measured regularly.
- Canasa may stain things it touches.
- Avoid becoming overheated.

POSSIBLE INTERACTION WITH OTHER DRUGS

GENERIC NAME OR DRUG CLASS	COMBINED EFFECT
None reported.	

POSSIBLE INTERACTION WITH OTHER SUBSTANCES

INTERACTS WITH	COMBINED EFFECT
Alcohol:	None expected.
Beverages:	None expected.
Cocaine:	None expected.
Foods:	None expected.
Marijuana:	None expected.
Tobacco:	None expected.

*See Glossary

METFORMIN

BRAND NAMES

Glucophage

BASIC INFORMATION

Habit forming? No
Prescription needed? Yes
Available as generic? Yes
Drug class: Antihyperglycemic, antidiabetic

USES

Treatment for hyperglycemia (excess sugar in the blood) that cannot be controlled by diet alone in patients with type II non-insulin-dependent diabetes mellitus (NIDDM).

DOSAGE & USAGE INFORMATION

How to take:
Tablet—Swallow with liquid.

When to take:
Usually 2 to 3 times a day as directed by doctor. Take with meals to lessen stomach irritation. Dosage may be increased on a weekly basis until maximum benefits are achieved.

Continued next column

If you forget a dose:
Take as soon as you remember. If it is almost time for the next dose, then skip the missed dose and wait for your next scheduled dose (don't double this dose).

What drug does:
Helps to lower blood sugar when it is too high. Treats the symptoms of diabetes, but does not cure it.

Time lapse before drug works:
May take several weeks for full effectiveness.

Don't take with:
Any other prescription or nonprescription drug without consulting your doctor or pharmacist.

OVERDOSE

SYMPTOMS:

- **Symptoms of lactic acidosis (acid in the blood)—chills, diarrhea, fatigue, muscle pain, sleepiness, slow heartbeat, breathing difficulty, unusual weakness.**
- **Symptoms of hypoglycemia (low blood sugar)—stomach pain, anxious feeling, cold sweats, chills, confusion, convulsions, cool pale skin, excessive hunger, nausea or vomiting, rapid heartbeat, nervousness, shakiness, unsteady walk, unusual weakness or tiredness, vision changes, unconsciousness.**

WHAT TO DO:

- **For symptoms of lactic acidosis, call doctor immediately.**
- **For mild low blood sugar symptoms, drink or eat something containing sugar right away.**
- **For more severe symptoms, dial 911 (emergency) for an ambulance or medical help or poison center 1-800-222-1222. Then give first aid immediately.**
- **See emergency information on inside covers.**

POSSIBLE ADVERSE REACTIONS OR SIDE EFFECTS

SYMPTOMS	WHAT TO DO
Life-threatening:	
In case of overdose or low blood sugar, see previous column.	
Common:	
• Stomach pain, diarrhea, vomiting.	Continue, but call doctor right away.
• Decreased appetite, changes in taste, gas, headache, weight loss, feeling of fullness or stomach discomfort, nausea.	Continue. Call doctor when convenient.
Infrequent:	
None expected.	
Rare:	
Lactic acidosis or severe low blood sugar (see symptoms under Overdose).	Discontinue. Call doctor right away or seek emergency help.

WARNINGS & PRECAUTIONS

Don't take if:
You are allergic to metformin.

Before you start, consult your doctor:

- If you have any kidney or liver disease or any heart or blood vessel disorder.
- If you have any chronic health problem.
- If you have an infection, illness or any condition that can cause low blood sugar.
- If you have a history of acid in the blood (metabolic acidosis or ketoacidosis).
- If you are allergic to any medication, food or other substance.

Over age 60:
No special problems expected. A lower starting dosage may be recommended by your doctor.

Pregnancy:
Decide with your doctor if drug benefits justify risks to unborn child. Risk category B (see page xviii).

Breast-feeding:
Drug passes into milk. Avoid drug or discontinue nursing until you finish medicine. Consult doctor for advice on maintaining milk supply.

Infants & children:
Safety and efficacy have not been established. Use only under close medical supervision.

Prolonged use:
- Schedule regular doctor visits to determine if the drug is continuing to be effective in controlling the diabetes and to check for any problems in kidney function.
- You will most likely require an antidiabetic medicine for the rest of your life.
- You will need to test your blood glucose levels several times a day, or for some, once to several times a week.

Skin & sunlight:
No special problems expected.

Driving, piloting or hazardous work:
No special problems expected.

Discontinuing:
Don't discontinue without consulting your doctor, even if you feel well. You can have diabetes without feeling any symptoms. Untreated diabetes can cause serious problems.

Others:
- Advise any doctor or dentist whom you consult that you take this medicine. Drug may interfere with the accuracy of some medical tests.
- Follow any special diet your doctor may prescribe. It can help control diabetes.
- Consult doctor if you become ill with vomiting or diarrhea.
- Use caution when exercising. Ask your doctor about an appropriate exercise program.
- Wear medical identification stating that you have diabetes and take this medication.
- Learn to recognize the symptoms of low blood sugar. You and your family need to know what to do if these symptoms occur.
- Have a glucagon kit and syringe in the event severe low blood sugar occurs. Carry a quick-acting sugar to treat symptoms of mild low blood sugar.
- High blood sugar (hyperglycemia) may occur with diabetes. Ask your doctor about symptoms to watch for and treatment steps to take.
- This drug may be discontinued temporarily prior to x-ray studies or some surgeries.
- Educate yourself about diabetes.

POSSIBLE INTERACTION WITH OTHER DRUGS

GENERIC NAME OR DRUG CLASS	COMBINED EFFECT
Amiloride	Increased metformin effect.
Calcium channel blockers*	Increased metformin effect.
Cimetidine	Increased metformin effect.
Dexfenfluramine	May require dosage change as weight loss occurs.
Digoxin	Increased metformin effect.
Dofetilide	Increased dofetilide effect.
Furosemide	Increased metformin effect.
Hyperglycemia-causing medications*	Increased risk of hyperglycemia.
Hypoglycemia-causing medications*	Increased risk of hypoglycemia.
Morphine	Increased metformin effect.
Procainamide	Increased metformin effect.
Quinidine	Increased metformin effect.
Quinine	Increased metformin effect.
Ranitidine	Increased metformin effect.

Continued on page 918

POSSIBLE INTERACTION WITH OTHER SUBSTANCES

INTERACTS WITH	COMBINED EFFECT
Alcohol:	Increased effect of metformin. Avoid excessive amounts.
Beverages:	None expected.
Cocaine:	None expected.
Foods:	None expected.
Marijuana:	None expected.
Tobacco:	None expected.

***See Glossary**

METHENAMINE

BRAND NAMES

Hip-Rex
Hiprex
Mandelamine
Urex

BASIC INFORMATION

Habit forming? No
Prescription needed? Yes
Available as generic? Yes
Drug class: Anti-infective (urinary)

USES

Suppresses chronic urinary tract infections.

DOSAGE & USAGE INFORMATION

How to take:

- Tablet—Swallow with liquid or food to lessen stomach irritation. If you can't swallow whole, crumble tablet and take with liquid or food. If enteric-coated tablet, swallow whole.
- Liquid form—Use a measuring spoon to ensure correct dose.
- Granules—Dissolve dose in 4 oz. of water. Drink all the liquid.

When to take:
At the same times each day.

If you forget a dose:
Take as soon as you remember up to 8 hours late. If more than 8 hours, wait for next scheduled dose (don't double this dose).

What drug does:
A chemical reaction in the urine changes methenamine into formaldehyde, which destroys certain bacteria.

Time lapse before drug works:
Continual use for 3 to 6 months.

Continued next column

OVERDOSE

SYMPTOMS:
Bloody urine, weakness, deep breathing, stupor, coma.
WHAT TO DO:

- **Dial 911 (emergency) for an ambulance or medical help or poison center 1-800-222-1222. Then give first aid immediately.**
- **See emergency information on inside covers.**

Don't take with:
Any other medicine without consulting your doctor or pharmacist.

POSSIBLE ADVERSE REACTIONS OR SIDE EFFECTS

SYMPTOMS	WHAT TO DO
Life-threatening: In case of overdose, see previous column.	
Common:	
• Rash.	Discontinue. Call doctor right away.
• Nausea, difficult urination.	Continue. Call doctor when convenient.
Infrequent:	
• Blood in urine.	Discontinue. Call doctor right away.
• Burning on urination, lower back pain.	Continue. Call doctor when convenient.
Rare: None expected.	

WARNINGS & PRECAUTIONS

Don't take if:
- You are allergic to methenamine.
- You have a severe impairment of kidney or liver function.
- Your urine cannot or should not be acidified (check with your doctor).

Before you start, consult your doctor:
- If you have had kidney or liver disease.
- If you plan to become pregnant within medication period.
- If you have had gout.

Over age 60:
Don't exceed recommended dose.

Pregnancy:
Decide with your doctor if drug benefits justify risk to unborn child. Risk category C (see page xviii).

Breast-feeding:
Drug passes into milk in small amounts. Consult doctor.

Infants & children:
Use only under medical supervision.

Prolonged use:
No problems expected.

Skin & sunlight:
No problems expected.

Driving, piloting or hazardous work:
No problems expected.

Discontinuing:
Don't discontinue without doctor's advice until you complete prescribed dose, even though symptoms diminish or disappear.

Others:
Requires an acid urine to be effective. Eat more protein foods, cranberries, cranberry juice with vitamin C, plums, prunes.

POSSIBLE INTERACTION WITH OTHER DRUGS

GENERIC NAME OR DRUG CLASS	COMBINED EFFECT
Antacids*	Decreased methenamine effect.
Carbonic anhydrase inhibitors*	Decreased methenamine effect.
Citrates*	Decreases effects of methenamine.
Diuretics, thiazide*	Decreased urine acidity.
Sodium bicarbonate	Decreased methenamine effect.
Sulfadoxine and pyrimethamine	Increased risk of kidney toxicity.
Sulfa drugs*	Possible kidney damage.

POSSIBLE INTERACTION WITH OTHER SUBSTANCES

INTERACTS WITH	COMBINED EFFECT
Alcohol:	Possible brain depression. Avoid or use with caution.
Beverages: Milk and other dairy products.	Decreased methenamine effect.
Cocaine:	None expected.
Foods: Citrus, cranberries, plums, prunes.	Increased methenamine effect.
Marijuana:	Drowsiness, muscle weakness or blood pressure drop.
Tobacco:	None expected.

***See Glossary**

METHOTREXATE

BRAND NAMES

Amethopterin
Folex
Folex PFS
Mexate
Mexate AQ
Rheumatrex
Trexall

BASIC INFORMATION

Habit forming? No
Prescription needed? Yes
Available as generic? Yes
Drug class: Antimetabolite, antipsoriatic

USES

- Treatment for some kinds of cancer.
- Treatment for psoriasis in patients with severe problems.
- Treatment for severe rheumatoid arthritis.

DOSAGE & USAGE INFORMATION

How to take:
- Tablet—Swallow with liquid.
- Injectable form—Is sometimes self-injected or used as an oral dose, consult doctor.

When to take:
At the same time each day.

If you forget a dose:
Skip the missed dose. Don't double the next dose.

What drug does:
Inhibits abnormal cell reproduction.

Time lapse before drug works:
May require 6 weeks for maximum effect.

Don't take with:
Any other medicine without consulting your doctor or pharmacist.

OVERDOSE

SYMPTOMS:
Headache, stupor, seizures.
WHAT TO DO:
- **Dial 911 (emergency) for an ambulance or medical help or poison center 1-800-222-1222. Then give first aid immediately.**
- **If patient is unconscious and not breathing, give mouth-to-mouth breathing. If there is no heartbeat, use cardiac massage and mouth-to-mouth breathing (CPR). Don't try to make patient vomit. If you can't get help quickly, take patient to nearest emergency facility.**
- **See emergency information on inside covers.**

POSSIBLE ADVERSE REACTIONS OR SIDE EFFECTS

SYMPTOMS	WHAT TO DO
Life-threatening:	
Hives, rash, intense itching, faintness soon after a dose (anaphylaxis).	Seek emergency treatment immediately.
Common:	
• Black stools or bloody vomit.	Discontinue. Seek emergency treatment.
• Sore throat, fever, mouth sores; chills; unusual bleeding or bruising.	Discontinue. Call doctor right away.
• Abdominal pain, nausea, vomiting.	Continue. Call doctor when convenient.
Infrequent:	
• Seizures.	Discontinue. Seek emergency treatment.
• Dizziness when standing after sitting or lying, drowsiness, headache, confusion, blurred vision, shortness of breath, joint pain, blood in urine, jaundice, diarrhea, red skin, back pain.	Discontinue. Call doctor right away.
• Cough, rash, sexual difficulties in males.	Continue. Call doctor when convenient.
• Acne, boils, hair loss, itchy skin.	Continue. Tell doctor at next visit.
Rare:	
• Convulsions.	Seek emergency treatment.
• Painful urination.	Discontinue. Seek emergency treatment.

WARNINGS & PRECAUTIONS

Don't take if:
You are allergic to any antimetabolite.

Before you start, consult your doctor:
- If you are alcoholic.
- If you have blood, liver or kidney disease.
- If you have colitis or peptic ulcer.
- If you have gout.
- If you have an infection.
- If you plan to become pregnant within 3 months.

Over age 60:
Adverse reactions and side effects may be more frequent and severe than in younger persons.

Pregnancy:
- Psoriasis—Risk to unborn child outweighs drug benefits. Don't use.
- Cancer—Consult doctor.
- Risk category X (see page xviii).

Breast-feeding:
Drug passes into milk. Avoid drug or discontinue nursing.

Infants & children:
Use only under special medical supervision.

Prolonged use:
- Adverse reactions more likely the longer drug is required.
- Talk to your doctor about the need for follow-up medical examinations or laboratory studies to check liver function, kidney function, complete blood counts (white blood cell count, platelet count, red blood cell count, hemoglobin, hematocrit).

Skin & sunlight:
May cause rash or intensify sunburn in areas exposed to sun or ultraviolet light (photosensitivity reaction). Avoid overexposure. Notify doctor if reaction occurs.

Driving, piloting or hazardous work:
Avoid if you feel dizzy, drowsy or confused. Otherwise, no problems expected.

Discontinuing:
Don't discontinue without doctor's advice until you complete prescribed dose, even though symptoms diminish or disappear. Some side effects may follow discontinuing. Report to doctor blurred vision, convulsions, confusion, persistent headache.

Others:
- Drink more water than usual to cause frequent urination.
- Don't give this medicine to anyone else for any purpose. It is a strong drug that requires close medical supervision.
- Report for frequent medical follow-up and laboratory studies.

POSSIBLE INTERACTION WITH OTHER DRUGS

GENERIC NAME OR DRUG CLASS	COMBINED EFFECT
Anticoagulants,* oral	Increased anti-coagulant effect.
Anticonvulsants,* hydantoin	Possible methotrexate toxicity.
Antigout drugs*	Decreased antigout effect. Toxic levels of methotrexate.
Anti-inflammatory drugs, nonsteroidal (NSAIDs)*	Possible increased methotrexate toxicity.
Asparaginase	Decreased methotrexate effect.
Bone marrow depressants*, other	Increased risk of bone marrow depression.
Clozapine	Toxic effect on bone marrow.
Diclofenac	May increase toxicity.
Etretinate	Increased chance of toxicity to liver.
Fluorouracil	Decreased methotrexate effect.
Folic acid	Possible decreased methotrexate effect.
Isoniazid	Increased risk of liver damage.
Leflunomide	Increased risk of side effects.
Leukovorin calcium	Decreased methotrexate toxicity.
Levamisole	Increased risk of bone marrow depression.
Oxyphenbutazone	Possible methotrexate toxicity.
Penicillins*	Increased risk of methotrexate toxicity.
Phenylbutazone	Possible methotrexate toxicity.

Continued on page 919

POSSIBLE INTERACTION WITH OTHER SUBSTANCES

INTERACTS WITH	COMBINED EFFECT
Alcohol:	Likely liver damage. Avoid.
Beverages:	Extra fluid intake decreases chance of methotrexate toxicity.
Cocaine:	Increased chance of methotrexate adverse reactions. Avoid.
Foods:	None expected.
Marijuana:	None expected.
Tobacco:	None expected.

***See Glossary**

METHYLDOPA

BRAND NAMES

Aldomet
Apo-Methyldopa
Dopamet
Novomedopa
Nu-Medopa

BASIC INFORMATION

Habit forming? No
Prescription needed? Yes
Available as generic? Yes
Drug class: Antihypertensive

USES

Reduces high blood pressure.

DOSAGE & USAGE INFORMATION

How to take:
Liquid or tablet—Swallow with liquid. If you can't swallow whole, crumble tablet and take with liquid or food.

When to take:
At the same times each day.

If you forget a dose:
Take as soon as you remember up to 2 hours late. If more than 2 hours, wait for next scheduled dose (don't double this dose).

What drug does:
Relaxes walls of small arteries to decrease blood pressure.

Time lapse before drug works:
Continual use for 2 to 4 weeks may be necessary to determine effectiveness.

Continued next column

OVERDOSE

SYMPTOMS:
Drowsiness; exhaustion; stupor; confusion; slow, weak pulse.
WHAT TO DO:
- **Dial 911 (emergency) for an ambulance or medical help or poison center 1-800-222-1222. Then give first aid immediately.**
- **If patient is unconscious and not breathing, give mouth-to-mouth breathing. If there is no heartbeat, use cardiac massage and mouth-to-mouth breathing (CPR). Don't try to make patient vomit. If you can't get help quickly, take patient to nearest emergency facility.**
- **See emergency information on inside covers.**

Don't take with:
Any other medicine without consulting your doctor or pharmacist.

POSSIBLE ADVERSE REACTIONS OR SIDE EFFECTS

SYMPTOMS	WHAT TO DO
Life-threatening:	
In case of overdose, see previous column.	
Common:	
Depression, sedation, nightmares, headache, drowsiness, weakness, stuffy nose, dry mouth, fluid retention, swollen feet or legs.	Continue. Call doctor when convenient.
Infrequent:	
• Fast heartbeat, fainting.	Discontinue. Call doctor right away.
• Insomnia, nausea, vomiting, diarrhea, constipation, foot and hand numbness and tingling.	Continue. Call doctor when convenient.
• Swollen breasts, diminished sex drive.	Continue. Tell doctor at next visit.
Rare:	
Rash, jaundice, dark urine, chills, breathing difficulty, unexplained fever, sore or "black" tongue, severe abdominal pain, decreased mental activity and memory impairment, facial paralysis, slow heartbeat, chest pain, swollen abdomen.	Discontinue. Call doctor right away.

WARNINGS & PRECAUTIONS

Don't take if:
You will have surgery within 2 months, including dental surgery, requiring general or spinal anesthesia.

Before you start, consult your doctor:
If you have liver disease.

Over age 60:
- Increased susceptibility to dizziness, unsteadiness, fainting, falling.
- Drug can produce or intensify Parkinson's disease.

Pregnancy:
No proven problems. Consult doctor. Risk category B (see page xviii).

Breast-feeding:
No proven problems. Consult doctor.

Infants & children:
Not used.

Prolonged use:
- May cause anemia.
- Severe edema (fluid retention).
- Talk to your doctor about the need for follow-up medical examinations or laboratory studies to check complete blood counts (white blood cell count, platelet count, red blood cell count, hemoglobin, hematocrit), blood pressure, liver function.

Skin & sunlight:
May cause rash or intensify sunburn in areas exposed to sun or ultraviolet light (photosensitivity reaction). Avoid overexposure. Notify doctor if reaction occurs.

Driving, piloting or hazardous work:
Don't drive or pilot aircraft until you learn how medicine affects you. Don't work around dangerous machinery. Don't climb ladders or work in high places. Danger increases if you drink alcohol or take medicine affecting alertness and reflexes, such as antihistamines, tranquilizers, sedatives, pain medicine, narcotics and mind-altering drugs.

Discontinuing:
Don't discontinue without consulting doctor. Dose may require gradual reduction if you have taken drug for a long time. Doses of other drugs may also require adjustment.

Others:
Avoid heavy exercise, exertion, sweating.

POSSIBLE INTERACTION WITH OTHER DRUGS

GENERIC NAME OR DRUG CLASS	COMBINED EFFECT
Amphetamines*	Decreased methyldopa effect.
Angiotensin-converting enzyme (ACE) inhibitors*	Possible excessive potassium in blood.
Anticoagulants*, oral	Increased anticoagulant effect.
Antidepressants, tricyclic*	Dangerous blood pressure rise. Decreased methyldopa effect.
Antihypertensives*	Increased antihypertensive effect.
Antivirals, HIV/AIDS*	Increased risk of pancreatitis.
Carteolol	Increased antihypertensive effect.
Clozapine	Toxic effect on the central nervous system.
Dapsone	Increased risk of adverse effect on blood cells.
Digitalis preparations*	Excessively slow heartbeat.
Diuretics, thiazide*	Increased methyldopa effect.
Ethinamate	Dangerous increased effects of ethinamate. Avoid combining.
Fluoxetine	Increased depressant effects of both drugs.
Guanfacine	May increase depressant effects of either drug.
Haloperidol	Increased sedation. Possibly dementia.
Isoniazid	Increased risk of liver damage.
Leucovorin	High alcohol content of leucovorin may cause adverse effects.
Levodopa	Increased effect of both drugs.
Loxapine	May increase toxic effects of both drugs.

Continued on page 919

POSSIBLE INTERACTION WITH OTHER SUBSTANCES

INTERACTS WITH	COMBINED EFFECT
Alcohol:	Increased sedation. Excessive blood pressure drop. Avoid.
Beverages:	None expected.
Cocaine:	Increased risk of heart block and high blood pressure.
Foods:	None expected.
Marijuana:	Possible fainting.
Tobacco:	Possible increased blood pressure.

*See Glossary

METHYLDOPA & THIAZIDE DIURETICS

GENERIC AND BRAND NAMES

METHYLDOPA & CHLOROTHIAZIDE
Aldoclor

METHYLDOPA & HYDROCHLOROTHIAZIDE
Aldoril
Novodoparil
PMS Dopazide

BASIC INFORMATION

Habit forming? No
Prescription needed? Yes
Available as generic? Yes
Drug class: Antihypertensive, diuretic (thiazide)

USES

- Controls, but doesn't cure, high blood pressure.
- Reduces fluid retention (edema).

DOSAGE & USAGE INFORMATION

How to take:
Tablet—Swallow with liquid. If you can't swallow whole, crumble tablet and take with liquid or food.

When to take:
At the same times each day.

If you forget a dose:
Take as soon as you remember up to 2 hours late. If more than 2 hours, wait for next scheduled dose (don't double this dose).

Continued next column

OVERDOSE

SYMPTOMS:
Drowsiness; exhaustion; cramps; weakness; stupor; confusion; slow, weak pulse; coma.
WHAT TO DO:
- **Dial 911 (emergency) for an ambulance or medical help or poison center 1-800-222-1222. Then give first aid immediately.**
- **If patient is unconscious and not breathing, give mouth-to-mouth breathing. If there is no heartbeat, use cardiac massage and mouth-to-mouth breathing (CPR). Don't try to make patient vomit. If you can't get help quickly, take patient to nearest emergency facility.**
- **See emergency information on inside covers.**

What drug does:
- Relaxes walls of small arteries to decrease blood pressure.
- Forces sodium and water excretion, reducing body fluid.
- Reduced body fluid and relaxed arteries lower blood pressure.

Time lapse before drug works:
Continual use for 2 to 4 weeks may be necessary to determine effectiveness.

Don't take with:
- Nonprescription drugs without consulting doctor.
- Any other medicine without consulting your doctor or pharmacist.

POSSIBLE ADVERSE REACTIONS OR SIDE EFFECTS

SYMPTOMS	WHAT TO DO
Life-threatening:	
Irregular heartbeat, weak pulse.	Discontinue. Seek emergency treatment.
Common:	
Depression, nightmares, drowsiness, weakness, stuffy nose, dry mouth, swollen feet and ankles, dizziness, sedation, increased thirst, muscle cramps.	Continue. Call doctor when convenient.
Infrequent:	
• Fast heartbeat, change in vision, abdominal pain, nervousness.	Discontinue. Call doctor right away.
• Insomnia, nausea, vomiting, diarrhea, headache, constipation.	Continue. Call doctor when convenient.
Rare:	
Rash, jaundice, dark urine, chills, breathing difficulty, hives, sore throat, fever, mouth sores, sore or "black" tongue, severe abdominal pain, decreased mental activity, memory impairment, facial paralysis, slow heartbeat, chest pain.	Discontinue. Call doctor right away.

WARNINGS & PRECAUTIONS

Don't take if:
- You are allergic to any thiazide diuretic drug.
- You will have surgery within 2 months, including dental surgery, requiring general or spinal anesthesia.

Before you start, consult your doctor:
- If you are allergic to any sulfa drug.
- If you have gout, liver, pancreas or kidney disorder.

Over age 60:
- Increased susceptibility to dizziness, unsteadiness, fainting, falling.
- Drug can produce or intensify Parkinson's disease.

Pregnancy:
Decide with your doctor if drug benefits justify risk to unborn child. Risk category C (see page xviii).

Breast-feeding:
Drug passes into milk. Avoid drug or discontinue nursing until you finish medicine. Consult doctor for advice on maintaining milk supply.

Infants & children:
Not recommended.

Prolonged use:
- May cause anemia.
- Severe edema (fluid retention).
- Talk to your doctor about the need for follow-up medical examinations or laboratory studies to check complete blood counts (white blood cell count, platelet count, red blood cell count, hemoglobin, hematocrit), blood pressure, liver function.

Skin & sunlight:
One or more drugs in this group may cause rash or intensify sunburn in areas exposed to sun or ultraviolet light (photosensitivity reaction). Avoid overexposure. Notify doctor if reaction occurs.

Driving, piloting or hazardous work:
Don't drive or pilot aircraft until you learn how medicine affects you. Don't work around dangerous machinery. Don't climb ladders or work in high places. Danger increases if you drink alcohol or take medicine affecting alertness and reflexes, such as antihistamines, tranquilizers, sedatives, pain medicine, narcotics and mind-altering drugs.

Discontinuing:
Don't discontinue without consulting doctor. Dose may require gradual reduction if you have taken drug for a long time. Doses of other drugs may also require adjustment.

Others:
- Hot weather and fever may cause dehydration and drop in blood pressure. Dose may require temporary adjustment. Weigh daily and report any unexpected weight decreases to your doctor.
- May cause rise in uric acid, leading to gout.
- May cause blood sugar rise in diabetics.
- Avoid heavy exercise, exertion, sweating.

POSSIBLE INTERACTION WITH OTHER DRUGS

GENERIC NAME OR DRUG CLASS	COMBINED EFFECT
Acebutolol	Increased antihypertensive effect. Dosages of both drugs may require adjustments.
Allopurinol	Decreased allopurinol effect.
Amphetamines*	Decreased methyldopa effect.
Angiotensin-converting enzyme (ACE) inhibitors*	Possible excessive potassium in blood.
Anticoagulants*, oral	Increased anticoagulant effect.
Antidepressants, tricyclic*	Dangerous changes in blood pressure. Avoid combination unless under medical supervision.

Continued on page 919

POSSIBLE INTERACTION WITH OTHER SUBSTANCES

INTERACTS WITH	COMBINED EFFECT
Alcohol:	Increased sedation. Excessive blood pressure drop. Avoid.
Beverages:	None expected.
Cocaine:	Increased risk of heart block and high blood pressure.
Foods: Licorice.	Excessive potassium loss that causes dangerous heart rhythms.
Marijuana:	May increase blood pressure.
Tobacco:	Possible increased blood pressure.

***See Glossary**

METHYLERGONOVINE

BRAND NAMES

Methergine
Methylergometrine

BASIC INFORMATION

Habit forming? No
Prescription needed? Yes
Available as generic? No
Drug class: Ergot preparation (uterine stimulant)

USES

Retards excessive post-delivery bleeding.

DOSAGE & USAGE INFORMATION

How to take:
Tablet—Swallow with liquid or food to lessen stomach irritation.

When to take:
At the same times each day.

If you forget a dose:
Don't take missed dose and don't double next one. Wait for next scheduled dose.

What drug does:
Causes smooth muscle cells of uterine wall to contract and surround bleeding blood vessels of relaxed uterus.

Time lapse before drug works:
Tablets—20 to 30 minutes.

Don't take with:
Any other medicine without consulting your doctor or pharmacist.

OVERDOSE

SYMPTOMS:
Vomiting, diarrhea, weak pulse, low blood pressure, dyspnea, angina, convulsions.
WHAT TO DO:

- **Dial 911 (emergency) for an ambulance or medical help or poison center 1-800-222-1222. Then give first aid immediately.**
- **If patient is unconscious and not breathing, give mouth-to-mouth breathing. If there is no heartbeat, use cardiac massage and mouth-to-mouth breathing (CPR). Don't try to make patient vomit. If you can't get help quickly, take patient to nearest emergency facility.**
- **See emergency information on inside covers.**

POSSIBLE ADVERSE REACTIONS OR SIDE EFFECTS

SYMPTOMS	WHAT TO DO
Life-threatening: In case of overdose, see previous column.	
Common:	
Nausea, vomiting, severe lower abdominal menstrual-like cramps.	Discontinue. Call doctor right away.
Infrequent:	
• Confusion, ringing in ears, diarrhea, muscle cramps.	Discontinue. Call doctor right away.
• Unusual sweating.	Continue. Call doctor when convenient.
Rare:	
Sudden, severe headache; shortness of breath; chest pain; numb, cold hands and feet.	Discontinue. Seek emergency treatment.

WARNINGS & PRECAUTIONS

Don't take if:
You are allergic to any ergot preparation.

Before you start, consult your doctor:
- If you have coronary artery or blood vessel disease.
- If you have liver or kidney disease.
- If you have high blood pressure.
- If you have postpartum infection.

Over age 60:
Not recommended.

Pregnancy:
Consult doctor. Risk category C (see page xviii).

Breast-feeding:
Drug passes into milk. Avoid drug or discontinue nursing until you finish medicine. Consult doctor for advice on maintaining milk supply.

Infants & children:
Not recommended.

Prolonged use:
Talk to your doctor about the need for follow-up medical examinations or laboratory studies to check blood pressure, ECG*.

Skin & sunlight:
No problems expected.

Driving, piloting or hazardous work:
No problems expected.

Discontinuing:
May be unnecessary to finish medicine. Follow doctor's instructions.

Others:
Drug should be used for short time only following childbirth or miscarriage.

POSSIBLE INTERACTION WITH OTHER DRUGS

GENERIC NAME OR DRUG CLASS	COMBINED EFFECT
Antianginals*	Possible vasospasm (peripheral and cardiac)
Ergot preparations*, other	Increased methyl-ergonovine effect.

POSSIBLE INTERACTION WITH OTHER SUBSTANCES

INTERACTS WITH	COMBINED EFFECT
Alcohol:	None expected.
Beverages:	None expected.
Cocaine:	None expected.
Foods:	None expected.
Marijuana:	None expected.
Tobacco:	Decreased methylergonovine effect. Don't smoke.

*See Glossary

METHYSERGIDE

BRAND NAMES

Sansert

BASIC INFORMATION

Habit forming? Yes
Prescription needed? Yes
Available as generic? No
Drug class: Vasoconstrictor

USES

Prevents migraine and other recurring vascular headaches. Not for acute attack.

DOSAGE & USAGE INFORMATION

How to take:
Tablet—Swallow with liquid or with food to lessen stomach irritation. If you can't swallow whole, crumble tablet and take with liquid or food.

When to take:
At the same times each day.

If you forget a dose:
Don't take missed dose. Wait for next scheduled dose (don't double this dose).

What drug does:
Blocks the action of serotonin, a chemical that constricts blood vessels.

Time lapse before drug works:
About 3 weeks.

Don't take with:
Any other medicine without consulting your doctor or pharmacist.

OVERDOSE

SYMPTOMS:
Nausea, vomiting, abdominal pain, severe diarrhea, lack of coordination, extreme thirst.
WHAT TO DO:
Overdose unlikely to threaten life. If person takes much larger amount than prescribed, call doctor, poison center 1-800-222-1222 or hospital emergency room for instructions.

POSSIBLE ADVERSE REACTIONS OR SIDE EFFECTS

SYMPTOMS	WHAT TO DO
Life-threatening: In case of overdose, see previous column.	
Common:	
• Itchy skin.	Discontinue. Call doctor right away.
• Nausea, vomiting, diarrhea, numbness or tingling of extremities, leg weakness, abdominal pain.	Continue. Call doctor when convenient.
• Drowsiness, constipation.	Continue. Tell doctor at next visit.
Infrequent:	
• Anxiety, agitation, hallucinations, unusually fast or slow heartbeat, dizziness.	Discontinue. Call doctor right away.
• Change in vision, nightmares, insomnia.	Continue. Call doctor when convenient.
Rare:	
• Extreme thirst, chest pain, shortness of breath, fever, pale or swollen extremities, leg cramps, lower back pain, side or groin pain, appetite loss, joint and muscle pain, rash, facial flush, painful or difficult urination.	Discontinue. Call doctor right away.
• Weight change, hair loss.	Continue. Tell doctor at next visit.

WARNINGS & PRECAUTIONS

Don't take if:
- You are allergic to any antiserotonin*.
- You plan to become pregnant within medication period.
- You have an infection.
- You have a heart or blood vessel disease.
- You have a chronic lung disease.
- You have a collagen (connective tissue) disorder.
- You have impaired liver or kidney function.

Before you start, consult your doctor:
- If you have been allergic to any ergot preparation.
- If you have had a peptic ulcer.

Over age 60:
Adverse reactions and side effects may be more frequent and severe than in younger persons.

Pregnancy:
Consult doctor. Risk category X (see page xviii).

Breast-feeding:
Drug probably passes into milk. Avoid drug or discontinue nursing until you finish medicine. Consult doctor for advice on maintaining milk supply.

Infants & children:
Not recommended.

Prolonged use:
- May cause fibrosis, a condition in which scar tissue is deposited on heart valves, in lung tissue, blood vessels and internal organs. After 6 months, decrease dose over 2 to 3 weeks. Then discontinue for at least 2 months for re-evaluation.
- Talk to your doctor about the need for follow-up medical examinations or laboratory studies to check retroperitoneal imaging*.

Skin & sunlight:
No problems expected.

Driving, piloting or hazardous work:
Avoid if you feel drowsy or dizzy. Otherwise, no problems expected.

Discontinuing:
- Don't discontinue without consulting doctor. Dose may require gradual reduction if you have taken drug for a long time. Doses of other drugs may also require adjustment.
- Probably should discontinue drug if you don't improve after 3 weeks use.

Others:
- Periodic laboratory tests for liver function and blood counts recommended.
- Potential for abuse.
- Some products contain tartrazine dye. Avoid, especially if you are allergic to aspirin.

POSSIBLE INTERACTION WITH OTHER DRUGS

GENERIC NAME OR DRUG CLASS	COMBINED EFFECT
Ergot preparations*	Unpredictable increased or decreased effect of either drug.
Narcotics*	Decreased narcotic effect.

POSSIBLE INTERACTION WITH OTHER SUBSTANCES

INTERACTS WITH	COMBINED EFFECT
Alcohol:	None expected. However, alcohol may trigger a migraine headache.
Beverages: Caffeine drinks.	Decreased methysergide effect.
Cocaine:	May make headache worse.
Foods:	None expected. Avoid foods to which you are allergic.
Marijuana:	No proven problems.
Tobacco:	Blood vessel constriction. Makes headache worse.

*See Glossary

METOCLOPRAMIDE

BRAND NAMES

Apo-Metoclop
Clopra
Emex
Maxeran
Octamide
Octamide PFS
Reclomide
Reglan

BASIC INFORMATION

Habit forming? No
Prescription needed? Yes
Available as generic? Yes
Drug class: Antiemetic, dopaminergic blocker

USES

- Relieves nausea and vomiting caused by chemotherapy and drug-related postoperative factors.
- Relieves symptoms of esophagitis and stomach swelling in people with diabetes.

DOSAGE & USAGE INFORMATION

How to take:
Tablet or syrup—Swallow with liquid or food to lessen stomach irritation.

When to take:
30 minutes before symptoms expected, up to 4 times a day.

If you forget a dose:
Take as soon as you remember up to 2 hours late. If more than 2 hours, wait for next scheduled dose (don't double this dose).

Continued next column

OVERDOSE

SYMPTOMS:
Severe drowsiness, muscle spasms, mental confusion, trembling, seizure, coma.
WHAT TO DO:
- **Dial 911 (emergency) for an ambulance or medical help or poison center 1-800-222-1222. Then give first aid immediately.**
- **If patient is unconscious and not breathing, give mouth-to-mouth breathing. If there is no heartbeat, use cardiac massage and mouth-to-mouth breathing (CPR). Don't try to make patient vomit. If you can't get help quickly, take patient to nearest emergency facility.**
- **See emergency information on inside covers.**

What drug does:
- Prevents smooth muscle in stomach from relaxing.
- Affects vomiting center in brain.

Time lapse before drug works:
30 to 60 minutes.

Don't take with:
Any other medicine without consulting your doctor or pharmacist.

POSSIBLE ADVERSE REACTIONS OR SIDE EFFECTS

SYMPTOMS	WHAT TO DO
Life-threatening: In case of overdose, see previous column.	
Common:	
Drowsiness, restlessness.	Continue. Call doctor when convenient.
Frequent	
Rash.	Continue. Call doctor when convenient.
Infrequent:	
• Wheezing, shortness of breath.	Discontinue. Call doctor right away.
• Dizziness; headache; insomnia; tender, swollen breasts; increased milk flow, menstrual changes; decreased sex drive.	Continue. Call doctor when convenient.
Rare:	
• Abnormal, involuntary movements of jaw, lips and tongue; depression; Parkinson's syndrome*.	Discontinue. Call doctor right away.
• Constipation, nausea, diarrhea, dry mouth.	Continue. Call doctor when convenient.

WARNINGS & PRECAUTIONS

Don't take if:
You are allergic to procaine, procainamide or metoclopramide.

Before you start, consult your doctor:
- If you have Parkinson's disease.
- If you have liver or kidney disease.
- If you have epilepsy.
- If you have bleeding from gastrointestinal tract or intestinal obstruction.
- If you will have surgery within 2 months, including dental surgery, requiring general or spinal anesthesia.

Over age 60:
Adverse reactions and side effects may be more frequent and severe than in younger persons.

Pregnancy:
No proven harm to unborn child. Avoid if possible. Consult doctor. Risk category B (see page xviii).

Breast-feeding:
Unknown effect. Consult doctor.

Infants & children:
Adverse reactions more likely to occur than in adults.

Prolonged use:
Adverse reactions including muscle spasms and trembling hands more likely to occur.

Skin & sunlight:
No problems expected.

Driving, piloting or hazardous work:
Don't drive or pilot aircraft until you learn how medicine affects you. Don't work around dangerous machinery. Don't climb ladders or work in high places. Danger increases if you drink alcohol or take medicine affecting alertness and reflexes, such as antihistamines, tranquilizers, sedatives, pain medicine, narcotics and mind-altering drugs.

Discontinuing:
May be unnecessary to finish medicine. Follow doctor's instructions.

Others:
No problems expected.

POSSIBLE INTERACTION WITH OTHER DRUGS

GENERIC NAME OR DRUG CLASS	COMBINED EFFECT
Acetaminophen	Increased absorption of acetaminophen.
Anticholinergics*	Decreased metoclopramide effect.
Aspirin	Increased absorption of aspirin.
Bromocriptine	Decreased bromocriptine effect.
Butyophenone	Increased chance of muscle spasm and trembling.
Central nervous system (CNS) depressants*	Excess sedation.
Clozapine	Toxic effect on the central nervous system.
Digitalis preparations*	Decreased absorption of digitalis.
Ethinamate	Dangerous increased effects of ethinamate. Avoid combining.
Fluoxetine	Increased depressant effects of both drugs.
Guanfacine	May increase depressant effects of either drug.
Insulin	Unpredictable changes in blood glucose. Dosages may require adjustment.
Leucovorin	High alcohol content of leucovorin may cause adverse effects.
Levodopa	Increased absorption of levodopa.
Lithium	Increased absorption of lithium.
Loxapine	May increase toxic effects of both drugs.
Methyprylon	Increased sedative effect, perhaps to dangerous level. Avoid.
Nabilone	Greater depression of central nervous system.

Continued on page 920

POSSIBLE INTERACTION WITH OTHER SUBSTANCES

INTERACTS WITH	COMBINED EFFECT
Alcohol:	Excess sedation. Avoid.
Beverages: Coffee.	Decreased metoclopramide effect.
Cocaine:	Decreased metoclopramide effect.
Foods:	None expected.
Marijuana:	Decreased metoclopramide effect.
Tobacco:	Decreased metoclopramide effect.

*See Glossary

METRONIDAZOLE

BRAND NAMES

Apo-Metronidazole
Flagyl
Helidac
Metizol
Metric 21
Metro Cream
Metro I.V.
Metrogel
Metrogel-Vaginal
Neo-Metric
Novonidazol
PMS Metronidazole
Protostat
Satric
Trikacide

BASIC INFORMATION

Habit forming? No
Prescription needed? Yes
Available as generic? Yes
Drug class: Antiprotozoal, antibacterial (antibiotic)

USES

- Treatment for infections susceptible to metronidazole, such as trichomoniasis and amebiasis.
- Treatment for bacterial infections.
- Topical—Treats acne rosacea (adult acne).
- Vaginal—Treats vaginal infections.
- Treatment (combined with other drugs) for duodenal ulcer associated with *Helicobacter pylori* infection.

DOSAGE & USAGE INFORMATION

How to take:
- Cream—Apply to affected area 3 times daily.
- Tablet—Swallow with liquid or food to lessen stomach irritation. If you can't swallow whole, crumble tablet and take with liquid or food.
- Topical gel—Apply thin layer to involved area.

When to take:
- At the same times each day.
- Gel—Apply twice a day.

Continued next column

OVERDOSE

SYMPTOMS:
Weakness, nausea, vomiting, diarrhea, confusion, seizures.
WHAT TO DO:
Overdose unlikely to threaten life. If person takes much larger amount than prescribed, call doctor, poison center 1-800-222-1222 or hospital emergency room for instructions.

If you forget a dose:
Take as soon as you remember up to 2 hours late. If more than 2 hours, wait for next scheduled dose (don't double this dose).

What drug does:
Kills organisms causing the infection.

Time lapse before drug works:
Begins in 1 hour. May require regular use for 10 days to cure infection.

Don't take with:
- Nonprescription medicines containing alcohol.
- Any other medicine without consulting your doctor or pharmacist.

POSSIBLE ADVERSE REACTIONS OR SIDE EFFECTS

SYMPTOMS	WHAT TO DO
Life-threatening:	
In case of overdose, see previous column.	
Common:	
Appetite loss, nausea, stomach pain, diarrhea, vomiting.	Continue. Call doctor when convenient.
Infrequent:	
• Dizziness, headache.	Continue. Call doctor when convenient.
• Numbness, tingling, weakness or pain in hands or feet.	Discontinue. Call doctor right away.
• Dark urine (will go away when drug is discontinued).	No action necessary.
Rare:	
• Metallic taste, unpleasant taste, dry mouth, vaginal irritation.	Continue. Call doctor when convenient.
• Unsteadiness or clumsiness; mood or mental changes; skin rash, hives, redness or itch; sore throat and fever; seizures; severe stomach or back pain.	Discontinue. Call doctor right away.

WARNINGS & PRECAUTIONS

Don't take if:
- You are allergic to metronidazole.
- You have had a blood cell or bone marrow disorder.

Before you start, consult your doctor:
- If you plan to become pregnant within medication period.
- If you have a brain or nervous system disorder.
- If you have liver or heart disease.
- If you drink alcohol.

Over age 60:
Adverse reactions and side effects may be more frequent and severe than in younger persons.

Pregnancy:
Consult doctor. Risk category B (see page xviii).

Breast-feeding:
Drug passes into milk. Avoid drug or discontinue nursing until you finish medicine. Consult doctor for advice on maintaining milk supply.

Infants & children:
Use in children for amoeba infection only under close medical supervision.

Prolonged use:
Talk to your doctor about the need for follow-up medical examinations or laboratory studies to check for giardiasis in stools.

Skin & sunlight:
No problems expected.

Driving, piloting or hazardous work:
Avoid if you feel dizzy or unsteady. Otherwise, no problems expected.

Discontinuing:
Don't discontinue without doctor's advice until you complete prescribed dose, even though symptoms diminish or disappear.

Others:
Avoid alcohol 12 hours before and *at least* 24 hours after treatment period with metronidazole.

POSSIBLE INTERACTION WITH OTHER DRUGS

GENERIC NAME OR DRUG CLASS	COMBINED EFFECT
Anticoagulants*, oral	Increased anti-coagulant effect. Possible bleeding or bruising.
Antihistamines, nonsedating	Serious heart rhythm problems with astemizole and terfenadine. Avoid.
Antivirals, HIV/AIDS*	Increased risk of peripheral neuropathy.
Cimetidine	Prolongs increased serum levels.
Disulfiram	Disulfiram reaction*. Avoid.
Nizatidine	Increased effect and toxicity of metoprolol.
Oxytetracycline	Decreased metronidazole effect.
Phenobarbital	Decreased metronidazole effect.
Phenytoin	Decreased metronidazole effect.

POSSIBLE INTERACTION WITH OTHER SUBSTANCES

INTERACTS WITH	COMBINED EFFECT
Alcohol:	Possible disulfiram reaction*. Avoid alcohol in *any* form or amount.
Beverages:	None expected.
Cocaine:	Decreased metron-idazole effect. Avoid.
Foods:	None expected.
Marijuana:	None expected.
Tobacco:	None expected.

*See Glossary

METYRAPONE

BRAND NAMES

Metopirone

BASIC INFORMATION

Habit forming? No
Prescription needed? Yes
Available as generic? No
Drug class: Antiadrenal

USES

- To diagnose the function of the pituitary gland.
- Treats Cushing's disease, a disorder characterized by higher than normal concentrations of cortisol (one of the hormones secreted by the adrenal glands) in the blood.

DOSAGE & USAGE INFORMATION

How to take:
- For medical testing purposes—Take the prescribed number of tablets with milk or food on the day before the scheduled test. On the day of the test, blood and urine studies will show the amount of hormones in your blood. Results of the test will help establish your diagnosis.
- For treatment of Cushing's syndrome—Swallow tablet with liquid. If you can't swallow whole, crumble tablet and take with liquid or food.

When to take:
- For medical testing—Take the prescribed number of tablets on the day before the scheduled test.
- For treatment of Cushing's disease—Take total daily amount in divided doses. Follow prescription directions carefully.

Continued next column

OVERDOSE

SYMPTOMS:
Nausea (severe), vomiting, diarrhea, abdominal pain, sudden weakness, irregular heartbeat.
WHAT TO DO:
- **Dial 911 (emergency) for an ambulance or medical help or poison center 1-800-222-1222. Then give first aid immediately.**
- **See emergency information on inside covers.**

If you forget a dose:
Take as soon as you remember up to 2 hours late. If more than 2 hours, wait for next scheduled dose (don't double this dose).

What drug does:
Prevents one of the chemical reactions in the production of cortisol by the adrenal glands.

Time lapse before drug works:
Approximately 1 hour.

Don't take with:
Cortisone*-like medicines for 48 hours prior to testing.

POSSIBLE ADVERSE REACTIONS OR SIDE EFFECTS

SYMPTOMS	WHAT TO DO?
Life-threatening: In case of overdose, see previous column.	
Common:	
Dizziness, headache, nausea.	Continue. Call doctor when convenient.
Infrequent:	
Drowsiness.	Continue. Call doctor when convenient.
Rare:	
Hair loss or excess growth, decreased appetite, confusion, acne (may begin or may worsen if already present).	Continue. Call doctor when convenient.

WARNINGS & PRECAUTIONS

Don't take if:
- You have adrenal insufficiency (Addison's disease).
- You have decreased pituitary function.

Before you start, consult your doctor:
- If you are allergic to metyrapone.
- If you have porphyria.

Over age 60:
No special problems expected.

Pregnancy:
Safety not established. Take only under careful supervision of medical professional. Risk category C (see page xviii).

Breast-feeding:
Drug may pass into milk, although controlled studies in humans have not been performed. Since the possibility exists, avoid nursing until you finish the medicine.

Infants & children:
No special problems expected.

Prolonged use:
No special problems expected.

Skin & sunlight:
No special problems expected.

Driving, piloting or hazardous work:
Don't drive or pilot aircraft until you learn how medicine affects you. Don't work around dangerous machinery. Don't climb ladders or work in high places. Danger increases if you drink alcohol or take medicine affecting alertness and reflexes.

Discontinuing:
No special problems expected.

Others:
Advise any doctor or dentist whom you consult that you take this medicine.

POSSIBLE INTERACTION WITH OTHER DRUGS

GENERIC NAME OR DRUG CLASS	COMBINED EFFECT
Antidiabetics, oral*	Increased risk of adverse reactions.
Contraceptives, oral*	Possible inaccurate test results.
Estrogens*	Possible inaccurate test results.
Insulin	Increased risk of adverse reactions.
Phenytoin	Possible inaccurate test results.

POSSIBLE INTERACTION WITH OTHER SUBSTANCES

INTERACTS WITH	COMBINED EFFECT
Alcohol:	None expected.
Beverages:	None expected.
Cocaine:	None expected.
Foods:	Increased appetite and absorption of nutrients, causing difficulty with weight control.
Marijuana:	None expected.
Tobacco:	None expected.

METYROSINE

BRAND NAMES

Demser

BASIC INFORMATION

Habit forming? No
Prescription needed? Yes
Available as generic? No
Drug class: Antihypertensive

USES

- Treatment of pheochromocytoma* (adrenal gland tumor) that causes high blood pressure.
- Preoperative medication for removal of the tumor.

DOSAGE & USAGE INFORMATION

How to take:
Capsules—Swallow with liquid. If you can't swallow whole, open capsule and take with liquid or food. Instructions to take on empty stomach mean 1 hour before or 2 hours after eating.

When to take:
- Usually 4 times a day, approximately 6 hours apart.
- If used before surgery, take for at least 5 to 7 days.

If you forget a dose:
Take as soon as you remember up to 2 hours late. If more than 2 hours, wait for next scheduled dose (don't double this dose).

What drug does:
Reduces blood pressure in patients with pheochromocytoma* by reducing synthesis of catecholamines*.

Time lapse before drug works:
2 to 3 days.

Continued next column

OVERDOSE

SYMPTOMS:
Confusion, sudden shortness of breath, hallucinations, seizures, coma.
WHAT TO DO:
- **Dial 911 (emergency) for an ambulance or medical help or poison center 1-800-222-1222. Then give first aid immediately.**
- **See emergency information on inside covers.**

Don't take with:
Any other medicines (including over-the-counter drugs such as cough and cold medicines, laxatives, antacids, diet pills, caffeine, nose drops or vitamins) without consulting your doctor.

POSSIBLE ADVERSE REACTIONS OR SIDE EFFECTS

SYMPTOMS	WHAT TO DO
Life-threatening:	
In case of overdose, see previous column.	
Common:	
• Severe diarrhea, tremors, drooling, speech difficulties.	Continue. Call doctor when convenient.
• Drowsiness.	Continue. Tell doctor at next visit.
Infrequent:	
Skin rash, sexual difficulties in males.	Continue. Call doctor when convenient.
Rare:	
• Shortness of breath, itching, bloody urine, muscle spasms, swollen feet.	Discontinue. Call doctor right away.
• Depression.	Continue. Call doctor when convenient.

WARNINGS & PRECAUTIONS

Don't take if:
You are allergic to metyrosine.

Before you start, consult your doctor:
- If you have liver disease.
- If you have mental depression.
- If you have Parkinson's disease.
- If you have kidney disease.

Over age 60:
Adverse reactions and side effects may be more frequent and severe than in younger persons. You may need smaller doses for shorter periods of time.

Pregnancy:
Decide with your doctor if drug benefits justify risk to unborn child. Risk category C (see page xviii).

Breast-feeding:
Not recommended. Consult doctor.

Infants & children:
No proven problems.

Prolonged use:
Talk to your doctor about the need for follow-up medical examinations or laboratory studies to check blood pressure, heart function, ECG*, kidney function and urinary catecholamine measurements.

Skin & sunlight:
No problems expected.

Driving, piloting or hazardous work:
Don't drive or pilot aircraft until you learn how medicine affects you. Don't work around dangerous machinery. Don't climb ladders or work in high places. Danger increases if you drink alcohol or take medicine affecting alertness and reflexes.

Discontinuing:
May experience increased energy and insomnia for a short period (2 to 7 days).

Others:
- Advise any doctor or dentist whom you consult that you take this medicine.
- May affect results in some medical tests.

POSSIBLE INTERACTION WITH OTHER DRUGS

GENERIC NAME OR DRUG CLASS	COMBINED EFFECT
Antidepressants, tricyclic*	Increased sedative effect of each.
Central nervous system (CNS) depressants*	Increased sedative effect.
Clozapine	Toxic effect on the central nervous system.
Phenothiazines*	Increased likelihood of toxic symptoms of each.
Sertraline	Increased depressive effects of both drugs.
Trimeprazine	Increased likelihood of toxic symptoms of each.

POSSIBLE INTERACTION WITH OTHER SUBSTANCES

INTERACTS WITH	COMBINED EFFECT
Alcohol:	May cause Parkinson's*-like disorder. Don't mix.
Beverages:	None expected.
Cocaine:	None expected.
Foods:	None expected.
Marijuana:	None expected.
Tobacco:	None expected.

***See Glossary**

MEXILETINE

BRAND NAMES

Mexitil

BASIC INFORMATION

Habit forming? No
Prescription needed? Yes
Available as generic? Yes
Drug class: Antiarrhythmic

USES

Stabilizes irregular heartbeat.

DOSAGE & USAGE INFORMATION

How to take:
Capsules—Swallow whole with food, milk or antacid to lessen stomach irritation.

When to take:
At the same times each day as directed by your doctor.

If you forget a dose:
Take as soon as you remember up to 4 hours late. If more than 4 hours, wait for next scheduled dose (don't double this dose).

What drug does:
Blocks the fast sodium channel in heart tissue.

Time lapse before drug works:
30 minutes to 2 hours.

Don't take with:
Any other medicine without consulting your doctor or pharmacist.

OVERDOSE

SYMPTOMS:
Nausea, vomiting, seizures, convulsions, cardiac arrest.
WHAT TO DO:

- **Dial 911 (emergency) for an ambulance or medical help or poison center 1-800-222-1222. Then give first aid immediately.**
- **See emergency information on inside covers.**

POSSIBLE ADVERSE REACTIONS OR SIDE EFFECTS

SYMPTOMS	WHAT TO DO
Life-threatening:	
Chest pain, shortness of breath, irregular or fast heartbeat.	Discontinue. Seek emergency treatment.
Common:	
Dizziness, anxiety, shakiness, unsteadiness when walking, heartburn, nausea, vomiting.	Discontinue. Call doctor right away.
Infrequent:	
• Sore throat, fever, mouth sores; blurred vision; confusion; constipation; diarrhea; headache; numbness or tingling in hands or feet; ringing in ears; unexplained bleeding or bruising; rash; slurred speech; insomnia; weakness; difficult swallowing.	Discontinue. Call doctor right away.
• Loss of taste.	Continue. Call doctor when convenient.
Rare:	
• Seizures.	Discontinue. Seek emergency treatment.
• Hallucinations, psychosis, memory loss, difficult breathing, swollen feet and ankles, hiccups, jaundice.	Discontinue. Call doctor right away.
• Hair loss, impotence.	Continue. Call doctor when convenient.

WARNINGS & PRECAUTIONS

Don't take if:
If you are allergic to mexiletine, lidocaine or tocainide.

Before you start, consult your doctor:
- If you have had liver or kidney disease or impaired kidney function.
- If you have had lupus.
- If you have a history of seizures.
- If you will have surgery within 2 months, including dental surgery, requiring general or spinal anesthesia.
- If you have heart disease or low blood pressure.

Over age 60:
Adverse reactions and side effects may be more frequent and severe than in younger persons. Ask doctor about smaller doses.

Pregnancy:
Decide with your doctor if drug benefits justify risk to unborn child. Risk category C (see page xviii).

Breast-feeding:
Drug passes into milk. Avoid drug or discontinue nursing until you finish medicine. Consult doctor for advice on maintaining milk supply.

Infants & children:
Use only under close medical supervision.

Prolonged use:
- May cause lupus*-like illness.
- Talk to your doctor about the need for follow-up medical examinations or laboratory studies to check ECG*, liver function.

Skin & sunlight:
No problems expected.

Driving, piloting or hazardous work:
Use caution if you feel dizzy or weak. Otherwise, no problems expected.

Discontinuing:
Don't discontinue without consulting doctor. Dose may require gradual reduction if you have taken drug for a long time. Doses of other drugs may also require adjustment.

Others:
No problems expected.

POSSIBLE INTERACTION WITH OTHER DRUGS

GENERIC NAME OR DRUG CLASS	COMBINED EFFECT
Cimetidine	Increased mexiletine effect and toxicity.
Encainide	Increased effect of toxicity on the heart muscle.
Nicardipine	Possible increased effect and toxicity of each drug.
Phenobarbital	Decreased mexiletine effect.
Phenytoin	Decreased mexiletine effect.
Propafenone	Increased effect of both drugs and increased risk of toxicity.
Rifampin	Decreased mexiletine effect.
Urinary acidifiers* (ammonium chloride, ascorbic acid, potassium or sodium phosphate)	May decrease effectiveness of medicine.
Urinary alkalizers* (acetazolamide, antacids with calcium or magnesium, citric acid, dichlorphenamide, methazolamide, potassium citrate, sodium bicarbonate, sodium citrate)	May slow elimination of mexiletine and cause need to adjust dosage.

POSSIBLE INTERACTION WITH OTHER SUBSTANCES

INTERACTS WITH	COMBINED EFFECT
Alcohol:	Causes irregular effectiveness of mexiletine. Avoid.
Beverages: Caffeine drinks, iced drinks.	Irregular heartbeat.
Cocaine:	Decreased mexiletine effect.
Foods:	None expected.
Marijuana:	Irregular heartbeat. Avoid.
Tobacco:	Dangerous combination. May lead to liver problems and reduce excretion of mexiletine.

*See Glossary

MIFEPRISTONE (RU-486)

BRAND NAMES

Mifeprex

BASIC INFORMATION

Habit forming? No
Prescription needed? Yes
Available as generic? No
Drug class: Abortifacient

USES

Terminates pregnancy in the early stages (up to 7 weeks or 49 days, since the beginning of the last menstrual period). Mifepristone is not approved for ending later pregnancies. Requires three trips to your doctor's office: day one for administration, day three for a second medication (if you are still pregnant) and day fourteen for follow-up and determination of the status of your pregnancy.

DOSAGE & USAGE INFORMATION

How to take:
Tablet—Taken on day one under strict compliance in the presence of your doctor. On day three misoprostol is taken in your doctor's office (if you are still pregnant).

When to take:
At your doctors office.

What drug does:
Mifepristone blocks a hormone (progesterone) needed for your pregnancy to continue.

If you forget a dose:
Medication is taken at your doctor's office.

Time lapse before drug works:
A few days to two weeks. If you are still pregnant after two weeks, your doctor will discuss other options you have including a surgical alternative to terminate your pregnancy.

Don't take with:
Any other prescription or nonprescription drug without consulting your doctor or pharmacist.

OVERDOSE

SYMPTOMS:
Symptoms are unknown.
WHAT TO DO:
Overdose unlikely to threaten life. If person takes much larger amount than prescribed, call doctor, poison center 1-800-222-1222 or hospital emergency room for instructions.

POSSIBLE ADVERSE REACTIONS OR SIDE EFFECTS

SYMPTOMS	WHAT TO DO
Life-threatening: None expected.	
Common: Nausea or vomiting, diarrhea, abdominal pain, back pain, dizziness, unusual tiredness or weakness, headache.	Call doctor if symptoms persist.
Infrequent:	
• Excessive and heavy vaginal bleeding.	Call doctor right away.
• Pale skin, troubled breathing, unusual bleeding or bruising, anxiety, upset stomach, acid indigestion, fever, insomnia, leg pain, increased clear or white vaginal discharge, shaking, stuffy nose, cough, fainting, genital itching or pain, chills or flu-like symptoms, sinusitis.	Call doctor if symptoms persist.
Rare: None expected.	

WARNINGS & PRECAUTIONS

Don't take if:
You are allergic to mifepristone or misoprostol.

Before you start, consult your doctor:
- If you have a history of adrenal failure.
- If you have a history of hemorrhagic (bleeding) disorders.
- If you have an ectopic pregnancy (a pregnancy outside the uterus).
- If you have any other medical problems.
- If you have anemia.
- If you have an in-place intra-uterine device (IUD).
- If you cannot easily get emergency medical help during the two weeks after you take the drug..
- If you have a family history of porphyria.

Over age 60:
Not used in this age group.

Pregnancy:
Mifepristone is used to terminate pregnancy.

Breast-feeding:
It is unknown if mifepristone is distributed into breast milk.Avoid drug or discontinue nursing until you finish medicine. Consult doctor for advice on maintaining milk supply.

Infants & children:
Safety and efficacy not established. Not used in this age group.

Prolonged use:
Not intended for prolonged use.

Skin & sunlight:
No problems expected.

Driving, piloting or hazardous work:
No problems expected.

Discontinuing:
Drug is administered in the presence of a licensed practitioner who has registered with the manufacturer.

Others:
- Prior to using this medication, you will be required to sign a statement that you have decided to end your pregnancy.
- Advise any doctor or dentist whom you consult that you take this medicine.
- The follow-up doctor visits are very important. Don't miss them.
- May affect the results in some medical tests.
- An ultrasonographic scan may be scheduled 14 days after mifepristone administration to confirm termination of pregnancy and assess bleeding.
- If you do not want to become pregnant again, start using a birth control method as soon as your pregnancy ends.
- If you are still pregnant after the two weeks, there may be birth defects if the pregnancy continues. Your doctor will discuss other options to end your pregnancy.

POSSIBLE INTERACTION WITH OTHER DRUGS

GENERIC NAME OR DRUG CLASS	COMBINED EFFECT
Anticoagulants*	Excessive bleeding.
Corticosteroids* (long term use)	Effects unknown. Avoid.
Enzyme inducers*	May decrease effect of mifepristone.
Enzyme inhibitors*	May increase effect of mifepristone.

POSSIBLE INTERACTION WITH OTHER SUBSTANCES

INTERACTS WITH	COMBINED EFFECT
Alcohol:	None expected. Best to avoid.
Beverages:	
Grapefruit juice	May increase effect of mifepristone.
Cocaine:	Unknown. Avoid.
Foods:	None expected.
Marijuana:	None expected.
Tobacco:	None expected.

***See Glossary**

MIGLITOL

BRAND NAMES

Glyset

BASIC INFORMATION

Habit forming? No
Prescription needed? Yes
Available as generic? No
Drug class: Antidiabetic

USES

Treatment for hyperglycemia (excess sugar in the blood) that cannot be controlled by diet alone in patients with type II non-insulin-dependent diabetes mellitus (NIDDM). May be used alone or in combination with other antidiabetic drugs.

DOSAGE & USAGE INFORMATION

How to take:
Tablet—Swallow with liquid. Take at the very beginning of a meal.

When to take:
Usually 3 times a day or as directed by doctor. Dosage may be increased at 4- to 8-week intervals until maximum benefits are achieved.

Continued next column

OVERDOSE

SYMPTOMS:

- **Will not produce hypoglycemia. May cause flatulence, diarrhea, abdominal pain. Unlikely to produce serious side effects.**
- **Symptoms of hypoglycemia—stomach pain, anxious feeling, cold sweats, chills, confusion, convulsions, cool pale skin, excessive hunger, nausea or vomiting, rapid heartbeat, nervousness, shakiness, unsteady walk, unusual weakness or tiredness, vision changes, unconsciousness.**

WHAT TO DO:

- **For mild low blood sugar symptoms, drink or eat something containing dextrose or glucose (fruits, honey, starches) right away.**
- **For more severe symptoms, dial 911 (emergency) for an ambulance or medical help or poison center 1-800-222-1222. Then give first aid immediately.**
- **See emergency information on inside covers.**

If you forget a dose:
And your meal is finished, then skip the missed dose and wait for your next meal and next scheduled dose (don't double this dose).

What drug does:
Impedes the digestion and absorption of arbohydrates and their subsequent conversion into glucose. This improves control of blood glucose and may reduce the complications of diabetes. However, miglitol does not cure diabetes.

Time lapse before drug works:
May take several weeks for full effectiveness.

Don't take with:
Any other prescription or nonprescription drug without consulting your doctor or pharmacist. All possible drug interactions have not been studied.

POSSIBLE ADVERSE REACTIONS OR SIDE EFFECTS

SYMPTOMS	WHAT TO DO
Life-threatening:	
In case of overdose or low blood sugar, see previous column.	
Common:	
Diarrhea, stomach cramps, gas, bloating feeling.	Continue. Call doctor when convenient.
Infrequent:	
Skin rash.	Continue. Call doctor when convenient.
Rare:	
Severe low blood sugar (see symptoms under Overdose).	Discontinue. Call doctor right away or seek emergency help.

WARNINGS & PRECAUTIONS

Don't take if:
You are allergic to miglitol.

Before you start, consult your doctor:
- If you have any kidney or liver disease or any heart or blood vessel disorder.
- If you have any chronic health problem.
- If you have an infection, illness or any condition that can cause low blood sugar.
- If you have a history of acid in the blood (metabolic acidosis or ketoacidosis).
- If you have inflammatory bowel disease or any other intestinal disorder.
- If you are allergic to any medication, food or other substance.

Over age 60:
No special problems expected.

Pregnancy:
Decide with your doctor if drug benefits justify risks to unborn child. Risk category B (see page xviii).

Breast-feeding:
Drug passes into milk. It is not recommended for use in nursing mothers.

Infants & children:
Safety and efficacy have not been established. Use only under close medical supervision.

Prolonged use:
- Schedule regular doctor visits to determine if the drug is continuing to be effective in controlling the diabetes and to check for any problems in kidney function.
- You will most likely require an antidiabetic medicine for the rest of your life.
- You will need to test your blood glucose levels several times a day, or for some, once to several times a week.

Skin & sunlight:
No special problems expected.

Driving, piloting or hazardous work:
No special problems expected.

Discontinuing:
Don't discontinue without consulting your doctor even if you feel well. You can have diabetes without feeling any symptoms. Untreated diabetes can cause serious problems.

Others:
- Advise any doctor or dentist whom you consult that you take this medicine.
- It may interfere with the accuracy of some medical tests.
- Follow any special diet your doctor may prescribe. It can help control diabetes.
- Consult doctor if you become ill with vomiting or diarrhea while taking this drug.
- Use caution when exercising. Ask your doctor about an appropriate exercise program.
- Wear medical identification stating that you have diabetes and take this medication.
- Learn to recognize the symptoms of low blood sugar. You and your family need to know what to do if these symptoms occur.
- Have a glucagon kit and syringe in the event severe low blood sugar occurs.
- High blood sugar (hyperglycemia) may occur with diabetes. Ask your doctor about symptoms to watch for and treatment steps to take.
- Educate yourself about diabetes.

POSSIBLE INTERACTION WITH OTHER DRUGS

GENERIC NAME OR DRUG CLASS	COMBINED EFFECT
Amylase (Pancreatic enzyme)	Decreased miglitol effect.
Antidiabetic agents, sulfonylurea	May cause hypoglycemia.
Charcoal, activated	Decreased miglitol effect.
Pancreatin (Pancreatic enzyme)	Decreased miglitol effect.
Propranolol	Decreased effect of propranolol.
Ranitidine	Decreased effect of ranitidine.

POSSIBLE INTERACTION WITH OTHER SUBSTANCES

INTERACTS WITH	COMBINED EFFECT
Alcohol:	May increase effect of miglitol. Avoid excessive amounts.
Beverages:	None expected.
Cocaine:	None expected. Best to avoid.
Foods:	None expected.
Marijuana:	None expected. Best to avoid.
Tobacco:	People with diabetes should not smoke.

MINOXIDIL

BRAND NAMES

Loniten

BASIC INFORMATION

Habit forming? No
Prescription needed? Yes
Available as generic? Yes
Drug class: Antihypertensive

USES

- Treatment for high blood pressure in conjunction with other drugs, such as beta-adrenergic blockers and diuretics.
- Treatment for congestive heart failure.
- Can stimulate hair growth.

DOSAGE & USAGE INFORMATION

How to take:
Tablet—Swallow with liquid. If you can't swallow whole, crumble tablet and take with liquid or food.

When to take:
At the same time each day, according to instructions on prescription label.

If you forget a dose:
Take as soon as you remember up to 2 hours late. If more than 2 hours, wait for next scheduled dose (don't double this dose).

What drug does:
Relaxes small blood vessels (arterioles) so blood can pass through more easily.

Time lapse before drug works:
2 to 3 hours for effect to begin; 3 to 7 days of continuous use may be necessary for maximum blood pressure response.

Don't take with:
Any other medicine without consulting your doctor or pharmacist.

OVERDOSE

SYMPTOMS:
Low blood pressure, fainting, chest pain, shortness of breath, coma.
WHAT TO DO:
- **Dial 911 (emergency) for an ambulance or medical help or poison center 1-800-222-1222. Then give first aid immediately.**
- **See emergency information on inside covers.**

POSSIBLE ADVERSE REACTIONS OR SIDE EFFECTS

SYMPTOMS	WHAT TO DO
Life-threatening:	
In case of overdose, see previous column.	
Common:	
• Excessive hair growth, flushed skin or redness.	Continue. Call doctor when convenient.
• Bloating.	Discontinue. Call doctor right away.
Infrequent:	
• Chest pain, irregular or slow heartbeat, shortness of breath, swollen feet or legs, rapid weight gain.	Discontinue. Call doctor right away.
• Numbness of hands, feet or face; headache; tender breasts; darkening of skin.	Continue. Call doctor when convenient.
Rare:	
Rash.	Discontinue. Call doctor right away.

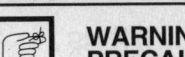

WARNINGS & PRECAUTIONS

Don't take if:
You are allergic to minoxidil.

Before you start, consult your doctor:
- If you have had recent stroke or heart attack or angina pectoris in past 3 weeks.
- If you have impaired kidney function.
- If you have pheochromocytoma*.

Over age 60:
Adverse reactions and side effects may be more frequent and severe than in younger persons.

Pregnancy:
Decide with your doctor if drug benefits justify risk to unborn child. Risk category C (see page xviii).

Breast-feeding:
Human studies not available. Avoid if possible. Consult doctor.

Infants & children:
Not recommended. Safety and dosage have not been established.

Prolonged use:
Request periodic blood examinations that include potassium levels.

Skin & sunlight:
May cause rash or intensify sunburn in areas exposed to sun or ultraviolet light (photosensitivity reaction). Avoid overexposure. Notify doctor if reaction occurs.

Driving, piloting or hazardous work:
Avoid if you become dizzy or faint. Otherwise, no problems expected.

Discontinuing:
Don't discontinue without consulting doctor. Dose may require gradual reduction if you have taken drug for a long time. Doses of other drugs may also require adjustment.

Others:
- Check pulse regularly. If it exceeds 20 or more beats per minute over your normal rate, consult doctor immediately.
- Check blood pressure frequently.

POSSIBLE INTERACTION WITH OTHER DRUGS

GENERIC NAME OR DRUG CLASS	COMBINED EFFECT
Anesthesia	Drastic blood pressure drop.
Antihypertensives*, other	Dosage adjustments may be necessary to keep blood pressure at desired level.
Carteolol	Increased anti-hypertensive effect.
Diuretics*	Dosage adjustments may be necessary to keep blood pressure at desired level.
Estrogens*	May increase blood pressure.
Guanadrel	Weakness and faintness when arising from bed or chair.
Guanethidine	Weakness and faintness when arising from bed or chair.
Lisinopril	Increased anti-hypertensive effect. Dosage of each may require adjustment.
Nicardipine	Blood pressure drop. Dosages may require adjustment.
Nimodipine	Dangerous blood pressure drop.
Nitrates*	Drastic blood pressure drop.
Sotalol	Increased anti-hypertensive effect.
Sympathomimetics*	Possible decreased minoxidil effect.
Terazosin	Decreased effectiveness of terazosin.

POSSIBLE INTERACTION WITH OTHER SUBSTANCES

INTERACTS WITH	COMBINED EFFECT
Alcohol:	Possible excessive blood pressure drop.
Beverages:	None expected.
Cocaine:	Increased risk of heart block and high blood pressure.
Foods: Salt substitutes.	Possible excessive potassium levels in blood.
Marijuana:	Increased dizziness.
Tobacco:	May decrease minoxidil effect. Avoid.

*See Glossary

MINOXIDIL (Topical)

BRAND NAMES

Dermal
Rogaine
Rogaine Extra Strength for Men
Rogaine for Men
Rogaine for Women

BASIC INFORMATION

Habit forming? No
Prescription needed? No
Available as generic? No
Drug class: Hair growth stimulant

USES

Treats hair loss on scalp from male and female pattern baldness (alopecia androgenetica).

DOSAGE & USAGE INFORMATION

How to use:
Topical solution

- Apply only to dry hair and scalp. With the provided applicator, apply the amount prescribed to the scalp area being treated. Begin in center of the treated area.
- Wash hands immediately after use.
- Don't use a blow dryer.
- If you are using at bedtime, wait 30 minutes after applying before retiring.

When to use:
Twice a day or as directed.

If you forget a dose:
Use as soon as you remember. No need to ever double the dose.

What drug does:
Stimulates hair growth by possibly dilating small blood capillaries, thereby providing more blood to hair follicles.

Time lapse before drug works:
Varies with individuals.

Don't use with:
Any other medicine without consulting your doctor or pharmacist.

OVERDOSE

SYMPTOMS:
None expected.
WHAT TO DO:
Not for internal use. If child accidentally swallows, call poison center 1-800-222-1222.

POSSIBLE ADVERSE REACTIONS OR SIDE EFFECTS

SYMPTOMS	WHAT TO DO
Life-threatening:	
Fast, irregular heartbeat (rare; represents too much absorbed into body).	Discontinue. Seek emergency treatment.
Common:	
None expected.	
Infrequent:	
Itching scalp; flaking, reddened skin.	Continue. Call doctor when convenient.
Rare:	
Burning scalp, skin rash, swollen face, headache, dizziness or fainting, hands and feet numb or tingling, rapid weight gain.	Discontinue. Call doctor right away.

WARNINGS & PRECAUTIONS

Don't use if:
You are allergic to minoxidil.

Before you start, consult your doctor:
- If you are allergic to anything.
- If you have heart disease or high blood pressure.
- If you have skin irritation or abrasion or severe sunburn (systemic absorption may be increased).

Over age 60:
No problems expected.

Pregnancy:
Decide with your doctor if drug benefits justify risk to unborn child. Risk category C (see page xviii).

Breast-feeding:
Don't use.

Infants & children:
Don't use.

Prolonged use:
No problems expected.

Skin & sunlight:
No problems expected.

Driving, piloting or hazardous work:
No problems expected.

Discontinuing:
No problems expected.

Others:
- Keep away from eyes, nose and mouth. Flush with plain water if accident occurs.
- New hair will drop out when you stop using minoxidil.
- Keep solution cool, but don't freeze.

POSSIBLE INTERACTION WITH OTHER DRUGS

GENERIC NAME OR DRUG CLASS	COMBINED EFFECT
Adrenocorticoids*, topical	May cause undesirable absorption of minoxidil.
Minoxidil, oral	Increased risk of toxicity.
Petrolatum, topical	May cause undesirable absorption of minoxidil.
Retinoids*, topical	May cause undesirable absorption of minoxidil.

POSSIBLE INTERACTION WITH OTHER SUBSTANCES

INTERACTS WITH	COMBINED EFFECT
Alcohol:	None expected.
Beverages:	None expected.
Cocaine:	None expected.
Foods:	None expected.
Marijuana:	None expected.
Tobacco:	None expected.

*See Glossary

MIRTAZAPINE

BRAND NAMES

Remeron
Remeron SolTab

BASIC INFORMATION

Habit forming? Not expected
Prescription needed? Yes
Available as generic? No
Drug class: Antidepressant

USES

Treats symptoms of mental depression.

DOSAGE & USAGE INFORMATION

How to take:
Tablet—Swallow with liquid. May be taken with or without food.

When to take:
At the same time each day, usually in the evening before bedtime.

If you forget a dose:
Take as soon as you remember up to 12 hours late. If more than 12 hours, wait for the next scheduled dose (don't double this dose).

What drug does:
The exact mechanism is unknown. It appears to block certain chemicals in the brain, which in turn helps production of other brain chemicals that play a role in helping to relieve symptoms of depression.

Time lapse before drug works:
Will take up to several weeks to show improvement of the depression symptoms.

Don't take with:
Any other prescription or nonprescription drug without consulting your doctor or pharmacist.

OVERDOSE

SYMPTOMS:
Drowsiness, disorientation, memory impairment, rapid heartbeat.
WHAT TO DO:

- **Dial 911 (emergency) for an ambulance or medical help or poison center 1-800-222-1222. Then give first aid immediately.**
- **See emergency information on inside covers.**

POSSIBLE ADVERSE REACTIONS OR SIDE EFFECTS

SYMPTOMS	WHAT TO DO
Life-threatening: None expected.	
Common:	
• Sleepiness, increased appetite, weight gain, dizziness, dry mouth, constipation, tiredness, increased thirst.	Continue. Call doctor when convenient.
• Abdominal pain, vomiting, joint pain, increased cough, rash, itching, agitation, anxiety, twitching, apathy.	Discontinue. Call doctor right away.
Infrequent:	
• Forgetfulness, lightheadedness.	Continue. Call doctor when convenient.
• Slow heartbeat, migraine, dehydration, weight loss, unusual weakness, pain in any part of the body, changes in menstrual periods, changes in vision or hearing, mouth sores, mood or mental changes, breathing difficulty, lack of coordination.	Discontinue. Call doctor right away.
Rare:	
• Muscle aches, strange dreams, headache.	Continue. Call doctor when convenient.
• Swelling of hands, feet or legs; infection (fever, chills, aches or pains, sore throat); swollen or discolored tongue; changes in urinary function; hives.	Discontinue. Call doctor right away.

WARNINGS & PRECAUTIONS

Don't take if:
You are allergic to mirtazapine.

Before you start, consult your doctor:
- If you have seizure disorder, heart disease, blood circulation problem or had a stroke.
- If you are dehydrated.
- If you have a history of drug dependence or drug abuse.
- If you have kidney or liver disease.
- If you have a history of mood disorders, such as mania, or thoughts of suicide.
- If you are allergic to any other medication, food or other substances.

Over age 60:
A lower starting dosage is usually recommended until a response is determined.

Pregnancy:
Decide with your doctor if drug benefits justify risk to unborn child. Risk category C (see page xviii).

Breast-feeding:
It is unknown if drug passes into milk. Avoid drug or discontinue nursing until you finish medicine. Consult doctor for advice on maintaining milk supply.

Infants & children:
Safety in children under age 18 has not been established.

Prolonged use:
Consult with your doctor on a regular basis while taking this drug to check your progress, to discuss any increase or changes in side effects and the need for continued treatment.

Skin & sunlight:
May cause a rash or intensify sunburn in areas exposed to sun or ultraviolet light (photosensitivity reaction). Avoid excessive sun exposure. Consult doctor if reaction occurs.

Driving, piloting or hazardous work:
Don't drive or pilot aircraft until you learn how medicine affects you. Don't work around dangerous machinery. Don't climb ladders or work in high places. Danger increases if you drink alcohol or take medicine affecting alertness and reflexes.

Discontinuing:
Consult doctor before discontinuing this drug.

Others:
- Get up slowly from a sitting or lying position to avoid dizziness, faintness or lightheadedness.
- Advise any doctor or dentist whom you consult that you take this medicine.
- Do not increase or reduce dosage without doctor's approval.

POSSIBLE INTERACTION WITH OTHER DRUGS

GENERIC NAME OR DRUG CLASS	COMBINED EFFECT
Benzodiazepines	Increased sedative effect. Avoid.
Monoamine oxidase, (MAO) inhibitors	Potentially life-threatening. Allow 14 days between use of 2 drugs.
Other medications	Complete studies have not been done to evaluate interactions with other drugs, but the potential exists for a variety of possible interactions. Consult doctor.

POSSIBLE INTERACTION WITH OTHER SUBSTANCES

INTERACTS WITH	COMBINED EFFECT
Alcohol:	Increased sedative affect. Avoid.
Beverages:	None expected.
Cocaine:	Unknown effect. Best to avoid.
Foods:	None expected.
Marijuana:	Unknown effect. Best to avoid.
Tobacco:	None expected.

MISOPROSTOL

BRAND NAMES

Arthrotec
Cytotec

BASIC INFORMATION

Habit forming? No
Prescription needed? Yes
Available as generic? No
Drug class: Antiulcer agent

USES

Prevents development of stomach ulcers in persons taking nonsteroidal anti-inflammatory drugs (NSAIDs), including aspirin.

DOSAGE & USAGE INFORMATION

How to take:
Tablets—Swallow with liquid. If you can't swallow whole, crumble tablet and take with liquid or food. Instructions to take on empty stomach mean 1 hour before or 2 hours after eating.

When to take:
Usually 4 times a day while awake, with or after meals and at bedtime.

If you forget a dose:
Take as soon as you remember up to 2 hours late. If more than 2 hours, wait for next scheduled dose (don't double this dose).

What drug does:
- Improves defense against peptic ulcers by strengthening natural defenses of the stomach lining.
- Decreases stomach acid production.

Time lapse before drug works:
10 to 15 minutes.

Don't take with:
Any other medicines (including over-the-counter drugs such as cough and cold medicines, laxatives, antacids, diet pills, caffeine, nose drops or vitamins) without consulting your doctor or pharmacist.

OVERDOSE

SYMPTOMS:
None expected.
WHAT TO DO:
Overdose unlikely to threaten life. If person takes much larger amount than prescribed, call doctor, poison center 1-800-222-1222 or hospital emergency room for instructions.

POSSIBLE ADVERSE REACTIONS OR SIDE EFFECTS

SYMPTOMS	WHAT TO DO
Life-threatening: None expected.	
Common: Abdominal pain, diarrhea.	Discontinue. Call doctor right away.
Infrequent: • Nausea or vomiting.	Continue. Call doctor when convenient.
• Constipation, headache.	Continue. Tell doctor at next visit.
Rare: • Gaseousness.	Continue. Tell doctor at next visit.
• Vaginal bleeding.	Discontinue. Call doctor right away.

WARNINGS & PRECAUTIONS

Don't take if:
- You are allergic to any prostaglandin*.
- You are pregnant or of child-bearing age.

Before you start, consult your doctor:
- If you have epilepsy.
- If you have heart disease.
- If you have blood vessel disease of any kind.

Over age 60:
No special problems expected.

Pregnancy:
- Risk to unborn child outweighs drug benefits. Don't use.
- May also lead to serious complications in pregnant women, including excessive bleeding and future infertility.
- Risk category X (see page xviii).

Breast-feeding:
Drug passes into milk. Avoid drug or discontinue nursing until you finish medicine. Consult doctor for advice on maintaining milk supply.

Infants & children:
Not recommended for children under 18.

Prolonged use:
Talk to your doctor about the need for follow-up medical examinations or laboratory studies to check gastric analysis.

Skin & sunlight:
No problems expected.

Driving, piloting or hazardous work:
Avoid if you feel confused, drowsy or dizzy.

Discontinuing:
No special problems expected.

Others:
Advise any doctor or dentist whom you consult that you take this medicine.

POSSIBLE INTERACTION WITH OTHER DRUGS

GENERIC NAME OR DRUG CLASS	COMBINED EFFECT
Antacids*, magnesium-containing	Severe diarrhea.

POSSIBLE INTERACTION WITH OTHER SUBSTANCES

INTERACTS WITH	COMBINED EFFECT
Alcohol:	Decreases misoprostol effect. Avoid.
Beverages: Caffeine-containing.	Decreases misoprostol effect. Avoid.
Cocaine:	Decreases misoprostol effect. Avoid.
Foods:	None expected.
Marijuana:	Decreases misoprostol effect. Avoid.
Tobacco:	Decreases misoprostol effect. Avoid.

*See Glossary

MITOTANE

BRAND NAMES

Lysodren   o,p´-DDD

BASIC INFORMATION

Habit forming? No
Prescription needed? Yes
Available as generic? No
Drug class: Antineoplastic, antiadrenal

USES

- Treatment for some kinds of cancer.
- Treatment of Cushing's disease.

DOSAGE & USAGE INFORMATION

How to take:
Tablet—Take with liquid after light meal. Don't drink fluid with meals. Drink extra fluids between meals. Avoid sweet and fatty foods.

When to take:
At the same time each day.

If you forget a dose:
Take as soon as you remember. Don't ever double dose.

What drug does:
Suppresses adrenal cortex to prevent manufacture of excess cortisone.

Time lapse before drug works:
2 to 3 weeks for full effect.

Don't take with:
Any other medicine without consulting your doctor or pharmacist.

OVERDOSE

SYMPTOMS:
Headache, vomiting blood, stupor, seizure.
WHAT TO DO:

- **Dial 911 (emergency) for an ambulance or medical help or poison center 1-800-222-1222. Then give first aid immediately.**
- **If patient is unconscious and not breathing, give mouth-to-mouth breathing. If there is no heartbeat, use cardiac massage and mouth-to-mouth breathing (CPR). Don't try to make patient vomit. If you can't get help quickly, take patient to nearest emergency facility.**
- **See emergency information on inside covers.**

POSSIBLE ADVERSE REACTIONS OR SIDE EFFECTS

SYMPTOMS	WHAT TO DO
Life-threatening:	
In case of overdose, see previous column.	
Common:	
• Darkened skin, appetite loss, nausea, vomiting.	Continue. Call doctor when convenient.
• Mental depression, drowsiness.	Continue. Tell doctor at next visit.
Infrequent:	
• Fever, chills, sore throat.	Discontinue. Seek emergency treatment.
• Unusual bleeding or bruising, difficult breathing.	Discontinue. Call doctor right away.
• Rash, hair loss, blurred vision, seeing double, cough, tiredness, weakness, dizziness when standing after sitting or lying down.	Continue. Call doctor when convenient.
Rare:	
Blood in urine.	Continue. Call doctor when convenient.

WARNINGS & PRECAUTIONS

Don't take if:
You are allergic to mitotane corticosteroids* or any antineoplastic drug.

Before you start, consult your doctor:
- If you have liver disease.
- If you have infection.

Over age 60:
Adverse reactions and side effects may be more frequent and severe than in younger persons.

Pregnancy:
Decide with your doctor whether drug benefits justify risk to unborn child. Risk category C (see page xviii).

Breast-feeding:
Unknown if drug passes into milk. Consult doctor.

Infants & children:
Use only under care of medical supervisors who are experienced in administering anticancer drugs.

Prolonged use:
Adverse reactions more likely the longer drug is required.

Skin & sunlight:
No problems expected.

Driving, piloting or hazardous work:
No problems expected.

Discontinuing:
- Don't discontinue without consulting doctor. Dose may require gradual reduction if you have taken drug for a long time. Doses of other drugs may also require adjustment.
- Some side effects may follow discontinuing. Report any new symptoms.

Others:
No problems expected.

POSSIBLE INTERACTION WITH OTHER DRUGS

GENERIC NAME OR DRUG CLASS	COMBINED EFFECT
Adrenocorticoids, systemic	Decreased adreno-corticoid effect.
Antidepressants*	Increased central nervous system depression.
Antihistamines*	Increased central nervous system depression.
Central nervous system (CNS) depressants*	Increased sedation.
Phenytoin	Possible increased metabolism.
Spironolactone	Decreased mitotane effect.
Warfarin	Decreased warfarin effect.

POSSIBLE INTERACTION WITH OTHER SUBSTANCES

INTERACTS WITH	COMBINED EFFECT
Alcohol:	Increased depression. Avoid.
Beverages:	None expected.
Cocaine:	Increased toxicity. Avoid.
Foods:	Reduced irritation in stomach.
Marijuana:	None expected.
Tobacco:	Increased possibility of lung toxicity.

*See Glossary

MODAFINIL

BRAND NAMES

Provigil

BASIC INFORMATION

Habit forming? Yes
Prescription needed? Yes
Available as generic? No
Drug class: Antinarcoleptic, central nervous system stimulant

USES

Treatment to help people who have narcolepsy to stay awake during the day. It does not cure narcolepsy.

DOSAGE & USAGE INFORMATION

How to take:
Tablet—Swallow with liquid. If you can't swallow whole, crumble tablet and take with liquid or food.

When to take:
At the same time each day, usually in the morning.

If you forget a dose:
Take as soon as you remember, until noon of the same day. If you don't remember until later, skip the missed dose to avoid problems getting to sleep. Return to your regular dosing schedule the next day. Do not double doses.

Continued next column

OVERDOSE

SYMPTOMS:
Overdose is unlikely to threaten life. Symptoms include agitation, increased blood pressure, increased heart rate and insomnia.
WHAT TO DO:
If person takes much larger amount than prescribed, call doctor, poison center 1-800-222-1222 or hospital emergency room for instructions.

What drug does:
Stimulates the central nervous system.

Time lapse before drug works:
2 to 4 hours.

Don't take with:
Any other medicine without consulting your doctor or pharmacist.

POSSIBLE ADVERSE REACTIONS OR SIDE EFFECTS

SYMPTOMS	WHAT TO DO
Life-threatening:	
None expected.	
Common:	
Anxiety, headache, nausea, nervousness trouble sleeping.	Continue. Call doctor when convenient.
Infrequent:	
• Vision changes, chills or fever, confusion, dizziness, fainting, increased thirst or urination, depression, memory or mood changes, shortness of breath, trouble in urinating, uncontrolled face, mouth and tongue movements.	Continue. Call doctor right away.
• Appetite changes, diarrhea, mouth dryness, skin dryness, skin flushing, muscle stiffness, stuffy or runny nose, skin tingling, trembling or shaking, vomiting.	Continue. Call doctor when convenient.
Rare:	
None expected.	

WARNINGS & PRECAUTIONS

Don't take if:
You are allergic to modafinil or any other central nervous system stimulants.

Before you start, consult your doctor:
- If you have heart disease or have had a heart attack.
- If you have had high blood pressure.
- If you have had liver or kidney disease.
- If you have a history of severe mental illness.

Over age 60:
Adverse reactions and side effects may be more frequent and severe than in younger persons.

Pregnancy:
Decide with your doctor if drug benefits justify risk to unborn child. Risk category C (see page xviii).

Breast-feeding:
It is unknown if modafinil is secreted in human milk; therefore, it should not be taken by nursing women and for one month after you stop using modafinil.

Infants & children:
Safety and efficacy in children younger than 16 years of age have not been established.

Prolonged use:
May lead to physical or mental dependence. Consult your doctor if any of the following signs of dependence occur:

A strong desire to continue taking this medication.
A need to increase the dose to receive the effects of the medicine.
Withdrawal side effects when you stop taking the medicine.

Skin & sunlight:
No problems expected.

Driving, piloting or hazardous work:
Don't drive or pilot aircraft until you learn how medicine affects you. Don't work around dangerous machinery. Don't climb ladders or work in high places. Danger increases if you drink alcohol or take medicine affecting alertness and reflexes such as antihistamines, tranquilizers or sedatives, pain medicine, narcotics and mind-altering drugs.

Discontinuing:
- Consult your doctor if any symptoms occur after discontinuing the medication.
- Dose may require gradual reduction if you have taken drug for a long time.
- Advise any doctor or dentist whom you consult that you take this medicine.

Others:
- If you are using a birth control method, such as pills or implants, they may not be as effective while taking modafinil and for up to one month after stopping modafinil.
- May affect the results in some medical tests.

POSSIBLE INTERACTION WITH OTHER DRUGS

GENERIC NAME OR DRUG CLASS	COMBINED EFFECT
Antidepressants, tricyclic*	Increased effect of antidepressant.
CNS stimulants*	Increased effect of stimulants.
Diazepam	Decreased diazepam effect.
Enzyme inducers*	Decreased modafinil effect.
Enzyme inhibitors*	Increased modafinil effect.
MAO inhibitors*	Unknown effect.
Mephenytoin	Mephenytoin dose may need adjustment.
Steroidal contraceptives	Decreased contraceptive effect.
Theophylline	Decreased theophylline effect.
Warfarin	Increased warfarin effect.

POSSIBLE INTERACTION WITH OTHER SUBSTANCES

INTERACTS WITH	COMBINED EFFECT
Alcohol:	Effects unknown. Avoid.
Beverages:	None expected.
Cocaine:	Effects unknown. Avoid.
Foods:	None expected.
Marijuana:	Effects unknown. Avoid.
Tobacco:	Interferes with absorption. Avoid.

*See Glossary

MOLINDONE

BRAND NAMES

Moban
Moban Concentrate

BASIC INFORMATION

Habit forming? No
Prescription needed? Yes
Available as generic? No
Drug class: Antipsychotic

USES

Treats severe emotional, mental or nervous problems.

DOSAGE & USAGE INFORMATION

How to take:
Tablet or solution—Swallow with liquid or food to lessen stomach irritation. If you can't swallow tablet whole, crumble and take with food or liquid.

When to take:
Follow instructions on prescription label. Doses should be evenly spaced. For example, 4 times a day means every 6 hours.

If you forget a dose:
Take as soon as you remember up to 2 hours late. If more than 2 hours, wait for next scheduled dose (don't double this dose).

What drug does:
Corrects an imbalance in nerve impulses from the brain.

Time lapse before drug works:
Some benefit seen within a week; 4 to 6 weeks for full benefit.

Don't take with:
- Antacid or medicine for diarrhea.
- Nonprescription drugs for cough, cold or allergy.

OVERDOSE

SYMPTOMS:
Stupor, convulsions, coma.
WHAT TO DO:
- **Dial 911 (emergency) for an ambulance or medical help or poison center 1-800-222-1222. Then give first aid immediately.**
- **See emergency information at end of book.**

POSSIBLE ADVERSE REACTIONS OR SIDE EFFECTS

SYMPTOMS	WHAT TO DO
Life-threatening:	
High fever, rapid pulse, profuse sweating, muscle rigidity, confusion and irritability, seizures.	Discontinue. Seek emergency treatment.
Common:	
Sedation, low blood pressure and dizziness.	Continue. Call doctor when convenient.
Infrequent:	
• Jerky or involuntary movements, especially of the face, lips, jaw, tongue; slow-frequency tremor of head or limbs, especially while moving; muscle rigidity, lack of facial expression and slow, inflexible movements	Discontinue. Call doctor right away.
• Pacing or restlessness; intermittent spasms of muscles of face, eyes, tongue, jaw, neck, body or limbs; dry mouth, blurred vision, constipation, difficulty urinating.	Continue. Call doctor when convenient.
Rare:	
Other symptoms not listed above.	Continue. Call doctor when convenient.

WARNINGS & PRECAUTIONS

Don't take if:
- You are allergic to any phenothiazine.
- You have a blood or bone marrow disease.

Before you start, consult your doctor:
- If you will have surgery within 2 months, including dental surgery, requiring general or spinal anesthesia.
- If you have asthma, emphysema or other lung disorder, glaucoma, prostate trouble, seizure disorders.
- If you take nonprescription ulcer medicine, asthma medicine or amphetamines.

Over age 60:
Adverse reactions and side effects may be more frequent and severe than in younger persons. More likely to develop involuntary movement of jaws, lips, tongue; chewing. Report this to your doctor immediately. Early treatment can help.

Pregnancy:
Decide with your doctor if drug benefits justify risk to unborn child. Risk category C (see page xviii).

Breast-feeding:
Safety not established. Consult doctor.

Infants & children:
Don't give to children younger than 2.

Prolonged use:
- May lead to tardive dyskinesia (involuntary movement of jaws, lips, tongue; chewing).
- Talk to your doctor about the need for follow-up medical examinations or laboratory studies to check kidney function, eyes.

Skin & sunlight:
Avoid getting overheated. The drug affects body temperature and sweating.

Driving, piloting or hazardous work:
Don't drive or pilot aircraft until you learn how medicine affects you. Don't work around dangerous machinery. Don't climb ladders or work in high places. Danger increases if you drink alcohol or take medicine affecting alertness and reflexes.

Discontinuing:
- Nervous and mental disorders—Don't discontinue without doctor's advice until you complete prescribed dose, even though symptoms diminish or disappear.
- Notify your doctor if any of the following occurs—Uncontrollable movements of tongue, arms and legs; lip smacking.

Others:
Advise any doctor or dentist whom you consult that you take this medicine.

POSSIBLE INTERACTION WITH OTHER DRUGS

GENERIC NAME OR DRUG CLASS	COMBINED EFFECT
Anticholinergics*	Increased anticholinergic effect.
Antidepressants, tricyclic*	Increased molindone effect.
Antihistamines*	Increased antihistamine effect.
Appetite suppressants*	Decreased appetite suppressant effect.
Beta-adrenergic blocking agents*	Increased tranquilizer effect.
Bupropion	Increased risk of seizures.
Central nervous system (CNS) depressants*	Increased depressive effects of both drugs.
Clozapine	Toxic effect on the central nervous system.
Extrapyramidal reaction-causing medications*	Increased frequency and severity of extrapyramidal effects.
Fluoxetine	Increased depressant effects of both drugs.
Guanethidine	Decreased guanethidine effect.
Guanfacine	May increase depressant effects of either drug.
Leucovorin	High alcohol content of leucovorin may cause adverse effects.
Levodopa	Decreased levodopa effect.
Loxapine	May increase toxic effects of both drugs.
Mind-altering drugs*	Increased effect of mind-altering drugs.

Continued on page 920

POSSIBLE INTERACTION WITH OTHER SUBSTANCES

INTERACTS WITH	COMBINED EFFECT
Alcohol:	Dangerous oversedation.
Beverages:	None expected.
Cocaine:	Decreased molindone effect. Avoid.
Foods:	None expected.
Marijuana:	Drowsiness. May increase antinausea effect.
Tobacco:	None expected.

*See Glossary

MONOAMINE OXIDASE (MAO) INHIBITORS

GENERIC AND BRAND NAMES

PHENELZINE	TRANYLCYPROMINE
Nardil	Parnate

BASIC INFORMATION

Habit forming? No
Prescription needed? Yes
Available as generic? No
Drug class: MAO (monoamine oxidase) inhibitor, antidepressant

USES

- Treatment for depression and panic disorder.
- Prevention of vascular or tension headaches.

DOSAGE & USAGE INFORMATION

How to take:
Tablet—Swallow with liquid. If you can't swallow whole, crumble tablet and take with liquid or food.

When to take:
At the same times each day.

If you forget a dose:
Take as soon as you remember up to 2 hours late. If more than 2 hours, wait for next scheduled dose (don't double this dose).

What drug does:
Inhibits nerve transmissions in brain that may cause depression.

Time lapse before drug works:
4 to 6 weeks for maximum effect.

Continued next column

OVERDOSE

SYMPTOMS:
Restlessness, agitation, excitement, fever, confusion, dizziness, heartbeat irregularities, hallucinations, sweating, breathing difficulties, insomnia, irritability, convulsions, coma.
WHAT TO DO:
- **Dial 911 (emergency) for an ambulance or medical help or poison center 1-800-222-1222. Then give first aid immediately.**
- **See emergency information at end of book.**

Don't take with:
- Nonprescription diet pills; nose drops; medicine for asthma, cough, cold or allergy; medicine containing caffeine or alcohol.
- Foods containing tyramine*. Life-threatening elevation of blood pressure may result.
- Any other medicine without consulting your doctor or pharmacist.

POSSIBLE ADVERSE REACTIONS OR SIDE EFFECTS

SYMPTOMS	WHAT TO DO
Life-threatening:	
In case of overdose, see previous column. Also see above regarding dangers associated with tyramine.	
Common:	
• Fatigue, weakness.	Continue. Call doctor when convenient.
• Dizziness when changing position, restlessness, tremors, dry mouth, constipation, difficult urination, blurred vision, "sweet tooth."	Continue. Tell doctor at next visit.
Infrequent:	
• Fainting, enlarged pupils, severe headache, chest pain, rapid or pounding heartbeat.	Discontinue. Seek emergency treatment.
• Hallucinations, insomnia, nightmares, diarrhea, swollen feet or legs, joint pain.	Continue. Call doctor when convenient.
• Diminished sex drive.	Continue. Tell doctor at next visit.
Rare:	
Rash, nausea, vomiting, stiff neck, jaundice, fever, increased sweating, dark urine, slurred speech, staggering gait.	Discontinue. Call doctor right away.

WARNINGS & PRECAUTIONS

Don't take if:
- You are allergic to any MAO inhibitor.
- You have heart disease, congestive heart failure, heart rhythm irregularities or high blood pressure.
- You have liver or kidney disease.

Before you start, consult your doctor:
- If you are alcoholic.
- If you have had a stroke.

- If you have diabetes, epilepsy, asthma, overactive thyroid, schizophrenia, Parkinson's disease, adrenal gland tumor.
- If you will have surgery within 2 months, including dental surgery, requiring general or spinal anesthesia.

Over age 60:
Not recommended. Adverse effects more likely.

Pregnancy:
Decide with your doctor if drug benefits justify risk to unborn child. Risk category C (see page xviii).

Breast-feeding:
Safety not established. Consult doctor.

Infants & children:
Not recommended. Consult doctor.

Prolonged use:
- May be toxic to liver.
- Talk to your doctor about the need for follow-up medical examinations or laboratory studies to check blood pressure, liver function.

Skin & sunlight:
No special problems expected.

Driving, piloting or hazardous work:
Don't drive or pilot aircraft until you learn how medicine affects you. Don't work around dangerous machinery. Don't climb ladders or work in high places. Danger increases if you drink alcohol or take medicine affecting alertness and reflexes.

Discontinuing:
- Don't discontinue without doctor's advice until you complete prescribed dose, even though symptoms diminish or disappear.
- Follow precautions regarding foods, drinks and other medicines for 2 weeks after discontinuing.
- Adverse symptoms caused by this medicine may occur even after discontinuation. If you develop any of the symptoms listed under Overdose, notify your doctor immediately.

Others:
- May affect blood sugar levels in patients with diabetes.
- Advise any doctor or dentist whom you consult about the use of this medicine.
- Fever may indicate that MAO inhibitor dose requires adjustment.

POSSIBLE INTERACTION WITH OTHER DRUGS

GENERIC NAME OR DRUG CLASS	COMBINED EFFECT
Amphetamines*	Blood pressure rise to life-threatening level.
Anticholinergics*	Increased anticholinergic effect.
Anticonvulsants*	Changed seizure pattern.
Antidepressants, tricyclic*	Blood pressure rise to life-threatening level. Possible fever, convulsions, delirium.
Antidiabetic agents, oral* and insulin	Excessively low blood sugar.
Antihypertensives*	Excessively low blood pressure.
Beta-adrenergic blocking agents*	Possible blood pressure rise if MAO inhibitor is discontinued after simultaneous use with acebutolol.
Bupropion	Increased risk of side effects.
Buspirone	Very high blood pressure.
Caffeine	Irregular heartbeat or high blood pressure.
Carbamazepine	Fever, seizures. Avoid.

Continued on page 920

POSSIBLE INTERACTION WITH OTHER SUBSTANCES

INTERACTS WITH	COMBINED EFFECT
Alcohol:	Increased sedation to dangerous level.
Beverages:	
Caffeine drinks.	Irregular heartbeat or high blood pressure.
Drinks containing tyramine*.	Blood pressure rise to life-threatening level.
Cocaine:	Overstimulation. Possibly fatal.
Foods:	
Foods containing tyramine*.	Blood pressure rise to life-threatening level.
Marijuana:	Overstimulation. Avoid.
Tobacco:	None expected.

***See Glossary**

MORICIZINE

BRAND NAMES

Ethmozine

BASIC INFORMATION

Habit forming? No
Prescription needed? Yes
Available as generic? No
Drug class: Antiarrhythmic

USES

Treats severe heartbeat irregularities, primarily life-threatening ventricular tachycardia.

DOSAGE & USAGE INFORMATION

How to take:
Tablets—As directed, by mouth with water.

When to take:
When directed. The first dose of this medicine is usually given in an emergency room or in the hospital under continuous monitoring.

If you forget a dose:
Take as soon as you remember up to 4 hours late. If more than 4 hours, wait for next scheduled dose (don't double this dose).

What drug does:
Affects the electrical conduction system inside the heart.

Time lapse before drug works:
Promptly, but may require up to 2 hours for full effect.

Don't take with:
Any other medicine without consulting your doctor or pharmacist.

OVERDOSE

SYMPTOMS:
Fainting, chest pain, vomiting, lethargy, coma.
WHAT TO DO:
- **Dial 911 (emergency) for an ambulance or medical help or poison center 1-800-222-1222. Then give first aid immediately.**
- **See emergency information on inside covers.**

POSSIBLE ADVERSE REACTIONS OR SIDE EFFECTS

SYMPTOMS	WHAT TO DO
Life-threatening: In case of overdose, see previous column.	
Common:	
Dizziness.	Continue. Call doctor when convenient.
Infrequent:	
Chest pain; blurred vision; diarrhea; dry mouth; headache; numbness and tingling in arms, legs; nausea; abdominal pain.	Discontinue. Call doctor right away.
Rare:	
Sudden high fever.	Discontinue. Call doctor right away.

WARNINGS & PRECAUTIONS

Don't take if:
- You have pre-existing heart block.
- You have right bundle branch block.
- You are allergic to moricizine.

Before you start, consult your doctor:
- If you take any other prescription or nonprescription medicine.
- If you have liver or kidney disease.
- If you have any heart problems.

Over age 60:
No age-related adverse effects expected.

Pregnancy:
Consult doctor. Risk category B (see page xviii).

Breast-feeding:
Drug may pass into milk. Consult doctor.

Infants & children:
No special problems expected.

Prolonged use:
No special problems expected.

Skin & sunlight:
No special problems expected.

Driving, piloting or hazardous work:
Don't drive or pilot aircraft until you learn how medicine affects you. Don't work around dangerous machinery. Don't climb ladders or work in high places. Danger increases if you drink alcohol or take medicine affecting alertness and reflexes.

Discontinuing:
No special problems expected.

Others:
The first dose of this medication is usually given while the patient is being closely monitored in an intensive care setting with cardiac monitoring or in an emergency room.

POSSIBLE INTERACTION WITH OTHER DRUGS

GENERIC NAME OR DRUG CLASS	COMBINED EFFECT
Antiarrhythmics*, other	Possible increased effects of both drugs.
Cimetidine	Increased concentration of cimetidine in the blood.
Theophylline	Decreased effect of theophylline.

POSSIBLE INTERACTION WITH OTHER SUBSTANCES

INTERACTS WITH	COMBINED EFFECT
Alcohol:	Avoid.
Beverages:	None expected.
Cocaine:	Increased irregular heartbeat. Avoid.
Foods:	None expected.
Marijuana:	Possible increased irregular heartbeat. Avoid.
Tobacco:	Possible increased irregular heartbeat. Avoid.

*See Glossary

MUSCLE RELAXANTS, SKELETAL

GENERIC AND BRAND NAMES

CARISOPRODOL
- Rela
- Sodol
- Soma
- Soma Compound with Codeine
- Sopridol
- Soridol

CHLORPHENESIN
- Maolate

CHLORZOXAZONE
- Paraflex
- Parafon Forte

METAXALONE
- Skelaxin

METHOCARBAMOL
- Carbacot
- Delaxin
- Marbaxin
- Robamol
- Robaxin
- Robaxisal
- Robomol
- Skelex

BASIC INFORMATION

Habit forming? Possibly
Prescription needed? Yes
Available as generic? Yes, for some.
Drug class: Muscle relaxant

USES

Adjunctive treatment to rest, analgesics and physical therapy for muscle spasms.

DOSAGE & USAGE INFORMATION

How to take:
- Tablets—Swallow with liquid. If you can't swallow whole, crumble tablet and take with liquid or food. Instructions to take on empty stomach mean 1 hour before or 2 hours after eating.
- Extended-release tablets—Swallow whole with liquid. Don't crumble tablet.

When to take:
As needed, no more often than every 4 hours.

Continued next column

OVERDOSE

SYMPTOMS:
Nausea, vomiting, diarrhea, convulsions, headache. May progress to severe weakness, difficult breathing, sensation of paralysis, coma.

WHAT TO DO:
- **Dial 911 (emergency) for an ambulance or medical help or poison center 1-800-222-1222. Then give first aid immediately.**
- **See emergency information on inside covers.**

If you forget a dose:
Take as soon as you remember. Wait 4 hours for next dose (don't double this dose).

What drug does:
Blocks body's pain messages to brain. Also causes sedation.

Time lapse before drug works:
30 to 60 minutes.

Don't take with:
Any other medicine without consulting your doctor or pharmacist.

POSSIBLE ADVERSE REACTIONS OR SIDE EFFECTS

SYMPTOMS	WHAT TO DO
Life-threatening:	
Hives, rash, intense itching, faintness soon after a dose (anaphylaxis); extreme weakness, transient paralysis, temporary vision loss.	Seek emergency treatment immediately.
Common:	
• Drowsiness, dizziness.	Continue. Call doctor when convenient.
• Orange or red-purple urine.	No action necessary.
Infrequent:	
• Agitation, constipation or diarrhea, nausea, cramps, vomiting, wheezing, shortness of breath, headache, depression, muscle weakness, trembling, insomnia, uncontrolled eye movements, fainting.	Discontinue. Call doctor right away.
• Blurred vision.	Continue. Call Doctor when convenient.
Rare:	
• Black, tarry or bloody stool; convulsions.	Discontinue. Seek emergency treatment.
• Rash, hives, or itch; sore throat; fever; jaundice; tiredness; weakness; hiccups.	Discontinue. Call doctor right away.

WARNINGS & PRECAUTIONS

Don't take if:
- You are allergic to any skeletal muscle relaxant.
- You have porphyria.

Before you start, consult your doctor:
- If you have had liver or kidney disease.
- If you plan pregnancy within medication period.
- If you are allergic to tartrazine dye.
- If you suffer from depression.

Over age 60:
Adverse reactions and side effects may be more frequent and severe than in younger persons.

Pregnancy:
Safety not proven. Avoid if possible. Consult doctor. Risk category C (see page xviii).

Breast-feeding:
Drug may pass into milk. Avoid drug or discontinue nursing until you finish medicine. Consult doctor for advice on maintaining milk supply.

Infants & children:
Not recommended.

Prolonged use:
- Talk to your doctor about the need for follow-up medical examinations or laboratory studies to check liver function, kidney function, complete blood counts (white blood cell count, platelet count, red blood cell count, hemoglobin, hematocrit).
- Safety beyond 8 weeks of treatment not established.

Skin & sunlight:
No problems expected.

Driving, piloting or hazardous work:
Don't drive or pilot aircraft until you learn how medicine affects you. Don't work around dangerous machinery. Don't climb ladders or work in high places. Danger increases if you drink alcohol or take medicine affecting alertness and reflexes, such as antihistamines, tranquilizers, sedatives, pain medicine, narcotics and mind-altering drugs.

Discontinuing:
Don't discontinue without doctor's advice until you complete prescribed dose, even though symptoms diminish or disappear.

Others:
- May affect results in some medical tests.
- Advise any doctor or dentist whom you consult that you take this medicine.

POSSIBLE INTERACTION WITH OTHER DRUGS

GENERIC NAME OR DRUG CLASS	COMBINED EFFECT
Antidepressants*	Increased sedation.
Antihistamines*	Increased sedation.
Clozapine	Toxic effect on the central nervous system.
Central nervous system (CNS) depressants*	Increased depressive effects of both drugs.
Dronabinol	Increased effect of dronabinol on central nervous system. Avoid combination.
Mind-altering drugs*	Increased sedation.
Muscle relaxants*, others	Increased sedation.
Narcotics*	Increased sedation.
Sedatives*	Increased sedation.
Sertraline	Increased depressive effects of both drugs.
Sleep inducers*	Increased sedation.
Tranquilizers*	Increased sedation.

POSSIBLE INTERACTION WITH OTHER SUBSTANCES

INTERACTS WITH	COMBINED EFFECT
Alcohol:	Increased sedation.
Beverages:	None expected.
Cocaine:	Lack of coordination, increased sedation.
Foods:	None expected.
Marijuana:	Lack of coordination, drowsiness, fainting.
Tobacco:	None expected.

*See Glossary

NABILONE

BRAND NAMES

Cesamet

BASIC INFORMATION

Habit forming? No
Prescription needed? Yes
Available as generic? No
Drug class: Antiemetic

USES

- Treats nausea and vomiting.
- Prevents nausea and vomiting in patients receiving cancer chemotherapy.

DOSAGE & USAGE INFORMATION

How to take:
Capsule—Swallow with liquid. If you can't swallow whole, open capsule and take with liquid or food.

When to take:
At the same times each day, according to instructions on prescription label.

If you forget a dose:
Take as soon as you remember up to 2 hours late. If more than 2 hours, wait for next scheduled dose (don't double this dose).

What drug does:
Chemically related to marijuana, it probably regulates the vomiting control center in the brain.

Continued next column

OVERDOSE

SYMPTOMS:
Mood changes; confusion and delusions; hallucinations; mental depression; nervousness; breathing difficulty; fast, slow or pounding heartbeat; fainting.

WHAT TO DO:
- **Dial 911 (emergency) for an ambulance or medical help or poison center 1-800-222-1222. Then give first aid immediately.**
- **If patient is unconscious and not breathing, give mouth-to-mouth breathing. If there is no heartbeat, use cardiac massage and mouth-to-mouth breathing (CPR). Don't try to make patient vomit. If you can't get help quickly, take patient to nearest emergency facility.**
- **See emergency information on inside covers.**

Time lapse before drug works:
2 hours.

Don't take with:
Alcohol or any drug that depresses the central nervous system. See Central Nervous System (CNS) Depressants in the Glossary.

POSSIBLE ADVERSE REACTIONS OR SIDE EFFECTS

SYMPTOMS	WHAT TO DO
Life-threatening:	
Mood changes; fainting; hallucinations; fast, slow or pounding heartbeat; confusion and delusions; mental depression; nervousness; breathing difficulty.	Seek emergency treatment.
Common:	
Dry mouth.	Continue. Call doctor when convenient.
Infrequent:	
Clumsiness, mental changes, drowsiness, headache, false sense of well-being.	Discontinue. Call doctor right away.
Rare:	
Blurred vision, dizziness on standing, appetite loss, muscle pain.	Discontinue. Call doctor right away.

WARNINGS & PRECAUTIONS

Don't take if:
- You are allergic to nabilone or marijuana.
- You have schizophrenic, manic or depressive states.

Before you start, consult your doctor:
- If you have abused drugs or are dependent on them, including alcohol.
- If you have had high blood pressure or heart disease.
- If you have had impaired liver function.

Over age 60:
Adverse reactions and side effects may be more frequent and severe than in younger persons. You may need smaller doses for shorter periods of time.

Pregnancy:
Decide with your doctor whether drug benefits justify risk to unborn child. Risk category C (see page xviii).

Breast-feeding:
Drug passes into milk. Avoid drug or discontinue nursing until you finish medicine. Consult doctor for advice on maintaining milk supply.

Infants & children:
Not recommended for children 18 and younger. Use only under doctor's supervision.

Prolonged use:
- Avoid prolonged use. This medicine is intended to be used only during a cycle of cancer chemotherapy.
- Talk to your doctor about the need for follow-up medical examinations or laboratory studies to check blood pressure, heart function.

Skin & sunlight:
No problems expected.

Driving, piloting or hazardous work:
Don't drive or pilot aircraft until you learn how medicine affects you. Don't work around dangerous machinery. Don't climb ladders or work in high places. Danger increases if you drink alcohol or take medicine affecting alertness and reflexes.

Discontinuing:
No problems expected.

Others:
- Blood pressure should be measured regularly.
- Learn to count and recognize changes in your pulse.
- Get up from bed or chair slowly to avoid fainting.

POSSIBLE INTERACTION WITH OTHER DRUGS

GENERIC NAME OR DRUG CLASS	COMBINED EFFECT
Apomorphine	Decreased effect of apomorphine.
Central nervous system (CNS) depressants*, other	Greater depression of the central nervous system.

POSSIBLE INTERACTION WITH OTHER SUBSTANCES

INTERACTS WITH	COMBINED EFFECT
Alcohol:	Dangerous depression of the central nervous system. Avoid.
Beverages:	None expected.
Cocaine:	Decreased nabilone effect. Avoid.
Foods:	None expected.
Marijuana:	None expected.
Tobacco:	None expected.

*See Glossary

NAFARELIN

BRAND NAMES

Synarel

BASIC INFORMATION

Habit forming? No
Prescription needed? Yes
Available as generic? No
Drug class: Gonadotropin inhibitor

USES

- Treatment for endometriosis to relieve pain and reduce scattered implants of endometrial tissue.
- Treatment for central precocious puberty.

DOSAGE & USAGE INFORMATION

How to take:
Nasal spray—Follow instructions on package insert provided with your medicine.

When to take:
As directed by your doctor. Usually two times a day.

If you forget a dose:
Take as soon as you remember. Don't double this dose.

What drug does:
Reduces estrogen production by ovaries.

Time lapse before drug works:
May require 6 months for full effect.

Don't take with:
- Birth control pills.
- Nasal sprays to decongest the membranes in the nose.
- Any other medicine without consulting your doctor or pharmacist.

OVERDOSE

SYMPTOMS:
None expected.
WHAT TO DO:
Overdose unlikely to threaten life. If person takes much larger amount than prescribed, call doctor, poison center 1-800-222-1222 or hospital emergency room for instructions.

POSSIBLE ADVERSE REACTIONS OR SIDE EFFECTS

SYMPTOMS	WHAT TO DO
Life-threatening: None expected.	
Common: Hot flashes.	No action necessary.
Infrequent: Decreased sexual desire, vaginal dryness, headache, acne, swelling of hands and feet, reduction of breast size, weight gain, itchy scalp with flaking, muscle ache, nasal irritation.	Continue. Call doctor when convenient.
Rare: Insomnia, depression, weight loss.	Continue. Call doctor when convenient.

WARNINGS & PRECAUTIONS

Don't take if:
- You become pregnant.
- You have breast cancer.
- You are allergic to any of the ingredients in nafarelin.
- You have undiagnosed abnormal vaginal bleeding.

Before you start, consult your doctor:
- If you take birth control pills.
- If you have diabetes.
- If you have heart disease.
- If you have epilepsy.
- If you have kidney disease.
- If you have liver disease.
- If you have migraine headaches.
- If you need to use topical nasal decongestants.

Over age 60:
Adverse reactions and side effects may be more frequent and severe than in younger persons.

Pregnancy:
Risk to unborn child outweighs drug benefits. Don't use. Stop if you get pregnant. Consult doctor. Risk category X (see page xviii).

Breast-feeding:
Unknown whether medicine filters into milk. Consult doctor.

Infants & children:
Not recommended.

Prolonged use:
- Full effect requires prolonged use. Don't discontinue without consulting doctor.
- Talk to your doctor about the need for mammogram, follow-up medical examinations or laboratory studies to check liver function.

Skin & sunlight:
No special problems expected.

Driving, piloting or hazardous work:
No special problems expected.

Discontinuing:
Don't discontinue without consulting doctor. Menstrual periods may be absent for 2 to 3 months after discontinuation.

Others:
- May alter blood sugar levels in diabetic persons.
- Interferes with accuracy of laboratory tests to study pituitary gonadotropic and gonadal functions.
- Experience with nafarelin has been limited to women 18 years of age and older.
- Bone density decreases during treatment phase, but recovers following treatment.

POSSIBLE INTERACTION WITH OTHER DRUGS

GENERIC NAME OR DRUG CLASS	COMBINED EFFECT
Decongestant nasal sprays*	Decreased absorption of nafarelin.

POSSIBLE INTERACTION WITH OTHER SUBSTANCES

INTERACTS WITH	COMBINED EFFECT
Alcohol:	Excessive nervous system depression. Avoid.
Beverages: Caffeine drinks.	Rapid, irregular heartbeat. Avoid.
Cocaine:	May interfere with expected action of nafarelin. Avoid.
Foods:	None expected.
Marijuana:	May interfere with expected action of nafarelin. Avoid.
Tobacco:	Rapid, irregular heartbeat; increased leg cramps. Avoid.

*See Glossary

NALIDIXIC ACID

BRAND NAMES

NegGram

BASIC INFORMATION

Habit forming? No
Prescription needed? Yes
Available as generic? Yes
Drug class: Antimicrobial

USES

Treatment for urinary tract infections.

DOSAGE & USAGE INFORMATION

How to take:
- Tablet—Swallow with food or milk to lessen stomach irritation. If you can't swallow whole, crumble tablet and take with liquid or food.
- Liquid—Take with liquid or food.

When to take:
At the same times each day.

If you forget a dose:
Take as soon as you remember up to 2 hours late. If more than 2 hours, wait for next scheduled dose (don't double this dose).

What drug does:
Destroys bacteria susceptible to nalidixic acid.

Time lapse before drug works:
1 to 2 weeks.

Don't take with:
Any other medicine without consulting your doctor or pharmacist.

OVERDOSE

SYMPTOMS:
Lethargy, stomach upset, behavioral changes, hyperglycemia, psychosis, convulsions and stupor.
WHAT TO DO:
- **Dial 911 (emergency) for an ambulance or medical help or poison center 1-800-222-1222. Then give first aid immediately.**
- **If patient is unconscious and not breathing, give mouth-to-mouth breathing. If there is no heartbeat, use cardiac massage and mouth-to-mouth breathing (CPR). Don't try to make patient vomit. If you can't get help quickly, take patient to nearest emergency facility.**
- **See emergency information on inside covers.**

POSSIBLE ADVERSE REACTIONS OR SIDE EFFECTS

SYMPTOMS	WHAT TO DO
Life-threatening:	
Hives, rash, intense itching, faintness soon after a dose (anaphylaxis).	Seek emergency treatment immediately.
Common:	
Rash; itchy skin; decreased, blurred or double vision; halos around lights or excess brightness; changes in color vision; nausea; vomiting; diarrhea.	Discontinue. Call doctor right away.
Infrequent:	
• Dizziness, drowsiness, sensitivity to sun, headache.	Continue. Call doctor when convenient.
• Dark urine, hallucinations, mood changes.	Discontinue. Call doctor right away.
Rare:	
Paleness, sore throat or fever, severe abdominal pain, pale stool, unusual bleeding or bruising, jaundice, fatigue, weakness, seizures, psychosis, joint pain, numbness or tingling in hands or feet.	Discontinue. Call doctor right away.

WARNINGS & PRECAUTIONS

Don't take if:
- You are allergic to nalidixic acid.
- You have a seizure disorder (epilepsy, convulsions).

Before you start, consult your doctor:
- If you plan to become pregnant within medication period.
- If you have or have had kidney or liver disease.
- If you have impaired circulation of the brain (hardened arteries).
- If you have Parkinson's disease.
- If you have diabetes (drug may affect urine sugar tests).

Over age 60:
Adverse reactions and side effects may be more frequent and severe than in younger persons.

Pregnancy:
Consult doctor. Risk category B (see page xviii).

Breast-feeding:
Drug passes into milk. Avoid drug or discontinue nursing until you finish medicine. Consult doctor for advice on maintaining milk supply.

Infants & children:
Not recommended.

Prolonged use:
Talk to your doctor about the need for follow-up medical examinations or laboratory studies to check complete blood counts (white blood cell count, platelet count, red blood cell count, hemoglobin, hematocrit), liver function, kidney function.

Skin & sunlight:
May cause rash or intensify sunburn in areas exposed to sun or ultraviolet light (photosensitivity reaction). Avoid overexposure. Notify doctor if reaction occurs.

Driving, piloting or hazardous work:
Avoid if you feel drowsy, dizzy or have vision problems. Otherwise, no problems expected.

Discontinuing:
Don't discontinue without consulting doctor. Dose may require gradual reduction if you have taken drug for a long time. Doses of other drugs may also require adjustment.

Others:
Periodic blood counts and liver and kidney function tests recommended.

POSSIBLE INTERACTION WITH OTHER DRUGS

GENERIC NAME OR DRUG CLASS	COMBINED EFFECT
Antacids*	Decreased absorption of nalidixic acid.
Anticoagulants*, oral	Increased anticoagulant effect.
Calcium supplements*	Decreased effect of nalidixic acid.
Nitrofurantoin	Decreased effect of nalidixic acid.
Probenecid	Decreased effect of nalidixic acid.
Vitamin C (in large doses)	Increased effect of nalidixic acid.

POSSIBLE INTERACTION WITH OTHER SUBSTANCES

INTERACTS WITH	COMBINED EFFECT
Alcohol:	Impaired alertness, judgment and coordination.
Beverages:	None expected.
Cocaine:	Impaired judgment and coordination.
Foods:	None expected.
Marijuana:	Impaired alertness, judgment and coordination.
Tobacco:	None expected.

NALTREXONE

BRAND NAMES

Barr
ReVia

BASIC INFORMATION

Habit forming? No
Prescription needed? Yes
Available as generic? Yes
Drug class: Narcotic antagonist

USES

- Treats detoxified former narcotics addicts. It helps maintain a drug-free state.
- May be used to treat alcoholism (in conjunction with counseling).

DOSAGE & USAGE INFORMATION

How to take:
- *Don't take at all until detoxification has been accomplished.*
- Tablets—Swallow with liquid or food to lessen stomach irritation. If you can't swallow whole, crumble tablet and take with liquid or food.

When to take:
At the same time every day or every other day as directed.

If you forget a dose:
Follow detailed instructions from the one who prescribed for you.

What drug does:
Binds to opioid receptors in the central nervous system and blocks the effects of narcotic drugs.

Time lapse before drug works:
1 hour.

Don't take with:
- Narcotics.
- Any other medicine without consulting your doctor or pharmacist.

OVERDOSE

SYMPTOMS:
Seizures, coma.
WHAT TO DO:
- **Dial 911 (emergency) for an ambulance or medical help or poison center 1-800-222-1222. Then give first aid immediately.**
- **See emergency information at end of book.**

POSSIBLE ADVERSE REACTIONS OR SIDE EFFECTS

SYMPTOMS	WHAT TO DO
Life-threatening:	
Hallucinations, very fast heartbeat, fainting, breathing difficulties.	Seek emergency treatment immediately.
Common:	
Skin rash, chills, constipation, appetite loss, irritability, insomnia, anxiety, headache, nausea, vomiting.	Continue. Call doctor when convenient.
Infrequent:	
• Nosebleeds, joint pain.	Discontinue. Call doctor right away.
• Abdominal pain, blurred vision, confusion, earache, fever, depression, diarrhea, common cold symptoms.	Continue. Call doctor when convenient.
Rare:	
• Pain, tenderness or color change in feet.	Discontinue. Call doctor right away.
• Ringing in ears, swollen glands, decreased sex drive.	Continue. Call doctor when convenient.

WARNINGS & PRECAUTIONS

Don't take if:
- You don't have close medical supervision.
- You are currently dependent on drugs.
- You have severe liver disease.

Before you start, consult your doctor:
If you have mild liver disease.

Over age 60:
Adverse reactions and side effects may be more frequent and severe than in younger persons. You may need smaller doses for shorter periods of time.

Pregnancy:
Decide with your doctor whether drug benefits justify risk to unborn child. Risk category C (see page xviii).

Breast-feeding:
Safety not established. Consult doctor.

Infants & children:
Not recommended.

Prolonged use:
- Not recommended.
- Talk to your doctor about the need for follow-up medical examinations or laboratory studies to check kidney function.

Skin & sunlight:
No problems expected.

Driving, piloting or hazardous work:
Don't drive or pilot aircraft until you learn how medicine affects you. Don't work around dangerous machinery. Don't climb ladders or work in high places. Danger increases if you drink alcohol or take medicine affecting alertness and reflexes.

Discontinuing:
Don't discontinue without consulting doctor. Dose may require gradual reduction if you have taken drug for a long time. Doses of other drugs may also require adjustment.

Others:
- Probably not effective in treating people addicted to substances other than opium or morphine derivatives.
- Must be given under close supervision by people experienced in using naltrexone to treat addicts.
- Attempting to use narcotics to overcome effects of naltrexone may lead to coma and death.
- Advise any doctor or dentist whom you consult that you take this medicine.
- Withdraw from medication several days prior to expected surgery.

POSSIBLE INTERACTION WITH OTHER DRUGS

GENERIC NAME OR DRUG CLASS	COMBINED EFFECT
Narcotic medicines* (butorphanol, codeine, heroin, hydrocodone, hydromorphone, levorphanol, morphine, nalbuphine, opium, oxycodone, oxymorphone, paregoric, pentazocine, propoxyphene)	1. Precipitates withdrawal symptoms. May lead to cardiac arrest, coma and death (if naltrexone taken while person is dependent on these drugs). 2. If these drugs are taken while person is taking naltrexone, opioid effect (pain relief) will be blocked.
Isoniazid	Increased risk of liver damage.

POSSIBLE INTERACTION WITH OTHER SUBSTANCES

INTERACTS WITH	COMBINED EFFECT
Alcohol:	Unpredictable effects. Avoid.
Beverages:	None expected.
Cocaine:	Unpredictable effects. Avoid.
Foods:	None expected.
Marijuana:	Unpredictable effects. Avoid.
Tobacco:	None expected.

*See Glossary

NARCOTIC ANALGESICS

GENERIC AND BRAND NAMES

See complete list of generic and brand names in the *Generic and Brand Name Directory*, page 862.

BASIC INFORMATION

Habit forming? Yes
Prescription needed? Yes
Available as generic? Yes
Drug class: Narcotic

USES

Relieves pain and diarrhea; suppresses cough.

DOSAGE & USAGE INFORMATION

How to take:

- Tablet, capsule or extended-release tablet—Swallow with liquid. If you can't swallow whole, crumble tablet or open capsule and take with liquid or food. Do not crush or crumble extended release forms.
- Liquid form of morphine—Mix with fruit juice just before taking to improve taste.
- Syrup—Mix with one-half glass of water (4 oz.) before swallowing.
- Dispersible tablets—Stir into water or fruit juice just before taking each dose.
- Liquid forms—May need to be diluted with water before taking. Follow directions on label.
- Suppositories—Remove wrapper and moisten suppository with water. Gently insert into rectum, small end first.
- Transdermal—Follow instructions on prescription.

Continued next column

- Nasal—Follow package instructions.
- Transmucosal—Follow instructions on prescription.

When to take:
When needed. No more often than every 4 hours.

If you forget a dose:
Take as soon as you remember. Wait 4 hours for next dose.

What drug does:

- Blocks pain messages to brain and spinal cord.
- Reduces sensitivity of brain's cough control center.

Time lapse before drug works:
30 minutes.

Don't take with:
Any other medicine without consulting your doctor or pharmacist.

OVERDOSE

SYMPTOMS:
Deep sleep, slow breathing; slow pulse; respiratory arrest; flushed, warm skin; seizures; constricted pupils.

WHAT TO DO:

- **Dial 911 (emergency) for an ambulance or medical help or poison center 1-800-222-1222. Then give first aid immediately.**
- **If patient is unconscious and not breathing, give mouth-to-mouth breathing. If there is no heartbeat, use cardiac massage and mouth-to-mouth breathing (CPR). Don't try to make patient vomit. If you can't get help quickly, take patient to nearest emergency facility.**
- **See emergency information on inside covers.**

POSSIBLE ADVERSE REACTIONS OR SIDE EFFECTS

SYMPTOMS	WHAT TO DO
Life-threatening:	
Irregular or slow heartbeat, difficult breathing, wheezing.	Discontinue. Seek emergency treatment.
Common:	
Dizziness, drowsiness, tiredness, headache, lightheadedness, nausea or vomiting, stomach cramps, overexcitement.	Continue. Call doctor when convenient.
Infrequent:	
• Black, tarry stools; bloody or cloudy urine; painful or frequent urination; fast, slow or pounding heartbeat; hallucinations; breathing problems, wheezing; back or side pain; red dots on skin; red or flushed face; ringing or buzzing in ears; skin rash, hives or itching; sore throat; fever; face swelling; decreased urine; trembling; uncontrolled muscle movements; unusual bleeding or bruising; yellow skin or eyes.	Discontinue. Call doctor right away.
• Feeling depressed, pale stools.	Continue. Call doctor when convenient.

Rare:

Changes in vision, constipation, dry mouth, loss of appetite, restlessness, night-mares, trouble sleeping.	Discontinue. Call doctor when convenient.

WARNINGS & PRECAUTIONS

Don't take if:
- You are allergic to any narcotic.
- Diarrhea is due to toxic effect of drugs or poisons.

Before you start, consult your doctor:
- If you have impaired liver or kidney function.
- If you will have surgery within 2 months, including dental surgery, requiring general or spinal anesthesia.
- If you have asthma.

Over age 60:
More likely to be drowsy, dizzy, unsteady or constipated. Use only if absolutely necessary.

Pregnancy:
Risk factors vary for drugs in this group. See category list on page xviii and consult doctor.

Breast-feeding:
Drug filters into milk. May harm child. Avoid.

Infants & children:
Not recommended.

Prolonged use:
- With high doses and long-term use, can cause psychological and physical dependence (addiction).
- May cause chronic constipation.

Skin & sunlight:
No special problems expected.

Driving, piloting or hazardous work:
Don't drive or pilot aircraft until you learn how medicine affects you. Don't work around dangerous machinery. Don't climb ladders or work in high places. Danger increases if you drink alcohol or take medicine affecting alertness and reflexes, such as antihistamines, tranquilizers, sedatives, pain medicine, narcotics and mind-altering drugs.

Discontinuing:
- Discontinue in 2 days if symptoms don't improve. Report to the doctor any symptoms that develop after discontinuing, such as gooseflesh, irritability, insomnia, yawning, weakness, large eye pupils.
- If used for several weeks or more, consult doctor before discontinuing.

Others:
- Some products contain tartrazine dye. Avoid, especially if you are allergic to aspirin.
- Lying down after the first few doses may decrease unwanted effects of nausea, vomiting, lightheadedness or dizziness.

POSSIBLE INTERACTION WITH OTHER DRUGS

GENERIC NAME OR DRUG CLASS	COMBINED EFFECT
Analgesics*, other	Increased analgesic effect.
Anticoagulants*, oral	Possible increased anticoagulant effect.
Anticholinergics*	Increased anticholinergic effect.
Antidepressants*	Increased sedative effect.
Antihistamines*	Increased sedative effect.
Anti-inflammatory drugs, nonsteroidal (NSAIDs)*	Increased narcotic effect.
Butorphanol	Possibly precipitates withdrawal with chronic narcotic use.
Carbamazepine	Increased carba-mazepine effect possible with propoxyphene.
Carteolol	Increased narcotic effect. Dangerous sedation.

Continued on page 922

POSSIBLE INTERACTION WITH OTHER SUBSTANCES

INTERACTS WITH	COMBINED EFFECT
Alcohol:	Increased intoxicat-ing effect of alcohol. Avoid.
Beverages:	None expected.
Cocaine:	Increased toxic effects of cocaine. Avoid.
Foods:	None expected.
Marijuana:	Impaired physical and mental perfor-mance. Avoid.
Tobacco:	None expected.

*See Glossary

NARCOTIC ANALGESICS & ACETAMINOPHEN

GENERIC AND BRAND NAMES

See complete list of generic and brand names in the *Generic and Brand Name Directory*, page 862.

BASIC INFORMATION

Habit forming? Yes
Prescription needed? Yes
Available as generic? Yes
Drug class: Narcotic, analgesic, fever reducer

USES

Relieves pain.

DOSAGE & USAGE INFORMATION

How to take:

- Tablet or capsule—Swallow with liquid. If you can't swallow whole, crumble tablet or open capsule and take with liquid or food.
- Syrup—Mix with one-half glass of water (4 oz.) before swallowing.
- Liquid forms—May need to be diluted with water before taking. Follow directions on label.

When to take:
When needed. No more often than every 4 hours.

If you forget a dose:
Take as soon as you remember. Wait 4 hours for next dose.

Continued next column

OVERDOSE

SYMPTOMS:
Stomach upset; irritability; sweating, convulsions; deep sleep; slow breathing; slow pulse; flushed, warm skin; constricted pupils; coma.
WHAT TO DO:

- **Dial 911 (emergency) for an ambulance or medical help or poison center 1-800-222-1222. Then give first aid immediately.**
- **If patient is unconscious and not breathing, give mouth-to-mouth breathing. If there is no heartbeat, use cardiac massage and mouth-to-mouth breathing (CPR). Don't try to make patient vomit. If you can't get help quickly, take patient to nearest emergency facility.**
- **See emergency information on inside covers.**

What drug does:

- May affect hypothalamus—the part of the brain that helps regulate body heat and receives body's pain messages.
- Blocks pain messages to brain and spinal cord.
- Reduces sensitivity of brain's cough control center.

Time lapse before drug works:
15 to 30 minutes. May last 4 hours.

Don't take with:

- Other drugs with acetaminophen. Too much acetaminophen can damage liver and kidneys.
- Any other medicine without consulting your doctor or pharmacist.

POSSIBLE ADVERSE REACTIONS OR SIDE EFFECTS

SYMPTOMS	WHAT TO DO
Life-threatening:	
Irregular or slow heartbeat, difficult breathing, wheezing.	Discontinue. Seek emergency treatment.
Common:	
Dizziness, drowsiness, tiredness, headache, lightheadedness, nausea or vomiting, stomach cramps, overexcitement.	Continue. Call doctor when convenient.
Infrequent:	
• Black, tarry stools; bloody or cloudy urine; painful or frequent urination; fast, slow or pounding heartbeat; hallucinations; breathing problems, wheezing; back or side pain; red dots on skin; red or flushed face; ringing or buzzing in ears; skin rash, hives or itching; sore throat; fever; face swelling; decreased urine; trembling; uncontrolled muscle movements; unusual bleeding or bruising; yellow skin or eyes.	Discontinue. Call doctor right away.
• Feeling depressed, pale stools.	Continue. Call doctor when convenient.
Rare:	
Changes in vision, constipation, dry mouth, loss of appetite, restlessness, nightmares, trouble sleeping.	Discontinue. Call doctor when convenient.

WARNINGS & PRECAUTIONS

Don't take if:
- You are allergic to any narcotic or acetaminophen.
- Your symptoms don't improve after 2 days use. Call your doctor.

Before you start, consult your doctor:
- If you have bronchial asthma, kidney disease or liver damage.
- If you will have surgery within 2 months, including dental surgery, requiring general or spinal anesthesia.

Over age 60:
More likely to be drowsy, dizzy, unsteady or constipated. Don't exceed recommended dose. You can't eliminate drug as efficiently as younger persons. Use only if absolutely necessary.

Pregnancy:
Risk factors vary for drugs in this group. See category list on page xviii and consult doctor.

Breast-feeding:
Drug filters into milk. May harm child. Avoid.

Infants & children:
Not recommended.

Prolonged use:
- With high doses and long-term use, can cause psychological and physical dependence (addiction).
- May cause chronic constipation.

Skin & sunlight:
No problems expected.

Driving, piloting or hazardous work:
Don't drive or pilot aircraft until you learn how medicine affects you. Don't work around dangerous machinery. Don't climb ladders or work in high places. Danger increases if you drink alcohol or take medicine affecting alertness and reflexes, such as antihistamines, tranquilizers, sedatives, pain medicine, narcotics and mind-altering drugs.

Discontinuing:
- Discontinue in 2 days if symptoms don't improve. Report to your doctor any symptoms that develop after discontinuing, such as gooseflesh, irritability, insomnia, yawning, weakness, large eye pupils.
- If used for several weeks or more, consult doctor before discontinuing.

Others:
Lying down after the first few doses may decrease unwanted effects of nausea, vomiting, lightheadedness or dizziness.

POSSIBLE INTERACTION WITH OTHER DRUGS

GENERIC NAME OR DRUG CLASS	COMBINED EFFECT
Analgesics*, other	Increased analgesic effect.
Anticoagulants*, other	May increase anticoagulant effect. Prothrombin times should be monitored.
Anticholinergics*	Increased anticholinergic effect.
Antidepressants*	Increased sedative effect.
Antihistamines*	Increased sedative effect.
Carteolol	Increased narcotic effect. Dangerous sedation.
Mind-altering drugs*	Increased sedative effect.
Narcotics*, other	Increased narcotic effect.
Nitrates*	Excessive blood pressure drop.
Phenobarbital and other barbiturates*	Quicker elimination and decreased effect of acetaminophen.

Continued on page 923

POSSIBLE INTERACTION WITH OTHER SUBSTANCES

INTERACTS WITH	COMBINED EFFECT
Alcohol:	Increased intoxicating effect of alcohol. Long-term use may cause toxic effect in liver. Avoid.
Beverages:	None expected.
Cocaine:	Increased toxic effects of cocaine. Avoid.
Foods:	None expected.
Marijuana:	Impaired physical and mental performance. Avoid.
Tobacco:	None expected.

***See Glossary**

NARCOTIC ANALGESICS & ASPIRIN

GENERIC AND BRAND NAMES

See complete list of generic and brand names in the *Generic and Brand Name Directory*, page 862.

BASIC INFORMATION

Habit forming? Yes
Prescription needed? Yes
Available as generic? Yes
Drug class: Narcotic, analgesic, anti-inflammatory (nonsteroidal)

USES

Reduces pain, fever, inflammation.

DOSAGE & USAGE INFORMATION

How to take:
Tablet or capsule—Swallow with liquid. If you can't swallow whole, crumble tablet or open capsule and take with liquid or food.

When to take:
When needed. No more often than every 4 hours.

If you forget a dose:
Take as soon as you remember. Wait 4 hours for next dose.

Continued next column

OVERDOSE

SYMPTOMS:
Ringing in ears; nausea; vomiting; dizziness; fever; deep sleep; slow breathing; slow pulse; flushed, warm skin; constricted pupils; hallucinations; convulsions; coma.
WHAT TO DO:
- **Dial 911 (emergency) for an ambulance or medical help or poison center 1-800-222-1222. Then give first aid immediately.**
- **If patient is unconscious and not breathing, give mouth-to-mouth breathing. If there is no heartbeat, use cardiac massage and mouth-to-mouth breathing (CPR). Don't try to make patient vomit. If you can't get help quickly, take patient to nearest emergency facility.**
- **See emergency information on inside covers.**

What drug does:
- Affects hypothalamus, the part of the brain which regulates temperature by dilating small blood vessels in skin.
- Prevents clumping of platelets (small blood cells) so blood vessels remain open.
- Decreases prostaglandin effect.
- Suppresses body's pain messages.
- Reduces sensitivity of brain's cough control center.

Time lapse before drug works:
30 minutes.

Don't take with:
- Tetracyclines. Space doses 1 hour apart.
- Any other medicine without consulting your doctor or pharmacist.

POSSIBLE ADVERSE REACTIONS OR SIDE EFFECTS

SYMPTOMS	WHAT TO DO
Life-threatening:	
Irregular or slow heartbeat, difficult breathing, wheezing.	Discontinue. Seek emergency treatment.
Common:	
Dizziness, drowsiness, tiredness, headache, lightheadedness, nausea or vomiting, stomach cramps, overexcitement.	Continue. Call doctor when convenient.
Infrequent:	
• Black, tarry stools; bloody or cloudy urine; painful or frequent urination; fast, slow or pounding heartbeat; hallucinations; breathing problems, wheezing; back or side pain; red dots on skin; red or flushed face; ringing or buzzing in ears; skin rash, hives or itching; sore throat; fever; face swelling; decreased urine; trembling; uncontrolled muscle movements; unusual bleeding or bruising; yellow skin or eyes.	Discontinue. Call doctor right away.
• Feeling depressed, pale stools.	Continue. Call doctor when convenient.
Rare:	
Changes in vision, constipation, dry mouth, loss of appetite, restlessness, nightmares, trouble sleeping.	Discontinue. Call doctor when convenient.

WARNINGS & PRECAUTIONS

Don't take if:
- You are allergic to any narcotic or subject to any substance abuse.
- You have a peptic ulcer of stomach or duodenum or a bleeding disorder.

Before you start, consult your doctor:
- If you have impaired liver or kidney function, asthma or nasal polyps.
- If you have had stomach or duodenal ulcers, gout.
- If you will have surgery within 2 months, including dental surgery, requiring general or spinal anesthesia.

Over age 60:
- More likely to be drowsy, dizzy, unsteady or constipated. Use only if absolutely necessary.
- More likely to cause hidden bleeding in stomach or intestines. Watch for dark stools.

Pregnancy:
Risk factors vary for drugs in this group. See category list on page xviii and consult doctor.

Breast-feeding:
Drug passes into milk and may harm child. Avoid drug or discontinue nursing until you finish medicine. Consult doctor for advice on maintaining milk supply.

Infants & children:
Not recommended.

Prolonged use:
- With high doses and long-term use, can cause psychological and physical dependence (addiction).
- May cause chronic constipation.

Skin & sunlight:
No special problems expected.

Driving, piloting or hazardous work:
Don't drive or pilot aircraft until you learn how medicine affects you. Don't work around dangerous machinery. Don't climb ladders or work in high places. Danger increases if you drink alcohol or take medicine affecting alertness and reflexes, such as antihistamines, tranquilizers, sedatives, pain medicine, narcotics and mind-altering drugs.

Discontinuing:
- Discontinue in 2 to 3 days if symptoms don't improve. Report to your doctor any symptoms that develop after discontinuing, such as gooseflesh, irritability, insomnia, yawning, weakness, large eye pupils.
- If used for several weeks or more, consult doctor before discontinuing.

Others:
- Aspirin can complicate surgery; illness; pregnancy, labor and delivery.
- Urine tests for blood sugar may be inaccurate
- Lying down after the first few doses may decrease unwanted effects of nausea, vomiting, lightheadedness or dizziness.
- Don't use if medicine has a strong vinegar-like odor. This means the aspirin is breaking down.

POSSIBLE INTERACTION WITH OTHER DRUGS

GENERIC NAME OR DRUG CLASS	COMBINED EFFECT
Acebutolol	Decreased anti-hypertensive effect of acebutolol.
Adrenocorticoids, systemic	Increased risk of ulcers. Increased adrenocorticoid effect.
Alendonate	Increased risk of stomach irritation.
Allopurinol	Decreased allopurinol effect.
Angiotensin-converting enzyme (ACE) inhibitors*	Decreased effect of ACE inhibitor.
Antacids*	Decreased aspirin effect.
Anticoagulants*, oral	Increased anticoagulant effect. Abnormal bleeding.
Antidepressants*	Increased sedative effect.
Antidiabetics*, oral	Low blood sugar.

Continued on page 923

POSSIBLE INTERACTION WITH OTHER SUBSTANCES

INTERACTS WITH	COMBINED EFFECT
Alcohol:	Possible stomach irritation and bleeding. Increased intoxicating effect of alcohol. Avoid.
Beverages:	None expected.
Cocaine:	Decreased cocaine toxic effects. Avoid.
Foods:	None expected.
Marijuana:	Impaired physical and mental performance. Avoid.
Tobacco:	None expected.

***See Glossary**

NATAMYCIN (Ophthalmic)

BRAND NAMES

Natacyn
Pimaricin

BASIC INFORMATION

Habit forming? No
Prescription needed? Yes
Available as generic? No
Drug class: Antifungal (ophthalmic)

USES

Treats fungus infections of the eye.

DOSAGE & USAGE INFORMATION

How to use:
Eye drops
- Wash hands.
- Apply pressure to inside corner of eye with middle finger.
- Tilt head backward. Pull lower lid away from eye with index finger of the same hand.
- Drop eye drops into pouch and close eye. Don't blink.
- Continue pressure for 1 minute after placing medicine in eye.
- Keep eyes closed for 1 to 2 minutes.
- Don't touch applicator tip to any surface (including the eye). If you accidentally touch tip, clean with warm soap and water.
- Keep container tightly closed.
- Keep drops cool, but don't freeze.
- Wash hands immediately after using.

When to use:
As directed. Usually 1 drop in eye every 1 or 2 hours for 3 or 4 days, then every 3 to 4 hours.

If you forget a dose:
Use as soon as you remember.

What drug does:
Changes cell membrane of fungus causing loss of essential constituents of fungus cell.

Continued next column

OVERDOSE

SYMPTOMS:
None expected.
WHAT TO DO:
Not intended for internal use. If child accidentally swallows, call poison center 1-800-222-1222.

Time lapse before drug works:
Starts to work immediately. May require 2 weeks or more to cure infection.

Don't use with:
Other eye drops without consulting your eye doctor.

POSSIBLE ADVERSE REACTIONS OR SIDE EFFECTS

SYMPTOMS	WHAT TO DO
Life-threatening:	
None expected.	
Common:	
None expected.	
Infrequent:	
Eye irritation not present before using natamycin.	Discontinue. Call doctor right away.
Rare:	
None expected.	

WARNINGS & PRECAUTIONS

Don't use if:
You are allergic to natamycin or any antifungal medicine*.

Before you start, consult your doctor:
If you have allergies to any substance.

Over age 60:
No problems expected.

Pregnancy:
Decide with your doctor if drug benefits justify risk to unborn child. Risk category C (see page xviii).

Breast-feeding:
No problems expected, but check with doctor.

Infants & children:
No problems expected.

Prolonged use:
May cause eye irritation.

Skin & sunlight:
No problems expected.

Driving, piloting or hazardous work:
No problems expected.

Discontinuing:
Don't discontinue without consulting your eye doctor.

Others:
Notify doctor if condition doesn't improve within 1 week.

POSSIBLE INTERACTION WITH OTHER DRUGS

GENERIC NAME OR DRUG CLASS	COMBINED EFFECT
Clinically significant interactions with oral or injected medicines unlikely.	

POSSIBLE INTERACTION WITH OTHER SUBSTANCES

INTERACTS WITH	COMBINED EFFECT
Alcohol:	None expected.
Beverages:	None expected.
Cocaine:	None expected.
Foods:	None expected.
Marijuana:	None expected.
Tobacco:	None expected.

***See Glossary**

NEDOCROMIL

BRAND NAMES

Tilade

BASIC INFORMATION

Habit forming? No
Prescription needed? Yes
Available as generic? No
Drug class: Antiasthmatic (anti-inflammatory)

USES

For maintenance treatment of mild to moderate asthma. Not used to treat an active asthma attack.

DOSAGE & USAGE INFORMATION

How to take:
Inhaler–Follow instructions on the metered-dose inhaler pack.

When to take:
At the same times each day. Initial treatment is usually 2 inhalations 4 times a day. After symptoms subside, dosage may be reduced by your doctor.

If you forget a dose:
Take as soon as you remember up to 2 hours late. If more than 2 hours, wait for next scheduled dose (don't double this dose).

What drug does:
Inhibits inflammatory cells associated with asthma. Inhibits reflex reactions to irritants and to exercise and cold.

Time lapse before drug works:
2 to 4 days, but may require several weeks to achieve maximum effectiveness.

Don't take with:
Any other prescription or nonprescription drug without consulting your doctor.

OVERDOSE

SYMPTOMS:
None expected.
WHAT TO DO:
Overdose unlikely to threaten life. If person takes much larger amount than prescribed, call doctor, poison center 1-800-222-1222 or hospital emergency room for instructions.

POSSIBLE ADVERSE REACTIONS OR SIDE EFFECTS

SYMPTOMS	WHAT TO DO
Life-threatening: None expected.	
Common: Unpleasant taste.	No action necessary.
Infrequent:	
• Headache, nausea, throat irritation, cough, runny nose or stuffy nose.	Continue. Call doctor when convenient.
• Increased bronchospasm (increased wheezing, tightness in chest, difficulty in breathing).	Discontinue. Call doctor right away.
Rare: None expected.	

WARNINGS & PRECAUTIONS

Don't take if:
You are allergic to nedocromil.

Before you start, consult your doctor:
No problems expected.

Over age 60:
No problems expected.

Pregnancy:
Decide with your doctor if drug benefits outweigh risks to unborn child. Risk category C (see page xviii).

Breast-feeding:
Not known if drug passes into milk. Consult with your doctor.

Infants & children:
Give only under close medical supervision, especially to children younger than age 12.

Prolonged use:
No problems expected.

Skin & sunlight:
No problems expected.

Driving, piloting or hazardous work:
No problems expected.

Discontinuing:
No problems expected. Don't discontinue abruptly without talking to your doctor.

Others:
- Advise any doctor or dentist whom you consult that you take this medicine.
- May affect the results in some medical tests.

POSSIBLE INTERACTION WITH OTHER DRUGS

GENERIC NAME OR DRUG CLASS	COMBINED EFFECT
None expected.	

POSSIBLE INTERACTION WITH OTHER SUBSTANCES

INTERACTS WITH	COMBINED EFFECT
Alcohol:	None expected.
Beverages:	None expected.
Cocaine:	None expected.
Foods:	None expected.
Marijuana:	None expected.
Tobacco:	None expected.

*See Glossary

NEFAZODONE

BRAND NAMES

Serzone

BASIC INFORMATION

Habit forming? No
Prescription needed? Yes
Available as generic? No
Drug class: Antidepressant (phenylpiperazine)

USES

Treats symptoms of mental depression.

DOSAGE & USAGE INFORMATION

How to take:
Tablet—Swallow with liquid. May be taken with or without food.

When to take:
At the same times each day. The prescribed dosage may be increased weekly until maximum benefits are achieved.

If you forget a dose:
Take as soon as you remember up to 2 hours late. If more than 2 hours, wait for the next scheduled dose (don't double this dose).

What drug does:
The exact mechanism is unknown. It appears to block reuptake of serotonin and norepinephrine (stimulating chemicals in the brain that play a role in emotions and psychological disturbances).

Time lapse before drug works:
Will take up to several weeks to relieve the depression.

Don't take with:
Any other medication without consulting your doctor or pharmacist.

OVERDOSE

SYMPTOMS:
Drowsiness, nausea, vomiting, low blood pressure (faintness, weakness, dizziness, lightheadedness) or increased severity of adverse reactions.
WHAT TO DO:
- **Dial 911 (emergency) for an ambulance or medical help or poison center 1-800-222-1222. Then give first aid immediately.**
- **See emergency information at end of book.**

POSSIBLE ADVERSE REACTIONS OR SIDE EFFECTS

SYMPTOMS	WHAT TO DO
Life-threatening: In case of overdose, see previous column.	
Common:	
• Clumsiness or unsteadiness, blurred vision or other vision changes, fainting, lightheadedness, ringing in the ears, skin rash or itching.	Discontinue. Call doctor right away.
• Strange dreams, constipation or diarrhea, dry mouth, heartburn, fever, chills, flushing or feeling warm, headache, increased appetite, insomnia, coughing, tingling or prickly sensations, sore throat, trembling, drowsiness, confusion or agitation, memory lapses.	Continue. Call doctor when convenient.
Infrequent:	
• Tightness in chest; trouble breathing; wheezing; eye pain; combination of nausea, vomiting, diarrhea and stomach pain.	Discontinue. Call doctor right away.
• Joint pain, breast pain, increased thirst.	Continue. Call doctor when convenient.
Rare:	
• Face swelling, hives, muscle pain or stiffness, chest pain, fast heartbeat, mood or mental changes, difficulty speaking, hallucinations, uncontrolled excited behavior, twitching, ear pain, increased hearing sensitivity, bleeding or bruising, irritated red eyes, eyes sensitive to light, pain in back or side, swollen glands, problems with urination.	Discontinue. Call doctor right away.
• Unusual tiredness or weakness, false sense of well-being, menstrual changes, change in sexual desire or function.	Continue. Call doctor when convenient.

WARNINGS & PRECAUTIONS

Don't use if:
You are allergic to nefazodone or trazodone (phenylpiperazine antidepressants).

Before you start, consult your doctor:
- If you have a seizure disorder, heart disease or blood circulation problem or have had a stroke.
- If you are dehydrated.
- If you have a history of drug dependence or drug abuse.
- If you have a history of mood disorders, such as mania, or thoughts of suicide.
- If you are allergic to any medication, food or other substances.

Over age 60:
A lower starting dosage is usually recommended until a response is determined.

Pregnancy:
Decide with your doctor if drug benefits justify risk to unborn child. Risk category C (see page xviii).

Breast-feeding:
It is unknown if drug passes into milk. Avoid drug or discontinue nursing until you finish medicine. Consult doctor for advice on maintaining milk supply.

Infants & children:
Safety in children under age 18 has not been established.

Prolonged use:
Consult with your doctor on a regular basis while taking this drug to check your progress and to discuss any increase or changes in side effects and the need for continued treatment.

Skin & sunlight:
May cause a rash or intensify sunburn in areas exposed to sun or ultraviolet light (photosensitivity reaction). Avoid excess sun exposure and use sunscreen. Consult doctor if reaction occurs.

Driving, piloting or hazardous work:
Don't drive or pilot aircraft until you learn how medicine affects you. Don't work around dangerous machinery. Don't climb ladders or work in high places. Danger increases if you drink alcohol or take medicine affecting alertness and reflexes.

Discontinuing:
Don't discontinue this drug without consulting doctor. Dosage may require a gradual reduction before stopping.

Others:
- Get up slowly from a sitting or lying position to avoid dizziness, faintness or lightheadedness.
- May affect the results of some medical tests.
- Advise any doctor or dentist whom you consult that you take this medicine.
- Take medicine only as directed. Do not increase or reduce dosage without doctor's approval.

POSSIBLE INTERACTION WITH OTHER DRUGS

GENERIC NAME OR DRUG CLASS	COMBINED EFFECT
Alprazolam	Increased effect of alprazolam.
Antihistamines, nonsedating	Serious heart rhythm problems with astemizole or terfenadine. Avoid.
Antihypertensives*	Possible too-low blood pressure.
Astemizole	Serious heart problems. Avoid.
Central nervous system (CNS) depressants*	Increased sedation. Avoid.
Digoxin	Increased digoxin effect.
Haloperidol	Unknown effect. May need dosage adjustment.
Monoamine oxidase (MAO) inhibitors*	Potentially life-threatening. Allow 14 days between use of 2 drugs.
Propranolol	Unknown effect. May need dosage adjustment of both drugs.
Selective serotonin reuptake inhibitors*	Potentially life-threatening serotonin syndrome (see Glossary). Avoid.

Continued on page 924

POSSIBLE INTERACTION WITH OTHER SUBSTANCES

INTERACTS WITH	COMBINED EFFECT
Alcohol:	Increased sedative affect. Avoid.
Beverages:	None expected.
Cocaine:	Unknown. Avoid.
Foods:	None expected.
Marijuana:	Unknown. Best to avoid.
Tobacco:	None expected.

***See Glossary**

NEOMYCIN (Oral)

BRAND NAMES

Mycifradin

BASIC INFORMATION

Habit forming? No
Prescription needed? Yes
Available as generic? Yes
Drug class: Antibacterial

USES

- Clears intestinal tract of germs prior to surgery.
- Treats some causes of diarrhea.
- Lowers blood cholesterol.
- Lessens symptoms of hepatic coma.

DOSAGE & USAGE INFORMATION

How to take:
Tablet—Swallow with liquid or food to lessen stomach irritation. If you can't swallow whole, crumble tablet and take with liquid or food.

When to take:
According to directions on prescription.

If you forget a dose:
Take as soon as you remember up to 2 hours late. If more than 2 hours, wait for next scheduled dose (don't double this dose).

What drug does:
Kills germs susceptible to neomycin.

Time lapse before drug works:
2 to 3 days.

Continued next column

OVERDOSE

SYMPTOMS:
Loss of hearing, difficulty breathing, respiratory paralysis.
WHAT TO DO:

- **Dial 911 (emergency) for an ambulance or medical help or poison center 1-800-222-1222. Then give first aid immediately.**
- **If patient is unconscious and not breathing, give mouth-to-mouth breathing. If there is no heartbeat, use cardiac massage and mouth-to-mouth breathing (CPR). Don't try to make patient vomit. If you can't get help quickly, take patient to nearest emergency facility.**
- **See emergency information on inside covers.**

Don't take with:
Any other medicine without consulting your doctor or pharmacist.

POSSIBLE ADVERSE REACTIONS OR SIDE EFFECTS

SYMPTOMS	WHAT TO DO
Life-threatening:	
In case of overdose, see previous column.	
Common:	
Sore mouth or rectum, nausea, vomiting.	Continue. Call doctor when convenient.
Infrequent:	
None expected.	
Rare:	
Clumsiness, dizziness, rash, hearing loss, ringing or noises in ear, frothy stools, gaseousness, decreased frequency of urination, diarrhea.	Discontinue. Call doctor right away.

WARNINGS & PRECAUTIONS

Don't take if:
You are allergic to neomycin or any aminoglycoside*.

Before you start, consult your doctor:
- If you will have surgery within 2 months, including dental surgery, requiring general or spinal anesthesia.
- If you have hearing loss or loss of balance secondary to 8th cranial nerve disease.
- If you have intestinal obstruction.
- If you have myasthenia gravis, Parkinson's disease, kidney disease, ulcers in intestines.

Over age 60:
Adverse reactions and side effects may be more frequent and severe than in younger persons.

Pregnancy:
Risk to unborn child outweighs drug benefits. Don't use. Risk category D (see page xviii).

Breast-feeding:
Avoid if possible. Effect unknown. Consult doctor.

Infants & children:
Give only under close medical supervision.

Prolonged use:
- Adverse effects more likely.
- Talk to your doctor about the need for follow-up medical examinations or laboratory studies to check hearing, kidney function.

Skin & sunlight:
No problems expected.

Driving, piloting or hazardous work:
No problems expected.

Discontinuing:
May be unnecessary to finish medicine. Follow doctor's instructions.

Others:
No problems expected.

POSSIBLE INTERACTION WITH OTHER DRUGS

GENERIC NAME OR DRUG CLASS	COMBINED EFFECT
Aminoglycosides*	Increased chance of toxic effect on hearing, kidneys, muscles.
Beta carotene	Decreased absorption of beta carotene.
Capreomycin	Increased chance of toxic effects on hearing, kidneys.
Cephalothin	Increased chance of toxic effect on kidneys.
Cisplatin	Increased chance of toxic effects on hearing, kidneys.
Ethacrynic acid	Increased chance of toxic effects on hearing, kidneys.
Furosemide	Increased chance of toxic effects on hearing, kidneys.
Mercaptomerin	Increased chance of toxic effects on hearing, kidneys.
Penicillins*	Decreased antibiotic effect.
Tiopronin	Increased risk of toxicity to kidneys.
Vancomycin	Increased chance of toxic effects on hearing, kidneys.

POSSIBLE INTERACTION WITH OTHER SUBSTANCES

INTERACTS WITH	COMBINED EFFECT
Alcohol:	Increased chance of toxicity. Avoid.
Beverages:	None expected.
Cocaine:	Increased chance of toxicity. Avoid.
Foods:	None expected.
Marijuana:	Increased chance of toxicity. Avoid.
Tobacco:	None expected.

***See Glossary**

NEOMYCIN (Topical)

BRAND NAMES

Myciguent

BASIC INFORMATION

Habit forming? No
Prescription needed? No
Available as generic? Yes
Drug class: Antibacterial (topical)

USES

Treats skin infections that may accompany burns, superficial boils, insect bites or stings, skin ulcers, minor surgical wounds.

DOSAGE & USAGE INFORMATION

How to take:

- Cream, lotion, ointment—Bathe and dry area before use. Apply small amount and rub gently.
- May cover with gauze or bandage if desired.

When to take:
3 or 4 times daily, or as directed by doctor.

If you forget a dose:
Use as soon as you remember.

What drug does:
Kills susceptible bacteria by interfering with bacterial DNA and RNA.

Time lapse before drug works:
Begins first day. May require treatment for a week or longer to cure infection.

Don't take with:
Any other medicine without consulting your doctor or pharmacist.

OVERDOSE

SYMPTOMS:
None expected.
WHAT TO DO:

- **Not for internal use. If child accidentally swallows, call poison control center.**
- **Dial 911 (emergency) for an ambulance or medical help or poison center 1-800-222-1222. Then give first aid immediately.**
- **See emergency information on inside covers.**

POSSIBLE ADVERSE REACTIONS OR SIDE EFFECTS

SYMPTOMS	WHAT TO DO
Life-threatening: None expected.	
Common: None expected.	
Infrequent: Itching, swollen, red skin.	Discontinue. Call doctor right away.
Rare: None expected.	

WARNINGS & PRECAUTIONS

Don't take if:
You are allergic to neomycin or any topical medicine.

Before you start, consult your doctor:
If any lesions on the skin are open sores.

Over age 60:
No problems expected.

Pregnancy:
Consult doctor. Risk category C (see page xviii).

Breast-feeding:
No problems expected, but check with doctor.

Infants & children:
No problems expected, but check with doctor.

Prolonged use:
No problems expected, but check with doctor.

Skin & sunlight:
No special problems expected.

Driving, piloting or hazardous work:
No problems expected, but check with doctor.

Discontinuing:
No problems expected, but check with doctor.

Others:
- Heat and moisture in bathroom medicine cabinet can cause breakdown of medicine. Store someplace else.
- Keep medicine cool, but don't freeze.

POSSIBLE INTERACTION WITH OTHER DRUGS

GENERIC NAME OR DRUG CLASS	COMBINED EFFECT
Any other topical medication	Hypersensitivity reactions more likely to occur.

POSSIBLE INTERACTION WITH OTHER SUBSTANCES

INTERACTS WITH	COMBINED EFFECT
Alcohol:	None expected.
Beverages:	None expected.
Cocaine:	None expected.
Foods:	None expected.
Marijuana:	None expected.
Tobacco:	None expected.

NIACIN (Vitamin B-3, Nicotinic Acid, Nicotinamide)

BRAND AND GENERIC NAMES

Advicor
Endur-Acin
Nia-Bid
Niac
Niacels
Niacin
Niacor
Nico-400
Nicobid
Nicolar
Nicotinex
Nicotinyl alcohol
Papulex
Roniacol
Ronigen
Rycotin
Slo-Niacin
Span-Niacin
Tega-Span
Tri-B3

There are numerous other multiple vitamin-mineral supplements available. Check labels.

BASIC INFORMATION

Habit forming? No
Prescription needed?
Tablets: No
Liquid, capsules: Yes
Available as generic? Yes
Drug class: Vitamin supplement, vasodilator, antihyperlipidemic

USES

- Replacement for niacin lost due to inadequate diet.
- Treatment for vertigo (dizziness) and ringing in ears.
- Prevention of premenstrual headache.
- Reduction of blood levels of cholesterol and triglycerides.
- Treatment for pellagra.

OVERDOSE

SYMPTOMS:
Body flush, nausea, vomiting, abdominal cramps, diarrhea, weakness, lightheadedness, fainting, sweating.
WHAT TO DO:
Overdose unlikely to threaten life. If person takes much larger amount than prescribed, call doctor, poison center 1-800-222-1222 or hospital emergency room for instructions.

DOSAGE & USAGE INFORMATION

How to take:
- Tablet, capsule or liquid—Swallow with liquid or food to lessen stomach irritation.
- Extended-release tablets or capsules—Swallow each dose whole.

When to take:
At the same times each day.

If you forget a dose:
Take as soon as you remember. Wait 4 hours for next dose.

What drug does:
- Corrects niacin deficiency.
- Dilates blood vessels.
- In large doses, decreases cholesterol production.

Time lapse before drug works:
15 to 20 minutes.

Don't take with:
Any other medicine without consulting your doctor or pharmacist.

POSSIBLE ADVERSE REACTIONS OR SIDE EFFECTS

SYMPTOMS	WHAT TO DO
Life-threatening:	
None expected.	
Common:	
Dry skin.	Continue. Call doctor when convenient.
Infrequent:	
• Upper abdominal pain, diarrhea.	Discontinue. Call doctor right away.
• Headache, dizziness, faintness, temporary numbness and tingling in hands and feet.	Continue. Call doctor when convenient.
• "Hot" feeling, flush.	No action necessary.
Rare:	
Rash, itching, jaundice, double vision, weakness and faintness when arising from bed or chair.	Discontinue. Call doctor right away.

NIACIN (Vitamin B-3, Nicotinic Acid, Nicotinamide)

WARNINGS & PRECAUTIONS

Don't take if:
You are allergic to niacin or any niacin-containing vitamin mixtures.

Before you start, consult your doctor:
- If you have sensitivity to tartrazine dye.
- If you have diabetes.
- If you have gout.
- If you have gallbladder or liver disease.
- If you have impaired liver function.
- If you have active peptic ulcer.

Over age 60:
Response to drug cannot be predicted. Dose must be individualized.

Pregnancy:
Consult doctor. Risk category C (see page xviii).

Breast-feeding:
Studies inconclusive. Consult doctor.

Infants & children:
- Use only under supervision.
- Keep vitamin-mineral supplements out of children's reach.

Prolonged use:
- May cause impaired liver function.
- Talk to your doctor about the need for follow-up medical examinations or laboratory studies to check liver function, blood sugar.

Skin & sunlight:
No problems expected.

Driving, piloting or hazardous work:
Avoid if you feel dizzy or faint. Otherwise, no problems expected.

Discontinuing:
May be unnecessary to finish medicine. Follow doctor's instructions.

Others:
- A balanced diet should provide all the niacin a healthy person needs and make supplements unnecessary. Best sources are meat, eggs and dairy products.
- Store in original container in cool, dry, dark place. Bathroom medicine chest too moist.
- Obesity reduces effectiveness.
- Some nicotinic acid products contain tartrazine dye. Read labels carefully if sensitive to tartrazine.

POSSIBLE INTERACTION WITH OTHER DRUGS

GENERIC NAME OR DRUG CLASS	COMBINED EFFECT
Antidiabetics*	Decreased antidiabetic effect.
Beta-adrenergic blocking agents*	Excessively low blood pressure.
Dexfenfluramine	May require dosage change as weight loss occurs.
HMG-CoA reductase inhibitors*	Increased risk of muscle or kidney problems.
Mecamylamine	Excessively low blood pressure.
Methyldopa	Excessively low blood pressure.
Probenecid	Decreased effect of probenecid.
Sulfinpyrazone	Decreased effect of sulfinpyrazone.

POSSIBLE INTERACTION WITH OTHER SUBSTANCES

INTERACTS WITH	COMBINED EFFECT
Alcohol:	Excessively low blood pressure. Use caution.
Beverages:	None expected.
Cocaine:	Increased flushing.
Foods:	None expected.
Marijuana:	None expected.
Tobacco:	Decreased niacin effect.

*See Glossary

NICOTINE

BRAND NAMES

Habitrol
Nicoderm
Nicoderm CQ
Nicorette
Nicorette DS
Nicotrol
Nicotrol NS

BASIC INFORMATION

Habit Forming? Yes
Prescription needed? No
Available as generic? Yes, for some
Drug class: Antismoking agent

USES

Treatment aid to giving up smoking. Nicotine replacement is to be used in conjunction with a medically supervised, behavioral modification program for smoking cessation.

DOSAGE & USAGE INFORMATION

How to use:
- Skin patch—Apply to clean, nonhairy site on the trunk or upper outer arm. Fold old patch in half (sticky sides together) and dispose of where children and pets cannot get to it.
- Chewing gum—Chew gum pieces slowly and intermittently (chew several times, then place between cheek and gum) for best effect.
- Nasal spray—Spray one or two sprays in each nostril.

When to use:
- Skin patch—Daily. Remove old patch and apply new patch to new location on the skin.
- Chewing gum—When there is an urge to smoke, chew the gum for about 30 minutes.
- Nasal spray—Hourly, or as directed. Dosage adjustments should be made as needed.
- For all—Always follow product's directions.

Continued next column

OVERDOSE

SYMPTOMS:
Early symptoms—Nausea, vomiting, severe diarrhea, increased mouth watering, abdominal pain, cold sweat, severe headache, dizziness, confusion, vision and hearing changes. Late symptoms—Irregular or fast pulse, fainting, breathing difficulty, convulsions.
WHAT TO DO:
- **Dial 911 (emergency) for an ambulance or medical help or poison center 1-800-222-1222. Then give first aid immediately.**
- **See emergency information on inside covers.**

If you forget a dose:
- Skin patch—Remove old patch and apply new patch as soon as you remember, then return to regular schedule.
- Chewing gum or nasal spray—Use as soon as you remember (don't double dosages).

What drug does:
Delivers a supply of nicotine to the body for relief of smoking withdrawal symptoms (irritability, headache, nervousness, drowsiness, fatigue). Reduces craving for cigarettes.

Time lapse before drug works:
Minutes to hours depending on type of product.

Don't take with:
Other prescription or nonprescription drugs without consulting your doctor or pharmacist.

POSSIBLE ADVERSE REACTIONS OR SIDE EFFECTS

SYMPTOMS	WHAT TO DO
Life-threatening: In case of overdose, see previous column.	
Common:	
• Skin patch—itching, redness, burning or skin rash at site of patch. • Chewing gum—dental problems, sore mouth or throat, belching, mouth watering. • Nasal spray—runny nose, watering eyes, throat irritation, sneezing and cough.	Continue. Call doctor when convenient.
Infrequent:	
Diarrhea, dizziness, indigestion, nervousness, strange dreams, muscle aches, nausea, constipation, increased cough, tiredness, irritability, changes in menstruation, insomnia, headache, increase in sweating.	Continue. Call doctor when convenient.
Rare:	
• Allergic reaction (swelling, hives, rash, itching, vomiting, irregular or fast heartbeat); symptoms of overdose occur (high doses of nicotine can cause toxic effects, even in people who are nicotine tolerant).	Discontinue. Call doctor right away.
• Hiccups or hoarsenss with chewing gum.	Continue. Call doctor when convenient.

WARNINGS & PRECAUTIONS

Don't take if:
You are allergic to nicotine or any of the components in the skin patch.

Before you start, consult your doctor:
- If you are pregnant.
- If you have a skin disorder; mouth, throat, dental or TMJ disorder; long-term nasal disorder (allergy, hay fever, sinusitis, polyps) or asthma.
- If you have cardiovascular or peripheral vascular disease or high blood pressure.
- If you have liver or kidney disease.
- If you have hyperthyroidism, insulin-dependent diabetes, pheochromocytoma, peptic ulcer disease or endocrine disorder.

Over age 60:
Adverse reactions and side effects may be more frequent and severe than in younger persons.

Pregnancy:
Tobacco smoke and nicotine are harmful to the fetus. The specific effects of nicotine from these drugs are unknown. Discuss the risks of both with your doctor. Risk category varies for drugs in this group (see page xviii).

Breast-feeding:
Drug passes into breast milk. Avoid drug or discontinue nursing until you finish medicine. Consult doctor for advice on maintaining milk supply.

Infants & children:
Not recommended.

Prolonged use:
Treatment may take several months. Nicotine replacement therapy is not intended for long-term use.

Skin & sunlight:
No problems expected.

Driving, piloting or hazardous work:
Avoid if you feel dizzy or lightheaded. Otherwise, no problems expected.

Discontinuing:
Adverse reactions and side effects related to nicotine withdrawal may continue for some time after discontinuing.

Others:
- Advise any doctor or dentist whom you consult that you take this medicine.
- May affect results of some medical tests.
- Keep both the used and unused skin patches out of the reach of children and pets. Dispose of old patches according to directions.
- For full benefit from this treatment and to decrease risk of side effects, stop cigarette smoking as soon as you begin treatment.

POSSIBLE INTERACTION WITH OTHER DRUGS

GENERIC NAME OR DRUG CLASS	COMBINED EFFECT
Acetaminophen	Increased effect of acetaminophen.
Beta-adrenergic blocking agents*	Increased effect of beta blocker.
Bronchodilators, xanthine* (except dyphylline)	Increased broncho-dilator effect.
Imipramine	Increased effect of imipramine.
Insulin & insulin lispro	May require insulin dosage adjustment.
Isoproterenol	Decreased effect of isoproterenol.
Oxazepam	Increased effect of oxazepam.
Pentazocine	Increased effect of pentazocine.
Phenylephrine	Decreased effect of phenylephrine.
Propoxyphene	Increased effect of propoxyphene.
Theophylline	Increased effect of theophylline.

POSSIBLE INTERACTION WITH OTHER SUBSTANCES

INTERACTS WITH	COMBINED EFFECT
Alcohol:	Increased cardiac irritability. Avoid.
Beverages:	None expected.
Cocaine:	Increased cardiac irritability. Avoid.
Foods:	None expected.
Marijuana:	Increased toxic effects. Avoid.
Tobacco:	Increased adverse effects of nicotine. Must avoid.

*See Glossary

NIMODIPINE

BRAND NAMES

Nimotop

BASIC INFORMATION

Habit Forming? No
Prescription needed? Yes
Available as generic? No
Drug class: Calcium channel blocker

USES

Helps repair the damage caused by a ruptured blood vessel in the head (also called ruptured aneurysm or subarachnoid hemorrhage).
Note: Unlike other calcium channel blockers, nimodipine is not used for angina or high blood pressure.

DOSAGE & USAGE INFORMATION

How to take:
Capsule—Swallow with liquid.

When to take:
Results are best if you begin taking within 96 hours after bleeding into the brain begins. Continue taking for 21 days or as directed by your physician.

If you forget a dose:
Take as soon as you remember up to 2 hours late. If more than 2 hours, wait for next scheduled dose (don't double this dose).

What drug does:
This is a calcium channel blocking drug that crosses easily from blood vessels into the brain, where it prevents spasms of the brain's arteries.

Continued next column

OVERDOSE

SYMPTOMS:
Unusally fast or unusually slow heartbeat, loss of consciousness, cardiac arrest.
WHAT TO DO:

- **Dial 911 (emergency) for an ambulance or medical help or poison center 1-800-222-1222. Then give first aid immediately.**
- **If patient is unconscious and not breathing, give mouth-to-mouth breathing. If there is no heartbeat, use cardiac massage and mouth-to-mouth breathing (CPR). Don't try to make patient vomit. If you can't get help quickly, take patient to nearest emergency facility.**
- **See emergency information on inside covers.**

Time lapse before drug works:
1 to 2 hours.

Don't take with:
Any other medicine without consulting your doctor or pharmacist.

POSSIBLE ADVERSE REACTIONS OR SIDE EFFECTS

SYMPTOMS	WHAT TO DO
Life-threatening: In case of overdose, see previous column.	
Common:	
Tiredness, flushing, swelling of feet, ankles and abdomen.	Continue. Tell doctor at next visit.
Infrequent:	
• Unusually fast or unusually slow heartbeat, wheezing, cough, shortness of breath.	Discontinue. Call doctor right away.
• Dizziness; numbness or tingling in hands or feet; difficult urination.	Continue. Call doctor when convenient.
• Nausea, constipation.	Continue. Tell doctor at next visit.
Rare:	
• Transient blindness, increased angina, chest pain.	Discontinue. Seek emergency treatment.
• Fainting, fever, rash, jaundice, depression, psychosis.	Discontinue. Call doctor right away.
• Pain and swelling in joints, hair loss, vivid dreams.	Continue. Call doctor when convenient.
• Headache.	Continue. Tell doctor at next visit.

WARNINGS & PRECAUTIONS

Don't take if:

- You are allergic to any calcium channel blocking drug*.
- You have very low blood pressure.

Before you start, consult your doctor:

- If you have kidney or liver disease.
- If you have high blood pressure.
- If you have heart disease other than coronary artery disease.

Over age 60:
Adverse reactions and side effects may be more frequent and severe than in younger persons.

Pregnancy:
Decide with your doctor if drug benefits justify risk to unborn child. Risk category C (see page xviii).

Breast-feeding:
Safety not established. Avoid if possible. Consult doctor.

Infants & children:
Not recommended.

Prolonged use:
Talk to your doctor about the need for follow-up medical examinations or laboratory studies to check blood pressure, liver function, kidney function, ECG*.

Skin & sunlight:
No special problems expected.

Driving, piloting or hazardous work:
Avoid if you feel dizzy. Otherwise, no problems expected.

Discontinuing:
Don't discontinue without doctor's advice until you complete prescribed dose, even though symptoms diminish or disappear.

Others:

- Learn to check your own pulse rate. If it drops to 50 beats per minute or lower, don't take nimodipine until you consult your doctor.
- Drug may lower blood sugar level if daily dose is more than 60 mg.

POSSIBLE INTERACTION WITH OTHER DRUGS

GENERIC NAME OR DRUG CLASS	COMBINED EFFECT
Angiotensin-converting enzyme (ACE) inhibitors*	Possible excessive potassium in blood. Dosages may need adjustment.
Antiarrhythmics*	Possible increased effect and toxicity of each drug.
Anticoagulants*, oral	Possible increased anticoagulant effect.
Anticonvulsants, hydantoin*	Increased anti-convulsant effect.
Antihypertensives*	Blood pressure changes. Dosage may need adjustment.
Beta-adrenergic blocking agents* (oral or ophthalmic)	Possible irregular heartbeat. May worsen congestive heart failure.
Betaxolol eye drops	May cause increased effect of nimodipine on heart function.
Calcium (large doses)	Possible decreased nimodipine effect.
Carbamazepine	May increase carbamazepine effect and toxicity.
Cimetidine	Possible increased nimodipine effect and toxicity.
Cyclosporine	Increased cyclosporine toxicity.
Disopyramide	May cause dangerously slow, fast or irregular heartbeat.
Diuretics*	Dangerous blood pressure drop.
Levobutanol eye drops	May cause increased effect of nimodipine on heart function.
Lithium	Possible decreased lithium effect.
Nicardipine	Possible increased effect and toxicity of each drug.
Phenytoin	Possible decreased nimodipine effect.
Quinidine	Increased quinidine effect.
Rifampin	Decreased nimodipine effect.

Continued on page 924

POSSIBLE INTERACTION WITH OTHER SUBSTANCES

INTERACTS WITH	COMBINED EFFECT
Alcohol:	Dangerously low blood pressure. Avoid.
Beverages:	None expected.
Cocaine:	Possible irregular heartbeat. Avoid.
Foods:	None expected.
Marijuana:	Possible irregular heartbeat. Avoid.
Tobacco:	Possible rapid heartbeat. Avoid.

***See Glossary**

NITRATES

GENERIC AND BRAND NAMES

See complete list of generic and brand names in the *Generic and Brand Name Directory*, page 862.

BASIC INFORMATION

Habit forming? No
Prescription needed? Yes
Available as generic? Yes
Drug class: Antianginal (nitrate)

USES

- Reduces frequency and severity of angina attacks.
- Treats congestive heart failure.

DOSAGE & USAGE INFORMATION

How to take:

- Extended-release tablets or capsules—Swallow each dose whole with liquid.
- Chewable tablet—Chew tablet at earliest sign of angina, and hold in mouth for 2 minutes.
- Regular tablet or capsule—Swallow whole with liquid. Don't crush, chew or open.
- Buccal tablets (Nitrogard)—Allow to dissolve inside of mouth.
- Translingual spray (Nitrolingual)—Spray under tongue according to instructions enclosed with prescription.
- Ointment—Apply as directed.
- Patches—Apply to skin according to package instructions.
- Sublingual tablets—Place under tongue every 3 to 5 minutes at earliest sign of angina. If you don't have complete relief with 3 or 4 tablets, call doctor.

Continued next column

OVERDOSE

SYMPTOMS:
Dizziness; blue fingernails and lips; feeling of pressure in head, fever, fainting; shortness of breath; weak, fast heartbeat; convulsions.
WHAT TO DO:

- **Dial 911 (emergency) for an ambulance or medical help or poison center 1-800-222-1222. Then give first aid immediately.**
- **See emergency information on inside covers.**

When to take:

- Swallowed tablets—Take at the same times each day, 1 or 2 hours after meals.
- Sublingual tablets or spray—At onset of angina.
- Ointment—Follow prescription directions.
- Patches—According to physician's instructions.

If you forget a dose:
Take as soon as you remember up to 2 hours late. If more than 2 hours, wait for next scheduled dose (don't double this dose).

What drug does:
Relaxes blood vessels, increasing blood flow to heart muscle.

Time lapse before drug works:

- Sublingual tablets and spray—1 to 3 minutes.
- Other forms—15 to 30 minutes. Will not stop an attack, but may prevent attacks.

Don't take with:
Any other medicine without consulting your doctor or pharmacist.

POSSIBLE ADVERSE REACTIONS OR SIDE EFFECTS

SYMPTOMS	WHAT TO DO
Life-threatening:	
In case of overdose, see previous column.	
Common:	
Headache, flushed face and neck, dry mouth, nausea, vomiting.	Continue. Tell doctor at next visit.
Infrequent:	
• Fainting, rapid heartbeat.	Discontinue. Call doctor right away.
• Restlessness, blurred vision, dizziness.	Continue. Call doctor when convenient.
Rare:	
• Rash.	Discontinue. Call doctor right away.
• Severe irritation, peeling.	Continue. Call doctor when convenient.

WARNINGS & PRECAUTIONS

Don't take if:
You are allergic to nitrates, including nitroglycerin.

Before you start, consult your doctor:

- If you are taking nonprescription drugs.
- If you plan to become pregnant within medication period.
- If you have glaucoma.

- If you have reacted badly to any vasodilator drug.
- If you drink alcoholic beverages or smoke marijuana.

Over age 60:
Adverse reactions and side effects may be more frequent and severe than in younger persons.

Pregnancy:
Decide with your doctor if drug benefits justify risk to unborn child. Risk category C (see page xviii).

Breast-feeding:
Effect unknown. Consult your doctor.

Infants & children:
Not recommended.

Prolonged use:
- Drug may become less effective and require higher doses.
- Talk to your doctor about the need for follow-up medical examinations or laboratory studies to check blood pressure, heart rate.

Skin & sunlight:
No problems expected.

Driving, piloting or hazardous work:
Don't drive or pilot aircraft until you learn how medicine affects you. Don't work around dangerous machinery. Don't climb ladders or work in high places. Danger increases if you drink alcohol or take medicine affecting alertness and reflexes.

Discontinuing:
Except for sublingual tablets, don't discontinue without doctor's advice until you complete prescribed dose, even though symptoms diminish or disappear.

Others:
- If discomfort is not caused by angina, nitrate medication will not bring relief. Call doctor if discomfort persists.
- Periodic urine and laboratory blood studies of white cell counts recommended if you take nitrates.
- Keep sublingual tablets in original container. Always carry them with you, but keep from body heat if possible.
- Sublingual tablets produce a burning, stinging sensation when placed under the tongue. Replace supply if no burning or stinging is noted.
- To avoid development of tolerance, drug-free intervals of 10 hours are sufficient.

POSSIBLE INTERACTION WITH OTHER DRUGS

GENERIC NAME OR DRUG CLASS	COMBINED EFFECT
Anticholinergics*	Increased internal eye pressure.
Antihypertensives*	Excessive blood pressure drop.
Beta-adrenergic blocking agents*	Excessive blood pressure drop.
Calcium channel blockers*	Decreased blood pressure.
Carteolol	Possible excessive blood pressure drop.
Guanfacine	Increased effects of both drugs.
Narcotics*	Excessive blood pressure drop.
Phenothiazines*	May decrease blood pressure.
Sildenafil	Increased effect of nitrates.
Sympathomimetics*	Possible reduced effects of both medicines.

POSSIBLE INTERACTION WITH OTHER SUBSTANCES

INTERACTS WITH	COMBINED EFFECT
Alcohol:	Excessive blood pressure drop.
Beverages:	None expected.
Cocaine:	Reduced effectiveness of nitrates.
Foods:	None expected.
Marijuana:	Decreased nitrate effect.
Tobacco:	Decreased nitrate effect.

***See Glossary**

NITROFURANTOIN

BRAND NAMES

Apo-Nitrofurantoin
Cyantin
Furadantin
Furalan
Furaloid
Furan
Furanite
Furantoin
Furatine
Furaton
Macrobid
Macrodantin
Nephronex
Nifuran
Nitrex
Nitrofan
Nitrofor
Nitrofuracot
Novofuran
Ro-Antoin
Sarodant
Trantoin
Urotoin

BASIC INFORMATION

Habit forming? No
Prescription needed? Yes
Available as generic? Yes
Drug class: Antimicrobial, antibacterial (antibiotic)

USES

Treatment for urinary tract infections.

DOSAGE & USAGE INFORMATION

How to take:

- Tablet or capsule—Swallow with food or milk to lessen stomach irritation. If you can't swallow whole, crumble tablet or open capsule and take with liquid or food.
- Extended-release capsule—Swallow with liquid. Do not open capsule.
- Liquid—Shake well and take with food. Use a measuring spoon to ensure accuracy.

When to take:
At the same times each day.

If you forget a dose:
Take as soon as you remember up to 2 hours late. If more than 2 hours, wait for next scheduled dose (don't double this dose).

Continued next column

OVERDOSE

SYMPTOMS:
Nausea, vomiting, abdominal pain, diarrhea.
WHAT TO DO:
Overdose unlikely to threaten life. If person takes much larger amount than prescribed, call doctor, poison center 1-800-222-1222 or hospital emergency room for instructions.

What drug does:
Prevents susceptible bacteria in the urinary tract from growing and multiplying.

Time lapse before drug works:
1 to 2 weeks.

Don't take with:
Any other medicine without consulting your doctor or pharmacist.

POSSIBLE ADVERSE REACTIONS OR SIDE EFFECTS

SYMPTOMS	WHAT TO DO
Life-threatening:	
Hives, rash, intense itching, faintness soon after a dose (anaphylaxis).	Seek emergency treatment immediately.
Common:	
• Diarrhea, appetite loss, nausea, vomiting, chest pain, cough, difficult breathing, chills or unexplained fever, abdominal pain.	Discontinue. Call doctor right away.
• Rusty-colored or brown urine.	No action necessary.
Infrequent:	
• Rash, itchy skin, numbness, tingling or burning of face or mouth, fatigue, weakness.	Discontinue. Call doctor right away.
• Dizziness, headache, drowsiness, paleness (in children), discolored teeth (from liquid form).	Continue. Call doctor when convenient.
Rare:	
Jaundice.	Discontinue. Call doctor right away.

WARNINGS & PRECAUTIONS

Don't take if:
- You are allergic to nitrofurantoin.
- You have impaired kidney function.
- You drink alcohol.

Before you start, consult your doctor:
- If you are prone to allergic reactions.
- If you are pregnant and within 2 weeks of delivery.
- If you have had kidney disease, lung disease, anemia, nerve damage, or G6PD* deficiency (a metabolic deficiency).
- If you have diabetes. Drug may affect urine sugar tests.

Over age 60:
Adverse reactions and side effects may be more frequent and severe than in younger persons.

Pregnancy:
Consult doctor. Risk category B (see page xviii).

Breast-feeding:
Drug passes into milk. Avoid drug or discontinue nursing until you finish medicine. Consult doctor for advice on maintaining milk supply.

Infants & children:
Don't give to infants younger than 1 month. Use only under medical supervision for older children.

Prolonged use:
- Chest pain, cough, shortness of breath.
- Talk to your doctor about the need for follow-up medical examinations or laboratory studies to check liver function, lung function.

Skin & sunlight:
No problems expected.

Driving, piloting or hazardous work:
Avoid if you feel dizzy or drowsy. Otherwise, no problems expected.

Discontinuing:
Don't discontinue without consulting doctor. Dose may require gradual reduction if you have taken drug for a long time. Doses of other drugs may also require adjustment.

Others:
Periodic blood counts, liver function tests, and chest x-rays recommended.

POSSIBLE INTERACTION WITH OTHER DRUGS

GENERIC NAME OR DRUG CLASS	COMBINED EFFECT
Antivirals, HIV/AIDS*	Increased risk of pancreatitis and peripheral neuropathy.
Hemolytics*, other	Increased risk of toxicity.
Nalidixic acid	Decreased nitrofurantoin effect.
Neurotoxic medicines*	Increased risk of damage to nerve cells.
Probenecid	Increased nitrofurantoin effect.
Sulfinpyrazone	Possible nitrofurantoin toxicity.

POSSIBLE INTERACTION WITH OTHER SUBSTANCES

INTERACTS WITH	COMBINED EFFECT
Alcohol:	Possible disulfiram reaction*. Avoid.
Beverages:	None expected.
Cocaine:	None expected.
Foods:	None expected.
Marijuana:	None expected.
Tobacco:	None expected.

*See Glossary

NON-NUCLEOSIDE REVERSE TRANSCRIPTASE INHIBITORS

GENERIC AND BRAND NAMES

DELAVIRDINE
Rescriptor
EFAVIRENZ
Sustiva
NEVIRAPINE
Viramune

BASIC INFORMATION

Habit forming? No
Prescription needed? Yes
Available as generic? No
Drug class: Antiviral, HIV and AIDS

USES

For treatment of HIV and AIDS patients. Used in combination with one or more of the other AIDS drugs. May be used to prevent HIV transmission.

DOSAGE & USAGE INFORMATION

How to take:
- Oral suspension—Swallow with liquid.
- Tablet—Swallow with liquid. May be taken with or without food. Efavirenz should not be taken with a high fat meal.

When to take:
At the same time each day. At the start of treatment, one tablet is taken daily for 2 weeks and then increased to 2 tablets daily. This helps to decrease risk of side effects.

If you forget a dose:
Twice-a-day dose—Take as soon as you remember up to 2 hours late. If more than 2 hours, wait for next scheduled dose (don't double this dose).

What drug does:
Interferes with HIV replication. It helps slow the progress of HIV disease, but does not cure it.

Continued next column

OVERDOSE

SYMPTOMS:
Swelling, extreme tiredness, fever, insomnia, rash, dizziness, vomiting, feeling of movement.
WHAT TO DO:
Overdose unlikely to threaten life. If person takes much larger amount than prescribed, call doctor, poison center 1-800-222-1222 or hospital emergency room for instructions.

Time lapse before drug works:
May require several weeks or months before full benefits are apparent.

Don't take with:
Any other prescription or nonprescription drugs without consulting your doctor or pharmacist. This is very important with these anitiviral drugs.

POSSIBLE ADVERSE REACTIONS OR SIDE EFFECTS

SYMPTOMS	WHAT TO DO
Life-threatening:	
Severe skin rash.	Discontinue. Call doctor right away or get emergency help.
Common:	
Mild to moderate skin rash, chills,. fever, sore throat.	Discontinue. Call doctor right away.
Infrequent:	
• Fever, blistering skin, mouth sores, aching joints or muscles, eye inflammation, unusual tiredness.	Continue, but call doctor right away.
• Headache, nausea, diarrhea burning or tingling feeling, numbness, sleepiness, loss of appetite, constipation, mood or mental changes, intense dreams, anxiety, difficulty concentrating.	Continue. Call doctor when convenient.
Rare:	
• Yellow skin or eyes, dark urine, heart palpitations, thoughts of suicide.	Discontinue. Call doctor right away.
• Any other unusual symptoms that occur (may be due to the illness, this drug or other drugs being taken).	Continue, but call doctor right away.

NON-NUCLEOSIDE REVERSE TRANSCRIPTASE INHIBITORS

WARNINGS & PRECAUTIONS

Don't take if:
You are allergic to non-nucleoside reverse transcriptase inhibitors.

Before you start, consult your doctor:
- If you are allergic to any medicine, food or other substance, or have a family history of allergies.
- If you have kidney or liver disease.

Over age 60:
Though medical studies are incomplete, the adverse reactions and side effects may be more frequent and severe than in younger persons.

Pregnancy:
Decide with your doctor if drug benefits justify risk to unborn child. Risk category C (see page xviii).

Breast-feeding:
Drug passes into milk. Avoid drug or discontinue nursing until you finish medicine. Consult doctor for advice on maintaining milk supply.

Infants & children:
Safety and efficacy have not been established. Use only under close medical supervision.

Prolonged use:
- Long-term effects have not been established.
- Talk to your doctor about frequent blood counts and liver function studies.

Skin & sunlight:
No problems expected.

Driving, piloting or hazardous work:
Don't drive or pilot aircraft until you learn how medicine affects you. Don't work around dangerous machinery. Don't climb ladders or work in high places. Danger increases if you drink alcohol or take medicine affecting alertness and reflexes, such as antihistamines, tranquilizers, sedatives, pain medicines, narcotics and mind-altering drugs.

Discontinuing:
Don't discontinue without doctor's advice until you complete prescribed dose, even though symptoms diminish or disappear.

Others:
- Advise any doctor or dentist whom you consult that you take this medicine.
- Consult your doctor if any signs of infection develop (fever, chills, sore throat, intestinal problems, etc.).
- If a rash does occur when the drug is first started, it is vital to consult your doctor.
- Do not increase dosage without doctor's approval.

POSSIBLE INTERACTION WITH OTHER DRUGS

GENERIC NAME OR DRUG CLASS	COMBINED EFFECT
Amphetamines	May require dosage adjustment of amphetamine.
Antacids	Take 1-2 hours apart.
Benzodiazepines	May require dosage adjustment of benzodiazepine.
Calcium channel blockers	May require dosage adjustment of calcium channel blocker.
Carbamazepine	Decreased antiviral drug effect.
Clarithromycin	Interaction effects vary.
Contraceptives, oral*	Decreased contraceptive effect. Use alternative birth control method.
Didanosine	Take at least 1 hour apart.
Ergot preparations*	May require dosage adjustment of ergot drug.
Fluoxetine	Increased antiviral effect.
Histamine H2 receptor antagonists	May require dosage adjustment of antiviral drug.

POSSIBLE INTERACTION WITH OTHER SUBSTANCES

INTERACTS WITH	COMBINED EFFECT
Alcohol:	None expected.
Beverages:	None expected.
Cocaine:	Unknown effect. Best to avoid.
Foods:	None expected.
Marijuana:	Unknown effect. Best to avoid.
Tobacco:	None expected.

***See Glossary**

NUCLEOSIDE REVERSE TRANSCRIPTASE INHIBITORS

GENERIC AND BRAND NAMES

ABACAVIR
- Trizivir
- Ziagen

DIDANOSINE
- Videx

LAMIVUDINE
- 3TC
- Combivir
- Epivir
- Trizivir

STAVUDINE
- d4T

ZALCITABINE
- ddC
- Hivid

ZIDOVUDINE
- Apo-Zidovudine
- AZT
- Combivir
- Novo-AZT
- Retrovir
- Trizivir

BASIC INFORMATION

Habit forming? No
Prescription needed? Yes
Available as generic? No
Drug class: Antiviral

USES

- Treats human immunodeficiency virus (HIV).
- Treats acquired immunodeficiency syndrome (AIDS).

DOSAGE & USAGE INFORMATION

How to take:
- Didanosine tablets—Chew or manually crumble tablet. If crumble tablet, mix with at least 1 oz. of water and swallow immediately.
- Tablets or capsules—Swallow with water.
- Syrup—Measure correct dosage with a specially marked measuring device.
- Buffered didanosine for oral solution—Follow instructions on label. Swallow immediately after mixing.

Continued next column

OVERDOSE

SYMPTOMS:
Seizures, severe nausea and vomiting, extreme tiredness or weakness, increase in bruising or bleeding, loss of coordination, involuntary eye movements.

WHAT TO DO:
- **Dial 911 (emergency) for an ambulance or medical help or poison center 1-800-222-1222. Then give first aid immediately.**
- **See emergency information on inside covers.**

When to take:
At the same time each day, according to instructions on prescription label. Follow directions on label for taking with or without food.

If you forget a dose:
Take as soon as you remember up to 2 hours late. If more than 2 hours, wait for next scheduled dose (don't double this dose).

What drug does:
Suppresses replication of human immunodeficiency virus.

Time lapse before drug works:
Depends on the progress of the disease.

Don't take with:
Any other medicine without consulting your doctor or pharmacist.

POSSIBLE ADVERSE REACTIONS OR SIDE EFFECTS

SYMPTOMS	WHAT TO DO
Life-threatening: In case of overdose, see previous column.	
Common:	
• Tingling, numbness and burning in the feet and ankles (peripheral neuropathy).	Discontinue. Call doctor right away.
• Headache, anxiety, restlessness, digestive disturbances, diarrhea.	Continue. Call doctor when convenient.
Infrequent:	
• Unusual tiredness and weakness, fever, chills, sore throat, unusual bleeding or bruising, yellow skin and eyes, skin rash, pale skin, muscle or joint pain, mouth or throat sores, stomach pain, nausea and vomiting.	Discontinue. Call doctor right away.
• Lack of strength or energy, difficulty sleeping, discolored nails.	Continue. Call doctor when convenient.
Rare:	
Seizures, mood or mental changes, confusion.	Discontinue. Call doctor right away.

WARNINGS & PRECAUTIONS

Don't take if:
You are allergic to antivirals for HIV and AIDS.

NUCLEOSIDE REVERSE TRANSCRIPTASE INHIBITORS

Before you start, consult your doctor:
- If you have a history of alcoholism.
- If you have hypertriglyceridemia, anemia, gout, phenylketonuria or pancreatitis.
- If you have any condition requiring sodium restriction.
- If you have liver or kidney disease.
- If you have peripheral neuropathy.

Over age 60:
No special problems expected.

Pregnancy:
Risk factors vary for drugs in this group. See category list on page xviii and consult doctor.

Breast-feeding:
Unknown effects. Consult doctor.

Infants & children:
May cause depigmentation of the retina. Children should have eye exams every 3 to 6 months to check for vision changes.

Prolonged use:
Talk with your doctor about the need for follow-up medical examination or laboratory studies to check blood serum and uric acid levels.

Skin & sunlight:
No special problems expected.

Driving, piloting or hazardous work:
Don't drive or pilot aircraft until you learn how medicine affects you. Don't work around dangerous machinery. Don't climb ladders or work in high places. Danger increases if you drink alcohol or take medicine affecting alertness and reflexes, such as antihistamines, tranquilizers, sedatives, pain medicines, narcotics and mind-altering drugs.

Discontinuing:
Don't discontinue without consulting doctor. Dose may require gradual reduction if you have taken drug for a long time. Doses of other drugs may require adjustment.

Others:
- Advise any doctor or dentist whom you consult that you take this medicine.
- Avoid sexual intercourse or use condoms to help prevent the transmission of HIV. Don't share needles or equipment for injections with other persons.
- The drugs in this group may be combined for treatment. This increases the risk of side effects such as peripheral neuropathy.
- Numerous medical studies are ongoing concerning the use of these and other anti-HIV drugs. Full safety and effectiveness are still being determined.

POSSIBLE INTERACTION WITH OTHER DRUGS

GENERIC NAME OR DRUG CLASS	COMBINED EFFECT
Antacids*, aluminum- or magnesium-containing	Decreased effect of zalcitabine.
Bone marrow depressants*, other	Drugs may need dosage changes.
Cimetidine	Increased effect of zalcitabine and zidovudine.
Clarithromycin	Decreased effect of zidovudine.
Dapsone	Increased risk of peripheral neuropathy. Reduced absorption of both drugs.
Fluoroquinolones	Decreased antibiotic effect.
Gancyclovir	Increased toxicity of both drugs. Use with caution.
Itraconazole	Decreased absorption of itraconazole.
Ketoconazole	Decreased effect of ketoconazole.
Pancreatitus-associated drugs*	Increased risk of pancreatitus with didanosine.
Peripheral neuropathy-associated drugs*	Increased risk of peripheral neuropathy.

Continued on page 924

POSSIBLE INTERACTION WITH OTHER SUBSTANCES

INTERACTS WITH	COMBINED EFFECT
Alcohol:	Increased chance of pancreatitis or peripheral neuropathy.
Beverages:	None expected.
Cocaine:	None expected.
Foods:	None expected.
Marijuana:	None expected.
Tobacco:	None expected.

***See Glossary**

NUCLEOTIDE REVERSE TRANSCRIPTASE INHIBITORS

GENERIC AND BRAND NAMES

TENOFOVIR
Viread

BASIC INFORMATION

Habit forming? No
Prescription needed? Yes
Available as generic? No
Drug class: Antiviral

USES

Treats human immunodeficiency virus (HIV). and acquired immunodeficiency syndrome (AIDS). Used in combination with other antiretroviral agents. Does not cure or prevent HIV or AIDS.

DOSAGE & USAGE INFORMATION

How to take:
Tablets —Swallow with water. Take with a meal.

When to take:
At the same time each day, according to instructions on prescription label.

If you forget a dose:
Take as soon as you remember. If it is almost time for the next dose, wait for next scheduled dose (don't double this dose).

What drug does:
Suppresses replication of human immunodeficiency virus.

Time lapse before drug works:
Depends on the progress of the disease.

Don't take with:
Any other medicine without consulting your doctor or pharmacist.

OVERDOSE

SYMPTOMS:
Unknown effects.
WHAT TO DO:
If person takes much larger amount than prescribed, call doctor, poison center 1-800-222-1222 or hospital emergency room for instructions.

POSSIBLE ADVERSE REACTIONS OR SIDE EFFECTS

SYMPTOMS	WHAT TO DO
Life-threatening: None expected.	
Common: Vomiting, lack or loss of strength.	Continue. Call doctor when convenient.
Infrequent: Gaseousness, weight loss, diarrhea.	Continue. Call doctor when convenient.
Rare: Breathing fast or shallow, shortness of breath, unusual tiredness, sleepiness, stomach discomfort, loss of appetite, muscle cramping or pain, overall feeling of discomfort, any unusual symptoms.	Continue, but call doctor right away.

WARNINGS & PRECAUTIONS

Don't take if:
You are allergic to tenofovir.

Before you start, consult your doctor:
If you have liver or kidney disease.

Over age 60:
Studies have not been done in this age group.

Pregnancy:
Consult your doctor. Risk category B (see page xviii).

Breast-feeding:
It is unknown if drug passes into milk. It is not recommended that HIV-infected mothers breast-feed if other options are available. Consult your doctor.

Infants & children:
Safety and efficacy have not been established. use only with close medical supervision.

Prolonged use:
- Talk with your doctor about the need for follow-up medical examination or laboratory studies to check drug's effectiveness.
- Long-term effects of this drug are unknown. Studies are ongoing.

Skin & sunlight:
No special problems expected.

Driving, piloting or hazardous work:
No problems expected.

Discontinuing:
Don't discontinue without consulting doctor.

Others:
- Advise any doctor or dentist whom you consult that you take this medicine.
- Avoid sexual intercourse or use condoms to help prevent the transmission of HIV. Don't share needles or equipment for injections with other persons.
- This drug is combined with others for optimum treatment. This increases the risk of side effects or adverse reactions.
- Numerous medical studies are ongoing concerning the use of these and other anti-HIV drugs. Full safety and effectiveness are still being determined.

POSSIBLE INTERACTION WITH OTHER DRUGS

GENERIC NAME OR DRUG CLASS	COMBINED EFFECT
Antivirals for herpes virus	Increased effect of tenofovir.
Didanosine	Increased effect of didanosine. Take tenofovir 2 hours before or 1 hour after didanosine.

POSSIBLE INTERACTION WITH OTHER SUBSTANCES

INTERACTS WITH	COMBINED EFFECT
Alcohol:	None expected.
Beverages:	None expected.
Cocaine:	None expected. Best to avoid.
Foods:	None expected.
Marijuana:	None expected. Best to avoid.
Tobacco:	None expected.

*See Glossary

NYSTATIN

BRAND NAMES

Dermacomb
Myco II
Mycobiotic II
Mycogen II
Mycolog II
Mycostatin
Myco-Triacet II
Mykacet
Mykacet II
Mytrex
Nadostine
Nilstat
Nystaform
Nystex
Tristatin II

BASIC INFORMATION

Habit forming? No
Prescription needed? Yes
Available as generic? Yes
Drug class: Antifungal

USES

Treatment of fungus infections of the mouth or vagina that are susceptible to nystatin.

DOSAGE & USAGE INFORMATION

How to take:

- Tablet—Swallow with liquid. If you can't swallow whole, crumble tablet and take with liquid or food.
- Ointment, cream or lotion—Use as directed by doctor and label.
- Liquid—Take as directed. Instruction varies by preparation.
- Lozenges—Take as directed on label.

When to take:
At the same time each day.

If you forget a dose:
Take as soon as you remember up to 2 hours late. If more than 2 hours, wait for next scheduled dose (don't double this dose).

Continued next column

OVERDOSE

SYMPTOMS:
Mild overdose may cause nausea, vomiting, diarrhea.
WHAT TO DO:
Overdose unlikely to threaten life. If person takes much larger amount than prescribed, call doctor, poison center 1-800-222-1222 or hospital emergency room for instructions.

What drug does:
Prevents growth and reproduction of fungus.

Time lapse before drug works:
Begins immediately. May require 3 weeks for maximum benefit, depending on location and severity of infection.

Don't take with:
Any other medicine without consulting your doctor or pharmacist.

POSSIBLE ADVERSE REACTIONS OR SIDE EFFECTS

SYMPTOMS	WHAT TO DO
Life-threatening: None expected.	
Common: (at high doses) Nausea, stomach pain, vomiting, diarrhea.	Discontinue. Call doctor right away.
Infrequent: Mild irritation, itch at application site.	Discontinue. Call doctor right away.
Rare: None expected.	

WARNINGS & PRECAUTIONS

Don't take if:
You are allergic to nystatin.

Before you start, consult your doctor:
If you plan to become pregnant within medication period.

Over age 60:
No problems expected.

Pregnancy:
No proven harm to unborn child. Avoid if possible. Consult doctor. Risk category B (see page xviii).

Breast-feeding:
No proven problems. Consult doctor.

Infants & children:
No problems expected.

Prolonged use:
No problems expected.

Skin & sunlight:
No problems expected.

Driving, piloting or hazardous work:
No problems expected.

Discontinuing:
Don't discontinue without doctor's advice until you complete prescribed dose, even though symptoms diminish or disappear.

Others:
No problems expected.

POSSIBLE INTERACTION WITH OTHER DRUGS

GENERIC NAME OR DRUG CLASS	COMBINED EFFECT
None reported.	

POSSIBLE INTERACTION WITH OTHER SUBSTANCES

INTERACTS WITH	COMBINED EFFECT
Alcohol:	None expected.
Beverages:	None expected.
Cocaine:	None expected.
Foods:	None expected.
Marijuana:	None expected.
Tobacco:	None expected.

OLANZAPINE

BRAND NAMES

Zyprexa

BASIC INFORMATION

Habit forming? No
Prescription needed? Yes
Available as generic? No
Drug class: Antipsychotic

USES

Treatment for symptoms of schizophrenia, acute mania and other psychotic disorders.

DOSAGE & USAGE INFORMATION

How to take:
Tablet—Swallow with liquid. May be taken with or without food.

When tc take:
Once a day at the same time each day. The prescribed dosage may be increased over the first few days of use.

If you forget a dose:
Take as soon as you remember. If it is almost time for the next dose, wait for the next scheduled dose (don't double this dose).

What drug does:
The exact mechanism is unknown. It appears to alleviate symptoms of schizophrenia by blocking certain nerve impulses between nerve cells.

Time lapse before drug works:
One to 7 days. Further increases in the dosage amount may be necessary to relieve symptoms for some patients.

Don't take with:
Any other medication without consulting your doctor or pharmacist. All possible drug interactions have not been studied.

OVERDOSE

SYMPTOMS:
Drowsiness and slurred speech; other symptoms may occur that were not observed in medical studies of the drug.
WHAT TO DO:
If person takes much larger amount than prescribed, call doctor, poison center 1-800-222-1222 or hospital emergency room for instructions.

POSSIBLE ADVERSE REACTIONS OR SIDE EFFECTS

SYMPTOMS	WHAT TO DO
Life-threatening:	
High fever, rapid pulse, profuse sweating, muscle rigidity, confusion and irritability, seizures (neuroleptic malignant syndrome - rare).	Discontinue. Seek emergency treatment.
Common:	
• Dizziness, difficulty in speaking or swallowing, shaking hands and fingers, trembling, vision problems, weakness, lightheadedness when arising from a sitting or lying position.	Continue. Call doctor right away.
• Drowsiness, constipation, weight gain, agitation, insomnia, headache, nervousness, runny nose, anxiety, dry mouth, personality disorder, arm or leg stiffness.	Continue. Call doctor when convenient.
Infrequent:	
• Jerky or involuntary movements, especially of the face, lips, jaw, tongue; chest pain, fast heartbeat.	Continue. Call doctor right away.
• Fever, flu-like symptoms, twitching, mood or mental changes, speech unclear, swollen feet or ankles, appetite increased, cough, saliva increased, muscle tightness, muscle spasms (face, neck, back), joint pain, nausea or vomiting, sore throat, thirstiness, incontinence, abdominal pain.	Continue. Call doctor when convenient.
Rare:	
• Breathing difficulty.	Discontinue. Call doctor right away.
• Swollen face, rash, confusion, decreased sex drive, menstrual changes, sluggishness.	Continue. Call doctor when convenient.

WARNINGS & PRECAUTIONS

Don't take if:
You are allergic to olanzapine

Before you start, consult your doctor:
- If you have liver disease, heart disease or a blood vessel disorder.
- If you have Alzheimer's.
- If you have a history of breast cancer.
- If you have intestinal blockage.
- If you are subject to dehydration or low body temperature.
- If you have a history of drug abuse/dependence.
- If you have glaucoma.
- If you have prostate problems.
- If you are allergic to any medication, food or other substance.
- If you have a history of seizures.

Over age 60:
Adverse reactions and side effects may be more severe than in younger persons. A lower starting dosage is usually recommended until a response is determined.

Pregnancy:
Decide with your doctor if drug benefits justify any possible risk to unborn child. Risk category C (see page xviii).

Breast-feeding:
It is unknown if drug passes into milk. It is not recommended for nursing mothers.

Infants & children:
Safety in children under age 18 has not been established. Use only under close medical supervision.

Prolonged use:
Consult with your doctor on a regular basis while taking this drug to check your progress or to discuss any increase or changes in side effects and the need for continued treatment. Long term effectiveness has not been established.

Skin & sunlight:
- May cause rash or intensify sunburn in areas exposed to sun or ultraviolet light (photosensitivity reaction). Use sunscreen and avoid overexposure. Notify doctor if reaction occurs.
- Hot temperatures, exercise, and hot baths can increase risk of heatstroke. Drug may affect body's ability to maintain normal temperature.

Driving, piloting or hazardous work:
Don't drive or pilot aircraft until you learn how medicine affects you. Don't work around dangerous machinery. Don't climb ladders or work in high places. Danger increases if you drink alcohol or take medicine affecting alertness and reflexes.

Discontinuing:
Don't discontinue this drug without consulting doctor. Dosage may require a gradual reduction before stopping.

Others:
- Get up slowly from a sitting or lying position to avoid any dizziness, faintness or lightheadedness.
- Advise any doctor or dentist whom you consult that you take this medicine.
- Take medicine only as directed. Do not increase or reduce dosage without doctor's approval.
- Doctor may need to monitor enzymes in liver to ensure liver functions are not affected by medication.

POSSIBLE INTERACTION WITH OTHER DRUGS

GENERIC NAME OR DRUG CLASS	COMBINED EFFECT
Anticholinergics*, other	Increased risk of side effects.
Antihypertensives*	Increased effect of antihypertensive.
Carbamazepine	Decreased effect of olanzapine.
Central nervous system (CNS) depressants*, other	Increased sedative effect.
Enzyme inducers*	May decrease olanzapine effect.
Enzyme inhibitors*	May increase olanzapine effect.
Dopamine agonists*	May decrease effect of dopamine agonist.
Hepatotoxics*	Increased risk of liver problems.
Levodopa	May decrease levodopa effect.

POSSIBLE INTERACTION WITH OTHER SUBSTANCES

INTERACTS WITH	COMBINED EFFECT
Alcohol:	Increased sedation and dizziness. Avoid.
Beverages:	None expected.
Cocaine:	Effect not known. Best to avoid.
Foods:	None expected.
Marijuana:	Effect not known. Best to avoid.
Tobacco:	Decreased olanzapine effect. Avoid.

OLSALAZINE

BRAND NAMES

Dipentum

BASIC INFORMATION

Habit forming? No
Prescription needed? Yes
Available as generic? No
Drug class: Inflammatory bowel disease suppressant

USES

To maintain remission of ulcerative colitis. Generally prescribed when intolerance to sulfasalazine exists.

DOSAGE & USAGE INFORMATION

How to take:
Capsule—Swallow with liquid or food to lessen stomach irritation. If you can't swallow whole, open capsule and take with liquid or food.

When to take:
Usually twice a day, or as directed on prescription label.

If you forget a dose:
- Take as soon as possible.
- Skip if it is almost time for next dose.
- Don't double next dose.
- Notify your doctor if there are questions.

What drug does:
Inhibits prostaglandin production in the colon.

Time lapse before drug works:
1 hour.

Don't take with:
Any other medicine without consulting your doctor or pharmacist.

OVERDOSE

SYMPTOMS:
None expected.
WHAT TO DO:
Overdose unlikely to threaten life. If person takes much larger amount than prescribed, call doctor, poison center 1-800-222-1222 or hospital emergency room for instructions.

POSSIBLE ADVERSE REACTIONS OR SIDE EFFECTS

SYMPTOMS	WHAT TO DO
Life-threatening:	
Fever, sore throat, paleness, unusual bleeding (representing effect on blood, a rare complication).	Seek emergency treatment.
Common:	
Diarrhea, appetite loss, nausea, vomiting.	Continue. Call doctor when convenient.
Infrequent:	
Mood changes, sleeplessness, headache.	Continue. Call doctor when convenient.
Rare:	
Skin eruption (acne-like), muscle aches.	Continue. Call doctor when convenient.

WARNINGS & PRECAUTIONS

Don't take if:
- You are allergic to aspirin or any other salicylate.
- You are allergic to mesalamine.

Before you start, consult your doctor:
- If you have kidney disease.
- If you are taking any other prescription or nonprescription medicine.

Over age 60:
No special problems expected.

Pregnancy:
Decide with your doctor if drug benefits justify risk to unborn child. Risk category C (see page xviii).

Breast-feeding:
Unknown effects. Consult doctor.

Infants & children:
Effect not documented. Consult your family doctor or pediatrician.

Prolonged use:
Follow through with full prescribed course of treatment.

Skin & sunlight:
No special problems expected.

Driving, piloting or hazardous work:
Don't drive or pilot aircraft until you learn how medicine affects you. Don't work around dangerous machinery. Don't climb ladders or work in high places. Danger increases if you drink alcohol or take medicine affecting alertness and reflexes.

Discontinuing:
Don't discontinue without consulting doctor. Dose may require gradual reduction if you have taken drug for a long time. Doses of other drugs may also require adjustment.

Others:
Request your doctor to check blood counts and kidney function on a regular basis.

POSSIBLE INTERACTION WITH OTHER DRUGS

GENERIC NAME OR DRUG CLASS	COMBINED EFFECT

None expected since olsalazine is not appreciably absorbed from the gastrointestinal tract into the bloodstream.

POSSIBLE INTERACTION WITH OTHER SUBSTANCES

INTERACTS WITH	COMBINED EFFECT
Alcohol:	Increased risk of gastrointestinal upset and/or bleeding.
Beverages: Highly spiced beverages.	Will irritate underlying condition that olsalazine treats.
Cocaine:	Avoid.
Foods: Highly spiced foods.	Will irritate underlying condition that olsalazine treats.
Marijuana:	Avoid.
Tobacco:	Will irritate underlying condition that olsalazine treats. Avoid.

ORLISTAT

BRAND NAMES

Xenical

BASIC INFORMATION

Habit forming? No
Prescription needed? Yes
Available as generic? No
Drug class: Antiobesity, lipase inhibitor

USES

Treatment for obesity and weight loss. To be used in conjunction with a reduced-calorie diet. Treatment with this drug is not recommended for cosmetic weight loss.

DOSAGE & USAGE INFORMATION

How to take:
Capsule—Swallow with liquid, If you can't swallow, whole open capsule and take with liquid.

When to take:
With or shortly following meals (containing fats) up to three times daily.

If you forget a dose:
Skip the missed dose and return to your regular dosing schedule. Do not double dose.

What drug does:
Blocks some of the normal absorption of fats from the intestines, causing them to be excreted in the feces.

Time lapse before drug works:
Several months or longer for maximum benefit.

Don't take with:
Any other medicine without consulting your doctor or pharmacist.

OVERDOSE

SYMPTOMS:
None expected.
WHAT TO DO:
Overdose unlikely to threaten life. If person takes much larger amount than prescribed, call doctor, poison center 1-800-222-1222 or hospital emergency room for instructions.

POSSIBLE ADVERSE REACTIONS OR SIDE EFFECTS

SYMPTOMS	WHAT TO DO
Life-threatening: None expected.	
Common:	
• Flu-like symptoms, runny nose, congestion, sneezing, sore throat, cough, fever.	Continue. Call doctor when convenient.
• Abdominal pain, oily bowel movements, inability to hold bowel movements, immediate need to have bowel movements, gas with leaky bowel movements, oily spotting of underwear, headaches.	Continue. Call doctor if symptoms persist.
Infrequent:	
• Cough, troubled breathing, tightness in chest, wheezing.	Discontinue. Call doctor right away.
• Anxiety, back pain, menstrual irregularities, rectal pain or discomfort, tooth or gum problems.	Continue. Call doctor if symptoms persist.
Rare:	
• Diarrhea, hearing changes, pain in ear, bloody or cloudy urine, difficult or painful urination, frequent urge to urinate.	Discontinue. Call doctor right away.
• Joint pain, dizziness, dry skin, fatigue, insomnia, muscle pain, nausea, skin rash, vomiting.	Continue. Call doctor if symptoms persist.

WARNINGS & PRECAUTIONS

Don't take if:
- You are allergic to orlistat.
- You have been diagnosed with malabsorption.
- You have cholestasis.

Before you start, consult your doctor:
- If you are allergic to any foods or dyes.
- If you are taking any other medications or dietary supplements for weight loss.
- If you have a history of anorexia or bulimia.
- If you have kidney stones or gallbladder problems.
- If you are pregnant or are planning to become pregnant.

Over age 60:
Adverse reactions and side effects may be more frequent and severe than in younger persons.

Pregnancy:
Not recommended for use during pregnancy. Risk category B (see page xviii).

Breast-feeding:
It is unknown if orlistat passes into milk. Avoid drug or discontinue nursing until you finish medicine. Consult doctor for advice on maintaining milk supply.

Infants & children:
Not recommended for persons under 18 years of age.

Prolonged use:
Talk to your doctor about the need for follow-up medical examinations or laboratory studies.

Skin & sunlight:
No problems expected.

Driving, piloting or hazardous work:
No special problems expected.

Discontinuing:
Don't discontinue without doctor's advice.

Others:
- Expect to start with small doses and increase gradually to lessen frequency and severity of adverse reactions.
- Orlistat may interefere with your body's absorption of certain vitamins; therefore, you should take a multivitamin supplement daily, two hours before or after taking orlistat.
- Orlistat may affect the results of some medical tests.
- During treatment, you should be on a nutritionally balanced reduced-calorie diet that contains no more than 30 percent of calories from fat.
- Patients with diabetes may require a reduced dosage of oral hypoglycemic medicine or insulin due to weight loss.
- Advise any doctor or dentist whom you consult that you take this medicine.

POSSIBLE INTERACTION WITH OTHER DRUGS

GENERIC NAME OR DRUG CLASS	COMBINED EFFECT
Cyclosporine	Unknown effect. Monitor closely.
Pravastatin	Increased pravastatin effect.
Vitamins A,D, E, K	Decreased vitamin effect.
Warfarin	Increased warfarin effect.

POSSIBLE INTERACTION WITH OTHER SUBSTANCES

INTERACTS WITH	COMBINED EFFECT
Alcohol:	None expected.
Beverages:	None expected.
Cocaine:	Effects unknown Avoid.
Foods:	None expected.
Marijuana:	Effects unknown Avoid.
Tobacco:	None expected.

ORPHENADRINE

BRAND NAMES

Banflex
Blanex
Disipal
Flexagin
Flexain
Flexoject
Flexon
K-Flex
Marflex
Myolin
Myotrol
Neocyten
Noradex
Norflex
O-Flex
Orflagen
Orfro
Orphenate
Tega-Flex

BASIC INFORMATION

Habit forming? Possibly
Prescription needed?
U.S.: Yes
Canada: No
Available as generic? Yes
Drug class: Muscle relaxant, anticholinergic, antihistamine, antiparkinsonism

USES

- Reduces discomfort of muscle strain.
- Relieves symptoms of Parkinson's disease.
- Adjunctive treatment to rest, analgesics and physical therapy for muscle spasms.

DOSAGE & USAGE INFORMATION

How to take:
- Tablet—Swallow with liquid. If you can't swallow whole, crumble tablet and take with liquid or food.
- Extended-release tablet—Swallow whole. Do not crumble.

When to take:
At the same times each day.

Continued next column

If you forget a dose:
Take as soon as you remember up to 6 hours late. If more than 6 hours, wait for next scheduled dose (don't double this dose).

What drug does:
Sedative and analgesic effects reduce spasm and pain in skeletal muscles.

Time lapse before drug works:
1 to 2 hours.

Don't take with:
Any other medicine without consulting your doctor or pharmacist.

OVERDOSE

SYMPTOMS:
Fainting, confusion, blurred vision, difficulty swallowing, difficulty breathing, decreased urination, widely dilated pupils, rapid heartbeat, rapid pulse, paralysis, convulsions, coma.
WHAT TO DO:
- **Dial 911 (emergency) for an ambulance or medical help or poison center 1-800-222-1222. Then give first aid immediately.**
- **See emergency information on inside covers.**

POSSIBLE ADVERSE REACTIONS OR SIDE EFFECTS

SYMPTOMS	WHAT TO DO
Life-threatening:	
Extreme weakness; transient paralysis; temporary loss of vision; hives, rash, intense itching, faintness soon after a dose (anaphylaxis).	Seek emergency treatment immediately.
Common:	
None expected.	
Infrequent:	
• Weakness, headache, dizziness, agitation, drowsiness, tremor, confusion, rapid or pounding heartbeat, depression, hearing loss.	Discontinue. Call doctor right away.
• Dry mouth, nausea, vomiting, constipation, urinary hesitancy or retention, abdominal pain, muscle weakness.	Continue. Call doctor when convenient.
Rare:	
Rash, itchy skin, blurred vision, hallucinations.	Discontinue. Call doctor right away.

WARNINGS & PRECAUTIONS

Don't take if:
- You are allergic to orphenadrine.
- You are allergic to tartrazine dye.

Before you start, consult your doctor:
- If you have glaucoma.
- If you have myasthenia gravis.
- If you have difficulty emptying bladder.
- If you have had heart disease or heart rhythm disturbance.
- If you have had a peptic ulcer.
- If you have prostate enlargement.

Over age 60:
Adverse reactions and side effects may be more frequent and severe than in younger persons.

Pregnancy:
Decide with your doctor if drug benefits justify risk to unborn child. Risk category C (see page xviii).

Breast-feeding:
No proven problems. Consult doctor.

Infants & children:
Not recommended for children younger than 12.

Prolonged use:
- Increased internal eye pressure.
- Talk to your doctor about the need for follow-up medical examinations or laboratory studies to check complete blood counts (white blood cell count, platelet count, red blood cell count, hemoglobin, hematocrit), liver function, kidney function.

Skin & sunlight:
No problems expected.

Driving, piloting or hazardous work:
Don't drive or pilot aircraft until you learn how medicine affects you. Don't work around dangerous machinery. Don't climb ladders or work in high places. Danger increases if you drink alcohol or take medicine affecting alertness and reflexes, such as antihistamines, tranquilizers, sedatives, pain medicine, narcotics and mind-altering drugs.

Discontinuing:
May be unnecessary to finish medicine. Follow doctor's instructions.

Others:
No problems expected.

POSSIBLE INTERACTION WITH OTHER DRUGS

GENERIC NAME OR DRUG CLASS	COMBINED EFFECT
Anticholinergics*	Increased anticholinergic effect.
Antidepressants, tricyclic*	Increased sedation.
Antihistamines*	Increased sedation.
Attapulgite	Decreased orphenadrine effect.
Carteolol	Decreased antihistamine effect.
Chlorpromazine	Hypoglycemia (low blood sugar).
Cisapride	Decreased orphenadrine effect.
Contraceptives, oral*	Decreased contraceptive effect.
Griseofulvin	Decreased griseofulvin effect.
Levodopa	Increased levodopa effect. (Improves effectiveness in treating Parkinson's disease).
Nabilone	Greater depression of central nervous system.
Nitrates*	Increased internal eye pressure.
Nizatidine	Increased nizatidine effect.
Phenylbutazone	Decreased phenylbutazone effect.
Potassium supplements*	Increased possibility of intestinal ulcers with oral potassium tablets.
Propoxyphene	Possible confusion, nervousness, tremors.

POSSIBLE INTERACTION WITH OTHER SUBSTANCES

INTERACTS WITH	COMBINED EFFECT
Alcohol:	Increased drowsiness. Avoid.
Beverages:	None expected.
Cocaine:	Decreased orphenadrine effect. Avoid.
Foods:	None expected.
Marijuana:	Increased drowsiness, mouth dryness, muscle weakness, fainting.
Tobacco:	None expected.

*See Glossary

ORPHENADRINE, ASPIRIN & CAFFEINE

BRAND NAMES

N3 Gesic
N3 Gesic Forte
Norgesic
Norgesic Forte
Norphadrine
Norphadrine Forte
Orphenagesic
Orphenagesic Forte

BASIC INFORMATION

Habit forming? Yes
Prescription needed? Yes
Available as generic? No
Drug class: Stimulant, vasoconstrictor, muscle relaxant, analgesic, anti-inflammatory (nonsteroidal)

USES

- Reduces discomfort of muscle strain.
- Reduces pain, fever, inflammation.
- Relieves swelling, stiffness, joint pain.
- Treats drowsiness and fatigue.

DOSAGE & USAGE INFORMATION

How to take:
Tablet—Swallow with liquid. If you can't swallow whole, crumble and take with liquid or food.

When to take:
At the same times each day.

If you forget a dose:
Take as soon as you remember up to 2 hours late. If more than 2 hours, wait for next scheduled dose (don't double this dose).

What drug does:
- Sedative and analgesic effects reduce spasm and pain in skeletal muscles.
- Affects hypothalamus, the part of the brain which regulates temperature by dilating small blood vessels in skin.

Continued next column

- Prevents clumping of platelets (small blood cells) so blood vessels remain open.
- Decreases prostaglandin effect.
- Suppresses body's pain messages.
- Constricts blood vessel walls.
- Stimulates central nervous system.

Time lapse before drug works:
1 hour.

Don't take with:
- Tetracyclines. Space doses 1 hour apart.
- Nonprescription drugs without consulting doctor.
- Any other medicine without consulting your doctor or pharmacist.

OVERDOSE

SYMPTOMS:
Fainting, confusion, widely dilated pupils, rapid pulse, ringing in ears, nausea, vomiting, dizziness, fever, deep and rapid breathing, excitement, rapid heartbeat, hallucinations, coma.

WHAT TO DO:
- **Dial 911 (emergency) for an ambulance or medical help or poison center 1-800-222-1222. Then give first aid immediately.**
- **See emergency information on inside covers.**

POSSIBLE ADVERSE REACTIONS OR SIDE EFFECTS

SYMPTOMS	WHAT TO DO
Life-threatening:	
Hives, rash, intense itching, wheezing, faintness soon after a dose (anaphylaxis), convulsions, fever.	Seek emergency treatment immediately.
Common:	
• Nausea, vomiting, abdominal cramps, nervousness, urgent urination, low blood sugar (hunger, anxiety, cold sweats, rapid pulse).	Discontinue. Call doctor right away.
• Ringing in ears, indigestion, heartburn, insomnia.	Continue. Call doctor when convenient.
Infrequent:	
• Weakness, headache, dizziness, drowsiness, agitation, tremor, confusion, irregular heartbeat, hearing loss, diarrhea, hallucinations.	Discontinue. Call doctor right away.
• Dry mouth, constipation.	Continue. Call doctor when convenient.
Rare:	
• Black or bloody vomit.	Discontinue. Seek emergency treatment.
• Change in vision; blurred vision; black, bloody or tarry stool; bloody urine; dilated pupils; uncontrolled movement of hands; sore throat; fever.	Discontinue. Call doctor right away.

WARNINGS & PRECAUTIONS

Don't take if:
- You need to restrict sodium in your diet. Buffered effervescent tablets and sodium salicylate are high in sodium.
- Aspirin has a strong vinegar-like odor, which means it has decomposed.
- You have a peptic ulcer of stomach or duodenum, a bleeding disorder, heart disease.
- You are allergic to any stimulant or orphenadrine.

Before you start, consult your doctor:
- If you have had stomach or duodenal ulcers, gout, heart disease or heart rhythm disturbance, peptic ulcer.
- If you have asthma, nasal polyps, irregular heartbeat, hypoglycemia (low blood sugar), epilepsy, glaucoma, myasthenia gravis, difficulty emptying bladder, prostate enlargement.

Over age 60:
- More likely to cause hidden bleeding in stomach or intestines. Watch for dark stools.
- Adverse reactions and side effects may be more frequent and severe than in younger persons.

Pregnancy:
Risk to unborn child outweighs drug benefits. Don't use. Risk category D (see page xviii).

Breast-feeding:
Drug passes into milk. Avoid drug or discontinue nursing until you finish medicine. Consult doctor for advice on maintaining milk supply.

Infants & children:
- Overdose frequent and severe. Keep bottles out of children's reach.
- Consult doctor before giving to persons under age 18 who have fever and discomfort of viral illness, especially chicken pox and influenza. Probably increases risk of Reye's syndrome.
- Not recommended for children under 12.

Prolonged use:
- Kidney damage. Periodic kidney function test recommended.
- Stomach ulcers more likely.
- Increased internal eye pressure.
- Talk to your doctor about the need for follow-up medical examinations or laboratory studies to check liver function, complete blood counts (white blood cell count, platelet count, red blood cell count, hemoglobin, hematocrit).

Skin & sunlight:
No special problems expected.

Driving, piloting or hazardous work:
Don't drive or pilot aircraft until you learn how medicine affects you. Don't work around dangerous machinery. Don't climb ladders or work in high places. Danger increases if you drink alcohol or take medicine affecting alertness and reflexes, such as antihistamines, tranquilizers, sedatives, pain medicine, narcotics and mind-altering drugs.

Discontinuing:
- For chronic illness—Don't discontinue without doctor's advice until you complete prescribed dose, even though symptoms diminish or disappear.
- May be unnecessary to finish medicine if you take it for a short-term illness. Follow doctor's instructions.

Others:
- Aspirin can complicate surgery; illness; pregnancy, labor and delivery.
- For arthritis, don't change dose without consulting doctor.
- Urine tests for blood sugar may be inaccurate.
- May produce or aggravate fibrocystic breast disease in women.

POSSIBLE INTERACTION WITH OTHER DRUGS

GENERIC NAME OR DRUG CLASS	COMBINED EFFECT
Acebutolol	Decreased antihypertensive effect of acebutolol.

Continued on page 924

POSSIBLE INTERACTION WITH OTHER SUBSTANCES

INTERACTS WITH	COMBINED EFFECT
Alcohol:	Possible stomach irritation and bleeding, increased drowsiness. Avoid.
Beverages: Caffeine drinks.	Increased caffeine effect.
Cocaine:	Decreased orphenadrine effect. Overstimulation. Avoid.
Foods:	None expected.
Marijuana:	Increased effect of drugs. May lead to dangerous, rapid heartbeat. Increased dry mouth. Avoid.
Tobacco:	Increased heartbeat. Avoid.

***See Glossary**

OXCARBAZEPINE

BRAND NAMES

Trileptal

BASIC INFORMATION

Habit forming? No
Prescription needed? Yes
Available as generic? No
Drug class: Anticonvulsant, antiepileptic

USES

Treatment for partial (focal) epileptic seizures. May be used alone or in combination with other antiepileptic drugs.

DOSAGE & USAGE INFORMATION

How to take:
Tablet–Swallow with liquid. May be taken with or without food.

When to take:
Your doctor will determine the best schedule. Dosages will be increased rapidly over the first few days of use. Further increases may be necessary to achieve maximum benefits.

If you forget a dose:
Take as soon as you remember. If it is almost time for the next dose, skip the missed dose and wait for your next scheduled dose (don't double this dose).

What drug does:
The exact mechanism is unknown. The anticonvulsant action may result from an altered transport of brain amino acids. Amino acids play an important part in chemical reactions within the cells.

Time lapse before drug works:
May take several weeks for effectiveness.

Don't take with:
Any other prescription or nonprescription drug without consulting your doctor or pharmacist.

OVERDOSE

SYMPTOMS:
Double vision, slurred speech, drowsiness, tiredness, diarrhea.
WHAT TO DO:
Overdose unlikely to threaten life. If person takes much larger amount than prescribed, call doctor, poison center 1-800-222-1222 or hospital emergency room for instructions.

POSSIBLE ADVERSE REACTIONS OR SIDE EFFECTS

SYMPTOMS	WHAT TO DO
Life-threatening: None expected.	
Common:	
• Cough with fever and sneezing and sore throat, clumsiness, vision changes, dizziness, crying, depression, false sense of well-being, spinning sensation, uncontrolled eye movement, feeling of constant movement of self or surroundings.	Continue, but call doctor right away.
• Runny or stuffy nose, nausea or vomiting, sleepiness.	Continue. Call doctor when convenient.
Infrequent:	
• Blurred vision, cloudy or bloody urine, urination (decreased or increased, painful, urgent), confusion, falling, bruising, ill feeling, thirstiness, hoarseness, vaginal itching, heartbeat irregularities, facial pain, memory loss, coordination problems, trembling, shortness of breath, unusual tiredness or weakness.	Continue, but call doctor right away.
• Sour stomach, acne, changes in taste, dry mouth, constipation or diarrhea, heartburn, sweating, feeling of warmth in face or chest, back pain, belching, bloody nose.	Continue. Call doctor when convenient.
Rare:	
Sore or bleeding lips, chills, chest pain, irritability, hives or itching, muscle or joint pain, nervousness, rectal bleeding, peeling or blistering skin, sores in mouth, swollen legs, purple spots on skin, burning feeling in chest or stomach.	Continue, but call, doctor right away.

WARNINGS & PRECAUTIONS

Don't take if:
You are allergic to oxcarbazepine or carbamazepine.

Before you start, consult your doctor:
- If you have a history of kidney disease.
- If you have hyponatremia (too little sodium in the body).
- If you are allergic to any medication, food or other substance.
- If you have any other medical problems.

Over age 60:
No special problems expected.

Pregnancy:
Decide with your doctor if drug benefits justify risks to unborn child. Risk category C (see page xviii).

Breast-feeding:
Drug passes into milk. Avoid drug or discontinue nursing until you finish medicine. Consult doctor for advice on maintaining milk supply.

Infants & children:
No special problems expected for children over age four.

Prolonged use:
No special problems expected. Follow-up laboratory blood studies may be recommended by your doctor.

Skin & sunlight:
No problems expected.

Driving, piloting or hazardous work:
Don't drive or pilot aircraft until you learn how medicine affects you. Don't work around dangerous machinery. Don't climb ladders or work in high places. Danger increases if you drink alcohol or take other medicines affecting alertness and reflexes such as antihistamines, tranquilizers, sedatives, pain medicine, narcotics and mind-altering drugs.

Discontinuing:
Don't discontinue without doctor's approval due to risk of increased seizure activity. The dosage may need to be gradually decreased before stopping the drug completely.

Others:
- Advise any doctor or dentist whom you consult that you take this medicine.
- The effectiveness of oral contraceptives that contain estrogen may be reduced. Talk to your doctor about other forms of birth control
- Oxcarbazepine may be used with other anticonvulsant drugs and additional side effects may occur. If they do, discuss them with your doctor.
- This medicine alone may cause drowsiness, dizziness, or lightheadedness, especially when getting up from a sitting or lying position.

POSSIBLE INTERACTION WITH OTHER DRUGS

GENERIC NAME OR DRUG CLASS	COMBINED EFFECT
Anticonvulsants*, other	Increase risk of side effects.
Contraceptives, oral*	Decreased effect of contraceptive.
CNS Depressants* (antihistamines, sleeping pills, tranquilizers and sedatives)	Increased sedative effect.
Felodipine	Decreased effect of felodipine.
Verapamil	Decreased effect of verapamil.

POSSIBLE INTERACTION WITH OTHER SUBSTANCES

INTERACTS WITH	COMBINED EFFECT
Alcohol:	Increased sedative effect. Avoid.
Beverages:	None expected.
Cocaine:	Unknown effect. Avoid.
Foods:	None expected.
Marijuana:	Unknown effect. Avoid.
Tobacco:	None expected.

*See Glossary

OXTRIPHYLLINE & GUAIFENESIN

BRAND NAMES

Brondecon
Brondelate
Choledyl
Expectorant

BASIC INFORMATION

Habit forming? No
Prescription needed? Yes
Available as generic? Yes
Drug class: Bronchodilator (xanthine), cough/cold preparation

USES

- Treatment for bronchial asthma symptoms.
- Loosens mucus in respiratory passages from allergies and infections.

DOSAGE & USAGE INFORMATION

How to take:
Tablet or elixir—Swallow with liquid. If you can't swallow tablet whole, crumble and take with liquid or food.

When to take:
Most effective taken on empty stomach 1 hour before or 2 hours after eating. However, may take with food to lessen stomach upset.

If you forget a dose:
Take as soon as you remember up to 2 hours late. If more than 2 hours, wait for next scheduled dose (don't double this dose).

What drug does:
- Relaxes and expands bronchial tubes.
- Increases production of watery fluids to thin mucus so it can be coughed out or absorbed.

Time lapse before drug works:
15 to 30 minutes.

Don't take with:
- Any stimulant.
- Any other medicine without consulting your doctor or pharmacist.

OVERDOSE

SYMPTOMS:
Restlessness, irritability, confusion, delirium, convulsions, rapid pulse, nausea, vomiting, coma.
WHAT TO DO:
- **Dial 911 (emergency) for an ambulance or medical help or poison center 1-800-222-1222. Then give first aid immediately.**
- **See emergency information on inside covers.**

POSSIBLE ADVERSE REACTIONS OR SIDE EFFECTS

SYMPTOMS	WHAT TO DO
Life-threatening:	
Difficult breathing, irregular or fast heartbeat.	Discontinue. Seek emergency treatment.
Common:	
Headache, irritability, nervousness, restlessness, insomnia, nausea, vomiting, abdominal pain, drowsiness.	Continue. Call doctor when convenient.
Infrequent:	
• Hives, rash, red or flushed façe, diarrhea, heartburn, muscle twitching.	Discontinue. Call doctor right away.
• Dizziness, lightheadedness, appetite loss.	Continue. Call doctor when convenient.
Rare:	
None expected.	

WARNINGS & PRECAUTIONS

Don't take if:
- You are allergic to any cough or cold preparation containing guaifenesin or any bronchodilator.
- You have an active peptic ulcer.

Before you start, consult your doctor:
- If you have had impaired kidney or liver function.
- If you have gastritis, peptic ulcer, high blood pressure or heart disease.
- If you take medication for gout.

Over age 60:
Adverse reactions and side effects may be more frequent and severe than in younger persons. For drug to work, you must drink 8 to 10 glasses of fluid per day.

Pregnancy:
Decide with your doctor if drug benefits justify risk to unborn child. Risk category C (see page xviii).

Breast-feeding:
Drug passes into milk. Avoid drug or discontinue nursing until you finish medicine. Consult doctor for advice on maintaining milk supply.

Infants & children:
Use only under medical supervision.

Prolonged use:
- Stomach irritation.
- Talk to your doctor about the need for follow-up medical examinations or laboratory studies to check serum oxtriphylline levels, lung function.

Skin & sunlight:
No problems expected.

Driving, piloting or hazardous work:
Avoid if lightheaded or dizzy. Otherwise, no problems expected.

Discontinuing:
May be unnecessary to finish medicine. Follow doctor's instructions.

Others:
No problems expected.

POSSIBLE INTERACTION WITH OTHER DRUGS

GENERIC NAME OR DRUG CLASS	COMBINED EFFECT
Allopurinol	Decreased allopurinol effect.
Anticoagulants,* oral	Possible risk of bleeding.
Ephedrine	Increased effect of both drugs.
Epinephrine	Increased effect of both drugs.
Erythromycins*	Increased bronchodilator effect.
Furosemide	Increased furosemide effect.
Lincomycins*	Increased bronchodilator effect.
Lithium	Decreased lithium effect.
Probenecid	Decreased effect of both drugs.
Propranolol	Decreased bronchodilator effect.
Rauwolfia alkaloids*	Rapid heartbeat.
Sulfinpyrazone	Decreased sulfin pyrazone effect.
Troleandomycin	Increased bronchodilator effect.

POSSIBLE INTERACTION WITH OTHER SUBSTANCES

INTERACTS WITH	COMBINED EFFECT
Alcohol:	None expected.
Beverages:	
Caffeine drinks.	Nervousness and insomnia.
Other.	You must drink 8 to 10 glasses of fluid per day for drug to work.
Cocaine:	Excess stimulation. Avoid.
Foods:	None expected.
Marijuana:	Slightly increased antiasthmatic effect of bronchodilator.
Tobacco:	Decreased bronchodilator effect and harmful for all conditions requiring bronchodilator treatment. Avoid.

*See Glossary

OXYBUTYNIN

BRAND NAMES

Ditropan

BASIC INFORMATION

Habit forming? No
Prescription needed? Yes
Available as generic? Yes
Drug class: Antispasmodic (urinary tract)

USES

Reduces spasms of urinary bladder and urethra that cause symptoms of frequent urination, urgency, night-time urination and incontinence.

DOSAGE & USAGE INFORMATION

How to take:
Tablets or syrup—Swallow with water.

When to take:
At the same time every day. Do not take with food unless instructed to do so by doctor.

If you forget a dose:
Take as soon as you remember up to 2 hours late. If more than 2 hours, wait for next scheduled dose. Don't double this dose.

What drug does:
Blocks nerve impulses at parasympathetic nerve endings, preventing muscle contractions and gland secretions of organs involved.

Time lapse before drug works:
30 minutes to 1 hour.

Don't take with:
Any other medicine without consulting your doctor or pharmacist.

OVERDOSE

SYMPTOMS:
Unsteadiness, confusion, dizziness, severe drowsiness, fast heartbeat, fever, red face, hallucinations, difficult breathing.
WHAT TO DO:
Overdose unlikely to threaten life. If person takes much larger amount than prescribed, call doctor, poison center 1-800-222-1222 or hospital emergency room for instructions.

POSSIBLE ADVERSE REACTIONS OR SIDE EFFECTS

SYMPTOMS	WHAT TO DO
Life-threatening: In case of overdose, see previous column.	
Common:	
Constipation; decreased sweating; drowsiness; dryness of mouth, nose and throat.	Continue. Call doctor when convenient.
Infrequent:	
Difficult swallowing, decreased sexual ability, headache, difficult urination, sensitivity to light, nausea, vomiting, insomnia, tiredness.	Continue. Call doctor when convenient.
Rare:	
Skin rash, eye pain, blurred vision.	Discontinue. Call doctor right away.

WARNINGS & PRECAUTIONS

Don't take if:
- You are allergic to any anticholinergic.
- You have trouble with stomach bloating.
- You have difficulty emptying your bladder completely.
- You have narrow-angle glaucoma.
- You have severe ulcerative colitis.

Before you start, consult your doctor:
- If you have open-angle glaucoma.
- If you have angina or fast heartbeat.
- If you have chronic bronchitis or asthma.
- If you have hiatal hernia; liver, kidney or thyroid disease; enlarged prostate or myasthenia gravis.
- If you will have surgery within 2 months, including dental surgery, requiring general or spinal anesthesia.

Over age 60:
Adverse reactions and side effects may be more frequent and severe than in younger persons. You may require smaller doses for shorter periods of time.

Pregnancy:
No proven harm to unborn child, but avoid if possible. Consult doctor. Risk category B (see page xviii).

Breast-feeding:
Unknown effect. Consult doctor.

Infants & children:
Not recommended for children under 5.

Prolonged use:
Side effects more likely.

Skin & sunlight:
No special problems expected.

Driving, piloting or hazardous work:
Don't drive or pilot aircraft until you learn how medicine affects you. Don't work around dangerous machinery. Don't climb ladders or work in high places. Danger increases if you drink alcohol or take medicine affecting alertness and reflexes.

Discontinuing:
May be unnecessary to finish medicine. Follow doctor's instructions.

Others:
Advise any doctor or dentist whom you consult that you take this medicine.

POSSIBLE INTERACTION WITH OTHER DRUGS

GENERIC NAME OR DRUG CLASS	COMBINED EFFECT
Anticholinergics*	Increased effect of oxybutynin.
Central nervous system (CNS) depressants*	Increased sedative effect.

POSSIBLE INTERACTION WITH OTHER SUBSTANCES

INTERACTS WITH	COMBINED EFFECT
Alcohol:	Increased sedative effect.
Beverages:	None expected.
Cocaine:	Excessively rapid heartbeat. Avoid.
Foods:	None expected.
Marijuana:	Drowsiness and dry mouth.
Tobacco:	None expected.

OXYMETAZOLINE (Nasal)

BRAND NAMES

See complete list of brand names in the *Generic and Brand Name Directory*, page 862.

BASIC INFORMATION

Habit forming? No
Prescription needed? No
Available as generic? Yes
Drug class: Sympathomimetic

USES

Relieves congestion of nose, sinuses and throat from allergies and infections.

DOSAGE & USAGE INFORMATION

How to take:
Nasal solution, nasal spray—Use as directed on label. Avoid contamination. Don't use same container for more than 1 person.

When to take:
When needed, no more often than every 4 hours.

If you forget a dose:
Take as soon as you remember. Wait 4 hours for next dose.

What drug does:
Constricts walls of small arteries in nose, sinuses and eustachian tubes.

Time lapse before drug works:
5 to 30 minutes. May last 8 to 12 hours.

Continued next column

OVERDOSE

SYMPTOMS:
Headache, sweating, anxiety, agitation, rapid and irregular heartbeat (rare occurrence with systemic absorption).
WHAT TO DO:

- **Dial 911 (emergency) for an ambulance or medical help or poison center 1-800-222-1222. Then give first aid immediately.**
- **If patient is unconscious and not breathing, give mouth-to-mouth breathing. If there is no heartbeat, use cardiac massage and mouth-to-mouth breathing (CPR). If you can't get help quickly, take patient to nearest emergency facility.**
- **See emergency information on inside covers.**

Don't take with:

- Nonprescription drugs for allergy, cough or cold without consulting doctor.
- Any other medicine without consulting your doctor or pharmacist.

POSSIBLE ADVERSE REACTIONS OR SIDE EFFECTS

SYMPTOMS	WHAT TO DO
Life-threatening: In case of overdose, see previous column.	
Common: None expected.	
Infrequent:	
Burning, dry or stinging nasal passages.	Continue. Call doctor when convenient.
Rare:	
Rebound congestion (increased runny or stuffy nose); headache, insomnia, nervousness (may occur with systemic absorption).	Discontinue. Call doctor right away.

WARNINGS & PRECAUTIONS

Don't take if:
You are allergic to oxymetazoline or other nasal spray.

Before you start, consult your doctor:
- If you have heart disease or high blood pressure.
- If you have diabetes.
- If you have overactive thyroid.
- If you have taken MAO inhibitors in past 2 weeks.
- If you have glaucoma.

Over age 60:
Adverse reactions and side effects may be more frequent and severe than in younger persons.

Pregnancy:
Consult doctor. Risk category C (see page xviii).

Breast-feeding:
No proven problems. Consult doctor.

Infants & children:
Don't give to children younger than 2.

Prolonged use:
Drug may lose effectiveness, cause increased congestion (rebound effect*) and irritate nasal membranes.

Skin & sunlight:
No problems expected.

Driving, piloting or hazardous work:
No problems expected.

Discontinuing:
May be unnecessary to finish medicine. Follow doctor's instructions.

Others:
Don't use for more than 3 days in a row.

POSSIBLE INTERACTION WITH OTHER DRUGS

GENERIC NAME OR DRUG CLASS	COMBINED EFFECT
Antidepressants, tricyclic*	Possible rise in blood pressure.
Butorphanol	Delays start of butorphanol effect.
Maprotiline	Possible increased blood pressure.

POSSIBLE INTERACTION WITH OTHER SUBSTANCES

INTERACTS WITH	COMBINED EFFECT
Alcohol:	None expected.
Beverages: Caffeine drinks.	Nervousness or insomnia.
Cocaine:	High risk of heart-beat irregularities and high blood pressure.
Foods:	None expected.
Marijuana:	Overstimulation. Avoid.
Tobacco:	None expected.

*See Glossary

PACLITAXEL

BRAND NAMES

Taxol

BASIC INFORMATION

Habit forming? No
Prescription needed? Yes
Available as generic? No
Drug class: Antineoplastic

USES

Treats ovarian cancer, breast cancer and some lung cancers.

DOSAGE & USAGE INFORMATION

How to take:
Injection–Administered only by a doctor or under the supervision of a doctor.

When to take:
Your doctor will determine the schedule. Usually the drug is infused over a 24-hour period at 21-day intervals. Other drugs may be given prior to paclitaxel injection to help prevent adverse effects.

If you forget a dose:
Not a concern since drug is administered by a doctor.

What drug does:
Interferes with the growth of cancer cells, which are eventually destroyed.

Time lapse before drug works:
Results may not show for several weeks or months.

Don't take with:
Any other prescription or nonprescription drug without consulting your doctor.

OVERDOSE

SYMPTOMS:
None expected.
WHAT TO DO:
Overdose is unlikely. You will be monitored by medical personnel during the time of the infusion.

POSSIBLE ADVERSE REACTIONS OR SIDE EFFECTS

SYMPTOMS	WHAT TO DO
Life-threatening:	
Anaphylactic reaction soon after an injection (hives, rash, intense itching, faintness, breathing difficulty).	Emergency care will be provided.
Common:	
• Paleness, tiredness, flushing of face, skin rash or itching, shortness of breath, fever, chills, cough or hoarseness, back or side pain, difficult or painful urination, unusual bleeding or bruising, black or tarry stools, blood in stool or urine, pinpoint red spots on skin, bleeding gums, delayed wound healing.	Call doctor right away.
• Pain in joints or muscles; diarrhea; nausea and vomiting; numbness, burning or tingling in hands or feet.	Call doctor when convenient.
• Loss of hair (should regrow after treatment completed).	No action necessary.
Infrequent:	
Heart rhythm disturbances, chest pain.	Call doctor right away.
Rare:	
Pain or redness at injection site, mouth or lip sores.	Call doctor right away.

WARNINGS & PRECAUTIONS

Don't take if:
You are allergic to paclitaxel.

Before you start, consult your doctor:
- If you have an infection or any other medical problem.
- If you have or recently had chickenpox or herpes zoster (shingles).
- If you have heart problems.
- If you are pregnant or if you plan to become pregnant.
- If you have had radiation therapy or previously taken anticancer drugs.

Over age 60:
No problems expected.

Pregnancy:
Animal studies show fetal abnormalities and increased risk of abortion. Discuss with your doctor whether drug benefits justify risk to unborn child. Risk category D (see page xviii).

Breast-feeding:
Not known if drug passes into milk. Avoid drug or discontinue nursing until you finish medicine. Consult doctor for advice on maintaining milk supply.

Infants & children:
Safety and effectiveness of use in children not established.

Prolonged use:
Not recommended for long-term use.

Skin & sunlight:
No problems expected.

Driving, piloting or hazardous work:
Avoid if you feel side effects such as nausea and vomiting.

Discontinuing:
Your doctor will determine the schedule.

Others:
- Advise any doctor or dentist whom you consult that you take this medicine.
- May affect the results in some medical tests.
- Do not have any immunizations (vaccinations) without doctor's approval. Other household members should not take oral polio vaccine. It could pass the polio virus on to you. Avoid any contact with persons who have taken oral polio vaccine.
- Possible delayed effects (including some types of cancers) may occur months to years after use. Your doctor should discuss with you all risks involving this drug.
- You will have increased risk of infections. Take extra precautions (handwashing), and avoid people with infections. Avoid crowds if possible. Contact your doctor immediately if you develop signs or symptoms of infection.
- Use care in the use of toothbrushes, dental floss and toothpicks. Talk to your medical doctor before you have dental work done.
- Do not touch your eyes or the inside of your nose without carefully washing your hands first.
- Avoid activities (e.g., contact sports) that could cause bruising or injury.
- Avoid cutting yourself when using a safety razor, fingernail or toenail clippers.

POSSIBLE INTERACTION WITH OTHER DRUGS

GENERIC NAME OR DRUG CLASS	COMBINED EFFECT
Blood dyscrasia-causing medicines*	Increased risk of paclitaxel toxicity.
Bone marrow depressants,* (other)	Increased risk of paclitaxel toxicity.

POSSIBLE INTERACTION WITH OTHER SUBSTANCES

INTERACTS WITH	COMBINED EFFECT
Alcohol:	None expected.
Beverages:	None expected.
Cocaine:	None expected.
Foods:	None expected.
Marijuana:	None expected.
Tobacco:	None expected.

***See Glossary**

PANCREATIN, PEPSIN, BILE SALTS, HYOSCYAMINE, ATROPINE, SCOPOLAMINE & PHENOBARBITAL

BRAND NAMES

Donnazyme

BASIC INFORMATION

Habit forming? Yes
Prescription needed? Yes
Available as generic? No
Drug class: Digestant, sedative, anticholinergic

USES

- Replaces deficient digestive enzymes.
- Sometimes used to relieve indigestion.

DOSAGE & USAGE INFORMATION

How to take:
Tablet—Swallow with liquid or food to lessen stomach irritation. If you can't swallow whole, crumble tablet and take with food or liquid.

When to take:
With or after meals.

If you forget a dose:
Skip it and resume schedule. Don't double dose.

What drug does:
Blocks nerve impulses at parasympathetic nerve endings, preventing smooth muscle contraction and gland secretions.

Time lapse before drug works:
30 to 60 minutes.

Continued next column

OVERDOSE

SYMPTOMS:
Hallucinations, excitement, breathing difficulty, irregular heartbeat (too fast or too slow), fainting, collapse, coma.
WHAT TO DO:
- **Dial 911 (emergency) for an ambulance or medical help or poison center 1-800-222-1222. Then give first aid immediately.**
- **See emergency information on inside covers.**

Don't take with:
Any medicine that will decrease mental alertness or reflexes, such as alcohol, other mind-altering drugs, cough/cold medicines, antihistamines, allergy medicine, sedatives, tranquilizers (sleeping pills or "downers"), barbiturates, seizure medicine, narcotics, other prescription medicine for pain, muscle relaxants, anesthetics.

POSSIBLE ADVERSE REACTIONS OR SIDE EFFECTS

SYMPTOMS	WHAT TO DO
Life-threatening: In case of overdose, see previous column.	
Common:	
• Constipation, decreased sweating, headache.	Discontinue. Call doctor right away.
• Drowsiness, dry mouth, frequent urination.	Continue. Call doctor when convenient.
Infrequent:	
• Blurred vision.	Discontinue. Call doctor right away.
• Diminished sex drive, swallowing difficulty, sensitivity to light, insomnia.	Continue. Call doctor when convenient.
Rare:	
• Jaundice; unusual bleeding or bruising; swollen feet and ankles; abdominal pain; sore throat, fever, mouth sores; rash; hives; vomiting; joint pain; eye pain; diarrhea; blood in urine.	Discontinue. Call doctor right away.
• Unusual tiredness.	Continue. Call doctor when convenient.

WARNINGS & PRECAUTIONS

Don't take if:
- You are allergic to any of the drugs in this combination.
- You have trouble with stomach bloating, difficulty emptying your bladder completely, narrow-angle glaucoma, severe ulcerative colitis, porphyria.

PANCREATIN, PEPSIN, BILE SALTS, HYOSCYAMINE, ATROPINE, SCOPOLAMINE & PHENOBARBITAL

Before you start, consult your doctor:
- If you have open-angle glaucoma, angina, chronic bronchitis or asthma, liver disease, hiatal hernia, enlarged prostate, myasthenia gravis, epilepsy, kidney or liver damage, anemia, chronic pain.
- If you will have surgery within 2 months, including dental surgery, requiring general or spinal anesthesia.

Over age 60:
Adverse reactions and side effects may be more frequent and severe than in younger persons

Pregnancy:
Decide with your doctor if drug benefits justify risk to unborn child. Risk category C (see page xviii).

Breast-feeding:
Drug passes into milk. Avoid drug or discontinue nursing until you finish medicine. Consult doctor for advice on maintaining milk supply.

Infants & children:
Use only under medical supervision.

Prolonged use:
- Chronic constipation, possible fecal impaction.
- May cause addiction, anemia, chronic intoxication.
- May lower body temperature, making exposure to cold temperatures hazardous.

Skin & sunlight:
One or more drugs in this group may cause rash or intensify sunburn in areas exposed to sun or ultraviolet light (photosensitivity reaction). Avoid overexposure. Notify doctor if reaction occurs..

Driving, piloting or hazardous work:
Don't drive or pilot aircraft until you learn how medicine affects you. Don't work around dangerous machinery. Don't climb ladders or work in high places. Danger increases if you drink alcohol or take medicine affecting alertness and reflexes, such as antihistamines, tranquilizers, sedatives, pain medicine, narcotics and mind-altering drugs.

Discontinuing:
- May be unnecessary to finish medicine. Follow doctor's instructions.
- If you develop withdrawal symptoms of hallucinations, agitation or sleeplessness after discontinuing, call doctor right away.

Others:
- Potential for abuse.
- Enzyme deficiencies probably better treated with identified separate substances rather than a mixture of components.

POSSIBLE INTERACTION WITH OTHER DRUGS

GENERIC NAME OR DRUG CLASS	COMBINED EFFECT
Adrenocorticoids, systemic	Possible glaucoma.
Amantadine	Increased atropine effect.
Antacids*	Decreased absorption of scopolamine.
Anticholinergics*, other	Increased anticholinergic effect.
Anticoagulants*, oral	Decreased anticoagulant effect.
Antidepressants, tricyclic*	Decreased antidepressant effect. Possible dangerous oversedation.
Antidiabetics*, oral	Increased phenobartital effect.
Antihistamines*	Increased atropine effect.
Anti-inflammatory drugs, nonsteroidal (NSAIDs)*	Decreased antiinflammatory effects.

Continued on page 925

POSSIBLE INTERACTION WITH OTHER SUBSTANCES

INTERACTS WITH	COMBINED EFFECT
Alcohol:	Possible fatal oversedation. Avoid.
Beverages:	None expected.
Cocaine:	Excessively rapid heartbeat. Avoid.
Foods:	None expected.
Marijuana:	Excessive sedation, drowsiness and dry mouth.
Tobacco:	May increase stomach acidity, decreasing the effectiveness of the drug. Avoid.

*See Glossary

PANCRELIPASE

BRAND NAMES

Cotazym
Cotazym E.C.S.
Cotazym-65B
Cotazym-S
Enzymase-16
Ilozyme
Ku-Zyme HP
Lipancreatin
Pancoate
Pancrease
Pancrease MT4
Pancrease MT10
Pancrease MT16
Protilase
Ultrase MT 12
Ultrase MT 20
Ultrase MT 24
Viokase
Zymase

BASIC INFORMATION

Habit forming? No
Prescription needed? Yes
Available as generic? Yes
Drug class: Enzyme (pancreatic)

USES

- Replaces pancreatic enzyme lost due to surgery or disease.
- Treats fatty stools (steatorrhea).

DOSAGE & USAGE INFORMATION

How to take:
- Tablets, capsules or delayed-release capsules—Swallow whole. Do not take with milk or milk products.
- Powder—Sprinkle on liquid or soft food.

When to take:
Before meals.

If you forget a dose:
Take as soon as you remember up to 2 hours late. If more than 2 hours, wait for next scheduled dose (don't double this dose).

What drug does:
Enhances digestion of proteins, carbohydrates and fats.

Continued next column

OVERDOSE

SYMPTOMS:
Shortness of breath, wheezing, diarrhea.
WHAT TO DO:
Overdose unlikely to threaten life. If person takes much larger amount than prescribed, call doctor, poison center 1-800-222-1222 or hospital emergency room for instructions.

Time lapse before drug works:
30 minutes.

Don't take with:
Any other medicine without consulting your doctor or pharmacist.

POSSIBLE ADVERSE REACTIONS OR SIDE EFFECTS

SYMPTOMS	WHAT TO DO
Life-threatening: None expected.	
Common: None expected.	
Infrequent: Diarrhea, asthma.	Discontinue. Call doctor right away.
Rare:	
• Rash, hives, blood in urine, swollen feet or legs, abdominal cramps.	Discontinue. Call doctor right away.
• Nausea, joint pain.	Continue. Call doctor when convenient.

WARNINGS & PRECAUTIONS

Don't take if:
You are allergic to pancreatin, pancrelipase, or pork.

Before you start, consult your doctor:
If you take any other medicines.

Over age 60:
Adverse reactions and side effects may be more frequent and severe than in younger persons.

Pregnancy:
Decide with your doctor if drug benefits justify risk to unborn child. Risk category C (see page xviii).

Breast-feeding:
Drug may pass into milk. Avoid drug or discontinue nursing until you finish medicine. Consult doctor for advice on maintaining milk supply.

Infants & children:
Give under close medical supervision only.

Prolonged use:
No additional problems expected.

Skin & sunlight:
No problems expected.

Driving, piloting or hazardous work:
No problems expected.

Discontinuing:
Don't discontinue without consulting doctor. Dose may require gradual reduction if you have taken drug for a long time. Doses of other drugs may also require adjustment.

Others:
If you take powder form, avoid inhaling.

POSSIBLE INTERACTION WITH OTHER DRUGS

GENERIC NAME OR DRUG CLASS	COMBINED EFFECT
Calcium carbonate antacids*	Decreased effect of pancrelipase.
Iron supplements	Decreased iron absorption.
Magnesium hydroxide antacids*	Decreased effect of pancrelipase.

POSSIBLE INTERACTION WITH OTHER SUBSTANCES

INTERACTS WITH	COMBINED EFFECT
Alcohol:	Unknown.
Beverages: Milk.	Decreased effect of pancrelipase.
Cocaine:	Unknown.
Foods: Ice cream, milk products.	Decreased effect of pancrelipase.
Marijuana:	Decreased absorption of pancrelipase.
Tobacco:	Decreased absorption of pancrelipase.

*See Glossary

PANTOTHENIC ACID (Vitamin B-5)

BRAND AND GENERIC NAMES

CALCIUM PANTOTHENATE | **Dexol T.D.**

An ingredient in numerous multiple vitamin-mineral supplements. Check labels.

BASIC INFORMATION

Habit forming? No
Prescription needed? No
Available as generic? Yes
Drug class: Vitamin supplement

USES

Prevents and treats vitamin B-5 deficiency.

DOSAGE & USAGE INFORMATION

How to take:
Tablet—Swallow with liquid.

When to take:
At the same times each day.

If you forget a dose:
Take as soon as you remember, then resume regular schedule.

What drug does:
Acts as co-enzyme in carbohydrate, protein and fat metabolism.

Time lapse before drug works:
15 to 20 minutes.

Don't take with:
- Levodopa—Small amounts of pantothenic acid will nullify levodopa effect. Carbidopa-levodopa combination not affected by this interaction.
- Any other medicine without consulting your doctor or pharmacist.

OVERDOSE

SYMPTOMS:
None expected.
WHAT TO DO:
Overdose unlikely to threaten life.

POSSIBLE ADVERSE REACTIONS OR SIDE EFFECTS

SYMPTOMS	WHAT TO DO
Life-threatening:	
None expected.	
Common:	
Heartburn.	Discontinue. Seek emergency treatment.
Infrequent:	
Cramps.	Discontinue Call doctor right away.
Rare:	
Rash, hives, difficult breathing.	Discontinue. Seek emergency treatment.

WARNINGS & PRECAUTIONS

Don't take if:
You are allergic to pantothenic acid.

Before you start, consult your doctor:
If you have hemophilia.

Over age 60:
No problems expected.

Pregnancy:
Risk factor not designated. See category list on page xviii and consult doctor.

Breast-feeding:
Don't exceed recommended dose. Consult doctor.

Infants & children:
Don't exceed recommended dose.

Prolonged use:
Large doses for more than 1 month may cause toxicity.

Skin & sunlight:
No problems expected.

Driving, piloting or hazardous work:
No problems expected.

Discontinuing:
No problems expected.

Others:
Regular pantothenic acid supplements are recommended if you take chloramphenicol, cycloserine, ethionamide, hydralazine, immunosuppressants*, isoniazid or penicillamine. These decrease pantothenic acid absorption and can cause anemia or tingling and numbness in hands and feet.

POSSIBLE INTERACTION WITH OTHER DRUGS

GENERIC NAME OR DRUG CLASS	COMBINED EFFECT
None significant.	

POSSIBLE INTERACTION WITH OTHER SUBSTANCES

INTERACTS WITH	COMBINED EFFECT
Alcohol:	None expected.
Beverages:	None expected.
Cocaine:	None expected.
Foods:	None expected.
Marijuana:	None expected.
Tobacco:	May decrease pantothenic acid absorption. Decreased pantothenic acid effect.

***See Glossary**

PAPAVERINE

BRAND NAMES

Cerespan
Genabid
Pavabid
Pavabid Plateau Caps
Pavacot
Pavagen
Pavarine
Pavased
Pavatine
Pavatym
Paverolan

BASIC INFORMATION

Habit forming? No
Prescription needed? Yes
Available as generic? Yes
Drug class: Vasodilator

USES

- May improve circulation in the extremities or brain.
- Injected into penis to produce erections.

DOSAGE & USAGE INFORMATION

How to take:
- Tablet—Swallow with liquid or food to lessen stomach irritation. If you can't swallow whole, crumble tablet and take with liquid or food.
- Extended-release capsules—Swallow whole with liquid.
- Injections to penis—Follow doctor's instructions.

When to take:
At the same times each day.

If you forget a dose:
Take as soon as you remember up to 2 hours late. If more than 2 hours, wait for next scheduled dose (don't double this dose).

What drug does:
Relaxes and expands blood vessel walls, allowing better distribution of oxygen and nutrients.

Continued next column

OVERDOSE

SYMPTOMS:
Weakness, fainting, flush, sweating, stupor, irregular heartbeat.
WHAT TO DO:
- **Dial 911 (emergency) for an ambulance or medical help or poison center 1-800-222-1222. Then give first aid immediately.**
- **See emergency information on inside covers.**

Time lapse before drug works:
30 to 60 minutes.

Don't take with:
- Nonprescription drugs without consulting doctor.
- Any other medicine without consulting your doctor or pharmacist.

POSSIBLE ADVERSE REACTIONS OR SIDE EFFECTS

SYMPTOMS	WHAT TO DO
Life-threatening: None expected.	
Common:	
• Drowsiness, dizziness, headache, flushed face, stomach irritation, indigestion, nausea, mild constipation.	Continue. Call doctor when convenient.
• Dry mouth, throat.	Continue. Tell doctor at next visit.
Infrequent:	
Rash, itchy skin, blurred or double vision, weakness, fast heartbeat.	Discontinue. Call doctor right away.
Rare:	
Jaundice.	Discontinue. Call doctor right away.

WARNINGS & PRECAUTIONS

Don't take if:
You are allergic to papaverine.

Before you start, consult your doctor:
- If you plan to become pregnant within medication period.
- If you have had a heart attack, heart disease, angina or stroke.
- If you have Parkinson's disease.

Over age 60:
Adverse reactions and side effects may be more frequent and severe than in younger persons.

Pregnancy:
Decide with your doctor if drug benefits justify risk to unborn child. Risk category C (see page xviii).

Breast-feeding:
Drug may filter into milk. May harm child. Avoid.

Infants & children:
Not recommended.

Prolonged use:
No problems expected.

Skin & sunlight:
No problems expected.

Driving, piloting or hazardous work:
Don't drive or pilot aircraft until you learn how medicine affects you. Don't work around dangerous machinery. Don't climb ladders or work in high places. Danger increases if you drink alcohol or take medicine affecting alertness and reflexes, such as antihistamines, tranquilizers, sedatives, pain medicine, narcotics and mind-altering drugs.

Discontinuing:
May be unnecessary to finish medicine. If drug does not help in 1 to 2 weeks, consult doctor about discontinuing.

Others:
- Periodic liver function tests recommended.
- Internal eye pressure measurements recommended if you have glaucoma.

POSSIBLE INTERACTION WITH OTHER DRUGS

GENERIC NAME OR DRUG CLASS	COMBINED EFFECT
Levodopa	Decreased levodopa effect.
Narcotics*	Increased sedation.
Pain relievers*	Increased sedation.
Pergolide	Decreased pergolide effect.
Sedatives*	Increased sedation.
Sympathomimetics*	Reversal of the effect of papaverine.
Tranquilizers*	Increased sedation.

POSSIBLE INTERACTION WITH OTHER SUBSTANCES

INTERACTS WITH	COMBINED EFFECT
Alcohol:	None expected.
Beverages:	None expected.
Cocaine:	Decreased papaverine effect.
Foods:	None expected.
Marijuana:	None expected.
Tobacco:	Decrease in papaverine's dilation of blood vessels.

*See Glossary

PARALDEHYDE

BRAND NAMES

Paral

BASIC INFORMATION

Habit forming? Yes
Prescription needed? Yes
Available as generic? Yes
Drug class: Anticonvulsant

USES

- Treats convulsions.
- Treats toxic symptoms caused by drugs that may produce convulsions.

DOSAGE & USAGE INFORMATION

How to take:

- Follow doctor's instructions.
- May be given orally, rectally or by injection into a muscle.

When to take:
Follow doctor's instructions.

If you forget a dose:
Take as soon as you remember up to 2 hours late. If more than 2 hours, wait for next scheduled dose (don't double this dose).

What drug does:
Depresses central nervous system.

Time lapse before drug works:

- Oral—30 minutes to 1 hour.
- Rectal—2 to 3 hours.

Don't take with:
Any other medicines (including over-the-counter drugs such as cough and cold medicines, laxatives, antacids, diet pills, caffeine, nose drops or vitamins) without consulting your doctor.

OVERDOSE

SYMPTOMS:
Decreased urination, breathing difficulty, confusion, slow heartbeat, weakness.
WHAT TO DO:

- **Dial 911 (emergency) for an ambulance or medical help or poison center 1-800-222-1222. Then give first aid immediately.**
- **See emergency information on inside covers.**

POSSIBLE ADVERSE REACTIONS OR SIDE EFFECTS

SYMPTOMS	WHAT TO DO
Life-threatening: In case of overdose, see previous column.	
Common:	
• Skin rash, jaundice (yellow skin and eyes).	Discontinue. Call doctor right away.
• Drowsiness, nausea, halitosis.	Continue. Call doctor when convenient.
Infrequent:	
Clumsiness, dizziness, headache.	Continue. Call doctor when convenient.
Rare:	
Abdominal cramps.	Continue. Call doctor when convenient.

WARNINGS & PRECAUTIONS

Don't take if:
You know you are allergic to paraldehyde.

Before you start, consult your doctor:
- If you have chronic lung disease.
- If you have history of drug abuse.
- If you have liver disease.
- If you have peptic ulcer.
- If you have colitis.

Over age 60:
No special problems expected.

Pregnancy:
Decide with your doctor if drug benefits justify risk to unborn child. Risk category C (see page xviii).

Breast-feeding:
Effect not documented. Consult your doctor.

Infants & children:
No special problems expected.

Prolonged use:
- May be habit forming.
- Talk to your doctor about the need for follow-up medical examinations or laboratory studies to check liver function.

Skin & sunlight:
No problems expected.

Driving, piloting or hazardous work:
Avoid if you feel confused, drowsy or dizzy.

Discontinuing:
May develop withdrawal symptoms, such as: convulsions, hallucinations, sweating, muscle cramps, nausea or vomiting, trembling. If you experience any of these, notify your doctor right away.

Others:
- Advise any doctor or dentist whom you consult that you take this medicine.
- May affect results in some medical tests.
- Strong odor of paraldehyde on breath lasts for 24 hours.

POSSIBLE INTERACTION WITH OTHER DRUGS

GENERIC NAME OR DRUG CLASS	COMBINED EFFECT
Addictive drugs*	Increased risk of addiction.
Central nervous system (CNS) depressants*, other	Possible oversedation. Avoid simultaneous use.
Disulfiram	Increased paraldehyde effect. Avoid simultaneous use.
Sertraline	Increased depressive effects of both drugs.

POSSIBLE INTERACTION WITH OTHER SUBSTANCES

INTERACTS WITH	COMBINED EFFECT
Alcohol:	Dangerous sedation. Avoid.
Beverages:	None expected.
Cocaine:	None expected.
Foods:	None expected.
Marijuana:	None expected.
Tobacco:	None expected.

*See Glossary

PARAGORIC

BRAND NAMES

Brown Mixture
Camphorated Opium Tincture
Kapectolin with Paregoric
Parapectolin

BASIC INFORMATION

Habit forming? Yes
Prescription needed? Yes
Available as generic? Yes
Drug class: Narcotic, antidiarrheal

USES

Reduces intestinal cramps and diarrhea.

DOSAGE & USAGE INFORMATION

How to take:
Drops or liquid—Dilute dose in beverage before swallowing.

When to take:
As needed for diarrhea, no more often than every 4 hours.

If you forget a dose:
Take as soon as you remember. Wait 4 hours for next dose.

What drug does:
Anesthetizes surface membranes of intestines and blocks nerve impulses.

Time lapse before drug works:
2 to 6 hours.

Don't take with:
Any other medicine without consulting your doctor or pharmacist.

OVERDOSE

SYMPTOMS:
Deep sleep; slow breathing; slow pulse; flushed, warm skin; constricted pupils.
WHAT TO DO:

- **Dial 911 (emergency) for an ambulance or medical help or poison center 1-800-222-1222. Then give first aid immediately.**
- **If patient is unconscious and not breathing, give mouth-to-mouth breathing. If there is no heartbeat, use cardiac massage and mouth-to-mouth breathing (CPR). Don't try to make patient vomit. If you can't get help quickly, take patient to nearest emergency facility.**
- **See emergency information on inside covers.**

POSSIBLE ADVERSE REACTIONS OR SIDE EFFECTS

SYMPTOMS	WHAT TO DO
Life-threatening: In case of overdose, see previous column.	
Common: Dizziness, flushed face, unusual tiredness, difficult urination.	Continue. Call doctor when convenient.
Infrequent: Severe constipation, abdominal pain, vomiting.	Discontinue. Call doctor right away.
Rare: • Hives, rash, itchy skin, slow heartbeat, irregular breathing.	Discontinue. Call doctor right away.
• Depression.	Continue. Call doctor when convenient.

WARNINGS & PRECAUTIONS

Don't take if:
You are allergic to any narcotic*.

Before you start, consult your doctor:
If you have impaired liver or kidney function.

Over age 60:
More likely to be drowsy, dizzy, unsteady or constipated.

Pregnancy:
Risk factor varies with length of pregnancy. See category list on page xviii and consult doctor.

Breast-feeding:
Drug filters into milk. May depress infant. Avoid.

Infants & children:
Use only under medical supervision.

Prolonged use:
Causes psychological and physical dependence.

Skin & sunlight:
No problems expected.

Driving, piloting or hazardous work:
Don't drive or pilot aircraft until you learn how medicine affects you. Don't work around dangerous machinery. Don't climb ladders or work in high places. Danger increases if you drink alcohol or take medicine affecting alertness and reflexes, such as antihistamines, tranquilizers, sedatives, pain medicine, narcotics and mind-altering drugs.

Discontinuing:
May be unnecessary to finish medicine. Follow doctor's instructions.

Others:
Great potential for abuse.

POSSIBLE INTERACTION WITH OTHER DRUGS

GENERIC NAME OR DRUG CLASS	COMBINED EFFECT
Analgesics*	Increased analgesic effect.
Anticholinergics*	Increased risk of constipation.
Antidepressants*	Increased sedation.
Antidiarrheal preparations*	Increased sedative effect. Avoid.
Antihistamines*	Increased sedation.
Central nervous system (CNS) depressants*	Increased central nerve system depression.
Naloxone	Decreased paregoric effect.
Naltrexone	Decreased paregoric effect.
Narcotics*, other	Increased narcotic effect.

POSSIBLE INTERACTION WITH OTHER SUBSTANCES

INTERACTS WITH	COMBINED EFFECT
Alcohol:	Increases alcohol's intoxicating effect. Avoid.
Beverages:	None expected.
Cocaine:	None expected.
Foods:	None expected.
Marijuana:	Impairs physical and mental performance.
Tobacco:	None expected.

*See Glossary

PEDICULICIDES (Topical)

GENERIC AND BRAND NAMES

LINDANE
- GBH
- G-Well
- Kwellada
- Kwildane
- PMS Lindane

MALATHION
- Derbac
- Ovide

PERMETHRIN
- Acticin
- Elimite Cream
- Nix Cream Rinse

PYRETHRINS & PIPERONYL BUTOXIDE
- A-200 Gel
- A-200 Shampoo
- Barc
- Blue
- Lice-Enz Foam And Comb Lice Killing Shampoo Kit
- Pyrinyl
- R&C
- TISIT
- TISIT Blue
- Triple X

BASIC INFORMATION

Habit forming? No
Prescription needed? Yes
Available as generic? Yes, some
Drug class: Pediculicide, scabicide

USES

- Treats scabies and lice infections of skin or scalp.
- Cream and lotion treats scabies.
- Shampoo treats lice infections.

OVERDOSE

SYMPTOMS:
Rarely (toxic effects from too much absorbed through skin)—Vomiting, muscle cramps, dizziness, seizure, rapid heartbeat.
WHAT TO DO:
- **Not for internal use. If child accidentally swallows, call poison center 1-800-222-1222.**
- **Dial 911 (emergency) for an ambulance or medical help. Then give first aid immediately.**
- **See emergency information on inside covers.**

DOSAGE & USAGE INFORMATION

How to use:
- All household members should be examined for infection and treated if infected.
- Read directions on product for proper application technique and length of time to leave on the body.
- Wear plastic gloves when you apply. Use care not to apply more than directed. Avoid contact with eyes, nose and mouth. Flush eyes with water if product gets in the eyes.
- Bathe before applying. Wash hands after applying.
- Use in well-ventilated room.

When to use:
As directed on package.

If you forget a dose:
Use as soon as you remember.

What drug does:
Absorbed into bodies of lice and scabies organisms, killing them.

Time lapse before drug works:
Cream or lotion requires 8 to 12 hours contact with skin.

Don't use with:
Other medicines for scabies or lice.

POSSIBLE ADVERSE REACTIONS OR SIDE EFFECTS

SYMPTOMS	WHAT TO DO
Life-threatening	
None expected.	
Common	
None expected.	
Infrequent	
None expected.	
Rare	
• Skin irritation or rash.	Discontinue. Call doctor right away.
• Skin itch that continues 1 week to several weeks after treatment.	Call doctor when convenient.

WARNINGS & PRECAUTIONS

Don't use if:
You are allergic to any medicine with lindane, pyrethrins or piperonyl butoxide.

Before you start, consult your doctor:
- If you are allergic to anything that touches your skin.
- If you are using any other medicines, creams, lotions or oils.

Over age 60:
Adverse reactions and side effects may be more frequent and severe than in younger persons. Ask doctor about smaller doses.

Pregnancy:
Risk factors vary for drugs in this group. See category list on page xviii and consult doctor.

Breast-feeding:
Effect unknown. Avoid if possible. Consult doctor.

Infants & children:
More likely to be toxic. Use only under close medical supervision.

Prolonged use:
Not recommended. Avoid.

Skin & sunlight:
No problems expected, but check with doctor.

Driving, piloting or hazardous work:
No problems expected, but check with doctor.

Discontinuing:
No problems expected, but check with doctor.

Others:
- Don't use on open sores or wounds.
- Put on freshly dry cleaned or washed clothing after treatment.
- After treatment, boil all bed sheets, covers and towels before using.
- Store items that can't be washed or cleaned in plastic bags for 2 weeks.
- Avoid inhaling or swallowing drug.
- Thoroughly clean house.
- Wash combs and hairbrushes in hot soapy water. Don't share with others.
- Even after successful treatment, itching can continue due to remaining inflammation in the skin. This should not be confused with a reinfection. Consult doctor if you are unsure.

POSSIBLE INTERACTION WITH OTHER DRUGS

GENERIC NAME OR DRUG CLASS	COMBINED EFFECT
Antimyasthenics*	Excessive absorption and chance of toxicity (with malathion only).
Cholinesterase inhibitors*	Excessive absorption and chance of toxicity (with malathion only).

POSSIBLE INTERACTION WITH OTHER SUBSTANCES

INTERACTS WITH	COMBINED EFFECT
Alcohol:	None expected.
Beverages:	None expected.
Cocaine:	None expected.
Foods:	None expected.
Marijuana:	None expected.
Tobacco:	None expected.

***See Glossary**

PEMOLINE

BRAND NAMES

Cylert
Cylert Chewable

BASIC INFORMATION

Habit forming? Yes
Prescription needed? Yes
Available as generic? No
Drug class: Central nervous system stimulant

USES

Decreases overactivity and lengthens attention span in children with attention-deficit hyperactivity disorder (ADHD). It is used as part of the total management plan that includes educational, social and psychological treatment.

DOSAGE & USAGE INFORMATION

How to take:
- Tablet—Swallow with liquid or food to lessen stomach irritation. If you can't swallow whole, crumble tablet and take with liquid or food.
- Chewable tablets—Chew well before swallowing.

When to take:
Daily in the morning.

Continued next column

OVERDOSE

SYMPTOMS:
Agitation, confusion, fast heartbeat, hallucinations, severe headache, high fever with sweating, large pupils, muscle twitching or trembling, uncontrolled eye or body movements, vomiting.
WHAT TO DO:
- **Dial 911 (emergency) for an ambulance or medical help or poison center 1-800-222-1222. Then give first aid immediately.**
- **If patient is unconscious and not breathing, give mouth-to-mouth breathing. If there is no heartbeat, use cardiac massage and mouth-to-mouth breathing (CPR). Don't try to make patient vomit. If you can't get help quickly, take patient to nearest emergency facility.**
- **See emergency information at end of book.**

If you forget a dose:
Take as soon as you remember up to 2 hours late. If more than 2 hours, wait for next scheduled dose (don't double this dose).

What drug does:
Stimulates brain to improve alertness, concentration and attention span. Calms the hyperactive child.

Time lapse before drug works:
- 1 month or more for maximum effect on child.
- 30 minutes to stimulate adults.

Don't take with:
Any other medicine without consulting your doctor or pharmacist.

POSSIBLE ADVERSE REACTIONS OR SIDE EFFECTS

SYMPTOMS	WHAT TO DO
Life-threatening: In case of overdose, see previous column.	
Common: Trouble sleeping, loss of appetite, weight loss.	Continue. Call doctor when convenient.
Infrequent: Irritability, depression dizziness, headache, drowsiness, skin rash, stomach ache.	Continue. Call doctor when convenient.
Rare: Yellow skin or eyes; symptoms of overdose (agitation, confusion, fast heartbeat, hallucinations, severe headache, high fever with sweating, large pupils, muscle twitching or trembling, uncontrolled eye or body movements, vomiting).	Discontinue. Call doctor right away.

WARNINGS & PRECAUTIONS

Don't take if:
You are allergic to pemoline.

Before you start, consult your doctor:
- If you have liver disease.
- If you have kidney disease.
- If patient is younger than 6 years.
- If there is marked emotional instability.

Over age 60:
Adverse reactions and side effects may be more frequent and severe than in younger persons.

Pregnancy:
No proven harm to unborn child. Avoid if possible. Consult doctor. Risk category B (see page xviii).

Breast-feeding:
Effect unknown. Consult doctor.

Infants & children:
Use only under close medical supervision.

Prolonged use:
- Rare possibility of physical growth retardation.
- Talk to your doctor about the need for follow-up medical examinations or laboratory studies to check liver function, growth charts.

Skin & sunlight:
No problems expected.

Driving, piloting or hazardous work:
Don't drive or pilot aircraft until you learn how medicine affects you. Don't work around dangerous machinery. Don't climb ladders or work in high places. Danger increases if you drink alcohol or take medicine affecting alertness and reflexes, such as antihistamines, tranquilizers, sedatives, pain medicine, narcotics and mind-altering drugs.

Discontinuing:
- Don't discontinue without consulting doctor. Dose may require gradual reduction if you have taken drug for a long time. Doses of other drugs may also require adjustment.
- If you notice any of the following symptoms after discontinuing, notify your doctor: mental depression (severe), tiredness or weakness.

Others:
- Dose must be carefully adjusted by doctor. Don't give more or less than prescribed dose.
- Be sure you and the doctor discuss benefits and risks of this drug before starting.
- Consult doctor if no improvement is noticed after 1 month of drug use.
- Advise any doctor or dentist whom you consult about the use of this medicine.

POSSIBLE INTERACTION WITH OTHER DRUGS

GENERIC NAME OR DRUG CLASS	COMBINED EFFECT
Anticonvulsants*	Dosage adjustment for anticonvulsant may be necessary.
Central nervous system (CNS) stimulants*, other	May increase toxic effects of both drugs.

POSSIBLE INTERACTION WITH OTHER SUBSTANCES

INTERACTS WITH	COMBINED EFFECT
Alcohol:	More chance of depression. Avoid.
Beverages: Caffeine drinks.	Overstimulation. Avoid.
Cocaine:	Convulsions or excessive nervousness.
Foods:	None expected.
Marijuana:	Unknown.
Tobacco:	Unknown.

***See Glossary**

PENICILLAMINE

BRAND NAMES

Cuprimine
Depen

BASIC INFORMATION

Habit forming? No
Prescription needed? Yes
Available as generic? No
Drug class: Chelating agent, antirheumatic, antidote (heavy metal)

USES

- Treatment for rheumatoid arthritis.
- Prevention of kidney stones.
- Treatment for heavy metal poisoning.

DOSAGE & USAGE INFORMATION

How to take:
Tablets or capsules—With liquid on an empty stomach 1 hour before or 2 hours after eating.

When to take:
At the same times each day.

If you forget a dose:
- 1 dose a day—Take as soon as you remember up to 12 hours late. If more than 12 hours, wait for next scheduled dose (don't double this dose).
- More than 1 dose a day—Take as soon as you remember up to 2 hours late. If more than 2 hours, wait for next scheduled dose (don't double this dose).

Continued next column

OVERDOSE

SYMPTOMS:
Ulcers, sores, convulsions, coughing up blood, coma.
WHAT TO DO:
- **Dial 911 (emergency) for an ambulance or medical help or poison center 1-800-222-1222. Then give first aid immediately.**
- **See emergency information on inside covers.**

What drug does:
- Combines with heavy metals so kidney can excrete them.
- Combines with cysteine (amino acid found in many foods) to prevent cysteine kidney stones.
- May improve protective function of some white blood cells against rheumatoid arthritis.

Time lapse before drug works:
2 to 3 months.

Don't take with:
Any other medicine without consulting your doctor or pharmacist.

POSSIBLE ADVERSE REACTIONS OR SIDE EFFECTS

SYMPTOMS	WHAT TO DO
Life-threatening:	
In case of overdose, see previous column.	
Common:	
Rash, itchy skin, swollen lymph glands, appetite loss, nausea, diarrhea, vomiting, decreased taste.	Discontinue. Call doctor right away.
Infrequent:	
Sore throat, fever, unusual bruising, swollen feet or legs, bloody or cloudy urine, weight gain, fatigue, weakness, joint pain.	Discontinue. Call doctor right away.
Rare:	
Double or blurred vision; pain; ringing in ears; ulcers, sores, white spots in mouth; difficult breathing; coughing up blood; jaundice; abdominal pain; skin blisters; peeling skin.	Discontinue. Call doctor right away.

WARNINGS & PRECAUTIONS

Don't take if:
- You are allergic to penicillamine.
- You have severe anemia.

Before you start, consult your doctor:
- If you have kidney disease.
- If you are allergic to any pencillin antibiotic.

Over age 60:
More likely to damage blood cells and kidneys.

Pregnancy:
Decide with your doctor if drug benefits justify risk to unborn child. Risk category C (see page xviii).

Breast-feeding:
Safety not established. Consult doctor.

Infants & children:
Use only under medical supervision.

Prolonged use:
- May damage blood cells, kidney, liver.
- Talk to your doctor about the need for follow-up medical examinations or laboratory studies to check complete blood counts (white blood cell count, platelet count, red blood cell count, hemoglobin, hematocrit), kidney function, liver function.

Skin & sunlight:
No problems expected.

Driving, piloting or hazardous work:
No problems expected.

Discontinuing:
No problems expected.

Others:
Request laboratory studies on blood and urine every 2 weeks. Kidney and liver function studies recommended every 6 months.

POSSIBLE INTERACTION WITH OTHER DRUGS

GENERIC NAME OR DRUG CLASS	COMBINED EFFECT
Gold compounds*	Damage to blood cells and kidney.
Immuno-suppressants*	Damage to blood cells and kidney.
Iron supplements*	Decreased effect of penicillamine. Wait 2 hours between doses.
Pyridoxine (vitamin B-6)	Increased need for pyridoxine.

POSSIBLE INTERACTION WITH OTHER SUBSTANCES

INTERACTS WITH	COMBINED EFFECT
Alcohol:	Increased side effects of penicillamine.
Beverages:	None expected.
Cocaine:	Increased side effects of penicillamine.
Foods:	Possible decreased penicillamine effect due to decreased absorption.
Marijuana:	Increased side effects of penicillamine.
Tobacco:	None expected.

***See Glossary**

PENICILLINS

GENERIC AND BRAND NAMES

See complete list of generic and brand names in the *Generic and Brand Name Directory*, page 862.

BASIC INFORMATION

Habit forming? No
Prescription needed? Yes
Available as generic? Yes
Drug class: Antibacterial

USES

Treatment of bacterial infections that are susceptible to penicillin, including lower respiratory tract infections, otitis media, sinusitis, skin and skin structure infections, urinary tract infections, gastrointestinal disorders, ulcers, endocarditis, pharyngitis. Different penicillins treat different kinds of infections.

DOSAGE & USAGE INFORMATION

How to take:

- Tablet or capsule—Swallow with liquid on an empty stomach 1 hour before or 2 hours after eating. You may take amoxicillin, penicillin V, pivampicillin or pivmecillinam on a full stomach.
- Chewable tablet—Chew or crush before swallowing.
- Oral suspension—Measure each dose with an accurate measuring device (not a household teaspoon). Store according to instructions.

When to take:
Follow instructions on prescription label, or take as directed by doctor. The number of doses, the time between doses and the length of treatment will depend on the problem being treated.

If you forget a dose:
Take as soon as you remember, then continue regular schedule. If it is almost time for the next dose, wait for that dose (don't double that dose).

Continued next column

OVERDOSE

SYMPTOMS:
Severe diarrhea, nausea or vomiting.
WHAT TO DO:
Overdose unlikely to threaten life. If person takes much larger amount than prescribed, call doctor, poison center 1-800-222-1222 or hospital emergency room for instructions.

What drug does:
Destroys susceptible bacteria. Does not kill viruses (e.g., colds or influenza), fungi or parasites.

Time lapse before drug works:
May be several days before medicine affects infection.

Don't take with:
Any other medicine without consulting your doctor or pharmacist.

POSSIBLE ADVERSE REACTIONS OR SIDE EFFECTS

SYMPTOMS	WHAT TO DO
Life-threatening:	
Hives, rash, intense itching, shortness of breath, faintness soon after a dose (anaphylaxis).	Seek emergency treatment immediately.
Common:	
Nausea, vomiting or diarrhea (all mild); sore mouth or tongue; white patches in mouth or on tongue; vaginal itching or discharge; stomach pain.	Continue. Call doctor when convenient.
Infrequent:	
None expected.	
Rare:	
Unexplained bleeding or bruising, weakness, sore throat, fever, severe abdominal cramps, diarrhea (watery and severe), convulsions.	Discontinue. Call doctor right away.

WARNINGS & PRECAUTIONS

Don't take if:
You are allergic to penicillins* or cephalosporins*. A life-threatening reaction may occur.

Before you start, consult your doctor:
- If you are allergic to any substance or drug.
- If you have mononucleosis.
- If you have congestive heart failure.
- If you have high blood pressure or any bleeding disorder.
- If you have cystic fibrosis.
- If you have kidney disease or a stomach or intestinal disorder.

Over age 60:
No special problems expected.

Pregnancy:
Consult doctor. Risk category B (see page xviii).

Breast-feeding:
Drug passes into milk. Child may become sensitive to penicillins and have allergic reactions to penicillin drugs. Discuss risks and benefits with your doctor.

Infants & children:
No special problems expected.

Prolonged use:
- You may become more susceptible to infections caused by germs not responsive to penicillins.
- Talk to your doctor about the need for follow-up medical examinations or laboratory studies.

Skin & sunlight:
No problems expected.

Driving, piloting or hazardous work:
Usually not dangerous. Most hazardous reactions likely to occur a few minutes after taking penicillin.

Discontinuing:
Don't discontinue without doctor's advice until you complete prescribed dose, even though symptoms diminish or disappear.

Others:
- Urine sugar test for diabetes may show false positive result.
- If your symptoms don't improve within a few days (or if they worsen), call your doctor.
- Don't take medicines for diarrhea without your doctor's approval.
- Birth control pills may not be effective. Use additional birth control methods.

POSSIBLE INTERACTION WITH OTHER DRUGS

GENERIC NAME OR DRUG CLASS	COMBINED EFFECT
Chloramphenicol	Decreased effect of both drugs.
Cholestyramine	May decrease penicillin effect.
Colestipol	May decrease penicillin effect.
Contraceptives, oral*	Impaired contraceptive efficiency.
Erythromycins*	Decreased effect of both drugs.
Methotrexate	Increased risk of methotrexate toxicity.
Probenecid	Increased effect of all penicillins.
Sodium benzoate & sodium phenylacetate	May reduce effect of sodium benzoate & sodium phenylacetate.
Sulfonamides*	Decreased penicillin effect.
Tetracyclines*	Decreased effect of both drugs.

POSSIBLE INTERACTION WITH OTHER SUBSTANCES

INTERACTS WITH	COMBINED EFFECT
Alcohol:	Occasional stomach irritation.
Beverages:	None expected.
Cocaine:	None expected.
Foods: Acidic fruits or juices, aged cheese, wines, syrups (if taken with penicillin G).	Decreased antibiotic effect.
Marijuana:	None expected.
Tobacco:	None expected.

*See Glossary

PENICILLINS & BETA-LACTAMASE INHIBITORS

GENERIC AND BRAND NAMES

AMOXICILLIN & CLAVULANATE	**Augmentin** **Clavulin**

BASIC INFORMATION

Habit forming? No
Prescription needed? Yes
Available as generic? No
Drug class: Antibacterial

USES

Treatment of bacterial infections that are susceptible to penicillin and beta-lactamase inhibitors, including lower respiratory tract infections, otitis media, sinusitis, skin and skin structure infections, urinary tract infections.

DOSAGE & USAGE INFORMATION

How to take:

- Tablet—Swallow with liquid on a full or empty stomach. Taking with food may lessen any stomach irritation.
- Chewable tablet—Chew or crush before swallowing.
- Oral suspension—Measure each dose with an accurate measuring device (not a household teaspoon).

When to take:
Follow instructions on prescription label, or take as directed by doctor. Normally the drug is taken every 8 hours for 7 to 10 days.

If you forget a dose:
Take as soon as you remember, then continue regular schedule. If it is almost time for the next dose, wait for that dose (don't double it).

Continued next column

OVERDOSE

SYMPTOMS:
Severe diarrhea, nausea or vomiting.
WHAT TO DO:
Overdose unlikely to threaten life. If person takes much larger amount than prescribed, call doctor, poison center 1-800-222-1222 or hospital emergency room for instructions.

What drug does:
Destroys susceptible bacteria. Does not kill viruses, fungi or parasites. Beta-lactamase inhibitors increase penicillin's effectiveness by inactivating beta-lactamase (a substance in some bacteria which destroys the penicillin).

Time lapse before drug works:
May be several days before medicine affects infection.

Don't take with:
Any other medicine without consulting your doctor or pharmacist.

POSSIBLE ADVERSE REACTIONS OR SIDE EFFECTS

SYMPTOMS	WHAT TO DO
Life-threatening:	
Hives, rash, intense itching, shortness of breath, faintness soon after a dose (anaphylaxis).	Seek emergency treatment immediately.
Common:	
Nausea, vomiting or diarrhea (all mild); sore mouth or tongue; white patches in mouth or on tongue; vaginal itching or discharge; stomach pain.	Continue. Call doctor when convenient.
Infrequent:	
None expected.	
Rare:	
Unexplained bleeding or bruising, weakness, sore throat, fever, severe abdominal cramps, diarrhea (watery and severe), convulsions.	Discontinue. Call doctor right away.

PENICILLINS & BETA-LACTAMASE INHIBITORS

WARNINGS & PRECAUTIONS

Don't take if:
You are allergic to penicillins or cephalosporins. Life-threatening reaction may occur.

Before you start, consult your doctor:
- If you are allergic to any substance or drug.
- If you have mononucleosis.
- If you have congestive heart failure.
- If you have high blood pressure or any bleeding disorder.
- If you have cystic fibrosis.
- If you have kidney disease or a stomach or intestinal disorder.

Over age 60:
No special problems expected.

Pregnancy:
Consult doctor. Risk category B (see page xviii).

Breast-feeding:
Drug passes into milk. Child may become sensitive to penicillins and have allergic reactions to penicillin drugs. Avoid penicillin or discontinue nursing until you finish medicine. Consult doctor for advice on maintaining milk supply.

Infants & children:
No special problems expected.

Prolonged use:
- You may become more susceptible to infections caused by germs not responsive to penicillins.
- Talk to your doctor about the need for follow-up medical examinations or laboratory studies to check SGPT*, SGOT*.

Skin & sunlight:
No problems expected.

Driving, piloting or hazardous work:
Usually not dangerous. Most hazardous reactions likely to occur a few minutes after taking.

Discontinuing:
Don't discontinue without doctor's advice until you complete prescribed dose, even though symptoms diminish or disappear.

Others:
- Urine sugar test for diabetes may show false positive result.
- If your symptoms don't improve within a few days (or if they worsen), call your doctor.
- Don't take for diarrhea without your doctor's approval.
- Birth control pills may not be effective. Use additional birth control methods.

POSSIBLE INTERACTION WITH OTHER DRUGS

GENERIC NAME OR DRUG CLASS	COMBINED EFFECT
Chloramphenicol	Decreased effect of both drugs.
Cholestyramine	May decrease penicillin effect.
Colestipol	May decrease penicillin effect.
Contraceptives, oral*	Impaired contraceptive efficiency.
Erythromycins*	Decreased effect of both drugs.
Methotrexate	Increased risk of methotrexate toxicity.
Probenecid	Increased effect of all penicillins.
Sodium benzoate & sodium phenylacetate	May reduce effect of sodium benzoate & sodium phenylacetate.
Tetracyclines*	Decreased effect of both drugs.

POSSIBLE INTERACTION WITH OTHER SUBSTANCES

INTERACTS WITH	COMBINED EFFECT
Alcohol:	Occasional stomach irritation.
Beverages:	None expected.
Cocaine:	None expected.
Foods:	None expected.
Marijuana:	None expected.
Tobacco:	None expected.

PENTAMIDINE

BRAND NAMES

NebuPent
Pentacarinat
Pneumopent

BASIC INFORMATION

Habit forming? No
Prescription needed? Yes
Available as generic? No
Drug class: Antiprotozoal

USES

- Treats pneumocystis carinii, which is common in AIDS patients.
- Treats some tropical diseases such as leishmaniasis, African sleeping sickness and others.

DOSAGE & USAGE INFORMATION

How to take:
Inhalation—Follow package instructions.

When to take:
According to doctor's instructions.

If you forget a dose:
Not likely to happen.

What drug does:
Interferes with RNA and DNA of infecting organisms.

Time lapse before drug works:
30 minutes to 1 hour.

Don't take with:
Any other medicines (including over-the-counter drugs such as cough and cold medicines, laxatives, antacids, diet pills, caffeine, nose drops or vitamins) without consulting your doctor.

OVERDOSE

SYMPTOMS:
None expected.
WHAT TO DO:
Overdose unlikely to threaten life. If person takes much larger amount than prescribed, call doctor, poison center 1-800-222-1222 or hospital emergency room for instructions.

POSSIBLE ADVERSE REACTIONS OR SIDE EFFECTS

SYMPTOMS	WHAT TO DO
Life-threatening: Unconsciousness, rapid pulse, cold sweats.	Seek emergency treatment immediately.
Common: Chest pain or congestion; wheezing; coughing; difficulty in breathing; skin rash; pain, dryness or sensation of lump in throat.	Discontinue. Call doctor right away.
Infrequent: • Abdomen or back pain, nausea, vomiting, anxiety, cold sweats, chills, headache, appetite changes, decreased urination, unusual tiredness.	Discontinue. Call doctor right away.
• Bitter or metallic taste.	No action necessary.
Rare: None expected.	

WARNINGS & PRECAUTIONS

Don't take if:
You know you are allergic to pentamidine.

Before you start, consult your doctor:
If you have asthma.

Over age 60:
Adverse reactions and side effects may be more frequent and severe than in younger persons. You may need smaller doses for shorter periods of time.

Pregnancy:
Decide with your doctor if drug benefits justify risk to unborn child. Risk category C (see page xviii).

Breast-feeding:
Unknown effects. Not recommended. Consult doctor.

Infants & children:
Unknown effects. Consult doctor.

Prolonged use:
Talk to your doctor about the need for follow-up medical examinations or laboratory studies to check blood sugar; blood pressure; kidney, liver and heart function; complete blood counts (white blood cell count, platelet count, red blood cell count, hemoglobin, hematocrit); ECG* and serum calcium.

Skin & sunlight:
No problems expected.

Driving, piloting or hazardous work:
Avoid if you feel confused, drowsy or dizzy.

Discontinuing:
No special problems expected.

Others:
- Advise any doctor or dentist whom you consult that you take this medicine.
- May affect results in some medical tests.
- Avoid exposure to people who have infectious diseases.
- To help decrease bitter taste in mouth, dissolve a hard candy after taking medicine.
- Consult your doctor for additional information on the injectable form of this drug.

POSSIBLE INTERACTION WITH OTHER DRUGS

GENERIC NAME OR DRUG CLASS	COMBINED EFFECT
None reported with inhalation form of drug.	

POSSIBLE INTERACTION WITH OTHER SUBSTANCES

INTERACTS WITH	COMBINED EFFECT
Alcohol:	Increased likelihood of adverse reactions. Avoid.
Beverages:	None expected.
Cocaine:	Increased likelihood of adverse reactions. Avoid.
Foods:	None expected.
Marijuana:	Increased likelihood of adverse reactions. Avoid.
Tobacco:	Increased likelihood of adverse reactions. Avoid.

*See Glossary

PENTOXIFYLLINE

BRAND NAMES

Trental

BASIC INFORMATION

Habit forming? No
Prescription needed? Yes
Available as generic? Yes
Drug class: Hemorrheologic agent

USES

Reduces pain in legs caused by poor circulation.

DOSAGE & USAGE INFORMATION

How to take:
Extended-release tablets—Swallow whole with water and food.

When to take:
At mealtimes. Taking with food decreases the likelihood of irritating the stomach to cause nausea.

If you forget a dose:
Take as soon as you remember up to 3 hours late. If more than 3 hours, wait for next scheduled dose (don't double this dose).

What drug does:
- Reduces "stickiness" of red blood cells and improves flexibility of the red cells.
- Improves blood flow through blood vessels.

Time lapse before drug works:
1 hour. Several weeks for full effect on circulation.

Don't take with:
- Tobacco or medicines to treat hypertension.
- Any other medicine without consulting your doctor or pharmacist.

OVERDOSE

SYMPTOMS:
Drowsiness, flushed face, fainting, nervousness, convulsions, coma.
WHAT TO DO:
- **Dial 911 (emergency) for an ambulance or medical help or poison center 1-800-222-1222. Then give first aid immediately.**
- **See emergency information on inside covers.**

POSSIBLE ADVERSE REACTIONS OR SIDE EFFECTS

SYMPTOMS	WHAT TO DO
Life-threatening:	
Chest pain, irregular heartbeat.	Discontinue. Seek emergency treatment.
Common:	
None expected.	
Infrequent:	
• Dizziness, headache, nausea, vomiting. low blood pressure, nosebleed, swollen feet and ankles, viral-like syndrome, nasal congestion, laryngitis, rash, itchy skin, blurred vision, abdominal pain.	Discontinue. Call doctor right away.
• Insomnia, nervousness, red eyes.	Continue. Call doctor when convenient.
Rare:	
None expected.	

WARNINGS & PRECAUTIONS

Don't take if:
You are allergic to pentoxifylline.

Before you start, consult your doctor:
- If you are allergic to caffeine, theophylline, theobromine, aminophyllin, dyphyllin, oxtriphylline, theobromine.
- If you have angina.
- If you have liver or kidney disease.

Over age 60:
Adverse reactions and side effects may be more frequent and severe than in younger persons. Ask doctor about smaller doses.

Pregnancy:
Decide with your doctor if drug benefits justify risk to unborn child. Risk category C (see page xviii).

Breast-feeding:
Drug passes into milk. Avoid drug or discontinue nursing until you finish medicine. Consult doctor for advice on maintaining milk supply.

Infants & children:
Not recommended.

Prolonged use:
No problems expected.

Skin & sunlight:
No problems expected.

Driving, piloting or hazardous work:
Wait to see if drug causes drowsiness or dizziness. If none, no problems expected.

Discontinuing:
No problems expected.

Others:
Don't smoke.

POSSIBLE INTERACTION WITH OTHER DRUGS

GENERIC NAME OR DRUG CLASS	COMBINED EFFECT
Anticoagulants*, oral	Possible decreased effect of anticoagulant.
Antihypertensives*	Possible increased effect of hypertensive medication.

POSSIBLE INTERACTION WITH OTHER SUBSTANCES

INTERACTS WITH	COMBINED EFFECT
Alcohol:	Unknown. Best to avoid.
Beverages: Coffee, tea or other caffeine-containing beverages.	May decrease effectiveness of pentoxifylline.
Cocaine:	Reduced effect of pentoxifylline.
Foods:	None expected.
Marijuana:	Decreased effect of pentoxifylline.
Tobacco:	Decreased effect of pentoxifylline. Avoid.

*See Glossary

PERGOLIDE

BRAND NAMES

Permax

BASIC INFORMATION

Habit forming? No
Prescription needed? Yes
Available as generic? No
Drug class: Antidyskinetic

USES

Treats Parkinson's disease when used together with levodopa or carbidopa.

DOSAGE & USAGE INFORMATION

How to take:
Tablets—Swallow with liquid. If you can't swallow whole, crumble tablet and take with liquid or food. Instructions to take on empty stomach mean 1 hour before or 2 hours after eating.

When to take:
Follow doctor's instructions. Usually 3 times a day.

If you forget a dose:
Take as soon as you remember up to 2 hours late. If more than 2 hours, wait for next scheduled dose (don't double this dose).

What drug does:
- Stimulates dopamine receptors in the central nervous system to make them more active.
- Lowers the required dosage of carbidopa and levodopa.

Time lapse before drug works:
Not documented.

Don't take with:
Any other medicines (including over-the-counter drugs such as cough and cold medicines, laxatives, antacids, diet pills, caffeine, nose drops or vitamins) without consulting your doctor or pharmacist.

OVERDOSE

SYMPTOMS:
None expected.
WHAT TO DO:
Overdose unlikely to threaten life. If person takes much larger amount than prescribed, call doctor, poison center 1-800-222-1222 or hospital emergency room for instructions.

POSSIBLE ADVERSE REACTIONS OR SIDE EFFECTS

SYMPTOMS	WHAT TO DO
Life-threatening:	
Seizures, chest pain, shortness of breath.	Seek emergency treatment immediately.
Common:	
• Confusion; hallucinations; painful urination; unusual movements of face, head, hands andtongue.	Discontinue. Seek emergency treatment.
• Abdominal pain, constipation, dizziness, nasal stuffiness.	Continue. Call doctor when convenient.
Infrequent:	
Chills, diarrhea, dry mouth, appetite loss, facial swelling, increased sex drive.	Continue. Call doctor when convenient.
Rare:	
Weakness, vision changes, fainting, increased sweating, nausea and vomiting.	Discontinue. Seek emergency treatment.

WARNINGS & PRECAUTIONS

Don't take if:
You are allergic to pergolide or any ergot preparation*.

Before you start, consult your doctor:
- If you have heartbeat irregularities.
- If you have hallucinations.

Over age 60:
No special problems expected.

Pregnancy:
Consult doctor. Risk category B (see page xviii).

Breast-feeding:
Not recommended. Pergolide can prevent lactation. Consult doctor.

Infants & children:
Effect not documented. Consult your doctor.

Prolonged use:
Request frequent blood pressure checks.

Skin & sunlight:
No problems expected.

Driving, piloting or hazardous work:
Don't drive or pilot aircraft until you learn how medicine affects you. Don't work around dangerous machinery. Don't climb ladders or work in high places. Danger increases if you drink alcohol or take medicine affecting alertness and reflexes.

Discontinuing:
No special problems expected.

Others:
- Advise any doctor or dentist whom you consult that you take this medicine.
- May affect results in some medical tests.

POSSIBLE INTERACTION WITH OTHER DRUGS

GENERIC NAME OR DRUG CLASS	COMBINED EFFECT
Chlorprothixene	Decreased pergolide effect.
Droperidol	Decreased pergolide effect.
Flupenthixol	Decreased pergolide effect.
Haloperidol	Decreased pergolide effect.
Hypotension-causing drugs*	Increased hypotension effect.
Loxapine	Decreased pergolide effect.
Methyldopa	Decreased pergolide effect.
Metoclopropamide	Decreased pergolide effect.
Molindone	Decreased pergolide effect.
Papaverine	Decreased pergolide effect.
Phenothiazines*	Decreased pergolide effect.
Reserpine	Decreased pergolide effect.
Sertraline	Increased depressive effects of both drugs.
Thiothixene	Decreased pergolide effect.

POSSIBLE INTERACTION WITH OTHER SUBSTANCES

INTERACTS WITH	COMBINED EFFECT
Alcohol:	Increased likelihood of adverse reactions. Avoid.
Beverages:	None expected.
Cocaine:	Increased likelihood of adverse reactions. Avoid.
Foods:	None expected.
Marijuana:	Increased likelihood of adverse reactions. Avoid.
Tobacco:	None expected.

*See Glossary

PHENAZOPYRIDINE

BRAND NAMES

Azo-Cheragan
Azo-Gantrisin
Azo-Standard
Baridium
Eridium
Geridium
Phen-Azo
Phenazodine
Pyrazodine
Pyridiate
Pyridium
Pyronium
Urodine
Urogesic
Viridium

BASIC INFORMATION

Habit forming? No
Prescription needed? Yes
Available as generic? Yes
Drug class: Analgesic (urinary)

USES

Relieves pain of lower urinary tract irritation, as in cystitis, urethritis or prostatitis. Relieves symptoms only. Phenazopyridine alone does not cure infections.

DOSAGE & USAGE INFORMATION

How to take:
Tablet—Swallow with liquid or food to lessen stomach irritation.

When to take:
At the same times each day.

If you forget a dose:
Take as soon as you remember up to 2 hours late. If more than 2 hours, wait for next scheduled dose (don't double this dose).

What drug does:
Anesthetizes lower urinary tract. Relieves pain, burning, pressure and urgency to urinate.

Time lapse before drug works:
1 to 2 hours.

OVERDOSE

SYMPTOMS:
Shortness of breath, weakness.
WHAT TO DO:
Overdose unlikely to threaten life. If person takes much larger amount than prescribed, call doctor, poison center 1-800-222-1222 or hospital emergency room for instructions.

Don't take with:
Any other medicine without consulting your doctor or pharmacist.

POSSIBLE ADVERSE REACTIONS OR SIDE EFFECTS

SYMPTOMS	WHAT TO DO
Life-threatening: In case of overdose, see previous column.	
Common:	
Red-orange urine.	No action necessary.
Infrequent:	
Indigestion, fatigue, weakness, dizziness, abdominal pain.	Continue. Call doctor when convenient.
Rare:	
• Rash, jaundice, bluish skin color.	Discontinue. Call doctor right away.
• Headache.	Continue. Call doctor when convenient.

WARNINGS & PRECAUTIONS

Don't take if:
- You have hepatitis.
- You are allergic to any urinary analgesic.

Before you start, consult your doctor:
If you have kidney or liver disease.

Over age 60:
Adverse reactions and side effects may be more frequent and severe than in younger persons.

Pregnancy:
No proven harm to unborn child. Avoid if possible. Consult doctor. Risk category B (see page xviii).

Breast-feeding:
Effect unknown. Consult doctor.

Infants & children:
Not recommended.

Prolonged use:
- Orange or yellow skin.
- Anemia. Occasional blood studies recommended.

Skin & sunlight:
No problems expected.

Driving, piloting or hazardous work:
No problems expected.

Discontinuing:
May be unnecessary to finish medicine. Follow doctor's instructions.

Others:
No problems expected.

POSSIBLE INTERACTION WITH OTHER DRUGS

GENERIC NAME OR DRUG CLASS	COMBINED EFFECT
None significant.	

POSSIBLE INTERACTION WITH OTHER SUBSTANCES

INTERACTS WITH	COMBINED EFFECT
Alcohol:	None expected.
Beverages:	None expected.
Cocaine:	None expected.
Foods:	None expected.
Marijuana:	None expected.
Tobacco:	None expected.

PHENOTHIAZINES

GENERIC AND BRAND NAMES

See complete list of generic and brand names in the *Generic and Brand Name Directory*, page 862.

BASIC INFORMATION

Habit forming? No
Prescription needed? Yes
Available as generic? Yes, for some.
Drug class: Tranquilizer, antiemetic (phenothiazine)

USES

- Reduces anxiety, agitation.
- Stops nausea, vomiting, hiccups.

DOSAGE & USAGE INFORMATION

How to take:
- Tablet or extended-release capsule—Swallow with liquid or food to lessen stomach irritation.
- Suppositories—Remove wrapper and moisten suppository with water. Gently insert into rectum, pointed end first.
- Drops or liquid—Dilute dose in beverage.

When to take:
- Nervous and mental disorders—Take at the same times each day.
- For other uses, take as directed by your doctor.

If you forget a dose:
Nervous and mental disorders—Take up to 2 hours late. If more than 2 hours, wait for next scheduled dose (don't double this dose).

What drug does:
- Suppresses brain centers that control abnormal emotions and behavior.
- Suppresses brain's vomiting center.

Continued next column

OVERDOSE

SYMPTOMS:
Stupor, convulsions, coma.
WHAT TO DO:
- **Dial 911 (emergency) for an ambulance or medical help or poison center 1-800-222-1222. Then give first aid immediately.**
- **See emergency information at end of book.**

Time lapse before drug works:
Some benefit seen within a week; takes 4 to 6 weeks for full effect.

Don't take with:
- Antacid or medicine for diarrhea.
- Nonprescription drug for cough, cold or allergy.
- Any other medicine without consulting your doctor or pharmacist.

POSSIBLE ADVERSE REACTIONS OR SIDE EFFECTS

SYMPTOMS	WHAT TO DO
Life-threatening:	
High fever, rapid pulse, profuse sweating, muscle rigidity, confusion and irritability, seizures.	Discontinue. Seek emergency treatment.
Common:	
Dry mouth, blurred vision, constipation, difficulty urinating; sedation, dizziness, low blood pressure.	Continue. Call doctor when convenient.
Infrequent:	
• Continuous jerky or involuntary movements, especially of the face, lips, jaw, tongue; slow-frequency tremor of head or limbs, especially while moving; muscle rigidity, lack of facial expression and slow, inflexible movements.	Discontinue. Call doctor right away.
• Pacing or restlessness; intermittent spasms of muscles of face, eyes, tongue, jaw, neck, body or limbs; jaundice (yellow skin or eyes).	Continue. Call doctor when convenient.
Rare:	
Other symptoms not listed above.	Continue. Call doctor when convenient.

WARNINGS & PRECAUTIONS

Don't take if:
- You are allergic to any phenothiazine.
- You have a blood or bone marrow disease.

Before you start, consult your doctor:
- If you will have surgery within 2 months, including dental surgery, requiring general or spinal anesthesia.
- If you have asthma, emphysema or other lung disorder; glaucoma; or prostate trouble.
- If you take nonprescription ulcer medicine, asthma medicine or amphetamines.

Over age 60:
Adverse reactions and side effects may be more frequent and severe than in younger persons. More likely to develop involuntary movement of jaws, lips, tongue; chewing. Report this to your doctor immediately. Early treatment can help.

Pregnancy:
Risk factors vary for drugs in this group. See category list on page xviii and consult doctor.

Breast-feeding:
Drug passes into milk. Avoid drug or discontinue nursing until you finish medicine. Consult doctor for advice on maintaining milk supply.

Infants & children:
- Don't give to children younger than 2.
- Children more likely than adults to develop adverse reactions from these drugs.

Prolonged use:
May lead to tardive dyskinesia (involuntary movement of jaws, lips, tongue; chewing).

Skin & sunlight:
- One or more drugs in this group may cause rash or intensify sunburn in areas exposed to sun or ultraviolet light (photosensitivity reaction). Use sunscreen and avoid overexposure. Notify doctor if reaction occurs. Sensitivity may remain for 3 months after discontinuing drug.
- Avoid getting overheated or chilled. These drugs affect body temperature and sweating.

Driving, piloting or hazardous work:
Don't drive or pilot aircraft until you learn how medicine affects you. Don't work around dangerous machinery. Don't climb ladders or work in high places. Danger increases if you drink alcohol or take medicine affecting alertness and reflexes.

Discontinuing:
- Nervous and mental disorders—Don't discontinue without doctor's advice until you complete prescribed dose, even though symptoms diminish or disappear.
- Other disorders—Follow doctor's instructions about discontinuing.
- Adverse reactions may occur after drug is discontinued. Consult doctor if new symptoms develop, such as dizziness, nausea, stomach pain, trembling or tardive dyskinesia*.

Others:
- To relieve mouth dryness, chew or suck sugarless gum, candy, or ice.
- Avoid getting the liquid form of the drug on the skin. It may cause a skin rash or irritation.
- Advise any doctor or dentist whom you consult that you take this medicine.

POSSIBLE INTERACTION WITH OTHER DRUGS

GENERIC NAME OR DRUG CLASS	COMBINED EFFECT
Anticholinergics*	Increased phenothiazine effect
Anticonvulsants*	Increased risk of seizures. May need to increase dosage of anticonvulsant.
Antidepressants, tricyclic*	Increased anti-depressant effect.
Antihistamines*	Increased antihistamine effect.
Antihypertensives*	Severe low blood pressure.
Appetite suppressants*	Decreased appetite suppressant effect.
Bupropion	Increased risk of seizures.

Continued on page 926

POSSIBLE INTERACTION WITH OTHER SUBSTANCES

INTERACTS WITH	COMBINED EFFECT
Alcohol:	Dangerous oversedation. Avoid
Beverages:	None expected.
Cocaine:	Decreased phenothiazine effect. Avoid.
Foods:	None expected.
Marijuana:	Drowsiness. May increase antinausea effect.
Tobacco:	None expected.

***See Glossary**

PHENYLEPHRINE

BRAND NAMES

See complete list of brand names in the *Generic and Brand Name Directory*, page 862.

BASIC INFORMATION

Habit forming? No
Prescription needed? No
Available as generic? Yes
Drug class: Sympathomimetic, decongestant

USES

- Temporary relief of congestion of nose, sinuses and throat caused by allergies, colds or sinusitis.
- Treats congestion of eustachian tubes caused by middle ear infections.

DOSAGE & USAGE INFORMATION

How to take:

- Nasal drops or spray—Wash hands before use. Blow nose gently, and then use the drops or spray according to instructions on the label.
- Combination drug products—Use according to label directions. Phenylephrine is the decongestant ingredient in many combination cough, cold and hay fever remedies.

When to take:
As needed, no more often than every 4 hours.

If you forget a dose:
Take when you remember. Wait 4 hours for next dose. Never double a dose.

What drug does:
Narrows blood vessel walls of nose, sinus and throat tissues, enlarging airways.

Time lapse before drug works:
5 to 30 minutes.

Continued next column

OVERDOSE

SYMPTOMS:
Headache, heart palpitations, vomiting, blood pressure rise, slow and forceful pulse.
WHAT TO DO:

- **Dial 911 (emergency) for an ambulance or medical help or poison center 1-800-222-1222. Then give first aid immediately.**
- **See emergency information on inside covers.**

Don't take with:
Nonprescription drugs for asthma, cough, cold, allergy, appetite suppressants, sleeping pills or drugs containing caffeine without consulting doctor.

POSSIBLE ADVERSE REACTIONS OR SIDE EFFECTS

SYMPTOMS	WHAT TO DO
Life-threatening: In case of overdose, see previous column.	
Common: Burning, dryness, stinging inside nose; headache.	Continue. Call doctor when convenient.
Infrequent: None expected.	
Rare: Unusual sweating, fast or pounding heartbeat, nervousness, insomnia (all symptoms of too much being absorbed into body).	Discontinue. Call doctor right away.

WARNINGS & PRECAUTIONS

Don't take if:
You are allergic to any sympathomimetic.

Before you start, consult your doctor:
- If you have high blood pressure.
- If you have heart disease.
- If you have diabetes.
- If you have overactive thyroid.
- If you have taken MAO inhibitors in past 2 weeks.

Over age 60:
Adverse reactions and side effects may be more frequent and severe than in younger persons.

Pregnancy:
Decide with your doctor if drug benefits justify risk to unborn child. Risk category C (see page xviii).

Breast-feeding:
Drug passes into milk. Avoid drug or discontinue nursing until you finish medicine. Consult doctor for advice on maintaining milk supply.

Infants & children:
Use only under close supervision.

Prolonged use:
- Rebound* congestion and chemical irritation of nasal membranes.
- May cause functional dependence.
- Talk to your doctor about the need for follow-up medical examinations or laboratory studies to check blood pressure, ECG*.

Skin & sunlight:
No problems expected.

Driving, piloting or hazardous work:
No problems expected.

Discontinuing:
May be unnecessary to finish medicine. Follow label or doctor's instructions.

Others:
- Call the doctor if symptoms worsen or new symptoms develop with use of this medicine.
- Heed all warnings on the product label.

POSSIBLE INTERACTION WITH OTHER DRUGS

GENERIC NAME OR DRUG CLASS	COMBINED EFFECT
Antidepressants, tricyclic*	Increased phenylephrine effect.
Guanadrel	Heart or blood pressure problems. Avoid.
Guanethidine	Heart or blood pressure problems. Avoid.
Maprotiline	Dangerous blood pressure rise. Don't use within 14 days.
Monoamine oxidase (MAO) inhibitors*	Dangerous blood pressure rise. Don't use within 14 days.
Nicotine	Decreased effect of phenylephrine.

POSSIBLE INTERACTION WITH OTHER SUBSTANCES

INTERACTS WITH	COMBINED EFFECT
Alcohol:	None expected.
Beverages: Caffeine drinks.	Excess brain stimulation.
Cocaine:	Excess brain stimulation.
Foods:	None expected.
Marijuana:	None expected.
Tobacco:	None expected.

*See Glossary

PHENYLEPHRINE (Ophthalmic)

BRAND NAMES

Ak-Dilate
Ak-Nefrin
Dilatair
Dionephrine
I-Phrine
Isopto Frin
Minims Phenylephrine
Mydfrin
Neofrin
Neo-Synephrine
Ocugestrin
Ocu-Phrin
Phenoptic
Prefrin Liquifilm
Relief Eye Drops for Red Eyes
Spersaphrine

BASIC INFORMATION

Habit forming? No
Prescription needed? Yes, some strengths
Available as generic? No
Drug class: Mydriatic, decongestant (ophthalmic)

USES

- High-concentration drops—Dilates pupils.
- Low-concentration drops (available without prescription)—Relieves minor eye irritations caused by colds, hay fever, dust, wind, swimming, sun, smog, hard contact lenses, eye strain, smoke.

DOSAGE & USAGE INFORMATION

How to use:
Eye drops
- Wash hands.
- Apply pressure to inside corner of eye with middle finger.
- Continue pressure for 1 minute after placing medicine in eye.
- Tilt head backward. Pull lower lid away from eye with index finger of the same hand.
- Drop eye drops into pouch and close eye. Don't blink.
- Keep eyes closed for 1 to 2 minutes.
- Don't touch applicator tip to any surface (including the eye). If you accidentally touch tip, clean with warm soap and water.
- Keep container tightly closed.

Continued next column

OVERDOSE

SYMPTOMS:
None expected.
WHAT TO DO:
Not intended for internal use. If child accidentally swallows, call poison center 1-800-222-1222.

- Keep cool, but don't freeze.
- Wash hands immediately after using.

When to use:
As directed on label.

If you forget a dose:
Use as soon as you remember.

What drug does:
Acts on small blood vessels to make them constrict.

Time lapse before drug works:
15 to 90 minutes.

Don't use with:
- Other eye drops or ointment without consulting your eye doctor.
- Antidepressants*, guanadrel, guanethidine, maprotiline, pargyline, any monoamine oxidase (MAO) inhibitor*.

POSSIBLE ADVERSE REACTIONS OR SIDE EFFECTS

SYMPTOMS	WHAT TO DO
Life-threatening:	
None expected, unless you use much more than directed.	Discontinue. Call doctor right away.
Common:	
None expected.	
Infrequent:	
Burning or stinging eyes, headache, eyes more sensitive to light, watery eyes, eye irritation not present before.	Continue. Call doctor when convenient.
Rare:	
None expected, unless too much gets absorbed. If so, symptoms will be paleness, dizziness, tremor, increased sweating, irregular or fast heartbeat.	Discontinue. Call doctor right away.

PHENYLEPHRINE (Ophthalmic)

WARNINGS & PRECAUTIONS

Don't use if:
- You are allergic to phenylephrine.
- You have glaucoma.

Before you start, consult your doctor:
- If you have heart disease with irregular heartbeat, high blood pressure, diabetes.
- If you take antidepressants*, guanadrel, guanethidine, maprotiline, pargyline, any monoamine oxidase (MAO) inhibitor*.

Over age 60:
Adverse reactions and side effects may be more frequent and severe than in younger persons. Ask doctor about smaller doses.

Pregnancy:
Decide with your doctor if drug benefits justify risk to unborn child. Risk category C (see page xviii).

Breast-feeding:
Safety not established. Consult doctor.

Infants & children:
Use only under close medical supervision.

Prolonged use:
Avoid if possible.

Skin & sunlight:
No special problems expected.

Driving, piloting or hazardous work:
No problems expected.

Discontinuing:
No problems expected.

Others:
Consult doctor if condition doesn't improve in 3 to 4 days.

POSSIBLE INTERACTION WITH OTHER DRUGS

GENERIC NAME OR DRUG CLASS	COMBINED EFFECT
Clinically significant interactions with oral or injected medicines unlikely.	

POSSIBLE INTERACTION WITH OTHER SUBSTANCES

INTERACTS WITH	COMBINED EFFECT
Alcohol:	None expected.
Beverages:	None expected.
Cocaine:	None expected.
Foods:	None expected.
Marijuana:	None expected.
Tobacco:	None expected.

*See Glossary

PILOCARPINE (Oral)

BRAND NAMES

Salagen

BASIC INFORMATION

Habit forming? No
Prescription needed? Yes
Available as generic? No
Drug class: Cholinergic

USES

Treatment for dry mouth caused by radiation treatment of patients with cancer of the head or neck of patients with Sjogren's syndrome.

DOSAGE & USAGE INFORMATION

How to take:
Tablets—Follow doctor's directions. May require dosing several times a day.

When to take:
At the same times each day.

If you forget a dose:
Take as soon as you remember. If it is almost time for your next dose, skip the missed dose and return to your regular dosing schedule (don't double this dose).

What drug does:
Stimulates the salivary glands to increase their secretions.

Time lapse before drug works:
20-60 minutes.

Don't take with:
Any other medicine without consulting your doctor or pharmacist.

OVERDOSE

SYMPTOMS:
Stomach cramps or pain, diarrhea, severe nausea or vomiting, rapid heartbeat, chest pain, confusion, fainting, bad headache, severe shortness of breath, unusual trembling or shaking, visual problems.
WHAT TO DO:

- **If person takes much larger amount than prescribed, call doctor, poison center 1-800-222-1222 or hospital emergency room for instructions.**
- **If symptoms are severe or critical, dial 911 (emergency) for an ambulance or medical help. Then give first aid immediately.**

POSSIBLE ADVERSE REACTIONS OR SIDE EFFECTS

SYMPTOMS	WHAT TO DO
Life-threatening: In case of overdose, see previous column.	
Common: Runny nose, cough, fever, chills, diarrhea, indigestion, nausea, tiredness or weakness, warm feeling, sweating, skin flushing or red, urinary frequency, joint pain or muscle aches.	Continue. Call doctor when convenient.
Infrequent:	
• Swelling (ankles, feet, face or fingers), rapid heartbeat, visual problems, bloody nose, vomiting.	Discontinue. Call doctor right away.
• Trembling or shaking, trouble with swallowing, voice change, headache.	Continue. Call doctor when convenient.
Rare: None expected.	

WARNINGS & PRECAUTIONS

Don't take if:
You are allergic to pilocarpine (ophthalmic or oral) or have uncontrolled asthma.

Before you start, consult your doctor:
- If you have gallbladder problems.
- If you have iritis or glaucoma.
- If you have had heart or blood vessel disease.
- If you have asthma.
- If you have any cognitive or psychiatric problem.
- If you have or have had, kidney disease.
- If you have been told you have a tendency for retinal detachment or have retinal disease.
- If you have peptic ulcer disease.

Over age 60:
No problems expected.

Pregnancy:
Decide with your doctor if drug benefits justify risk to unborn child. Risk category C (see page xviii).

Breast-feeding:
It is unknown if pilocarpine passes into breast milk. Avoid drug or discontinue nursing until you finish medicine. Consult doctor for advice on maintaining milk supply.

Infants & children:
Safety and efficacy has not been established in children.

Prolonged use:
If no improvement is seen after twelve weeks of using this medicine, consult doctor.

Skin & sunlight:
No problems expected.

Driving, piloting or hazardous work:
May cause visual disturbances, especially at night. Don't drive or pilot aircraft until you learn how medicine affects you. Don't work around dangerous machinery. Don't climb ladders or work in high places. Danger increases if you drink alcohol or take medicine affecting alertness and reflexes.

Discontinuing:
Consult doctor before discontinuing.

Others:
- Advise any doctor or dentist whom you consult that you take this medicine.
- Since this drug causes sweating, be sure to drink plenty of fluids.

POSSIBLE INTERACTION WITH OTHER DRUGS

GENERIC NAME OR DRUG CLASS	COMBINED EFFECT
Anticholinergics*	Decreased effect of both drugs.
Antiglaucoma agents*	Increased antiglaucoma effect.
Antiglaucoma, beta blockers	Increased risk of side effects.
Beta adrenergic blocking agents	Increased risk of side effects.
Bethanechol	Increased risk of side effects.
Cholinergics*, other	Increased effect of both drugs.

POSSIBLE INTERACTION WITH OTHER SUBSTANCES

INTERACTS WITH	COMBINED EFFECT
Alcohol:	None expected.
Beverages:	None expected.
Cocaine:	None expected. Best to avoid.
Foods:	None expected.
Marijuana:	None expected. Best to avoid.
Tobacco:	None expected.

*See Glossary

POTASSIUM SUPPLEMENTS

GENERIC AND BRAND NAMES

See complete list of generic and brand names in the *Generic and Brand Name Directory*, page 862.

BASIC INFORMATION

Habit forming? No
Prescription needed? Yes
Available as generic? Yes
Drug class: Mineral supplement (potassium), electrolyte replenisher, antihyperthyroid.

USES

- Treatment for potassium deficiency due to diuretics, cortisone or digitalis medicines.
- Treatment for hypercalcemia due to cancer.
- Treats overactive thyroid disease.
- Treats iodine deficiency.
- Treatment for low potassium associated with some illnesses.

DOSAGE & USAGE INFORMATION

How to take:
- Tablet or capsule—Take as directed on label.
- Effervescent tablets, granules, powder or liquid—Dilute dose in water.

When to take:
At the same time each day, preferably with food or immediately after meals.

If you forget a dose:
Take as soon as you remember. Don't double next dose.

What drug does:
Preserves or restores normal function of nerve cells, thyroid, heart and skeletal muscle cells and kidneys, as well as stomach juice secretions.

Time lapse before drug works:
30 minutes to 2 hours. Full benefit may require 12 to 24 hours.

Continued next column

OVERDOSE

SYMPTOMS:
Paralysis of arms and legs, irregular heart-beat, blood pressure drop, convulsions, coma, cardiac arrest.
WHAT TO DO:
- **Dial 911 (emergency) for an ambulance or medical help or poison center 1-800-222-1222. Then give first aid immediately.**
- **See emergency information on inside covers.**

Don't take with:
Any other medicine without consulting your doctor or pharmacist.

POSSIBLE ADVERSE REACTIONS OR SIDE EFFECTS

SYMPTOMS	WHAT TO DO
Life-threatening: In case of overdose, see previous column.	
Common:	
• Skin rash, swollen salivary glands.	Discontinue. Call doctor right away.
• Diarrhea, nausea abdominal pain.	Continue. Call doctor when convenient.
Infrequent:	
Bone and joint pain, numbness or tingling in hands or feet, vomiting, dizziness.	Discontinue. Call doctor right away.
Rare:	
Confusion; irregular heartbeat; difficult breathing; unusual fatigue; weakness; heaviness of legs; hemorrhage, perforation with enteric-coated tablets (rarely with wax matrix tablets); esophageal ulceration with tablets; bloody stools.	Discontinue. Call doctor right away.

WARNINGS & PRECAUTIONS

Don't take if:
- You are allergic to any potassium supplement.
- You have acute or chronic kidney disease.

Before you start, consult your doctor:
- If you have Addison's disease or familial periodic paralysis.
- If you have heart disease.
- If you have intestinal blockage.
- If you have a stomach ulcer.
- If you use diuretics.
- If you have high blood pressure.
- If you have kidney disease.
- If you have pancreatitis.
- If you use heart medicine.
- If you use laxatives or have chronic diarrhea.
- If you use salt substitutes or low-salt milk.

Over age 60:
Observe dose schedule strictly. Potassium balance is critical. Deviation above or below normal can have serious results.

Pregnancy:
Consult with your doctor before taking potassium supplements, as they may pose a significant risk to your unborn child. Risk category D (see page xviii).

Breast-feeding:
Drug passes into milk. Avoid drug or discontinue nursing until you finish medicine. Consult doctor for advice on maintaining milk supply.

Infants & children:
Use only under doctor's supervision.

Prolonged use:
- Talk to your doctor about the need for follow-up medical examinations or laboratory studies to check serum potassium levels.
- If burning mouth, headache or salivation occur, discontinue and call doctor.

Skin & sunlight:
No problems expected.

Driving, piloting or hazardous work:
Don't drive or pilot aircraft until you learn how medicine affects you. Don't work around dangerous machinery. Don't climb ladders or work in high places. Danger increases if you drink alcohol or take medicine affecting alertness and reflexes.

Discontinuing:
Don't discontinue without consulting doctor. Dose may require gradual reduction if you have taken drug for a long time. Doses of other drugs may also require adjustment.

Others:
- Overdose or underdose serious. Frequent EKGs and laboratory blood studies to measure serum electrolytes and kidney function recommended.
- Prolonged diarrhea may call for increased dosage of potassium.
- Advise any doctor or dentist you consult that you take this medicine.
- Serious injury may necessitate temporary decrease in potassium.
- Some products contain tartrazine dye. Avoid, especially if you are allergic to aspirin.

POSSIBLE INTERACTION WITH OTHER DRUGS

GENERIC NAME OR DRUG CLASS	COMBINED EFFECT
Adrenocorticoids, systemic	Decreased potassium effect.
Amiloride	Dangerous rise in blood potassium.
Angiotensin-converting enzyme (ACE) inhibitors*	Possible increased potassium effect.
Antacids*	May decrease potassium absorption.
Anticholinergics, other*	Increased possibility of intestinal ulcers, which sometimes occur with oral potassium tablets.
Anti-inflammatory drugs, nonsteroidal (NSAIDs)*	Increased risk of stomach irritation.
Antithyroid drugs*	Excessive effect of antithyroid drugs.
Beta-adrenergic blocking agents*	Increased potassium levels.
Calcium	Decreased potassium effect.
Cortisone drugs*	Increased fluid retention.
Digitalis preparations*	Possible irregular heartbeat.
Diuretics, thiazide or loop*	Decreased potassium effect.
Laxatives*	Possible decreased potassium effect.
Lithium	Increased chance of producing a thyroid goiter.
Losartan	Increased potassium levels.

Continued on page 926

POSSIBLE INTERACTION WITH OTHER SUBSTANCES

INTERACTS WITH	COMBINED EFFECT
Alcohol:	None expected.
Beverages:	
• Salty drinks such as tomato juice, commercial thirst quenchers.	Increased fluid retention.
• Low-salt milk or salt substitutes.	Increased potassium levels.
Cocaine:	May cause irregular heartbeat.
Foods: Salty foods.	Increased fluid retention.
Marijuana:	May cause irregular heartbeat.
Tobacco:	None expected.

PRIMAQUINE

GENERIC NAMES

PRIMAQUINE

BASIC INFORMATION

Habit forming? No
Prescription needed? Yes
Available as generic? Yes
Drug class: Antiprotozoal (antimalarial)

USES

- Treats some forms of malaria.
- Prevents relapses of some forms of malaria.
- Treats pneumocystis carinii pneumonia (used in combination with clindamycin).

DOSAGE & USAGE INFORMATION

How to take:
Tablets—Take with meals or antacids to minimize stomach irritation.

When to take:
At the same time each day, according to instructions on prescription label.

If you forget a dose:
Take as soon as you remember up to 2 hours late. If more than 2 hours, wait for next scheduled dose. Don't double this dose.

What drug does:
Alters the properties of DNA in malaria organisms to prevent them from multiplying.

Time lapse before drug works:
2 to 3 hours.

Don't take with:
Any other medicine without consulting your doctor or pharmacist.

OVERDOSE

SYMPTOMS:
None expected.
WHAT TO DO:
Overdose unlikely to threaten life. If person takes much larger amount than prescribed, call doctor, poison center 1-800-222-1222 or hospital emergency room for instructions.

POSSIBLE ADVERSE REACTIONS OR SIDE EFFECTS

SYMPTOMS	WHAT TO DO
Life-threatening: None expected.	
Common: None expected.	
Infrequent: Dark urine; back, leg or stomach pain; appetite loss; pale skin; fever.	Discontinue. Call doctor right away.
Rare: Blue fingernails, lips and skin; dizziness; difficult breathing; extraordinary tiredness; sore throat; fever.	Discontinue. Call doctor right away.

WARNINGS & PRECAUTIONS

Don't take if:
- You have G6PD* deficiency.
- You are hypersensitive to primaquine.

Before you start, consult your doctor:
If you are Black, Oriental, Asian or of Mediterranean origin.

Over age 60:
No special problems expected.

Pregnancy:
Decide with your doctor if drug benefits justify risk to unborn child. Risk category C (see page xviii).

Breast-feeding:
Effect unknown. Consult doctor.

Infants & children:
No special problems expected.

Prolonged use:
No special problems expected.

Skin & sunlight:
No special problems expected.

Driving, piloting or hazardous work:
No special problems expected.

Discontinuing:
No special problems expected.

Others:
- If you are Black, Asian, Oriental or of Mediterranean origin, insist on a test for G6PD* deficiency before taking this medicine.
- Advise any doctor or dentist whom you consult that you take this medicine.

POSSIBLE INTERACTION WITH OTHER DRUGS

GENERIC NAME OR DRUG CLASS	COMBINED EFFECT
Hemolytics*, other	Increased risk of serious side effects affecting the blood.
Quinacrine	Increased toxic effects of primaquine.

POSSIBLE INTERACTION WITH OTHER SUBSTANCES

INTERACTS WITH	COMBINED EFFECT
Alcohol:	Possible liver toxicity. Avoid.
Beverages:	None expected.
Cocaine:	None expected.
Foods:	None expected.
Marijuana:	None expected.
Tobacco:	None expected.

*See Glossary

PRIMIDONE

BRAND NAMES

Apo-Primidone
Myidone
Mysoline
PMS Primadone
Sertan

BASIC INFORMATION

Habit forming? No
Prescription needed? Yes
Available as generic? Yes
Drug class: Anticonvulsant

USES

Prevents some forms of epileptic seizures.

DOSAGE & USAGE INFORMATION

How to take:

- Tablet—Swallow with liquid. If you can't swallow whole, crumble tablet and take with liquid or food.
- Liquid—If desired, dilute dose in beverage before swallowing.

When to take:
Daily in regularly spaced doses, according to doctor's prescription.

If you forget a dose:
Take as soon as you remember up to 2 hours late. If more than 2 hours, wait for next scheduled dose (don't double this dose).

What drug does:
Probably inhibits repetitious spread of impulses along nerve pathways.

Continued next column

OVERDOSE

SYMPTOMS:
Slow, shallow breathing; weak, rapid pulse; confusion, deep sleep, coma.
WHAT TO DO:

- **Dial 911 (emergency) for an ambulance or medical help or poison center 1-800-222-1222. Then give first aid immediately.**
- **If patient is unconscious and not breathing, give mouth-to-mouth breathing. If there is no heartbeat, use cardiac massage and mouth-to-mouth breathing (CPR). Don't try to make patient vomit. If you can't get help quickly, take patient to nearest emergency facility.**
- **See emergency information on inside covers.**

Time lapse before drug works:
2 to 3 weeks.

Don't take with:
Any other medicine without consulting your doctor or pharmacist.

POSSIBLE ADVERSE REACTIONS OR SIDE EFFECTS

SYMPTOMS	WHAT TO DO
Life-threatening: In case of overdose, see previous column.	
Common:	
• Difficult breathing.	Discontinue. Call doctor right away.
• Confusion, change in vision.	Continue. Call doctor when convenient.
• Clumsiness, dizziness, drowsiness.	Continue. Tell doctor at next visit.
Infrequent:	
• Unusual excitement, particularly in children; nausea; vomiting.	Discontinue. Call doctor right away.
• Headache, fatigue, weakness.	Continue. Call doctor when convenient.
Rare:	
• Rash or hives, appetite loss, acute psychosis, hair loss, fever, joint pain.	Discontinue. Call doctor right away.
• Swollen eyelids or legs.	Continue. Call doctor when convenient.
• Decreased sexual ability.	Continue. Tell doctor at next visit.

WARNINGS & PRECAUTIONS

Don't take if:

- You are allergic to any barbiturate.
- You have had porphyria.

Before you start, consult your doctor:

- If you have had liver, kidney or lung disease or asthma.
- If you have lupus.

Over age 60:
Adverse reactions and side effects may be more frequent and severe than in younger persons.

Pregnancy:
Consult doctor. Risk category D (see page xviii).

Breast-feeding:
Drug filters into milk. May harm child. Avoid. Consult doctor.

Infants & children:
Use only under medical supervision.

Prolonged use:
- Enlarged lymph and thyroid glands.
- Anemia.
- Rickets in children and osteomalacia (insufficient calcium to bones) in adults.
- Talk to your doctor about the need for follow-up medical examinations or laboratory studies to check complete blood counts (white blood cell count, platelet count, red blood cell count, hemoglobin, hematocrit), liver function, kidney function.

Skin & sunlight:
No special problems expected.

Driving, piloting or hazardous work:
Don't drive or pilot aircraft until you learn how medicine affects you. Don't work around dangerous machinery. Don't climb ladders or work in high places. Danger increases if you drink alcohol or take medicine affecting alertness and reflexes.

Discontinuing:
Don't discontinue abruptly or without doctor's advice until you complete prescribed dose, even though symptoms diminish or disappear.

Others:
- Tell doctor if you become ill or injured and must interrupt dose schedule.
- Periodic laboratory blood tests of drug level recommended.

POSSIBLE INTERACTION WITH OTHER DRUGS

GENERIC NAME OR DRUG CLASS	COMBINED EFFECT
Adrenocorticoids, systemic	Decreased adreno-corticoid effect.
Anticoagulants*, oral	Decreased primidone effect.
Anticonvulsants*, other	Changed seizure pattern.
Antidepressants*	Increased anti-depressant effect.
Antihistamines*	Increased sedation effect of primidone.
Aspirin	Decreased aspirin effect.
Carbamazepine	Unpredictable increase or decrease of primidone effect.
Carbonic anhydrase inhibitors*	Possible decreased primidone effect.
Central nervous system (CNS) depressants*	Increased CNS depressant effects.
Contraceptives, oral*	Decreased contraceptive effect.
Cyclosporine	Decreased cyclosporine effect.
Digitalis preparations*	Decreased digitalis effect.
Disulfiram	Possible increased primidone effect.
Estrogens*	Decreased estrogen effect.
Griseofulvin	Possible decreased griseofulvin effect.
Isoniazid	Decreased primidone effect.
Lamotrigine	Decreased lamotrigine effect.
Leucovorin (large dose)	May counteract anti-convulsant effect of primidone.
Loxapine	Decreased anti-convulsant effect of primidone.
Metronidazole	Possible decreased metronidazole effect.
Mind-altering drugs*	Increased effect of mind-altering drug.
Monoamine oxidase (MAO) inhibitors*	Increased sedation effect of primidone.
Nabilone	Greater depression of central nervous system.

Continued on page 926

POSSIBLE INTERACTION WITH OTHER SUBSTANCES

INTERACTS WITH	COMBINED EFFECT
Alcohol:	Dangerous sedative effect. Avoid.
Beverages:	None expected.
Cocaine:	Decreased primidone effect.
Foods:	Possible need for more vitamin D.
Marijuana:	Decreased anti-convulsant effect of primidone. Drowsiness, unsteadiness.
Tobacco:	None expected.

PROBENECID

BRAND NAMES

Benemid
Benuryl
Probalan

BASIC INFORMATION

Habit forming? No
Prescription needed? Yes
Available as generic? Yes
Drug class: Antigout

USES

- Treats chronic gout.
- Increases blood levels of penicillins and cephalosporins.

DOSAGE & USAGE INFORMATION

How to take:
Tablet—Swallow with liquid or food to lessen stomach irritation. If you can't swallow whole, crumble tablet and take with liquid or food.

When to take:
At the same time each day.

If you forget a dose:
Take as soon as you remember up to 12 hours late. If more than 12 hours, wait for next scheduled dose (don't double this dose).

What drug does:
- Forces kidneys to excrete uric acid.
- Reduces amount of penicillin excreted in urine.

Time lapse before drug works:
May require several months of regular use to prevent acute gout.

Don't take with:
- Nonprescription drugs containing aspirin or caffeine.
- Any other medicine without consulting your doctor or pharmacist.

OVERDOSE

SYMPTOMS:
Breathing difficulty, severe nervous agitation, vomiting, seizures, convulsions, delirium, coma.
WHAT TO DO:
- **Dial 911 (emergency) for an ambulance or medical help or poison center 1-800-222-1222. Then give first aid immediately.**
- **See emergency information on inside covers.**

POSSIBLE ADVERSE REACTIONS OR SIDE EFFECTS

SYMPTOMS	WHAT TO DO
Life-threatening:	
In case of overdose, see previous column.	
Common:	
Headache, appetite loss, nausea, vomiting.	Continue. Call doctor when convenient.
Infrequent:	
• Blood in urine, low back pain. worsening gout.	Discontinue. Call doctor right away.
• Dizziness, flushed face, itchy skin.	Continue. Call doctor when convenient.
• Painful or frequent urination, sore gums.	Continue. Tell doctor at next visit.
Rare:	
Sore throat, fever and chills; difficult breathing; unusual bleeding or bruising; red, painful joint; jaundice; foot, leg or face swelling.	Discontinue. Call doctor right away.

WARNINGS & PRECAUTIONS

Don't take if:
- You are allergic to any uricosuric*.
- You have acute gout.
- Patient is younger than 2.

Before you start, consult your doctor:
- If you have had kidney stones or kidney disease.
- If you have a peptic ulcer.
- If you have bone marrow or blood cell disease.
- If you are undergoing chemotherapy for cancer.

Over age 60:
Adverse reactions and side effects may be more frequent and severe than in younger persons.

Pregnancy:
Consult doctor. Risk category B (see page xviii).

Breast-feeding:
Effect unknown. Consult doctor.

Infants & children:
Not recommended.

Prolonged use:
- Possible kidney damage.
- Talk to your doctor about the need for follow-up medical examinations or laboratory studies to check serum uric acid, urine uric acid.

Skin & sunlight:
No problems expected.

Driving, piloting or hazardous work:
Avoid if you feel dizzy. Otherwise, no problems expected.

Discontinuing:
Don't discontinue without consulting doctor. Dose may require gradual reduction if you have taken drug for a long time. Doses of other drugs may also require adjustment.

Others:
If signs of gout attack develop while taking medicine, consult doctor.

POSSIBLE INTERACTION WITH OTHER DRUGS

GENERIC NAME OR DRUG CLASS	COMBINED EFFECT
Allopurinol	Increased effect of each drug.
Anticoagulants*, oral	Increased anti-coagulant effect.
Anti-inflammatory drugs, nonsteroidal (NSAIDs)*	Increased toxic risk.
Aspirin	Decreased probenecid effect.
Bismuth subsalicylate	Decreased probenecid effect.
Cephalosporins*	Increased cephalosporin effect.
Ciprofloxacin	May cause kidney dysfunction.
Dapsone	Increased dapsone effect. Increased toxicity.
Diclofenac	Increased diclofenac effect.
Diuretics, thiazide*	Decreased probenecid effect.
Hypoglycemics, oral*	Increased hypo-glycemic effect.
Indomethacin	Increased adverse effects of indomethacin.
Ketoprofen	Increased risk of ketoprofen toxicity.
Loracarbef	Increased loracarbef effect.
Methotrexate	Increased methotrexate toxicity.
Nitrofurantoin	Incresed effect of nitrofurantoin.
Para-aminosalicylic acid	Increased effect of para-aminosalicylic acid.
Penicillins*	Enhanced penicillin effect.
Pyrazinamide	Decreased probenecid effect.
Salicylates*	Decreased probenecid effect.
Sodium benzoate & sodium phenylacetate	May reduce effect of sodium benzoate & sodium phenylacetate.
Sulfa drugs*	Slows elimination. May cause harmful accumulation of sulfa.
Thioguanine	More likelihood of toxicity of both drugs.
Valacyclovir	Increased valacyclovir effect.
Zidovudine	Increased zidovudine toxicity risk.

POSSIBLE INTERACTION WITH OTHER SUBSTANCES

INTERACTS WITH	COMBINED EFFECT
Alcohol:	Decreased probenecid effect.
Beverages: Caffeine drinks.	Loss of probenecid effectiveness.
Cocaine:	None expected.
Foods:	None expected.
Marijuana:	Daily use—Decreased probenecid effect.
Tobacco:	None expected.

*See Glossary

PROBENECID & COLCHICINE

BRAND NAMES

Col Benemid
Col-Probenecid
Proben-C

BASIC INFORMATION

Habit forming? No
Prescription needed? Yes
Available as generic? Yes
Drug class: Antigout

USES

- Increases blood levels of penicillins and cephalosporins.
- Relieves joint pain, inflammation, swelling from gout.
- Also used for familial Mediterranean fever, dermatitis herpetiformis.

DOSAGE & USAGE INFORMATION

How to take:
Tablet—Swallow with liquid or food to lessen stomach irritation. If you can't swallow whole, crumble tablet and take with liquid or food.

When to take:
At the same time each day.

If you forget a dose:
Take as soon as you remember up to 12 hours late. If more than 12 hours, wait for next scheduled dose (don't double this dose).

What drug does:
- Forces kidneys to excrete uric acid.
- Reduces amount of penicillin excreted in urine.
- Decreases acidity of joint tissues and prevents deposits of uric acid crystals.

Time lapse before drug works:
12 to 48 hours.

Continued next column

OVERDOSE

SYMPTOMS:
Breathing difficulty, severe nervous agitation, convulsions, bloody urine, diarrhea, vomiting, muscle weakness, fever, stupor, seizures, delirium, coma.

WHAT TO DO:
- **Dial 911 (emergency) for an ambulance or medical help or poison center 1-800-222-1222. Then give first aid immediately.**
- **See emergency information on inside covers.**

Don't take with:
- Nonprescription drugs containing aspirin or caffeine.
- Any other medicine without consulting your doctor or pharmacist.

POSSIBLE ADVERSE REACTIONS OR SIDE EFFECTS

SYMPTOMS	WHAT TO DO
Life-threatening: Blood in urine; convulsions; severe muscle weakness; difficult breathing; burning feeling of stomach, throat or skin; worsening gout.	Discontinue. Seek emergency treatment.
Common: Diarrhea, headache, abdominal pain.	Discontinue. Call doctor right away.
Infrequent: • Back pain; painful, difficult urination.	Discontinue. Call doctor right away.
• Dizziness, red or flushed face, urgent urination, sore gums, hair loss.	Continue. Call doctor when convenient.
Rare: Sudden decrease in urine output; nausea; vomiting; mood change; fever; chills; diarrhea; jaundice; numbness or tingling in hands or feet; rash; sore throat, fever, mouth sores; swollen face, feet and ankles; unexplained bleeding or bruising; weight gain or loss; low white or red blood cells.	Discontinue. Call doctor right away.

WARNINGS & PRECAUTIONS

Don't take if:
You are allergic to any uricosuric* or colchicine.

Before you start, consult your doctor:
- If you have had kidney stones, kidney disease, heart or liver disease, peptic ulcers or ulcerative colitis.
- If you have bone marrow or blood cell disease.
- If you will have surgery within 2 months, including dental surgery, requiring general or spinal anesthesia.
- If you are undergoing chemotherapy for cancer.

Over age 60:
Adverse reactions and side effects may be more frequent and severe than in younger persons. Colchicine has a narrow margin of safety for people in this age group.

Pregnancy:
Risk factor varies with length of pregnancy. See category list on page xviii and consult doctor.

Breast-feeding:
No problems expected, but consult doctor.

Infants & children:
Not recommended.

Prolonged use:
- Possible kidney damage.
- Permanent hair loss.
- Anemia. Request blood counts.
- Numbness or tingling in hands and feet.
- Talk to your doctor about the need for follow-up medical examinations or laboratory studies to check serum uric acid, urine uric acid.

Skin & sunlight:
No problems expected.

Driving, piloting or hazardous work:
Don't drive or pilot aircraft until you learn how medicine affects you. Don't work around dangerous machinery. Don't climb ladders or work in high places. Danger increases if you drink alcohol or take medicine affecting alertness and reflexes, such as antihistamines, tranquilizers, sedatives, pain medicine, narcotics and mind-altering drugs.

Discontinuing:
- May be unnecessary to finish medicine. Follow doctor's instructions.
- Stop taking if severe digestive upsets occur before symptoms are relieved.

Others:
- If signs of gout attack develop while taking medicine, consult doctor.
- Limit each course of treatment to 8 mg. Don't exceed 3 mg per 24 hours.
- May decrease sperm count in males.

POSSIBLE INTERACTION WITH OTHER DRUGS

GENERIC NAME OR DRUG CLASS	COMBINED EFFECT
Acetohexamide	Increased acetohexamide effect.
Allopurinol	Increased effect of each drug.
Anticoagulants*, oral	Irregular effect on anticoagulation, sometimes increased, sometimes decreased. Follow prothrombin times.
Antidepressants*	Oversedation.
Antihistamines*	Oversedation.
Antihypertensives*	Decreased antihypertensive effect.
Anti-inflammatory drugs, nonsteroidal (NSAIDs)*	Increased toxic risk.
Appetite suppressants*	Increased appetite suppressant effect.
Bismuth subsalicylate	Decreased probenecid effect.
Cephalosporins*	Increased cephalosporin effect.
Dapsone	Increased dapsone effect. Increased toxicity.
Diclofenac	Increased diclofenac effect.
Diuretics, thiazide*	Decreased probenecid effect.
Indomethacin	Increased adverse effects of indomethacin.
Ketoprofen	Increased effect of ketoprofen toxicity.

Continued on page 927

POSSIBLE INTERACTION WITH OTHER SUBSTANCES

INTERACTS WITH	COMBINED EFFECT
Alcohol:	Decreased probenecid effect.
Beverages:	
Caffeine drinks.	Loss of probenecid effectiveness.
Herbal teas.	Increased colchicine effect. Avoid.
Cocaine:	Overstimulation. Avoid.
Foods:	None expected.
Marijuana:	Decreased colchicine and probenecid effect.
Tobacco:	None expected.

*See Glossary

PROCAINAMIDE

BRAND NAMES

Procan SR
Promine
Pronestyl
Pronestyl SR

BASIC INFORMATION

Habit forming? No
Prescription needed? Yes
Available as generic? Yes
Drug class: Antiarrhythmic

USES

Stabilizes irregular heartbeat.

DOSAGE & USAGE INFORMATION

How to take:
- Tablet or capsule—Swallow with liquid.
- Extended-release tablets—Swallow each dose whole. Do not crush them.

When to take:
Best taken on empty stomach, 1 hour before or 2 hours after meals. If necessary, may be taken with food or milk to lessen stomach upset.

If you forget a dose:
Take as soon as you remember up to 2 hours late (4 hours for extended-release tablets). If more than 2 hours, wait for next scheduled dose (don't double this dose).

What drug does:
Slows activity of pacemaker (rhythm control center of heart) and delays transmission of electrical impulses.

Time lapse before drug works:
30 to 60 minutes.

Don't take with:
Any other medicine without consulting your doctor or pharmacist.

OVERDOSE

SYMPTOMS:
Fast and irregular heartbeat, confusion, stupor, decreased blood pressure, fainting, cardiac arrest.
WHAT TO DO:
- **Dial 911 (emergency) for an ambulance or medical help or poison center 1-800-222-1222. Then give first aid immediately.**
- **See emergency information on inside covers.**

POSSIBLE ADVERSE REACTIONS OR SIDE EFFECTS

SYMPTOMS	WHAT TO DO
Life-threatening:	
Hives, rash, intense itching, faintness soon after dose (anaphylaxis); convulsions.	Seek emergency treatment immediately.
Common:	
Diarrhea, appetite loss, nausea, vomiting, bitter taste.	Continue. Call doctor when convenient.
Infrequent:	
Joint pain, painful breathing, dizziness.	Discontinue. Call doctor right away.
Rare:	
• Hallucinations, depression, confusion, psychosis, itchy skin, rash, sore throat, fever, jaundice, unusual bleeding or bruising.	Discontinue. Call doctor right away.
• Headache, fatigue.	Continue. Call doctor when convenient.

WARNINGS & PRECAUTIONS

Don't take if:
- You are allergic to procainamide.
- You have myasthenia gravis.

Before you start, consult your doctor:
- If you are allergic to local anesthetics that end in "caine."
- If you have had liver or kidney disease or impaired kidney function.
- If you have had lupus.
- If you take digitalis preparations*.
- If you will have surgery within 2 months, including dental surgery, requiring general or spinal anesthesia.

Over age 60:
Adverse reactions and side effects may be more frequent and severe than in younger persons.

Pregnancy:
Decide with your doctor if drug benefits justify risk to unborn child. Risk category C (see page xviii).

Breast-feeding:
No proven problems. Consult doctor.

Infants & children:
Not recommended.

Prolonged use:
- May cause lupus*-like illness.
- Talk to your doctor about the need for follow-up medical examinations or laboratory studies to check ANA titers*, blood pressure, complete blood counts (white blood cell count, platelet count, red blood cell count, hemoglobin, hematocrit).

Skin & sunlight:
No problems expected.

Driving, piloting or hazardous work:
Use caution if you feel dizzy or weak. Otherwise, no problems expected.

Discontinuing:
Don't discontinue without doctor's advice until you complete prescribed dose, even though symptoms diminish or disappear.

Others:
- Some products contain tartrazine dye. Avoid, especially if you are allergic to aspirin.
- May affect results of some medical tests.

POSSIBLE INTERACTION WITH OTHER DRUGS

GENERIC NAME OR DRUG CLASS	COMBINED EFFECT
Acetazolamide	Increased procainamide effect.
Ambenonium	Decreased ambenonium effect.
Aminoglycosides*	Possible severe muscle weakness, impaired breathing.
Antiarrhythmics*, other	Increased likelihood of adverse reactions with either drug. Possible increased effect of both drugs.
Anticholinergics*	Increased anti-cholinergic effect.
Antihypertensives*	Increased anti-hypertensive effect.
Antimyasthenics*	Decreased anti-myasthenic effect.
Cimetidine	Increased procainamide effect.
Cisapride	Decreased procainamide effect.
Metformin	Increased metformin effect.

POSSIBLE INTERACTION WITH OTHER SUBSTANCES

INTERACTS WITH	COMBINED EFFECT
Alcohol:	None expected.
Beverages: Caffeine drinks, iced drinks.	Irregular heartbeat.
Cocaine:	Decreased procainamide effect.
Foods:	None expected.
Marijuana:	None expected.
Tobacco:	Decreased procainamide effect.

*See Glossary

PROCARBAZINE

BRAND NAMES

Matulane
Natulan

BASIC INFORMATION

Habit forming? No
Prescription needed? Yes
Available as generic? No
Drug class: Antineoplastic

USES

Treatment for some kinds of cancer.

DOSAGE & USAGE INFORMATION

How to take:
Capsule—Swallow with liquid after light meal. Don't drink fluids with meals. Drink extra fluids between meals. Avoid sweet or fatty foods.

When to take:
At the same time each day.

If you forget a dose:
Take as soon as you remember. Don't double dose ever.

What drug does:
Inhibits abnormal cell reproduction. Procarbazine is an alkylating agent* and an MAO inhibitor.

Time lapse before drug works:
Up to 6 weeks for full effect.

Don't take with:
Any other medicine without consulting your doctor or pharmacist.

OVERDOSE

SYMPTOMS:
Restlessness, agitation, fever, convulsions, bleeding.
WHAT TO DO:

- **Dial 911 (emergency) for an ambulance or medical help or poison center 1-800-222-1222. Then give first aid immediately.**
- **If patient is unconscious and not breathing, give mouth-to-mouth breathing. If there is no heartbeat, use cardiac massage and mouth-to-mouth breathing (CPR). Don't try to make patient vomit. If you can't get help quickly, take patient to nearest emergency facility.**
- **See emergency information on inside covers.**

POSSIBLE ADVERSE REACTIONS OR SIDE EFFECTS

SYMPTOMS	WHAT TO DO
Life-threatening:	
In case of overdose, see previous column.	
Common:	
• Nausea, vomiting, decreased urination, numbness or tingling in hands or feet, hair loss, rapid or pounding heartbeat, shortness of breath.	Discontinue. Call doctor right away.
• Fatigue, weakness, confusion.	Continue. Call doctor when convenient.
• Dizziness when changing position, dry mouth, inflamed tongue, constipation, difficult urination.	Continue. Tell doctor at next visit.
Infrequent:	
• Fainting.	Discontinue. Seek emergency treatment.
• Severe headache; abnormal bleeding or bruising; muscle, joint or chest pain, enlarged eye pupils; black, tarry stools; bloody urine.	Discontinue. Call doctor right away.
• Hallucinations, insomnia, nightmares, diarrhea, swollen feet or legs, nervousness, eyes sensitive to light, cough or hoarseness, mouth sores depression.	Continue. Call doctor when convenient.
• Diminished sex drive.	Continue. Tell doctor at next visit.
Rare:	
Rash, stiff neck, jaundice, fever, sore throat, vomiting blood, wheezing.	Discontinue. Call doctor right away.

WARNINGS & PRECAUTIONS

Don't take if:

- You are allergic to any MAO inhibitor.
- You have heart disease, congestive heart failure, heart rhythm irregularities or high blood pressure.
- You have liver or kidney disease.

Before you start, consult your doctor:

- If you are alcoholic.
- If you have asthma.

- If you have had a stroke.
- If you have diabetes or epilepsy.
- If you have overactive thyroid.
- If you have schizophrenia.
- If you have Parkinson's disease.
- If you have adrenal gland tumor.
- If you will have surgery within 2 months, including dental surgery, requiring general or spinal anesthesia.

Over age 60:
Not recommended.

Pregnancy:
Consult doctor. Risk category D (see page xviii).

Breast-feeding:
Safety not established. Consult doctor.

Infants & children:
Not recommended.

Prolonged use:
- May be toxic to liver.
- Talk to your doctor about the need for follow-up medical examinations or laboratory studies to check complete blood counts (white blood cell count, platelet count, red blood cell count, hemoglobin, hematocrit), bone marrow, kidney function.

Skin & sunlight:
No special problems expected.

Driving, piloting or hazardous work:
Don't drive or pilot aircraft until you learn how medicine affects you. Don't work around dangerous machinery. Don't climb ladders or work in high places. Danger increases if you drink alcohol or take medicine affecting alertness and reflexes.

Discontinuing:
- Don't discontinue without doctor's advice until you complete prescribed dose, even though symptoms diminish or disappear.
- Follow precautions regarding foods, drinks and other medicines for 2 weeks after discontinuing.

Others:
- May affect blood sugar levels in patients with diabetes.
- Advise any doctor or dentist whom you consult that you take this drug.

POSSIBLE INTERACTION WITH OTHER DRUGS

GENERIC NAME OR DRUG CLASS	COMBINED EFFECT
Amphetamines*	Blood pressure rise to life-threatening level.
Anticonvulsants*, oral	Changed seizure pattern.
Antidepressants, tricyclic*	Blood pressure rise to life-threatening level.
Antidiabetics*, oral and insulin	Excessively low blood sugar.
Antihistamines*	Increased sedation.
Barbiturates*	Increased sedation.
Bone marrow depressants*	Increased toxicity to bone marrow.
Buspirone	Elevated blood pressure.
Caffeine	Irregular heartbeat or high blood pressure.
Carbamazepine	Fever, seizures. Avoid.
Central nervous system (CNS) depressants*	Increased CNS depression.
Clozapine	Toxic effect on bone marrow and central nervous system.
Cyclobenzaprine	Fever, seizures. Avoid.
Dextromethorphan	Fever, hypertension.

Continued on page 927

POSSIBLE INTERACTION WITH OTHER SUBSTANCES

INTERACTS WITH	COMBINED EFFECT
Alcohol:	Increased sedation to dangerous level. Disulfiram-like reaction*.
Beverages:	
Caffeine drinks.	Irregular heartbeat or high blood pressure.
Drinks containing tyramine*.	Blood pressure rise to life-threatening level.
Cocaine:	Overstimulation. Possibly fatal.
Foods:	
Foods containing tyramine*.	Blood pressure rise to life-threatening level.
Marijuana:	Overstimulation. Avoid.
Tobacco:	None expected.

*See Glossary

PROGESTINS

GENERIC AND BRAND NAMES

See complete list of generic and brand names in the *Generic and Brand Name Directory,* page 862.

BASIC INFORMATION

Habit forming? No
Prescription needed? Yes
Available as generic? Yes, for some.
Drug class: Female sex hormone (progestin)

USES

- Treatment for menstrual or uterine disorders caused by progestin imbalance.
- Contraceptive (when combined with estrogens in birth control pills).
- Treatment for cancer of breast and uterus.
- Treatment for toxic sleep apnea.
- Treatment for female hormone imbalance.
- Megestrol is used for treatment of weight loss in AIDS and cancer patients.
- Treatment for female infertility caused by progesterone deficiency.
- Treatment for hyperplasia.

DOSAGE & USAGE INFORMATION

How to take:

- Capsule—Swallow with liquid. Do not crush, chew or break.
- Tablet—Swallow with liquid or food to lessen stomach irritation. You may crumble tablet.
- Injection—Under doctor's supervision.
- Oral suspension—Follow package instructions.

When to take:
At the same time each day.

If you forget a dose:

- Treatment for menstrual disorders—Take up to 2 hours late. If more than 2 hours, wait for next dose (don't double this dose).
- Contraceptive—Consult your doctor. You may need to use another birth control method until next period.

Continued next column

OVERDOSE

SYMPTOMS:
Nausea, vomiting, fluid retention, breast discomfort or enlargement, vaginal bleeding.
WHAT TO DO:
Overdose unlikely to threaten life. If person takes much larger amount than prescribed, call doctor, poison center 1-800-222-1222 or hospital emergency room for instructions.

What drug does:

- Creates a uterine lining similar to that of pregnancy that prevents bleeding.
- Suppresses a pituitary gland hormone responsible for ovulation.
- Stimulates cervical mucus, which stops sperm penetration and prevents pregnancy.
- Mechanism that produces weight gain is unknown. Appears to stimulate appetite and metabolism without fluid retention.

Time lapse before drug works:

- Menstrual disorders—24 to 48 hours.
- Contraception—3 weeks.
- Cancer—May require 2 to 3 months regular use for maximum benefit.

Don't take with:
Any other medicine without consulting your doctor or pharmacist.

POSSIBLE ADVERSE REACTIONS OR SIDE EFFECTS

SYMPTOMS	WHAT TO DO
Life-threatening:	
Blood clot in leg, brain or lung; hives, rash, intense itching, faintness soon after a dose (anaphylaxis).	Seek emergency treatment immediately.
Common:	
Appetite or weight changes, swollen feet or ankles, unusual tiredness or weakness, menstrual cycle changes.	Continue. Tell doctor at next visit.
Infrequent:	
• Prolonged vaginal bleeding, pain in calf.	Discontinue. Call doctor right away.
• Depression.	Continue. Call doctor when convenient.
• Acne, increased facial or body hair, nausea, tender breasts, headache, enlarged clitoris.	Continue. Tell doctor at next visit.
Rare:	
• Rash, stomach or side pain, jaundice, fever, vision changes.	Discontinue. Call doctor right away.
• Amenorrhea*, hair loss, insomnia, brown skin spots, voice change.	Continue. Call doctor when convenient.

WARNINGS & PRECAUTIONS

Don't take if:
- You are allergic to any progestin hormone.
- You may be pregnant.
- You have liver or gallbladder disease.
- You have had thrombophlebitis, embolism or stroke.
- You have unexplained vaginal bleeding.
- You have had breast or uterine cancer.

Before you start, consult your doctor:
- If you have heart or kidney disease.
- If you have diabetes.
- If you have a seizure disorder.
- If you suffer migraines.
- If you are easily depressed.

Over age 60:
No special problems expected.

Pregnancy:
Risk factors vary for drugs in this group. See category list on page xviii and consult doctor.

Breast-feeding:
Drug passes into milk. Avoid drug or discontinue nursing until you finish medicine. Consult doctor for advice on maintaining milk supply.

Infants & children:
Use only for female children under medical supervision.

Prolonged use:
No problems expected.

Skin & sunlight:
No problems expected.

Driving, piloting or hazardous work:
No problems expected.

Discontinuing:
Consult doctor. This medicine stays in the body and causes fetal abnormalities. Wait at least 3 months before becoming pregnant.

Others:
- Patients with diabetes must be monitored closely.
- Symptoms of blood clot in leg, brain or lung are: chest, groin, leg pain; sudden, severe headache; loss of coordination; vision change; shortness of breath; slurred speech.
- May affect results in some medical tests.
- Advise any doctor or dentist whom you consult that you take this medicine.

POSSIBLE INTERACTION WITH OTHER DRUGS

GENERIC NAME OR DRUG CLASS	COMBINED EFFECT
Bromocriptine	Decreased bromocriptine effect.
Dofetilide	Increased risk of heart problems.
Hypoglycemics, oral*	Decreased oral hypoglycemic effect.
Insulin	Decreased insulin effect.
Phenobarbital	Decreased progestin effect.
Phenothiazines*	Increased phenothiazine effect.
Phenylbutazone	Decreased progestin effect.
Rifampin	Decreased contraceptive effect.

POSSIBLE INTERACTION WITH OTHER SUBSTANCES

INTERACTS WITH	COMBINED EFFECT
Alcohol:	None expected.
Beverages:	None expected.
Cocaine:	Decreased progestin effect.
Foods: Salt.	Fluid retention.
Marijuana:	Possible menstrual irregularities or bleeding between periods.
Tobacco: All forms.	Possible blood clots in lung, brain, legs. Avoid.

*See Glossary

PROGUANIL

BRAND NAMES

Malarone
Paludrine

BASIC INFORMATION

Habit forming? No
Prescription needed? Yes
Available as generic? No
Drug class: Antimalarial

USES

Prevents and treats malaria.

DOSAGE & USAGE INFORMATION

How to take:
Tablet—Swallow whole with liquid after meals.

When to take:
At the same time each day.

If you forget a dose:
Take as soon as you remember, however, if it is almost time for the next dose, skip the missed dose and return to your normal schedule (don't double this dose).

What drug does:
Exact mechanism unknown.

Time lapse before drug works:
1 to 2 weeks.

Don't take with:
Any other prescription or nonprescription drug without consulting your doctor or pharmacist.

OVERDOSE

SYMPTOMS:
Abdominal pain, blood in urine, lower back pain, pain or burning on urination, vomiting.
WHAT TO DO:
If person takes much larger amount than prescribed, call doctor, poison center 1-800-222-1222 or hospital emergency room for instructions.

POSSIBLE ADVERSE REACTIONS OR SIDE EFFECTS

SYMPTOMS	WHAT TO DO
Life-threatening: None expected.	
Common: Abdominal pain, back pain, coughing, diarrhea, fever, headache, itching, loss of strength, nausea, muscle pain, sore throat, sneezing, vomiting.	Continue. Call doctor if symptoms persist.
Infrequent: Acid or sour stomach, belching, dizziness, flu-like symptoms, heartburn, indigestion, loss of appetite, weight loss, temporary hair loss.	Continue. Call doctor if symptoms persist.
Rare: Skin rash or itching	Continue. Call doctor when convenient.

WARNINGS & PRECAUTIONS

Don't take if:
You are allergic to proguanil.

Before you start, consult your doctor:
- If you are pregnant or breast-feeding.
- If you have kidney problems.

Over age 60:
No problems expected.

Pregnancy:
Pregnancy increases the risk of death and disability. Decide with your doctor whether drug benefits justify risk to unborn child. Risk category C (see page xviii). Folate supplements should be taken by pregnant women while taking proguanil.

Breast-feeding:
Drug passes into milk. Avoid drug or discontinue nursing until you finish medicine. Consult doctor for advice on maintaining milk supply.

Infants & children:
Not expected to cause different side effects in children than it does in adults.

Prolonged use:
Not intended for long term use.

Skin & sunlight:
No problems expected.

Driving, piloting or hazardous work:
Don't drive or pilot aircraft until you learn how medicine affects you. Don't work around dangerous machinery. Don't climb ladders or work in high places. Danger increases if you drink alcohol or take medicine affecting alertness and reflexes, such as antihistamines, tranquilizers, sedatives, pain medicine, narcotics and mind-altering drugs.

Discontinuing:
Don't discontinue without doctor's advice until you complete the prescribed dosage.

Others:
Advise any doctor or dentist whom you consult that you take this medicine. Persons of Asian or African descent metabolize this drug rapidly, therefore the drug may not reach effective blood levels for protection against malaria.

POSSIBLE INTERACTION WITH OTHER DRUGS

GENERIC NAME OR DRUG CLASS	COMBINED EFFECT
None expected	

POSSIBLE INTERACTION WITH OTHER SUBSTANCES

INTERACTS WITH	COMBINED EFFECT
Alcohol:	None expected.
Beverages:	None expected.
Cocaine:	None expected.
Foods:	None expected.
Marijuana:	None expected.
Tobacco:	None expected.

PROPAFENONE

BRAND NAMES

Rhythmol

BASIC INFORMATION

Habit forming? No
Prescription needed? Yes
Available as generic? No
Drug class: Antiarrhythmic

USES

Treats severe heartbeat irregularities (life-threatening ventricular rhythm disturbances).

DOSAGE & USAGE INFORMATION

How to take:
Tablet—Swallow with liquid or food to lessen stomach irritation. If you can't swallow whole, crumble tablet and take with liquid or food.

When to take:
At the same time each day, according to instructions on prescription label.

If you forget a dose:
Take as soon as you remember up to 2 hours late. If more than 2 hours, wait for next scheduled dose. Don't double this dose.

What drug does:
Slows electrical activity in the heart to decrease the excitability of the heart muscle.

Time lapse before drug works:
3-1/2 hours to 1 week for full effect. Begins working almost immediately.

Don't take with:
Any other medicine (including nonprescription drugs such as cough and cold medicines, nose drops, vitamins, laxatives, antacids, diet pills, or caffeine) without consulting your doctor or pharmacist.

OVERDOSE

SYMPTOMS:
Very rapid heart rate that is also irregular.
WHAT TO DO:
Overdose unlikely to threaten life. If person takes much larger amount than prescribed, call doctor, poison center 1-800-222-1222 or hospital emergency room for instructions.

POSSIBLE ADVERSE REACTIONS OR SIDE EFFECTS

SYMPTOMS	WHAT TO DO
Life-threatening:	
Severe chest pain, severe shortness of breath	Seek emergency treatment.
Common:	
• Faster or more irregular heartbeat.	Discontinue. Call doctor right away.
• Taste change, dizziness.	Continue. Call doctor when convenient.
Infrequent:	
• Blurred vision, skin rash.	Discontinue. Call doctor right away.
• Constipation, diarrhea.	Continue. Call doctor when convenient.
• Dry mouth, nausea.	Continue. Tell doctor at next visit.
Rare:	
Fever, chills, trembling, joint pain, slow heartbeat.	Discontinue. Call doctor right away.

WARNINGS & PRECAUTIONS

Don't take if:
You are allergic to propafenone.

Before you start, consult your doctor:
- If you have asthma or bronchospasm.
- If you have congestive heart failure.
- If you have liver disease or kidney disease.
- If you have a recent history of heart attack.
- If you have a pacemaker.

Over age 60:
More likely to have decreased kidney function and require dosage modification.

Pregnancy:
Decide with your doctor if drug benefits justify risk to unborn child. Risk category C (see page xviii).

Breast-feeding:
No proven problems. Consult doctor.

Infants & children:
Safety and efficacy not established.

Prolonged use:
Don't discontinue without consulting doctor. Dose may require gradual reduction if you have taken drug for a long time. Dosages of other drugs may also require adjustment.

Skin & sunlight:
No special problems expected.

Driving, piloting or hazardous work:
Don't drive or pilot aircraft until you learn how medicine affects you. Don't work around dangerous machinery. Don't climb ladders or work in high places. Danger increases if you drink alcohol or take medicine affecting alertness and reflexes.

Discontinuing:
Don't discontinue without consulting doctor. Dose may require gradual reduction if you have taken drug for a long time. Doses of other drugs may also require adjustment.

Others:
- Advise any doctor or dentist whom you consult that you take this medicine, especially if you are to be anesthetized.
- Report changes in symptoms to your doctor and return for periodic visits to check progress.
- Carry or wear a medical I.D. card or bracelet.

POSSIBLE INTERACTION WITH OTHER DRUGS

GENERIC NAME OR DRUG CLASS	COMBINED EFFECT
Anesthetics, local (e.g., prior to dental procedures)	May increase risk of side effects.
Antiarrhythmics*, other	Increased risk of adverse reactions.
Beta-adrenergic blocking agents*	Increased beta blocker effect.
Digitalis preparations*	Increased digitalis absorption. May require decreased dosage of digitalis preparation.
Doxepin (topical)	Increased risk of toxicity of both drugs.
Warfarin	Increased warfarin effect.

POSSIBLE INTERACTION WITH OTHER SUBSTANCES

INTERACTS WITH	COMBINED EFFECT
Alcohol:	Unpredictable effect on heartbeat. Avoid.
Beverages: Caffeine drinks.	Increased heartbeat irregularity. Avoid.
Cocaine:	Increased heartbeat irregularity. Avoid.
Foods:	None expected.
Marijuana:	Increased heartbeat irregularity. Avoid.
Tobacco:	Increased heartbeat irregularity. Avoid.

***See Glossary**

PROPANTHELINE

BRAND NAMES

Pro-Banthine
Propanthel

BASIC INFORMATION

Habit forming? No
Prescription needed?
High strength: Yes
Low strength: No
Available as generic? Yes
Drug class: Antispasmodic, anticholinergic

USES

Reduces spasms of digestive system, bladder and urethra.

DOSAGE & USAGE INFORMATION

How to take:
Tablet—Swallow with liquid or food to lessen stomach irritation.

When to take:
30 minutes before meals (unless directed otherwise by doctor).

If you forget a dose:
Take as soon as you remember up to 2 hours late. If more than 2 hours, wait for next scheduled dose (don't double this dose).

What drug does:
Blocks nerve impulses at parasympathetic nerve endings, preventing muscle contractions and gland secretions of organs involved.

Time lapse before drug works:
15 to 30 minutes.

Don't take with:
Any other medicine without consulting your doctor or pharmacist.

OVERDOSE

SYMPTOMS:
Dilated pupils, blurred vision, rapid pulse and breathing, dizziness, fever, hallucinations, confusion, slurred speech, agitation, flushed face, convulsions, coma.
WHAT TO DO:
- **Dial 911 (emergency) for an ambulance or medical help or poison center 1-800-222-1222. Then give first aid immediately.**
- **See emergency information on inside covers.**

POSSIBLE ADVERSE REACTIONS OR SIDE EFFECTS

SYMPTOMS	WHAT TO DO
Life-threatening:	
Hives, rash, intense itching, faintness soon after a dose (anaphylaxis).	Seek emergency treatment immediately.
Common:	
• Confusion, delirium, rapid heartbeat.	Discontinue. Call doctor right away.
• Nausea, vomiting, decreased sweating.	Continue. Call doctor when convenient.
• Constipation, loss of taste.	Continue. Tell doctor at next visit.
• Dry ears, nose, throat, mouth.	No action necessary.
Infrequent:	
• Headache, difficult urination, nasal congestion, altered taste, impotence.	Continue. Call doctor when convenient.
• Lightheadedness.	Discontinue. Call doctor right away.
Rare:	
Rash or hives, eye pain, blurred vision.	Discontinue. Call doctor right away.

WARNINGS & PRECAUTIONS

Don't take if:
- You are allergic to any anticholinergic.
- You have trouble with stomach bloating.
- You have difficulty emptying your bladder completely.
- You have narrow-angle glaucoma.
- You have severe ulcerative colitis.

Before you start, consult your doctor:
- If you have open-angle glaucoma.
- If you have angina.
- If you have chronic bronchitis or asthma.
- If you have hiatal hernia.
- If you have liver, kidney or thyroid disease.
- If you have enlarged prostate.
- If you have myasthenia gravis.
- If you have peptic ulcer.
- If you will have surgery within 2 months, including dental surgery, requiring general or spinal anesthesia.

Over age 60:
Adverse reactions and side effects may be more frequent and severe than in younger persons.

Pregnancy:
Decide with your doctor whether drug benefits justify risk to unborn child. Risk category C (see page xviii).

Breast-feeding:
Drug passes into milk and decreases milk flow. Avoid drug or discontinue nursing until you finish medicine. Consult doctor for advice on maintaining milk supply.

Infants & children:
Use only under medical supervision.

Prolonged use:
Chronic constipation, possible fecal impaction. Consult doctor immediately.

Skin & sunlight:
No problems expected.

Driving, piloting or hazardous work:
Use disqualifies you for piloting aircraft. Otherwise, no problems expected.

Discontinuing:
May be unnecessary to finish medicine. Follow doctor's instructions.

Others:
Advise any doctor or dentist whom you consult that you take this medicine.

POSSIBLE INTERACTION WITH OTHER DRUGS

GENERIC NAME OR DRUG CLASS	COMBINED EFFECT
Adrenocorticoids, systemic	Possible glaucoma.
Amantadine	Increased propantheline effect.
Antacids*	Decreased propantheline effect.
Anticholinergics*, other	Increased propantheline effect.
Antidepressants, tricyclic*	Increased propantheline effect. Increased sedation.
Antidiarrhea preparations*	Reduced propantheline effect.
Antihistamines*	Increased propantheline effect.
Attapulgite	Decreased propantheline effect.
Buclizine	Increased propantheline effect.
Digitalis preparations*	Possible decreased absorption of digitalis.
Haloperidol	Increased internal eye pressure.
Ketoconazole	Decreased ketoconazole effect.
Meperidine	Increased propantheline effect.
Methylphenidate	Increased propantheline effect.
Molindone	Increased anti-cholinergic effect.
Monoamine oxidase (MAO) inhibitors*	Increased propantheline effect.
Nitrates*	Increased internal eye pressure.
Nizatidine	Increased nizatidine effect.
Orphenadrine	Increased propantheline effect.
Phenothiazines*	Increased propantheline effect.
Pilocarpine	Loss of pilocarpine effect in glaucoma treatment.
Potassium supplements*	Increased possibility of intestinal ulcers with oral potassium tablets.
Quinidine	Increased propantheline effect.
Sedatives* or central nervous system (CNS) depressants*	Increased sedative effect of both drugs.
Vitamin C	Decreased propantheline effect. Avoid large doses of vitamin C.

POSSIBLE INTERACTION WITH OTHER SUBSTANCES

INTERACTS WITH	COMBINED EFFECT
Alcohol:	None expected.
Beverages:	None expected.
Cocaine:	Excessively rapid heartbeat. Avoid.
Foods:	None expected.
Marijuana:	Drowsiness and dry mouth.
Tobacco:	None expected.

*See Glossary

PROTEASE INHIBITORS

GENERIC AND BRAND NAMES

AMPRENAVIR
  Agenerase
INDINAVIR
  Crixivan
LOPINAVIR
  Kaletra
NELFINAVIR
  Viracept
RITONAVIR
  Kaletra
  Norvir
SAQUINAVIR
  Fortovase
  Invirase

BASIC INFORMATION

Habit forming? No
Prescription needed? Yes
Available as generic? No
Drug class: Protease inhibitor

USES

Used in combination with other drugs as a treatment for advanced HIV infection in selected patients. Does not cure HIV infection.

DOSAGE & USAGE INFORMATION

How to take:

- Tablet or capsule—Swallow with liquid. Take with food or meal to enhance drug's absorption. Take indinavir 1 hour before or 2 hours after eating. Your doctor may recommend additional methods to help the body absorb the drug.
- Liquid ritonavir—Swallow with chocolate milk or liquid nutritional supplement to disguise unpleasant taste.

When to take:
At the same times each day, according to instructions on prescription label.

If you forget a dose:
Take as soon as you remember up to 2 hours late. If more than 2 hours, wait for next scheduled dose (don't double this dose).

Continued next column

What drug does:
Blocks an enzyme called protease that is vital to the final stages of HIV replication (reproduction). Blocking protease causes HIV to make copies of itself that can't infect new cells.

Time lapse before drug works:
It will take weeks to months of treatment with the drug to determine the benefits of this therapy.

Don't take with:
Any other medicine without consulting your doctor or pharmacist. This includes any nonprescription medication.

OVERDOSE

SYMPTOMS:
Unknown effect.
WHAT TO DO:
Overdose unlikely to threaten life. If person takes much larger amount than prescribed, call doctor, poison center 1-800-222-1222 or hospital emergency room for instructions.

POSSIBLE ADVERSE REACTIONS OR SIDE EFFECTS

SYMPTOMS	WHAT TO DO
Life-threatening: None expected.	
Common: Diarrhea, abdominal discomfort, nausea, sores on mouth, dizziness, dry mouth, tiredness, appetite loss.	Continue. Call doctor when convenient.
Infrequent: Rash, muscle or joint pain, headache, abdominal pain, weakness, back pain, numbness or tingling in hands or feet, tingling around mouth.	Continue. Call doctor when convenient.
Rare:	
• Confusion, yellow skin or eyes, severe skin reaction, lack of coordination, seizures. Watch for warning signs of hyperglycemia or diabetes (increased thirst and hunger, unexplained weight loss, increased urination, fatigue and dry itchy skin).	Continue, but call doctor right away.
• Other symptoms not listed. They may be drug-associated or infection-associated.	Continue. Call doctor when convenient.

Note: Additional adverse reactions and side effects are often caused by other HIV medications that are used in combination with protease inhibitors.

WARNINGS & PRECAUTIONS

Don't take if:
You are allergic to protease inhibitors.

Before you start, consult your doctor:
- If you have liver or kidney disease
- If you have diabetes or hypertension.
- If you have peripheral neuropathy*.
- If you have any questions or concerns about the drug. Protease inhibitors are a new class of anti-HIV drugs that are still undergoing medical testing. Ask your doctor about new or additional information regarding adverse reactions, side effects, drug interactions, absorption problems, effectiveness and long-term use.

Over age 60:
No special problems expected.

Pregnancy:
Risk factors vary for drugs in this group. See category list on page xviii and consult doctor.

Breast-feeding:
It is unknown if drug passes into milk. Breast-feeding not recommended in HIV-infected women.

Infants & children:
Nelfinavir and ritonavir have been approved for use in children 2 to 13.

Prolonged use:
- The effects of long-term use are unknown.
- Medical studies have shown that HIV can become resistant to the effects of these drugs.

Skin & sunlight:
No special problems expected.

Driving, piloting or hazardous work:
Don't drive or pilot aircraft until you learn how medicine affects you. Don't work around dangerous machinery. Don't climb ladders or work in high places. Danger increases if you drink alcohol or take medicine affecting alertness and reflexes.

Discontinuing:
Don't discontinue without consulting doctor.

Others:
- Advise any doctor or dentist whom you consult that you take this medicine.
- These drugs have not been shown to reduce the risk of transmitting HIV to others through sexual contact. Avoid sexual activities or use condoms to help prevent the transmission of HIV. In addition, don't share needles or equipment for injections with other persons.
- These drugs may cause or aggravate diabetes or hypertension.

POSSIBLE INTERACTION WITH OTHER DRUGS

GENERIC NAME OR DRUG CLASS	COMBINED EFFECT
Anticonvulsants*	Decreased effect of ritonavir.
Astemizole	Serious heart rhythm problems. Avoid.
Contraceptives, oral	Decreased contraceptive effect with ritonavir.
Dexamethasone	Decreased effect of ritonavir.
Dofetilide	Increased dofetilide effect.
Enzyme inducers*	Decreased effect of protease inhibitor.
Enzyme inhibitors*	Increased effect of enzyme inhibitor.
Non-nucleoside reverse transcriptase inhibitors	May require dosage adjustment of protease inhibitor.
Rifabutin	Decreased effect of protease inhibitor.
Rifampin	Decreased effect of protease inhibitor.
Numerous other drugs	Unknown effect. Consult doctor.

POSSIBLE INTERACTION WITH OTHER SUBSTANCES

INTERACTS WITH	COMBINED EFFECT
Alcohol:	None expected.
Beverages:	None expected.
Cocaine:	Problems not known. Best to avoid.
Foods:	None expected.
Marijuana:	Problems not known. Best to avoid.
Tobacco:	Decreased effect of ritonavir.

*See Glossary

PROTECTANT (Ophthalmic)

GENERIC AND BRAND NAMES

HYDROXYPROPYL CELLULOSE
- **Lacrisert**

HYDROXYPROPYL METHYL-CELLULOSE
- **Artificial Tears**
- **Bion Tears**
- **Eye Lube**
- **Gonak**
- **Goniosoft**
- **Goniosol**
- **Isopto Alkaline**
- **Isopto Plain**
- **Isopto Tears**
- **Just Tears**
- **Lacril**
- **Methocel**
- **Moisture Drops**
- **Nature's Tears**
- **Ocutears**
- **Tearisol**
- **Tears Naturale**
- **Tears Naturale Free**
- **Tears Naturale II**
- **Tears Renewed**
- **Ultra Tears**

BASIC INFORMATION

Habit forming? No
Prescription needed? Yes
Available as generic? Yes, for some
Drug class: Protectant (ophthalmic), artificial tears

USES

- Relieves eye dryness and irritation caused by inadequate flow of tears.
- Moistens contact lenses and artificial eyes.

OVERDOSE

SYMPTOMS:
None expected.
WHAT TO DO:
Not intended for internal use. If child accidentally swallows, call poison center 1-800-222-1222.

DOSAGE & USAGE INFORMATION

How to use:
Eye drops
- Wash hands.
- Apply pressure to inside corner of eye with middle finger.
- Continue pressure for 1 minute after placing medicine in eye.
- Tilt head backward. Pull lower lid away from eye with index finger of the same hand.
- Drop eye drops into pouch and close eye. Don't blink.
- Keep eyes closed for 1 to 2 minutes.
- Don't touch applicator tip to any surface (including the eye). If you accidentally touch tip, clean with warm soap and water.
- Keep container tightly closed.
- Keep cool, but don't freeze.
- Wash hands immediately after using.

When to use:
As directed. Usually every 3 or 4 hours.

If you forget a dose:
Use as soon as you remember.

What drug does:
- Stabilizes and thickens tear film.
- Lubricates and protects eye.

Time lapse before drug works:
2 to 10 minutes.

Don't use with:
Other eye drops without consulting your doctor.

POSSIBLE ADVERSE REACTIONS OR SIDE EFFECTS

SYMPTOMS	WHAT TO DO
Life-threatening	
None expected.	
Common	
None expected.	
Infrequent	
Eye irritation not present before using artificial tears.	Discontinue. Call doctor right away.
Rare	
None expected.	

WARNINGS & PRECAUTIONS

Don't use if:
You are allergic to any artificial tears.

Before you start, consult your doctor:
If you use any other eye drops.

Over age 60:
No problems expected.

Pregnancy:
Risk factor not designated. See category list on page xviii and consult doctor.

Breast-feeding:
No problems expected, but check with doctor.

Infants & children:
Don't use.

Prolonged use:
Don't use for more than 3 or 4 days.

Skin & sunlight:
No problems expected.

Driving, piloting or hazardous work:
No problems expected.

Discontinuing:
May not need all the medicine in container. If symptoms disappear, stop using.

Others:
Check with your doctor if eye irritation continues or becomes worse.

POSSIBLE INTERACTION WITH OTHER DRUGS

GENERIC NAME OR DRUG CLASS	COMBINED EFFECT

Clinically significant interactions with oral or injected medicines unlikely.

POSSIBLE INTERACTION WITH OTHER SUBSTANCES

INTERACTS WITH	COMBINED EFFECT
Alcohol:	None expected.
Beverages:	None expected.
Cocaine:	None expected.
Foods:	None expected.
Marijuana:	None expected.
Tobacco:	None expected.

PROTON PUMP INHIBITORS

GENERIC AND BRAND NAMES

ESOMEPRAZOLE
Nexium
LANSPORAZOLE
Prevacid
OMEPRAZOLE
Losec
Prilosec
PANTOPRAZOLE
Pantoloc
Protonix
RABEPRAZOLE
Aciphex

BASIC INFORMATION

Habit forming? No
Prescription needed? Yes
Available as generic? No
Drug class: Antiulcer agent, proton pump inhibitor

USES

- Treats gastroesophageal reflux (splashing of stomach acid from the stomach up onto the lower end of the esophagus).
- Treats ulcers in the stomach and duodenum.
- Treats any disorder associated with excess production of stomach acid (such as Zollinger-Ellison syndrome).

DOSAGE & USAGE INFORMATION

How to take:
- Delayed-release and extended-release capsules—Swallow whole. Do not crush, chew or break open.
- Delayed release oral suspension—Follow instructions on product.
- Tablets (enteric coated)—Swallow with liquid.

When to take:
Once daily, immediately before a meal (preferably breakfast), unless otherwise directed by your doctor. With once-a-day dosing, it is important to take the medicine on schedule.

Continued next column

OVERDOSE

SYMPTOMS:
Severe drowsiness, seizures, breathing difficulty, decreased body temperature.
WHAT TO DO:
- **Dial 911 (emergency) for an ambulance or medical help or poison center 1-800-222-1222. Then give first aid immediately.**
- **See emergency information on inside covers.**

If you forget a dose:
Take as soon as you remember. If it is almost time for the next dose, wait for next scheduled dose (don't double this dose).

What drug does:
Inhibits secretion of stomach acid.

Time lapse before drug works:
1 to 3 hours.

Don't take with:
Any other medicine without consulting your doctor or pharmacist.

POSSIBLE ADVERSE REACTIONS OR SIDE EFFECTS

SYMPTOMS	WHAT TO DO
Life-threatening: In case of overdose, see previous column.	
Common:	
Diarrhea, stomach pain.	Continue. Call doctor when convenient.
Infrequent:	
Nausea, loss of appetite, headache, heartburn, muscle pain, skin rash, drowsiness.	Continue. Call doctor when convenient.
Rare:	
Weakness or unusual tiredness; sore throat and fever; sores on mouth; unusual bleeding or bruising; cloudy or bloody urine; difficult, frequent or painful urination.	Discontinue. Call doctor right away.

WARNINGS & PRECAUTIONS

Don't take if:
You are allergic to any of these medications.

Before you start, consult your doctor:
- If you are allergic to any medicines, foods or other substances.
- If you have or have had liver disease.
- If you have a stomach infection.

Over age 60:
No special problems expected.

Pregnancy:
Risk factors may vary for drugs in this group. See category list on page xviii and consult doctor.

Breast-feeding:
Safety not established. Best to avoid or discontinue nursing until you finish medicine. Consult doctor for advice on maintaining milk supply.

Infants & children:
Safety not established. Consult doctor.

Prolonged use:
The length of treatment can run from 4 to 8 weeks or may be indefinite. Though your symptoms may improve in 1 to 2 weeks, your doctor will determine when healing is complete.

Skin & sunlight:
No special problems expected.

Driving, piloting or hazardous work:
No special problems expected.

Discontinuing:
Don't discontinue without consulting doctor until you complete prescribed dose, even though symptoms diminish or disappear

Others:
- Advise any doctor or dentist whom you consult that you take this medicine.
- If directed by your doctor, it is permissible and sometimes helpful to take with antacids* to relieve upper abdominal pain. Antacids may be used more than once daily if needed.
- May affect results of some medical tests.

POSSIBLE INTERACTION WITH OTHER DRUGS

GENERIC NAME OR DRUG CLASS	COMBINED EFFECT
Anticoagulants* (warfarin, coumadin, indandione derivatives)	Increased anticoagulant effect with omeprazole.
Diazepam	Increased effect of diazepam with omeprazole.
Phenytoin	Increased effect of phenytoin with omeprazole.
Sucralfate	Decreased effect of lansoprazole. Take it 30 minutes before sucralfate.
Theophylline	May require dosage adjustment of theophylline with lansoprazole.

POSSIBLE INTERACTION WITH OTHER SUBSTANCES

INTERACTS WITH	COMBINED EFFECT
Alcohol:	None expected.
Beverages:	None expected.
Cocaine:	None expected.
Foods:	None expected.
Marijuana:	None expected.
Tobacco:	None expected.

*See Glossary

PSEUDOEPHEDRINE

BRAND NAMES

See complete list of brand names in the *Generic and Brand Name Directory*, page 862.

BASIC INFORMATION

Habit forming? No
Prescription needed?
U.S.: High strength—Yes
Low strength—No
Canada: No
Available as generic? Yes
Drug class: Sympathomimetic, decongestant

USES

Reduces congestion of nose, sinuses, eustachian tubes and throat from allergies and infections.

DOSAGE & USAGE INFORMATION

How to take:
- Tablet or capsule—Swallow with liquid. You may chew or crush tablet or open capsule.
- Extended-release tablet or capsule—Swallow each dose whole.
- Syrup—Take as directed on label.
- Drops—Place directly on tongue and swallow.
- Oral solution—Take as direced on label.
- Combination products—Follow instructions on label.

When to take:
- At the same times each day.
- To prevent insomnia, take last dose of day a few hours before bedtime.

If you forget a dose:
Take up to 2 hours late. If more than 2 hours, wait for next dose (don't double this dose).

Continued next column

OVERDOSE

SYMPTOMS:
Nervousness, restlessness, headache, rapid or irregular heartbeat, sweating, nausea, vomiting, anxiety, confusion, delirium, muscle tremors, convulsions, hallucinations.
WHAT TO DO:
- **Dial 911 (emergency) for an ambulance or medical help or poison center 1-800-222-1222. Then give first aid immediately.**
- **See emergency information on inside covers.**

What drug does:
Decreases blood volume in nasal tissues, shrinking tissues and enlarging airways.

Time lapse before drug works:
15 to 20 minutes.

Don't take with:
- Nonprescription drugs with caffeine without consulting doctor.
- Any other medicine without consulting your doctor or pharmacist.

POSSIBLE ADVERSE REACTIONS OR SIDE EFFECTS

SYMPTOMS	WHAT TO DO
Life-threatening:	
In case of overdose, see previous column.	
Common:	
None expected.	
Infrequent:	
• Nausea or vomiting, irregular or slow heartbeat, difficult breathing, unusually fast or pounding heartbeat, painful or difficult urination, increased sweating, trembling.	Discontinue. Call doctor right away.
• Agitation, insomnia, dizziness, headache, shakiness, weakness, paleness.	Continue. Call doctor when convenient.
Rare:	
Hallucinations, seizures.	Discontinue. Seek emergency treatment.

WARNINGS & PRECAUTIONS

Don't take if:
You are allergic to any sympathomimetic drug.

Before you start, consult your doctor:
- If you have overactive thyroid or diabetes.
- If you have taken any monoamine oxidase (MAO) inhibitor* in past 2 weeks.
- If you take digitalis preparations or have high blood pressure or heart disease.
- If you will have surgery within 2 months, including dental surgery, requiring general or spinal anesthesia.
- If you have urination difficulty.

Over age 60:
Adverse reactions and side effects may be more frequent and severe than in younger persons.

Pregnancy:
No proven harm to unborn child. Avoid if possible. Consult doctor. Risk category B (see page xviii).

Breast-feeding:
Drug passes into milk. Avoid drug or discontinue nursing until you finish medicine. Consult doctor for advice on maintaining milk supply.

Infants & children:
Keep dose low or avoid.

Prolonged use:
No proven problems.

Skin & sunlight:
No problems expected.

Driving, piloting or hazardous work:
Avoid if you feel dizzy. Otherwise, no problems expected.

Discontinuing:
May be unnecessary to finish medicine. Follow doctor's instructions.

Others:
- Call the doctor if symptoms worsen or new symptoms develop with use of this medicine.
- Heed all warnings on the product label.

POSSIBLE INTERACTION WITH OTHER DRUGS

GENERIC NAME OR DRUG CLASS	COMBINED EFFECT
Antidepressants, tricyclic*	Increased risk of heart toxicity or severe headaches.
Antihypertensives*	Decreased anti-hypertensive effect.
Beta-adrenergic blocking agents*	Decreased effect of both drugs.
Calcium supplements*	Increased pseudo-ephedrine effect.
Digitalis preparations*	Irregular heartbeat.
Epinephrine	Increased epinephrine effect. Excessive heart stimulation and blood pressure increase.
Ergot preparations*	Serious blood pressure rise.
Guanadrel	Decreased effect of both drugs.
Guanethidine	Decreased effect of both drugs.
Linezolid	Possible increased blood pressure.
Methyldopa	Possible increased blood pressure.
Monoamine oxidase (MAO) inhibitors*	Increased pseudo-ephedrine effect.
Nitrates*	Possible decreased effects of both drugs.
Phenothiazines*	Possible increased pseudoephedrine toxicity. Possible decreased pseudo-ephedrine effect.
Rauwolfia	Decreased rauwolfia effect.
Sympathomimetics*, other	Increased pseudo-ephedrine effect.
Terazosin	Decreased effective-ness of terazosin.

POSSIBLE INTERACTION WITH OTHER SUBSTANCES

INTERACTS WITH	COMBINED EFFECT
Alcohol:	None expected.
Beverages: Caffeine drinks.	Nervousness or insomnia.
Cocaine:	High risk of heart-beat irregularities and high blood pressure.
Foods:	None expected.
Marijuana:	Rapid heartbeat.
Tobacco:	None expected.

*See Glossary

PSORALENS

GENERIC AND BRAND NAMES

METHOXSALEN
- Oxsoralen
- Oxsoralen Topical
- Oxsoralen Ultra
- UltraMOP

TRIOXSALEN
- Trisoralen

BASIC INFORMATION

Habit forming? No
Prescription needed? Yes
Available as generic? No
Drug class: Repigmenting agent (psoralen)

USES

- Repigmenting skin affected with vitiligo (absence of skin pigment).
- Treatment for psoriasis, when other treatments haven't helped.
- Treatment for mycosis fungoides.

DOSAGE & USAGE INFORMATION

How to take or apply:
- Tablet or capsule—Swallow with liquid or food to lessen stomach irritation.
- Topical—As directed by doctor.

When to take or apply:
2 to 4 hours before exposure to sunlight or sunlamp.

If you forget a dose:
Take as soon as you remember. Delay sun exposure for at least 2 hours after taking.

What drug does:
Helps pigment cells when used in conjunction with ultraviolet light.

Time lapse before drug works:
- For vitiligo, 6 to 9 months.
- For psoriasis, 10 weeks or longer.
- For tanning, 3 to 4 days.

Don't take with:
Any other medicine that causes skin sensitivity to sun. Ask pharmacist.

OVERDOSE

SYMPTOMS:
Blistering skin, swelling feet and legs.
WHAT TO DO:
Overdose unlikely to threaten life. If person takes much larger amount than prescribed, call doctor, poison center 1-800-222-1222 or hospital emergency room for instructions.

POSSIBLE ADVERSE REACTIONS OR SIDE EFFECTS

SYMPTOMS	WHAT TO DO
Life-threatening:	
None expected.	
Common:	
• Increased skin sensitivity to sun.	Always protect from overexposure.
• Increased eye sensitivity to sunlight.	Always protect with wrap-around sunglasses.
• Nausea.	Continue. Call doctor when convenient.
Infrequent:	
• Skin red and sore.	Discontinue. Call doctor right away.
• Dizziness, headache, depression, leg cramps, insomnia.	Continue. Call doctor when convenient.
Rare:	
Hepatitis with jaundice, blistering and peeling.	Discontinue. Call doctor right away.

WARNINGS & PRECAUTIONS

Don't take if:
- You are allergic to any other psoralen.
- You are unwilling or unable to remain under close medical supervision.

Before you start, consult your doctor:
- If you have heart or liver disease.
- If you have allergy to sunlight.
- If you have cataracts.
- If you have albinism.
- If you have lupus erythematosis, porphyria, chronic infection, skin cancer or peptic ulcer.
- If you will have surgery within 2 months, including dental surgery, requiring general or spinal anesthesia.
- If you have skin cancer.

Over age 60:
Adverse reactions and side effects may be more frequent and severe than in younger persons.

Pregnancy:
Risk factors vary for drugs in this group. See category list on page xviii and consult doctor.

Breast-feeding:
Drug may pass into milk. Avoid drug or discontinue nursing until you finish medicine. Consult doctor for advice on maintaining milk supply.

Infants & children:
Not recommended.

Prolonged use:
- Increased chance of toxic effects.
- Talk to your doctor about the need for follow-up medical examinations or laboratory studies to check ANA titers*, complete blood counts (white blood cell count, platelet count, red blood cell count, hemoglobin, hematocrit), liver function, kidney function, eyes.

Skin & sunlight:
- One or more drugs in this group may cause rash or intensify sunburn in areas exposed to sun or ultraviolet light (photosensitivity reaction). Avoid overexposure. Notify doctor if reaction occurs.
- Too much can burn skin. Cover skin for 24 hours before and 8 hours following treatments.

Driving, piloting or hazardous work:
No problems expected. Protect eyes and skin from bright light.

Discontinuing:
Skin may remain sensitive for some time after treatment stops. Use extra protection from sun.

Others:
- Use sunblock on lips.
- Don't use just to make skin tan.
- Don't use hard gelatin capsules interchangeably with soft gelatin capsules.

POSSIBLE INTERACTION WITH OTHER DRUGS

GENERIC NAME OR DRUG CLASS	COMBINED EFFECT
Photosensitizing medications*	Greatly increased likelihood of extreme sensitivity to sunlight.

POSSIBLE INTERACTION WITH OTHER SUBSTANCES

INTERACTS WITH	COMBINED EFFECT
Alcohol:	May increase chance of liver toxicity.
Beverages: Lime drinks.	Avoid—toxic.
Cocaine:	Increased chance of toxicity. Avoid.
Foods: Those containing furocoumarin (limes, parsley, figs, parsnips, carrots, celery, mustard).	May cause toxic reaction to psoralens.
Marijuana:	Increased chance of toxicity. Avoid.
Tobacco:	May cause uneven absorption of medicine. Avoid.

*See Glossary

PYRIDOXINE (Vitamin B-6)

BRAND NAMES

Beesix
Hexa-Betalin
Pyroxine
Rodex
Vitabec 6
Numerous other multiple vitamin-mineral supplements. Check labels.

BASIC INFORMATION

Habit forming? No
Prescription needed?
High strength: Yes
Low strength: No
Available as generic? Yes
Drug class: Vitamin supplement

USES

- Prevention and treatment of pyridoxine deficiency.
- Treatment of some forms of anemia.
- Treatment of INH (isonicotinic acid hydrozide), cycloserine poisoning.

DOSAGE & USAGE INFORMATION

How to take:
- Tablets—Swallow with liquid.
- Extended-release capsules—Swallow each dose whole with liquid.

When to take:
At the same times each day.

If you forget a dose:
Take as soon as you remember, then resume regular schedule.

What drug does:
Acts as co-enzyme in carbohydrate, protein and fat metabolism.

Time lapse before drug works:
15 to 20 minutes.

Don't take with:
- Levodopa—Small amounts of pyridoxine will nullify levodopa effect. Carbidopa-levodopa combination not affected by this interaction.
- Any other medicine without consulting your doctor or pharmacist.

OVERDOSE

SYMPTOMS:
None expected.
WHAT TO DO:
Overdose unlikely to threaten life.

POSSIBLE ADVERSE REACTIONS OR SIDE EFFECTS

SYMPTOMS	WHAT TO DO
Life-threatening: None expected.	
Common: None expected.	
Infrequent: Nausea, headache.	Discontinue. Call doctor right away.
Rare: Numbness or tingling in hands or feet (large doses).	Discontinue. Call doctor right away.

WARNINGS & PRECAUTIONS

Don't take if:
You are allergic to pyridoxine.

Before you start, consult your doctor:
If you are pregnant or breast-feeding.

Over age 60:
No problems expected.

Pregnancy:
Don't exceed recommended dose. Consult doctor. Risk category A (see page xviii).

Breast-feeding:
Don't exceed recommended dose. Consult doctor.

Infants & children:
Don't exceed recommended dose.

Prolonged use:
Large doses for more than 1 month may cause toxicity.

Skin & sunlight:
No problems expected.

Driving, piloting or hazardous work:
No problems expected.

Discontinuing:
No problems expected.

Others:
- Advise any doctor or dentist whom you consult that you take this medicine.
- Regular pyridoxine supplements recommended if you take chloramphenicol, cycloserine, ethionamide, hydralazine, immunosuppressants, isoniazid or penicillamine. These decrease pyridoxine absorption and can cause anemia or tingling and numbness in hands and feet.

POSSIBLE INTERACTION WITH OTHER DRUGS

GENERIC NAME OR DRUG CLASS	COMBINED EFFECT
Contraceptives, oral*	Decreased pyridoxine effect.
Cycloserine	Decreased pyridoxine effect.
Estrogens*	Decreased pyridoxine effect.
Ethionamide	Decreased pyridoxine effect.
Hydralazine	Decreased pyridoxine effect.
Hypnotics, barbiturates*	Decreased hypnotic effect.
Immuno-suppressants*	Decreased pyridoxine effect.
Isoniazid	Decreased pyridoxine effect.
Levodopa	Decreased levodopa effect.
Penicillamine	Decreased pyridoxine effect.
Phenobarbital	Possible decreased phenobarbital effect.
Phenytoin	Decreased phenytoin effect.

POSSIBLE INTERACTION WITH OTHER SUBSTANCES

INTERACTS WITH	COMBINED EFFECT
Alcohol:	None expected.
Beverages:	None expected.
Cocaine:	None expected.
Foods:	None expected.
Marijuana:	None expected.
Tobacco:	May decrease pyridoxine absorption. Decreased pyridoxine effect.

*See Glossary

QUETIAPINE

BRAND NAMES

Seroquel

BASIC INFORMATION

Habit forming? No
Prescription needed? Yes
Available as generic? No
Drug class: Antipsychotic

USES

Treatment for symptoms of schizophrenia and other psychotic disorders.

DOSAGE & USAGE INFORMATION

How to take:
Tablet—Swallow with liquid. May be taken with or without food.

When to take:
As directed by your doctor—2 to 3 times a day at the same times each day. The prescribed dosage may be increased over the first few days of use.

If you forget a dose:
Take as soon as you remember. If it is almost time for the next dose, wait for the next scheduled dose (don't double this dose).

What drug does:
The exact mechanism is unknown. It appears to alleviate symptoms of schizophrenia by blocking certain nerve impulses between nerve cells.

Time lapse before drug works:
One to 7 days. Further increases in the dosage amount may be necessary to relieve symptoms for some patients.

Don't take with:
Any other medication without consulting your doctor or pharmacist. All possible drug interactions have not been studied.

OVERDOSE

SYMPTOMS:
Drowsiness and slurred speech; other symptoms may occur that were not observed in medical studies of the drug.
WHAT TO DO:
If person takes much larger amount than prescribed, call doctor, poison center 1-800-222-1222 or hospital emergency room for instructions.

POSSIBLE ADVERSE REACTIONS OR SIDE EFFECTS

SYMPTOMS	WHAT TO DO
Life-threatening:	
High fever, rapid pulse, profuse sweating, muscle rigidity, confusion and irritability, seizures (neuroleptic malignant syndrome —rare).	Discontinue. Seek emergency treatment.
Common:	
• Dizziness, difficulty in speaking or swallowing, shaking hands and fingers, trembling, vision problems, weakness, lightheadedness when arising from a sitting or lying position.	Continue. Call doctor right away.
• Drowsiness, constipation, weight gain, agitation, insomnia, headache, nervousness, runny nose, anxiety, dry mouth, personality disorder, arm or leg stiffness.	Continue. Call doctor when convenient.
Infrequent:	
• Jerky or involuntary movements, especially of the face, lips, jaw, tongue; chest pain, fast heartbeat.	Continue. Call doctor right away.
• Fever, flu-like symptoms, twitching, mood or mental changes, speech unclear, swollen feet or ankles, appetite increased, cough, saliva increased, muscle tightness, muscle spasms (face, neck, back), joint pain, nausea or vomiting, sore throat, thirstiness, incontinence, abdominal pain.	Continue. Call doctor when convenient.
Rare:	
• Breathing difficulty.	Discontinue. Call doctor right away.
• Swollen face, rash, confusion, decreased sex drive, menstrual changes, sluggishness.	Continue. Call doctor when convenient.

WARNINGS & PRECAUTIONS

Don't take if:
You are allergic to quetiapine

Before you start, consult your doctor:
- If you have liver disease, heart disease or a blood vessel disorder.
- If you have Alzheimer's.
- If you have a history of breast cancer.
- If you have intestinal blockage.
- If you are subject to dehydration or low body temperature.
- If you have a history of drug abuse or dependence.
- If you have glaucoma or cataracts.
- If you have prostate problems.
- If you are allergic to any medication, food or other substance.
- If you have a history of seizures.

Over age 60:
Adverse reactions and side effects may be more severe than in younger persons. A lower starting dosage is usually recommended until a response is determined.

Pregnancy:
Decide with your doctor if drug benefits justify any possible risk to unborn child. Risk category C (see page xviii).

Breast-feeding:
It is unknown if drug passes into milk. It is not recommended for nursing mothers.

Infants & children:
Safety in children under age 18 has not been established. Use only under close medical supervision.

Prolonged use:
- Consult with your doctor on a regular basis while taking this drug to check your progress or to discuss any increase or changes in side effects and the need for continued treatment. Long term effectiveness has not been established.
- Get eyes examined every 6 months.

Skin & sunlight:
- May cause rash or intensify sunburn in areas exposed to sun or ultraviolet light (photosensitivity reaction). Use sunscreen and avoid overexposure. Notify doctor if reaction occurs.
- Advise any doctor or dentist whom you consult that you take this medicine.
- Hot temperatures, exercise, and hot baths can increase risk of heatstroke. Drug may affect body's ability to maintain normal temperature.

Driving, piloting or hazardous work:
Don't drive or pilot aircraft until you learn how medicine affects you. Don't work around dangerous machinery. Don't climb ladders or work in high places. Danger increases if you drink alcohol or take medicine affecting alertness and reflexes.

Discontinuing:
Don't discontinue this drug without consulting doctor. Dosage may require a gradual reduction before stopping.

Others:
- Get up slowly from a sitting or lying position to avoid any dizziness, faintness or lightheadedness.
- Advise any doctor or dentist whom you consult that you take this medicine.
- Take medicine only as directed. Do not increase or reduce dosage without doctor's approval.

POSSIBLE INTERACTION WITH OTHER DRUGS

GENERIC NAME OR DRUG CLASS	COMBINED EFFECT
Central nervous system (CNS) depressants*, other	Increased sedative effect.
Enzyme inhibitors*	May increase quetiapine effect.
Enzyme inducers*	Decreased quetiapine effect.
Phenytoin	Decreased quetiapine effect.
Thioridazine	Decreased quetiapine effect.

POSSIBLE INTERACTION WITH OTHER SUBSTANCES

INTERACTS WITH	COMBINED EFFECT
Alcohol:	Increased sedation and dizziness. Avoid.
Beverages:	None expected.
Cocaine:	Effect not known. Best to avoid.
Foods:	None expected.
Marijuana:	Effect not known. Best to avoid.
Tobacco:	None expected.

*See Glossary

QUINACRINE

BRAND NAMES

Atabrine

BASIC INFORMATION

Habit forming? No
Prescription needed? Yes
Available as generic? Yes
Drug class: Antiprotozoal

USES

- Treats disease caused by the intestinal parasite *Giardia lamblia.*
- Treats mild to moderate discoid lupus erythematosus.

DOSAGE & USAGE INFORMATION

How to take:
Tablets—Swallow with full glass of water, tea or fruit juice. If you can't swallow whole, crumble tablet and mix with jam or chocolate syrup.

When to take:
After meals.

If you forget a dose:
Take as soon as you remember up to 2 hours late. If more than 2 hours, wait for next scheduled dose (don't double this dose).

What drug does:
Destroys *Giardia lamblia* parasites in the gastrointestinal system.

Continued next column

OVERDOSE

SYMPTOMS:
Severe abdominal cramps, convulsions, severe diarrhea, fainting, irregular heartbeat, restlessness.
WHAT TO DO:
- **Dial 911 (emergency) for an ambulance or medical help or poison center 1-800-222-1222. Then give first aid immediately.**
- **If patient is unconscious and not breathing, give mouth-to-mouth breathing. If there is no heartbeat, use cardiac massage and mouth-to-mouth breathing (CPR). Don't try to make patient vomit. If you can't get help quickly, take patient to nearest emergency facility.**
- **See emergency information on inside covers.**

Time lapse before drug works:
1 day.

Don't take with:
Any other medicine without consulting your doctor or pharmacist.

POSSIBLE ADVERSE REACTIONS OR SIDE EFFECTS

SYMPTOMS	WHAT TO DO
Life-threatening:	
In case of overdose, see previous column.	
Common:	
• Dizziness, nausea, headache.	Discontinue. Call doctor right away.
• Yellow eyes, skin, urine (due to dye-like characteristics of quinacrine).	Report to doctor, but no action necessary.
Infrequent:	
• Mild abdominal cramps; mild diarrhea; appetite loss; skin rash, itching or peeling.	Discontinue. Call doctor right away.
• Mood changes.	Continue. Call doctor when convenient.
Rare:	
Hallucinations, nightmares.	Discontinue. Call doctor right away.

WARNINGS & PRECAUTIONS

Don't take if:
You are allergic to quinacrine.

Before you start, consult your doctor:
- If you have porphyria.
- If you have had psoriasis.
- If you have a history of severe mental disorders.
- If you are on a low-salt, low-sugar or other special diet.

Over age 60:
No special problems.

Pregnancy:
Decide with your doctor whether drug benefits justify risk to unborn child. Treatment best begun after child has been delivered. Risk category C (see page xviii).

Breast-feeding:
Effect unknown. Consult doctor.

Infants & children:
Children tolerate quinacrine poorly. Quinacrine may cause vomiting due to bitter taste. Try crushing tablets in jam, honey or chocolate syrup.

Prolonged use:
- Can cause eye problems, liver disease, aplastic anemia. Don't use for more than 5 days.
- Talk to your doctor about the need for follow-up medical examinations or laboratory studies to check stools for giardiasis.

Skin & sunlight:
No problems expected.

Driving, piloting or hazardous work:
Don't drive or pilot aircraft until you learn how medicine affects you. Don't work around dangerous machinery. Don't climb ladders or work in high places. Danger increases if you drink alcohol or take medicine affecting alertness and reflexes, such as antihistamines, tranquilizers, sedatives, pain medicine, narcotics and mind-altering drugs.

Discontinuing:
Don't discontinue before 5 days without consulting doctor.

Others:
- Advise any doctor or dentist whom you consult that you take this medicine.
- Request 3 stool exams several days apart.

POSSIBLE INTERACTION WITH OTHER DRUGS

GENERIC NAME OR DRUG CLASS	COMBINED EFFECT
Primaquine	Decreased effect of primaquine.

POSSIBLE INTERACTION WITH OTHER SUBSTANCES

INTERACTS WITH	COMBINED EFFECT
Alcohol:	Increased adverse effects of both. Avoid.
Beverages:	None expected.
Cocaine:	None expected.
Foods:	None expected.
Marijuana:	None expected.
Tobacco:	None expected.

QUINIDINE

BRAND NAMES

Apo-Quinidine
Cardioquin
Cin-Quin
Duraquin
Novoquinidin
Quinaglute Dura-Tabs
Quinalan
Quinate
Quinidex Extentabs
Quinora

BASIC INFORMATION

Habit forming? No
Prescription needed?
U.S.: Yes
Canada: No
Available as generic? Yes
Drug class: Antiarrhythmic

USES

- Corrects heart rhythm disorders.
- May be used in treatment of malaria.

DOSAGE & USAGE INFORMATION

How to take:
- Tablet or capsule—Swallow with liquid or food to lessen stomach irritation.
- Extended-release tablets—Swallow each dose whole. Don't crush them.

When to take:
At the same times each day.

If you forget a dose:
Take as soon as you remember up to 2 hours late. If more than 2 hours, wait for next scheduled dose (don't double this dose).

Continued next column

OVERDOSE

SYMPTOMS:
Confusion, severe blood pressure drop, lethargy, breathing difficulty, fainting, seizures, coma.
WHAT TO DO:
- **Dial 911 (emergency) for an ambulance or medical help or poison center 1-800-222-1222. Then give first aid immediately.**
- **If patient is unconscious and not breathing, give mouth-to-mouth breathing. If there is no heartbeat, use cardiac massage and mouth-to-mouth breathing (CPR). Don't try to make patient vomit. If you can't get help quickly, take patient to nearest emergency facility.**
- **See emergency information on inside covers.**

What drug does:
Delays nerve impulses to the heart to regulate heartbeat.

Time lapse before drug works:
2 to 4 hours.

Don't take with:
Any other medicine without consulting your doctor or pharmacist.

POSSIBLE ADVERSE REACTIONS OR SIDE EFFECTS

SYMPTOMS	WHAT TO DO
Life-threatening:	
Hives, rash, intense itching, faintness soon after a dose (anaphylaxis); wheezing.	Seek emergency treatment immediately.
Common:	
Bitter taste, diarrhea, nausea, vomiting, appetite loss, abdominal pain.	Discontinue. Call doctor right away.
Infrequent:	
• Dizziness, lightheadedness, fainting, headache, confusion, rash, change in vision, difficult breathing, rapid heartbeat.	Discontinue. Call doctor right away.
• Ringing in ears.	Continue. Call doctor when convenient.
Rare:	
• Unusual bleeding or bruising, difficulty or pain on swallowing, fever, joint pain, jaundice, hepatitis.	Discontinue. Call doctor right away.
• Weakness.	Continue. Call doctor when convenient.

WARNINGS & PRECAUTIONS

Don't take if:
- You are allergic to quinidine.
- You have an active infection.

Before you start, consult your doctor:
About any drug you take, including nonprescription drugs.

Over age 60:
Adverse reactions and side effects may be more frequent and severe than in younger persons.

Pregnancy:
Decide with your doctor if drug benefits justify risk to unborn child. Risk category C (see page xviii).

Breast-feeding:
Drug filters into milk. May harm child. Consult doctor.

Infants & children:
No problems expected.

Prolonged use:
Talk to your doctor about the need for follow-up studies to check complete blood counts (white blood cell count, platelet count, red blood cell count,hemoglobin, hematocrit), liver function, kidney function, serum potassium levels, ECG*.

Skin & sunlight:
May cause rash or intensify sunburn in areas exposed to sun or ultraviolet light (photosensitivity reaction). Avoid overexposure. Notify doctor if reaction occurs.

Driving, piloting or hazardous work:
Don't drive or pilot aircraft until you learn how medicine affects you. Don't work around dangerous machinery. Don't climb ladders or work in high places. Danger increases if you drink alcohol or take medicine affecting alertness and reflexes, such as antihistamines, tranquilizers, sedatives, pain medicine, narcotics and mind-altering drugs.

Discontinuing:
Don't discontinue without doctor's advice until you complete prescribed dose, even though symptoms diminish or disappear.

Others:
Advise any doctor or dentist whom you consult that you take this medicine.

POSSIBLE INTERACTION WITH OTHER DRUGS

GENERIC NAME OR DRUG CLASS	COMBINED EFFECT
Alkalizers, urinary*	Slows quinidine elimination, increasing its effect and toxicity.
Antacids	Take at least 2 hours apart.
Antiarrhythmics*	May increase or decrease effect or toxicity of quinidine.
Anticoagulants*, oral	Possible increased anticoagulant effect.
Anticonvulsants, hydantoin	Decreased effect of quinidine.
Antidepressants, tricyclic	Increased risk of heart rhythm problems.
Beta-adrenergic blocking agents*	May slow heartbeat excessively.
Cimetidine	Increased quinidine effect.
Digitalis preparations*	May slow heartbeat excessively. Dose adjustments may be needed.
Doxepin (topical)	Increased risk of toxicity of both drugs.
Encainide	Possible irregular heartbeat.
Enzyme inhibitors*	Increased effect of quinidine.
Erythromycin	Possible irregular heartbeat.
Flecainide	Possible irregular heartbeat.
Haloperidol	Possible irregular heartbeat.
Mefloquine	Possible irregular heartbeat. Avoid.
Metformin	Increased metformin effect.
Nicardipine	Possible increased effect and toxicity of each drug.
Nifedipine	Possible decreased quinidine effect.
Nimodipine	Increased quinidine effect.
Phenobarbital	Decreased quinidine effect.
Phenothiazines*	Possible increased quinidine effect.
QT interval prolongation-causing drugs*	Heartbeat irregularities.

POSSIBLE INTERACTION WITH OTHER SUBSTANCES

INTERACTS WITH	COMBINED EFFECT
Alcohol:	None expected.
Beverages: Caffeine drinks.	Causes rapid heartbeat. Use sparingly.
Cocaine:	Irregular heartbeat. Avoid.
Foods:	None expected.
Marijuana:	Can cause fainting.
Tobacco:	Irregular heartbeat. Avoid.

*See Glossary

QUININE

BRAND NAMES

Legatrin
NovoQuinine
Quin-260
Quin-amino
Quinamm
Quindan
Quiphile
Q-Vel

BASIC INFORMATION

Habit forming? No
Prescription needed?
High strength: Yes
Low strength: No
Available as generic? Yes
Drug class: Antiprotozoal

USES

- Treatment or prevention of malaria.
- Relief of muscle cramps.

DOSAGE & USAGE INFORMATION

How to take:
Tablet or capsule—Swallow with liquid or food to lessen stomach irritation.

When to take:
- Prevention—At the same time each day, usually at bedtime.
- Treatment—At the same times each day in evenly spaced doses.

If you forget a dose:
- Prevention—Take as soon as you remember up to 12 hours late. If more than 12 hours, wait for next scheduled dose (don't double this dose).
- Treatment—Take as soon as you remember up to 2 hours late. If more than 2 hours, wait for next scheduled dose (don't double this dose).

Continued next column

OVERDOSE

SYMPTOMS:
Severe impairment of vision and hearing; severe nausea, vomiting, diarrhea; shallow breathing, fast heartbeat; apprehension, confusion, delirium.
WHAT TO DO:
Dial 911 (emergency) for an ambulance or medical help or poison center 1-800-222-1222. Then give first aid immediately.

What drug does:
- Reduces contractions of skeletal muscles.
- Increases blood flow.
- Interferes with genes in malaria micro-organisms.

Time lapse before drug works:
May require several days or weeks for maximum effect.

Don't take with:
Any other medicine without consulting your doctor or pharmacist.

POSSIBLE ADVERSE REACTIONS OR SIDE EFFECTS

SYMPTOMS	WHAT TO DO
Life-threatening:	
In case of overdose, see previous column.	
Common:	
• Blurred vision or change in vision, eyes sensitive to light.	Discontinue. Call doctor right away.
• Dizziness, headache, abdominal discomfort, mild nausea, vomiting, diarrhea.	Continue. Call doctor when convenient.
• Ringing or buzzing in ears, impaired hearing.	Continue. Tell doctor at next visit.
Infrequent:	
Rash, hives, itchy skin, difficult breathing.	Discontinue. Call doctor right away.
Rare:	
Sore throat, fever, unusual bleeding or bruising, unusual tiredness or weakness, angina.	Discontinue. Call doctor right away.

WARNINGS & PRECAUTIONS

Don't take if:
You are allergic to quinine or quinidine.

Before you start, consult your doctor:
- If you plan to become pregnant within medication period.
- If you have asthma.
- If you have eye disease, hearing problems or ringing in the ears.
- If you have heart disease.
- If you have myasthenia gravis.

Over age 60:
Adverse reactions and side effects may be more frequent and severe than in younger persons.

Pregnancy:
Risk to unborn child outweighs drug benefits. Don't use. Risk category X (see page xviii).

Breast-feeding:
Drug filters into milk. May harm child. Consult doctor.

Infants & children:
Use only under medical supervision.

Prolonged use:
May develop headache, blurred vision, nausea, temporary hearing loss, but seldom need to discontinue because of these symptoms.

Skin & sunlight:
May cause rash or intensity sunburn in areas exposed to sun or ultraviolet light (photosensitivity reaction). Avoid overexposure. Notify doctor if reaction occurs.

Driving, piloting or hazardous work:
Avoid if you feel dizzy or have blurred vision. Otherwise, no problems expected.

Discontinuing:
Don't discontinue without doctor's advice until you complete prescribed dose, even though symptoms diminish or disappear.

Others:
- Advise any doctor or dentist whom you consult that you take this medicine.
- Don't confuse with quinidine, a medicine for heart rhythm problems.

POSSIBLE INTERACTION WITH OTHER DRUGS

GENERIC NAME OR DRUG CLASS	COMBINED EFFECT
Alkalizers*, urinary	Possible toxic effects of quinine.
Antacids* (with aluminum hydroxide)	Decreased quinine effect.
Anticoagulants*, oral	Increased anti-coagulant effect.
Dapsone	Increased risk of adverse effect on blood cells.
Digitalis	Possible increased digitalis effect.
Digoxin	Possible increased digoxin effect.
Mefloquine	Increased risk of heartbeat irregularities.
Metformin	Increased metformin effect.
Quinidine	Possible toxic effects of quinine.

POSSIBLE INTERACTION WITH OTHER SUBSTANCES

INTERACTS WITH	COMBINED EFFECT
Alcohol:	None expected.
Beverages:	None expected.
Cocaine:	None expected.
Foods:	None expected.
Marijuana:	None expected.
Tobacco:	None expected.

***See Glossary**

RALOXIFENE

BRAND NAMES

Evista

BASIC INFORMATION

Habit forming? No
Prescription needed? Yes
Available as generic? No
Drug class: Osteoporosis postmenopausal, prophylactic

USES

- Prevents and treats osteoporosis in postmenopausal women.
- Lowers low-density lipoprotein (LDL) cholesterol blood levels.
- Does not treat hot flashes of menopause.

DOSAGE & USAGE INFORMATION

How to take:
Tablets—Swallow with water, with or without food. If you can't swallow whole, crumble tablet and take with liquid or food.

When to take:
At the same time each day.

If you forget a dose:
Take as soon as you remember up to 12 hours late. If more than 12 hours, wait for next scheduled dose (don't double this dose).

What drug does:
Has estrogen-like effects on bone and increases bone mineral density.

Time lapse before drug works:
Up to twelve months.

Don't take with:
Any other prescription or nonprescription drug without consulting your doctor or pharmacist.

OVERDOSE

SYMPTOMS:
None reported.
WHAT TO DO:
Overdose unlikely to threaten life. If person takes much larger amount than prescribed, call doctor, poison center 1-800-222-1222 or hospital emergency room for instructions.

POSSIBLE ADVERSE REACTIONS OR SIDE EFFECTS

SYMPTOMS	WHAT TO DO
Life-threatening:	
Blood clot formation.	Discontinue. Seek emergency treatment immediately.
Common:	
• Chest pain; bloody or cloudy urine; burning or painful urination; frequent urge to urinate; infection; cold- or flu-like symptoms; leg cramping; skin rash; swelling of hands, ankle or feet; vaginal itching.	Discontinue. Call doctor right away.
• Joint or muscle pain, swollen joints, gas, upset stomach, vomiting, hot flashes, insomnia, white vaginal discharge, depression, sweating, unexplained weight gain.	Continue. Call doctor if symptoms persist.
Infrequent:	
Abdominal pain, diarrhea, loss of appetite, nausea, weakness, migraine headache, difficulty breathing, fever, congestion.	Discontinue. Call doctor right away.
Rare:	
None expected.	

WARNINGS & PRECAUTIONS

Don't take if:

- You are allergic to raloxifene.
- You are scheduled for surgery within 72 hours.

Before you start, consult your doctor:

- If you have any other medical problem.
- If you plan to become pregnant within the medication period.
- If you have or have had a history of blood clot formation.
- If you have or have had cancer or tumors.
- If you have liver disease.

Over age 60:
Adverse reactions and side effects in older adults have been similar to those experienced by women who have just undergone menopause.

Pregnancy:
Use of raloxifene is not recommended during pregnancy. Risk category X (see page xviii).

Breast-feeding:
Unknown whether drug passes into milk and is not recommended during breast-feeding. Presently raloxifene is to be used in post-menopausal women only.

Infants & children:
Not recommended for this age group.

Prolonged use:
No problems expected. Your doctor should periodically evaluate your response to the drug and adjust the dose if necessary.

Skin & sunlight:
No problems expected.

Driving, piloting or hazardous work:
No problems expected.

Discontinuing:
Don't discontinue without consulting doctor.

Others:

- Advise any doctor or dentist whom you consult that you take this medicine.
- In addition to taking the drug, weight-bearing exercise and adequate intake of calcium and vitamin D are essential in preventing bone loss. Periods of prolonged activity may worsen your condition. Daily dietary supplements of elemental calcium and vitamin D may be recommended by your doctor.
- May help lower low-density lipoprotein (LDL) cholesterol levels.

POSSIBLE INTERACTION WITH OTHER DRUGS

GENERIC NAME OR DRUG CLASS	COMBINED EFFECT
Cholestyramine	Lessens the effect of raloxifene.
Estrogens	Not recommended for use with raloxifene.
Protein bound drugs*	Caution is recommended; consult doctor before taking any of these in conjunction with raloxifene.
Warfarin	May lessen the effect of warfarin.

POSSIBLE INTERACTION WITH OTHER SUBSTANCES

INTERACTS WITH	COMBINED EFFECT
Alcohol:	None expected.
Beverages:	None expected.
Cocaine:	Effects unknown. Avoid.
Foods:	None expected.
Marijuana:	Effects unknown. Avoid.
Tobacco:	None expected.

***See Glossary**

RAUWOLFIA ALKALOIDS

GENERIC AND BRAND NAMES

See complete list of generic and brand names in the *Generic and Brand Name Directory*, page 862.

BASIC INFORMATION

Habit forming? No
Prescription needed? Yes
Available as generic? Yes
Drug class: Antihypertensive, tranquilizer (rauwolfia alkaloid)

USES

- Treatment for high blood pressure.
- Tranquilizer for mental and emotional disturbances.

DOSAGE & USAGE INFORMATION

How to take:
Tablet or timed-release capsule—Swallow with liquid or food to lessen stomach irritation. If you can't swallow whole, crumble tablet or open capsule and take with liquid or food.

When to take:
At the same times each day.

If you forget a dose:
Take as soon as you remember up to 2 hours late. If more than 2 hours, wait for next scheduled dose (don't double this dose).

What drug does:
- Interferes with nerve impulses and relaxes blood vessel muscles, reducing blood pressure.
- Suppresses brain centers that control emotions.

Time lapse before drug works:
3 weeks continual use required to determine effectiveness.

Continued next column

OVERDOSE

SYMPTOMS:
Drowsiness; slow, weak pulse; slow, shallow breathing; diarrhea; coma; flush; low body temperature; pinpoint pupils.
WHAT TO DO:
- **Dial 911 (emergency) for an ambulance or medical help or poison center 1-800-222-1222. Then give first aid immediately.**
- **See emergency information on inside covers.**

Don't take with:
Any other medicine without consulting your doctor or pharmacist.

POSSIBLE ADVERSE REACTIONS OR SIDE EFFECTS

SYMPTOMS	WHAT TO DO
Life-threatening: In case of overdose, see previous column.	
Common:	
• Depression, dizziness.	Continue. Call doctor when convenient.
• Headache, faintness, drowsiness, lethargy, red eyes, stuffy nose, impotence, diminished sex drive, diarrhea, dry mouth.	Continue. Tell doctor at next visit.
Infrequent:	
• Black stool; bloody vomit; chest pain; shortness of breath; irregular or slow heartbeat; stiffness in muscles, bones, joints.	Discontinue. Call doctor right away.
• Trembling hands, foot and leg swelling.	Continue. Call doctor when convenient.
Rare:	
• Rash or itchy skin, sore throat, fever, abdominal pain, nausea, vomiting, unusual bleeding or bruising, jaundice.	Discontinue. Call doctor right away.
• Painful urination, nightmares.	Continue. Call doctor when convenient.

WARNINGS & PRECAUTIONS

Don't take if:
You are allergic to any rauwolfia alkaloid.

Before you start, consult your doctor:
- If you have been depressed.
- If you have had peptic ulcer, ulcerative colitis or gallstones.
- If you have epilepsy.
- If you will have surgery within 2 months, including dental surgery, requiring general or spinal anesthesia.

Over age 60:
Adverse reactions and side effects may be more frequent and severe than in younger persons.

Pregnancy:
Decide with your doctor whether drug benefits justify risk to unborn child. Risk category C (see page xviii).

Breast-feeding:
Drug passes into milk. Avoid drug or discontinue nursing until you finish medicine. Consult doctor for advice on maintaining milk supply.

Infants & children:
Not recommended.

Prolonged use:
- Causes cancer in laboratory animals. Consult your doctor if you have a family or personal history of cancer.
- Talk to your doctor about the need for follow-up medical examinations or laboratory studies.

Skin & sunlight:
No problems expected.

Driving, piloting or hazardous work:
Avoid if you feel drowsy, dizzy or faint. Otherwise, no problems expected.

Discontinuing:
Don't discontinue without consulting doctor. Dose may require gradual reduction if you have taken drug for a long time. Doses of other drugs may also require adjustment.

Others:
- Advise any doctor or dentist whom you consult that you take this medicine.
- Consult your doctor if you do isometric exercises. These raise blood pressure. Drug may intensify blood pressure rise.

POSSIBLE INTERACTION WITH OTHER DRUGS

GENERIC NAME OR DRUG CLASS	COMBINED EFFECT
Anticoagulants*, oral	Unpredictable increased or decreased effect of anticoagulant.
Anticonvulsants*	Serious change in seizure pattern.
Antidepressants*	Increased anti-depressant effect.
Antihistamines*	Increased anti-histamine effect.
Antihypertensives*, other	Increased rauwolfia effect.
Aspirin	Decreased aspirin effect.
Beta-adrenergic blocking agents*	Increased rauwolfia alkaloid effect. Excessive sedation.
Carteolol	Increased anti-hypertensive effect.
Central nervous system (CNS) depressants*	Increased CNS depression.
Clozapine	Toxic effect on the central nervous system.
Digitalis preparations*	Possible irregular heartbeat.
Dronabinol	Increased effects of both drugs. Avoid.
Ethinamate	Dangerous increased effects of ethinamate. Avoid combining.
Fluoxetine	Increased depressant effects of both drugs.
Guanfacine	May increase depressant effects of either medicine.
Leucovorin	High alcohol content of leucovorin may cause adverse effects.
Levodopa	Decreased levodopa effect.

Continued on page 928

POSSIBLE INTERACTION WITH OTHER SUBSTANCES

INTERACTS WITH	COMBINED EFFECT
Alcohol:	Increased intoxication. Use with extreme caution.
Beverages: Carbonated drinks.	Decreased rauwolfia alkaloid effect.
Cocaine:	Increased risk of heart block and high blood pressure.
Foods: Spicy foods.	Possible digestive upset.
Marijuana:	Occasional use—Mild drowsiness. Daily use—Moderate drowsiness, low blood pressure, depression.
Tobacco:	None expected.

*See Glossary

RESERPINE, HYDRALAZINE & HYDROCHLOROTHIAZIDE

BRAND NAMES

Cam-Ap-Es
Cherapas
Ser-A-Gen
Seralazide
Serpazide
Tri-Hydroserpine
Unipres

BASIC INFORMATION

Habit forming? No
Prescription needed? Yes
Available as generic? Yes
Drug class: Antihypertensive

USES

- Treatment for high blood pressure and congestive heart failure.
- Reduces fluid retention (edema).

DOSAGE & USAGE INFORMATION

How to take:
Tablet—Swallow with liquid. If you can't swallow whole, crumble and take with liquid or food.

When to take:
At the same times each day.

If you forget a dose:
Take as soon as you remember up to 2 hours late. If more than 2 hours, wait for next scheduled dose (don't double this dose).

What drug does:
- Interferes with nerve impulses and relaxes blood vessels, reducing blood pressure.
- Suppresses brain centers that control emotions.
- Forces sodium and water excretion, reducing body fluid. Reduced body fluid and relaxed arteries lower blood pressure.

Time lapse before drug works:
Regular use for several weeks may be necessary to determine drug's effectiveness.

Continued next column

OVERDOSE

SYMPTOMS:
Drowsiness; slow, shallow breathing; pinpoint pupils; diarrhea; flush; low body temperature; rapid, weak heartbeat; fainting; extreme weakness; cold, sweaty skin; cramps, coma.
WHAT TO DO:
- **Dial 911 (emergency) for an ambulance or medical help or poison center 1-800-222-1222. Then give first aid immediately.**
- **See emergency information on inside covers.**

Don't take with:
- Nonprescription drugs containing alcohol without consulting doctor.
- Any other medicine without consulting your doctor or pharmacist.

POSSIBLE ADVERSE REACTIONS OR SIDE EFFECTS

SYMPTOMS	WHAT TO DO
Life-threatening:	
Rapid or irregular heartbeat, weak pulse, fainting, black stool, black or bloody vomit, chest pain.	Discontinue. Seek emergency treatment.
Common:	
• Nausea, vomiting.	Discontinue. Call doctor right away.
• Headache, diarrhea, drowsiness, runny nose, appetite loss.	Continue. Call doctor when convenient.
Infrequent:	
• Blurred vision, chest pain, abdominal pain, rash, hives, joint pain.	Discontinue. Call doctor right away.
• Dizziness; mood change; headache; dry mouth; weakness; tiredness; weight gain or loss; eyes red, watery, irritated; confusion; constipation; red or flushed face; joint stiffness; depression; anxiety; foot and leg swelling.	Continue. Call doctor when convenient.
Rare:	
• Jaundice; unexplained bleeding or bruising; sore throat, fever, mouth sores; weakness and faintness when arising from bed or chair.	Discontinue. Call doctor right away.
• Numbness, tingling, burning feeling in feet and hands; nasal congestion; impotence; nightmares.	Continue. Call doctor when convenient.

WARNINGS & PRECAUTIONS

Don't take if:
You are allergic to any rauwolfia alkaloid, hydralazine, any thiazide diuretic drug*, or tartrazine dye.

RESERPINE, HYDRALAZINE & HYDROCHLOROTHIAZIDE

Before you start, consult your doctor:
- If you have been depressed.
- If you have had peptic ulcer, ulcerative colitis, gallstones, kidney disease or impaired kidney function, lupus or a stroke.
- If you have epilepsy, gout; liver, pancreas or kidney disorder.
- If you feel pain in chest, neck or arms on physical exertion.
- If you are allergic to any sulfa drug*.
- If you will have surgery within 2 months, including dental surgery, requiring general or spinal anesthesia.

Over age 60:
Adverse reactions and side effects may be more frequent and severe than in younger persons, especially dizziness and excessive potassium loss.

Pregnancy:
Decide with your doctor if drug benefits justify risk to unborn child. Risk category C (see page xviii).

Breast-feeding:
Drug passes into milk. Avoid drug or discontinue nursing until you finish medicine. Consult doctor.

Infants & children:
Not recommended.

Prolonged use:
- Causes cancer in laboratory animals. Consult your doctor if you have a family or personal history of cancer.
- Possible psychosis.
- May cause lupus; numbness, tingling in hands or feet.
- Talk to your doctor about the need for follow-up medical examinations or laboratory studies.

Skin & sunlight:
One or more drugs in this group may cause rash or intensify sunburn in areas exposed to sun or ultraviolet light (photosensitivity reaction). Avoid overexposure. Notify doctor if reaction occurs.

Driving, piloting or hazardous work:
Don't drive or pilot aircraft until you learn how medicine affects you. Don't work around dangerous machinery. Don't climb ladders or work in high places. Danger increases if you drink alcohol or take medicine affecting alertness and reflexes.

Discontinuing:
Don't discontinue without consulting doctor. Dose may require gradual reduction if you have taken drug for a long time. Doses of other drugs may also require adjustment.

Others:
- Consult your doctor if you do isometric exercises. These raise blood pressure. Drug may intensify blood pressure rise.
- Vitamin B-6 supplement may be advisable. Consult doctor.
- Hot weather and fever may cause dehydration and drop in blood pressure. Dose may require temporary adjustment. Weigh daily and report any unexpected weight decreases to your doctor.
- Advise any doctor or dentist whom you consult that you take this medicine.
- May cause rise in uric acid, leading to gout.
- May cause blood sugar rise in diabetics.
- Some products contain tartrazine dye. Avoid, especially if you are allergic to aspirin.

POSSIBLE INTERACTION WITH OTHER DRUGS

GENERIC NAME OR DRUG CLASS	COMBINED EFFECT
Acebutolol	Possible increased effects of drugs.

Continued on page 928

POSSIBLE INTERACTION WITH OTHER SUBSTANCES

INTERACTS WITH	COMBINED EFFECT
Alcohol:	Increased intoxication. Avoid.
Beverages:	
Carbonated drinks.	Decreased rauwolfia alkaloids effect.
Cocaine:	Dangerous blood pressure rise. Avoid.
Foods:	
Spicy foods.	Possible digestive upset.
Licorice.	Excessive potassium loss that causes dangerous heart rhythms.
Marijuana:	Weakness on standing. May increase blood pressure. Occasional use—Mild drowsiness. Daily use—Moderate drowsiness, low blood pressure, depression.
Tobacco:	Possible angina attacks.

*See Glossary

RETINOIDS (Oral)

GENERIC AND BRAND NAMES

ACITRETIN
Soriatane

BASIC INFORMATION

Habit forming? No
Prescription needed? Yes
Available as generic? No
Drug class: Antipsoriatic

USES

- Treats psoriasis in patients who don't respond well to standard or usual treatment.
- Treats arthritic symptoms sometimes associated with psoriasis.
- Treats ichthyosis.

DOSAGE & USAGE INFORMATION

How to take:
Capsules—Swallow with liquid or food to lessen stomach irritation. If you can't swallow whole, open capsule and take with liquid or food.

When to take:
At the same time each day, according to instructions on prescription label.

If you forget a dose:
One dose a day—Take as soon as you remember, up to 12 hours late. If more than 12 hours, wait for next scheduled dose (don't double this dose).

What drug does:
- Mechanism of action on skin is unknown, but positive effects on the disease have been documented. It probably reduces the production of protein in the outer layers of skin. It is chemically related to tretinoin (Retin-A).
- Also functions as an anti-inflammatory agent.

Time lapse before drug works:
- 2 to 6 hours for effects to begin.
- Prolonged treatment, up to 2 to 4 weeks (sometimes with psoralens, ultraviolet light may be necessary to develop maximum benefit).

OVERDOSE

SYMPTOMS:
Unknown. If overdose is suspected, follow instructions below.
WHAT TO DO:
- **Dial 911 (emergency) for an ambulance or medical help or poison center 1-800-222-1222. Then give first aid immediately.**
- **See emergency information on inside covers.**

Don't take with:
Any other medicine without consulting your doctor or pharmacist.

POSSIBLE ADVERSE REACTIONS OR SIDE EFFECTS

SYMPTOMS	WHAT TO DO
Life-threatening: None expected.	
Common:	
• Bone and joint pain, stiffness, eye irritation or inflammation, unusual tiredness, muscle cramps, abdominal cramps, unusual bruising.	Discontinue. Call doctor right away.
• Dry skin, irritated or inflamed skin, hair thinning, dry eyes, mild nosebleed, mild headache, contact lens sensitivity, peeling of skin on hands or feet, thirstiness.	Continue. Call doctor when convenient.
Infrequent:	
• Blurred vision, hearing loss or other change in hearing, dark-colored urine, jaundice (yellow skin or eyes).	Discontinue. Call doctor right away.
• Dizziness, dry mouth, mild nausea, hair thinning, nail problems (redness, soreness or loosening), runny nose, lip symptoms (chapped, redness, sore, cracking, swelling), sore tongue.	Continue. Call doctor when convenient.
Rare:	
• Nausea and vomiting, severe and continuing headache.	Discontinue. Call doctor right away.
• Confusion, anxiety, depression, bleeding or inflamed gums.	Discontinue. Call doctor when convenient.

WARNINGS & PRECAUTIONS

Don't take if:
- If you are pregnant or expect to get pregnant in the future. Fetal abnormalities have occurred while using and after discontinuing the drug.
- If you are allergic to retinoids or parabens (used as preservative in gelatin capsule).

Before you start, consult your doctor:
- If you have heart or blood vessel disease.
- If you are allergic to any medication, food or other substance.
- If you have high plasma triglycerides.
- If you are an alcoholic.
- If you have diabetes mellitus.
- If you are a female of reproductive age.
- If you have kidney or liver disease.

Over age 60:
Adverse reactions and side effects may be more frequent and severe than in younger persons. You may need smaller doses for shorter periods of time.

Pregnancy:
Risk to unborn child outweighs drug benefits. Retinoids have caused major human fetal abnormalities. Don't use. Risk category X (see page xviii).

Breast-feeding:
Drug passes into milk. Avoid drug or discontinue nursing until you finish medicine. Consult doctor for advice on maintaining milk supply.

Infants & children:
Don't use.

Prolonged use:
- No problems expected if used for no more than 4 months per treatment session.
- Talk to your doctor about the need for follow-up medical examinations or laboratory studies to check blood lipids, liver function.

Skin & sunlight:
May cause rash or intensify sunburn in areas exposed to sun or ultraviolet light (photosensitivity reaction). Avoid overexposure. Notify doctor if reaction occurs.

Driving, piloting or hazardous work:
Don't drive or pilot aircraft until you learn how medicine affects you. Don't work around dangerous machinery. Don't climb ladders or work in high places. Danger increases if you drink alcohol or take medicine affecting alertness and reflexes.

Discontinuing:
Don't discontinue without consulting doctor. Dose may require gradual reduction if you have taken drug for a long time. Doses of other drugs may also require adjustment.

Others:
- Courses of treatment are usually limited to 4 months, and repeating, if necessary, after a 4-month rest period.
- It is strongly recommended to continue birth control indefinitely after treatment is stopped.
- Certain methods of birth control may fail while using this drug, including tubal ligation and progestin (minipill) preparations. Other birth control methods may be affected also. Use two different methods of birth control.
- Don't donate blood during treatment or for 3 years thereafter.
- Advise any doctor or dentist whom you consult that you take this medicine.
- May cause problem in controlling blood sugar.
- During early treatment, psoriasis may appear to worsen.
- May cause changes in cholesterol levels in blood. Laboratory blood studies should be obtained prior to and during treatment.
- May cause calcium deposits in tendons and ligaments.
- Women who take etretinate should never plan on pregnancy.

POSSIBLE INTERACTION WITH OTHER DRUGS

GENERIC NAME OR DRUG CLASS	COMBINED EFFECT
Abrasive soaps or cleaners	Excessive drying effect on skin.
Acne preparations*	Excessive drying effect on skin.
Any topical preparation containing alcohol such as after-shave lotions	Excessive drying effect on skin.
Carbamazepine	Decreased retinoid activity.

Continued on page 929

POSSIBLE INTERACTION WITH OTHER SUBSTANCES

INTERACTS WITH	COMBINED EFFECT
Alcohol:	May cause hypertriglyceridemia. Avoid.
Beverages: Milk.	Aids absorption of etretinate.
Cocaine:	None expected.
Foods: High-fat diet or milk products.	Aids absorption of etretinate.
Marijuana:	None expected.
Tobacco:	None expected.

***See Glossary**

RETINOIDS (Topical)

GENERIC AND BRAND NAMES

ADAPALENE
Differin
BEXAROTENE
Targretin
TAZAROTENE
Tazorac
TRETINOIN
Avita
Renova
Retin-A Cream
Retin-A Cream Regimen Kit
Retin-A Gel
Retin-A Gel Regimen Kit
TRETINOIN (Con't)
Retin-A Solution
Retinoic Acid
Solage
Stieva-A Cream
Stieva-A Cream Forte
Stieva-A Gel
Stieva-A Solution
Vesanoid
Vitamin A Acid Cream
Vitamin A Acid Gel

BASIC INFORMATION

Habit forming? No
Prescription needed? Yes
Available as generic? No
Drug class: Antiacne (topical), antipsoriatic

USES

- Treatment for acne, psoriasis, ichthyosis, keratosis, folliculitis, flat warts.
- Treatment for sun-damaged skin (wrinkles), mottled skin, rough skin and pigmented skin.
- Bexarotene treats skin cancer (cutaneous T cell lymphoma),
- Solage is a combination drug —tretinoin plus-mequinol (which is not covered in this topic).

DOSAGE & USAGE INFORMATION

How to use:
Wash skin with nonmedicated soap, pat dry, wait 20 minutes before applying.
- Cream or gel—Apply to affected areas with fingertips and rub in gently.

Continued next column

- Solution—Apply to affected areas with gauze pad or cotton swab. Avoid getting too wet so medicine doesn't drip into eyes or mouth, onto lips or inside nose.
- Follow manufacturer's directions on container.

When to use:
Apply once daily, usually in the evening before going to bed.

If you forget a dose:
Use as soon as you remember if it is still the same day. If more than 12 hours late, wait for the next dose (don't double this dose).

What drug does:
Helps control acne inflammation and prevent new acne outbreaks. Increases skin cell turnover so skin layer peels off more easily.

Time lapse before drug works:
May require 2 to 6 weeks for minimum benefit and 3 to 12 months for full benefit.

Don't use with:
Any other topical medicine without consulting your doctor or pharmacist.

OVERDOSE

SYMPTOMS:
None expected.
WHAT TO DO:
- **If person accidentally swallows drug, call doctor, poison center 1-800-222-1222 or hospital emergency room for instructions.**
- **See emergency information on inside covers.**

POSSIBLE ADVERSE REACTIONS OR SIDE EFFECTS

SYMPTOMS	WHAT TO DO
Life-threatening: None expected.	
Common:	
• Mild redness, itching, chapping, dryness of skin during first few weeks of use.	Depending on severity, may reduce frequency of use.
• Worsening of acne or psoriasis during first few weeks of use (due to action of the drug on previous unseen breakouts).	Expected effect. No action necessary.
Infrequent:	
Painful skin irritation, darkening or lightening of skin where treated.	Discontinue. Call doctor when convenient.
Rare: None expected.	

WARNINGS & PRECAUTIONS

Don't take if:
You are allergic to topical retinoids or any of the components of the gel product.

Before you start, consult your doctor:
- If you are using any other prescription or nonprescription medicine for the skin.
- If you are using abrasive skin cleansers or medicated cosmetics.

Over age 60:
No problems expected.

Pregnancy:
- Adapalene and tretinoin—Discuss with your doctor if benefits outweigh risks to unborn child. Risk category C (see page xx).
- Tazarotene—Risk to unborn child outweighs drug's benefits. Don't use. Risk category X (see page xviii).

Breast-feeding:
Effect unknown. Consult doctor.

Infants & children:
Not recommended.

Prolonged use:
No problems expected.

Skin & sunlight:
- May cause rash or intensify sunburn in areas exposed to sun or ultraviolet light. Avoid over-exposure. Notify doctor if reaction occurs.
- If you are normally exposed to considerable sunlight, use extra caution. Use broad spectrum of sunscreen on treated areas and wear protective clothing (e.g., hat).

Driving, piloting or hazardous work:
No problems expected.

Discontinuing:
- May be unnecessary to finish medicine. Discontinue when acne improves. For some patients, this medicine may be used indefinitely to control acne.
- If skin problem doesn't improve after first few weeks of use, consult doctor.

Others:
- Cold or windy weather may further irritate the skin. Avoid if possible.
- Products with a drying effect on the skin may cause irritation when used with retinoids. These include cosmetics, abrasive soaps and cleansers, astringents, and topical products that contain alcohol, spices or lime.
- Advise any doctor or dentist whom you consult that you use this medicine.
- Brand name Solage also contains the drug mequinol.
- Don't apply drug to skin area that has cuts, abrasions, a rash or is sunburned.

POSSIBLE INTERACTION WITH OTHER DRUGS

GENERIC NAME OR DRUG CLASS	COMBINED EFFECT
Antiacne topical preparations, other	Excessive skin irritation.
Cosmetics (medicated)	Severe skin irritation.
Insect repellents containing DEET	Repellent can be absorbed into skin.
Skin-peeling agents (salicylic acid, sulfur, resorcinol)	Excessive skin irritation.
Skin preparations with alcohol	Severe skin irritation.
Soaps or cleansers (abrasive)	Severe skin irritation.

POSSIBLE INTERACTION WITH OTHER SUBSTANCES

INTERACTS WITH	COMBINED EFFECT
Alcohol:	None expected.
Beverages:	None expected.
Cocaine:	None expected.
Foods:	None expected.
Marijuana:	None expected.
Tobacco:	None expected.

RIBAVIRIN

BRAND NAMES

Tribavirin
Virazid
Virazole

BASIC INFORMATION

Habit forming? No
Prescription needed? Yes
Available as generic? No
Drug class: Antiviral

USES

- Treats severe viral pneumonia.
- Treats respiratory syncytial virus (RSV) infections in hospitalized infants or children.
- Treats influenza A and B with some success.
- Does not treat other viruses such as the common cold.
- Rebetol brand is used to treat chronic hepatitis C when combined with another drug. The information in this chart does not include any facts about Rebetol. Your doctor will provide you the the information and instructions on Rebetol and will follow your therapy carefully.

DOSAGE & USAGE INFORMATION

How to take:
By inhalation of a fine mist through mouth. Requires a special sprayer attached to oxygen mask, face mask for infants or hood.

When to take:
As ordered by your doctor.

If you forget a dose:
Use as soon as you remember.

What drug does:
Kills virus or prevents its growth.

Time lapse before drug works:
Begins working in 1 hour. May require treatment for 12 to 18 hours per day for 3 to 7 days.

Don't take with:
Any other medicine without consulting your doctor or pharmacist.

OVERDOSE

SYMPTOMS:
None expected.
WHAT TO DO:
Overdose unlikely to threaten life. If person takes much larger amount than prescribed, call doctor, poison center 1-800-222-1222 or hospital emergency room for instructions.

POSSIBLE ADVERSE REACTIONS OR SIDE EFFECTS

SYMPTOMS	WHAT TO DO
Life-threatening:	
None expected.	
Common:	
None expected.	
Infrequent:	
• Unusual tireness or weakness.	Discontinue. Call doctor right away.
• Headache, insomnia, appetite loss, nausea.	Continue. Call doctor when convenient.
Rare:	
Skin irritation or rash.	Continue. Call doctor when convenient.

WARNINGS & PRECAUTIONS

Don't take if:
You are allergic to ribavirin.

Before you start, consult your doctor:
- If you are now on low-salt, low-sugar or any special diet.
- If you have severe anemia.

Over age 60:
Adverse reactions and side effects may be more frequent and severe than in younger persons. Ask doctor about smaller doses.

Pregnancy:
Risk to unborn child outweighs drug benefits. Don't use. Risk category X (see page xviii).

Breast-feeding:
Drug may pass into milk. Avoid drug or discontinue nursing until you finish medicine. Consult doctor for advice on maintaining milk supply.

Infants & children:
Use only under close medical supervision.

Prolonged use:
No problems expected.

Skin & sunlight:
No special problems expected.

Driving, piloting or hazardous work:
Don't drive or pilot aircraft until you learn how medicine affects you. Don't work around dangerous machinery. Don't climb ladders or work in high places. Danger increases if you drink alcohol or take medicine affecting alertness and reflexes, such as antihistamines, tranquilizers, sedatives, pain medicine, narcotics and mind-altering drugs.

Discontinuing:
Don't discontinue without consulting doctor. Dose may require gradual reduction if you have taken drug for a long time. Doses of other drugs may also require adjustment.

Others:
- Ribavirin is indicated for use in treatment of severe viral pneumonia caused by repiratory syncytial virus (RSV) in hospitalized infants and young children.
- Health care workers exposed to ribavirin may experience headache; eye itching, redness or swelling.
- Female health care workers who are pregnant or may become pregnant should avoid exposure to drug.
- The information in this chart does not cover or include the brand name Rebetol. Your doctor must provide that information for you.

POSSIBLE INTERACTION WITH OTHER DRUGS

GENERIC NAME OR DRUG CLASS	COMBINED EFFECT
Zidovudine	Decreased effect of ribavirin and zidovudine.

POSSIBLE INTERACTION WITH OTHER SUBSTANCES

INTERACTS WITH	COMBINED EFFECT
Alcohol:	None expected.
Beverages:	None expected.
Cocaine:	None expected.
Foods:	None expected.
Marijuana:	None expected.
Tobacco:	None expected.

RIBOFLAVIN (Vitamin B-2)

BRAND NAMES

Many multivitamin preparations. Check labels.

BASIC INFORMATION

Habit forming? No
Prescription needed? No
Available as generic? Yes
Drug class: Vitamin supplement

USES

- Dietary supplement to ensure normal growth and health.
- Dietary supplement to treat symptoms caused by deficiency of B-2: sores in mouth, eyes sensitive to light, itching and peeling skin.

DOSAGE & USAGE INFORMATION

How to take:
Tablet—Swallow with liquid or food to lessen stomach irritation. If you can't swallow whole, crumble tablet and take with liquid or food.

When to take:
At the same times each day.

If you forget a dose:
Take as soon as you remember. Resume regular schedule. Don't double dose.

What drug does:
Promotes normal growth and health.

Time lapse before drug works:
Requires continual intake.

Don't take with:
Any other medicine without consulting your doctor or pharmacist.

OVERDOSE

SYMPTOMS:
Dark urine, nausea, vomiting.
WHAT TO DO:
Overdose unlikely to threaten life. If person takes much larger amount than prescribed, call doctor, poison center 1-800-222-1222 or hospital emergency room for instructions.

POSSIBLE ADVERSE REACTIONS OR SIDE EFFECTS

SYMPTOMS	WHAT TO DO
Life-threatening:	
None expected.	
Common:	
Urine yellow in color.	No action necessary.
Infrequent:	
None expected.	
Rare:	
None expected.	

RIBOFLAVIN (Vitamin B-2)

WARNINGS & PRECAUTIONS

Don't take if:
- You are allergic to any B vitamin.
- You have chronic kidney failure.

Before you start, consult your doctor:
If you are pregnant or plan pregnancy.

Over age 60:
No problems expected.

Pregnancy:
Take within recommended guidelines. Consult doctor. Risk category A (see page xviii).

Breast-feeding:
Take within recommended guidelines. Consult doctor.

Infants & children:
Consult doctor.

Prolonged use:
No problems expected.

Skin & sunlight:
No problems expected.

Driving, piloting or hazardous work:
No problems expected.

Discontinuing:
No problems expected.

Others:
- Advise any doctor or dentist whom you consult that you take this medicine.
- A balanced diet should provide all the vitamin B-2 a healthy person needs and make supplements unnecessary during periods of good health. Best sources are milk, meats and green leafy vegetables.

POSSIBLE INTERACTION WITH OTHER DRUGS

GENERIC NAME OR DRUG CLASS	COMBINED EFFECT
Anticholinergics*	Possible increased riboflavin absorption.
Antidepressants, tricyclic*	Decreased riboflavin effect.
Phenothiazines*	Decreased riboflavin effect.
Probenecid	Decreased riboflavin effect.

POSSIBLE INTERACTION WITH OTHER SUBSTANCES

INTERACTS WITH	COMBINED EFFECT
Alcohol:	Prevents uptake and absorption of vitamin B-2.
Beverages:	None expected.
Cocaine:	None expected.
Foods:	None expected.
Marijuana:	None expected.
Tobacco:	Prevents absorption of vitamin B-2 and other vitamins and nutrients.

***See Glossary**

RIFAMYCINS

GENERIC AND BRAND NAMES

RIFAMPIN
- Rifadin
- Rifamate
- Rifampicin
- Rimactane

RIFAPENTINE
- Priftin

BASIC INFORMATION

Habit forming? No
Prescription needed? Yes
Available as generic? Yes
Drug class: Antibacterial, antitubercular

USES

Treatment for tuberculosis and other infections. Used in combination with other antitubercular medications.

DOSAGE & USAGE INFORMATION

How to take:
Capsule or tablet—Swallow with liquid or food. If you can't swallow whole, open capsule or crumble tablet and take with liquid or small amount of food. For child, mix with small amount of applesauce or jelly.

When to take:
1 hour before or 2 hours after a meal.

If you forget a dose:
Take as soon as you remember up to 2 hours late. If more than 2 hours, wait for next scheduled dose (don't double this dose).

What drug does:
Prevents multiplication of tuberculosis germs.

Continued next column

OVERDOSE

SYMPTOMS:
Slow, shallow breathing; weak, rapid pulse; cold, sweaty skin; coma.
WHAT TO DO:
- **Dial 911 (emergency) for an ambulance or medical help or poison center 1-800-222-1222. Then give first aid immediately.**
- **If patient is unconscious and not breathing, give mouth-to-mouth breathing. If there is no heartbeat, use cardiac massage and mouth-to-mouth breathing (CPR). Don't try to make patient vomit. If you can't get help quickly, take patient to nearest emergency facility.**
- **See emergency information on inside covers.**

Time lapse before drug works:
Usually 2 weeks. May require 1 to 2 years without missed doses for maximum benefit.

Don't take with:
Any other medicine without consulting your doctor or pharmacist.

POSSIBLE ADVERSE REACTIONS OR SIDE EFFECTS

SYMPTOMS	WHAT TO DO
Life-threatening: In case of overdose, see previous column.	
Common:	
• Diarrhea; reddish urine, stool, saliva, sweat and tears.	Continue. Call doctor when convenient.
• Blood in urine, joint pain, back or side pain, swelling of feet or legs.	Continue, but call doctor right away.
Infrequent:	
• Rash; flushed, itchy skin of face and scalp; blurred vision; difficulty breathing; nausea, vomiting; abdominal cramps; tiredness; bleeding or bruising.	Continue, but call doctor right away.
• Dizziness, unsteady gait, confusion, muscle or bone pain, heart-burn, flatulence, chills, headache, fever, mood or behavior changes.	Continue. Call doctor when convenient.
Rare:	
• Sore throat, mouth or tongue; jaundice.	Discontinue. Call doctor right away.
• Appetite loss, less urination.	Continue. Call doctor when convenient.

WARNINGS & PRECAUTIONS

Don't take if:
- You are allergic to any of the rifamycins.
- You wear soft contact lenses.

Before you start, consult your doctor:
If you are alcoholic or have liver disease.

Over age 60:
Adverse reactions and side effects may be more frequent and severe than in younger persons.

Pregnancy:
Decide with your doctor if drug benefits justify risk to unborn child. Risk category C (see page xviii).

Breast-feeding:
Effect unknown. Consult doctor.

Infants & children:
Use only under medical supervision.

Prolonged use:
- You may become more susceptible to infections caused by germs not responsive to rifamycins.
- Talk to your doctor about the need for follow-up medical examinations or laboratory studies to check liver function.

Skin & sunlight:
No problems expected.

Driving, piloting or hazardous work:
Don't drive or pilot aircraft until you learn how medicine affects you. Don't work around dangerous machinery. Don't climb ladders or work in high places. Danger increases if you drink alcohol or take medicine affecting alertness and reflexes, such as antihistamines, tranquilizers, sedatives, pain medicine, narcotics and mind-altering drugs.

Discontinuing:
Don't discontinue without doctor's advice until you complete prescribed dose, even though symptoms diminish or disappear.

Others:
- Reddish tears may discolor soft contact lenses.
- Advise any doctor or dentist you consult that you are using this medication.

POSSIBLE INTERACTION WITH OTHER DRUGS

GENERIC NAME OR DRUG CLASS	COMBINED EFFECT
Adrenocorticoids, systemic	Decreased adreno-corticoid effect.
Anticoagulants*, oral	Decreased anti-coagulant effect.
Antidepressants*, tricyclic	Decreased anti-depressant effect.
Antidiabetics*, oral	Decreased antidiabetic effect.
Antifungals*, azole	Decreased anti-fungal effect.
Barbiturates*	Decreased barbiturate effect.
Calcium channel* blockers	Decreased channel blocker effect.
Chloramphenicol	Decreased effect of both drugs.
Ciproflax	Decreased antibiotic effect.
Clarithromycin	Decreased antibiotic effect.
Clofibrate	Decreased clofibrate effect.
Clozapine	Toxic effect on bone marrow.
Contraceptives, oral*	Decreased contra-ceptive effect.
Cyclosporine	Decreased effect of both drugs.
Dapsone	Decreased dapsone effect.
Diazepam	Decreased diazepam effect.
Digitalis preparations*	Decreased digitoxin effect.
Disopyramide	Decreased disopyramide effect.
Doxycycline	Decreased antibiotic effect.
Estrogens* (including contraceptive pills)	Decreased effect of both drugs.
Haloperidol	Decreased haloperidol effect.
Hepatotoxics*	Increased risk of liver toxicity.
Isoniazid	Possible toxicity to liver.
Leflunomide	Increased risk of leflunomide toxicity.
Levothyroxine	Decreased levothyroxine effect.
Methadone	Decreased methadone effect.
Mexiletine	Decreased mexiletine effect.

Continued on page 929

POSSIBLE INTERACTION WITH OTHER SUBSTANCES

INTERACTS WITH	COMBINED EFFECT
Alcohol:	Possible toxicity to liver.
Beverages:	None expected.
Cocaine:	None expected.
Foods:	None expected.
Marijuana:	None expected.
Tobacco:	None expected.

*See Glossary

RILUZOLE

BRAND NAMES

Rilutek

BASIC INFORMATION

Habit forming? No
Prescription needed? Yes
Available as generic? No
Drug class: Amyotrophic lateral sclerosis therapy agent

USES

Treatment for amyotrophic lateral sclerosis (ALS or Lou Gehrig's disease), a motor neuron disorder that causes weakness and atrophy of the muscles. Riluzole may extend a patient's survival time and delay the need for surgery for complications. It does not cure the disorder.

DOSAGE & USAGE INFORMATION

How to take:
Tablet—Swallow with liquid. Instructions to take on an empty stomach mean 1 hour before or 2 hours after eating.

When to take:
Usually every 12 hours.

If you forget a dose:
Take as soon as you remember up to 6 hours late. If more than 6 hours, wait for the next dose (don't double this dose).

What drug does:
The cause of ALS is unknown and the exact mechanism of how the drug works is also unknown. It appears to decrease production of certain chemicals in the body and may affect some cellular activity that leads to the progressive weakness caused by the disorder.

Time lapse before drug works:
6 to 18 months for maximum benefits.

Don't take with:
Any other medicine without consulting your doctor or pharmacist.

OVERDOSE

SYMPTOMS:
None reported to date.
WHAT TO DO:
If person takes much larger amount than prescribed, call doctor, poison center 1-800-222-1222 or hospital emergency room for instructions.

POSSIBLE ADVERSE REACTIONS OR SIDE EFFECTS

SYMPTOMS	WHAT TO DO
Life-threatening: None expected.	
Common:	
• Difficulty breathing, abdominal pain, increased coughing, blood pressure increased.	Discontinue. Call doctor right away.
• Mouth has a burning, or tingling feeling, constipation, nausea, vomiting, dizziness, mild weakness, headache, diarrhea.	Continue. Call doctor when convenient.
Infrequent: Skin symptoms (redness, itching, scaling, bruising, oozing or thickening), fever, sore feet or legs, sores in mouth or on lips, fast heartbeat.	Discontinue. Call doctor right away.
Rare: Changes in vision, tightness in chest, wheezing, memory loss, mood changes, severe drowsiness, hallucinations, mental changes, swelling (face, hands, fingers, feet or legs), nosebleed, blood in urine, unusual bleeding, unusual tiredness or weakness, severe headache, pain in various parts of the body, eyes red or irritated, continued or painful penile erection, noisy breathing, loss of bladder control, hives.	Discontinue. Call doctor right away.

WARNINGS & PRECAUTIONS

Don't take if:
You are sensitive to riluzole.

Before you start, consult your doctor:
- If you are allergic to any medicine, food or other substance, or have a family history of allergies.
- If you have liver or kidney disease.

Over age 60:
No problems expected.

Pregnancy:
Decide with your doctor if drug benefits justify risk to unborn child. Risk category C (see page xviii).

Breast-Feeding:
Not recommended. Consult doctor.

Infants & children:
Not recommended for this age group.

Prolonged use:
Talk to your doctor about the need for follow-up medical examinations or laboratory studies to check liver function.

Skin & sunlight:
No problems expected.

Driving, piloting or hazardous work:
Don't drive or pilot aircraft until you learn how medicine affects you. Don't work around dangerous machinery. Don't climb ladders or work in high places. Danger increases if you drink alcohol or take other medicines affecting alertness and reflexes.

Discontinuing:
No problems expected.

Others:
- May affect the results of some medical tests.
- Use as directed. Don't increase or decrease dosage without doctor's approval.
- Advise any doctor or dentist whom you consult that you take this medicine.
- Call your doctor if you develop a fever.

POSSIBLE INTERACTION WITH OTHER DRUGS

GENERIC NAME OR DRUG CLASS	COMBINED EFFECT
Hepatotoxics*	Increased risk of adverse effects.
Other medications	Complete studies have not been done to evaluate interactions with other drugs, but the potential exists for a variety of possible interactions. Consult doctor.

POSSIBLE INTERACTION WITH OTHER SUBSTANCES

INTERACTS WITH	COMBINED EFFECT
Alcohol:	Increased risk of adverse effects.
Beverages:	None expected.
Cocaine:	Problems not known. Best to avoid.
Foods:	None expected.
Marijuana:	Problems not known. Best to avoid.
Tobacco:	May decrease riluzole effect.

***See Glossary**

RISPERIDONE

BRAND NAMES

Risperdal

BASIC INFORMATION

Habit forming? No
Prescription needed? Yes
Available as generic? No
Drug class: Antipsychotic

USES

Treats nervous, mental and emotional conditions. Helps in managing the signs and symptoms of schizophrenia.

DOSAGE & USAGE INFORMATION

How to take:

- Tablet—Swallow with liquid. May be taken with or without food.
- Oral solution—Dilute in 3 to 4 ounces of liquid (water, orange juice or low fat milk; don't use cola or tea).

When to take:
At the same times each day. The prescribed dosage will gradually be increased over the first few days of use.

If you forget a dose:
Take as soon as you remember. If it is almost time for the next dose, wait for the next scheduled dose (don't double this dose).

What drug does:
The exact mechanism is unknown. It appears to block certain nerve impulses between nerve cells.

Time lapse before drug works:
One to 7 days. A further increase in the dosage amount may be necessary to relieve symptoms for some patients.

Continued next column

OVERDOSE

SYMPTOMS:
Extreme drowsiness, rapid heartbeat, faintness, convulsions, excessive sweating, difficulty breathing, loss of muscular control.
WHAT TO DO:

- **Dial 911 (emergency) for an ambulance or medical help or poison center 1-800-222-1222. Then give first aid immediately.**
- **See emergency information at end of book.**

Don't take with:
Any other medication without consulting your doctor or pharmacist.

POSSIBLE ADVERSE REACTIONS OR SIDE EFFECTS

SYMPTOMS	WHAT TO DO
Life-threatening:	
High fever, rapid pulse, profuse sweating, muscle rigidity, confusion and irritability, seizures (malignant neuroleptic syndrome - rare).	Discontinue. Seek emergency treatment.
Common:	
Anxiety, drowsiness, dizziness, digestive problems, rash, sexual dysfunction.	Continue. Call doctor when convenient.
Infrequent:	
• Jerky or involuntary movements, especially of the face, lips, jaw, tongue (with higher doses only); slow-frequency tremor of head, face, or limbs, especially while moving; muscle rigidity, lack of facial expression and slow, inflexible movements.	Discontinue. Call doctor right away.
• Dry mouth, blurred vision, constipation, difficulty urinating; sedation, dizziness and low blood pressure; pacing or restlessness, intermittent spasms of muscles of face, eyes, tongue, jaw, neck, body or limbs.	Continue. Call doctor when convenient.
Rare:	
Other symptoms not listed above.	Continue. Call doctor when convenient.

WARNINGS & PRECAUTIONS

Don't take if:
You are allergic to risperidone.

Before you start, consult your doctor:
- If you have liver or kidney disease or heart disease.
- If you are allergic to any other medications.
- If you have a history of seizures.

Over age 60:
Adverse reactions and side effects may be more severe than in younger persons. A lower starting dosage is usually recommended until a response is determined.

Pregnancy:
Decide with your doctor if drug benefits justify any possible risk to unborn child. Risk category C (see page xviii).

Breast-feeding:
It is unknown if drug passes into milk. Avoid nursing until you finish medicine. Consult doctor for advice on maintaining milk supply.

Infants & children:
Safety in children under age 12 has not been established. Use only under close medical supervision.

Prolonged use:
Consult with your doctor on a regular basis while taking this drug to check your progress or to discuss any increase or changes in side effects and the need for continued treatment.

Skin & sunlight:
- May cause rash or intensify sunburn in areas exposed to sun or ultraviolet light (photosensitivity reaction). Use sunscreen and avoid overexposure. Notify doctor if reaction occurs.
- Hot temperatures and exercise, hot baths can increase risk of heatstroke. Drug may affect body's ability to maintain normal temperature.

Driving, piloting or hazardous work:
Don't drive or pilot aircraft until you learn how medicine affects you. Don't work around dangerous machinery. Don't climb ladders or work in high places. Danger increases if you drink alcohol or take medicine affecting alertness and reflexes.

Discontinuing:
Don't discontinue this drug without consulting doctor. Dosage may require a gradual reduction before stopping.

Others:
- Get up slowly from a sitting or lying position to avoid any dizziness, faintness or lightheadedness.
- Advise any doctor or dentist whom you consult that you take this medicine.
- Take medicine only as directed. Do not increase or reduce dosage without doctor's approval.

POSSIBLE INTERACTION WITH OTHER DRUGS

GENERIC NAME OR DRUG CLASS	COMBINED EFFECT
Antihypertensives*	Increased antihypertensive effect.
Carbamazepine	Decreased effect of risperidone.
Clozapine	Increased effect of risperidone.
Central nervous system (CNS) depressants*, other	Increased sedative effect.
Levodopa	May decrease levodopa effect.

POSSIBLE INTERACTION WITH OTHER SUBSTANCES

INTERACTS WITH	COMBINED EFFECT
Alcohol:	Increased sedative affect. Avoid.
Beverages:	None expected.
Cocaine:	Effect not known. Best to avoid.
Foods:	None expected.
Marijuana:	Effect not known. Best to avoid.
Tobacco:	None expected.

*See Glossary

RITODRINE

BRAND NAMES

Yutopar

BASIC INFORMATION

Habit forming? No
Prescription needed? Yes
Available as generic? Yes
Drug class: Labor inhibitor, beta-adrenergic stimulator

USES

Halts premature labor in pregnancies of 20 or more weeks.

DOSAGE & USAGE INFORMATION

How to take:
Tablet—Swallow with liquid or food to lessen stomach irritation. If you can't swallow whole, crumble tablet and take with liquid or food.

When to take:
Every 4 to 6 hours until term.

If you forget a dose:
Take as soon as you remember up to 2 hours late. If more than 2 hours, wait for next scheduled dose (don't double this dose).

What drug does:
Inhibits contractions of uterus (womb).

Time lapse before drug works:
30 to 60 minutes (oral form). Faster intravenously.

Don't take with:
Any other medicine without consulting your doctor or pharmacist.

OVERDOSE

SYMPTOMS:
Rapid, irregular heartbeat to 120 or more; shortness of breath.
WHAT TO DO:
- **Dial 911 (emergency) for an ambulance or medical help or poison center 1-800-222-1222. Then give first aid immediately.**
- **If patient is unconscious and not breathing, give mouth-to-mouth breathing. If there is no heartbeat, use cardiac massage and mouth-to-mouth breathing (CPR). Don't try to make patient vomit. If you can't get help quickly, take patient to nearest emergency facility.**
- **See emergency information on inside covers.**

POSSIBLE ADVERSE REACTIONS OR SIDE EFFECTS

SYMPTOMS	WHAT TO DO
Life-threatening:	
Hives, rash, intense itching, faintness soon after a dose (anaphylaxis).	Seek emergency treatment immediately.
Common:	
Irregular heartbeat, fast heartbeat.	Discontinue. Call doctor right away.
Infrequent:	
• Shortness of breath.	Discontinue. Call doctor right away.
• Nervousness, trembling, headache, nausea, vomiting.	Continue. Call doctor when convenient.
Rare:	
Rash, angina, jaundice.	Discontinue. Call doctor right away.

WARNINGS & PRECAUTIONS

Don't take if:
- You have heart disease.
- You have eclampsia.
- You have lung congestion.
- You have infection in the uterus.
- You have an overactive thyroid.
- You have a bleeding disorder.

Before you start, consult your doctor:
- If you have asthma.
- If you have diabetes.
- If you have high blood pressure.
- If you have pre-eclampsia.

Over age 60:
Not used.

Pregnancy:
Ritodrine crosses placenta, but animal studies show that it doesn't affect fetuses. Benefits versus risks must be assessed by you and your doctor. Risk category B (see page xviii).

Breast-feeding:
Not applicable.

Infants & children:
Not used.

Prolonged use:
Talk to your doctor about the need for follow-up medical examinations or laboratory studies to check blood sugar, ECG*, fluid and electrolytes.

Skin & sunlight:
No problems expected.

Driving, piloting or hazardous work:
Don't drive or pilot aircraft until you learn how medicine affects you. Don't work around dangerous machinery. Don't climb ladders or work in high places. Danger increases if you drink alcohol or take medicine affecting alertness and reflexes, such as antihistamines, tranquilizers, sedatives, pain medicine, narcotics and mind-altering drugs.

Discontinuing:
Don't discontinue without consulting doctor. Dose may require gradual reduction if you have taken drug for a long time. Doses of other drugs may also require adjustment.

Others:
None expected.

POSSIBLE INTERACTION WITH OTHER DRUGS

GENERIC NAME OR DRUG CLASS	COMBINED EFFECT
Adrenal corticosteroids*	Increased chance of fluid in lungs of mother. Avoid.
Anesthetics, general*	Possible cardiac arrhythmias or hypotension.
Beta-adrenergic blocking agents*	Decreased effect of ritodrine.
Diazoxide	Possible cardiac arrhythmias or hypotension.
Magnesium sulfate	Possible cardiac arrhythmias or hypotension.
Meperidine	Possible cardiac arrhythmias or hypotension.
Sympathomimetics*	Increased side effects of both.

POSSIBLE INTERACTION WITH OTHER SUBSTANCES

INTERACTS WITH	COMBINED EFFECT
Alcohol:	Increased adverse effects. Avoid.
Beverages:	None expected.
Cocaine:	Injury to fetus. Avoid.
Foods:	None expected.
Marijuana:	Injury to fetus. Avoid.
Tobacco:	Injury to fetus. Avoid.

***See Glossary**

SALICYLATES

GENERIC AND BRAND NAMES

See complete list of generic and brand names in the *Generic and Brand Name Directory*, page 862.

BASIC INFORMATION

Habit forming? No
Prescription needed? For some
Available as generic? Yes
Drug class: Analgesic, anti-inflammatory (nonsteroidal)

USES

- Reduces pain, fever, inflammation.
- Relieves swelling, stiffness, joint pain of arthritis or rheumatism.
- Decreases risk of myocardial infarction (aspirin only).

DOSAGE & USAGE INFORMATION

How to take:
- Tablet or capsule—Swallow with liquid.
- Extended-release tablets—Swallow each dose whole.
- Suppositories—Remove wrapper and moisten suppository with water. Gently insert into rectum, large end first.

When to take:
Pain, fever, inflammation—As needed, no more often than every 4 hours.

If you forget a dose:
- Pain, fever—Take as soon as you remember. Wait 4 hours for next dose.
- Arthritis—Take as soon as you remember up to 2 hours late. Return to regular schedule.

What drug does:
- Affects hypothalamus, the part of the brain that regulates temperature by dilating small blood vessels in skin.

Continued next column

- Prevents clumping of platelets (small blood cells) so blood vessels remain open.
- Decreases prostaglandin effect.
- Suppresses body's pain messages.

Time lapse before drug works:
30 minutes for pain, fever, arthritis.

Don't take with:
- Tetracyclines. Space doses 1 hour apart.
- Any other medicine without consulting your doctor or pharmacist.

OVERDOSE

SYMPTOMS:
Ringing in ears; nausea; vomiting; dizziness; fever; deep, rapid breathing; hallucinations; convulsions; coma.
WHAT TO DO:
- **Dial 911 (emergency) for an ambulance or medical help or poison center 1-800-222-1222. Then give first aid immediately.**
- **See emergency information on inside covers.**

POSSIBLE ADVERSE REACTIONS OR SIDE EFFECTS

SYMPTOMS	WHAT TO DO
Life-threatening:	
Hives, rash, intense itching, faintness soon after a dose (anaphylaxis); black or bloody vomit; blood in urine.	Seek emergency treatment immediately.
Common:	
• Nausea, vomiting, abdominal pain.	Discontinue. Seek emergency treatment.
• Heartburn, indigestion.	Continue. Call doctor when convenient.
• Ringing in ears.	Continue. Tell doctor at next visit.
Infrequent:	
None expected.	
Rare:	
• Black stools, unexplained fever.	Discontinue. Seek emergency treatment.
• Rash, hives, itchy skin, diminished vision, shortness of breath, wheezing, jaundice.	Discontinue. Call doctor right away.
• Drowsiness, headache.	Continue. Call doctor when convenient.

WARNINGS & PRECAUTIONS

Don't take if:
- You need to restrict sodium in your diet. Buffered effervescent tablets and sodium salicylate are high in sodium.
- Salicylates have a strong vinegar-like odor, which means they have decomposed.
- You have a bleeding disorder.

Before you start, consult your doctor:
- If you have had stomach or duodenal ulcers.
- If you have had gout.
- If you have asthma or nasal polyps.

Over age 60:
More likely to cause hidden bleeding in stomach or intestines. Watch for dark stools.

Pregnancy:
Risk factors vary for drugs in this group. See category list on page xviii and consult doctor.

Breast-feeding:
Drug passes into milk. Avoid drug or discontinue nursing until you finish medicine. Consult doctor for advice on maintaining milk supply.

Infants & children:
- Overdose frequent and severe. Keep bottles out of children's reach.
- Do not give to persons under age 18 who have fever and discomfort of viral illness, especially chicken pox and influenza. Probably increases risk of Reye's syndrome.

Prolonged use:
- Kidney damage. Periodic kidney function test recommended.
- Talk to your doctor about the need for follow-up medical examinations or laboratory studies to check liver function.

Skin & sunlight:
No special problems expected.

Driving, piloting or hazardous work:
No restrictions unless you feel drowsy.

Discontinuing:
For chronic illness—Don't discontinue without doctor's advice until you complete prescribed dose, even though symptoms diminish or disappear.

Others:
- Salicylates can complicate surgery, pregnancy, labor and delivery, and illness.
- Advise any doctor or dentist whom you consult that you take this medicine.
- For arthritis—Don't change dose without consulting doctor.
- Urine tests for blood sugar may be inaccurate.

POSSIBLE INTERACTION WITH OTHER DRUGS

GENERIC NAME OR DRUG CLASS	COMBINED EFFECT
Acetaminophen	Increased risk of kidney damage (with high, prolonged dose of each).
Adrenocorticoids, systemic	Decreased salicylate effect.
Allopurinol	Decreased allopurinol effect.
Angiotensin-converting enzyme (ACE) inhibitors*	Decreased ACE inhibitor effect.
Antacids*	Decreased salicylate effect.
Anticoagulants*, oral	Increased anti-coagulant effect. Abnormal bleeding.
Antidiabetics*, oral	Low blood sugar.
Anti-inflammatory drugs, nonsteroidal (NSAIDs)*	Risk of stomach bleeding and ulcers.
Aspirin, other	Likely salicylate toxicity.
Beta-adrenergic blocking agents*	Decreased anti-hypertensive effect.
Bismuth subsalicylate	Increased risk of salicylate toxicity.
Bumetanide	Decreased diuretic effect.
Calcium supplements*	Increased salicylate effect.
Carteolol	Decreased anti-hypertensive effect of carteolol.
Ethacrynic acid	Decreased diuretic effect.
Furosemide	Possible salicylate toxicity.
Gold compounds*	Increased likelihood of kidney damage.
Indomethacin	Risk of stomach bleeding and ulcers.
Insulin	Decreased blood sugar.

Continued on page 930

POSSIBLE INTERACTION WITH OTHER SUBSTANCES

INTERACTS WITH	COMBINED EFFECT
Alcohol:	Possible stomach irritation and bleeding. Avoid.
Beverages:	None expected.
Cocaine:	None expected.
Foods:	None expected.
Marijuana:	Possible increased pain relief, but marijuana may slow body's recovery. Avoid.
Tobacco:	None expected.

***See Glossary**

SCOPOLAMINE (Hyoscine)

BRAND NAMES

See complete list of brand names in the *Generic and Brand Name Directory*, page 862.

BASIC INFORMATION

Habit forming? No
Prescription needed?
High strength: Yes
Low strength: No
Available as generic? Yes
Drug class: Antispasmodic, anticholinergic

USES

- Reduces spasms of digestive system, bladder and urethra.
- Relieves painful menstruation.
- Prevents motion sickness.

DOSAGE & USAGE INFORMATION

How to take:
- Tablet or capsule—Swallow with liquid or food to lessen stomach irritation.
- Drops—Dilute dose in beverage.
- Skin discs—Clean application site. Change application sites with each dose.

When to take:
- Motion sickness—Apply disc 30 minutes before departure.
- Other uses—Take 30 minutes before meals (unless directed otherwise by doctor).

If you forget a dose:
Take up to 2 hours late. If more than 2 hours, wait for next dose (don't double this dose).

What drug does:
Blocks nerve impulses at parasympathetic nerve endings, preventing muscle contractions and gland secretions of organs involved.

Continued next column

OVERDOSE

SYMPTOMS:
Dilated pupils, blurred vision, rapid pulse and breathing, dizziness, fever, hallucinations, confusion, slurred speech, agitation, flushed face, convulsions, coma.
WHAT TO DO:
- **Dial 911 (emergency) for an ambulance or medical help or poison center 1-800-222-1222. Then give first aid immediately.**
- **See emergency information on inside covers.**

Time lapse before drug works:
15 to 30 minutes.

Don't take with:
Any other medicine without consulting your doctor or pharmacist.

POSSIBLE ADVERSE REACTIONS OR SIDE EFFECTS

SYMPTOMS	WHAT TO DO
Life-threatening:	
Hives, rash, intense itching, faintness soon after a dose (anaphylaxis).	Seek emergency treatment immediately.
Common:	
• Confusion, delirium, rapid heartbeat.	Discontinue. Call doctor right away.
• Nausea, vomiting, decreased sweating.	Continue. Call doctor when convenient.
• Constipation, loss of taste.	Continue. Tell doctor at next visit.
• Dryness in ears, nose, throat, mouth.	No action necessary.
Infrequent:	
• Headache, difficult urination, nasal congestion, altered taste.	Continue. Call doctor when convenient.
• Lightheadedness.	Discontinue. Call doctor right away.
Rare:	
Rash or hives; eye pain, blurred vision.	Discontinue. Call doctor right away.

WARNINGS & PRECAUTIONS

Don't take if:
- You are allergic to any anticholinergic.
- You have trouble with stomach bloating.
- You have difficulty emptying your bladder completely.
- You have narrow-angle glaucoma.
- You have severe ulcerative colitis.

Before you start, consult your doctor:
- If you have open-angle glaucoma, angina, chronic bronchitis or asthma, hiatal hernia, liver disease, enlarged prostate, myasthenia gravis, peptic ulcer, kidney or thyroid disease.
- If you will have surgery within 2 months, including dental surgery, requiring general or spinal anesthesia.

Over age 60:
Adverse reactions and side effects may be more frequent and severe than in younger persons.

Pregnancy:
Decide with your doctor whether drug benefits justify risk to unborn child. Risk category C (see page xviii).

Breast-feeding:
Drug passes into milk and decreases milk flow. Avoid drug or discontinue nursing until you finish medicine. Consult doctor for advice on maintaining milk supply.

Infants & children:
Use only under medical supervision.

Prolonged use:
Chronic constipation, possible fecal impaction. Consult doctor immediately.

Skin & sunlight:
No problems expected.

Driving, piloting or hazardous work:
Use disqualifies you for piloting aircraft. Don't drive until you learn how medicine affects you. Don't work around dangerous machinery. Don't climb ladders or work in high places.

Discontinuing:
May be unnecessary to finish medicine. Follow doctor's instructions.

Others:
Advise any doctor or dentist whom you consult that you take this medicine.

POSSIBLE INTERACTION WITH OTHER DRUGS

GENERIC NAME OR DRUG CLASS	COMBINED EFFECT
Adrenocorticoids, systemic	Possible glaucoma.
Amantadine	Increased scopolamine effect.
Antacids*	Decreased scopolamine effect.
Anticholinergics*, other	Increased scopolamine effect.
Antidepressants, tricyclic*	Increased scopolamine effect. Increased sedation.
Antidiarrheals*	Decreased scopolamine effect.
Antihistamines*	Increased scopolamine effect.
Attapulgite	Decreased scopolamine effect.
Buclizine	Increased scopolamine effect.
Clozapine	Toxic effect on the central nervous system.
Digitalis preparations*	Possible decreased absorption of scopolamine.
Encainide	Increased effect of toxicity on heart muscle.
Ethinamate	Dangerous increased effects of ethinamate. Avoid combining.
Fluoxetine	Increased depressant effects of both drugs.
Guanfacine	May increase depressant effects of either medicine.
Haloperidol	Increased internal eye pressure.
Ketoconazole	Decreased keto-conazole effect.
Leucovorin	High alcohol content of leucovorin may cause adverse effects.
Meperidine	Increased scopolamine effect.
Methylphenidate	Increased scopolamine effect.
Methyprylon	May increase seda-tive effect to danger-ous level. Avoid.
Molindone	Increased anti-cholinergic effect.
Monoamine oxidase (MAO) inhibitors*	Increased scopolamine effect.

Continued on page 930

POSSIBLE INTERACTION WITH OTHER SUBSTANCES

INTERACTS WITH	COMBINED EFFECT
Alcohol:	None expected.
Beverages:	None expected.
Cocaine:	Excessively rapid heartbeat. Avoid.
Foods:	None expected.
Marijuana:	Drowsiness, dry mouth.
Tobacco:	None expected.

SELECTIVE SEROTONIN REUPTAKE INHIBITORS (SSRIs)

GENERIC AND BRAND NAMES

CITALOPRAM
Celexa
FLUOXETINE
Prozac
Prozac Weekly
Sarafem
FLUVOXAMINE
Luvox
PAROXETINE
Paxil
SERTRALINE
Zoloft

BASIC INFORMATION

Habit forming? No
Prescription needed? Yes
Available as generic? No
Drug class: Antidepressant, antiobsessional agent, antianxiety agent.

USES

- Treatment for mental depression.
- Treatment for obsessive compulsive disorder.
- Fluoxetine is used for treatment of premenstrual dysphoric disorder (PMDD).*
- Fluoxetine and fluvoxamine treat bulimia.
- Paroxetine also treats anxiety and Post Traumatic Stress Disorder (PTSD).

DOSAGE & USAGE INFORMATION

How to take:
- Capsules or tablets—Swallow with water. May be taken with or without food. If you can't swallow whole, crumble tablet or open capsule and take with liquid or food.
- Oral solution—follow instructions on label.

When to take:
At the same time each day or weekly, usually in the am. Fluvoxamine dosage might be twice daily.

If you forget a dose:
Take as soon as you remember. If it is near the time of your next dose, skip the missed dose and resume normal schedule. Don't double this dose.

OVERDOSE

SYMPTOMS:
Dizziness, sweating, nausea, vomiting, tremor, heart rhythm disturbances. In rare cases, amnesia, coma and convulsions have occurred.
WHAT TO DO:
- **Dial 911 (emergency) for an ambulance or medical help or poison center 1-800-222-1222. Then give first aid immediately.**
- **See emergency information at end of book.**

What drug does:
Affects serotonin, one of the chemicals in the brain called neurotransmitters, that plays a role in emotions and psychological disturbances.

Time lapse before drug works:
1 to 4 weeks.

Don't take with:
Any other prescription or nonprescription drugs without consulting your doctor or pharmacist.

POSSIBLE ADVERSE REACTIONS OR SIDE EFFECTS

SYMPTOMS	WHAT TO DO
Life-threatening:	
Rash, itchy skin, breathing problems, chest pain (allergic reaction).	Seek emergency treatment immediately.
Common:	
Drowsiness, nausea, cough or hoarseness, lower back or side pain, sores on lips or mouth, constipation or diarrhea, headache, anxiety, changes in sexual desire or function, insomnia, dry mouth, unusual weakness or tiredness.	Continue. Call doctor when convenient
Infrequent:	
• Vision changes, confusion, apathy (lack of emotion), breathing difficulty, chills, black or tarry stools, fever, enlarged lymph glands, heart rhythm changes, vomiting, skin rash or itching.	Discontinue. Call doctor right away.
• Abdominal pain, loss of appetite, yawning, tingling, skin burning or prickly feeling, stuffy nose, change in sense of taste, tooth grinding, trembling, increased saliva, gas heartburn, sweating,. urinary changes, muscle or joint pain, menstrual changes, weight changes, loss of hair.	Continue. Call doctor when convenient.

SELECTIVE SEROTONIN REUPTAKE INHIBITORS (SSRIs)

Rare:

• Seizures (convulsions)	Discontinue. Seek emergency help.
• Abnormal bleeding breast tenderness or enlargement; red peeling skin, red or irritated eyes, sore throat, sudden body or facial spasms, dizziness, signs of low blood sugar (anxiety, chills, nervousness, difficulty concentrating), clumsiness,	Discontinue. Call doctor right away.

WARNINGS & PRECAUTIONS

Don't take if:
- You are allergic to any SSRI's.
- You currently take (or have taken in the last two weeks) a monoamine oxidase (MAO) inhibitor.

Before you start, consult your doctor:
- If you have any other medical problem.
- If you have had kidney or liver problems.
- If you have a history of seizure disorders.
- If you have a history of drug abuse or dependence.
- If you have a history of mood disorders, such as mania, or thoughts of suicide.
- If you are allergic to any medication, food or other substances.

Over age 60:
Adverse reactions and side effects may be more severe and frequent than in younger patients; dosage may need to be adjusted.

Pregnancy:
Decide with your doctor if drug benefits justify risk to unborn child. Risk category C (see page xviii).

Breast-feeding:
Drugs pass into milk. Avoid drug or discontinue nursing until you finish medicine. Consult doctor for advice on maintaining milk supply.

Infants & children:
Safety and effectiveness in children has not been established. Fluvoxamine not recommended for children under 8 years of age.

Prolonged use:
No problems expected. Your doctor should periodically evaluate your response to the drug and adjust the dose if necessary.

Skin & sunlight:
One or more drugs in this group may cause rash or intensify sunburn in areas exposed to sun or ultraviolet light (photosensitivity reaction). Avoid overexposure. Notify doctor if reaction occurs.

Driving, piloting or hazardous work:
Don't drive or pilot aircraft until you learn how medicine affects you. Don't work around dangerous machinery. Don't climb ladders or work in high places. Danger increases if you drink alcohol or take medicine affecting alertness and reflexes.

Discontinuing:
- Don't discontinue without consulting doctor. You may need to reduce the dose gradually to avoid side effects.
- After discontinuing the drug, call your doctor right away if any new or unusual symptoms develop (emotional or physical).

Others:
- Advise any doctor or dentist whom you consult that you take this medicine.
- Take medicine only as directed. Do not increase or reduce dosage without doctor's approval.

POSSIBLE INTERACTION WITH OTHER DRUGS

GENERIC NAME OR DRUG CLASS	COMBINED EFFECT
Anticoagulants, oral*	Increased risk of side effects of both drugs.
Antidepressants, tricyclic*	Increased risk of side effects.
Benzodiazepines*	Increased benzo-diazepine effect.
Bromocriptine	Increased risk of serotonin syndrome*.
Buspirone	Increased risk of serotonin syndrome*.

Continued on page 930

POSSIBLE INTERACTION WITH OTHER SUBSTANCES

INTERACTS WITH	COMBINED EFFECT
Alcohol:	Contributes to depression. Avoid.
Beverages:	None expected.
Cocaine:	Effects unknown. Avoid.
Foods:	None expected.
Marijuana:	Effects unknown. Avoid.
Tobacco:	None expected.

***See Glossary**

SELEGILINE

BRAND NAMES

Carbex
Eldepryl
Jumex
Jumexal
Juprenil
Movergan
Procythol
SD Deprenyl

BASIC INFORMATION

All the information in this chart applies only when selegiline is given with other drugs that treat Parkinson's disease.

Habit forming? No
Prescription needed? Yes
Available as generic? Yes
Drug class: Antidyskinetic

USES

- Treats Parkinson's disease *(paralysis agitans)* when given with levodopa or the combination of levodopa and carbidopa.
- Treats mental depression when taken alone.

DOSAGE & USAGE INFORMATION

How to take:
Tablets—Swallow with liquid. If you can't swallow whole, crumble tablet and take with liquid or food.

Continued next column

OVERDOSE

SYMPTOMS:
Mouth-opening difficulty; neck and heel muscle spasm; sweating; irregular, fast heartbeat; reflexes hyperactive; cold or clammy skin; chest pain; agitation; fainting; seizures; coma. Symptoms can develop 12 to 48 hours after ingestion.
WHAT TO DO:

- **Dial 911 (emergency) for an ambulance or medical help or poison center 1-800-222-1222. Then give first aid immediately.**
- **If patient is unconsciousness and not breathing, give mouth-to-mouth breathing. If there is no heartbeat, use cardiac massage and mouth-to-mouth breathing (CPR). Don't try to make patient vomit. If you can't get help quickly, take patient to nearest emergency facility.**
- **See emergency information on inside covers.**

When to take:
Usually taken at breakfast and lunch to minimize nausea or insomnia. Don't take after mid-afternoon.

If you forget a dose:
Take as soon as you remember up to 2 hours late. If more than 2 hours, wait for next scheduled dose (don't double this dose).

What drug does:
Inhibits action of monoamine oxidase Type B (MAO B), a major chemical enzyme in the brain. Doses higher than recommended can cause high blood pressure.

Time lapse before drug works:
2 hours.

Don't take with:

- Any foods containing tyramine, such as cheese; wine; beer; nonalcoholic beer; liqueurs; yeast extracts; bean pods; pickled or smoked fish, meat, chicken, turkey or other poultry; fermented sausage (summer sausage, salami, pepperoni); bologna; overripe fruit; caffeine.
- Any other medicines (including over-the-counter drugs such as cough and cold medicines, laxatives, antacids, diet pills, nose drops or vitamins) without consulting your doctor.

POSSIBLE ADVERSE REACTIONS OR SIDE EFFECTS

SYMPTOMS	WHAT TO DO
Life-threatening:	
• In case of overdose, see previous column.	
• Severe chest pain, enlarged pupils, heartbeat irregularities, severe nausea and vomiting, stiff neck.	Seek emergency treatment.
Common:	
• Mood changes, unusual or uncontrolled body movements, hallucinations, headache, lip smacking, difficult urination.	Discontinue. Call doctor right away.
• Abdominal pain, dizziness, dry mouth, insomnia, mild nausea.	Continue. Call doctor when convenient.
Infrequent:	
• Chest pain, heartbeat irregularities, wheezing, swollen feet, speech difficulty, bloody or black stools.	Discontinue. Seek emergency treatment.

• Constipation; anxiety; tiredness; eyelid spasm; unpleasant taste; blurred vision; leg pain; ringing ears; chills; skin rash; burning lips or mouth; drowsiness; frequent, decreased urination.	Continue. Call doctor when convenient.
Rare:	
Weight loss, heartburn, jaw clenching or teeth gnashing, impaired memory, uncontrolled body movements.	Continue. Call doctor when convenient.

WARNINGS & PRECAUTIONS

Don't take if:
You are allergic to selegiline.

Before you start, consult your doctor:
If you have a past medical history of peptic ulcer, profound dementia, severe psychosis, tardive dyskinesia, excessive tremor.

Over age 60:
Adverse reactions and side effects may be more frequent and severe than in younger persons. You may need smaller doses for shorter periods of time.

Pregnancy:
Decide with your doctor if drug benefits justify risk to unborn child. Risk category C (see page xviii).

Breast-feeding:
Unknown if drug passes into milk. Consult doctor.

Infants & children:
Not recommended.

Prolonged use:
Talk to your doctor about the need for follow-up medical examinations or laboratory studies to check complete blood counts (white blood cell count, platelet count, red blood cell count, hemoglobin, hematocrit), stomach x-rays.

Skin & sunlight:
May cause rash or intensify sunburn in areas exposed to sun or ultraviolet light (photosensitivity reaction). Avoid overexposure. Notify doctor if reaction occurs.

Driving, piloting or hazardous work:
Don't drive or pilot aircraft until you learn how medicine affects you. Don't work around dangerous machinery. Don't climb ladders or work in high places. Danger increases if you drink alcohol or take medicine affecting alertness and reflexes.

Discontinuing:
No special problems expected.

Others:
- Avoid sudden rises from lying-down or sitting positions.
- Advise any doctor or dentist whom you consult that you take this medicine.
- May affect results in some medical tests.

POSSIBLE INTERACTION WITH OTHER DRUGS

GENERIC NAME OR DRUG CLASS	COMBINED EFFECT
Caffeine (high doses)	Can cause same symptoms as tyramine-containing foods*. (See "Don't Take With" information block on previous page).
Fluoxetine	Increased risk of mental status changes.
Levodopa	Increased risk of adverse reactions.
Meperdine	Possibly severe drop in blood pressure. Avoid.
Narcotics*	Severe toxic reaction leading to seizures, coma, and/or death.

Continued on page 931

POSSIBLE INTERACTION WITH OTHER SUBSTANCES

INTERACTS WITH	COMBINED EFFECT
Alcohol:	Can cause severe toxicity. Avoid.
Beverages: Drinks containing large quantities of caffeine.	Can cause severe toxicity. Avoid.
Cocaine:	High blood pressure, rapid heartbeat. Avoid.
Foods: Tyramine-containing*. (See "Don't Take With" information block on previous page).	Severe toxicity, perhaps leading to death. *Carefully* avoid.
Marijuana:	Rapid heart rate. Avoid.
Tobacco:	Rapid heart rate. Avoid.

*See Glossary

SIBUTRAMINE

BRAND NAMES

Meridia

BASIC INFORMATION

Habit forming? Dependence possible
Prescription needed? Yes
Available as generic? No
Drug class: Appetite suppressant

USES

Treatment for obesity and maintenance of weight loss. The drug is to be used in conjunction with a reduced calorie diet and weight management program. Treatment with this drug is not recommended for "cosmetic" weight loss—that is when a person's height-to-weight ratio does not provide a medical reason for weight loss. Your doctor will help determine your body mass index (BMI), a method of measuring for obesity.

DOSAGE & USAGE INFORMATION

How to take:
Capsule–Swallow with liquid. It may be taken with or without food. Read instructions carefully that are provided with the prescription.

When to take:
Once a day usually in the morning.

If you forget a dose:
Take as soon as you remember. If it is almost time for the next dose, then skip the missed dose and wait for your next scheduled dose (don't double this dose).

What drug does:
Allows certain chemicals in the brain to act longer in controlling appetite regulating center.

Time lapse before drug works:
Weight loss should begin within 4 weeks.

Don't take with:
Any other prescription or non-prescription drug without consulting your doctor or pharmacist.

Continued next column

OVERDOSE

SYMPTOMS:
It is unknown what symptoms may occur. There is very limited experience with overdose.
WHAT TO DO:
If person takes much larger amount than prescribed, call doctor, poison center 1-800-222-1222 or hospital emergency room for instructions.

POSSIBLE ADVERSE REACTIONS OR SIDE EFFECTS

SYMPTOMS	WHAT TO DO
Life-threatening: None known.	
Common: Dry mouth, headache, constipation, insomnia (these symptoms usually go away with continued treatment).	Continue. Call doctor when convenient.
Infrequent:	
• Increase in blood pressure or heart rate.	Discontinue. Call doctor right away.
• Back pain, flu-like symptoms, stomach pain, increased appetite, nausea, heartburn, muscle aches, dizziness, nervousness, anxiety, depression, sore throat, runny nose.	Continue. Call doctor when convenient.
Rare: Chest pain, fainting, swelling of feet or ankles, allergic reaction including skin rash or hives, seizure, any other symptoms you are concerned about.	Discontinue. Call doctor right away.

WARNINGS & PRECAUTIONS

Don't take if:
- You are allergic to sibutramine.
- If you have a history of anorexia nervosa.

Before you start, consult your doctor:
- If you have a history of uncontrolled high blood pressure, any heart disorder, coronary artery disease, stroke (or symptoms of a stroke), seizures, or other medical problem.
- If you have any kidney or liver disorder.
- If organic causes of obesity have not been ruled out, such as hypothyroidism.
- If you have glaucoma.
- If you are allergic to any other medication, food or other substance.

Over age 60:
No special problems expected, but a lower starting dosage may be recommended.

Pregnancy:
Sibutramine is not recommended for pregnant women. Risk category C (see page xviii).

Breast-feeding:
It is unknown if drug passes into milk. Avoid drug or discontinue nursing until you finish medicine. Consult doctor for advice on maintaining milk supply.

Infants & children:
Safety and effectiveness in ages under 16 has not established.

Prolonged use:
- Schedule regular visits to your doctor to determine if drug is continuing to be effective in controlling weight and to monitor your blood pressure.
- The effectiveness and safety of taking this drug beyond one year have not been established.

Skin & sunlight:
No problems expected.

Driving, piloting or hazardous work:
Don't drive or pilot aircraft until you learn how medicine affects you. Don't work around dangerous machinery. Don't climb ladders or work in high places. Danger increases if you drink alcohol or take other medicines affecting alertness and reflexes.

Discontinuing:
Notify your doctor if any new symptoms occur after the drug is stopped.

Others:
- Advise any doctor or dentist whom you consult that you take this medicine.
- Use as directed. Don't increase or decrease dosage without doctor's approval.
- Notify your doctor if you don't lose at least 4 pounds in the first month of treatment.
- Other weight control agents have been associated with heart valve problems and primary pulmonary hypertension.
- Monitor blood pressure.

POSSIBLE INTERACTION WITH OTHER DRUGS

GENERIC NAME OR DRUG CLASS	COMBINED EFFECT
Appetite suppressants*, other	Unknown effect. Avoid.
Decongestants*	May cause increase in blood pressure or heart rate. Avoid.
Central nervous system (CNS) depressants*	Increased sedation. Avoid.
Erythromycin	Increased effect of sibutramine.
Ketoconazole	Increased effect of sibutramine.
Monoamine oxidase, (MAO) inhibitors	Potentially life-threatening. Allow 14 days between use of 2 drugs.
Serotonergic agents*, other	May cause serotonin syndrome*. Avoid.

POSSIBLE INTERACTION WITH OTHER SUBSTANCES

INTERACTS WITH	COMBINED EFFECT
Alcohol:	Increased sedation. Avoid.
Beverages:	None expected.
Cocaine:	Unknown effect. Best to avoid.
Foods:	None expected.
Marijuana:	Unknown effect. Best to avoid.
Tobacco:	None expected.

*See Glossary

SILDENAFIL CITRATE

BRAND NAMES

Viagra

BASIC INFORMATION

Habit forming? No
Prescription needed? Yes
Available as generic? No
Drug class: Impotence therapy

USES

Treats male sexual function (erection) problems.

DOSAGE & USAGE INFORMATION

How to take:
Tablets—Swallow with water. If you can't swallow whole, crumble tablet and take with liquid or food.

When to take:
Take one-half hour to four hours before sexual activity. Use only once daily.

If you forget a dose:
Does not apply.

What drug does:
Increases blood flow to the penis, resulting in an erection.

Time lapse before drug works:
One-half hour to one hour.

Don't take with:
Any other prescription or nonprescription drug without consulting your doctor or pharmacist.

OVERDOSE

SYMPTOMS:
Same as those listed under Possible Adverse Reactions or Side Effects, with increased likelihood.
WHAT TO DO:
If person takes much larger amount than prescribed, call doctor, poison center 1-800-222-1222 or hospital emergency room for instructions.

POSSIBLE ADVERSE REACTIONS OR SIDE EFFECTS

SYMPTOMS	WHAT TO DO
Life-threatening:	
Fatalities have been reported when used with nitrate medications.	
Common:	
Headache, flushing, stomach upset, nasal stuffiness.	Continue. Call doctor if symptoms persist.
Infrequent:	
• Pain or other urination problems, blurred vision, changes in color perception, sensitivity to light, skin rash, dizziness, prolonged erection (lasting more than 4 hours).	Discontinue. Call doctor right away.
• Diarrhea.	Continue. Call doctor if symptoms persist.
Rare:	
Chest pain, fainting, foot or ankle swelling.	Discontinue. Call doctor right away.

WARNINGS & PRECAUTIONS

Don't take if:
You are allergic to sildenafil citrate.

Before you start, consult your doctor:
- If you have any other medical problem.
- If you have heart problems.
- If you have a bleeding disorder (e.g., ulcer).
- If you have vision problems.
- If you have any physical abnormalities of the penis.
- If you have or have had liver or kidney disease.

Over age 60:
Adverse reactions and side effects, especially, may be more severe and frequent than in younger patients.

Pregnancy:
Not indicated for use in females. Risk category B (see page xviii).

Breast-feeding:
Not indicated for use in females.

Infants & children:
Safety and effectiveness of use in children not established. Not recommended.

Prolonged use:
Talk to your doctor about the need for follow-up medical examinations or laboratory studies to determine drug's effectiveness.

Skin & sunlight:
No problems expected.

Driving, piloting or hazardous work:
Avoid if you feel side effects such as nausea and vomiting.

Discontinuing:
Your doctor will determine the schedule.

Others:
- Advise any doctor or dentist whom you consult that you take this medicine.
- Consult doctor if there are any significant changes in your vision.
- Do not combine the drug with any other impotence therapy unless approved by your doctor.
- There are many causes of impotence. Your doctor should perform a complete exam before prescribing this medication.

POSSIBLE INTERACTION WITH OTHER DRUGS

GENERIC NAME OR DRUG CLASS	COMBINED EFFECT
Enzyme inhibitors*	Increased blood level of sildenafil.
Nitrates	Increased effect of nitrates. Do not use.
Rifampin	Decreased effect of sildenafil.

POSSIBLE INTERACTION WITH OTHER SUBSTANCES

INTERACTS WITH	COMBINED EFFECT
Alcohol:	May inhibit the effects of sildenafil.
Beverages:	Grapefruit juice may increase blood levels of sildenafil.
Cocaine:	Effects unknown. Avoid.
Foods:	Grapefruit juice may increase blood levels of sildenafil.
Marijuana:	Effects unknown. Avoid.
Tobacco:	None expected.

***See Glossary**

SIMETHICONE

BRAND NAMES

Degas
Di-Gel
Extra Strength Gas-X
Extra Strength Maalox Anti-Gas
Extra Strength Maalox GRF Gas Relief Formula
Flatulex
Gas Aid
Gas Relief
Gas-X
Gas-X Extra Strength
Gas-X with Maalox
Gelusil
Genasyme
Imodium Advanced
Maalox Anti-Gas
Maalox GRF Gas Relief Formula
Maximum Strength Mylanta Gas Relief
Maximum Strength Phazyme
Mygel
Mylanta Gas
Mylicon
Mylicon-80
Mylicon-125
Ovol
Ovol 40
Ovol-80
Phazyme
Phazyme 55
Phazyme 95
Riopan Plus

BASIC INFORMATION

Habit forming? No
Prescription needed? No
Available as generic? Yes, for some
Drug class: Antiflatulent

USES

- Treatment for retention of abdominal gas.
- Used prior to x-ray of abdomen to reduce gas shadows.

DOSAGE & USAGE INFORMATION

How to take:
- Tablet or capsule—Swallow with liquid.
- Liquid—Dissolve in water. Drink complete dose.
- Chewable tablets—Chew completely. Don't swallow whole.

When to take:
After meals and at bedtime.

Continued next column

What drug does:
Reduces surface tension of gas bubbles in stomach.

Time lapse before drug works:
10 minutes.

If you forget a dose:
Take when remembered if needed.

Don't take with:
Any other medicine without consulting your doctor or pharmacist.

OVERDOSE

SYMPTOMS:
None expected.
WHAT TO DO:
Overdose unlikely to threaten life. If person takes much larger amount than prescribed, call doctor, poison center 1-800-222-1222 or hospital emergency room for instructions.

POSSIBLE ADVERSE REACTIONS OR SIDE EFFECTS

SYMPTOMS	WHAT TO DO
Life-threatening: None expected.	
Common: None expected.	
Infrequent: None expected.	
Rare: None expected.	

WARNINGS & PRECAUTIONS

Don't take if:
You are allergic to simethicone.

Before you start, consult your doctor:
No problems expected.

Over age 60:
No problems expected.

Pregnancy:
Consult doctor. Risk category C (see page xviii).

Breast-feeding:
No problems expected. Consult doctor.

Infants & children:
Not recommended.

Prolonged use:
No problems expected.

Skin & sunlight:
No problems expected.

Driving, piloting or hazardous work:
No problems expected.

Discontinuing:
May be unnecessary to finish medicine. Discontinue when symptoms disappear.

Others:
No problems expected.

POSSIBLE INTERACTION WITH OTHER DRUGS

GENERIC NAME OR DRUG CLASS	COMBINED EFFECT
None significant.	

POSSIBLE INTERACTION WITH OTHER SUBSTANCES

INTERACTS WITH	COMBINED EFFECT
Alcohol:	None expected.
Beverages:	None expected.
Cocaine:	None expected.
Foods:	None expected.
Marijuana:	None expected.
Tobacco:	None expected.

SODIUM BICARBONATE

BRAND NAMES

Alka-Seltzer Effervescent Pain Reliever & Antacid
Alka-Seltzer Morning Relief
Arm & Hammer Pure Baking Soda
Bell/ans
Bromo-Seltzer
Citrocarbonate
Soda Mint

BASIC INFORMATION

Habit forming? No
Prescription needed? No
Available as generic? Yes
Drug class: Alkalizer, antacid

USES

- Treats metobolic acidosis.
- Alkalinizes urine to reduce uric acid kidney stones.
- Treats hyperacidity of the stomach that is present with indigestion, gastroesophageal reflux and peptic ulcer disease.

DOSAGE & USAGE INFORMATION

How to take:
- Tablets—Swallow with liquid. If you can't swallow whole, crumble tablet and take with liquid or food.
- Powder—Mix in a glass of water and drink.
- Effervescent sodium bicarbonate—Mix in a glass of cold water and drink.

When to take:
- For hyperacidity—1 to 3 hours after meals.
- For kidney stones—According to prescription instructions.

If you forget a dose:
Take as soon as you remember up to 2 hours late. If more than 2 hours, wait for next scheduled dose (don't double this dose).

Continued next column

OVERDOSE

SYMPTOMS:
Excessive swelling of feet and lower legs.
WHAT TO DO:
Overdose unlikely to threaten life. If person takes much larger amount than prescribed, call doctor, poison center 1-800-222-1222 or hospital emergency room for instructions.

What drug does:
- Buffers acid in the stomach.
- Increases excretion of bicarbonate in the urine to help dissolve uric acid stones.

Time lapse before drug works:
Works immediately, but the duration of effect is short.

Don't take with:
Nonprescription drugs without consulting doctor.

POSSIBLE ADVERSE REACTIONS OR SIDE EFFECTS

SYMPTOMS	WHAT TO DO
Life-threatening: None expected.	
Common: None expected.	
Infrequent:	
• Stomach cramps that continue.	Discontinue. Call doctor right away.
• Nausea, headache, appetite loss (with long-term use).	Continue. Call doctor when convenient.
Rare:	
Muscle pain or twitching, nervousness, breathing difficulty, mild swelling of feet or lower legs (with large doses).	Discontinue. Call doctor right away.

WARNINGS & PRECAUTIONS

Don't take if:
You are allergic to sodium bicarbonate.

Before you start, consult your doctor:
If you have heart disease, kidney disease or toxemia of pregnancy.

Over age 60:
Adverse reactions and side effects may be more frequent and severe than in younger persons.

Pregnancy:
May cause weight gain and swelling of feet and ankles. Avoid if you have high blood pressure. Consult doctor. Risk category C (see page xviii).

Breast-feeding:
No problems expected, but consult doctor.

Infants & children:
Not recommended. Safety and dosage have not been established.

Prolonged use:
Don't use for longer than prescribed or recommended. May cause sodium overload.

Skin & sunlight:
No special problems expected.

Driving, piloting or hazardous work:
No special problems expected.

Discontinuing:
May be unnecessary to finish medicine. Follow doctor's instructions.

Others:
- Heat and moisture in bathroom medicine cabinet can cause breakdown of medicine. Store someplace else.
- May interfere with the accuracy of some medical tests (especially acidosis and urinalysis tests).

POSSIBLE INTERACTION WITH OTHER DRUGS

GENERIC NAME OR DRUG CLASS	COMBINED EFFECT
Adrenocorticoids*	Sodium overload.
Cortisone	Sodium overload.
Ketoconazole	Decreased absorption of ketoconazole.
Mecamylamine	Increased mecamylamine effect.
Methenamine	Decreased methenamine effect.
Tetracyclines*	Greatly reduced absorption of tetracyclines.
Any other medicine	Decreased absorption of other medicine if taken within 1 to 2 hours oftaking sodium bicarbonate.

POSSIBLE INTERACTION WITH OTHER SUBSTANCES

INTERACTS WITH	COMBINED EFFECT
Alcohol:	Decreased effectiveness of sodium bicarbonate.
Beverages: Milk and milk products (large amounts).	Increased risk of side effects.
Cocaine:	None expected.
Foods:	None expected.
Marijuana:	None expected.
Tobacco:	Decreased effectiveness of sodium bicarbonate.

*See Glossary

SODIUM FLUORIDE

BRAND NAMES

Fluor-A-Day
Fluorident
Fluoritab
Fluorodex
Fluotic
Flura
Karidium
Listermint with Fluoride
Luride
Luride-SF
Pediaflor
Pedi-Dent
Solu-Flur

Numerous other multiple vitamin-mineral supplements. Check labels.

BASIC INFORMATION

Habit forming? No
Prescription needed? Yes, for some
Available as generic? Yes
Drug class: Mineral supplement (fluoride)

USES

- Reduces tooth cavities.
- Treats osteoporosis.

DOSAGE & USAGE INFORMATION

How to take:
- Tablet—Swallow with liquid or crumble tablet and take with liquid (not milk) or food.
- Liquid—Measure with dropper and take directly or with liquid.
- Chewable tablets—Chew slowly and thoroughly before swallowing.

When to take:
Usually at bedtime after teeth are thoroughly brushed.

Continued next column

OVERDOSE

SYMPTOMS:
Stomach cramps or pain, nausea, faintness, vomiting (possibly bloody), diarrhea, black stools, shallow breathing, muscle spasms, seizures, arrhythmias.

WHAT TO DO:
- **Dial 911 (emergency) for an ambulance or medical help or poison center 1-800-222-1222. Then give first aid immediately.**
- **See emergency information on inside covers.**

If you forget a dose:
Take as soon as you remember. Don't double a forgotten dose. Return to schedule.

What drug does:
Provides supplemental fluoride to combat tooth decay.

Time lapse before drug works:
8 weeks to provide maximum effect.

Don't take with:
Any other medicine simultaneously.

POSSIBLE ADVERSE REACTIONS OR SIDE EFFECTS

SYMPTOMS	WHAT TO DO
Life-threatening: In case of overdose, see previous column.	
Common: Constipation, appetite loss.	Continue. Call doctor when convenient.
Infrequent:	
• Rash.	Discontinue. Call doctor right away.
• Tooth discoloration.	Continue. Call doctor when convenient.
Rare:	
• Severe upsets (digestive) only with overdose.	Discontinue. Seek emergency treatment.
• Sores in mouth and lips, aching bones, stiffness.	Discontinue. Call doctor right away.

WARNINGS & PRECAUTIONS

Don't take if:
- Your water supply contains 0.7 parts fluoride per million. Too much fluoride stains teeth permanently.
- You are allergic to any fluoride-containing product.
- You have underactive thyroid.

Before you start, consult your doctor:
- If you have kidney disease.
- If you have ulcers.
- If you have joint pain.

Over age 60:
No problems expected.

Pregnancy:
Consult doctor. Risk category C (see page xviii).

Breast-feeding:
No problems expected. Consult doctor.

Infants & children:
No problems expected except accidental overdose. Keep vitamin-mineral supplements out of children's reach.

Prolonged use:
Excess may cause discolored teeth and decreased calcium in blood.

Skin & sunlight:
No problems expected.

Driving, piloting or hazardous work:
No problems expected.

Discontinuing:
No problems expected.

Others:
- Store in original plastic container. Fluoride decomposes glass.
- Some products contain tartrazine dye. Avoid, especially if you are allergic to aspirin.

POSSIBLE INTERACTION WITH OTHER DRUGS

GENERIC NAME OR DRUG CLASS	COMBINED EFFECT
Calcium supplements*	Decreased effect of calcium and fluoride.

POSSIBLE INTERACTION WITH OTHER SUBSTANCES

INTERACTS WITH	COMBINED EFFECT
Alcohol:	None expected.
Beverages:	
Milk.	Prevents absorption of fluoride. Space dose 2 hours before or after milk.
Cocaine:	None expected.
Foods:	None expected.
Marijuana:	None expected.
Tobacco:	None expected.

*See Glossary

STIMULANT MEDICATIONS

GENERIC AND BRAND NAMES

METHYLPHENIDATE
Concerta
Metadate CD
Metadate ER
Methylin ER
PMS Methylphenidate
Ritalin
Ritalin SR

DEXMETHYL-PHENIDATE
Focalin

BASIC INFORMATION

Habit forming? Yes
Prescription needed? Yes
Available as generic? Yes, for some
Drug class: Central nervous system stimulant, sympathomimetic

USES

- Decreases overactivity and lengthens attention span in children with attention-deficit hyperactivity disorder (ADHD). It is used as part of the total management plan that includes educational, social and psychological treatment.
- Treatment of depression in adults.
- Treatment for narcolepsy (uncontrollable attacks of sleepiness) and other disorders.

DOSAGE & USAGE INFORMATION

How to take:
- Tablet—Swallow with liquid or food to lessen stomach irritation. If you can't swallow whole, crumble tablet and take with liquid or small amount of food.

Continued next column

OVERDOSE

SYMPTOMS:
Rapid heartbeat, fever, confusion, vomiting, agitation, hallucinations, convulsions, coma.
WHAT TO DO:
- **Dial 911 (emergency) for an ambulance or medical help or poison center 1-800-222-1222. Then give first aid immediately.**
- **If patient is unconscious and not breathing, give mouth-to-mouth breathing. If there is no heartbeat, use cardiac massage and mouth-to-mouth breathing (CPR). Don't try to make patient vomit. If you can't get help quickly, take patient to nearest emergency facility.**
- **See emergency information at end of book.**

- Extended-release tablet—Swallow whole with liquid.

When to take:
- At the same times each day, preferably on an empty stomach.
- Take extended-release tablet in the morning. Regular tablet often taken at breakfast and lunch. Don't take late in evening.

If you forget a dose:
Take as soon as you remember up to 2 hours late. If more than 2 hours, wait for next scheduled dose (don't double this dose).

What drug does:
Stimulates brain to improve alertness, concentration and attention span. Calms the hyperactive child and improves the ability to focus.

Time lapse before drug works:
- 1 month or more for maximum effect on child.
- 30 minutes to stimulate adults.

Don't take with:
Any other medicine without consulting your doctor or pharmacist.

POSSIBLE ADVERSE REACTIONS OR SIDE EFFECTS

SYMPTOMS	WHAT TO DO
Life-threatening: In case of overdose, see previous column.	
Common: Nervousness, trouble sleeping, dizziness, nausea, appetite loss, headache, drowsiness, stomach pain, weight loss.	Continue. Call doctor when convenient.
Infrequent: Rash or hives; chest pain; fast, irregular heartbeat; unusual bruising; joint pain; psychosis; uncontrollable movements; unexplained fever.	Discontinue. Call doctor right away.
Rare: Blurred vision, other vision change, sore throat, unusual tiredness, convulsions.	Discontinue. Call doctor right away.

WARNINGS & PRECAUTIONS

Don't take if:
You are allergic to stimulant medications.

Before you start, consult your doctor:
- If you have epilepsy or have seizures.
- If you have high blood pressure, heart or liver problems.
- If you have glaucoma.
- If you take MAO inhibitors*.
- If you have emotional, depressive or psychotic problems or have motor tics.
- If you have a history of drug abuse.

Over age 60:
Adverse reactions and side effects may be more frequent and severe than in younger persons.

Pregnancy:
Decide with your doctor if drug benefits justify risk to unborn child. Risk category C (see page xviii).

Breast-feeding:
No proven problems. Consult doctor.

Infants & children:
Use only under medical supervision for children 6 or older. Don't give to child younger than 6.

Prolonged use:
- Rare possibility of physical growth retardation in children.
- Talk to your doctor about the need for follow-up medical examinations or laboratory studies to check blood pressure, complete blood counts (white blood cell count, platelet count, red blood cell count, hemoglobin, hematocrit), growth charts.

Skin & sunlight:
No problems expected.

Driving, piloting or hazardous work:
No problems expected.

Discontinuing:
Don't discontinue abruptly. Don't discontinue without doctor's advice until you complete prescribed dose, even though symptoms diminish or disappear. Report to your doctor any new symptoms of depression, unusual behavior, unusual weakness or tiredness.

Others:
- Dose must be carefully adjusted by doctor.
- Advise any doctor or dentist whom you consult about the use of this medicine.

POSSIBLE INTERACTION WITH OTHER DRUGS

GENERIC NAME OR DRUG CLASS	COMBINED EFFECT
Anticholinergics*	Increased anticholinergic effect.
Anticoagulants*, oral	Increased anti-coagulant effect.
Anticonvulsants*	Increased anticonvulsant effect.
Antidepressants, tricyclic*	Increased anti-depressant effect. Decreased stimulant medication effect.
Antihypertensives*	Decreased antihypertensive effect.
Central nervous system (CNS) stimulants*	Overstimulation.
Dextrothyroxine	Increased stimulant medication effect.
Guanethidine	Decreased guanethidine effect.
Monoamine oxidase (MAO) inhibitors*	Dangerous rise in blood pressure.
Pimozide	May mask the cause of tics.

POSSIBLE INTERACTION WITH OTHER SUBSTANCES

INTERACTS WITH	COMBINED EFFECT
Alcohol:	None expected.
Beverages: Caffeine drinks.	May raise blood pressure.
Cocaine:	High risk of heart-beat irregularities and high blood pressure.
Foods: Foods containing tyramine*.	May raise blood pressure.
Marijuana:	None expected.
Tobacco:	None expected.

*See Glossary

SUCRALFATE

BRAND NAMES

Carafate
Sulcrate
Sulcrate Suspension Plus

BASIC INFORMATION

Habit forming? No
Prescription needed? Yes
Available as generic? Yes
Drug class: Antiulcer agent

USES

- Treatment for duodenal and gastric ulcers.
- Used to relieve side effects of nonsteroidal anti-inflammatory therapy in rheumatoid arthritis.
- Treatment for gastroesophageal reflux disease (GERD).

DOSAGE & USAGE INFORMATION

How to take:
- Tablet—Take as directed on an empty stomach.
- Oral suspension—Follow instructions on package.

When to take:
1 hour before meals and at bedtime. Allow 2 hours to elapse before taking other prescription medicines.

If you forget a dose:
Take as soon as you remember up to 2 hours late. If more than 2 hours, wait for next scheduled dose (don't double this dose).

What drug does:
Covers ulcer site and protects from acid, enzymes and bile salts.

Time lapse before drug works:
Begins in 30 minutes. May require several days to relieve pain.

Don't take with:
Any other medicine without consulting your doctor or pharmacist.

OVERDOSE

SYMPTOMS:
None expected.
WHAT TO DO:
Overdose unlikely to threaten life. If person takes much larger amount than prescribed, call doctor, poison center 1-800-222-1222 or hospital emergency room for instructions.

POSSIBLE ADVERSE REACTIONS OR SIDE EFFECTS

SYMPTOMS	WHAT TO DO
Life-threatening: None expected.	
Common: Constipation.	Continue. Call doctor when convenient.
Infrequent: Dizziness, sleepiness, rash, itchy skin, abdominal pain, indigestion, vomiting, nausea, dry mouth, diarrhea.	Continue. Call doctor when convenient.
Rare: Back pain.	Continue. Call doctor when convenient.

WARNINGS & PRECAUTIONS

Don't take if:
You are allergic to sucralfate.

Before you start, consult your doctor:
- If you will have surgery within 2 months, including dental surgery, requiring general or spinal anesthesia.
- If you have gastrointestinal or kidney disease.

Over age 60:
Adverse reactions and side effects may be more frequent and severe than in younger persons.

Pregnancy:
No proven harm to unborn child. Avoid if possible. Consult doctor. Risk category B (see page xviii).

Breast-feeding:
Unknown effects. Consult doctor.

Infants & children:
Safety not established.

Prolonged use:
Request blood counts if medicine needed longer than 8 weeks.

Skin & sunlight:
No problems expected.

Driving, piloting or hazardous work:
Don't drive or pilot aircraft until you learn how medicine affects you. Don't work around dangerous machinery. Don't climb ladders or work in high places. Danger increases if you drink alcohol or take medicine affecting alertness and reflexes, such as antihistamines, tranquilizers, sedatives, pain medicine, narcotics and mind-altering drugs.

Discontinuing:
Don't discontinue without consulting doctor. Dose may require gradual reduction if you have taken drug for a long time. Doses of other drugs may also require adjustment.

Others:
No problems expected.

POSSIBLE INTERACTION WITH OTHER DRUGS

GENERIC NAME OR DRUG CLASS	COMBINED EFFECT
Anagrelide	May interfere with anagrelide absorption.
Antacids*	Take 1/2 hour before or after sucralfate.
Cimetidine	Possible decreased absorption of cimetidine if taken simultaneously.
Ciprofloxacin	Decreased absorption of ciprofloxacin. Take 2 hours before sucralfate.
Digoxin	Decreased absorption of digoxin. Take 2 hours before sucralfate.
Fluoroquinolones	Decreased fluoroquinolone effect.
Ketoconazole	Decreased ketoconazole effect.
Lansoprazole	Decreased effect of lansoprazole. Take it 30 minutes before sucralfate.
Norfloxacin	Decreased absorption of norfloxacin. Take 2 hours before sucralfate.
Ofloxacin	Decreased absorption of ofloxacin. Take 2 hours before sucralfate.
Phenytoin	Possible decreased absorption of phenytoin if taken simultaneously.
Tetracyclines*	Possible decreased absorption of tetracycline if taken simultaneously.
Theophylline	Decreased absorption of theophylline. Take 2 hours before sucralfate.
Vitamins A, D, E, K	Decreased vitamin absorption.

POSSIBLE INTERACTION WITH OTHER SUBSTANCES

INTERACTS WITH	COMBINED EFFECT
Alcohol:	Irritates ulcer. Avoid.
Beverages: Caffeine.	Irritates ulcer. Avoid.
Cocaine:	May make ulcer worse. Avoid.
Foods:	No problems expected.
Marijuana:	May make ulcer worse. Avoid.
Tobacco:	May make ulcer worse. Avoid.

*See Glossary

SULFADOXINE AND PYRIMETHAMINE

BRAND NAMES

Fansidar

BASIC INFORMATION

Habit forming? No
Prescription needed? Yes
Available as generic? No
Drug class: Antiprotozoal

USES

- Treats malaria *(plasmodium faciparum).*
- Helps prevent malaria when traveling to areas where it exists.
- Also used to prevent isosporiasis in patients with acquired immunodeficiency disease.

DOSAGE & USAGE INFORMATION

How to take:
Tablets—Swallow with liquid. If you can't swallow whole, crumble tablet and take with liquid or food. Instructions to take on empty stomach mean 1 hour before or 2 hours after eating.

When to take:
Follow doctor's instructions.

If you forget a dose:
Take as soon as you remember. If close to time for next dose, skip this one and wait for next scheduled dose. Don't double dose.

What drug does:
The sulfa component kills bacteria; the pyrimethamine works to kill malaria organisms in red blood cells or human tisue.

Time lapse before drug works:
2 to 6 hours.

Continued next column

OVERDOSE

SYMPTOMS:
Appetite loss, sore throat and fever, seizure, coma.
WHAT TO DO:
- **Dial 911 (emergency) for an ambulance or medical help or poison center 1-800-222-1222. Then give first aid immediately.**
- **See emergency information on inside front covers.**

Don't take with:
- Any other medicines (including over-the-counter drugs such as cough and cold medicines, laxatives, antacids, diet pills, caffeine, nose drops or vitamins) without consulting your doctor.
- Mefloquine.

POSSIBLE ADVERSE REACTIONS OR SIDE EFFECTS

SYMPTOMS	WHAT TO DO
Life-threatening: In case of overdose, see previous column.	
Common:	
Loss or change of taste; diarrhea; skin rash; pale skin; sore throat; sore, red tongue; mouth ulcers; fever; excessive bleeding; tiredness, light sensitivity.	Discontinue. Call doctor right away.
Infrequent:	
Aching joints, fever, skin blisters or peeling, jaundice (yellow skin and eyes).	Discontinue. Call doctor right away.
Rare:	
Bloody urine, burning on urination, back pain, swollen neck.	Discontinue. Call doctor right away.

SULFADOXINE AND PYRIMETHAMINE

WARNINGS & PRECAUTIONS

Don't take if:
You know you are allergic to sulfa drugs, furosemide, thiazide diuretics, carbonase anhydrase inhibitors.

Before you start, consult your doctor:
- If you have AIDS.
- If you have anemia, seizures, G6PD* deficiency, liver disease, porphyria, kidney disease.
- If you can't tolerate sulfa drugs.

Over age 60:
Adverse reactions and side effects may be more frequent and severe than in younger persons. You may need smaller doses for shorter periods of time.

Pregnancy:
Use birth control so you won't get pregnant while in an endemic malaria area. Should not be taken during pregnancy if it can possibly be avoided. Consult doctor. Risk category C (see page xviii).

Breast-feeding:
Drug passes into milk. Avoid drug or discontinue nursing until you finish medicine. Consult doctor for advice on maintaining milk supply.

Infants & children:
Don't use in infants under 2 months old.

Prolonged use:
Talk to your doctor about the need for follow-up medical examinations or laboratory studies to check complete blood counts (white blood cell count, platelet count, red blood cell count, hemoglobin, hematocrit) and urinalyses.

Skin & sunlight:
May cause rash or intensify sunburn in areas exposed to sun or ultraviolet light (photosensitivity reaction). Avoid overexposure. Notify doctor if reaction occurs.

Driving, piloting or hazardous work:
Avoid if you feel confused, drowsy or dizzy.

Discontinuing:
Don't discontinue for 4 to 6 weeks after you leave endemic malaria areas.

Others:
- Advise any doctor or dentist whom you consult that you take this medicine.
- May affect results in some medical tests.
- Sleep under mosquito netting while in endemic areas. Wear long-sleeved shirts and long pants.
- Report to your doctor if you develop any symptoms of illness while you take this medicine—even if the symptoms seem minor.

POSSIBLE INTERACTION WITH OTHER DRUGS

GENERIC NAME OR DRUG CLASS	COMBINED EFFECT
Anticoagulants*	Increased risk of toxicity.
Anticonvulsants*	Increased risk of toxicity.
Antidiabetics*	Increased risk of toxicity.
Bone marrow depressants*	Increased risk of bleeding or other toxic symptoms.
Clozapine	Toxic effect on the central nervous system.
Contraceptives, oral*	Reduced reliability of the pill.
Hepatotoxic medicines*	Increased risk of liver toxicity.
Methenamine	Increased risk of kidney toxicity.
Methotrexate	Increased risk of toxicity.
Zidovudine	Increased risk of liver toxicity.

POSSIBLE INTERACTION WITH OTHER SUBSTANCES

INTERACTS WITH	COMBINED EFFECT
Alcohol:	Nausea and vomiting. Avoid.
Beverages:	No special problems expected.
Cocaine:	Increased likelihood of adverse reactions or seizures. Avoid.
Foods:	No special problems expected.
Marijuana:	Increased likelihood of adverse reactions. Avoid.
Tobacco:	No special problems expected.

*See Glossary

SULFASALAZINE

BRAND NAMES

Azaline	Salazopyrin
Azulfidine	Salazosulfapyridine
Azulfidine En-Tabs	Salicylazosulfa-pyridine
PMS Sulfasalazine	S.A.S. Enteric-500
PMS Sulfasalazine EC	S.A.S.-500

BASIC INFORMATION

Habit forming? No
Prescription needed? Yes
Available as generic? Yes
Drug class: Sulfa (sulfonamide)

USES

- Treatment for ulceration and bleeding from ulcerative colitis.
- Treatment for rheumatoid arthritis for patients not responding to other treatments.

DOSAGE & USAGE INFORMATION

How to take:
- Tablet—Swallow with liquid. Instructions to take on empty stomach mean 1 hour before or 2 hours after eating.
- Liquid—Shake carefully before measuring.

When to take:
At the same times each day, evenly spaced.

If you forget a dose:
Take as soon as you remember up to 2 hours late. If more than 2 hours, wait for next scheduled dose (don't double this dose).

What drug does:
Anti-inflammatory action reduces tissue destruction in colon.

Time lapse before drug works:
2 to 5 days.

Don't take with:
Any other medicine without consulting your doctor or pharmacist.

OVERDOSE

SYMPTOMS:
Less urine, bloody urine, coma.
WHAT TO DO:
- **Dial 911 (emergency) for an ambulance or medical help or poison center 1-800-222-1222. Then give first aid immediately.**
- **See emergency information on inside covers.**

POSSIBLE ADVERSE REACTIONS OR SIDE EFFECTS

SYMPTOMS	WHAT TO DO
Life-threatening:	
In case of overdose, see previous column.	
Common:	
• Itchy skin, rash.	Discontinue. Call doctor right away.
• Headache, nausea, vomiting, diarrhea, appetite loss, skin sensitive to sun.	Continue. Call doctor when convenient.
• Orange urine or skin.	Continue. Tell doctor at next visit.
Infrequent:	
• Red, peeling or blistering skin; sore throat; fever; swallowing difficulty; unusual bruising; aching joints or muscles; jaundice.	Discontinue. Call doctor right away.
• Dizziness, tiredness, weakness, impotence.	Continue. Call doctor when convenient.
Rare:	
Painful urination; low back pain; numbness, tingling, burning feeling in feet and hands, bloody urine, neck swelling.	Discontinue. Call doctor right away.

WARNINGS & PRECAUTIONS

Don't take if:
You are allergic to any sulfa drug*.

Before you start, consult your doctor:
- If you are allergic to carbonic anhydrase inhibitors, oral antidiabetics or thiazide or loop diuretics.
- If you are allergic by nature.
- If you have liver or kidney disease.
- If you have porphyria.
- If you have developed anemia from use of any drug.

Over age 60:
Adverse reactions and side effects may be more frequent and severe than in younger persons.

Pregnancy:
Consult doctor. Risk category B (see page xviii).

Breast-feeding:
Drug passes into milk. Avoid drug or discontinue nursing until you finish medicine. Consult doctor for advice on maintaining milk supply.

Infants & children:
Don't give to infants younger than 2 years.

Prolonged use:
- May enlarge thyroid gland.
- You may become more susceptible to infections caused by germs not responsive to this drug.
- Request frequent blood counts, liver and kidney function studies.

Skin & sunlight:
May cause rash or intensify sunburn in areas exposed to sun or ultraviolet light (photosensitivity reaction). Avoid overexposure. Notify doctor if reaction occurs.

Driving, piloting or hazardous work:
Avoid if you feel dizzy. Otherwise, no problems expected.

Discontinuing:
Don't discontinue without doctor's advice until you complete prescribed dose, even though symptoms diminish or disappear.

Others:
- Drink 2 quarts of liquid each day to prevent adverse reactions.
- If you require surgery, tell anesthetist you take sulfa. Pentothal anesthesia should not be used.

POSSIBLE INTERACTION WITH OTHER DRUGS

GENERIC NAME OR DRUG CLASS	COMBINED EFFECT
Aminobenzoates	Possible decreased sulfa effect.
Antibiotics*	Decreased sulfa effect.
Anticoagulants*, oral	Increased anti-coagulant effect.
Anticonvulsants, hydantoin*	Toxic effect on brain.
Antidiabetics*	Toxic effect on brain.
Aspirin	Increased sulfa effect.
Calcium supplements*	Decreased sulfa effect.
Clozapine	Toxic effect on the central nervous system.
Digoxin	Decreased digoxin effect.
Hepatotoxic agents*	Increased liver toxicity.
Iron supplements*	Decreased sulfa effect.
Isoniazid	Possible anemia.
Mecamylamine	Decreased antibiotic effect.
Methenamine	Possible kidney blockage.
Methotrexate	Increased methotrexate effect.
Oxyphenbutazone	Increased sulfa effect.
Para-aminosalicylic acid	Decreased sulfa effect.
Penicillins*	Decreased penicillin effect.
Phenylbutazone	Increased sulfa effect.
Probenecid	Increased sulfa effect.
Sulfinpyrazone	Increased sulfa effect.
Sulfonureas*	May increase hypo-glycemic action.
Trimethoprim	Increased sulfa effect.
Vitamin C	Possible kidney damage. Avoid large doses of vitamin C.
Zidovudine	Increased risk of toxic effects of zidovudine.

POSSIBLE INTERACTION WITH OTHER SUBSTANCES

INTERACTS WITH	COMBINED EFFECT
Alcohol:	Increased alcohol effect.
Beverages: Less than 2 quarts of fluid daily.	Kidney damage.
Cocaine:	None expected.
Foods:	None expected.
Marijuana:	None expected.
Tobacco:	None expected.

*See Glossary

SULFINPYRAZONE

BRAND NAMES

Anturan
Anturane
Apo-Sulfinpyrazone
Novopyrazone

BASIC INFORMATION

Habit forming? No
Prescription needed? Yes
Available as generic? Yes
Drug class: Antigout

USES

- Treatment for chronic gout.
- May be prescribed to reduce the risk of recurrent heart attack.

DOSAGE & USAGE INFORMATION

How to take:
Tablet or capsule—Swallow with liquid or food to lessen stomach irritation. If you can't swallow whole, crumble tablet or open capsule and take with liquid or food.

When to take:
At the same times each day.

If you forget a dose:
Take as soon as you remember up to 2 hours late. If more than 2 hours, wait for next scheduled dose (don't double this dose).

Continued next column

OVERDOSE

SYMPTOMS:
Breathing difficulty, vomiting, imbalance, seizures, convulsions, coma.
WHAT TO DO:
- **Dial 911 (emergency) for an ambulance or medical help or poison center 1-800-222-1222. Then give first aid immediately.**
- **If patient is unconscious and not breathing, give mouth-to-mouth breathing. If there is no heartbeat, use cardiac massage and mouth-to-mouth breathing (CPR). Don't try to make patient vomit. If you can't get help quickly, take patient to nearest emergency facility.**
- **See emergency information on inside covers.**

What drug does:
Reduces uric acid level in blood and tissues by increasing amount of uric acid secreted in urine by kidneys.

Time lapse before drug works:
May require 6 months to prevent gout attacks.

Don't take with:
Any other medicine without consulting your doctor or pharmacist.

POSSIBLE ADVERSE REACTIONS OR SIDE EFFECTS

SYMPTOMS	WHAT TO DO
Life-threatening: In case of overdose, see previous column.	
Common: None expected.	
Infrequent:	
• Painful or difficult urination, worsening gout.	Discontinue. Call doctor right away.
• Rash, nausea, vomiting, abdominal pain, low back pain.	Continue. Call doctor when convenient.
Rare:	
• Black, bloody or tarry stools.	Discontinue. Seek emergency treatment.
• Sore throat; fever; unusual bleeding or bruising; red, painful joints; blood in urine; fatigue or weakness.	Discontinue. Call doctor right away.

WARNINGS & PRECAUTIONS

Don't take if:
- You are allergic to any uricosuric*.
- You have acute gout.
- You have active ulcers (stomach or duodenal), enteritis or ulcerative colitis.
- You have blood cell disorders.
- You are allergic to oxyphenbutazone or phenylbutazone.

Before you start, consult your doctor:
If you have kidney or blood disease.

Over age 60:
Adverse reactions and side effects may be more frequent and severe than in younger persons. You require lower dose because of decreased kidney function.

Pregnancy:
Decide with your doctor whether drug benefits justify risk to unborn child. Risk category C (see page xviii).

Breast-feeding:
Effect unknown. Consult doctor.

Infants & children:
Not recommended.

Prolonged use:
- Possible kidney damage.
- Talk to your doctor about the need for follow-up medical examinations or laboratory studies to check complete blood counts (white blood cell count, platelet count, red blood cell count, hemoglobin, hematocrit), kidney function, serum uric acid and urine uric acid.

Skin & sunlight:
No problems expected.

Driving, piloting or hazardous work:
No problems expected.

Discontinuing:
Don't discontinue without consulting doctor. Dose may require gradual reduction if you have taken drug for a long time. Doses of other drugs may also require adjustment.

Others:
- Drink 10 to 12 glasses of water each day you take this medicine.
- Periodic blood and urine laboratory tests recommended.

POSSIBLE INTERACTION WITH OTHER DRUGS

GENERIC NAME OR DRUG CLASS	COMBINED EFFECT
Allopurinol	Increased effect of each drug.
Anticoagulants*, oral	Increased anticoagulant effect.
Antidiabetics*, oral	Increased antidiabetic effect.
Aspirin	Bleeding tendency. Decreased sulfinpyrazone effect.
Bismuth subsalicylate	Decreased sulfinpyrazone effect.
Cephalosporins*	Increased risk of bleeding.
Cholestyramine	Decreased sulfinpyrazone effect.
Contraceptives, oral*	Increased bleeding between menstrual periods.
Diuretics*	Decreased sulfinpyrazone effect.
Nitrofurantoin	Increased risk of toxicity.
Penicillins*	Increased penicillin effect.
Salicylates*	Bleeding tendency. Decreased sulfinpyrazone effect.
Sulfa drugs*	Increased effect of sulfa drugs.
Thioguanine	May need increased dosage of sulfinpyrazone.

POSSIBLE INTERACTION WITH OTHER SUBSTANCES

INTERACTS WITH	COMBINED EFFECT
Alcohol:	Decreased sulfinpyrazone effect.
Beverages: Caffeine drinks.	Decreased sulfinpyrazone effect.
Cocaine:	None expected.
Foods:	None expected.
Marijuana:	Occasional use—None expected. Daily use—May increase blood level of uric acid.
Tobacco:	None expected.

*See Glossary

SULFONAMIDES

GENERIC AND BRAND NAMES

See complete list of generic and brand names in the *Generic and Brand Names Directory*, page 862.

BASIC INFORMATION

Habit forming? No
Prescription needed? Yes
Available as generic? Yes, for some
Drug class: Antibacterial (antibiotic), antiprotozoal, sulfa (sulfonamide)

USES

- Treatment of urinary tract and other infections.
- Sulfamethoxazole in combination with trimethoprim, may be used to treat bronchitis, certain types of pneumonia, skin infections, middle ear infections, intestinal tract infections and urinary tract infections.

DOSAGE & USAGE INFORMATION

How to take:
- Tablet—Swallow with liquid. Instructions to take on empty stomach mean 1 hour before or 2 hours after eating. Drink an extra amount of water daily so that urine output will be adequate.
- Liquid—Shake carefully before measuring.
- Other forms—Follow label instructions.

When to take:
At the same times each day, evenly spaced.

If you forget a dose:
Take as soon as you remember up to 2 hours late. If more than 2 hours, wait for next scheduled dose (don't double this dose).

What drug does:
Interferes with a nutrient (folic acid) necessary for growth and reproduction of bacteria. Will not attack viruses.

Continued next column

OVERDOSE

SYMPTOMS:
Less urine, bloody urine, stomach pain, lightheadedness, headache, drowsiness, coma.
WHAT TO DO:
- **Dial 911 (emergency) for an ambulance or medical help or poison center 1-800-222-1222. Then give first aid immediately.**
- **See emergency information on inside covers.**

Time lapse before drug works:
2 to 5 days to affect infection.

Don't take with:
Any other medicine without consulting your doctor or pharmacist.

POSSIBLE ADVERSE REACTIONS OR SIDE EFFECTS

SYMPTOMS	WHAT TO DO
Life-threatening:	
In case of overdose, see previous column.	
Common:	
• Itchy skin, rash.	Discontinue. Call doctor right away.
• Headache, nausea, vomiting, diarrhea, appetite loss, skin sensitive to sun, dizziness.	Continue. Call doctor when convenient.
Infrequent:	
• Red, peeling or blistering skin; sore throat; fever; swallowing difficulty; unusual bruising or bleeding; aching joints or muscles; yellow skin or eyes; pale skin.	Discontinue. Call doctor right away.
• Weakness or tiredness.	Continue. Call doctor when convenient.
Rare:	
Painful urination, low back pain, numbness, stomach pain, bloody diarrhea or urine, neck swelling, mood or behavior changes, increased or decreased urine output, thirst.	Discontinue. Call doctor right away.

WARNINGS & PRECAUTIONS

Don't take if:
You are allergic to any sulfa drug.

Before you start, consult your doctor:
- If you are allergic to carbonic anhydrase inhibitors, oral antidiabetics or diuretics (thiazide or loop).
- If you are allergic by nature.
- If you have liver or kidney disease.
- If you have glucose 6-phosphate dehydrogenase (G6PD) disease.
- If you have porphyria.
- If you have anemia or other blood problems.

Over age 60:
Adverse reactions and side effects may be more frequent and severe than in younger persons.

Pregnancy:
Decide with your doctor if drug benefits justify risk to unborn child. Risk category C (see page xviii).

Breast-feeding:
Drug passes into milk. Avoid drug or discontinue nursing until you finish medicine. Consult doctor for advice on maintaining milk supply.

Infants & children:
Don't give to infants younger than 2 months.

Prolonged use:
- You may become more susceptible to infections caused by germs not responsive to this drug.
- Drug may enlarge thyroid gland (rare).
- Talk to your doctor about the need for frequent blood counts, liver and kidney function studies.

Skin & sunlight:
May cause rash or intensify sunburn in areas exposed to sun or ultraviolet light (photosensitivity reaction). Avoid excess exposure. Notify doctor if reaction occurs.

Driving, piloting or hazardous work:
Avoid if you feel dizzy. Otherwise, no problems expected.

Discontinuing:
Don't discontinue without doctor's advice until you complete prescribed dose, even though symptoms diminish or disappear.

Others:
- Drink 2 quarts of liquid each day to prevent side effects or adverse reactions.
- Advise any doctor or dentist whom you consult that you take this medicine.
- If you require surgery, tell anesthetist you take sulfa. Pentothal anesthesia should not be used.

POSSIBLE INTERACTION WITH OTHER DRUGS

GENERIC NAME OR DRUG CLASS	COMBINED EFFECT
Aminobenzoate potassium	Possible decreased sulfonamide effect.
Anticoagulants*, oral	Increased anti-coagulant effect.
Anticonvulsants*, hydantoin	Increased anti-convulsant effect.
Antidiabetics*, oral	Increased anti-diabetic effect.
Bone marrow depressants*	Increased risk of side effects.
Contraceptives*, oral estrogen	Decreased contraceptive effect.
Cyclosporine	Decreased cyclosproine effect.
Hemolytics*, other	Increased risk of side effects.
Hepatotoxic agents*	Increased liver toxicity.
Mecamylamine	Decreased antibiotic effect.
Methenamine	Possible kidney blockage.
Methotrexate	Increased methotrexate effect.
Penicillins*	Decreased penicillin effect.
Phenylbutazone	Increased sulfonamide effect.
Probenecid	Increased sulfonamide effect.
Sulfinpyrazone	Increased sulfonamide effect.

POSSIBLE INTERACTION WITH OTHER SUBSTANCES

INTERACTS WITH	COMBINED EFFECT
Alcohol:	None expected.
Beverages: Inadequate fluid intake.	Increased risk of side effects.
Cocaine:	None expected.
Foods:	None expected.
Marijuana:	None expected.
Tobacco:	None expected.

*See Glossary

SULFONAMIDES & PHENAZOPYRIDINE

BRAND AND GENERIC NAMES

SULFAMETHOXAZOLE & PHENAZOPYRIDINE
- **Azo Gantanol**
- **Azo-Sulfamethoxazole**

SULFISOXAZOLE & PHENAZOPYRIDINE
- **Azo Gantrisin**
- **Azo-Sulfisoxazol**
- **Azo-Truxazole**
- **Sul-Azo**

BASIC INFORMATION

Habit forming? No
Prescription needed? Yes
Available as generic? Yes
Drug class: Analgesic (urinary), sulfonamide

USES

- Treats infections responsive to this drug.
- Relieves pain of lower urinary tract irritation, as in cystitis, urethritis or prostatitis.

DOSAGE & USAGE INFORMATION

How to take:
Tablet—Swallow with liquid. Instructions to take on empty stomach mean 1 hour before or 2 hours after eating.

When to take:
At the same times each day, after meals.

If you forget a dose:
Take as soon as you remember up to 2 hours late. If more than 2 hours, wait for next scheduled dose (don't double this dose).

What drug does:
- Interferes with a nutrient (folic acid) necessary for growth and reproduction of bacteria. Will not attack viruses.
- Anesthetizes lower urinary tract. Relieves pain, burning, pressure and urgency to urinate.

Continued next column

OVERDOSE

SYMPTOMS:
Less urine, bloody urine, shortness of breath, weakness, coma.
WHAT TO DO:
- **Dial 911 (emergency) for an ambulance or medical help or poison center 1-800-222-1222. Then give first aid immediately.**
- **See emergency information on inside covers.**

Time lapse before drug works:
2 to 5 days to affect infection.

Don't take with:
Any other medicine without consulting your doctor or pharmacist.

POSSIBLE ADVERSE REACTIONS OR SIDE EFFECTS

SYMPTOMS	WHAT TO DO
Life-threatening:	
In case of overdose, see previous column.	
Common:	
• Rash, itchy skin.	Discontinue. Call doctor right away.
• Dizziness, diarrhea, headache, appetite loss, nausea, vomiting, skin sensitive to sun.	Continue. Call doctor when convenient.
Infrequent:	
• Joint pain; swallowing difficulty; pale skin; blistering; peeling of skin; sore throat, fever, mouth sores; unexplained bleeding or bruising; jaundice.	Discontinue. Call doctor right away.
• Abdominal pain, indigestion, weakness, tiredness.	Continue. Call doctor when convenient.
Rare:	
Back pain; neck swelling; numbness, tingling, burning feeling in feet and hands; bloody urine; painful urination.	Discontinue. Call doctor right away.

WARNINGS & PRECAUTIONS

Don't take if:
- You are allergic to any sulfa drug or urinary analgesic.
- You have hepatitis.

Before you start, consult your doctor:
- If you are allergic to carbonic anhydrase inhibitors, oral antidiabetics or thiazide or loop diuretics.
- If you are allergic by nature.
- If you have liver or kidney disease, porphyria.
- If you have developed anemia from use of any drug.
- If you have G6PD* deficiency.

Over age 60:
Adverse reactions and side effects may be more frequent and severe than in younger persons.

Pregnancy:
Risk factors vary for drugs in this group. See category list on page xviii and consult doctor.

Breast-feeding:
Drug passes into milk. Avoid drug or discontinue nursing until you finish medicine. Consult doctor for advice on maintaining milk supply.

Infants & children:
Don't give to infants younger than 1 month.

Prolonged use:
- May enlarge thyroid gland.
- You may become more susceptible to infections caused by germs not responsive to this drug.
- Request frequent blood counts, liver and kidney function studies.
- Orange or yellow skin.
- Anemia. Occasional blood studies recommended.

Skin & sunlight:
One or more drugs in this group may cause rash or intensify sunburn in areas exposed to sun or ultraviolet light (photosensitivity reaction). Avoid overexposure. Notify doctor if reaction occurs.

Driving, piloting or hazardous work:
Avoid if you feel dizzy. Otherwise, no problems expected.

Discontinuing:
Don't discontinue without doctor's advice until you complete prescribed dose, even though symptoms diminish or disappear.

Others:
- Drink 2 quarts of liquid each day to prevent adverse reactions.
- If you require surgery, tell anesthetist you take sulfa.
- Will probably cause urine to be reddish orange. Requires no action.
- May stain fabrics.

POSSIBLE INTERACTION WITH OTHER DRUGS

GENERIC NAME OR DRUG CLASS	COMBINED EFFECT
Aminobenzoates	Possible decreased sulfa effect.
Anticoagulants*, oral	Increased anti-coagulant effect.
Anticonvulsants, hydantoin*	Toxic effect on brain.
Antidiabetics*	Toxic effect on brain.
Aspirin	Increased sulfa effect.
Clozapine	Toxic effect on the central nervous system.
Didanosine	Increased risk of pancreatitis.
Hepatotoxic agents*	Increased liver toxicity.
Isoniazid	Possible anemia.
Mecamylamine	Decreased antibiotic effect.
Methenamine	Possible kidney blockage.
Methotrexate	Increased methotrexate effect.
Oxyphenbutazone	Increased sulfa effect.
Para-aminosalicylic acid	Decreased sulfa effect.
Penicillins*	Decreased penicillin effect.
Phenylbutazone	Increased sulfa effect.
Probenecid	Increased sulfa effect.
Sulfinpyrazone	Increased sulfa effect.
Sulfonureas*	May increase hypo-glycemic action.
Trimethoprim	Increased sulfa effect.
Zidovudine	Increased risk of toxic effects of zidovudine.

POSSIBLE INTERACTION WITH OTHER SUBSTANCES

INTERACTS WITH	COMBINED EFFECT
Alcohol:	Increased alcohol effect.
Beverages: Less than 2 quarts of fluid daily.	Kidney damage.
Cocaine:	None expected.
Foods:	None expected.
Marijuana:	None expected.
Tobacco:	None expected.

*See Glossary

SULFONYLUREAS

GENERIC AND BRAND NAMES

See complete list of generic and brand names in the *Generic and Brand Name Directory*, page 862.

BASIC INFORMATION

Habit forming? No
Prescription needed? Yes
Available as generic? Yes, for some.
Drug class: Antidiabetic (oral), sulfonylurea

USES

- Treatment for diabetes in adults who can't control blood sugar by diet, weight loss and exercise.
- Treatment for diabetes insipidus (chlorpropamide).

DOSAGE & USAGE INFORMATION

How to take:
- Tablet—Swallow with liquid or food to lessen stomach irritation. If you can't swallow whole, crumble tablet and take with liquid or food.
- Extended-release tablet—Swallow whole with liquid. Do not crush or chew tablet.

When to take:
At the same times each day.

If you forget a dose:
Take as soon as you remember up to 2 hours late. If more than 2 hours, wait for next scheduled dose (don't double this dose).

What drug does:
Stimulates pancreas to produce more insulin. Insulin in blood forces cells to use sugar in blood.

Time lapse before drug works:
3 to 4 hours. May require 2 weeks for maximum benefit.

Don't take with:
Any other medicine without consulting your doctor or pharmacist.

OVERDOSE

SYMPTOMS:
Excessive hunger, nausea, anxiety, cool skin, cold sweats, drowsiness, rapid heartbeat, weakness, unconsciousness, coma.
WHAT TO DO:
- **Dial 911 (emergency) for an ambulance or medical help or poison center 1-800-222-1222. Then give first aid immediately.**
- **See emergency information on inside covers.**

POSSIBLE ADVERSE REACTIONS OR SIDE EFFECTS

SYMPTOMS	WHAT TO DO
Life-threatening: In case of overdose, see previous column.	
Common:	
• Dizziness.	Discontinue. Call doctor right away.
• Diarrhea, appetite loss, nausea, stomach pain, heartburn, constipation.	Continue. Call doctor when convenient.
Infrequent:	
• Low blood sugar (hunger, anxiety, cold sweats, rapid pulse), shortness of breath.	Discontinue. Seek emergency treatment.
• Headache.	Discontinue. Call doctor right away.
Rare:	
Fatigue, itchy skin or rash, sore throat, fever, ringing in ears, unusual bleeding or bruising, jaundice, edema, weakness, confusion.	Discontinue. Call doctor right away.

WARNINGS & PRECAUTIONS

Don't take if:
- You are allergic to any sulfonylurea.
- You have impaired kidney or liver function.

Before you start, consult your doctor:
- If you have a severe infection.
- If you have thyroid disease.
- If you take insulin.
- If you have heart disease.

Over age 60:
Dose usually smaller than for younger adults. Avoid episodes of low blood sugar because repeated ones can damage brain permanently.

Pregnancy:
Discuss any use of these drugs with your doctor. Risk factors vary for drugs in this group. See category list on page xviii and consult doctor.

Breast-feeding:
Drug filters into milk. May lower baby's blood sugar. Avoid.

Infants & children:
Don't give to infants or children.

Prolonged use:
- Adverse effects more likely.

- Talk to your doctor about the need for follow-up medical examinations or laboratory studies to check blood sugar, complete blood counts (white blood cell count, platelet count, redblood cell count, hemoglobin, hematocrit), eyes.

Skin and sunlight:
One or more drugs in this group may cause rash or intensify sunburn in areas exposed to sun or ultraviolet light (photosensitivity reaction). Avoid overexposure. Notify doctor if reaction occurs.

Driving, piloting or hazardous work:
No problems expected unless you develop hypoglycemia (low blood sugar). If so, avoid driving or hazardous activity.

Discontinuing:
Don't discontinue without consulting doctor. Dose may require gradual reduction if you have taken drug for a long time. Doses of other drugs may also require adjustment.

Others:
- Don't exceed recommended dose. Hypoglycemia (low blood sugar) may occur, even with proper dose schedule. You must balance medicine, diet and exercise.
- May affect results in some medical tests.
- Advise any doctor or dentist whom you consult that you take this medicine.

POSSIBLE INTERACTION WITH OTHER DRUGS

GENERIC NAME OR DRUG CLASS	COMBINED EFFECT
Adrenocorticoids, systemic	Decreased anti-diabetic effect.
Androgens*	Increased blood sugar lowering.
Anticoagulants*	Unpredictable prothrombin times.
Anticonvulsants, hydantoin*	Decreased blood sugar lowering.
Antifungals, azoles	Increased blood sugar lowering.
Anti-inflammatory nonsteriodal drugs (NSAIDs)*	Increased blood-sugar lowering.
Aspirin	Increased blood sugar lowering.
Beta-adrenergic blocking agents*	Increased blood sugar lowering. Possible increased difficulty in regulating blood sugar levels.
Bismuth subsalicylate	Increased insulin effect. May require dosage adjustment.
Chloramphenicol	Increased blood sugar lowering.
Cimetidine	Increased blood sugar lowering.
Clofibrate	Increased blood sugar lowering.
Contraceptives, oral*	Decreased blood sugar lowering.
Dapsone	Increased risk of adverse effect on blood cells.
Desmopressin	May increase desmopressin effect.
Dexfenfluramine	May require dosage change as weight loss occurs.
Dextrothyroxine	Antidiabetic may require adjustment.
Digoxin	Possible decreased digoxin effect.
Diuretics* (loop, thiazide)	Decreased blood sugar lowering.
Epinephrine	Increased blood sugar lowering.
Estrogens*	Increased blood sugar lowering.
Guanethidine	Unpredictable blood sugar lowering effect.
Hemolytics*	Increased risk of adverse effect on blood cells.

Continued on page 931

POSSIBLE INTERACTION WITH OTHER SUBSTANCES

INTERACTS WITH	COMBINED EFFECT
Alcohol:	Disulfiram reaction.* Avoid.
Beverages:	None expected.
Cocaine:	None expected.
Foods:	None expected.
Marijuana:	Decreased blood sugar lowering. Avoid.
Tobacco:	None expected.

***See Glossary**

TAMOXIFEN

BRAND NAMES

Alpha-Tamoxifen	**Novo-Tamoxifen**
Med Tamoxifen	**Tamofen**
Nolvadex	**Tamone**
Nolvadex-D	**Tamoplex**

BASIC INFORMATION

Habit forming? No
Prescription needed? Yes
Available as generic? No
Drug class: Antineoplastic

USES

- Treats advanced breast cancer.
- Can help prevent breast cancer in those at risk.

DOSAGE & USAGE INFORMATION

How to take:
- Tablets—Swallow with liquid. If you can't swallow whole, crumble tablet and take with liquid or food. Instructions to take on empty stomach mean 1 hour before or 2 hours after eating.
- Enteric-coated tablets—Swallow whole.

When to take:
Follow doctor's instructions.

If you forget a dose:
Skip the missed dose and return to regular schedule. Don't double dose.

What drug does:
Blocks uptake of estradiol and inhibits growth of cancer cells.

Time lapse before drug works:
- 4 to 10 weeks.
- With bone metastases—several months.

Continued next column

OVERDOSE

SYMPTOMS:
None expected.
WHAT TO DO:
Overdose unlikely to threaten life. If person takes much larger amount than prescribed, call doctor, poison center 1-800-222-1222 or hospital emergency room for instructions.

Don't take with:
Any other medicines (including over-the-counter drugs such as cough and cold medicines, laxatives, antacids, diet pills, caffeine, nose drops or vitamins) without consulting your doctor or pharmacist.

POSSIBLE ADVERSE REACTIONS OR SIDE EFFECTS

SYMPTOMS	WHAT TO DO
Life-threatening:	
Leg pain, shortness of breath.	Seek emergency treatment immediately.
Common:	
Hot flashes, nausea and vomiting, weight gain.	Continue. Call doctor when convenient.
Infrequent:	
Headache, dry skin, menstrual irregularities, vaginal itching.	Continue. Call doctor when convenient.
Rare:	
Blurred vision, confusion, sleepiness.	Discontinue. Call doctor right away.

WARNINGS & PRECAUTIONS

Don't take if:
You are allergic to tamoxifen.

Before you start, consult your doctor:
- If you have cataracts.
- If you have blood disorders.
- If you have high cholesterol.

Over age 60:
Adverse reactions and side effects may be more frequent and severe than in younger persons. You may need smaller doses for shorter periods of time.

Pregnancy:
Consult doctor. Risk category D (see page xviii).

Breast-feeding:
Effect not documented. Consult your doctor.

Infants & children:
Not intended for use in children.

Prolonged use:
Talk to your doctor about the need for follow-up medical examinations (especially pelvic exams) or laboratory studies to check complete blood counts (white blood cell count, platelet count, red blood cell count, hemoglobin, hematocrit) and serum calcium.

Skin & sunlight:
No problems expected.

Driving, piloting or hazardous work:
Avoid if you feel confused, drowsy or dizzy.

Discontinuing:
No special problems expected.

Others:
- Advise any doctor or dentist whom you consult that you take this medicine.
- May affect results in some medical tests.
- Be sure you and your doctor discuss all aspects of using this drug, and read all instructional materials.
- May make you more fertile. Talk to your doctor about using some type of birth control.

POSSIBLE INTERACTION WITH OTHER DRUGS

GENERIC NAME OR DRUG CLASS	COMBINED EFFECT
Antacids*	Decreased tamoxifen effect. Take 1 to 2 hours apart.
Cimetidine	Decreased tamoxifen effect.
Estrogens*	Decreased tamoxifen effect.
Famotidine	Decreased tamoxifen effect.
H_2 antagonist antihistamines*	Decreased tamoxifen effect.
Ranitidine	Decreased tamoxifen effect.

POSSIBLE INTERACTION WITH OTHER SUBSTANCES

INTERACTS WITH	COMBINED EFFECT
Alcohol:	None expected.
Beverages:	None expected.
Cocaine:	None expected.
Foods:	None expected.
Marijuana:	None expected.
Tobacco:	None expected.

***See Glossary**

TERPIN HYDRATE

BRAND NAMES

Prunicodeine
Terpin Hydrate and Codeine Syrup
Terpin-Dex

BASIC INFORMATION

Habit forming? Yes
Prescription needed? Yes
Available as generic? Yes
Drug class: Expectorant

USES

Decreases cough due to simple bronchial irritation.

DOSAGE & USAGE INFORMATION

How to take:
Follow each dose with 8 oz. water or food to decrease gastric distress. Works better in combination with a cool-air vaporizer.

When to take:
3 to 4 times each day, spaced at least 4 hours apart.

If you forget a dose:
Take as soon as you remember. Wait 4 hours for next dose.

What drug does:
Loosens mucus in bronchial tubes to make mucus easier to cough up.

Time lapse before drug works:
10 to 15 minutes.

Don't take with:
Any other medicine without consulting your doctor or pharmacist.

OVERDOSE

SYMPTOMS:
Nausea, drowsiness.
WHAT TO DO:
Overdose unlikely to threaten life. If person takes much larger amount than prescribed, call doctor, poison center 1-800-222-1222 or hospital emergency room for instructions.

POSSIBLE ADVERSE REACTIONS OR SIDE EFFECTS

SYMPTOMS	WHAT TO DO
Life-threatening: None expected.	
Common: None expected.	
Infrequent: Nausea, vomiting, abdominal pain.	Continue. Call doctor when convenient.
Rare: Symptoms of alcohol intoxication, especially in children.	Discontinue. Call doctor right away.

WARNINGS & PRECAUTIONS

Don't take if:
- You are allergic to terpin hydrate.
- You are a recovering or active alcoholic.

Before you start, consult your doctor:
If you plan to become pregnant within medication period.

Over age 60:
No problems expected.

Pregnancy:
Decide with your doctor if drug benefits justify risk to unborn child. Risk category C (see page xviii).

Breast-feeding:
Drug filters into milk. May harm child. Avoid.

Infants & children:
Use only under medical supervision.

Prolonged use:
Habit forming.

Skin & sunlight:
No problems expected.

Driving, piloting or hazardous work:
Don't drive or pilot aircraft until you learn how medicine affects you. Don't work around dangerous machinery. Don't climb ladders or work in high places. Danger increases if you drink alcohol or take medicine affecting alertness and reflexes, such as antihistamines, tranquilizers, sedatives, pain medicine, narcotics and mind-altering drugs.

Discontinuing:
May be unnecessary to finish medicine. Follow doctor's instructions.

Others:
- Exceeding recommended doses may cause intoxication; drug is 42.5% alcohol.
- Frequently combined with codeine, which increases hazards.

POSSIBLE INTERACTION WITH OTHER DRUGS

GENERIC NAME OR DRUG CLASS	COMBINED EFFECT
Antidepressants*	Increased sedation.
Antihistamines*	Increased sedation.
Central nervous system (CNS) depressants*	Increased sedative effect of both.
Disulfiram	Possible disulfiram reaction*.
Muscle relaxants*	Increased sedation.
Narcotics*	Increased sedation.
Sedatives*	Increased sedation.
Sleep inducers*	Increased sedation.
Tranquilizers*	Increased sedation.

POSSIBLE INTERACTION WITH OTHER SUBSTANCES

INTERACTS WITH	COMBINED EFFECT
Alcohol:	Contains alcohol. Increased sedative effect of both drugs. Avoid.
Beverages:	None expected.
Cocaine:	Unpredictable effect on nervous system. Avoid.
Foods:	None expected.
Marijuana:	Unpredictable effect on nervous system. Avoid.
Tobacco:	None expected.

*See Glossary

TESTOLACTONE

BRAND NAMES

Teslac

BASIC INFORMATION

Habit forming? No
Prescription needed? Yes
Available as generic? No
Drug class: Antineoplastic

USES

Treats advanced breast cancer.

DOSAGE & USAGE INFORMATION

How to take:
Tablets—Swallow with liquid. If you can't swallow whole, crumble tablet and take with liquid or food. Instructions to take on empty stomach mean 1 hour before or 2 hours after eating.

When to take:
Follow doctor's instructions.

If you forget a dose:
Take as soon as you remember up to 2 hours late. If more than 2 hours, wait for next scheduled dose (don't double this dose).

What drug does:
Inhibits growth of cancer cells.

Time lapse before drug works:
6 to 12 weeks.

Don't take with:
Any other medicines (including over-the-counter drugs such as cough and cold medicines, laxatives, antacids, diet pills, caffeine, nose drops or vitamins) without consulting your doctor.

OVERDOSE

SYMPTOMS:
None expected.
WHAT TO DO:
Overdose unlikely to threaten life. If person takes much larger amount than prescribed, call doctor, poison center 1-800-222-1222 or hospital emergency room for instructions.

POSSIBLE ADVERSE REACTIONS OR SIDE EFFECTS

SYMPTOMS	WHAT TO DO
Life-threatening: None expected.	
Common: Appetite loss.	Continue. Call doctor when convenient.
Infrequent: Diarrhea; swollen feet and legs; numb and tingling fingers, toes, face.	Continue. Call doctor when convenient.
Rare: Red tongue.	Continue. Call doctor when convenient.

WARNINGS & PRECAUTIONS

Don't take if:
You are allergic to testosterone.

Before you start, consult your doctor:
- If you have heart disease.
- If you have kidney disease.

Over age 60:
Adverse reactions and side effects may be more frequent and severe than in younger persons. You may need smaller doses for shorter periods of time.

Pregnancy:
Decide with your doctor if drug benefits justify risk to unborn child. Risk category C (see page xviii).

Breast-feeding:
Effect not documented. Consult your doctor.

Infants & children:
Not recommended.

Prolonged use:
Talk to your doctor about the need for follow-up medical examinations or laboratory studies to check serum calcium levels.

Skin & sunlight:
No problems expected.

Driving, piloting or hazardous work:
No problems expected.

Discontinuing:
No special problems expected.

Others:
- Advise any doctor or dentist whom you consult that you take this medicine.
- May affect results in some medical tests.

POSSIBLE INTERACTION WITH OTHER DRUGS

GENERIC NAME OR DRUG CLASS	COMBINED EFFECT
Anticoagulants*, oral	Increased anti-coagulant effect.

POSSIBLE INTERACTION WITH OTHER SUBSTANCES

INTERACTS WITH	COMBINED EFFECT
Alcohol:	None expected.
Beverages:	None expected.
Cocaine:	None expected.
Foods:	None expected.
Marijuana:	None expected.
Tobacco:	None expected.

***See Glossary**

TETRACYCLINES

GENERIC AND BRAND NAMES

See complete list of generic and brand names in the *Generic and Brand Name Directory*, page 862.

BASIC INFORMATION

Habit forming? No
Prescription needed? Yes
Available as generic? Yes
Drug class: Antibacterial, antiacne

USES

- Treatment for infections susceptible to any tetracycline. Will not cure virus infections such as colds or flu.
- Treatment for acne, ulcers. and used as diuretic.
- Treatment for dental bacterial infections.

DOSAGE & USAGE INFORMATION

How to take:
- Tablet or capsule—Take on empty stomach 1 hour before or 2 hours after eating. If you can't swallow whole, crumble tablet or open capsule and take with liquid or food.
- Delayed-release capsules—Swallow whole with liquid (don't take with milk).
- Dental product—Follow package instructions.
- Liquid—Shake well. Take with measuring spoon.

When to take:
At the same times each day, evenly spaced.

If you forget a dose:
Take as soon as you remember up to 2 hours late. If more than 2 hours, wait for next scheduled dose (don't double this dose).

What drug does:
Prevents germ growth and reproduction.

Time lapse before drug works:
- Infections—May require 5 days to affect infection.
- Acne—May require 4 weeks to affect acne.

Don't take with:
Any other medicine without consulting your doctor or pharmacist.

OVERDOSE

SYMPTOMS:
Severe nausea, vomiting, diarrhea.
WHAT TO DO:
Overdose unlikely to threaten life. If person takes much larger amount than prescribed, call doctor, poison center 1-800-222-1222 or hospital emergency room for instructions.

POSSIBLE ADVERSE REACTIONS OR SIDE EFFECTS

SYMPTOMS	WHAT TO DO
Life-threatening:	
Hives, rash, intense itching, faintness soon after a dose (anaphylaxis).	Seek emergency treatment immediately.
Common:	
• Mild stomach cramps, diarrhea, nausea or vomiting; dizziness, lightheadedness or unsteadiness (with minocycline).	Continue. Call doctor when convenient.
• Increased sensitivity to sunlight, tooth discoloration (in children age 8 and under).	Discontinue. Call doctor right away.
Infrequent:	
• Frequent or increased urination, excessive thirst, unusual tiredness or weakness (with demeclocycline); darker color or discoloration of skin and mucous membranes (with minocycline).	Discontinue. Call doctor right away.
• Sore mouth or tongue, rectal or genital itch.	Continue. Call doctor when convenient.
• Darkened tongue (will go away when drug is discontinued).	No action necessary.
Rare:	
Changes in vision, yellow skin or eyes, continued vomiting, severe stomach cramps, loss of appetite, ongoing headache, bulging fontanel (soft spot on head of infant).	Discontinue. Call doctor right away.

WARNINGS & PRECAUTIONS

Don't take if:
You are allergic to any tetracycline antibiotic.

Before you start, consult your doctor:
- If you have kidney or liver disease.
- If you have lupus.
- If you have myasthenia gravis.

Over age 60:
Dosage usually less than in younger adults. More likely to cause itching around rectum. Ask your doctor how to prevent it.

Pregnancy:
Risk to unborn child outweighs drug benefits. Don't use. Risk category D (see page xviii).

Breast-feeding:
Drug passes into milk. Avoid drug or discontinue nursing until you finish medicine. Consult doctor for advice on maintaining milk supply.

Infants & children:
May cause permanent teeth malformation or discoloration in children less than 8 years old. Don't use.

Prolonged use:
- You may become more susceptible to infections caused by germs not responsive to tetracycline.
- May cause rare problems in liver, kidney or bone marrow. Periodic laboratory blood studies, liver and kidney function tests recommended if you use drug a long time.

Skin & sunlight:
May cause rash or intensify sunburn in areas exposed to sun or ultraviolet light (photosensitivity reaction). Avoid overexposure. Notify doctor if reaction occurs.

Driving, piloting or hazardous work:
No problems expected.

Discontinuing:
Don't discontinue without doctor's advice until you complete prescribed dose, even though symptoms diminish or disappear.

Others:
- Avoid using outdated drug.
- May affect results in some medical tests.
- Birth control pills may not be effective. Use additional birth control method.

POSSIBLE INTERACTION WITH OTHER DRUGS

GENERIC NAME OR DRUG CLASS	COMBINED EFFECT
Antacids*	Decreased tetracycline effect.
Anticoagulants*, oral	Increased anti-coagulant effect.
Antivirals, HIV/AIDS*	Decreased antibiotic effect.
Bismuth subsalicylate	Decreased tetra-cycline absorption.
Calcium supplements*	Decreased tetracycline effect.
Cefixime	Decreased antibiotic effect of cefixime.
Cholestyramine or colestipol	Decreased tetracycline effect.
Contraceptives, oral*	Decreased contra-ceptive effect.
Desmopressin	Possible decreased desmopressin effect.
Digitalis preparations*	Increased digitalis effect.
Etretinate	Increased chance of adverse reactions of etretinate.
Lithium	Increased lithium effect.
Mineral supplements* (iron, calcium, magnesium, zinc)	Decreased tetracycline absorption. Separate doses by 1 to 2 hours.
Penicillins*	Decreased penicillin effect.
Sodium bicarbonate	Greatly reduced tetracycline absorption.
Tiopronin	Increased risk of toxicity to kidneys (except with doxycycline and minocycline).

Continued on page 932

POSSIBLE INTERACTION WITH OTHER SUBSTANCES

INTERACTS WITH	COMBINED EFFECT
Alcohol:	Possible liver damage. Avoid.
Beverages: Milk.	Decreased tetracy-cline absorption. Take dose 2 hours after or 1 hour before drinking.
Cocaine:	None expected.
Foods: Dairy products.	Decreased tetracycline absorption. Take dose 2 hours after or 1 hour before eating.
Marijuana:	No interactions expected, but marijuana may slow body's recovery. Avoid.
Tobacco:	None expected.

***See Glossary**

THEOPHYLLINE

BRAND NAMES

See complete list of brand names in the *Generic and Brand Name Directory*, page 862.

BASIC INFORMATION

Habit forming? No
Prescription needed? Yes
Available as generic? Yes
Drug class: Bronchodilator, expectorant

USES

- Treatment for bronchial asthma symptoms.
- Loosens mucus in respiratory passages.
- Relieves coughing, wheezing, shortness of breath.

DOSAGE & USAGE INFORMATION

How to take:
Tablet, capsule, elixir or syrup—Swallow with liquid.

When to take:
Most effective taken on empty stomach 1 hour before or 2 hours after eating. However, may take with food to lessen stomach upset.

If you forget a dose:
Take as soon as you remember up to 2 hours late. If more than 2 hours, wait for next scheduled dose (don't double this dose).

What drug does:
- Relaxes and expands bronchial tubes.
- Increases production of watery fluids to thin mucus so it can be coughed out or absorbed.

Time lapse before drug works:
15 to 30 minutes.

Don't take with:
Any other medicine without consulting your doctor or pharmacist.

OVERDOSE

SYMPTOMS:
Restlessness, irritability, confusion, hallucinations, drowsiness, mild weakness, nausea, vomiting blood, delirium, convulsions, rapid pulse, coma.
WHAT TO DO:
- **Dial 911 (emergency) for an ambulance or medical help or poison center 1-800-222-1222. Then give first aid immediately.**
- **See emergency information on inside covers.**

POSSIBLE ADVERSE REACTIONS OR SIDE EFFECTS

SYMPTOMS	WHAT TO DO
Life-threatening:	
Difficult breathing, uncontrollable heart rate, loss of consciousness.	Discontinue. Seek emergency treatment.
Common:	
• Headache, irritability, nervousness, restlessness, insomnia, drowsiness, nausea, vomiting.	Discontinue. Call doctor right away.
• Dizziness, lightheadedness, diarrhea, abdominal pain, heartburn.	Continue. Call doctor when convenient.
Infrequent:	
Skin rash or hives, red or flushed face, appetite loss, diarrhea.	Discontinue. Call doctor right away.
Rare:	
None expected.	

WARNINGS & PRECAUTIONS

Don't take if:
- You are allergic to any bronchodilator or cough or cold preparation containing guaifenesin.
- You have an active peptic ulcer.

Before you start, consult your doctor:
- If you have had impaired kidney or liver function.
- If you have gastritis, peptic ulcer, high blood pressure or heart disease.
- If you take medication for gout.

Over age 60:
Adverse reactions and side effects may be more frequent and severe than in younger persons. For drug to work, you must drink 8 to 10 glasses of fluid per day.

Pregnancy:
Decide with your doctor if drug benefits justify risk to unborn child. Risk category C (see page xviii).

Breast-feeding:
Drug passes into milk. Avoid drug or discontinue nursing until you finish medicine. Consult doctor for advice on maintaining milk supply.

Infants & children:
Use only under medical supervision.

Prolonged use:
Stomach irritation.

Skin & sunlight:
No problems expected.

Driving, piloting or hazardous work:
Avoid if lightheaded, drowsy or dizzy. Otherwise, no problems expected.

Discontinuing:
May be unnecessary to finish medicine. Follow doctor's instructions.

Others:
No problems expected.

POSSIBLE INTERACTION WITH OTHER DRUGS

GENERIC NAME OR DRUG CLASS	COMBINED EFFECT
Allopurinol	Decreased allopurinol effect.
Antiandrogens, nonsteroidal	Increased effect of theophylline.
Anticoagulants*, oral	Possible risk of bleeding.
Ciprofloxacin	Increased possibility of central nervous system poisoning, such as nausea, vomiting, restlessness, palpitations.
Clarithromycin	Increased concentration of theophylline.
Ephedrine	Increased effect of both drugs.
Epinephrine	Increased effect of both drugs.
Erythromycins*	Increased bronchodilator effect.
Finasteride	Decreased theophylline effect.
Furosemide	Increased furosemide effect.
Lincomycins*	Increased bronchodilator effect.
Lithium	Decreased lithium effect.
Moricizine	Decreased bronchodilator effect.
Nicotine	Increased bronchodilator effect.
Probenecid	Decreased effect of both drugs.
Propranolol	Decreased bronchodilator effect.
Rauwolfia alkaloids*	Rapid heartbeat.
Sulfinpyrazone	Decreased sulfinpyrazone effect.
Ticlopidine	Increased theophylline effect.
Troleandomycin	Increased bronchodilator effect.
Zafirlukast	May increase effect of zafirlukast.
Zileuton	Increased effect of zileuton.

POSSIBLE INTERACTION WITH OTHER SUBSTANCES

INTERACTS WITH	COMBINED EFFECT
Alcohol:	No proven problems.
Beverages:	You must drink 8 to 10 glasses of fluid per day for drug to work.
Caffeine drinks.	Nervousness and insomnia.
Cocaine:	Excess stimulation. Avoid.
Foods:	None expected.
Marijuana:	Slightly increased antiasthmatic effect of bronchodilator.
Tobacco:	Decreased bronchodilator effect. Cigarette smoking worsens all problems that this medicine treats. Avoid.

*See Glossary

THIAMINE (Vitamin B-1)

BRAND NAMES

Betalin S
Betaxin
Bewon
Biamine

Numerous other multiple vitamin-mineral supplements. Check labels.

BASIC INFORMATION

Habit forming? No
Prescription needed? No
Available as generic? Yes
Drug class: Vitamin supplement

USES

- Dietary supplement to promote normal growth, development and health.
- Treatment for beri-beri (a thiamine-deficiency disease).
- Dietary supplement for alcoholism, cirrhosis, overactive thyroid, infection, breast-feeding, absorption diseases, pregnancy, prolonged diarrhea, burns.

DOSAGE & USAGE INFORMATION

How to take:
Tablet or liquid—Swallow with beverage or food to lessen stomach irritation.

When to take:
At the same time each day.

If you forget a dose:
Take when remembered, then return to regular schedule.

What drug does:
- Promotes normal growth and development.
- Combines with an enzyme to metabolize carbohydrates.

Time lapse before drug works:
15 minutes.

Don't take with:
Any other medicine without consulting your doctor or pharmacist.

OVERDOSE

SYMPTOMS:
Increased severity of adverse reactions and side effects.
WHAT TO DO:
Overdose unlikely to threaten life. If person takes much larger amount than prescribed, call doctor, poison center 1-800-222-1222 or hospital emergency room for instructions.

POSSIBLE ADVERSE REACTIONS OR SIDE EFFECTS

SYMPTOMS	WHAT TO DO
Life-threatening:	
Hives, rash, intense itching, faintness soon after a dose (anaphylaxis) (injection only).	Seek emergency treatment immediately.
Common:	
None expected.	
Infrequent:	
None expected.	
Rare:	
• Wheezing.	Discontinue. Seek emergency treatment.
• Rash or itchy skin.	Discontinue. Call doctor right away.

WARNINGS & PRECAUTIONS

Don't take if:
You are allergic to any B vitamin.

Before you start, consult your doctor:
If you have liver or kidney disease.

Over age 60:
No problems expected.

Pregnancy:
Consult doctor. Risk category A (see page xviii).

Breast-feeding:
No problems expected in meeting child's normal daily requirements. Consult doctor.

Infants & children:
No problems expected.

Prolonged use:
No problems expected.

Skin & sunlight:
No problems expected.

Driving, piloting or hazardous work:
No problems expected.

Discontinuing:
No problems expected.

Others:
A balanced diet should provide enough thiamine for healthy people to make a supplement unnecessary. Best dietary sources of thiamine are whole-grain cereals and meats.

POSSIBLE INTERACTION WITH OTHER DRUGS

GENERIC NAME OR DRUG CLASS	COMBINED EFFECT
Barbiturates*	Decreased thiamine effect.

POSSIBLE INTERACTION WITH OTHER SUBSTANCES

INTERACTS WITH	COMBINED EFFECT
Alcohol:	None expected.
Beverages: Carbonates, citrates (additives listed on many beverage labels).	Decreased thiamine effect.
Cocaine:	None expected.
Foods: Carbonates, citrates (additives listed on many food labels).	Decreased thiamine effect.
Marijuana:	None expected.
Tobacco:	None expected.

*See Glossary

THIAZOLIDINEDIONES

GENERIC AND BRAND NAMES

PIOGLITAZONE
Actos

ROSIGLITAZONE
Avandia

BASIC INFORMATION

Habit forming? No
Prescription needed? Yes
Available as generic? No
Drug class: Antidiabetic

USES

Treatment for type II non-insulin-dependent diabetes mellitus (NIDDM). Rosiglitazone and pioglitazone may be used alone, with insulin or with other antidiabetic drugs.

DOSAGE & USAGE INFORMATION

How to take:
Tablet—Swallow with liquid. Take at mealtime. If you can't swallow whole, crumble tablet and take with liquid or food.

When to take:
Once a day or as directed by doctor. Dosage may be increased after several weeks.

If you forget a dose:
Wait for your next meal that same day and take dose then. If you forget until the next day, take that day's regular dose on schedule (don't double this dose).

Continued next column

OVERDOSE

SYMPTOMS:
Symptoms of hypoglycemia—stomach pain, anxious feeling, cold sweats, chills, confusion, convulsions, cool pale skin, excessive hunger, nausea or vomiting, rapid heartbeat, nervousness, shakiness, unsteady walk, unusual weakness or tiredness, vision changes, unconsciousness.
WHAT TO DO:
- **For mild low blood sugar symptoms, drink or eat something containing sugar right away.**
- **For more severe symptoms, dial 911 (emergency) for an ambulance or medical help or poison center 1-800-222-1222. Then give first aid immediately.**
- **See emergency information on inside covers.**

What drug does:
Lowers blood glucose by improving target cell response to insulin. However, thiazolidinediones do not cure diabetes.

Time lapse before drug works:
May take several weeks for full effectiveness.

Don't take with:
Any other prescription or nonprescription drug without consulting your doctor or pharmacist. All possible drug interactions have not been studied.

POSSIBLE ADVERSE REACTIONS OR SIDE EFFECTS

SYMPTOMS	WHAT TO DO
Life-threatening:	
In case of overdose or low blood sugar, see previous column.	
Common:	
• Pain in back or other body part, infection.	Continue. Call doctor right away.
• Headache, dizziness, nausea, unusual tiredness or weakness.	Continue. Call doctor when convenient.
Infrequent:	
Sore throat, runny nose, diarrhea.	Continue. Call doctor when convenient.
Rare:	
• Severe low blood sugar (see symptoms under Overdose).	Discontinue. Call doctor right away or seek emergency help.
• Liver problems including jaundice (yellow skin and eyes) and hepatitis that could lead to liver transplantation or death.	Discontinue. Call doctor right away.

WARNINGS & PRECAUTIONS

Don't take if:
You are allergic to any of the thiazolidinediones.

Before you start, consult your doctor:
- If you have liver disease or any heart disorder.
- If you have any chronic health problem.
- If you have a history of acid in the blood (metabolic acidosis or ketoacidosis).
- If you are allergic to any medication, food or other substance.

Over age 60:
No special problems expected.

Pregnancy:
Decide with your doctor if drug benefits justify risks to unborn child. Risk category B for troglitazone. Risk category C for pioglitazone and rosiglitazone (see page xviii).

Breast-feeding:
It is unknown if drug passes into milk. It is not recommended for use in nursing mothers.

Infants & children:
Safety and efficacy have not been established. Use only under close medical supervision.

Prolonged use:
- Schedule regular doctor visits to determine if the drug is continuing to be effective in controlling the diabetes and to check for any liver function problems.
- You will most likely require an antidiabetic medicine for the rest of your life.
- You will need to test your blood glucose levels several times a day, or for some, once to several times a week.

Skin & sunlight:
No special problems expected.

Driving, piloting or hazardous work:
No special problems expected.

Discontinuing:
Don't discontinue without consulting your doctor even if you feel well. You can have diabetes without feeling any symptoms. Untreated diabetes can cause serious problems.

Others:
- Use of these drugs may lead to liver problems. Currently, it is necessary to get liver function studies prior to starting the drug, then every other month for 6 months and periodically thereafter while on the drug.
- Advise any doctor or dentist whom you consult that you take this medicine. It may interfere with the accuracy of some medical tests.
- May cause ovulation to resume in some women with ovarian disorders. Discuss the need for nonhormonal contraception with your doctor.
- Follow any special diet your doctor may prescribe. It can help control diabetes.
- Consult doctor if you become ill with vomiting or diarrhea while taking this drug.
- Use caution when exercising. Ask your doctor about an appropriate exercise program.
- Wear medical identification stating that you have diabetes and take this medication.
- Learn to recognize the symptoms of low blood sugar. You and your family need to know what to do if these symptoms occur.
- Have a glucagon kit and syringe in the event severe low blood sugar occurs.
- Use of these drugs may raise both HDL and LDL cholesterol levels.
- High blood sugar (hyperglycemia) may occur with diabetes. Ask your doctor about symptoms to watch for and treatment steps to take.
- Educate yourself about diabetes.

POSSIBLE INTERACTION WITH OTHER DRUGS

GENERIC NAME OR DRUG CLASS	COMBINED EFFECT
Antidiabetic agents, sulfonylurea	May decrease fasting plasma glucose concentrations.
Cholestyramine	Decreased effect of troglitazone. Avoid.
Contraceptives, oral*	Decreased effect of contraceptive.
Cyclosporine	Decreased effect of cyclosporine.
HMG-CoA reductase inhibitors	Decreased effect of HMG-CoA reductase inhibitor.
Tacrolimus	Decreased effect of tacrolimus.

POSSIBLE INTERACTION WITH OTHER SUBSTANCES

INTERACTS WITH	COMBINED EFFECT
Alcohol:	No special problems. Avoid excessive amounts of alcohol.
Beverages:	None expected.
Cocaine:	No special problems. Best to avoid.
Foods:	None expected.
Marijuana:	No special problems. Best to avoid.
Tobacco:	People with diabetes should not smoke.

***See Glossary**

THIOGUANINE

BRAND NAMES

Lanvis

BASIC INFORMATION

Habit forming? No
Prescription needed? Yes
Available as generic? Yes
Drug class: Antineoplastic

USES

Treats some forms of leukemia.

DOSAGE & USAGE INFORMATION

How to take:
Tablets—Swallow with liquid. If you can't swallow whole, crumble tablet and take with liquid or food. Instructions to take on empty stomach mean 1 hour before or 2 hours after eating.

When to take:
According to doctor's instructions.

If you forget a dose:
Skip the missed dose and return to regular schedule. Don't double dose.

What drug does:
Interferes with growth of cancer cells.

Time lapse before drug works:
Varies greatly among patients.

Don't take with:
Any other medicines (including over-the-counter drugs such as cough and cold medicines, laxatives, antacids, diet pills, caffeine, nose drops or vitamins) without consulting your doctor.

OVERDOSE

SYMPTOMS:
None expected.
WHAT TO DO:
Overdose unlikely to threaten life. If person takes much larger amount than prescribed, call doctor, poison center 1-800-222-1222 or hospital emergency room for instructions.

POSSIBLE ADVERSE REACTIONS OR SIDE EFFECTS

SYMPTOMS	WHAT TO DO
Life-threatening:	
Black, tarry stools.	Discontinue. Seek emergency treatment.
Common:	
• Appetite loss, diarrhea, skin rash.	Continue. Call doctor when convenient.
• Nausea.	No action necessary.
Infrequent:	
Bloody urine; hoarseness or cough; fever or chills; lower back or side pain; painful or difficult urination; red spots on skin; unusual bleeding or bruising; joint pain; swollen feet and legs; unsteady gait.	Discontinue. Call doctor right away.
Rare:	
Mouth and lip sores; jaundice (yellow skin and eyes).	Discontinue. Call doctor right away.

WARNINGS & PRECAUTIONS

Don't take if:
- You are allergic to thioguanine.
- You have chicken pox or shingles.

Before you start, consult your doctor:
- If you have gout.
- If you have an infection.
- If you have kidney or liver disease.
- If you have had radiation or cancer chemotherapy within 6 weeks.

Over age 60:
Adverse reactions and side effects may be more frequent and severe than in younger persons. You may need smaller doses for shorter periods of time.

Pregnancy:
- Risk to unborn child outweighs drug benefits. Don't use.
- Don't use birth control pills for contraception.
- Risk category D (see page xviii).

Breast-feeding:
Drug may pass into milk. Avoid drug or discontinue nursing until you finish medicine. Consult doctor for advice on maintaining milk supply.

Infants & children:
No special problems expected.

Prolonged use:
- Increased likelihood of side effects.
- Talk to your doctor about the need for follow-up medical examinations or laboratory studies to check kidney and liver function, serum uric acid, and complete blood counts (white blood cell count, platelet count, red blood cell count, hemoglobin, hematocrit).

Skin & sunlight:
No problems expected.

Driving, piloting or hazardous work:
No problems expected.

Discontinuing:
Report to your doctor any of these symptoms that occur after discontinuing: black, tarry stools; bloody urine; hoarseness or cough; fever or chills; lower back or side pain; painful or difficult urination; red spots on skin; unusual bleeding or bruising.

Others:
- Advise any doctor or dentist whom you consult that you take this medicine.
- May affect results in some medical tests.
- Don't use birth control pills for contraception.

POSSIBLE INTERACTION WITH OTHER DRUGS

GENERIC NAME OR DRUG CLASS	COMBINED EFFECT
Antigout drugs*	May need increased antigout dosage.
Bone marrow depressants*, other	Increased risk of bone marrow depression.
Vaccines, live or killed	Increased risk of toxicity or reduced effectiveness of vaccine.
Zidovudine	More likelihood of toxicity of both drugs.

POSSIBLE INTERACTION WITH OTHER SUBSTANCES

INTERACTS WITH	COMBINED EFFECT
Alcohol:	Increased side effects.
Beverages:	None expected.
Cocaine:	Increased side effects.
Foods:	None expected.
Marijuana:	None expected.
Tobacco:	None expected.

***See Glossary**

THIOTHIXENE

BRAND NAMES

Navane
Thiothixene HCl Intensol

BASIC INFORMATION

Habit forming? No
Prescription needed? Yes
Available as generic? Yes
Drug class: Antipsychotic (thioxanthine)

USES

Reduces anxiety, agitation, psychosis.

DOSAGE & USAGE INFORMATION

How to take:
- Capsule—Swallow with liquid. If you can't swallow whole, open capsule and take with liquid or food.
- Syrup—Dilute dose in beverage before swallowing.

When to take:
At the same times each day.

If you forget a dose:
Take as soon as you remember up to 2 hours late. If more than 2 hours, wait for next scheduled dose (don't double this dose).

What drug does:
Corrects imbalance of nerve impulses.

Continued next column

OVERDOSE

SYMPTOMS:
Drowsiness, dizziness, weakness, muscle rigidity, twitching, tremors, confusion, dry mouth, blurred vision, rapid pulse, shallow breathing, low blood pressure, convulsions, coma.
WHAT TO DO:
- **Dial 911 (emergency) for an ambulance or medical help or poison center 1-800-222-1222. Then give first aid immediately.**
- **If patient is unconscious and not breathing, give mouth-to-mouth breathing. If there is no heartbeat, use cardiac massage and mouth-to-mouth breathing (CPR). Don't try to make patient vomit. If you can't get help quickly, take patient to nearest emergency facility.**
- **See emergency information at end of book.**

Time lapse before drug works:
3 weeks.

Don't take with:
Any other medicine without consulting your doctor or pharmacist.

POSSIBLE ADVERSE REACTIONS OR SIDE EFFECTS

SYMPTOMS	WHAT TO DO
Life-threatening:	
High fever, rapid pulse, profuse sweating, muscle rigidity, confusion and irritability, seizures.	Discontinue. Seek emergency treatment.
Common:	
• Jerky or involuntary movements, especially of the face, lips, jaw, tongue; slow-frequency tremor of head or limbs, especially while moving; muscle rigidity, lack of facial expression and slow, inflexible movements.	Discontinue. Call doctor right away.
• Pacing or restlessness; intermittent spasms of muscles of face, eyes, tongue, jaw, neck, body or limbs; dry mouth, blurred vision, constipation, difficulty urinating.	Continue. Call doctor when convenient.
Infrequent:	
• Sedation, low blood pressure and dizziness.	Continue. Call doctor when convenient.
• Other symptoms not listed above.	Continue. Call doctor when convenient.

WARNINGS & PRECAUTIONS

Don't take if:
- You are allergic to any thioxanthine or phenothiazine tranquilizer.
- You have serious blood disorder.
- You have Parkinson's disease.
- Patient is younger than 12.

Before you start, consult your doctor:
- If you have had liver or kidney disease.
- If you have epilepsy, glaucoma, prostate trouble.
- If you have high blood pressure or heart disease (especially angina).
- If you use alcohol daily.
- If you will have surgery within 2 months, including dental surgery, requiring general or spinal anesthesia.

Over age 60:
Adverse reactions and side effects may be more frequent and severe than in younger persons.

Pregnancy:
Decide with your doctor if drug benefits justify risk to unborn child. Risk category C (see page xviii).

Breast-feeding:
Studies inconclusive. Consult your doctor.

Infants & children:
Not recommended.

Prolonged use:
- Pigment deposits in lens and retina of eye.
- Involuntary movements of jaws, lips, tongue (tardive dyskinesia).
- Talk to your doctor about the need for follow-up medical examinations or laboratory studies to check complete blood counts (white blood cell count, platelet count, red blood cell count, hemoglobin, hematocrit), liver function, eyes.

Skin & sunlight:
- May cause rash or intensify sunburn in areas exposed to sun or ultraviolet light (photosensitivity reaction). Use sunscreen and avoid overexposure. Notify doctor if reaction occurs.
- Hot temperatures and exercise, hot baths can increase risk of heatstroke. Drug may affect body's ability to maintain normal temperature.

Driving, piloting or hazardous work:
Don't drive or pilot aircraft until you learn how medicine affects you. Don't work around dangerous machinery. Don't climb ladders or work in high places. Danger increases if you drink alcohol or take medicine affecting alertness and reflexes.

Discontinuing:
Don't discontinue without consulting doctor. Dose may require gradual reduction if you have taken drug for a long time. Doses of other drugs may also require adjustment.

Others:
- Advise any doctor or dentist whom you consult that you take this medicine.
- For dry mouth, suck sugarless hard candy or chew sugarless gum. If dry mouth persists, consult your dentist.

POSSIBLE INTERACTION WITH OTHER DRUGS

GENERIC NAME OR DRUG CLASS	COMBINED EFFECT
Anticonvulsants*	Change in seizure pattern.
Antidepressants, tricyclic*	Increased thiothixene effect. Excessive sedation.
Antihistamines*	Increased thiothixene effect. Excessive sedation.
Antihypertensives*	Excessively low blood pressure.
Barbiturates*	Increased thiothixene effect. Excessive sedation.
Bupropion	Increased risk of seizures.
Epinephrine	Excessively low blood pressure.
Guanethidine	Decreased guanethidine effect.
Levodopa	Decreased levodopa effect.
Mind-altering drugs*	Increased thiothixene effect. Excessive sedation.
Monoamine oxidase (MAO) inhibitors*	Excessive sedation.
Narcotics*	Increased thiothixene effect. Excessive sedation.

Continued on page 932

POSSIBLE INTERACTION WITH OTHER SUBSTANCES

INTERACTS WITH	COMBINED EFFECT
Alcohol:	Excessive brain depression. Avoid.
Beverages:	None expected.
Cocaine:	Decreased thiothixene effect. Avoid.
Foods:	None expected.
Marijuana:	Daily use—Fainting likely, possible psychosis.
Tobacco:	None expected.

***See Glossary**

THYROID HORMONES

GENERIC AND BRAND NAMES

LEVOTHYROXINE
- Eltroxin
- Levo-T
- Levothroid
- Levoxyl
- L-Thyroxine
- Synthroid

LIOTHYRONINE
- Cytomel

LIOTRIX
- Euthoid
- Thyrolar

THYROGLOBULIN
- Proloid

THYROID
- Armour Thyroid
- Thyrar
- Westhroid

BASIC INFORMATION

Habit forming? No
Prescription needed? Yes
Available as generic? Yes, for some
Drug class: Thyroid hormone

USES

Replacement for thyroid hormones lost due to deficiency.

DOSAGE & USAGE INFORMATION

How to take:
Tablet—Swallow with liquid.

When to take:
At the same time each day before a meal or on awakening.

If you forget a dose:
Take as soon as you remember up to 12 hours late. If more than 12 hours, wait for next scheduled dose (don't double this dose).

What drug does:
Increases cell metabolism rate.

Time lapse before drug works:
48 hours.

Continued next column

OVERDOSE

SYMPTOMS:
"Hot" feeling, heart palpitations, nervousness, sweating, hand tremors, insomnia, rapid and irregular pulse, headache, irritability, diarrhea, weight loss, muscle cramps, angina, congestive heart failure possible.
WHAT TO DO:
Overdose unlikely to threaten life. If person takes much larger amount than prescribed, call doctor, poison center 1-800-222-1222 or hospital emergency room for instructions.

Don't take with:
Any other medicine without consulting your doctor or pharmacist.

POSSIBLE ADVERSE REACTIONS OR SIDE EFFECTS

SYMPTOMS	WHAT TO DO
Life-threatening: In case of overdose, see previous column.	
Common: Tremor, headache, irritability, insomnia, appetite change, diarrhea, leg cramps, menstrual irregularities, fever, heat sensitivity, unusual sweating, weight loss, nervousness.	Continue. Call doctor when convenient.
Infrequent: Hives, rash, vomiting, chest pain, rapid and irregular heartbeat, shortness of breath.	Discontinue. Call doctor right away.
Rare: None expected.	

WARNINGS & PRECAUTIONS

Don't take if:
- You have had a heart attack within 6 weeks.
- You have no thyroid deficiency, but want to use this to lose weight.

Before you start, consult your doctor:
- If you have heart disease or high blood pressure.
- If you have diabetes.
- If you have Addison's disease, have had adrenal gland deficiency or use epinephrine, ephedrine or isoproterenol for asthma.

Over age 60:
More sensitive to thyroid hormone. May need smaller doses.

Pregnancy:
Considered safe if for thyroid deficiency only. Consult doctor. Risk category A (see page xviii).

Breast-feeding:
Present in milk. Consult doctor.

Infants & children:
Use only under medical supervision.

Prolonged use:
- No problems expected if dose is correct.
- Talk to your doctor about the need for follow-up medical examinations or laboratory studies to check thyroid, heart.

Skin & sunlight:
No problems expected.

Driving, piloting or hazardous work:
No problems expected.

Discontinuing:
Don't discontinue without consulting doctor. Dose may require gradual reduction if you have taken drug for a long time. Doses of other drugs may also require adjustment.

Others:
- Digestive upsets, tremors, cramps, nervousness, insomnia or diarrhea may indicate need for dose adjustment.
- Different brands can cause different results. Do not change brands without consulting doctor.
- Advise any doctor or dentist whom you consult that you take this medicine.

POSSIBLE INTERACTION WITH OTHER DRUGS

GENERIC NAME OR DRUG CLASS	COMBINED EFFECT
Adrenocorticoids, systemic	May require thyroid hormone dosage change.
Amphetamines*	Increased amphetamine effect.
Anticoagulants*, oral	Increased anti-coagulant effect.
Antidepressants, tricyclic*	Increased anti-depressant effect. Irregular heartbeat.
Antidiabetics*, oral or insulin	Antidiabetic may require adjustment.
Aspirin (large doses, continuous use)	Increased effect of thyroid hormone.
Barbiturates*	Decreased barbiturate effect.
Beta-adrenergic blocking agents*	Possible decreased effect of beta blocker.
Cholestyramine	Decreased effect of thyroid hormone.
Colestipol	Decreased effect of thyroid hormone.
Contraceptives, oral*	Decreased effect of thyroid hormone.
Digitalis preparations*	Decreased digitalis effect.
Ephedrine	Increased ephedrine effect.
Epinephrine	Increased epinephrine effect.
Estrogens*	Decreased effect of thyroid hormone.
Meglitinides	Increased blood sugar levels.
Methylphenidate	Increased methylphenidate effect.
Phenytoin	Possible decreased effect of thyroid hormone.
Sympathomimetics*	Increased risk of rapid or irregular heartbeat.

POSSIBLE INTERACTION WITH OTHER SUBSTANCES

INTERACTS WITH	COMBINED EFFECT
Alcohol:	None expected.
Beverages:	None expected.
Cocaine:	Excess stimulation. Avoid.
Foods:	None expected.
Marijuana:	None expected.
Tobacco:	None expected.

***See Glossary**

TICLOPIDINE

BRAND NAMES

Ticlid

BASIC INFORMATION

Habit forming? No
Prescription needed? Yes
Available as generic? No
Drug class: Platelet aggregation inhibitor

USES

Decreases the risk of stroke in patients who have warning signs of stroke or who have had strokes caused by blood clots.

DOSAGE & USAGE INFORMATION

How to take:
Tablets—Swallow with liquid. If you can't swallow whole, crumble tablet and take with liquid or food.

When to take:
Twice a day with food or as directed.

If you forget a dose:
Take as soon as you remember up to 2 hours late. If more than 2 hours, wait for next scheduled dose (don't double this dose).

What drug does:
Inhibits the clumping of platelets and thereby prevents blood clotting.

Time lapse before drug works:
2 hours.

Don't take with:
Any other drugs (particularly aspirin) without consulting doctor or pharmacist.

OVERDOSE

SYMPTOMS:
Bloody vomit or excessive bleeding from gums, nose or rectum.
WHAT TO DO:
Dial 911 (emergency) for an ambulance or medical help or poison center 1-800-222-1222. Then give first aid immediately.

POSSIBLE ADVERSE REACTIONS OR SIDE EFFECTS

SYMPTOMS	WHAT TO DO
Life-threatening: None expected.	
Common:	
• Diarrhea, elevated level of cholesterol in blood.	Continue. Call doctor when convenient.
• Nausea, skin rash, abdominal pain.	Discontinue. Call doctor right away.
Infrequent:	
• Unusual bleeding or bruising.	Discontinue. Seek emergency treatment.
• Headache.	Continue. Call doctor when convenient.
Rare:	
• Sore throat, mouth ulcers, fever, chills.	Discontinue. Seek emergency treatment.
• Dizziness, loss of appetite, gaseousness.	Continue. Call doctor when convenient.

WARNINGS & PRECAUTIONS

Don't take if:
- You are allergic to ticlopidine.
- You have reduced white blood cells (neutropenia).

Before you start, consult your doctor:
- If you have liver disease, kidney disease, peptic ulcers or diverticulitis.
- If you have any bleeding disorder.

Over age 60:
No special problems expected.

Pregnancy:
Use during pregnancy only if clearly needed. Consult doctor. Risk category B (see page xviii).

Breast-feeding:
Safety not established. Consult doctor.

Infants & children:
Not recommended. Safety has not been established.

Prolonged use:
No special problems expected.

Skin & sunlight:
No special problems expected.

Driving, piloting or hazardous work:
Don't drive or pilot aircraft until you learn how the medicine affects you. Don't work around dangerous machinery. Don't climb ladders or work in high places.

Discontinuing:
No special problems expected.

Others:
- Advise any doctor or dentist whom you consult that you take this medicine. This is particularly important if any surgery is scheduled.
- May affect results of some medical tests.
- Report any unusual bleeding to your doctor.

POSSIBLE INTERACTION WITH OTHER DRUGS

GENERIC NAME OR DRUG CLASS	COMBINED EFFECT
Antacids*	Decreased ticlopidine effect.
Aspirin	Increased effects of both drugs.
Digoxin	Slightly decreased digoxin effect.
Theophylline	Increased theophylline effect.

POSSIBLE INTERACTION WITH OTHER SUBSTANCES

INTERACTS WITH	COMBINED EFFECT
Alcohol:	Increased alcohol in blood. Avoid.
Beverages:	None expected.
Cocaine:	None expected.
Foods:	Best to take with foods to prevent stomach upset.
Marijuana:	None expected.
Tobacco:	None expected.

***See Glossary**

TIOPRONIN

BRAND NAMES

Capen	Thiola
Captimer	Thiosol
Epatiol	Tioglis
Mucolysin	Vincol
Sutilan	

BASIC INFORMATION

Habit forming? No
Prescription needed? Yes
Available as generic? No
Drug class: Antiurolithic

USES

Prevents the formation of kidney stones when there is too much cystine in the urine.

DOSAGE & USAGE INFORMATION

How to take:
Tablets—Swallow with liquid. If you can't swallow whole, crumble tablet and take with liquid or food. Instructions to take on empty stomach mean 1 hour before or 2 hours after eating.

When to take:
3 times daily (once approximately every 8 hours).

If you forget a dose:
Take as soon as you remember up to 2 hours late. If more than 2 hours, wait for next scheduled dose (don't double this dose).

What drug does:
Removes high levels of cystine from the body.

Time lapse before drug works:
Works immediately.

Continued next column

OVERDOSE

SYMPTOMS:
None expected. If massive overdose is suspected, follow instructions below.
WHAT TO DO:
- **Dial 911 (emergency) for an ambulance or medical help or poison center 1-800-222-1222. Then give first aid immediately.**
- **See emergency information on inside covers.**

Don't take with:
- Medicines that are known to cause kidney damage or depress bone marrow.
- Any other medicine without consulting your doctor or pharmacist.

POSSIBLE ADVERSE REACTIONS OR SIDE EFFECTS

SYMPTOMS	WHAT TO DO
Life-threatening:	
In case of overdose, see previous column	
Common:	
• Skin rash, itching skin, mouth sores, mouth ulcers.	Discontinue. Call doctor right away.
• Abdominal pain, gaseousness, diarrhea, nausea or vomiting.	Continue. Call doctor when convenient.
Infrequent:	
• Cloudy urine, chills, breathing difficulty, joint pain.	Discontinue. Call doctor right away.
• Impaired smell or taste.	Continue. Call doctor when convenient.
Rare:	
Coughing up blood, fever, unusual tiredness or weakness, double vision, muscle weakness.	Discontinue. Call doctor right away.

WARNINGS & PRECAUTIONS

Don't take if:
You are allergic to tiopronin or penicillamine.

Before you start, consult your doctor:
If you have had any of the following in the past:
- Agranulocytosis*
- Aplastic anemia*
- Thrombocytopenia*
- Impaired kidney function

Over age 60:
May require dosage adjustment if kidney function is impaired due to normal aging.

Pregnancy:
Decide with your doctor if drug benefits justify risk to unborn child. Risk category C (see page xviii).

Breast-feeding:
Drug passes into milk. Avoid or discontinue nursing until you finish medicine. Consult doctor for advice on maintaining milk supply.

Infants & children:
Safety not established. Consult doctor.

Prolonged use:
No special problems expected.

Skin & sunlight:
No special problems expected.

Driving, piloting or hazardous work:
Don't drive or pilot aircraft until you learn how medicine affects you. Don't work around dangerous machinery. Don't climb ladders or work in high places. Danger increases if you drink alcohol or take medicine affecting alertness and reflexes.

Discontinuing:
No special problems expected.

Others:
- Advise any doctor or dentist whom you consult that you take this medicine.
- May affect results of some medical tests.

POSSIBLE INTERACTION WITH OTHER DRUGS

GENERIC NAME OR DRUG CLASS	COMBINED EFFECT
Bone marrow depressants*	May increase possibility of toxic effects of tiopronin.
Medications toxic to kidneys (nephrotoxins*)	May increase possibility of toxic effects of tiopronin.

POSSIBLE INTERACTION WITH OTHER SUBSTANCES

INTERACTS WITH	COMBINED EFFECT
Alcohol:	None expected.
Beverages:	
Water.	Enhances effects of tiopronin. Drink 8 to 10 glasses daily.
Cocaine:	None expected.
Foods:	None expected.
Marijuana:	None expected.
Tobacco:	None expected.

***See Glossary**

TIZANIDINE

BRAND NAMES

Zanaflex

BASIC INFORMATION

Habit forming? No
Prescription needed? Yes
Available as generic? No
Drug class: Antispastic, muscle relaxant

USES

- Relieves muscle spasticity caused by diseases such as multiple sclerosis or injury to the spinal cord. It does not appear to improve muscle weakness.
- Relieves muscle spasticity caused by injury to spinal cord.

DOSAGE & USAGE INFORMATION

How to take:
Tablet—Swallow with liquid. It may be taken with or without food.

When to take:
Up to three times a day or as directed by your doctor.

If you forget a dose:
Take as soon as you remember up to 1 hour late. If more than 1 hour, wait for next scheduled dose (don't double this dose).

What drug does:
Slows nerve impulses that stimulate skeletal muscles, decreasing cramping.

Time lapse before drug works:
Within hours. Dosage may be increased over a several week period to achieve maximum effectiveness.

Don't take with:
Any other medicine without consulting your doctor or pharmacist. All possible drug interactions have not been studied.

OVERDOSE

SYMPTOMS:
Breathing difficulties, heartbeat irregularities; other symptoms may occur that were not observed in medical studies of the drug.
WHAT TO DO:
If person takes much larger amount than prescribed, call doctor, poison center 1-800-222-1222 or hospital emergency room for instructions.

POSSIBLE ADVERSE REACTIONS OR SIDE EFFECTS

SYMPTOMS	WHAT TO DO
Life-threatening: In case of overdose, see previous column.	
Common:	
• Nervousness, sensation changes (tingling, burning, prickling), skin sores, anxiety, tiredness or weakness, constipation, back pain, dizziness, dry mouth, depression, drowsiness, heartburn, lightheadedness when getting up from a sitting or lying position, increase in muscle spasm, muscle weakness, sore throat, runny nose, increased sweating.	Continue. Call doctor when convenient.
• Fever, liver problems, (weight loss, nausea, vomiting, yellow skin or eyes), pain or burning when urinating, involuntary movements, diarrhea, vomiting, stomach pain, speech problems.	Discontinue. Call doctor when convenient.
Infrequent:	
• Heartbeat irregularity, black or tarry stools, seizures, bloody vomit, fever and chills, fainting.	Discontinue. Call doctor right away
• Mental changes, mood changes, dry skin, swelling of hands or feet or other areas of the body, difficulty swallowing, migraine, neck pain, trembling or shaking, weight loss, joint or muscle pain, skin rash, feeling of coldness, puffy skin, weight gain, cough, white patches on tongue or in mouth, visual changes or eye pain.	Continue. Call doctor when convenient.
Rare:	
Other symptoms not mentioned above.	Continue. Call doctor when convenient.

WARNINGS & PRECAUTIONS

Don't take if:
You are allergic to tizanidine.

Before you start, consult your doctor:
- If you have liver disease.
- If you have kidney disease.
- If you are allergic to any medication, food or other substance.
- If you are taking an alpha-adrenergic blood pressure medicine.

Over age 60:
Adverse reactions and side effects may be more frequent and severe than in younger persons. Lower dosage may be recommended to start.

Pregnancy:
Decide with your doctor if drug benefits justify risk to unborn child. Risk category C (see page xviii).

Breast-feeding:
It is unknown if drug passes into milk. Avoid nursing or discontinue until you finish drug. Consult doctor.

Infants & children:
Safety and dosage have not been established.

Prolonged use:
Talk to your doctor about the need for liver function studies while using this drug.

Skin & sunlight:
No special problems expected.

Driving, piloting or hazardous work:
Don't drive or pilot aircraft until you learn how medicine affects you. Don't work around dangerous machinery. Don't climb ladders or work in high places. Danger increases if you drink alcohol or take medicine affecting alertness and reflexes, such as antihistamines, tranquilizers, sedatives, pain medicine, narcotics and mind-altering drugs.

Discontinuing:
Don't discontinue without consulting doctor.

Others:
- May interfere with the results in some medical tests.
- Get up slowly from a sitting or lying position to avoid any dizziness, faintness or lightheadedness.
- Advise any doctor or dentist whom you consult that you take this medicine.
- Take medicine only as directed. Do not increase or reduce dosage without doctor's approval.

POSSIBLE INTERACTION WITH OTHER DRUGS

GENERIC NAME OR DRUG CLASS	COMBINED EFFECT
Central nervous system (CNS) depressants *	Increased sedation.
Contraceptives, oral	Increased effect of tizanidine.
Hypotension-causing drugs*, other	Increased effect of hypotension.

POSSIBLE INTERACTION WITH OTHER SUBSTANCES

INTERACTS WITH	COMBINED EFFECT
Alcohol:	Increased sedation, low blood pressure. Avoid.
Beverages:	None expected.
Cocaine:	Increased spasticity. Avoid.
Foods:	None expected.
Marijuana:	Increased spasticity or sedation. Avoid.
Tobacco:	May interfere with absorption of medicine.

***See Glossary**

TOCAINIDE

BRAND NAMES

Tonocard

BASIC INFORMATION

Habit forming? No
Prescription needed? Yes
Available as generic? No
Drug class: Antiarrhythmic

USES

Stabilizes irregular heartbeat, particularly irregular contractions of the ventricles of the heart or a too rapid heart rate.

DOSAGE & USAGE INFORMATION

How to take:
Tablet—Swallow with food, water or milk. Dosage may need to be changed according to individual response.

When to take:
Take at regular times each day. For example, instructions to take 3 times a day means every 8 hours.

If you forget a dose:
Take as soon as you remember up to 4 hours late. If more than 4 hours, wait for next scheduled dose (don't double this dose).

What drug does:
Decreases excitability of cells of heart muscle.

Time lapse before drug works:
30 minutes to 2 hours.

Don't take with:
- Any other medicine without consulting your doctor or pharmacist.
- Wear identification information that states that you take this medicine so during an emergency a physician will know to avoid additional medicines that might be harmful or dangerous.

OVERDOSE

SYMPTOMS:
Convulsions, depressed breathing, cardiac arrest.
WHAT TO DO:
- **Dial 911 (emergency) for an ambulance or medical help or poison center 1-800-222-1222. Then give first aid immediately.**
- **See emergency information on inside covers.**

POSSIBLE ADVERSE REACTIONS OR SIDE EFFECTS

SYMPTOMS	WHAT TO DO
Life-threatening: In case of overdose, see previous column.	
Common:	
• Nausea, vomiting, lightheadedness, dizziness.	Discontinue. Call doctor right away.
• Appetite loss.	Continue. Call doctor when convenient.
Infrequent:	
• Trembling, headache.	Discontinue. Call doctor right away.
• Numbness or tingling in hands or feet.	Continue. Call doctor when convenient.
Rare:	
• Sore throat, unexplained bleeding or bruising, fever, chills, blurred vision, accelerated heart rate or more irregular heartbeat, cough, difficult breathing, wheezing, double vision, disorientation, shakiness, seizures, blisters.	Discontinue. Call doctor right away.
• Rash, swollen feet and ankles, unusual sweating.	Continue. Call doctor when convenient.

WARNINGS & PRECAUTIONS

Don't take if:
- You are allergic to tocainide or anesthetics whose names end in "caine."
- You have myasthenia gravis.

Before you start, consult your doctor:
- If you have congestive heart failure.
- If you are pregnant or plan to become pregnant.
- If you take anticancer drugs, trimethoprim, pyrimethamine, primaquine, phenylbutazone, penicillamine or oxyphenbutazone. These may affect blood cell production in bone marrow.
- If you take any other heart medicine such as digitalis, flucystosine, colchicine, chloramphenicol, beta-adrenergic blockers or azathioprine. These can worsen heartbeat irregularity.
- If you will have surgery within 2 months, including dental surgery, requiring general, local or spinal anesthesia.
- If you have liver or kidney disease.

Over age 60:
Adverse reactions and side effects may be more frequent and severe than in younger persons.

Pregnancy:
Decide with your doctor whether drug benefits justify risk to unborn child. Risk category C (see page xviii).

Breast-feeding:
Avoid if possible. Consult doctor.

Infants & children:
Not recommended. Safety and dosage have not been established.

Prolonged use:
Request periodic lab studies on blood, liver function, potassium levels, x-ray, ECG*.

Skin & sunlight:
No problems expected.

Driving, piloting or hazardous work:
Use caution if medicine causes you to feel dizzy or weak. Otherwise, no problems expected.

Discontinuing:
Don't discontinue without consulting doctor, even though symptoms diminish or disappear.

Others:
No problems expected.

POSSIBLE INTERACTION WITH OTHER DRUGS

GENERIC NAME OR DRUG CLASS	COMBINED EFFECT
Antiarrhythmics*, others	Increased possibility of adverse reactions from either drug.
Beta-adrenergic blocking agents*	Irregular heartbeat. May worsen congestive heart failure.
Bone marrow depressants*	Decreased production of blood cells in bone marrow.

POSSIBLE INTERACTION WITH OTHER SUBSTANCES

INTERACTS WITH	COMBINED EFFECT
Alcohol:	Possible irregular heartbeat. Avoid.
Beverages:	
Caffeine drinks, iced drinks.	Possible irregular heartbeat.
Cocaine:	Possible light-headedness, dizziness, quivering, convulsions.
Foods:	None expected.
Marijuana:	None expected.
Tobacco:	Possible irregular heartbeat.

***See Glossary**

TOLCAPONE

BRAND NAMES

Tasmar

BASIC INFORMATION

Habit forming? No
Prescription needed? Yes
Available as generic? No
Drug class: Antidyskinetic, antiparkinsonism

USES

Used in combination with levodopa and carbidopa for the treatment of the symptoms of Parkinson's disease.

DOSAGE & USAGE INFORMATION

How to take:
Tablets—Swallow with water, with or without food. If you can't swallow whole, crumble tablet and take with liquid or food.

When to take:
At the same time each day.

If you forget a dose:
Take as soon as possible. If it is almost time for your next dose, skip the missed dose and go back to your regular dosing schedule. Do not double doses.

What drug does:
Increases the blood levels of levodopa and carbidopa to restore the chemical balance necessary for normal nerve impulses.

Time lapse before drug works:
Up to two hours.

Don't take with:
Any other prescription or nonprescription drug without consulting your doctor.

OVERDOSE

SYMPTOMS:
Nausea, vomiting and dizziness.
WHAT TO DO:
Overdose unlikely to threaten life. If person uses much larger amount than prescribed, call doctor, poison center 1-800-222-1222 or hospital emergency room for instructions.

POSSIBLE ADVERSE REACTIONS OR SIDE EFFECTS

SYMPTOMS	WHAT TO DO
Life-threatening: None expected.	
Common:	
• Abdominal pain, loss of appetite, diarrhea, dizziness, twitching or unusual body movements, hallucinations, headache, fainting, sleeplessness, nausea, drowsiness, fainting, cough, fever, congestion, runny nose, sneezing, sore throat, vomiting.	Discontinue. Call doctor right away.
• Constipation, excessive dreaming, increased sweating, dry mouth.	Continue. Call doctor if symptoms persist.
• Change in urine color to bright yellow.	No action necessary.
Infrequent:	
• Chest pain, confusion, difficulty breathing, fatigue, falling, blood in urine, hyperactivity, flu-like symptoms, loss of balance control.	Discontinue. Call doctor right away.
• Heartburn, gas.	Continue. Call doctor if symptoms persist.
Rare:	
Agitation; joint pain; redness or swelling; burning feet; chest discomfort; low blood pressure; difficulty thinking or concentrating; muscle cramps; neck pain; burning, prickling or tingling sensations; sinus congestion; stiffness; bloody or cloudy urine; difficult or painful urination; frequent urge to urinate.	Discontinue. Call doctor right away.

WARNINGS & PRECAUTIONS

Don't take if:
- You have been diagnosed with liver problems.
- You are allergic to tolcapone or any other substances such as food preservatives or dyes.

Before you start, consult your doctor:
- If you have any other medical problem.
- If you suffer from hallucinations.
- If you have ever been diagnosed with kidney problems.
- If you have low blood pressure or are dizzy when getting up suddenly from a sitting or lying position.

Over age 60:
The risk of hallucinations (seeing, hearing or feeling things that are not there) may be increased in patients older than 75 years of age.

Pregnancy:
Decide with your doctor whether drug benefits justify risk to unborn child. Risk category C (see page xviii).

Breast-feeding:
It is not known if drug passes into milk. Avoid drugs or discontinue nursing until you finish medicine. Consult doctor for advice on maintaining milk supply.

Infants & children:
There is no identified potential use of tolcapone in children.

Prolonged use:
No problems expected.

Skin & sunlight:
No problems expected.

Driving, piloting or hazardous work:
Don't drive or pilot aircraft until you learn how medicine affects you. Don't work around dangerous machinery. Don't climb ladders or work in high places. Danger increases if you drink alcohol or take medicine affecting alertness and reflexes.

Discontinuing:
Because of the risk of liver failure, this drug should be stopped if no improvement in 3 weeks.

Others:
- Tolcapone has been indicated in several life-threatening cases of liver failure. This medication should not be used as a first-line treatment for Parkinson's disease.
- You will need frequent liver-function blood tests while you take this medicine.
- Advise any doctor or dentist whom you consult that you take this medicine.

POSSIBLE INTERACTION WITH OTHER DRUGS

GENERIC NAME OR DRUG CLASS	COMBINED EFFECT
Apomorphine	May require adjustment in dosage of apomorphine.
Desipramine	May increase incidence of adverse effects of tolcapone.
Dobutamine	May require adjustment in dosage of dobutamine.
Isoproterenol	May require adjustment in dosage of isoproterenol.
Methyldopa	May require adjustment in dosage of methyldopa.
Monoamine oxidase (MAO) inhibitor*	May reduce the effectiveness of the MAO inhibitor.
Warfarin	May require adjustment in dosage of warfarin.

POSSIBLE INTERACTION WITH OTHER SUBSTANCES

INTERACTS WITH	COMBINED EFFECT
Alcohol:	May increase incidence of hallucinations. Do not use.
Beverages:	None expected.
Cocaine:	May increase incidence of hallucinations. Do not use.
Foods:	None expected.
Marijuana:	May increase incidence of hallucinations. Do not use.
Tobacco:	None expected.

*See Glossary

TOLTERODINE

BRAND NAMES

Detrol
Detrol LA

BASIC INFORMATION

Habit forming? No
Prescription needed? Yes
Available as generic? No
Drug class: Antispasmodic

USES

Used to treat an overactive bladder with symptoms of urinary frequency, urgency or urge incontinence (inability to control bladder).

DOSAGE & USAGE INFORMATION

How to take:
Tablets—Swallow with water, with or without food. If you can't swallow whole, crumble tablet and take with liquid or food.

When to take:
At the same times each day.

If you forget a dose:
Take as soon as possible. If it is almost time for your next dose, skip the missed dose and go back to your regular dosing schedule. Do not double doses.

What drug does:
Decreases pressure on the bladder thereby easing the symptoms of overactive bladder.

Time lapse before drug works:
1 to 2 hours.

Don't take with:
Any other prescription or nonprescription drug without consulting your doctor.

OVERDOSE

SYMPTOMS:
Rapid breathing, dry mouth (anticholinergic effect).
WHAT TO DO:
Overdose unlikely to threaten life. If person uses much larger amount than prescribed, call doctor, poison center 1-800-222-1222 or hospital emergency room for instructions.

POSSIBLE ADVERSE REACTIONS OR SIDE EFFECTS

SYMPTOMS	WHAT TO DO
Life-threatening: None expected.	
Common:	
• Change in vision; difficult, burning or painful urination; frequent urge to urinate; bloody or cloudy urine.	Discontinue. Call doctor right away.
• Chest pain, dizziness, dry mouth, vomiting, abdominal pain, constipation, diarrhea, upset stomach, nausea, headache, flu-like symptoms, drowsiness, dry eyes.	Continue. Call doctor if symptoms persist.
• Flatulence (gas).	No action necessary.
Infrequent:	
Difficult urination, dizziness.	Continue. Call doctor if symptoms persist.
Rare: None expected.	

WARNINGS & PRECAUTIONS

Don't take if:
You are allergic to tolterodine.

Before you start, consult your doctor:
- If you have ever been diagnosed with urinary retention.
- If you have gastric retention.
- If you have glaucoma.
- If you have been diagnosed with liver or kidney disease.
- If you have any other medical problem.

Over age 60:
No problems expected.

Pregnancy:
Decide with your doctor whether drug benefits justify risk to unborn child. Risk category C (see page xviii).

Breast-feeding:
It is unknown if drug passes into milk. Avoid drug or discontinue nursing until you finish medicine. Consult doctor for advice on maintaining milk supply.

Infants & children:
Safety and efficacy have not been established in infants and children.

Prolonged use:
No problems expected.

Skin & sunlight:
No problems expected.

Driving, piloting or hazardous work:
Don't drive, pilot an aircraft or engage in any hazardous activities. Tolterodine can cause blurred vision.

Discontinuing:
Don't discontinue without consulting doctor.

Others:
- Advise any doctor or dentist whom you consult that you are taking this medication.
- Chew sugarless gum or suck on ice chips to relieve a dry mouth. Call your doctor or dentist if the dry mouth lasts longer than 2 weeks.

POSSIBLE INTERACTION WITH OTHER DRUGS

GENERIC NAME OR DRUG CLASS	COMBINED EFFECT
Enzyme inhibitors*	May require adjustment in dosage of tolterodine.

POSSIBLE INTERACTION WITH OTHER SUBSTANCES

INTERACTS WITH	COMBINED EFFECT
Alcohol:	None expected.
Beverages:	None expected.
Cocaine:	Effects unknown. Avoid.
Foods:	None expected.
Marijuana:	Effects unknown. Avoid.
Tobacco:	None expected.

*See Glossary

TOPIRAMATE

BRAND NAMES

Topamax

BASIC INFORMATION

Habit forming? No
Prescription needed? Yes
Available as generic? No
Drug class: Anticonvulsant, antiepileptic

USES

Treatment for partial (focal) epileptic seizures. May be used alone or in combination with other antiepileptic drugs.

DOSAGE & USAGE INFORMATION

How to take:

- Tablet–Swallow the tablets whole with a drink of water; do not crush or chew (the tablet has a bitter taste). May be taken with or without food and on a full or empty stomach.
- Sprinkle capsules–Can be swallowed whole or opened carefully and the contents sprinkled on a small amount of soft food, such as apple-sauce, pudding, ice cream, oatmeal, or yogurt. Swallow this mixture immediately. Do not chew or store for later use.

When to take:
Your doctor will determine the best schedule. Dosages will be increased rapidly over the first weeks of use. Further increases may be necessary to achieve maximum benefits.

If you forget a dose:
Take as soon as you remember. If it is almost time for the next dose, skip the missed dose and wait for your next scheduled dose (don't double this dose).

Continued next column

OVERDOSE

SYMPTOMS:
Slow or irregular heartbeat, confusion, dizziness, faintness, unusual tiredness or weakness, blue skin or fingernails, breathing difficulty, coma.
WHAT TO DO:

- **Dial 911 (emergency) for an ambulance or medical help or poison center 1-800-222-1222. Then give first aid immediately.**
- **See emergency information at end of book**

What drug does:
The exact mechanism of the anticonvulsant effect is unknown. It appears that it may block the spread of seizures rather than raise the seizure threshold like other anticonvulsants. Topiramate's anticonvulsant actions involve several mechanisms.

Time lapse before drug works:
May take several weeks for effectiveness.

Don't take with:
Any other prescription or nonprescription drug without consulting your doctor or pharmacist.

POSSIBLE ADVERSE REACTIONS OR SIDE EFFECTS

SYMPTOMS	WHAT TO DO
Life-threatening: In case of overdose, see previous column.	
Common:	
• Burning, prickling, or tingling sensations; clumsiness or unsteadiness; confusion; continuous, uncontrolled back-and -forth or rolling eye movements; dizziness; double vision or other vision problems; drowsiness; generalized slowing of mental and physical activity; memory problems; menstrual changes; menstrual pain; nervousness; speech or language problems; trouble in concentrating or paying attention; unusual tiredness or weakness.	Continue, but call doctor right away.
• Breast pain in women, nausea, tremor	Continue. Call doctor when convenient.
Infrequent:	
• Abdominal pain, fever, chills, sore throat, lessening of sensations or perception; loss of appetite; mood or mental changes (such as aggression, agitation, apathy, irritability, and depression) red, irritated, or bleeding gums; weight loss.	Continue, but call doctor right away.
• Back pain; chest pain; constipation; heartburn; hot flushes; increased sweating; leg pain.	Continue. Call doctor when convenient.

Rare:	
Eye pain, frequent or difficult urination, bloody urine, hearing loss, itching, unsteadiness, loss of bladder control, lower back or side pain, nosebleeds, pale skin, red or irritated eyes, ringing or buzzing in ears, skin rash, swelling, troubled breathing.	Continue, but call doctor right away.

WARNINGS & PRECAUTIONS

Don't take if:
You are allergic to topiramate.

Before you start, consult your doctor:
- If you have a history of liver disease.
- If you have kidney disease or kidney stones (nephrolithiasis).
- If you are allergic to any medication, food or other substance.
- If you have any other medical problems.

Over age 60:
No special problems expected.

Pregnancy:
Decide with your doctor if drug benefits justify risks to unborn child. Risk category C (see page xviii).

Breast-feeding:
It is unknown if drug passes into milk. Avoid drug or discontinue nursing until you finish medicine. Consult doctor for advice on maintaining milk supply.

Infants & children:
This medicine is approved for use from age 2 on. Dose is according to body weight. This medicine is not expected to cause different side effects or problems in children than it does in adults.

Prolonged use:
No special problems expected. Follow-up laboratory blood studies may be recommended by your doctor.

Skin & sunlight:
No problems expected.

Driving, piloting or hazardous work:
Don't drive or pilot aircraft until you learn how medicine affects you. Don't work around dangerous machinery. Don't climb ladders or work in high places. Danger increases if you drink alcohol or take other medicines affecting alertness and reflexes such as antihistamines, tranquilizers, sedatives, pain medicine, narcotics and mind-altering drugs.

Discontinuing:
Don't discontinue without doctor's approval due to risk of increased seizure activity. The dosage may need to be gradually decreased before stopping the drug completely.

Others:
- Advise any doctor or dentist whom you consult that you take this medicine.
- Drink plenty of fluids while taking topiramate. If you have had kidney stones in the past, this will help to reduce your chances of forming kidney stones.
- Topiramate may be used with other anticonvulsant drugs and additional side effects may also occur. If they do, discuss them with your doctor.

POSSIBLE INTERACTION WITH OTHER DRUGS

GENERIC NAME OR DRUG CLASS	COMBINED EFFECT
Anticonvulsants*, other	May decrease or increase effect of both drugs.
Carbonic anhydrase inhibitors*	Increased risk of kidney stones.
Contraceptives, oral*	Decreased effect of contraceptive.
CNS Depressants*	Increased sedative effect.
Digoxin	May decrease effect of digoxin.

POSSIBLE INTERACTION WITH OTHER SUBSTANCES

INTERACTS WITH	COMBINED EFFECT
Alcohol:	Increased sedative effect. Avoid.
Beverages:	None expected.
Cocaine:	Unknown effect. Avoid.
Foods:	None expected.
Marijuana:	Unknown effect. Avoid.
Tobacco:	None expected.

***See Glossary**

TOREMIFENE

BRAND NAMES

Fareston

BASIC INFORMATION

Habit forming? No
Prescription needed? Yes
Available as generic? No
Drug class: Antineoplastic

USES

Used to treat breast cancer in postmenopausal women.

DOSAGE & USAGE INFORMATION

How to take:
Tablets—Swallow with water, with or without food. If you can't swallow whole, crumble tablet and take with liquid or food.

When to take:
At the same time each day.

If you forget a dose:
Take as soon as possible. If it is almost time for your next dose, skip the missed dose and go back to your regular dosing schedule. Do not double doses.

What drug does:
Exact mechanism unknown. Appears to block growth-stimulating effects of estrogen in the tumor.

Time lapse before drug works:
4 to 6 weeks to determine effectiveness.

Don't take with:
Any other prescription or nonprescription drug without consulting your doctor.

OVERDOSE

SYMPTOMS:
Dizziness, headache, nausea and vomiting.
WHAT TO DO:
Overdose unlikely to threaten life. If person uses much larger amount than prescribed, call doctor, poison center 1-800-222-1222 or hospital emergency room for instructions.

POSSIBLE ADVERSE REACTIONS OR SIDE EFFECTS

SYMPTOMS	WHAT TO DO
Life-threatening:	
Pain or swelling of feet or lower legs, chest pain, shortness of breath.	Seek emergency treatment immediately.
Common:	
Hot flashes, nausea.	Continue. Call doctor if symptoms persist.
Infrequent:	
• Change in vaginal discharge, pain or feeling of pressure in pelvis, vaginal bleeding, confusion, increased urination, loss of appetite, unusual tiredness, changes in vision.	Continue. Call doctor right away.
• Dizziness, dry eyes, bone pain, vomiting.	Continue. Call doctor if symptoms persist.
Rare:	
None expected.	

WARNINGS & PRECAUTIONS

Don't take if:
- You are allergic to toremifene.
- You have a history of blood clots or have been diagnosed with thromboembolic disease.

Before you start, consult your doctor:
- If you have any other medical problem.
- If you have any blood or bleeding disorder.
- If you have ever been diagnosed with endometrial hyperplasia (unusual growth of the lining of the uterus).
- If you have a tumor that has spread to your bone.

Over age 60:
No problems expected.

Pregnancy:
Consult doctor. Risk category D (see page xviii).

Breast-feeding:
Drug may pass into milk. Avoid drug or discontinue nursing until you finish medicine. Consult doctor about maintaining milk supply.

Infants & children:
There is no identified potential use of toremifene in children.

Prolonged use:
Talk to your doctor about the need for follow-up laboratory studies to check complete blood count, blood calcium concentrations and liver function.

Skin & sunlight:
Avoid prolonged or extended exposure to direct sunlight and/or artificial sunlight while using this medication.

Driving, piloting or hazardous work:
No problems expected.

Discontinuing:
Don't discontinue without consulting doctor.

Others:
- Advise any doctor or dentist you consult that you are taking this medication.
- May interfere with the accuracy of some medical tests.

POSSIBLE INTERACTION WITH OTHER DRUGS

GENERIC NAME OR DRUG CLASS	COMBINED EFFECT
Anticoagulants	May increase time it takes blood to clot.
Diuretics, thiazide	Possible increased calcium.
Enzyme inducers*	May lessen the effect of toremifene.
Enzyme inhibitors*	May increase the effect of toremifene.

POSSIBLE INTERACTION WITH OTHER SUBSTANCES

INTERACTS WITH	COMBINED EFFECT
Alcohol:	None expected.
Beverages:	None expected.
Cocaine:	Effects unknown. Avoid.
Foods:	None expected.
Marijuana:	Effects unknown. Avoid.
Tobacco:	None expected.

*See Glossary

TRAMADOL

BRAND NAMES

Ultracet
Ultram

BASIC INFORMATION

Habit forming? No
Prescription needed? Yes
Available as generic? No
Drug class: Analgesic

USES

Treatment for moderate to moderately severe pain.

DOSAGE & USAGE INFORMATION

How to take:
Tablet—Swallow with liquid. May be taken with or without food.

When to take:
Every 4 to 6 hours as needed for pain.

If you forget a dose:
Take as soon as you remember. Wait at least 4 hours before the next dose.

What drug does:
The mode of action is not fully understood. It appears to block pain messages to the brain and spinal cord.

Time lapse before drug works:
Within 60 minutes.

Don't take with:
Any other medication without consulting your doctor or pharmacist.

OVERDOSE

SYMPTOMS:
Breathing difficulty, seizures.
WHAT TO DO:

- **Dial 911 (emergency) for an ambulance or medical help or poison center 1-800-222-1222. Then give first aid immediately.**
- **See emergency information on inside covers.**

POSSIBLE ADVERSE REACTIONS OR SIDE EFFECTS

SYMPTOMS	WHAT TO DO
Life-threatening: In case of overdose, see previous column.	
Common: Constipation, nausea, headache, drowsiness, clumsiness.	Continue. Call doctor when convenient.
Infrequent:	
• Constant urge to urinate or inability to urinate, blurred vision.	Discontinue. Call doctor right away.
• Loss of appetite, stomach pain, dry mouth, weakness, confusion, sweating, diarrhea, gas, hot flashes, heartburn, tiredness, flushing or redness of skin, nervousness, trouble sleeping.	Continue. Call doctor when convenient.
Rare: Balancing difficulty, skin reaction (itching, redness and swelling), memory problems, shortness of breath, difficulty performing tasks, hallucinations, dizziness or lightheadedness when getting up from a sitting or lying position, sensations in hands and feet (burning, tingling, pain, weakness, trembling or shaking), faintness, fast heartbeat.	Discontinue. Call doctor right away.

WARNINGS & PRECAUTIONS

Don't take if:
You are allergic to tramadol or narcotic medications.

Before you start, consult your doctor:
- If you have a seizure disorder.
- If you have kidney or liver disease.
- If you have a history of drug dependence or drug abuse, including alcohol abuse.
- If you have respiratory problems.

Over age 60:
Patients over age 75 usually require a dosage adjustment.

Pregnancy:
Decide with your doctor if drug benefits justify risk to unborn child. Risk category C (see page xviii).

Breast-feeding:
Drug passes into milk. Avoid drug or discontinue nursing until you finish medicine. Consult doctor for advice on maintaining milk supply.

Infants & children:
Safety in children under age 16 has not been established.

Prolonged use:
- Consult with your doctor on a regular basis while using this drug.
- Can cause drug dependence, addiction and withdrawal symptoms.

Skin & sunlight:
No special problems expected.

Driving, piloting or hazardous work:
Don't drive or pilot aircraft until you learn how medicine affects you. Don't work around dangerous machinery. Don't climb ladders or work in high places. Danger increases if you drink alcohol or take medicine affecting alertness and reflexes.

Discontinuing:
If you have taken this drug for a long time, consult with your doctor before discontinuing.

Others:
- Don't increase dosage or frequency of use without your doctor's approval.
- Advise any doctor or dentist whom you consult that you take this medicine.

POSSIBLE INTERACTION WITH OTHER DRUGS

GENERIC NAME OR DRUG CLASS	COMBINED EFFECT
Carbamazepine	Decreased effect of tramadol.
Central nervous system (CNS) depressants*	Increased sedation.
Monoamine oxidase (MAO) inhibitors*	Increased risk of seizures.
Narcotics*	Increased sedation.
Phenothiazines*	Increased sedation.
Quinidine	Unknown effect. May require dosage adjustment.
Tranquilizers*	Increased sedation.

POSSIBLE INTERACTION WITH OTHER SUBSTANCES

INTERACTS WITH	COMBINED EFFECT
Alcohol:	Increased sedation. Avoid.
Beverages:	None expected.
Cocaine:	Unknown effect. Best to avoid.
Foods:	None expected.
Marijuana:	Unknown effect. Best to avoid.
Tobacco:	None expected.

***See Glossary**

TRAZODONE

BRAND NAMES

Desyrel
Trialodine
Trazon

BASIC INFORMATION

Habit forming? No
Prescription needed? Yes
Available as generic? Yes
Drug class: Antidepressant (nontricyclic)

USES

- Treats mental depression.
- Treats anxiety.
- Helps promote sleep.
- Treats some types of chronic pain.

DOSAGE & USAGE INFORMATION

How to take:
Tablet—Swallow with liquid or food to lessen stomach irritation. If you can't swallow whole, crumble tablet and take with liquid or food.

When to take:
According to prescription directions. Bedtime dose usually higher than other doses.

If you forget a dose:
Take as soon as you remember up to 2 hours late. If more than 2 hours, wait for next scheduled dose (don't double this dose).

What drug does:
Inhibits serotonin* uptake in brain cells.

Continued next column

OVERDOSE

SYMPTOMS:
Fainting, irregular heartbeat, respiratory arrest, chest pain, seizures, coma.
WHAT TO DO:
- **Dial 911 (emergency) for an ambulance or medical help or poison center 1-800-222-1222. Then give first aid immediately.**
- **If patient is unconscious and not breathing, give mouth-to-mouth breathing. If there is no heartbeat, use cardiac massage and mouth-to-mouth breathing (CPR). Don't try to make patient vomit. If you can't get help quickly, take patient to nearest emergency facility.**
- **See emergency information at end of book.**

Time lapse before drug works:
2 to 4 weeks for full effect.

Don't take with:
Any other medicine without consulting your doctor or pharmacist.

POSSIBLE ADVERSE REACTIONS OR SIDE EFFECTS

SYMPTOMS	WHAT TO DO
Life-threatening: In case of overdose, see previous column.	
Common:	
Drowsiness.	Continue. Call doctor when convenient.
Infrequent:	
• Prolonged penile erections that may be very painful (priapism).	Seek emergency treatment immediately.
• Tremor, fainting, incoordination, blood pressure rise or drop, rapid heartbeat, shortness of breath.	Discontinue. Call doctor right away.
• Disorientation, confusion, fatigue, dizziness on standing, headache, nervousness, rash, itchy skin, blurred vision, ringing in ears, dry mouth, bad taste, diarrhea, nausea, vomiting, constipation, aching, menstrual changes, diminished sex drive, nightmares, vivid dreams.	Continue. Call doctor when convenient.
Rare:	
Unusual excitement	Discontinue. Call doctor right away.

WARNINGS & PRECAUTIONS

Don't take if:
- You are allergic to trazodone.
- You are thinking about suicide.

Before you start, consult your doctor:
- If you have heart rhythm problem.
- If you have any heart disease.
- If you will have surgery within 2 months, including dental surgery, requiring general or spinal anesthesia.
- If you have bipolar (manic-depressive) disorder.
- If you have liver or kidney disease.

Over age 60:
Adverse reactions and side effects may be more frequent and severe than in younger persons.

Pregnancy:
Decide with your doctor if drug benefits justify risk to unborn child. Risk category C (see page xviii).

Breast-feeding:
Drug passes into milk. Avoid drug or discontinue nursing until you finish medicine. Consult doctor for advice on maintaining milk supply.

Infants & children:
Not recommended.

Prolonged use:
See your doctor for occasional blood counts, especially if you have fever and sore throat.

Skin & sunlight:
May cause rash or intensity sunburn in areas exposed to sun or ultraviolet light (photosensitivity reaction). Use sunscreen and avoid overexposure. Notify doctor if reaction occurs.

Driving, piloting or hazardous work:
Don't drive or pilot aircraft until you learn how medicine affects you. Don't work around dangerous machinery. Don't climb ladders or work in high places. Danger increases if you drink alcohol or take medicine affecting alertness and reflexes, such as antihistamines, tranquilizers, sedatives, pain medicine, narcotics and mind-altering drugs.

Discontinuing:
Don't discontinue without consulting doctor. Dose may require gradual reduction if you have taken drug for a long time. Doses of other drugs may also require adjustment.

Others:
- Electroconvulsive therapy* should be avoided. Combined effect is unknown.
- Advise any doctor or dentist whom you consult that you take this medicine.
- For dry mouth, suck on sugarless hard candy or chew sugarless gum.

POSSIBLE INTERACTION WITH OTHER DRUGS

GENERIC NAME OR DRUG CLASS	COMBINED EFFECT
Antidepressants*, other	Excess drowsiness.
Antihistamines*	Excess drowsiness.
Antihypertensives*	Possible too-low blood pressure. Avoid.
Barbiturates*	Too-low blood pressure and drowsiness. Avoid.
Bupropion	Increased risk of seizures.
Central nervous system (CNS) depressants*	Increased sedation.
Digoxin	Possible increased digitalis level in blood.
Guanabenz	Increased effects of both medicines.
Monoamine oxidase (MAO) inhibitors*	May add to toxic effect of each.
Narcotics*	Excess drowsiness.
Phenytoin	Possible increased phenytoin level in blood.

POSSIBLE INTERACTION WITH OTHER SUBSTANCES

INTERACTS WITH	COMBINED EFFECT
Alcohol:	Excess sedation. Avoid.
Beverages: Caffeine.	May add to heartbeat irregularity. Avoid.
Cocaine:	May add to heartbeat irregularity. Avoid.
Foods:	None expected.
Marijuana:	May add to heartbeat irregularity. Avoid.
Tobacco:	May add to heartbeat irregularity. Avoid.

*See Glossary

TRIAZOLAM

BRAND NAMES

Apo-Triazo
Halcion
Novo-Triolam
Nu-Triazo

BASIC INFORMATION

Habit forming? Yes
Prescription needed? Yes
Available as generic? Yes
Drug class: Sedative-hypnotic agent

USES

- Treatment for insomnia (short term).
- Prevention or treatment of transient insomnia associated with sudden sleep schedule changes, such as travel across several time zones.

DOSAGE & USAGE INFORMATION

How to take:
Tablet—Swallow with liquid. If you can't swallow whole, crumble tablet and take with liquid or food.

When to take:
At the same time each day, according to instructions on prescription label. You should be in bed when you take your dose.

If you forget a dose:
Take as soon as you remember up to 2 hours late. If more than 2 hours, wait for next scheduled dose (don't double this dose).

Continued next column

OVERDOSE

SYMPTOMS:
Drowsiness, weakness, tremor, stupor, coma.
WHAT TO DO:
- **Dial 911 (emergency) for an ambulance or medical help or poison center 1-800-222-1222. Then give first aid immediately.**
- **If patient is unconscious and not breathing, give mouth-to-mouth breathing. If there is no heartbeat, use cardiac massage and mouth-to-mouth breathing (CPR). Don't try to make patient vomit. If you can't get help quickly, take patient to nearest emergency facility.**
- **See emergency information at end of book.**

What drug does:
Affects limbic system of brain, the part that controls emotions.

Time lapse before drug works:
Within 30 minutes.

Don't take with:
Any prescription or nonprescription drugs without consulting your doctor or pharmacist.

POSSIBLE ADVERSE REACTIONS OR SIDE EFFECTS

SYMPTOMS	WHAT TO DO
Life-threatening: In case of overdose, see previous column.	
Common:	
Clumsiness, drowsiness, dizziness.	Continue. Call doctor when convenient.
Infrequent:	
• Amnesia, hallucinations, confusion, depression, irritability, rash, itch, vision changes, sore throat, fever, chills, dry mouth.	Discontinue. Call doctor right away.
• Constipation or diarrhea, nausea, vomiting, difficult urination, vivid dreams, behavior changes, abdominal pain, headache.	Continue. Call doctor when convenient.
Rare:	
• Slow heartbeat, breathing difficulty.	Discontinue. Seek emergency treatment.
• Mouth, throat ulcers; jaundice.	Discontinue. Call doctor right away.
• Decreased sex drive.	Continue. Call doctor when convenient.

WARNINGS & PRECAUTIONS

Don't take if:
- You are allergic to any benzodiazepine.
- You have myasthenia gravis.
- You are an active or recovering alcoholic.
- Patient is younger than 6 months.

Before you start, consult your doctor:
- If you have liver, kidney or lung disease.
- If you have diabetes, epilepsy or porphyria.
- If you have glaucoma.

Over age 60:
Adverse reactions and side effects may be more frequent and severe than in younger persons. You may need smaller doses for shorter periods of time. You may develop agitation, rage or a "hangover" effect.

Pregnancy:
Risk to unborn child outweighs drug benefits. Don't use. Risk category X (see page xviii).

Breast-feeding:
Drug may pass into milk. Avoid drug or discontinue nursing until you finish medicine. Consult doctor for advice on maintaining milk supply.

Infants & children:
Not recommended.

Prolonged use:
May impair liver function.

Skin & sunlight:
No problems expected.

Driving, piloting or hazardous work:
Don't drive or pilot aircraft until you learn how medicine affects you. Don't work around dangerous machinery. Don't climb ladders or work in high places. Danger increases if you drink alcohol or take medicine affecting alertness and reflexes.

Discontinuing:
Don't discontinue without consulting doctor. Dose may require gradual reduction if you have taken drug for a long time. Doses of other drugs may also require adjustment.

Others:
- Hot weather, heavy exercise and profuse sweating may reduce excretion and cause overdose.
- Blood sugar may rise in diabetics, requiring insulin adjustment.
- Don't use for insomnia more than 4-7 days.
- Advise any doctor or dentist whom you consult that you take this medicine.
- Triazolam has a very short duration of action in the body.

POSSIBLE INTERACTION WITH OTHER DRUGS

GENERIC NAME OR DRUG CLASS	COMBINED EFFECT
Anticonvulsants*	Change in seizure frequency or severity.
Antidepressants*	Increased sedative effects of both drugs.
Antihistamines*	Increased sedative effects of both drugs.
Antihypertensives*	Excessively low blood pressure.
Central nervous system (CNS) depressants*, other	Increased central nervous system depression.
Cimetidine	Increased triazolam effect. May be dangerous.
Clozapine	Toxic effect on the central nervous system.
Contraceptives, oral*	Increased triazolam effect and toxicity.
Disulfiram	Increased triazolam effect and toxicity.
Erythromycins*	Increased triazolam effect and toxicity.
Isoniazid	Increased triazolam effect and toxicity.
Ketoconazole	Increased triazolam effect and toxicity.
Levodopa	Possible decreased levodopa effect and toxicity.
Molindone	Increased tranquilizer effect.
Monoamine oxidase (MAO) inhibitors*	Convulsions, deep sedation, rage.
Narcotics*	Increased sedative effects of both drugs.
Nefazodone	Increased effects of both drugs.

Continued on page 932

POSSIBLE INTERACTION WITH OTHER SUBSTANCES

INTERACTS WITH	COMBINED EFFECT
Alcohol:	Heavy sedation or amnesia. Avoid.
Beverages: Grapefruit juice	Increased triazolam effect.
Cocaine:	Decreased triazolam effect.
Foods:	None expected.
Marijuana:	Heavy sedation. Avoid.
Tobacco:	Decreased triazolam effect.

***See Glossary**

TRILOSTANE

BRAND NAMES

Modrastane

BASIC INFORMATION

Habit forming? No
Prescription needed? Yes
Available as generic? No
Drug class: Antiadrenal

USES

Temporary treatment of Cushing's syndrome until surgery on adrenals or radiation to pituitary gland can be performed.

DOSAGE & USAGE INFORMATION

How to take:
Capsules—Swallow with liquid. If you can't swallow whole, open capsule and take with liquid or food. Instructions to take on empty stomach mean 1 hour before or 2 hours after eating.

When to take:
Follow doctor's instructions.

If you forget a dose:
Take as soon as you remember up to 2 hours late. If more than 2 hours, wait for next scheduled dose (don't double this dose).

What drug does:
Decreases function of the adrenal cortex.

Time lapse before drug works:
8 hours.

Don't take with:
Any other medicines (including over-the-counter drugs such as cough and cold medicines, laxatives, antacids, diet pills, caffeine, nose drops or vitamins) without consulting your doctor.

OVERDOSE

SYMPTOMS:
None expected.
WHAT TO DO:
Overdose unlikely to threaten life. If person takes much larger amount than prescribed, call doctor, poison center 1-800-222-1222 or hospital emergency room for instructions.

POSSIBLE ADVERSE REACTIONS OR SIDE EFFECTS

SYMPTOMS	WHAT TO DO
Life-threatening:	
None expected.	
Common:	
Diarrhea, abdominal pain.	Discontinue. Call doctor right away.
Infrequent:	
Muscle ache, bloating, watery eyes, nausea, increased salivation, flushing, burning mouth or nose.	Continue. Call doctor when convenient.
Rare:	
Darkening skin, tiredness, appetite loss, depression, skin rash, vomiting.	Continue. Call doctor when convenient.

WARNINGS & PRECAUTIONS

Don't take if:
You know you are allergic to trilostane.

Before you start, consult your doctor:
- If you have an infection.
- If you will have surgery while taking.
- If you have a head injury.
- If you have kidney disease.

Over age 60:
Adverse reactions and side effects may be more frequent and severe than in younger persons. You may need smaller doses for shorter periods of time.

Pregnancy:
Risk to unborn child outweighs drug benefits. Don't use. Risk category X (see page xviii).

Breast-feeding:
Safety not established. Consult doctor.

Infants & children:
Effect not documented. Consult your pediatrician.

Prolonged use:
- Not intended for prolonged use.
- Talk to your doctor about the need for follow-up medical examinations or laboratory studies to check serum electrolytes and urinary 17 - hydroxycorticosteroid.

Skin & sunlight:
No problems expected.

Driving, piloting or hazardous work:
Avoid if you feel confused, drowsy or dizzy.

Discontinuing:
No special problems expected.

Others:
- Advise any doctor or dentist whom you consult that you take this medicine.
- May affect results in some medical tests.

POSSIBLE INTERACTION WITH OTHER DRUGS

GENERIC NAME OR DRUG CLASS	COMBINED EFFECT
Aminoglutethimide	Too much decrease in adrenal function.
Mitotane	Too much decrease in adrenal function.

POSSIBLE INTERACTION WITH OTHER SUBSTANCES

INTERACTS WITH	COMBINED EFFECT
Alcohol:	None expected.
Beverages:	None expected.
Cocaine:	None expected.
Foods:	None expected.
Marijuana:	None expected.
Tobacco:	None expected.

***See Glossary**

TRIMETHOBENZAMIDE

BRAND NAMES

Arrestin
Benzacot
Bio-Gan
Stemetic
Tebamide
Tegamide
T-Gen
Ticon
Tigan
Tiject-20
Triban
Tribenzagan

BASIC INFORMATION

Habit forming? No
Prescription needed? Yes
Available as generic? Yes
Drug class: Antiemetic

USES

Reduces nausea and vomiting.

DOSAGE & USAGE INFORMATION

How to take:

- Capsule—Swallow with liquid. If you can't swallow whole, open capsule and take with liquid or food.
- Suppositories—Remove wrapper and moisten suppository with water. Gently insert larger end into rectum. Push well into rectum with finger.

When to take:
When needed, no more often than label directs.

If you forget a dose:
Take when you remember. Wait as long as label directs for next dose.

Continued next column

OVERDOSE

SYMPTOMS:
Confusion, convulsions, coma.
WHAT TO DO:

- **Dial 911 (emergency) for an ambulance or medical help or poison center 1-800-222-1222. Then give first aid immediately.**
- **If patient is unconscious and not breathing, give mouth-to-mouth breathing. If there is no heartbeat, use cardiac massage and mouth-to-mouth breathing (CPR). Don't try to make patient vomit. If you can't get help quickly, take patient to nearest emergency facility.**
- **See emergency information on inside covers.**

What drug does:
Exact mechanism unknown. Possibly blocks nerve impulses to brain's vomiting centers.

Time lapse before drug works:
20 to 40 minutes.

Don't take with:
Any other prescription or nonprescription drugs without consulting doctor.

POSSIBLE ADVERSE REACTIONS OR SIDE EFFECTS

SYMPTOMS	WHAT TO DO
Life-threatening: In case of overdose, see previous column.	
Common: Drowsiness.	Continue. Call doctor when convenient.
Infrequent: Rash, blurred vision, diarrhea, dizziness, headache, muscle cramps, unusual tiredness.	Discontinue. Call doctor right away.
Rare: Seizures, tremor, depression, sore throat, fever, repeated vomiting, back pain, yellow skin or eyes, body spasm (head and heels bent backward and body bowed forward).	Discontinue. Call doctor right away.

WARNINGS & PRECAUTIONS

Don't take if:

- You are allergic to trimethobenzamide.
- You are allergic to local anesthetics and have suppository form.

Before you start, consult your doctor:
If you have reacted badly to antihistamines.

Over age 60:
More susceptible to low blood pressure and sedative effects of this drug.

Pregnancy:
Decide with your doctor if drug benefits justify risk to unborn child. Risk category C (see page xviii).

Breast-feeding:
Effect unknown. Avoid if possible. Consult doctor.

Infants & children:
- Injectable form not recommended.
- Avoid during viral infections. Drug may contribute to Reye's syndrome.

Prolonged use:
- Damages blood cell production of bone marrow.
- Causes Parkinson's-like symptoms of tremors, rigidity.

Skin & sunlight:
No special problems expected.

Driving, piloting or hazardous work:
- Use disqualifies you for piloting aircraft.
- Don't drive until you learn how medicine affects you. Don't work around dangerous machinery. Don't climb ladders or work in high places. Danger increases if you drink alcohol or take medicine affecting alertness and reflexes, such as antihistamines, tranquilizers, sedatives, pain medicine, narcotics and mind-altering drugs.

Discontinuing:
May be unnecessary to finish medicine. Follow doctor's instructions.

Others:
No problems expected.

POSSIBLE INTERACTION WITH OTHER DRUGS

GENERIC NAME OR DRUG CLASS	COMBINED EFFECT
Antidepressants*	Increased sedative effect.
Antihistamines*	Increased sedative effect.
Barbiturates*	Increased effect of both drugs.
Belladonna	Increased effect of both drugs.
Cholinergics*	Increased effect of both drugs.
Clozapine	Toxic effect on the central nervous system.
Ethinamate	Dangerous increased effects of ethinamate. Avoid combining.
Fluoxetine	Increased depressant effects of both drugs.
Guanfacine	May increase depressant effects of either medicine.
Leucovorin	High alcohol content of leucovorin may cause adverse effects.
Methyprylon	May increase sedative effect to dangerous level. Avoid.
Mind-altering drugs*	Increased effect of mind-altering drug.
Nabilone	Greater depression of central nervous system.
Narcotics*	Increased sedative effect.
Ototoxic medications*	May mask the symptoms of ototoxicity.
Phenothiazines*	Increased effect of both drugs.
Sedatives*	Increased sedative effect.
Sertraline	Increased depressive effects of both drugs.
Sleep inducers*	Increased effect of sleep inducer.
Tranquilizers*	Increased sedative effect.

POSSIBLE INTERACTION WITH OTHER SUBSTANCES

INTERACTS WITH	COMBINED EFFECT
Alcohol:	Oversedation. Avoid.
Beverages:	None expected.
Cocaine:	None expected.
Foods:	None expected.
Marijuana:	Increased antinausea effect.
Tobacco:	None expected.

***See Glossary**

TRIMETHOPRIM

BRAND NAMES

Apo-Sulfatrim
Apo-Sulfatrim DS
Bactrim
Bactrim DS
Bethaprim
Cotrim
Cotrim DS
Co-trimaxizole
Novotrimel
Novotrimel DS
Nu-Cotrimox
Nu-Cotrimox DS
Proloprim
Protrin
Roubac
Septra
Septra DS
SMZ-TMP
Sulfamethoprim
Sulfamethoprim DS
Sulfaprim
Sulfaprim DS
Sulfatrim
Sulfatrim DS
Sulfoxaprim
Sulfoxaprim DS
Sulmeprim
Triazole
Triazole DS
Trimeth-Sulfa
Trimpex
Trisulfam
Uroplus DS
Uroplus SS

BASIC INFORMATION

Habit forming? No
Prescription needed? Yes
Available as generic? Yes
Drug class: Antimicrobial (antibacterial)

USES

- Treats urinary tract infections susceptible to trimethoprim.
- Helps prevent recurrent urinary tract infections if taken once a day.
- Treats pneumocystis carinii pneumonia.

DOSAGE & USAGE INFORMATION

How to take:

- Tablet—Swallow with liquid or food to lessen stomach irritation. If can't swallow whole, crush or crumble tablet and take with food or liquid.
- Oral suspension (in combination with sulfamethoxazole)—Follow directions on label.

Continued next column

OVERDOSE

SYMPTOMS:
Nausea, vomiting, diarrhea.
WHAT TO DO:
Overdose unlikely to threaten life. If person takes much larger amount than prescribed, call doctor, poison center 1-800-222-1222 or hospital emergency room for instructions.

When to take:
Space doses evenly in 24 hours to keep constant amount in urine.

If you forget a dose:
Take as soon as possible. Wait 5 to 6 hours before next dose. Then return to regular schedule.

What drug does:
Stops harmful bacterial germs from multiplying. Will not kill viruses.

Time lapse before drug works:
2 to 5 days.

Don't take with:
Any other medicine without consulting your doctor or pharmacist.

POSSIBLE ADVERSE REACTIONS OR SIDE EFFECTS

SYMPTOMS	WHAT TO DO
Life-threatening: None expected.	
Common: None expected.	
Infrequent: Diarrhea, nausea, vomiting, stomach cramps, headache.	Continue. Call doctor when convenient.
Rare: Blue fingernails, lips and skin; difficult breathing; sore throat; fever; anemia; jaundice; unusual bleeding or bruising; unusual tiredness or weakness; skin changes (rash, itch, redness, blisters, peeling or loosening); aching joints or muscles.	Discontinue. Call doctor right away.

WARNINGS & PRECAUTIONS

Don't take if:
- You are allergic to trimethoprim or any sulfa drug*.
- You are anemic due to folic acid deficiency.

Before you start, consult your doctor:
If you have had liver or kidney disease.

Over age 60:
- Reduced liver and kidney function may require reduced dose.
- More likely to have severe anal and genital itch.
- Increased susceptibility to anemia.

Pregnancy:
Decide with your doctor whether drug benefits justify risk to unborn child. Risk category C (see page xviii).

Breast-feeding:
No proven harm to unborn child. Avoid if possible. Consult doctor.

Infants & children:
Use under medical supervision only.

Prolonged use:
- Anemia.
- Talk to your doctor about the need for follow-up medical examinations or laboratory studies to check complete blood counts (white blood cell count, platelet count, red blood cell count, hemoglobin, hematocrit).

Skin & sunlight:
May cause rash or intensify sunburn in areas exposed to sun or ultraviolet light (photosensitivity reaction). Avoid overexposure. Notify doctor if reaction occurs.

Driving, piloting or hazardous work:
No problems expected.

Discontinuing:
Don't discontinue without doctor's advice until you complete prescribed dose, even though symptoms diminish or disappear.

Others:
No problems expected.

POSSIBLE INTERACTION WITH OTHER DRUGS

GENERIC NAME OR DRUG CLASS	COMBINED EFFECT
Anticonvulsants*	Increased risk of anemia.
Bone marrow depressants*	Increased possibility of bone marrow supression.
Folate antagonists*, other	Increased risk of anemia.
Metformin	Increased metformin effect.
Phenytoin	Increased phenytoin effect.

POSSIBLE INTERACTION WITH OTHER SUBSTANCES

INTERACTS WITH	COMBINED EFFECT
Alcohol:	Increased alcohol effect with Bactrim or Septra.
Beverages:	None expected.
Cocaine:	None expected.
Foods:	None expected.
Marijuana:	None expected.
Tobacco:	None expected.

*See Glossary

TRIPTANS

GENERIC AND BRAND NAMES

ALMOTRIPTAN	**RIZATRIPTAN**
Axert	Maxalt
FROVATRIPTAN	**SUMATRIPTAN**
Frova	Imitrex
NARATRIPTAN	**ZOLMITRIPTAN**
Amerge	Zomig
	Zomig-ZMT

BASIC INFORMATION

Habit forming? No
Prescription needed? Yes
Available as generic? No
Drug class: Antimigraine

USES

- Treatment for acute migraine headaches not relieved by other medications (aspirin, acetaminophen and other nonsteroidal anti-inflammatory drugs). Does not prevent migraines.
- Treatment for cluster headaches.

DOSAGE & USAGE INFORMATION

How to take:

- Injection (sumatriptan—self-administered)—Inject under the skin (subcutaneous) of the outer thigh or outer upper arm. Follow your doctor's instructions and written package instructions for proper injection technique and method for disposal of the cartridges.
- Tablets—Swallow whole with liquid. Do not crush, break or chew tablet.
- Orally disintegrating tablet—Place on tongue, let it dissolve and swallow with saliva.
- Wafers (rizatriptan)—Place on tongue to dissolve and be swallowed with saliva.
- Nasal spray (sumatriptan)—One spray into one nostril as a single dose.

Continued next column

OVERDOSE

SYMPTOMS:
Convulsions, tremor, swelling of arms and legs, breathing difficulty, chest pain, paralysis, skin and hair loss, scab formation at injection site.
WHAT TO DO:

- **Dial 911 (emergency) for an ambulance or medical help or poison center 1-800-222-1222. Then give first aid immediately.**
- **See emergency information on inside covers.**

When to take:

- At the first sign of a migraine (aura or pain). After you administer, lie down in a quiet, dark room to increase effectiveness of drug.
- An additional dose may be helpful if the migraine returns. Do not exceed the prescribed quantity or frequency. Do not use additional dose if first dose does not bring substantial relief.
- Zolmitriptan tablets should not be taken until pain actually begins.
- If cluster headache, follow doctor's directions.

If you forget a dose:
Triptans are not taken on a routine schedule. They should be taken at the onset of your migraine.

What drug does:
Helps relieve headache pain and associated symptoms of migraine (nausea, vomiting, sensitivity to light and sound). It helps constrict dilated blood vessels that may contribute to development of migraines.

Time lapse before drug works:

- Oral dosage (tablets/wafers)—within 30 minutes.
- Injection—usually within 10 minutes for headache pain and within 20 minutes for associated nausea, vomiting and sensitivity to light and sound.

Don't take with:

- Ergotamine-containing medicines. Delay 24 hours.
- Any other medication without consulting your doctor or pharmacist.

POSSIBLE ADVERSE REACTIONS OR SIDE EFFECTS

SYMPTOMS	WHAT TO DO
Life-threatening: In case of overdose, see previous column.	
Common:	
Burning, pain, or redness at sumatriptan injection site; nausea or vomiting (may be from migraine or from drug); drowsiness or dizziness.	May readminister. Call doctor when convenient.
Infrequent:	
Sensation of burning, warmth, numbness, cold or tingling; discomfort of jaw, mouth, throat, nose or sinuses; dizziness; drowsiness; flushing; light-headedness; muscle aches, cramps, stiffness or weakness; anxiety; tiredness; vision changes; feeling of illness.	May readminister. Call doctor when convenient.

Rare:	
Pain, pressure or tightness in the chest; difficulty swallowing; irregular heartbeat.	Discontinue. Seek emergency help.

WARNINGS & PRECAUTIONS

Don't take if:
- You are allergic to any triptans.
- You have angina pectoris, a history of myocardial infarction or myocardial ischemia, Prinzmetal's angina, uncontrolled hypertension (high blood pressure).

Before you start, consult your doctor:
- If you have heart rhythm problems or coronary artery disease.
- If you have had a cerebrovascular accident (stroke).
- If you have liver or kidney disease.
- If you have controlled hypertension (high blood pressure).

Over age 60:
No problems expected.

Pregnancy:
Decide with your doctor whether drug benefits justify risk to unborn child. Risk category C (see page xviii).

Breast-feeding:
Unknown effects. Decide with your doctor whether drug benefits justify possible risk.

Infants & children:
Not recommended for patients under age 18.

Prolonged use:
Long-term effects unknown. As a precaution, do not use sumatriptan more often than every 5-7 days or as directed by your doctor.

Skin & sunlight:
No special problems expected.

Driving, piloting or hazardous work:
Avoid if you feel drowsy or dizzy. Otherwise no problems expected.

Discontinuing:
No problems expected. Talk to your doctor if you have plans to discontinue use of drug.

Others:
- Advise any doctor or dentist whom you consult that you take this medicine.
- May affect results in some medical tests (rare).
- Follow your doctor's recommendation of any additional treatment for prevention of migraines.
- Sensitivity to light is a symptom of migraine and is not drug-related.

POSSIBLE INTERACTION WITH OTHER DRUGS

GENERIC NAME OR DRUG CLASS	COMBINED EFFECT
Antidepressants*	Adverse effects unknown. Avoid.
Dihydroergotamine	Increased vasoconstriction. Delay 24 hours between drugs.
Ergotamine	Increased vasoconstriction. Delay 24 hours between drugs.
Furazolidone	Adverse effects unknown. Avoid.
Lithium	Adverse effects unknown. Avoid.
Monoamine oxidase (MAO) inhibitors*	Adverse effects unknown. Avoid.
Procarbazine	Adverse effects unknown. Avoid.
Selegiline	Adverse effects unknown. Avoid.

POSSIBLE INTERACTION WITH OTHER SUBSTANCES

INTERACTS WITH	COMBINED EFFECT
Alcohol:	No interaction known, but alcohol aggravates migraines. Avoid.
Beverages:	None expected.
Cocaine:	None expected.
Foods:	None expected.
Marijuana:	None expected.
Tobacco:	None expected.

***See Glossary**

URSODIOL

BRAND NAMES

Actigall
Ursofalk

BASIC INFORMATION

Habit forming? No
Prescription needed? Yes
Available as generic? No
Drug class: Anticholelithic

USES

- Dissolves cholesterol gallstones in selected patients who either can't tolerate surgery or don't require surgery for other reasons. Not used when surgery is clearly indicated.
- Prevention of gallstone formation during rapid weight loss.
- Treatment for primary biliary cirrhosis.

DOSAGE & USAGE INFORMATION

How to take:
Capsules—Swallow with liquid or food to lessen stomach irritation. If you can't swallow whole, open capsule and take with liquid or food.

When to take:
With meals, 2 or 3 times a day according to your doctor's instructions.

If you forget a dose:
Take as soon as you remember up to 2 hours late. If more than 2 hours, wait for next scheduled time. Don't double this dose.

What drug does:
Decreases secretion of cholesterol into bile by suppressing production and secretion of cholesterol by the liver. Ursodiol will not help gallstone problems unless the gallstones are made of cholesterol. It works best when the stones are small.

Time lapse before drug works:
Unpredictable. Varies among patients.

Continued next column

OVERDOSE

SYMPTOMS:
Severe diarrhea.
WHAT TO DO:
Overdose not expected to threaten life. If person takes much larger amount than prescribed, call doctor, poison center 1-800-222-1222 or hospital emergency room for instructions.

Don't take with:
Any other medicine without consulting your doctor or pharmacist.

POSSIBLE ADVERSE REACTIONS OR SIDE EFFECTS

SYMPTOMS	WHAT TO DO
Life-threatening: None expected.	
Common: None expected.	
Infrequent: None expected.	
Rare: Diarrhea.	Continue. Call doctor when convenient.

WARNINGS & PRECAUTIONS

Don't take if:
You can't tolerate other bile acids.

Before you start, consult your doctor:
- If you have complications of gallstones, such as infection or obstruction of the bile ducts.
- If you have had pancreatitis.
- If you have had chronically impaired liver function.
- If you take any other medicines for any reason.

Over age 60:
No special problems expected.

Pregnancy:
Consult doctor. Risk category B (see page xviii).

Breast-feeding:
Unknown, but no documented problems. Consult doctor.

Infants & children:
Not recommended. Adequate studies have not been performed.

Prolonged use:
- No special problems expected.
- Talk to your doctor about the need for follow-up medical examinations or laboratory studies to check kidney function.

Skin & sunlight:
No problems expected.

Driving, piloting or hazardous work:
Don't pilot aircraft until you learn how medicine affects you. Don't work around dangerous machinery. Don't climb ladders or work in high places. Danger increases if you drink alcohol or take medicine affecting alertness and reflexes, such as antihistamines, tranquilizers, sedatives, pain medicine, narcotics and mind-altering drugs.

Discontinuing:
Don't discontinue without consulting doctor.

Others:
Plan regular visits to your doctor while you take ursodiol. Have ultrasound and liver function studies done at appropriate intervals. Liver damage is unlikely, but theoretically could happen.

POSSIBLE INTERACTION WITH OTHER DRUGS

GENERIC NAME OR DRUG CLASS	COMBINED EFFECT
Antacids* (aluminum-containing)	Decreased absorption of ursodiol.
Cholestyramine	Decreased absorption of ursodiol.
Clofibrate	Decreased effect of ursodiol.
Colestipol	Decreased absorption of ursodiol.
Estrogens*	Decreased effect of ursodiol.
Progestins	Decreased effect of ursodiol.

POSSIBLE INTERACTION WITH OTHER SUBSTANCES

INTERACTS WITH	COMBINED EFFECT
Alcohol:	None expected, unless you have impaired liver function from alcohol abuse.
Beverages:	None expected.
Cocaine:	None expected.
Foods:	None expected.
Marijuana:	None expected.
Tobacco:	None reported. However, tobacco may possibly impair intestinal absorption from the intestinal tract. Better to avoid.

*See Glossary

VALPROIC ACID

GENERIC AND BRAND NAMES

Depakene   Myproic Acid

BASIC INFORMATION

Habit forming? No
Prescription needed? Yes
Available as generic? Yes
Drug class: Anticonvulsant

USES

- Treatment of various types of epilepsy.
- Treatment for bipolar (manic-depressive) disorder.

DOSAGE & USAGE INFORMATION

How to take:
Capsule or syrup—Swallow with liquid or food to lessen stomach irritation.

When to take:
Once a day.

If you forget a dose:
Take as soon as you remember. Don't ever double dose.

What drug does:
Increases concentration of gamma aminobutyric acid, which inhibits nerve transmission in parts of brain.

Time lapse before drug works:
1 to 4 hours, but full effect may take weeks.

Don't take with:
Any other medicine without consulting your doctor or pharmacist.

OVERDOSE

SYMPTOMS:
Coma
WHAT TO DO:

- **Dial 911 (emergency) for an ambulance or medical help or poison center 1-800-222-1222. Then give first aid immediately.**
- **If patient is unconscious and not breathing, give mouth-to-mouth breathing. If there is no heartbeat, use cardiac massage and mouth-to-mouth breathing (CPR). Don't try to make patient vomit. If you can't get help quickly, take patient to nearest emergency facility.**
- **See emergency information at end of book.**

POSSIBLE ADVERSE REACTIONS OR SIDE EFFECTS

SYMPTOMS	WHAT TO DO
Life-threatening:	
In case of overdose, see previous column.	
Common:	
Loss of appetite, indigestion, nausea, vomiting, abdominal cramps, diarrhea, tremor, unusual weight gain or loss, menstrual changes in girls.	Continue. Call doctor when convenient.
Infrequent:	
Clumsiness, or unsteadiness, constipation, skin rash, dizziness, drowsiness, unusual excitement or irritability.	Continue. Call doctor when convenient.
Rare:	
Mood or behavior changes; continued nausea, vomiting and appetite loss; increase in number of seizures; swelling of face, feet or legs; yellow skin or eyes; tiredness or weakness; back-and-forth eye movements (nystagmus); seeing double or seeing spots; severe stomach cramps; unusual bleeding or bruising.	Continue, but call doctor right away.

WARNINGS & PRECAUTIONS

Don't take if:
You are allergic to valproic acid.

Before you start, consult your doctor:

- If you have blood, kidney or liver disease.
- If you will have surgery within 2 months, including dental surgery, requiring general or spinal anesthesia.

Over age 60:
Adverse reactions and side effects may be more frequent and severe than in younger persons.

Pregnancy:
Risk to unborn child exists. Use only if benefits of drug greatly exceed fetal risk. Risk category D (see page xviii).

Breast-feeding:
Drug passes into milk. Avoid drug or discontinue nursing until you finish medicine. Consult doctor for advice on maintaining milk supply.

Infants & children:
Use under close medical supervision only.

Prolonged use:
Request periodic blood tests, liver and kidney function tests. These tests are necessary for safe and effective use.

Skin & sunlight:
No problems expected.

Driving, piloting or hazardous work:
Don't drive or pilot aircraft until you learn how medicine affects you. Don't work around dangerous machinery. Don't climb ladders or work in high places. Danger increases if you drink alcohol or take medicine affecting alertness and reflexes, such as antihistamines, tranquilizers, sedatives, pain medicine, narcotics and mind-altering drugs.

Discontinuing:
Don't discontinue without consulting doctor. Dose may require gradual reduction if you have taken drug for a long time. Doses of other drugs may also require adjustment.

Others:
Advise any doctor or dentist whom you consult that you take this drug.

POSSIBLE INTERACTION WITH OTHER DRUGS

GENERIC NAME OR DRUG CLASS	COMBINED EFFECT
Anticoagulants*, oral	Increased chance of bleeding.
Anticonvulsants*	Unpredictable. May require increase or decrease in dosage of valproic acid or other anticonvulsant.
Anti-inflammatory drugs, nonsteroidal* (NSAIDs)	Increased risk of bleeding problems.
Antivirals, HIV/AIDS*	Increased risk of pancreatitis.
Carbamazepine	Decreased valproic acid effect.
Central nervous system (CNS) depressants*	Increased sedative effect.
Clonazepam	May prolong seizure.
Felbamate	Increased side effects and adverse reactions of valproic acid.
Hepatotoxics*	Increased risk of liver toxicity.
Lamotrigine	Increased lamotrigine effect. Possibly decrease effect valproic acid.
Levocarnitine	Decreased levocarnitine. Patients taking valproic acid may need to take the supplement levocarnitine.
Phenobarbital	Increased phenobarbital levels; possibly toxic or beneficial effect.
Phenytoin	Unpredictable. Dose may require adjustment.
Primidone	Increased primidone effect. Possible toxicity.
Salicylates*	Increased effect of valproic acid.
Sertraline	Increased depressive effects of both drugs.
Sodium benzoate & sodium phenylacetate	May reduce effect of sodium benzoate & sodium phenylacetate.

Continued on page 932

POSSIBLE INTERACTION WITH OTHER SUBSTANCES

INTERACTS WITH	COMBINED EFFECT
Alcohol:	Deep sedation. Avoid.
Beverages:	None expected.
Cocaine:	Increased brain sensitivity. Avoid.
Foods:	None expected.
Marijuana:	Increased brain sensitivity. Avoid.
Tobacco:	Decreased valproic acid effect.

***See Glossary**

VANCOMYCIN

BRAND NAMES

Vancocin

BASIC INFORMATION

Habit forming? No
Prescription needed? Yes
Available as generic? Yes
Drug class: Antibacterial

USES

- Treats colitis when caused by *clostridium* infections.
- Treats some forms of severe diarrhea.

DOSAGE & USAGE INFORMATION

How to take:

- Capsules—Swallow with liquid. If you can't swallow whole, open capsule and take with liquid or food. Instructions to take on empty stomach mean 1 hour before or 2 hours after eating.
- Oral solution—Use the calibrated measuring device. Swallow with other liquid to prevent nausea.
- There is also an injectable form. This information applies to the oral form only.

When to take:
According to doctor's instructions. Usually every 6 hours.

If you forget a dose:
Take as soon as you remember up to 2 hours late. If more than 2 hours, wait for next scheduled dose (don't double this dose).

What drug does:
Kills bacterial cells.

Time lapse before drug works:
None. Works right away. This medicine is not absorbed to a great extent through the intestinal tract.

Continued next column

OVERDOSE

SYMPTOMS:
None expected.
WHAT TO DO:
Overdose unlikely to threaten life. If person takes much larger amount than prescribed, call doctor, poison center 1-800-222-1222 or hospital emergency room for instructions.

Don't take with:
Any other medicines (including over-the-counter drugs such as cough and cold medicines, laxatives, antacids, diet pills, caffeine, nose drops or vitamins) without consulting your doctor.

POSSIBLE ADVERSE REACTIONS OR SIDE EFFECTS

SYMPTOMS	WHAT TO DO
Life-threatening: None expected.	
Common: Bitter taste.	Continue. Tell doctor at next visit.
Infrequent: Nausea or vomiting.	Continue. Call doctor when convenient.
Rare: Hearing loss, ears ringing or buzzing.	Discontinue. Call doctor right away.

WARNINGS & PRECAUTIONS

Don't take if:
You are allergic to vancomycin.

Before you start, consult your doctor:
- If you have hearing problems.
- If you have severe kidney disease.
- If you have intestinal obstruction.

Over age 60:
Adverse reactions and side effects may be more frequent and severe than in younger persons. You may need smaller doses for shorter periods of time.

Pregnancy:
Consult doctor. Risk category B (see page xviii).

Breast-feeding:
No special problems expected. Consult doctor.

Infants & children:
No special problems expected.

Prolonged use:
Talk to your doctor about the need for follow-up medical examinations or laboratory studies to check hearing acuity, kidney function, vancomycin serum concentration and urinalyses.

Skin & sunlight:
No problems expected.

Driving, piloting or hazardous work:
No problems expected.

Discontinuing:
No special problems expected.

Others:
- Advise any doctor or dentist whom you consult that you take this medicine.
- May affect results in some medical tests.

POSSIBLE INTERACTION WITH OTHER DRUGS

GENERIC NAME OR DRUG CLASS	COMBINED EFFECT
Cholestyramine	Decreased therapeutic effect of vancomycin.
Colestipol	Decreased therapeutic effect of vancomycin.
Metformin	Increased metformin effect.
Nephrotoxics*	Increased risk of liver toxicity.

POSSIBLE INTERACTION WITH OTHER SUBSTANCES

INTERACTS WITH	COMBINED EFFECT
Alcohol:	None expected.
Beverages:	None expected.
Cocaine:	None expected.
Foods:	None expected.
Marijuana:	None expected.
Tobacco:	None expected.

*See Glossary

VENLAFAXINE

BRAND NAMES

Effexor

BASIC INFORMATION

Habit forming? Not known
Prescription needed? Yes
Available as generic? No
Drug class: Antidepressant (bicyclic)

USES

- Treats mental depression.
- Treats anxiety disorder.

DOSAGE & USAGE INFORMATION

How to use:
- Tablet—Swallow with liquid and take with food to lessen stomach irritation.
- Extended-release capsule—Swallow with liquid and take with food to lessen stomach irritation. Do not open, crush or chew capsule.

When to use:
At the same times each day (usually with meals or with a snack).

If you forget a dose:
Take as soon as you remember up to 2 hours late. If more than 2 hours, wait for the next scheduled dose (don't double this dose).

What drug does:
Increases the amount of certain chemicals in the brain that are required for the transmission of messages between nerve cells.

Time lapse before drug works:
Begins in 1 to 3 weeks, but may take 4 to 6 weeks for maximum benefit.

Don't take with:
Any other medication without consulting your doctor or pharmacist.

OVERDOSE

SYMPTOMS:
May cause no symptoms, or there may be extreme drowsiness, convulsions or rapid heartbeat.
WHAT TO DO:
- **Dial 911 (emergency) for an ambulance or medical help or poison center 1-800-222-1222. Then give first aid immediately.**
- **See emergency information at end of book.**

POSSIBLE ADVERSE REACTIONS OR SIDE EFFECTS

SYMPTOMS	WHAT TO DO
Life-threatening: In case of overdose, see previous column.	
Common:	
• Fast heartbeat, blurred vision, increased blood pressure.	Discontinue. Call doctor right away.
• Stomach pain, gas, insomnia or drowsiness, dizziness, decreased sexual drive, impotence, nausea or vomiting, headache, diarrhea or constipation, dryness of mouth, skin flushing, rash, loss of appetite, unusual tiredness, weakness, strange dreams, sweating, tremors, nervousness, headache.	Continue. Call doctor when convenient.
Infrequent:	
• Lightheadedness or faintness when arising from a sitting or lying position, mood or behavior changes, mental changes, difficulty urinating.	Continue. Call doctor when convenient.
• Weight loss or gain, changes in taste, ringing in ears.	Continue. Tell doctor at next visit.
Rare:	
Seizures.	Discontinue. Seek emergency help.

WARNINGS & PRECAUTIONS

Don't take if:
You are allergic to venlafaxine.

Before you start, consult your doctor:
- If you have liver or kidney disease.
- If you have high blood pressure.
- If you have thoughts about suicide.
- If you are allergic to any other medications.
- If you have a history of seizures.

Over age 60:
Adverse reactions and side effects may be more severe than in younger persons.

Pregnancy:
Decide with your doctor if drug benefits justify any possible risk to unborn child. Risk category C (see page xviii).

Breast-feeding:
It is unknown if drug passes into milk. Avoid nursing until you finish medicine. Consult doctor for advice on maintaining milk supply.

Infants & children:
Safety in children under age 18 has not been established. Use only under close medical supervision.

Prolonged use:
Consult with your doctor on a regular basis while taking this drug to check your progress, to monitor your blood pressure and to determine the need for continued treatment.

Skin & sunlight:
No special problems expected.

Driving, piloting or hazardous work:
Don't drive or pilot aircraft until you learn how medicine affects you. Don't work around dangerous machinery. Don't climb ladders or work in high places. Danger increases if you drink alcohol or take medicine affecting alertness and reflexes.

Discontinuing:
Don't discontinue this drug without consulting doctor. Dosage may require a gradual reduction before stopping.

Others:
- Get up slowly from a sitting or lying position to avoid any dizziness, faintness or lightheadedness.
- Advise any doctor or dentist whom you consult that you take this medicine.
- Take medicine only as directed. Do not increase or reduce dosage without doctor's approval.

POSSIBLE INTERACTION WITH OTHER DRUGS

GENERIC NAME OR DRUG CLASS	COMBINED EFFECT
Antidepressants*, other	Increased sedative effect. Not recommended.
Central nervous system (CNS) depressants*, other	Increased sedative effect.
Cimetidine	Increased risk of adverse reactions.
Monoamine oxidase (MAO) inhibitors*	Increased risk and severity of adverse reactions. Allow 14 days between use of the two drugs.

POSSIBLE INTERACTION WITH OTHER SUBSTANCES

INTERACTS WITH	COMBINED EFFECT
Alcohol:	Increased sedative affect. Avoid.
Beverages:	None expected.
Cocaine:	Effect not known. Best to avoid.
Foods:	None expected.
Marijuana:	Effect not known. Best to avoid.
Tobacco:	None expected.

*See Glossary

VITAMIN A

BRAND NAMES

Acon
Afaxin
Alphalin
Aquasol A
Dispatabs
Sust-A

Numerous multiple vitamin-mineral supplements. Check labels.

BASIC INFORMATION

Habit forming? No
Prescription needed? No
Available as generic? Yes
Drug class: Vitamin supplement

USES

- Dietary supplement to ensure normal growth and health, especially of eyes and skin.
- Beta carotene form decreases severity of sun exposure in patients with porphyria.

DOSAGE & USAGE INFORMATION

How to take:
- Drops or capsule—Swallow with liquid. If you can't swallow whole, open capsule and take with liquid or food.
- Oral solution—Swallow with liquid.
- Tablet—Swallow with liquid.

When to take:
At the same time each day.

If you forget a dose:
Take as soon as you remember, then resume regular schedule.

What drug does:
- Prevents night blindness.
- Promotes normal growth and health.

Continued next column

OVERDOSE

SYMPTOMS:
Increased adverse reactions and side effects. Jaundice (rare, but may occur with large doses), malaise, vomiting, irritability, bleeding gums, seizures, double vision, peeling skin.
WHAT TO DO:
If person takes much larger amount than prescribed, call doctor, poison center 1-800-222-1222 or hospital emergency room for instructions.

Time lapse before drug works:
Requires continual intake.

Don't take with:
Any other medicine without consulting your doctor or pharmacist.

POSSIBLE ADVERSE REACTIONS OR SIDE EFFECTS

SYMPTOMS	WHAT TO DO
Life-threatening: In case of overdose, see previous column.	
Common: None expected.	
Infrequent: Confusion; dizziness; drowsiness; headache; irritability; dry, cracked lips; peeling skin; hair loss; sensitvity to light.	Continue. Call doctor when convenient.
Rare: • Bulging soft spot on baby's head, double vision, bone or joint pain, abdominal pain, frequent urination, vomiting.	Discontinue. Call doctor right away.
• Diarrhea, appetite loss, nausea.	Continue. Call doctor when convenient.

WARNINGS & PRECAUTIONS

Don't take if:
You have chronic kidney failure.

Before you start, consult your doctor:
If you have any kidney disorder.

Over age 60:
No problems expected.

Pregnancy:
Risk factor determined by length of pregnancy and dosage amount. See category list on page xviii and consult doctor.

Breast-feeding:
No problems expected. Consult doctor.

Infants & children:
- Avoid large doses.
- Keep vitamin-mineral supplements out of children's reach.

Prolonged use:
No problems expected.

Skin & sunlight:
No special problems expected.

Driving, piloting or hazardous work:
No problems expected.

Discontinuing:
Don't discontinue without doctor's advice until you complete prescribed dose, even though symptoms diminish or disappear.

Others:
- Don't exceed dose. Too much over a long time may be harmful.
- A balanced diet should provide all the vitamin A a healthy person needs and prevent need for supplements. Best sources are liver, yellow-orange fruits and vegetables, dark-green, leafy vegetables, milk, butter and margarine.

POSSIBLE INTERACTION WITH OTHER DRUGS

GENERIC NAME OR DRUG CLASS	COMBINED EFFECT
Anticoagulants*	Increased anticoagulant effect with large doses (over 10,000 I.U.) of vitamin A.
Calcium supplements*	Decreased vitamin effect.
Cholestyramine	Decreased vitamin A absorption.
Colestipol	Decreased vitamin absorption.
Contraceptives, oral*	Increased vitamin A levels.
Etretinate	Increased risk of toxic effects.
Isotretinoin	Increased risk of toxic effect of each.
Mineral oil (long-term)	Decreased vitamin A absorption.
Neomycin	Decreased vitamin absorption.
Vitamin A derivatives, other	Increased toxicity risk.
Vitamin E (excess dose)	Vitamin A depletion.

POSSIBLE INTERACTION WITH OTHER SUBSTANCES

INTERACTS WITH	COMBINED EFFECT
Alcohol:	None expected.
Beverages:	None expected.
Cocaine:	None expected.
Foods:	None expected.
Marijuana:	None expected.
Tobacco:	None expected.

*See Glossary

VITAMIN B-12 (Cyanocobalamin)

GENERIC AND BRAND NAMES

CYANOCOBALAMIN
Anocobin
Bedoz
Berubigen
Betalin 12
Cyanabin
Kaybovite
Kaybovite-1000
Redisol
Rubion
Rubramin
Rubramin-PC

HYDROXOCOBAL-AMIN
Acti-B-12
Alpha Redisol
Alphamin
Codroxomin
Droxomin

Numerous other multiple vitamin-mineral supplements.

BASIC INFORMATION

Habit forming? No
Prescription needed? Yes, for some
Available as generic? Yes
Drug class: Vitamin supplement

USES

- Dietary supplement for normal growth, development and health.
- Treatment for nerve damage.
- Treatment for pernicious anemia.
- Treatment and prevention of vitamin B-12 deficiencies in people who have had stomach or intestines surgically removed.
- Prevention of vitamin B-12 deficiency in strict vegetarians and persons with absorption diseases.

DOSAGE & USAGE INFORMATION

How to take:
- Tablets—Swallow with liquid.
- Injection—Follow doctor's directions.

When to take:
- Oral—At the same time each day.
- Injection—Follow doctor's directions.

If you forget a dose:
Take when remembered. Don't double next dose. Resume regular schedule.

What drug does:
Acts as enzyme to promote normal fat and carbohydrate metabolism and protein synthesis.

Time lapse before drug works:
15 minutes.

Don't take with:
Any other medicine without consulting your doctor or pharmacist.

OVERDOSE

SYMPTOMS:
Increased adverse reactions and side effects.
WHAT TO DO:
Overdose unlikely to threaten life. If person takes much larger amount than prescribed, call doctor, poison center 1-800-222-1222 or hospital emergency room for instructions.

POSSIBLE ADVERSE REACTIONS OR SIDE EFFECTS

SYMPTOMS	WHAT TO DO
Life-threatening:	
Hives, rash, intense itching, faintness soon after a dose (anaphylaxis).	Seek emergency treatment immediately.
Common:	
None expected.	
Infrequent:	
None expected.	
Rare:	
• Itchy skin, wheezing.	Discontinue. Call doctor right away.
• Diarrhea.	Continue. Call doctor when convenient.

VITAMIN B-12 (Cyanocobalamin)

WARNINGS & PRECAUTIONS

Don't take if:
You have Leber's disease (optic nerve atrophy).

Before you start, consult your doctor:
- If you have gout.
- If you have heart disease.

Over age 60:
Don't take more than 100 mg per day unless prescribed by your doctor.

Pregnancy:
Risk factor determined by length of pregnancy and dosage amount. See category list on page xviii and consult doctor.

Breast-feeding:
Effect unknown. Consult doctor.

Infants & children:
No problems expected.

Prolonged use:
No problems expected.

Skin & sunlight:
No problems expected.

Driving, piloting or hazardous work:
No problems expected.

Discontinuing:
Don't discontinue without doctor's advice until you complete prescribed dose, even though symptoms diminish or disappear.

Others:
- A balanced diet should provide all the vitamin B-12 a healthy person needs and make supplements unnecessary. Best sources are meat, fish, egg yolk and cheese.
- Tablets should be used only for diet supplements. All other uses of vitamin B-12 require injections.
- Don't take large doses of vitamin C (1,000 mg or more per day) unless prescribed by your doctor.

POSSIBLE INTERACTION WITH OTHER DRUGS

GENERIC NAME OR DRUG CLASS	COMBINED EFFECT
Anticonvulsants*	Decreased absorption of vitamin B-12.
Chloramphenicol	Decreased vitamin B-12 effect.
Cholestyramine	Decreased absorption of vitamin B-12.
Cimetidine	Decreased absorption of vitamin B-12.
Colchicine	Decreased absorption of vitamin B-12.
Famotidine	Decreased absorption of vitamin B-12.
H_2 antagonists*	Decreased absorption of vitamin B-12.
Neomycin	Decreased absorption of vitamin B-12.
Para-aminosalicylic acid	Decreased effects of para-aminosalicyclic acid.
Potassium (extended-release forms)	Decreased absorption of vitamin B-12.
Ranitidine	Decreased absorption of vitamin B-12.
Vitamin C (ascorbic acid)	Destroys vitamin B-12 if taken at same time. Take 2 hours apart.

POSSIBLE INTERACTION WITH OTHER SUBSTANCES

INTERACTS WITH	COMBINED EFFECT
Alcohol:	Decreased absorption of vitamin B-12.
Beverages:	None expected.
Cocaine:	None expected.
Foods:	None expected.
Marijuana:	None expected.
Tobacco:	None expected.

*See Glossary

VITAMIN C (Ascorbic Acid)

BRAND NAMES

Ascorbicap
Cecon
Cemill
Cenolate
Cetane
Cevalin
Cevi-Bid
Ce-Vi-Sol
Cevita
C-Span
Flavorcee
Redoxon
Sunkist

Numerous other multiple vitamin-mineral supplements.

BASIC INFORMATION

Habit forming? No
Prescription needed? No
Available as generic? Yes
Drug class: Vitamin supplement

USES

- Prevention and treatment of scurvy and other vitamin C deficiencies.
- Treatment of anemia.
- Maintenance of acid urine.

DOSAGE & USAGE INFORMATION

How to take:
- Tablets, capsules, liquid—Swallow with 8 oz. water.
- Extended-release tablets—Swallow whole.
- Drops—Squirt directly into mouth or mix with liquid or food.
- Chewable tablets—Chew well before swallowing.

When to take:
1, 2 or 3 times per day, as prescribed on label.

If you forget a dose:
Take as soon as you remember, then return to regular schedule.

Continued next column

OVERDOSE

SYMPTOMS:
Diarrhea, vomiting, dizziness.
WHAT TO DO:
Overdose unlikely to threaten life. If person takes much larger amount than prescribed, call doctor, poison center 1-800-222-1222 or hospital emergency room for instructions.

What drug does:
- May help form collagen.
- Increases iron absorption from intestine.
- Contributes to hemoglobin and red blood cell production in bone marrow.

Time lapse before drug works:
1 week.

Don't take with:
Any other medicine without consulting your doctor or pharmacist.

POSSIBLE ADVERSE REACTIONS OR SIDE EFFECTS

SYMPTOMS	WHAT TO DO
Life-threatening: None expected.	
Common: None expected.	
Infrequent:	
• Mild diarrhea, nausea, vomiting.	Discontinue. Call doctor right away.
• Flushed face.	Continue. Call doctor when convenient.
Rare:	
• Kidney stones with high doses, anemia, abdominal pain.	Discontinue. Call doctor right away.
• Headache.	Continue. Tell doctor at next visit.

WARNINGS & PRECAUTIONS

Don't take if:
You are allergic to vitamin C.

Before you start, consult your doctor:
- If you have sickle-cell or other anemia.
- If you have had kidney stones.
- If you have gout.

Over age 60:
Don't take more than 1000 mg per day unless prescribed by your doctor.

Pregnancy:
Risk factor determined by length of pregnancy and dosage amount. See category list on page xviii and consult doctor.

Breast-feeding:
Avoid large doses. Consult doctor.

Infants & children:
- Avoid large doses.
- Keep vitamin-mineral supplements out of children's reach.

Prolonged use:
Large doses for longer than 2 months may cause kidney stones.

Skin & sunlight:
No problems expected.

Driving, piloting or hazardous work:
No problems expected.

Discontinuing:
No problems expected.

Others:
- Store in cool, dry place.
- May cause inaccurate tests for sugar in urine or blood in stool.
- May cause crisis in patients with sickle-cell anemia.
- A balanced diet should provide all the vitamin C a healthy person needs and make supplements unnecessary. Best sources are citrus, strawberries, cantaloupe and raw peppers.
- Don't take large doses of vitamin C (1,000 mg or more per day) unless prescribed by your doctor.
- Some products contain tartrazine dye. Avoid, if allergic (especially aspirin hypersensitivity).

POSSIBLE INTERACTION WITH OTHER DRUGS

GENERIC NAME OR DRUG CLASS	COMBINED EFFECT
Amphetamines*	Possible decreased amphetamine effect.
Anticholinergics*	Possible decreased anticholinergic effect.
Anticoagulants*, oral	Possible decreased anticoagulant effect.
Antidepressants, tricyclic (TCA)*	Possible decreased antidepressant effect.
Aspirin	Decreased vitamin C effect and salicylate excretion.
Barbiturates*	Decreased vitamin C effect. Increased barbiturate effect.
Cellulose sodium phosphate	Decreased vitamin C effect.
Contraceptives, oral*	Decreased vitamin C effect.
Estrogens*	Increased likelihood of adverse effects from estrogen with 1 g or more of vitamin C per day.
Iron supplements*	Increased iron absorption.
Mexiletine	Possible decreased effectiveness of mexiletine.
Quinidine	Possible decreased quinidine effect.
Salicylates*	Decreased vitamin C effect and salicylate excretion. May lead to salicylate toxicity.
Tranquilizers* (phenothiazine)	May decrease phenothiazine effect if no vitamin C deficiency exists.

POSSIBLE INTERACTION WITH OTHER SUBSTANCES

INTERACTS WITH	COMBINED EFFECT
Alcohol:	None expected.
Beverages:	None expected.
Cocaine:	None expected.
Foods:	None expected.
Marijuana:	None expected.
Tobacco:	Increased requirement for vitamin C.

***See Glossary**

VITAMIN D

GENERIC AND BRAND NAMES

ALFACALCIDOL
One-Alpha
CALCIFEDOL
Calderol
DIHYDROTACHY-STEROL
DHT
DHT Intensol
Hytakerol
DOXERCALCIFEROL
Hectorol
ERGOCALCIFEROL
Calciferol
Drisdol
Osto Forte
Radiostol
Radiostol Forte

BASIC INFORMATION

Habit forming? No
Prescription needed?
Low strength: No
High strength: Yes
Available as generic? Yes
Drug class: Vitamin supplement

USES

- Dietary supplement.
- Prevention of rickets (bone disease).
- Treatment for hypocalcemia (low blood calcium) in kidney disease.
- Treatment for postoperative muscle contractions.
- Daily supplement for people who must use sunscreen daily.

DOSAGE & USAGE INFORMATION

How to take:
- Tablet, capsule or liquid—Swallow with liquid.
- Drops—Dilute dose in beverage.
- Injection—Take under doctor's supervision.

Continued next column

OVERDOSE

SYMPTOMS:
Severe stomach pain, nausea, vomiting, weight loss; bone and muscle pain; increased urination, cloudy urine; mood or mental changes (possible psychosis); high blood pressure, irregular heartbeat; eye irritation or light sensitivity; itchy skin.
WHAT TO DO:
Overdose unlikely to threaten life. If person takes much larger amount than prescribed, call doctor, poison center 1-800-222-1222 or hospital emergency room for instructions.

When to take:
As directed, usually once a day at the same time each day.

If you forget a dose:
Take up to 12 hours late. If more than 12 hours, wait for next dose (don't double this dose).

What drug does:
- Maintains growth and health.
- Prevents rickets.
- Essential so body can use calcium and phosphate.

Time lapse before drug works:
2 hours. May require 2 to 3 weeks of continual use for maximum effect.

Don't take with:
Nonprescription drugs or drugs in Interaction column without consulting doctor.

POSSIBLE ADVERSE REACTIONS OR SIDE EFFECTS

SYMPTOMS	WHAT TO DO
Life-threatening:	
In case of overdose, see previous column.	
Common:	
None expected.	
Infrequent:	
Headache, metallic taste in mouth, thirst, dry mouth, constipation, appetite loss, nausea, vomiting, weakness, cloudy urine, sensitivity to light.	Continue. Call doctor when convenient.
Rare:	
• Increased urination, pink eye, psychosis, severe abdominal pain, fever.	Discontinue. Call doctor right away.
• Muscle pain, bone pain, diarrhea.	Continue. Tell doctor when convenient.

WARNINGS & PRECAUTIONS

Don't take if:
You are allergic to medicine containing vitamin D.

Before you start, consult your doctor:
- If you plan to become pregnant while taking vitamin D.
- If you have epilepsy.
- If you have heart or blood-vessel disease.
- If you have kidney disease.

Over age 60:
Adverse reactions and side effects may be more frequent and severe than in younger persons.

Pregnancy:
Risk factor determined by length of pregnancy and dosage amount. See category list on page xviii and consult doctor.

Breast-feeding:
No problems expected, but consult doctor.

Infants & children:
- Avoid large doses.
- Keep vitamins out of children's reach.

Prolonged use:
- No problems expected.
- Talk to your doctor about the need for follow-up medical examinations or laboratory studies to check kidney function, liver function, serum calcium.

Skin & sunlight:
No special problems expected.

Driving, piloting or hazardous work:
No problems expected.

Discontinuing:
Don't discontinue without doctor's advice until you complete prescribed dose, even though symptoms diminish or disappear.

Others:
- Don't exceed dose. Too much over a long time may be harmful.
- A balanced diet should provide all the vitamin D a healthy person needs and make supplements unnecessary. Best sources are fish and vitamin D-fortified milk and bread.
- Some products contain tartrazine dye. Avoid, if allergic (especially aspirin hypersensitivity).
- Sunscreen prevents the body from manufacturing vitamin D from sunshine. Take supplementary vitamin D if you use sunscreen daily. Ask doctor for dosage.

POSSIBLE INTERACTION WITH OTHER DRUGS

GENERIC NAME OR DRUG CLASS	COMBINED EFFECT
Antacids* (magnesium-containing)	Possible excess magnesium.
Anticonvulsants, hydantoin*	Decreased vitamin D effect.
Calcium (high doses)	Excess calcium in blood.
Calcium channel blockers*	Possible decreased effect of calcium channel blockers.
Calcium supplements*	Excessive absorption of vitamin D.
Cholestyramine	Decreased vitamin D effect.
Colestipol	Decreased vitamin D absorption.
Cortisone	Decreased vitamin D effect.
Digitalis preparations*	Heartbeat irregularities.
Diuretics, thiazide*	Possible increased calcium.
Mineral oil	Decreased vitamin D effect.
Neomycin	Decreased vitamin D absorption.
Nicardipine	Decreased nicardipine effect.
Phenobarbital	Decreased vitamin D effect.
Phosphorus preparations*	Accumulation of excess phosphorus.
Rifampin	Possible decreased vitamin D effect.
Vitamin D, other	Possible toxicity.

POSSIBLE INTERACTION WITH OTHER SUBSTANCES

INTERACTS WITH	COMBINED EFFECT
Alcohol:	None expected.
Beverages:	None expected.
Cocaine:	None expected.
Foods:	None expected.
Marijuana:	None expected.
Tobacco:	None expected.

*See Glossary

VITAMIN E

BRAND NAMES

Aquasol E
Chew-E
Eprolin
Epsilan-M
Pheryl-E
Viterra E

Numerous other multiple vitamin-mineral supplements. Check labels.

BASIC INFORMATION

Habit forming? No
Prescription needed? No
Available as generic? Yes
Drug class: Vitamin supplement

USES

- Dietary supplement to promote normal growth, development and health.
- Treatment and prevention of vitamin E deficiency, especially in premature or low-birth-weight infants.
- Treatment for fibrocystic disease of the breast.
- Treatment for circulatory problems to the lower extremities.
- Treatment for sickle-cell anemia.
- Treatment for lung toxicity from air pollution.

DOSAGE & USAGE INFORMATION

How to take:

- Tablet or capsule—Swallow with liquid or food to lessen stomach irritation.
- Drops—Dilute dose in beverage before swallowing or squirt directly into mouth.
- Injection—Take under doctor's supervision.

When to take:
At the same times each day.

If you forget a dose:
Take when you remember. Don't double next dose.

What drug does:

- Promotes normal growth and development.
- Prevents oxidation in body.

Continued next column

OVERDOSE

SYMPTOMS:
Nausea, vomiting, fatigue.
WHAT TO DO:
Overdose unlikely to threaten life. If person takes much larger amount than prescribed, call doctor, poison center 1-800-222-1222 or hospital emergency room for instructions.

Time lapse before drug works:
Not determined.

Don't take with:
Any other medicine without consulting your doctor or pharmacist.

POSSIBLE ADVERSE REACTIONS OR SIDE EFFECTS

SYMPTOMS	WHAT TO DO
Life-threatening: None expected.	
Common: Breast enlargement, dizziness, headache.	Continue. Call doctor when convenient.
Infrequent: Nausea, abdominal pain, muscle aches, pain in lower legs, fever, tiredness, weakness.	Continue. Call doctor when convenient.
Rare: Blurred vision, diarrhea.	Discontinue. Call doctor right away.

WARNINGS & PRECAUTIONS

Don't take if:
You are allergic to vitamin E.

Before you start, consult your doctor:
- If you have had blood clots in leg veins (thrombophlebitis).
- If you have liver disease.

Over age 60:
No problems expected. Avoid excessive doses.

Pregnancy:
No problems expected with normal daily requirements. Don't exceed prescribed dose. Consult doctor.

Breast-feeding:
No problems expected. Consult doctor.

Infants & children:
Use only under medical supervision.

Prolonged use:
Toxic accumulation of vitamin E. Don't exceed recommended dose.

Skin & sunlight:
No problems expected.

Driving, piloting or hazardous work:
No problems expected.

Discontinuing:
No problems expected.

Others:
A balanced diet should provide all the vitamin E a healthy person needs and make supplements unnecessary. Best sources are vegetable oils, whole-grain cereals, liver.

POSSIBLE INTERACTION WITH OTHER DRUGS

GENERIC NAME OR DRUG CLASS	COMBINED EFFECT
Anticoagulants*, oral	Increased anti-coagulant effect.
Cholestyramine	Decreased vitamin E absorption.
Colestipol	Decreased vitamin E absorption.
Iron supplements*	Possible decreased effect of iron supplement in patients with iron-deficiency anemia. Decreased vitamin E effect in healthy persons.
Mineral oil	Decreased vitamin E effect.
Neomycin	Decreased vitamin E absorption.
Vitamin A	Recommended dose of vitamin E—Increased benefit and decreased toxicity of vitamin A. Excess dose of vitamin E—Vitamin A depletion.

POSSIBLE INTERACTION WITH OTHER SUBSTANCES

INTERACTS WITH	COMBINED EFFECT
Alcohol:	None expected.
Beverages:	None expected.
Cocaine:	None expected.
Foods:	None expected.
Marijuana:	None expected.
Tobacco:	None expected.

*See Glossary

VITAMIN K

GENERIC AND BRAND NAMES

MENADIOL
Synkayvite

PHYTONADIONE
Mephyton

BASIC INFORMATION

Habit forming? No
Prescription needed? No
Available as generic? Yes
Drug class: Vitamin supplement

USES

- Dietary supplement.
- Treatment for bleeding disorders and malabsorption diseases due to vitamin K deficiency.
- Treatment for hemorrhagic disease of the newborn.
- Treatment for bleeding due to overdose of oral anticoagulants.

DOSAGE & USAGE INFORMATION

How to take:

- Usually given by injection in hospital or doctor's office.
- Tablet—Swallow with liquid. If you can't swallow whole, crumble tablet and take with liquid or food.

When to take:
At the same time each day.

If you forget a dose:
Take as soon as you remember up to 12 hours late. If more than 12 hours, wait for next scheduled dose (don't double this dose).

What drug does:

- Promotes growth, development and good health.
- Supplies a necessary ingredient for blood clotting.

Time lapse before drug works:
15 to 30 minutes to support blood clotting.

Don't take with:
Any other medicine without consulting your doctor or pharmacist.

OVERDOSE

SYMPTOMS:
Nausea, vomiting.
WHAT TO DO:
Overdose unlikely to threaten life. If person takes much larger amount than prescribed, call doctor, poison center 1-800-222-1222 or hospital emergency room for instructions.

POSSIBLE ADVERSE REACTIONS OR SIDE EFFECTS

SYMPTOMS	WHAT TO DO
Life-threatening: None expected.	
Common: None expected.	
Infrequent: Unusual taste, face flushing.	Continue. Call doctor when convenient.
Rare: Rash, hives.	Discontinue. Call doctor right away.

WARNINGS & PRECAUTIONS

Don't take if:

- You are allergic to vitamin K.
- You have G6PD* deficiency.
- You have liver disease.

Before you start, consult your doctor:
If you are pregnant.

Over age 60:
No problems expected.

Pregnancy:
Risk factor determined by length of pregnancy and dosage amount. See category list on page xviii and consult doctor.

Breast-feeding:
No problems expected. Consult doctor.

Infants & children:
Phytonadione is the preferred form for hemorrhagic disease of the newborn.

Prolonged use:
Talk to your doctor about the need for follow-up medical examinations or laboratory studies to check prothrombin time.

Skin & sunlight:
No problems expected.

Driving, piloting or hazardous work:
No problems expected.

Discontinuing:
No problems expected.

Others:

- Tell all doctors and dentists you consult that you take this medicine.
- Don't exceed dose. Too much over a long time may be harmful.
- A balanced diet should provide all the vitamin K a healthy person needs and make supplements unnecessary. Best sources are green, leafy vegetables, meat or dairy products.

POSSIBLE INTERACTION WITH OTHER DRUGS

GENERIC NAME OR DRUG CLASS	COMBINED EFFECT
Anticoagulants*, oral	Decreased anti-coagulant effect.
Cholestyramine	Decreased vitamin K effect.
Colestipol	Decreased vitamin K absorption.
Dapsone	Increased risk of adverse effect on blood cells.
Mineral oil (long-term)	Vitamin K deficiency.
Neomycin	Decreased vitamin K absorption.
Sulfa drugs*	Vitamin K deficiency.

POSSIBLE INTERACTION WITH OTHER SUBSTANCES

INTERACTS WITH	COMBINED EFFECT
Alcohol:	None expected.
Beverages:	None expected.
Cocaine:	None expected.
Foods:	None expected.
Marijuana:	None expected.
Tobacco:	None expected.

*See Glossary

VITAMINS & FLUORIDE

GENERIC AND BRAND NAMES

Adeflor
Cari-Tab
Mulvidren-F
Poly-Vi-Flor
Tri-Vi-Flor
Vi-Daylin/F
Vi-Penta F

Also available in the forms of multiple vitamins & fluoride; vitamins A, D & C & fluoride.

BASIC INFORMATION

Habit forming? No
Prescription needed? Yes
Available as generic? No
Drug class: Vitamins, minerals

USES

- Reduces incidence of tooth cavities (fluoride). Children who need supplements should take until age 16.
- Prevents deficiencies of vitamin included in formula (some contain multiple vitamins whose content varies among products; others contain only vitamins A, D and C).

DOSAGE & USAGE INFORMATION

How to take:
- Chewable tablets—Chew or crush before swallowing.
- Oral liquid—Measure with specially marked dropper. May mix with food, fruit juice, cereal.

When to take:
- Bedtime or with or just after meals.
- If at bedtime, brush teeth first.

Continued next column

OVERDOSE

SYMPTOMS:
Minor overdose—Black, brown or white spots on teeth.
Massive overdose—Shallow breathing, black or tarry stools, bloody vomit.
WHAT TO DO:
- **Dial 911 (emergency) for an ambulance or medical help or poison center 1-800-222-1222. Then give first aid immediately.**
- **See emergency information on inside covers.**

If you forget a dose:
Take as soon as you remember up to 2 hours late. If more than 2 hours, wait for next scheduled dose (don't double this dose).

What drug does:
Provides supplemental fluoride to combat tooth decay.

Time lapse before drug works:
8 weeks to provide maximum benefit.

Don't take with:
- Other medicine simultaneously.
- Any other medicine without consulting your doctor or pharmacist.

POSSIBLE ADVERSE REACTIONS OR SIDE EFFECTS

SYMPTOMS	WHAT TO DO
Life-threatening:	
Fainting, bloody vomit, bloody or black stool, breathing difficulty.	Discontinue. Seek emergency treatment.
Common:	
White, black or brown spots on teeth; nausea; vomiting.	Discontinue. Call doctor right away.
Infrequent:	
• Drowsiness; abdominal pain; increased salivation; watery eyes; weight loss; sore throat, fever, mouth sores; constipation; bone pain; rash; muscle stiffness; weakness; tremor; agitation.	Discontinue. Call doctor right away.
• Diarrhea.	Continue. Call doctor when convenient.
Rare:	
None expected.	

WARNINGS & PRECAUTIONS

Don't take if:

- Your water supply contains 0.7 parts fluoride per million. Too much fluoride stains teeth permanently.
- You are allergic to any fluoride-containing product.
- You have underactive thyroid.

Before you start, consult your doctor or dentist:
For proper dosage.

Over age 60:
No problems expected.

Pregnancy:
Risk factor determined by length of pregnancy and dosage amount. See category list on page xviii and consult doctor.

Breast-feeding:
No problems expected. Consult doctor.

Infants & children:
No problems expected in children over 3 years of age except in case of accidental overdose. Keep vitamin-mineral supplements out of children's reach.

Prolonged use:
Excess may cause discolored teeth and decreased calcium in blood.

Skin & sunlight:
No problems expected.

Driving, piloting or hazardous work:
No problems expected.

Discontinuing:
No problems expected.

Others:

- Store in original plastic container. Fluoride decomposes glass.
- Check with dentist once or twice a year to keep cavities at a minimum. Topical applications of fluoride may also be helpful.
- Fluoride probably not necessary if water contains about 1 part per million of fluoride or more. Check with health department.
- Don't freeze.
- Don't keep outdated medicine.

POSSIBLE INTERACTION WITH OTHER DRUGS

GENERIC NAME OR DRUG CLASS	COMBINED EFFECT
Anticoagulants*	Decreased effect of anticoagulant.
Iron supplements*	Decreased effect of any vitamin E if present in multivitamin product.
Vitamin A	May lead to vitamin A toxicity if vitamin A is in combination.
Vitamin D	May lead to vitamin D toxicity if vitamin D is in combination.

POSSIBLE INTERACTION WITH OTHER SUBSTANCES

INTERACTS WITH	COMBINED EFFECT
Alcohol:	None expected.
Beverages:	
Milk.	Prevents absorption of fluoride. Space dose 2 hours before or after milk.
Cocaine:	None expected.
Foods:	None expected.
Marijuana:	None expected.
Tobacco:	None expected.

*See Glossary

XYLOMETAZOLINE

BRAND NAMES

Chlorohist-LA
Inspire
Neo-Synephrine II Long Acting Nasal Spray Adult Strength
Neo-Synephrine II Long Acting Nose Drops Adult Strength
Otrivin Decongestant Nose Drops
Otrivin Nasal Drops
Otrivin Nasal Spray
Otrivin Pediatric Decongestant Nose Drops
Otrivin Pediatric Nasal Drops
Otrivin Pediatric Nasal Spray
Otrivin with M-D Pump

BASIC INFORMATION

Habit forming? No
Prescription needed? No
Available as generic? Yes
Drug class: Sympathomimetic

USES

Relieves congestion of nose, sinuses and throat from allergies and infections.

DOSAGE & USAGE INFORMATION

How to take:
Nasal solution, nasal spray—Use as directed on label. Avoid contamination. Don't use same container for more than 1 person.

When to take:
When needed, no more often than every 4 hours.

Continued next column

OVERDOSE

SYMPTOMS:
Headache, sweating, anxiety, agitation, rapid and irregular heartbeat (rare occurrence with systemic absorption).

WHAT TO DO:
- **Dial 911 (emergency) for an ambulance or medical help or poison center 1-800-222-1222. Then give first aid immediately.**
- **If patient is unconscious and not breathing, give mouth-to-mouth breathing. If there is no heartbeat, use cardiac massage and mouth-to-mouth breathing (CPR). If you can't get help quickly, take patient to nearest emergency facility.**
- **See emergency information on inside covers.**

If you forget a dose:
Take as soon as you remember. Wait 4 hours for next dose.

What drug does:
Constricts walls of small arteries in nose, sinuses and eustachian tubes.

Time lapse before drug works:
5 to 30 minutes.

Don't take with:
- Nonprescription drugs for allergy, cough or cold without consulting doctor.
- Any other medicine without consulting your doctor or pharmacist.

POSSIBLE ADVERSE REACTIONS OR SIDE EFFECTS

SYMPTOMS	WHAT TO DO
Life-threatening:	
In case of overdose, see previous column.	
Common:	
None expected.	
Infrequent:	
Burning, dry or stinging nasal passages.	Continue. Call doctor when convenient.
Rare:	
Rebound congestion (increased runny or stuffy nose); headache, insomnia, nervousness (may occur with systemic absorption).	Discontinue. Call doctor when convenient.

WARNINGS & PRECAUTIONS

Don't take if:
You are allergic to any sympathomimetic nasal spray.

Before you start, consult your doctor:
- If you have heart disease or high blood pressure.
- If you have diabetes.
- If you have overactive thyroid.
- If you have taken a monoamine oxidase (MAO) inhibitor* in past 2 weeks.
- If you have glaucoma.

Over age 60:
Adverse reactions and side effects may be more frequent and severe than in younger persons.

Pregnancy:
Decide with your doctor if drug benefits justify risk to unborn child. Risk category C (see page xviii).

Breast-feeding:
No proven problems. Consult doctor.

Infants & children:
Don't give to children younger than 2.

Prolonged use:
Drug may lose effectiveness, cause increased congestion (rebound effect*) and irritate nasal membranes.

Skin & sunlight:
No problems expected.

Driving, piloting or hazardous work:
No problems expected.

Discontinuing:
May be unnecessary to finish medicine. Follow doctor's instructions.

Others:
No problems expected.

POSSIBLE INTERACTION WITH OTHER DRUGS

GENERIC NAME OR DRUG CLASS	COMBINED EFFECT
Antidepressants, tricyclic*	Possible increased blood pressure.
Maprotiline	Possible increased blood pressure.
Monoamine oxidase (MAO) inhibitors*	Possible increased blood pressure.

POSSIBLE INTERACTION WITH OTHER SUBSTANCES

INTERACTS WITH	COMBINED EFFECT
Alcohol:	None expected.
Beverages: Caffeine drinks.	Nervousness or insomnia.
Cocaine:	High risk of heart-beat irregularities and high blood pressure.
Foods:	None expected.
Marijuana:	Overstimulation. Avoid.
Tobacco:	None expected.

*See Glossary

YOHIMBINE

BRAND NAMES

Actibine
Aphrodyne
Baron-X
Dayto Himbin
PMS-Yohimbine
Prohim
Thybine
Yocon
Yohimar
Yohimex
Yoman
Yovital

BASIC INFORMATION

Habit forming? No
Prescription needed? Yes
Available as generic? Yes
Drug class: Impotence therapy

USES

Treatment for men who are unable to have sexual intercourse (impotent). It may be helpful for some, but not all, men who suffer sexual dysfunction.

DOSAGE & USAGE INFORMATION

How to use:
Tablet—Swallow with liquid. May be taken with or without food.

When to use:
At the same times each day.

If you forget a dose:
Take as soon as you remember up to 4 hours late. If more than 4 hours, wait for next scheduled dose (don't double this dose).

What drug does:
It is unknown exactly how the drug works. It appears to increase the supply of certain body chemicals that can help produce erections.

Time lapse before drug works:
May take 2 to 3 weeks.

Don't take with:
Any other prescription or nonprescription drug without consulting your doctor or pharmacist.

OVERDOSE

SYMPTOMS:
May produce increases in heart rate and blood pressure, lack of coordination, trembling.
WHAT TO DO:
Overdose unlikely to threaten life. If person takes much larger amount than prescribed, call doctor, poison center 1-800-222-1222 or hospital emergency room for instructions.

POSSIBLE ADVERSE REACTIONS OR SIDE EFFECTS

SYMPTOMS	WHAT TO DO
Life-threatening: None expected.	
Common: None expected.	
Infrequent:	
• Rapid heartbeat, increased blood pressure.	Discontinue. Call doctor right away.
• Headache, dizziness, restlessness, irritability, nervousness, anxiety, insomnia, muscle aches.	Continue. Call doctor when convenient.
Rare:	
Nausea, vomiting, flushed skin, sweating, tremor.	Continue. Call doctor when convenient.

WARNINGS & PRECAUTIONS

Don't take if:
- You have an allergy to yohimbine or any rauwolfia alkaloids*.
- You have angina pectoris.
- You have heart disease or high blood pressure.
- You have impaired kidney function.

Before you start, consult your doctor:
- If you suffer from depression.
- If you have any psychiatric disorder.
- If you have liver disease.
- If you have allergies to any medications, foods or other substances.

Over age 60:
Studies have not shown any specific problems. Discuss possible benefits and risk factors with your doctor.

Pregnancy:
Not used in females.

Breast-feeding:
Not used in females.

Infants & children:
Not used in this age group.

Prolonged use:
Effects of long-term use are unknown. Visit your doctor regularly while using this drug to check its effectiveness, as well as your blood pressure and heart rate.

Skin & sunlight:
No special problems expected.

Driving, piloting or hazardous work:
Avoid if you experience any side effects (especially dizziness).

Discontinuing:
No special problems expected.

Others:
- Follow your doctor's instructions for using this drug. Don't take it more often or increase the dosage without your doctor's approval. It will increase the risk of high blood pressure and rapid heartbeat.
- Advise any doctor or dentist whom you consult that you take this medicine.

POSSIBLE INTERACTION WITH OTHER DRUGS

GENERIC NAME OR DRUG CLASS	COMBINED EFFECT
Antidepressants*	Decreased effect of antidepressant.
Antihypertensives*	Decreased effect of antihypertensive.

POSSIBLE INTERACTION WITH OTHER SUBSTANCES

INTERACTS WITH	COMBINED EFFECT
Alcohol:	Decreased yohimbine effect. Avoid.
Beverages:	None expected.
Cocaine	Effect unknown. Best to avoid.
Foods:	None expected.
Marijuana:	Effect unknown. Best to avoid.
Tobacco:	None expected.

*See Glossary

ZALEPLON

BRAND NAMES

Sonata

BASIC INFORMATION

Habit forming? Yes
Prescription needed? Yes
Available as generic? No
Drug class: Anti-insomnia, hypnotic, sedative

USES

Short-term treatment for insomnia (trouble sleeping).

DOSAGE & USAGE INFORMATION

How to take:
Capsule—Swallow with liquid. If you can't swallow whole, open capsule and take with liquid or food.

When to take:
Take immediately before bedtime. Ensure that you can get at least 4 hours of rest after taking your medication. Zaleplon may be taken with or without food; however, if taken after a heavy or fatty meal, it may not work as fast as it should.

If you forget a dose:
Skip the missed dose and return to your regular dosing schedule. Do not double dose.

Continued next column

OVERDOSE

SYMPTOMS:
Clumsiness, unsteadiness, stupor, severe dizziness or fainting, troubled breathing and sluggishness.
WHAT TO DO:

- **Dial 911 (emergency) for an ambulance or medical help or poison center 1-800-222-1222. Then give first aid immediately.**
- **If patient is unconscious and not breathing, give mouth-to-mouth breathing. If there is no heartbeat, use cardiac massage and mouth-to-mouth breathing (CPR). If you can't get help quickly, take patient to nearest emergency facility.**
- **See emergency information on inside covers.**

What drug does:
Acts as a central nervous system depressant, decreasing sleep problems such as trouble falling asleep, waking up too often during the night and waking up too early in the morning.

Time lapse before drug works:
Within 2 hours.

Don't take with:
Any other medicine without consulting your doctor or pharmacist.

POSSIBLE ADVERSE REACTIONS OR SIDE EFFECTS

SYMPTOMS	WHAT TO DO
Life-threatening:	
None expected.	
Common:	
Dizziness, headache, muscle pain, nausea.	Continue. Call doctor when convenient.
Infrequent:	
• Anxiety, vision problems, not feeling like oneself.	Discontinue. Call doctor right away.
• Abdominal pain; burning, prickling or tingling; constipation, cough, dry mouth, eye pain, fever, indigestion, arthritis, amnesia, skin rash, menstrual pain, nervousness, sensitive hearing, tightness in chest, trembling or shaking, unusual weakness, depression or tiredness, wheezing.	Continue. Call doctor if symptoms persist.
Rare:	
• Nosebleed, hallucinations.	Discontinue. Call doctor right away.
• Loss of appetite, back pain, chest pain, ear pain, general feeling of discomfort, sense of smell difficulty, swelling, rapid weight gain, sensitivity of skin and eyes to sunlight, skin rash, redness, burning, sunburn.	Continue. Call doctor if symptoms persist.

WARNINGS & PRECAUTIONS

Don't take if:
You have had an allergic reaction to zaleplon.

Before you start, consult your doctor:
- If you have a history of alcohol or drug abuse.
- If you have impaired kidney or liver function.
- If you are pregnant or nursing.
- If you have been diagnosed with clinical depression.

Over age 60:
Adverse reactions and side effects may be more frequent and severe than in younger persons.

Pregnancy:
Decide with your doctor whether drug benefits justify risk to unborn child. Risk category C (see page xviii).

Breast-feeding:
Drug passes into milk. Avoid drug or discontinue nursing until you finish medicine. Consult doctor for advice on maintaining milk supply.

Infants & children:
Not recommended.

Prolonged use:
Not intended for long term use.

Skin & sunlight:
No problems expected.

Driving, piloting or hazardous work:
Don't drive or pilot aircraft, work around dangerous machinery, climb ladders or work in high places for at least 4 hours after taking this medication. Danger increases if you drink alcohol or take medicine affecting alertness and reflexes, such as antihistamines, tranquilizers, sedatives, pain medicine, narcotics and mind-altering drugs.

Discontinuing:
Dose may require gradual reduction. If drug has been taken for a long time, consult doctor before discontinuing. You may have trouble sleeping for the first few nights after you stop taking zaleplon.

Others:
Advise any doctor or dentist whom you consult that you take this medicine.

POSSIBLE INTERACTION WITH OTHER DRUGS

GENERIC NAME OR DRUG CLASS	COMBINED EFFECT
Antidepressants, tricyclic*	Increased effect of either drug. Avoid.
Enzyme inducers*	Decreased zaleplon effect.
Central nervous system (CNS) depressants*	May increase effect of depressant.
Enzyme inhibitors*	Increased zaleplon effect.

POSSIBLE INTERACTION WITH OTHER SUBSTANCES

INTERACTS WITH	COMBINED EFFECT
Alcohol:	Increased sedation. Avoid.
Beverages:	None expected.
Cocaine:	None expected.
Foods:	None expected.
Marijuana:	Increased sedation. Avoid.
Tobacco:	None expected.

*See Glossary

ZINC SUPPLEMENTS

GENERIC AND BRAND NAMES

ZINC ACETATE
Galzin
ZINC GLUCONATE
Orazinc
ZINC SULFATE
Egozinc
PMS Egozinc
Verazinc
Zinc-220
Zincate

BASIC INFORMATION

Habit forming? No
Prescription needed? No
Available as generic? Yes
Drug class: Nutritional supplement (mineral)

USES

- Treats zinc deficiency that may lead to growth retardation, appetite loss, changes in taste or smell, skin eruptions, slow wound healing, decreased immune function, diarrhea or impaired night vision.
- In absence of a deficiency, is used to treat burns, eating disorders, liver disorders, prematurity in infants, intestinal diseases, parasitism, kidney disorders, skin disorders and stress.
- May be useful as a supplement for those who are breast-feeding or pregnant (under a doctor's supervision).
- Zinc acetate is used for treatment of Wilson's disease.

DOSAGE & USAGE INFORMATION

How to take:
Tablet or capsule—Swallow with liquid. If you can't swallow whole, crumble tablet or open capsule and take with liquid or food.

When to take:
At the same time each day, according to a doctor's instructions or the package label.

Continued next column

OVERDOSE

SYMPTOMS:
Dizziness, yellow eyes and skin, shortness of breath, chest pain, vomiting.
WHAT TO DO:
- **Have patient drink lots of water.**
- **Dial 911 (emergency) for an ambulance or medical help or poison center 1-800-222-1222. Then give first aid immediately.**

If you forget a dose:
Take as soon as you remember up to 2 hours late. If more than 2 hours, wait for next scheduled dose (don't double this dose).

What drug does:
Required by the body for the utilization of many enzymes, nucleic acids and proteins and for cell growth.

Time lapse before drug works:
2 hours.

Don't take with:
Any other nonprescription or prescription medicine without consulting doctor or pharmacist.

POSSIBLE ADVERSE REACTIONS OR SIDE EFFECTS

SYMPTOMS	WHAT TO DO
Life-threatening:	
In case of overdose, see previous column.	
Common:	
None expected.	
Infrequent:	
None expected.	
Rare:	
• Indigestion, heartburn, nausea and vomiting (only with large doses).	Continue. Call doctor when convenient.
• Fever, chills, sore throat, ulcers in throat or mouth, unusual tiredness or weakness (only with large doses).	Discontinue. Call doctor right away.

WARNINGS & PRECAUTIONS

Don't take if:
You are allergic to zinc.

Before you start, consult your doctor:
If you are pregnant or breast-feeding.

Over age 60:
No special problems expected. Nutritional supplements may be helpful if the diet is restricted in any way.

Pregnancy:
Adequate zinc intake is important. Risk factor not designated. See category list on page xviii and consult doctor.

Breast-feeding:
Adequate zinc intake important. Consult a doctor.

Infants & children:
Normal daily requirements vary with age. Consult a doctor.

Prolonged use:
No special problems expected.

Skin & sunlight:
No special problems expected.

Driving, piloting or hazardous work:
No special problems expected.

Discontinuing:
No special problems expected.

Others:
The best natural sources of zinc are red meats, oysters, herring, peas and beans.

POSSIBLE INTERACTION WITH OTHER DRUGS

GENERIC NAME OR DRUG CLASS	COMBINED EFFECT
Copper supplements	Inhibited absorption of copper.
Diuretics, thiazide*	Increased need for zinc.
Folic acid	Increased need for zinc.
Iron supplements*	Increased need for zinc.
Tetracyclines*	Decreased absorption of tetracycline if taken within 2 hours of each other.

POSSIBLE INTERACTION WITH OTHER SUBSTANCES

INTERACTS WITH	COMBINED EFFECT
Alcohol:	May increase need for zinc.
Beverages:	None expected.
Cocaine:	None expected.
Foods: High-fiber.	May decrease zinc absorption.
Marijuana:	None expected.
Tobacco:	May increase need for zinc.

***See Glossary**

ZIPRASIDONE

BRAND NAMES

Geodon

BASIC INFORMATION

Habit forming? No
Prescription needed? Yes
Available as generic? No
Drug class: Antipsychotic

USES

Treatment for schizophrenia.

DOSAGE & USAGE INFORMATION

How to take:
Capsule—Swallow with liquid. Should be taken with food. Do not chew capsule.

When to take:
At the same times each day. The prescribed dosage may gradually be increased over the first few days or weeks of use.

If you forget a dose:
Take as soon as you remember. If it is almost time for the next dose, wait for the next scheduled dose (don't double this dose).

What drug does:
The exact mechanism is unknown. It appears to block certain nerve impulses between nerve cells.

Time lapse before drug works:
One to 7 days. A further increase in the dosage amount may be necessary to relieve symptoms for some patients.

Don't take with:
Any other medication without consulting your doctor or pharmacist.

OVERDOSE

SYMPTOMS:
Extreme drowsiness, sleepiness, slurring of speech, high blood pressure.
WHAT TO DO:

- **If symptoms appear serious or severe, dial 911 (emergency) for an ambulance or medical help or poison center 1-800-222-1222. Then give first aid immediately.**
- **See emergency information at end of book.**

POSSIBLE ADVERSE REACTIONS OR SIDE EFFECTS

SYMPTOMS	WHAT TO DO
Life-threatening: In case of overdose, see previous column.	
Common: Constipation or diarrhea, indigestion or heartburn, weight gain, rash, belching, stomach pain, nausea, drowsiness, dizziness, restlessness, feeling weak or a loss of strength, lack of muscle and balance control, coordination problems, trouble in speaking, drooling, twisting body movements of face, neck and back), arms and legs or muscles feel stiff, muscles tremble, shuffling walk.	Continue. Call doctor when convenient.
Infrequent: Appetite loss and weight loss, runny or stuffy nose, dry mouth, sneezing, vision changes, red and itchy skin, dystonia (unable to move eyes, eyelid twitching, eyes blinking more, tongue wants to stick out, trouble in breathing or speaking or swallowing), muscles feel tight or ache, feel faint upon standing after sitting or lying.	Continue, but call doctor right away.
Rare: Faintness, persistent and painful erection, heartbeat (irregular, fast or pounding), palpitations, convulsions.	Discontinue. Call doctor right away.

WARNINGS & PRECAUTIONS

Don't take if:
You are allergic to ziprasidone.

Before you start, consult your doctor:
- If you have liver or kidney disease.
- If you have heart disease, heart rhythm problems, QT prolongation, heart failure, or recent heart attack.
- If you have a history of seizures.
- If the patient has Alzheimer's.
- If you have tardive dyskinesia.
- If you have hypokalemia (low potassium) or hypomagnesemia (low magnesium).
- If you have neuroleptic malignant syndrome (serious or fatal problems may occur).

Over age 60:
Adverse reactions and side effects may be more severe than in younger persons. A lower starting dosage is usually recommended until a response is determined.

Pregnancy:
Decide with your doctor if drug benefits justify any possible risk to unborn child. Risk category C (see page xviii).

Breast-feeding:
It is unknown if drug passes into milk. Avoid nursing until you finish medicine. Consult doctor for advice on maintaining milk supply.

Infants & children:
Safety and efficacy has not been established. Use only under close medical supervision.

Prolonged use:
Consult with your doctor on a regular basis while taking this drug to check your progress or to discuss any increase or changes in side effects and the need for continued treatment. Also to check blood levels of potassium and magnesium and to monitor you for any heart problems.

Skin & sunlight:
Hot temperatures and exercise, hot baths can increase risk of heatstroke. Drug may affect body's ability to maintain normal temperature.

Driving, piloting or hazardous work:
Don't drive or pilot aircraft until you learn how medicine affects you. Don't work around dangerous machinery. Don't climb ladders or work in high places. Danger increases if you drink alcohol or take medicine affecting alertness and reflexes.

Discontinuing:
Don't discontinue this drug without consulting doctor. Dosage may require a gradual reduction before stopping.

Others:
- Get up slowly from a sitting or lying position to avoid dizziness, faintness or lightheadedness.
- Advise any doctor or dentist whom you consult that you take this medicine.
- Take medicine only as directed. Do not increase or reduce dosage without doctor's approval.

POSSIBLE INTERACTION WITH OTHER DRUGS

GENERIC NAME OR DRUG CLASS	COMBINED EFFECT
Antihypertensives*	Increased antihypertensive effect.
Carbamazepine	Decreased effect of ziprasidone.
Central nervous system (CNS) depressants*	Increased sedative effect. Increased effect of ziprasidone.
Central nervous system (CNS) stimulants	Unknown effect. Avoid.
Dopamine agonists*	Decreased effect of dopamine agonist.
Enzyme inhibitors*	Increased effect of ziprasidone.
Levodopa	May decrease levodopa effect.
QT interval prolongation-causing drugs*	Heart rhythm problems. Avoid.

POSSIBLE INTERACTION WITH OTHER SUBSTANCES

INTERACTS WITH	COMBINED EFFECT
Alcohol:	Increased sedative affect. Avoid.
Beverages:	None expected.
Cocaine:	Effect not known. Best to avoid.
Foods:	None expected.
Marijuana:	Effect not known. Best to avoid.
Tobacco:	None expected.

*See Glossary

ZOLPIDEM

BRAND NAMES

Ambien

BASIC INFORMATION

Habit forming? Yes
Prescription needed? Yes
Available as generic? No
Drug class: Sedative-hypnotic agent

USES

Short-term (less than 2 weeks) treatment for insomnia.

DOSAGE & USAGE INFORMATION

How to take:
Tablets—Swallow with liquid.

When to take:
Take immediately before bedtime. For best results, do not take with a meal or immediately after eating a meal.

If you forget a dose:
Take as soon as you remember. Take drug only when you are able to get 7 to 8 hours of sleep before your daily activity begins. Do not exceed prescribed dosage.

What drug does:
Acts as a central nervous system depressant, decreasing sleep problems such as trouble falling asleep, waking up too often during the night and waking up too early in the morning.

Time lapse before drug works:
Within 1 to 2 hours.

Don't take with:
Any other prescription or nonprescription drug without consulting your doctor or pharmacist.

OVERDOSE

SYMPTOMS:
Drowsiness, weakness, stupor, coma.
WHAT TO DO:

- **Dial 911 (emergency) for an ambulance or medical help or poison center 1-800-222-1222. Then give first aid immediately.**
- **If patient is unconscious and not breathing, give mouth-to-mouth breathing. If there is no heartbeat, use cardiac massage and mouth-to-mouth breathing (CPR). If you can't get help quickly, take patient to nearest emergency facility.**
- **See emergency information at end of book.**

POSSIBLE ADVERSE REACTIONS OR SIDE EFFECTS

SYMPTOMS	WHAT TO DO
Life-threatening:	
In case of overdose, see previous column.	
Common:	
Daytime drowsiness, lightheadedness, dizziness, clumsiness, headache, diarrhea, nausea.	Continue. Call doctor when convenient.
Infrequent:	
Dry mouth, muscle aches or pain, tiredness, indigestion, joint pain, memory problems.	Continue. Call doctor when convenient.
Rare:	
Behavioral changes, agitation, confusion, hallucinations, worsening of depression, bloody or cloudy urine, painful or difficult urination, increased urge to urinate, skin rash or hives, itching.	Discontinue. Call doctor right away.

WARNINGS & PRECAUTIONS

Don't take if:
You are allergic to zolpidem.

Before you start, consult your doctor:
- If you have respiratory problems.
- If you have kidney or liver disease.
- If you suffer from depression.
- If you are an active or recovering alcoholic or substance abuser.

Over age 60:
Adverse reactions and side effects may be more frequent and severe than in younger persons. You may need smaller doses for shorter periods of time.

Pregnancy:
Consult doctor. Risk category B (see page xviii).

Breast-feeding:
Drug passes into milk. Avoid drug or discontinue nursing until you finish medicine. Consult doctor for advice on maintaining milk supply.

Infants & children:
Not recommended for patients under age 18.

Prolonged use:
Not recommended for long-term usage. Don't take for longer than 1 to 2 weeks unless under doctor's supervision.

Skin & sunlight:
No special problems expected.

Driving, piloting or hazardous work:
Don't drive or pilot aircraft until you learn how medicine affects you. Don't work around dangerous machinery. Don't climb ladders or work in high places. Danger increases if you drink alcohol or take other medicines affecting alertness and reflexes.

Discontinuing:
- Don't discontinue without consulting doctor. Dose may require gradual reduction if you have taken drug for a long time.
- You may have sleeping problems for 1 or 2 nights after stopping drug.

Others:
- Advise any doctor or dentist whom you consult that you take this medicine.
- Don't take drug if you are traveling on an overnight airplane trip of less than 7 or 8 hours. A temporary memory loss may occur (traveler's amnesia).

POSSIBLE INTERACTION WITH OTHER DRUGS

GENERIC NAME OR DRUG CLASS	COMBINED EFFECT
Central nervous system (CNS) depressants*	Increased sedative effect. Avoid.
Chlorpromazine	Increased sedative effect. Avoid.
Imipramine	Increased sedative effect. Avoid.

POSSIBLE INTERACTION WITH OTHER SUBSTANCES

INTERACTS WITH	COMBINED EFFECT
Alcohol:	Increased sedation. Avoid.
Beverages:	None expected.
Cocaine:	None expected.
Foods:	Decreased sedative effect if taken with a meal or right after a meal.
Marijuana:	None expected.
Tobacco:	None expected.

*See Glossary

ZONISAMIDE

BRAND NAMES

Zonegran

BASIC INFORMATION

Habit forming? No
Prescription needed? Yes
Available as generic? No
Drug class: Anticonvulsant, antiepileptic

USES

Treatment for partial (focal) epileptic seizures. May be used alone or in combination with other antiepileptic drugs.

DOSAGE & USAGE INFORMATION

How to take:
Capsule–Swallow with liquid. Do not break or chew capsule. May be taken with or without food and on a full or empty stomach.

When to take:
Your doctor will determine the best schedule. Dosages will be increased rapidly over the first weeks of use. Further increases may be necessary to achieve maximum benefits.

If you forget a dose:
Take as soon as you remember. If it is almost time for the next dose, skip the missed dose and wait for your next scheduled dose (don't double this dose).

What drug does:
The exact mechanism is unknown. Studies have suggested different ways in which the drug provides anticonvulsant activity.

Time lapse before drug works:
May take several weeks for effectiveness.

Don't take with:
Any other prescription or nonprescription drug without consulting your doctor or pharmacist.

OVERDOSE

SYMPTOMS:
Slow or irregular heartbeat, confusion, dizziness, faintness, unusual tiredness or weakness, blue skin or fingernails, breathing difficulty, coma.
WHAT TO DO:
- **Dial 911 (emergency) for an ambulance or medical help or poison center 1-800-222-1222. Then give first aid immediately.**
- **See emergency information at end of book.**

POSSIBLE ADVERSE REACTIONS OR SIDE EFFECTS

SYMPTOMS	WHAT TO DO
Life-threatening:	
In case of overdose, see previous column.	
Common:	
• Unsteady walk, shakiness.	Continue, but call doctor right away.
• Sleepiness, dizziness, anxiety, restlessness, loss of appetite.	Continue. Call doctor when convenient.
Infrequent:	
• Agitation, delusions, hallucinations, bruising of the skin, depression, unusual mood or mental changes, double vision.	Continue, but call doctor right away.
• Constipation or diarrhea, heartburn, dry mouth, flu-like symptoms (chills, fever, headache, aching muscles and joints), problems with speech, difficulty in concentrating, sour stomach, belching, back and forth eye movement, nausea, runny or stuffy nose, tingling or burning sensations.	Continue. Call doctor when convenient.
Rare:	
Other symptoms.	Continue. Call doctor when convenient.

WARNINGS & PRECAUTIONS

Don't take if:
You are allergic to zonisamide or any other sulfonamides.*

Before you start, consult your doctor:
- If you have a history of liver disease.
- If you have renal failure (inability of the kidneys to function properly).
- If you are allergic to any medication, food or other substance.
- If you have any other medical problems.

Over age 60:
No special problems expected.

Pregnancy:
Decide with your doctor if drug benefits justify risks to unborn child. Risk category C (see page xviii).

Breast-feeding:
Drug passes into milk. Avoid drug or discontinue nursing until you finish medicine. Consult doctor for advice on maintaining milk supply.

Infants & children:
Zonisamide has not been studied in children under age 16. Use only under medical supervision.

Prolonged use:
No special problems expected. Follow-up laboratory blood studies may be recommended by your doctor.

Skin & sunlight:
No problems expected.

Driving, piloting or hazardous work:
Don't drive or pilot aircraft until you learn how medicine affects you. Don't work around dangerous machinery. Don't climb ladders or work in high places. Danger increases if you drink alcohol or take other medicines affecting alertness and reflexes such as antihistamines, tranquilizers, sedatives, pain medicine, narcotics and mind-altering drugs.

Discontinuing:
Don't discontinue without doctor's approval due to risk of increased seizure activity. The dosage may need to be gradually decreased before stopping the drug completely.

Others:
- Advise any doctor or dentist whom you consult that you take this medicine.
- Zonisamide may be used with other anticonvulsant drugs and additional side effects may also occur. If they do, discuss them with your doctor.
- May alter some laboratory tests.

POSSIBLE INTERACTION WITH OTHER DRUGS

GENERIC NAME OR DRUG CLASS	COMBINED EFFECT
Anticonvulsants*, other	Decreased effect of zonisamide.
CNS Depressants*	Increased sedative effect.

POSSIBLE INTERACTION WITH OTHER SUBSTANCES

INTERACTS WITH	COMBINED EFFECT
Alcohol:	Increased sedative effect. Decreased effect of zonisamide. Avoid.
Beverages:	None expected.
Cocaine:	Unknown effect. Avoid.
Foods:	None expected.
Marijuana:	Unknown effect. Avoid.
Tobacco:	None expected.

*See Glossary

Generic and Brand Name Directory

How to Read the Lists Below

The following drugs are alphabetized by generic name or drug class name, shown in large capital letters. The generic names and brand names that follow each title in this list are the complete list referred to on the drug chart. Generic names are in all capital letters on these lists; brand names are lower case.

Some main headings, such as *ADRENOCORTICOIDS (Systemic)* (a drug class name on page 14), are followed by generic names, which are numbered, and then by brand names, each of which is followed by a superscript number. By matching numbers, you can determine the generic drug(s) in each brand-name drug. For example, under *ADRENOCORTICOIDS (Systemic)*, the brand-name drug Aristocort[8] contains the generic drug *TRIAMCINOLONE*, which is numbered 8.

Other main heads below, such as *ACETAMINOPHEN*, are simple generic names, followed by brand-name drugs containing that generic drug.

ACETAMINOPHEN

Abenol
Acephen
Aceta
Acetaminophen Uniserts
Aclophen
Actamin
Actamin Extra
Actamin Super
Actifed A
Actifed Plus
Actifed Plus Caplets
Actimol
Advanced Formula Dristan Caplets
Alba-Temp 300
Allerest No-Drowsiness
All-Nite Cold Formula
Amaphen
Aminofen
Aminofen Max
Anacin-3
Anacin-3 Extra Strength
Anolor 300
Anoquan
Anuphen
Apacet Capsules
Apacet Elixir
Apacet Extra Strength Caplets
Apacet Extra Strength Tablets
Apacet Oral Solution
Apacet Regular Strength Tablets
APAP
Apo-Acetaminophen
Arcet
Aspirin Free Anacin Maximum Strength Caplets
Aspirin Free Anacin Maximum Strength Tablets
Aspirin Free Bayer Select Maximum Strength Headache Plus Caplets
Aspirin-Free Excedrin Caplets
Atasol Caplets
Atasol Drops
Atasol Forte
Atasol Forte Caplets
Atasol Forte Tablets
Atasol Oral Solution
Atasol Tablets
Bancap
Banesin
Bayer Select Chest Cold Tablets
Bayer Select Flu Relief Caplets
Bayer Select Head and Chest Cold Caplets
Bayer Select Head Cold Caplets
Bayer Select Maximum Strength Pain Relief Formula
Bayer Select Maximum Strength Sinus Pain Relief Caplets
Bayer Select Night Time Cold Caplets
Benadryl Allergy/Sinus Headache Caplets
Benadryl Cold
Benadryl Cold Nighttime Liquid
Benadryl Plus
Beta-Phed
Bromo-Seltzer
Bucet
Buffets
Calmylin Cough & Cold
Campain
Children's Anacin 3
Children's Panadol
Children's Tylenol Cold
Children's Tylenol Cold Multi-Symptom Plus Cough
Children's Tylenol Soft Chews
Children's Tylenol Suspension Liquid
Children's Ty-Tab
Co-Apap
Codimal
Coldrine
Colrex Compound
Comtrex
Comtrex A/S Caplets
Comtrex Cough Formula
Comtrex Daytime Caplets
Comtrex Daytime Maximum Strength Cold and Flu Relief
Comtrex Daytime Maximum Strength Cold, Cough and Flu Relief
Comtrex Hot Flu Relief
Comtrex Multi-Symptom Hot Flu Relief
Comtrex Multi-Symptom Non-Drowsy Caplets
Comtrex Nighttime
Comtrex Nighttime Maximum Strength Cold and Flu Relief
Comtrex Nighttime Maximum Strength Cold, Cough and Flu Relief
Comtrex Sore Throat Relief
Conacetol
Conar-A
Congespirin
Congespirin for Children Cold Tablets
Congespirin for Children Liquid Cold Medicine
Congestant D
Contac Allergy/Sinus Day Caplets
Contac Allergy/Sinus Night Caplets
Contac Maximum Strength Sinus Caplets
Contac Night Caplets
Contac Non-Drowsy Formula Sinus Caplets
Contac Severe Cold Formula
Contac Severe Cold Formula Night Strength
CoTylenol Cold Medication
Dapa
Datril Extra Strength
DayCare
DayQuil Liquicaps
DayQuil Non-Drowsy Cold/Flu
DayQuil Non-Drowsy Cold/Flu Liquicaps
DayQuil Non-Drowsy Sinus Pressure and Pain Relief Caplets
Dolanex
Dolmar
Dorcol Children's Fever and Pain Reducer
Dristan AF
Dristan AF Plus
Dristan Cold and Flu
Dristan Cold Caplets
Dristan Cold Maximum Strength Caplets
Dristan Cold Multi-Symptom Formula
Dristan Juice Mix-in Cold, Flu, and Cough

Drixoral Cold and Flu
Drixoral Plus
Drixoral Sinus
Duoprin
Duradyne
Endolor
Esgic
Esgic Plus
Excedrin Caplets
Excedrin Extra Strength Caplets
Excedrin Extra Strength Tablets
Excedrin Migraine
Exdol
Exdol Strong
Ezol
Febridyne
Femcet
Fendol
Feverall Children's
Feverall Infants'
Feverall Junior Strength
Feverall Sprinkle Caps
Fioricet
Gelpirin
Gemnisyn
Genapap
Genapap Children's Elixir
Genapap Children's Tablets
Genapap Extra Strength
Genapap Infants'
Genapap Regular Strength Tablets
Gendecon
Gen-D-phen
Genebs
Genebs Extra Strength
Genebs Regular Strength Tablets
Genex
Genite
Goody's Extra Strength Tablets
Goody's Headache Powders
Halenol
Halenol Extra Strength
Histagesic Modified
Histosal
Hycomine Compound
Improved Sino-Tuss
Infants' Anacin-3
Infants' Apacet
Infants' Genapap
Infants' Panadol
Infants' Tylenol Suspension Drops
Isopap
Kolephrin
Kolephrin/DM Caplets
Liquiprin Children's Elixir
Liquiprin Infants' Drops
Mapap Cold Formula
Maximum Strength Tylenol Allergy Sinus Caplets
Maximum Strength Tylenol Flu Gelcaps
Meda Cap
Meda Tab
Medi-Flu
Medi-Flu Caplets
Medigesic
Myapap Elixir
Naldegesic
ND-Gesic
Neocitrin Colds and Flu Calorie Reduced
NeoCitrin Extra Strength Colds and Flu
NeoCitrin Extra Strength Sinus
Neopap
Nighttime Pamprin
NyQuil Hot Therapy
NyQuil Liquicaps
NyQuil Nighttime Colds Medicine
Nytcold Medicine
Nytime Cold Medicine Liquid
Omnicol
Oraphen-PD
Ornex Maximum Strength Caplets
Ornex No Drowsiness Caplets
Pacaps
Panadol
Panadol Extra Strength
Panadol Junior Strength Caplets
Panadol Maximum Strength Caplets
Panadol Maximum Strength Tablets
Panex
Panex 500
Paracetamol
Parafon Forte
Pedric
Pertussin All Night PM
Phenapap Sinus Headache & Congestion
Phenaphen
Phrenilin
Phrenilin Forte
Presalin
Redutemp
Remcol-C
Repan
Rhinogesic
Rid-A-Pain Compound
Robigesic
Robitussin Honey Flu
Robitussin Night Relief
Robitussin Night Relief Colds Formula Liquid
Rounox
S-A-C
Salphenyl
Sedapap
Semcet
Simplet
Sinarest No Drowsiness
Sinarest Sinus
Sine-Aid
Sine-Aid Maximum Strength
Sine-Aid Maximum Strength Caplets
Sine-Aid Maximum Strength Gelcaps
Sine-Off Maximum Strength Allergy/Sinus Formula Caplets
Sine-Off Maximum Strength No Drowsiness Formula Caplets
Singlet
Sinubid
Sinus Excedrin Extra Strength
Sinus Excedrin Extra Strength Caplets
Sinus Excedrin No Drowsiness
Sinus Excedrin No Drowsiness Caplets
Sinus Relief
Sinutab
Sinutab Extra Strength
Sinutab II Maximum Strength
Sinutab Maximum Strength Sinus Allergy
Sinutab Maximum Strength Sinus Allergy Caplets
Sinutab Maximum Strength without Drowsiness
Sinutab Maximum Strength without Drowsiness Caplets
Sinutab No Drowsiness
Sinutab No Drowsiness Extra Strength
Sinutab Regular
Sinutrex Extra Strength
Snaplets-FR
St. Joseph Aspirin Free Fever Reducer for Children
Sudafed Cold & Cough Liquid Caps
Sudafed Severe Cold Formula Caplets
Sudafed Sinus Maximum Strength
Sudafed Sinus Maximum Strength Caplets
Summit
Supac
Super-Anahist
Suppap
Tapanol
Tapanol Extra Strength
Tapar
Tavist Allergy/Sinus/Headache
Tempra
Tempra Caplets
Tempra Chewable Tablets
Tempra Double Strength
Tempra Drops
Tempra D.S.
Tempra Infants
Tempra Syrup
Tencet
Tenol
Tenol PlusTheraFlu Maximum Strength
Non-Drowsy Formula Flu, Cold and Cough Medicine
TheraFlu Nighttime Maximum Strength
TheraFlu/Flu & Cold
TheraFlu/Flu, Cold & Cough
Thera-Hist
Triad
Triaminic Sore Throat Formula
Triaprin
Tricom Tablets
Trigesic
Tri-Pain
Two-Dyne
Ty-Cold Cold Formula
Tylenol
Tylenol Allergy Sinus Gelcaps
Tylenol Allergy Sinus NightTime Maximum Strength Caplets
Tylenol Arthritis Extended Relief
Tylenol Caplets
Tylenol Children's Chewable Tablets
Tylenol Children's Elixir
Tylenol Children's Suspension Liquid
Tylenol Cold and Flu

Tylenol Cold and Flu No
Drowsiness Powder
Tylenol Cold Medication
Tylenol Cold Medication,
Non-Drowsy
Tylenol Cold Night Time
Tylenol Cold No Drowsiness
Formula Gelcaps
Tylenol Cough
Tylenol Cough with Decongestant
Tylenol Extra Strength
Tylenol Infants' Drops
Tylenol Junior Strength
Tylenol Junior Strength
Chewable Tablets
Tylenol Maximum Strength
Cough
Tylenol Maximum Strength Flu
Gelcaps
Tylenol Maximum Strength
Gelcaps
Tylenol Regular Strength Caplets
Tylenol Regular Strength Tablets
Tylenol Sinus Maximum Strength
Tylenol Sinus Maximum Strength
Caplets
Tylenol Sinus Medication
Tylenol Sinus Medication Extra
Strength
Tylenol Sore Throat
Tylenol Sore Maximum Strength
Ty-Pap
Ultracet
Valadol
Valadol Liquid
Valorin
Valorin Extra
Vanquis
Vicks 44 Cold, Flu and Cough
Liqui-Caps
Vicks 44M Cough, Cold and Flu
Relief
Vicks 44M Cough, Cold and Flu
Relief LiquiCaps
Vicks Dayquil Liquicaps
Vicks Formula 44M Multi-
Symptom Cough Mixture
Vicks NyQuil Multi-Symptom
Cold/Flu Relief
Vicks NyQuil Multi-Symptom
LiquiCaps
Women's Tylenol Menstrual
Relief Caplets

ADRENOCORTICOIDS (Systemic)

GENERIC NAMES
1. BETAMETHASONE
2. BUDESONIDE
3. CORTISONE
4 DEXAMETHASONE
5 HYDROCORTISONE (Cortisol)
6. METHYLPREDNISOLONE
7 PREDNISOLONE
8 PREDNISONE
9. TRIAMCINOLONE

BRAND NAMES
Apo-Prednisone[8]
Aristocort[9]
Betnelan[1]
Betnesol[1]
Celestone[1]
Cortef5
Cortenema5
Cortifoam5
Cortone3
Cortone Acetate3
Decadron4
Delta-Cortef7
Deltasone[8]
Deronil[4]
Dexasone[4]
Dexone 0.5[4]
Dexone 0.75[4]
Dexone 1.5[4]
Dexone 4[4]
Entocort EC[2]
Hexadrol[4]
Hydeltrasol[7]
Hydrocortone[5]
Kenacort[9]
Kenacort Diacetate[9]
Medrol[6]
Meprolonel[6]
Meticorten[8]
Mymethasone[4]
Nor-Pred-TBA[7]
Oradexon[4]
Orasone 1[8]
Orasone 5[8]
Orasone 10[8]
Orasone 20[8]
Orasone 50[8]
Pediapred[7]
Predisone Intensol[8]
Prednicen-M[8]
Prelone[7]
Sterapred DS[8]
Solurex[4]
Solurex LA[4]
Winpred[8]

ADRENOCORTICOIDS (Topical)

GENERIC NAMES
1. ALCLOMETASONE (Topical)
2. AMCINONIDE (Topical)
3. BECLOMETHASONE (Topical)
4. BETAMETHASONE (Topical)
5. CLOBETASOL (Topical)
6. CLOBETASONE (Topical)
7. CLOCORTOLONE (Topical)
8. CORTISOL
9. DESONIDE (Topical)
10. DESOXIMETASONE (Topical)
11. DEXAMETHASONE (Topical)
12. DIFLORASONE (Topical)
13. DIFLUCORTOLONE (Topical)
14. FLUMETHASONE (Topical)
15. FLUOCINOLONE (Topical)
16. FLUOCINONIDE (Topical)
17. FLURANDRENOLIDE (Topical)
18. FLUTICASONE
19. HALCINONIDE (Topical)
20. HALOBETASOL
21. HYDROCORTISONE (Dental)
22. HYDROCORTISONE (Topical)
23. METHYLPREDNISOLONE
24. MOMETASONE (Topical)
25. PREDNICARBATE
26. TRIAMCINOLONE (Dental)
27. TRIAMCINOLONE (Topical)

BRAND NAMES
9-1-1[22]
Aclovate[1]
Acticort-100[22]
Adcortyl[27]
Aeroseb-Dex[11]
Aeroseb-HC[22]
Ala-Cort[22]
Ala-Scalp HP[22]
Allercort[22]
Alphaderm[22]
Alphatrex[4]
Anucort-HC[22]
Anusol-HC[22]
Anusol-HC 2.5%[22]
Aristocort[27]
Aristocort A[27]
Aristocort C[27]
Aristocort D[27]
Aristocort R[27]
Bactine[22]
Barriere-HC[22]
Beben[4]
Beta HC[22]
Betacort Scalp Lotion[4]
Betaderm[4]
Betaderm Scalp Lotion[4]
Betamethacot[4]
Betatrex[4]
Beta-Val[4]
Betnovate[4]
Betnovate 1/2[4]
Bio-Syn[15]
CaldeCORT Anti-Itch[22]
CaldeCORT-Light[22]
Carmol-HC[22]
Celestoderm-V[4]
Celestoderm-V/2[4]
Cetacort[22]
Cloderm[7]
Cordran[17]
Cordran SP[17]
Cormax[5]
Cortacet[22]
Cortaid[22]
Cortaid FastStick[22]
Cortate[22]
Cort-Dome[22]
Cort-Dome High Potency[22]
Cortef[22]
Cortef Feminine Itch[22]
Corticaine[22]
Corticreme[22]
Cortifair[22]
Cortiment-10[22]
Cortiment-40[22]
Cortoderm[22]
Cortril[22]
Cultivate[18]
Cyclocort[2]
Decaderm[11]
Decadron[11]
Decaspray[11]
Delacort[22]
Delta-Tritex[27]
Demarest DriCort[22]
Dermabet[4]
Dermacomb[27]
Dermacort[22]
DermAtop[25]
DermiCort[22]
Dermovate[5]
Dermovate Scalp Application[5]

Dermtex HC[22]
DesOwen[9]
Diprolene[4]
Diprolene AF[4]
Diprosone[4]
Drenison[17]
Drenison-1/4[17]
Ectosone[4]
Ectosone Regular[4]
Ectosone Scalp Lotion[4]
Efcortelan[22]
Elocom[24]
Elocon[24]
Emo-Cort[22]
Emo-Cort Scalp Solution[22]
Epifoam[8]
Eumovate[6]
Fludroxycortide[17]
Fluocet[15]
Fluocin[16]
Fluoderm[15]
Fluolar[15]
Fluonid[15]
Fluonide[15]
Flurosyn[15]
Flutex[27]
Foille Cort[22]
Gly-Cort[22]
Gynecort[22]
Gynecort 10[22]
Halciderm[19]
Halog[19]
Halog E[19]
Hi-Cor 1.0[22]
Hi-Cor 2.5[22]
Hyderm[22]
Hydro-Tex[22]
Hytone[22]
Kenac[27]
Kenalog[27]
Kenalog in Orabase[27]
Kenalog-H[27]
Kenonel[27]
Lacticare-HC[22]
Lanacort[22]
Lanacort 10[22]
Lemoderm[22]
Licon[16]
Lidemol[16]
Lidex[16]
Lidex-E[16]
Locacorten[14]
Locoid[22]
Lotrisone[4]
Lyderm[16]
Maxiflor[12]
Maximum Strength Cortaid[22]
Maxivate[4]
Metaderm Mild[4]
Metaderm Regular[4] (Topical)
Metosyn[16]
Metosyn FAPG[16]
My Cort[22]
Nerisone[13]
Nerisone Oily[13]
Novobetamet[4]
Novohydrocort[22]
Nutracort[22]
Olux[5]
Orabase HCA[22]
Oracort[27]
Oralone[27]
Pandel[22]
Penecort[22]
Pentacort[22]
Pharma-Cort[22]
Prevex B[4]
Prevex HC[4]
Propaderm[3]
Psorcon[12]
Rederm[22]
Rhulicort[22]
Sarna HC[22]
Sential[22]
S-T Cort[22]
Synacort[22]
Synalar[15]
Synalar HP[15]
Synamol[15]
Synemol[15]
Teladar[4]
Temovate[5]
Temovate E[5]
Temovate Emollient[5]
Temovate Gel[5]
Temovate Scalp Application[5]
Texacort[22]
Topicort[10]
Topicort LP[10]
Topicort Mild[10]
Topilene[4]
Topisone[4]
Topsyn[16]
Triacet[27]
Triaderm[27]
Trianide Mild[27]
Trianide Regular[27]
Triderm[27]
Tridesilon[9]
Trymex[27]
Ultravate[20]
Unicort[22]
Uticort[4]
Valisone[4]
Valisone Reduced Strength[4]
Valisone Scalp Lotion[4]
Valnac[4]
Vioform-Hydrocortisone Lotion[22]
Westcort[22]

Some of these brands are available as oral medicine. Look under specific generic name for each brand.

ANDROGENS

GENERIC NAMES

1. ETHYLESTRENOL
2. FLUOXYMESTERONE
3. METHYLTESTOSTERONE
4. NANDROLONE
5. OXANDROLONE
6. OXYMETHOLONE
7. STANOZOLOL
8. TESTOSTERONE

BRAND NAMES

Anabolin[4]
Anabolin LA 100[4]
Anadrol-50[6]
Anapolon 50[6]
Andro 100[8]
Andro-Cyp 100[8]
Andro-Cyp 200[8]
Androderm[8]
Androgel[8]
Android-10[3]
Android-25[3]
Android-T[8]
Andro-LA 200[8]
Androlone[4]
Andronaq-50[8]
Andronaq-LA[8]
Andronate 100[8]
Andronate 200[8]
Andropository 100[8]
Andryl 200[8]
Deca-Durabolin[4]
Delatest[8]
Delatestryl[8]
Dep Andro 100[8]
Dep Andro 200[8]
Depotest[8]
Depo-Testosterone[8]
Durabolin[4]
Durabolin-50[4]
Duratest 100[8]
Duratest-200[8]
Durathate 200[8]
Everone[8]
Halotestin[2]
Histerone-50[8]
Histerone-100[8]
Hybolin Decanoate[4]
Hybolin-Improved[4]
Kabolin[4]
Malogen[8]
Malogex[8]
Maxibolin[4]
Metandren[3]
Nandrobolic[4]
Nandrobolic L.A.[4]
Neo-Durabolic[4]
Ora-Testryl[2]
Oreton[3]
T-Cypionate[8]
Testa-C[8]
Testamone 100[8]
Testaqua[8]
Testex[8]
Testoderm with Adhesive[8]
Testoject-50[8]
Testoject-LA[8]
Testone L.A.[8]
Testred[3]
Testred-Cypionate 200[8]
Testrin P.A.[8]
Virilon[3]
Virolon IM[3]
Winstrol[7]

ANDROGENS & ESTROGENS

GENERIC NAMES

1. CONJUGATED ESTROGENS & METHYLTESTOSTERONE
2. DIETHYLSTILBESTROL (DES) & METHYLTESTOSTERONE
3. ESTERIFIED ESTROGENS & METHYLTESTOSTERONE
4. FLUOXYMESTERONE & ETHINYL ESTRADIOL
5. TESTOSTERONE & ESTRADIOL

BRAND NAMES

Andrest 90-4[5]
Andro-Estro 90-4[5]
Androgyn L.A[5]
Climacteron[5]

De-Comberol[5]
Deladumone[5]
Delatestadiol[5]
Dep-Androgyn[5]
Depo-Testadiol[5]
Depotestogen[5]
Duo-Cyp[5]
Duo-Gen L.A.[5]
Duogex L.A.[5]
Dura-Dumone 90/4[5]
Duratestin[5]
Estratest[3]
Estratest H.S.[3]
Halodrin[4]
Menoject L.A.[5]
Neo-Pause[5]
OB[5]
Premarin with Methyltestosterone[1]
Teev[5]
Tes Est Cyp[5]
Test-Estro Cypionate[5]
Tylosterone[2]
Valertest No. 1[5]
Valertest No. 2[5]

ANESTHETICS (Topical)

GENERIC NAMES

1. BENZOCAINE
2. BENZOCAINE & MENTHOL
3. BUTAMBEN
4. DIBUCAINE
5. LIDOCAINE
6. LIDOCAINE & PRILOCAINE
7. PRAMOXINE
8. TETRACAINE
9. TETRACAINE & MENTHOL

BRAND NAMES

Americaine[1]
Amercaine Topical Anesthetic First Aid Ointment[1]
Amerçaine Topical Anesthetic Spray[1]
Benzocol[2]
Butesin Picrate[3]
Butyl Aminobenzoate[2]
Cinchocaine[4]
Dermoplast[2]
Emla [6]
Endocaine[1]
Ethyl Aminobenzoate[1]
Lagol[1]
Lidoderm[5]
Lignocaine[5]
Nupercainal Cream[4]
Nupercainal Ointment[4]
Pontocaine Cream[8]
Pontocaine Ointment[9]
Pramegel[7]
Prax[7]
Tronothane[7]
Unguentine[1]
Unguentine Plus[1]
Unguentine Spray[1]
Xylocaine[5]

ANGIOTENSIN-CONVERTING ENZYME (ACE) INHIBITORS

GENERIC NAMES

1. BENAZEPRIL
2. CAPTOPRIL
3. ENALAPRIL
4. FOSINOPRIL
5. LISINOPRIL
6. MOEXIPRIL
7. PERINDOPRIL
8. QUINAPRIL
9. RAMIPRIL
10. TRANDOLAPRIL

BRAND NAMES

Accupril[8]
Aceon[7]
Altace[9]
Apo-Capto[2]
Capoten[2]
Lexxel[3]
Lotensin[1]
Lotrel[1]
Mavik[10]
Monopril[4]
Novo-Captoril[2]
Prinivil[5]
Syn-Captopril[2]
Tarka[10]
Teczem[3]
Uniretic[6]
Univasc[6]
Vasotec[3]
Zestril[5]

ANGIOTENSIN-CONVERTING ENZYME (ACE) INHIBITORS & HYDROCHLOROTHIAZIDE

GENERIC NAMES

1. CAPTOPRIL & HYDROCHLOROTHIAZIDE
2. ENALAPRIL & HYDROCHLOROTHIAZIDE
3. LISINOPRIL & HYDROCHLOROTHIAZIDE
4. QUINAPRIL & HYDROCHLOROTHIAZIDE

BRAND NAMES

Accuretic[4]
Capozide[1]
Prinzide[3]
Vaseretic[2]
Zestoretic[3]

ANTACIDS

GENERIC NAMES

1. ALUMINA & MAGNESIA
2. ALUMINA & MAGNESIUM CARBONATE
3. ALUMINA & MAGNESIUM TRISILICATE
4. ALUMINA, MAGNESIA, & CALCIUM CARBONATE
5. ALUMINA, MAGNESIA, & SIMETHICONE
6. ALUMINA, MAGNESIUM CARBONATE, & CALCIUM CARBONATE
7. ALUMINA, MAGNESIUM TRISILICATE, & SODIUM BICARBONATE
8. ALUMINUM CARBONATE, BASIC
9. ALUMINUM HYDROXIDE
10. CALCIUM & MAGNESIUM CARBONATES
11. CALCIUM CARBONATE
12. CALCIUM CARBONATE & MAGNESIA
13. CALCIUM CARBONATE & MAGNESIUM HYDROXIDE
14. CALCIUM CARBONATE & SIMETHICONE
15. CALCIUM CARBONATE, MAGNESIA, & SIMETHICONE
16. CALCIUM, MAGNESIUM CARBONATES & MAGNESIUM OXIDE
17. DIHYDROXYALUMINUM AMINOACETATE
18. DIHYDROXYALUMINUM AMINOACETATE, MAGNESIA, & ALUMINA
19. DIHYDROXYALUMINUM SODIUM CARBONATE
20. MAGALDRATE
21. MAGALDRATE & SIMETHICONE
22. MAGNESIUM CARBONATE & SODIUM BICARBONATE
23. MAGNESIUM HYDROXIDE
24. MAGNESIUM OXIDE
25. MAGNESIUM TRISILICATE, ALUMINA, & MAGNESIA

BRAND NAMES

Advanced Formula Di-Gel[15]
Alamag[1]
Algenic Alka[2]
Algenic Alka Improved[2]
Algicon[9]
Alka-Mints[11]
Alkets[11]
Alkets Extra Strength[11]
Almacone[5]
Almacone II[5]
Alma-Mag #4 Improved[5]
Alma-Mag Improved[5]
AlternaGEL[9]
Alu-Cap[9]
Aludrox[5]
Alu-Tab[9]
Amitone[12]
Amphojel[9]
Amphojel 500[1]
Amphojel Plus[4]
AntaGel[5]
AntaGel-II[5]
Basaljel[9]
Calglycine[11]
Camalox[4]
Chooz[11]
Dialume[9]
Di-Gel[5]
Diovol Ex[1]
Diovol Plus[5]
Duracid[9]
Equilet[11]
Foamicon[3]
Gas-X with Maalox[14]
Gaviscon[2]

Gaviscon Extra Strength Relief Formula[9]
Gaviscon-2[7]
Gelusil[5]
Gelusil Extra-Strength[1]
Genalac[11]
Genaton[2]
Genaton Extra Strength[22]
Glycate[11]
Kudrox Double Strength[5]
Losopan[20]
Losopan Plus[21]
Lowsium[20]
Lowsium Plus[21]
Maalox[1]
Maalox HRF[2]
Maalox Plus[5]
Maalox Plus, Extra Strength[5]
Maalox TC[1]
Magnalox[5]
Magnalox Plus[5]
Magnatril[9]
Mag-Ox 400[24]
Mallamint[11]
Maox[24]
Marblen[10]
Mi-Acid[5]
Mi-Acid Double Strength[5]
Mintox[1]
Mintox Extra Strength[5]
Mygel[5]
Mygel II[5]
Mylagen[5]
Mylagen II[5]
Mylanta[5]
Mylanta Calci Tabs[12]
Mylanta Double Strength[5]
Mylanta Double Strength Plain[5]
Mylanta Gelcaps[10]
Mylanta Night Time Strength[9]
Mylanta Plain[5]
Mylanta-2 Extra Strength[5]
Mylanta-II[5]
Nephrox[9]
Neutralca-S[1]
Pepcid Complete[13]
Phillips' Milk of Magnesia[23]
Riopan[20]
Riopan Extra Strength[20]
Riopan Plus[21]
Riopan Plus Double Strength[21]
Riopan Plus Extra Strength[21]
Rolaids[12]
Rolaids Calcium Rich[11]
Rolaids Sodium Free[11]
Rulox[1]
Rulox No. 1[1]
Rulox No. 2[1]
Rulox Plus[5]
Simaal 2 Gel[5]
Simaal Gel[5]
Tempo[6]
Titralac[11]
Titralac Plus[11]
Triconsil[7]
Tums[11]
Tums E-X[11]
Tums Liquid Extra Strength[11]
Tums Liquid Extra Strength with Simethicone[14]
Univol[1]
Uro-Mag[24]

ANTIBACTERIALS (Ophthalmic)

GENERIC NAMES
1. CHLORAMPHENICOL
2. CHLORTETRACYCLINE
3. CIPROFLOXACIN
4. ERYTHROMYCIN (Ophthalmic)
5. GENTAMICIN (Ophthalmic)
6. NEOMYCIN
7. NEOMYCIN, POLYMIXIN B & BACITRACIN
8. NEOMYCIN, POLYMIXIN B & CORTISOL
9. NEOMYCIN, POLYMIXIN B & GRAMICIDIN
10. NEOMYCIN, POLYMIXIN B & HYDROCORTISONE
11. NORFLOXACIN (Ophthalmic)
12. OFLOXACIN (Ophthalmic)
13. POLYMYXIN B
14. SULFACETAMIDE (Ophthalmic)
15. SULFISOXAZOLE (Ophthalmic)
16. SULFONAMIDES (Ophthalmic)
17. TETRACYCLINE (Ophthalmic)
18. TOBRAMYCIN (Ophthalmic)

BRAND NAMES
Achromycin[17]
Aerosporin[13]
Ak-Chlor Ophthalmic Ointment[1]
Ak-Chlor Ophthalmic Solution[14]
Ak-Spore[13]
Ak-Sulf[14]
Aktob[18]
Alcomicin[5]
Aureomycin[2]
Bio-Triple[13]
Bleph-10[14]
Cetamide[14]
Chibroxin[11]
Chloracol Ophthalmic Solution (Ophthalmic)[1]
Chlorofair Ophthalmic Ointment[1]
Chlorofair Ophthalmic Solution[1]
Chloromycetin Ophthalmic Ointment[1]
Chloromycetin Ophthalmic Solution[1]
Chloroptic Ophthalmic Solution[1]
Chloroptic S.O.P.[1]
Ciloxan[3]
Cortisporin-Ophthalmic[13]
Econochlor Ophthalmic Ointment[1]
Econochlor Ophthalmic Solution[1]
Fenicol Ophthalmic Ointment[1]
Gantrisin[15]
Garamycin[5]
Genoptic[5]
Gentacidin[5]
Gentafair[5]
Gentak[5]
Gentrasul[5]
I-Chlor Ophthalmic Solution[1]
Ilotycin[4]
I-Sulfacet[14]
Mycitracin[13]
Neociden Ophthalmic Ointment[7]
Neociden Ophthalmic Solution[9]
Neosporin[13]
Neosporin Ophthalmic Solution[13]
Neotal[13]
Neotricin[13]
Ocu-Chlor Ophthalmic Ointment[1]
Ocu-Chlor Ophthalmic Solution[1]
Ocuflox[12]
Ocu-Mycin[13]
Ocu-Spor-B[13]
Ocu-Spor-G[13]
Ocusporin[13]
Ocu-Sul-10[14]
Ocu-Sul-15[14]
Ocu-Sul-30[14]
Ocusulf-10[14]
Ocutricin[13]
Ophthacet[14]
Ophthalmic
Ophthochlor Ophthalmic Solution[1]
Ophtho-Chloram Ophthalmic Solution[1]
Pentamycetin[10]
Pentamycetin Ophthalmic Ointment[10]
Pentamycetin Ophthalmic Solution[10]
P.N. Ophthalmic[13]
Regasporin[7]
Sodium Sulamyd[14]
Sopamycetin Ophthalmic Ointment[10]
Sopamycetin Ophthalmic Solution[10]
Spectro-Chlor Ophthalmic Ointment[1]
Spectro-Chlor Ophthalmic Solution[1]
Spectro-Genta[5]
Spectro-Sporin[13]
Spectro-Sulf[14]
Steri-Units Sulfacetamide[14]
Sulf-10[14]
Sulfair[14]
Sulfair 10[14]
Sulfair 15[14]
Sulfair Forte[14]
Sulfamide[14]
Sulfex[14]
Sulten-10[14]
Tobradex[18]
Tobrex[18]
Tribiotic[13]
Tri-Ophthalmic[13]
Triple Antibiotic[9]
Tri-Thalmic[13]

ANTICHOLINERGICS

GENERIC NAMES
1. ANISOTROPINE
2. ATROPINE
3. HOMATROPINE
4. ISOPROPAMIDE
5. MEPENZOLATE
6. METHANTHELINE
7. METHSCOPOLAMINE
8. OXYPHENCYCLIMINE
9. PIRENZEPINE
10. TRIDIHEXETHYL

BRAND NAMES
AH-Chew[7]
Banthine[6]
Baycodan[3]

Cantil[5]
Codan[3]
D.A. Chewable[7]
Dallergy[3]
Dallergy Caplets[3]
Darbid[4]
Daricon[8]
Dura-Vent/DA[7]
Extendryl[7]
Extendryl JR[7]
Extendryl SR[7]
Gastrozepin[9]
Homapin[3]
Hycodan[3]
Hydromet[3]
Hydropane6
OMNIhist L.A.[7]
Pamine[7]
Pathilon[10]
Prehist D[7]
Tussigon[3]
Valpin 50[1]

ANTIDEPRESSANTS, TRICYCLIC

GENERIC NAMES
1. AMITRYPTILINE
2. AMOXAPINE
3. CLOMIPRAMINE
4. DESIPRAMINE
5. DOXEPIN
6. IMIPRAMINE
7. NORTRIPTYLINE
8. PERPHENAZINE & AMITRYPTILINE
9. PROTRIPTYLINE
10. TRIMIPRAMINE

BRAND NAMES
Adapin[5]
Anafranil[3]
Apo-Amitriptyline[1]
Apo-Imipramine[6]
Apo-Trimip[10]
Asendin[2]
Aventyl[7]
Elavil[1]
Elavil Plus[8]
Endep[1]
Etrafon[8]
Etrafon-A[8]
Etrafon-D[8]
Etrafon-F[8]
Etrafon-Forte[8]
Impril[6]
Levate[1]
Norfranil[6]
Norpramin[4]
Novo-Doxepin[5]
Novopramine [6]
Novo-Tripramine[10]
Novotriptyn[1]
Pamelor[7]
PMS Amitriptyline[1]
PMS Impramine[6]
PMS Levazine[8]
Rhotrimine[10]
Sinequan[5]
Surmontil[10]
Tipramine[6]
Tofranil[6]
Tofranil-PM[6]
Triadapin[5]
Triavil[8]
Triptil[9]
Vivactil[9]

ANTIDYSKINETICS

GENERIC NAMES
1. BENZTROPINE
2. BIPERIDEN
3. COMTAN
4. ETHOPROPAZINE
5. PIMOZIDE
6. PRAMIPEXOLE
7. PROCYCLIDINE
8. ROPINIROLE
9. TRIHEXYPHENIDYL

BRAND NAMES
Akineton[2]
Apo-Benztropine[1]
Apo-Trihex[4]
Artane[9]
Artane Sequels[9]
Cogentin[1]
Comtan[3]
Kemadrin[7]
Mirapex[6]
Orap[5]
Parsidol[4]
Parsitan[4]
PMS Benztropine[1]
PMS Procyclidine[7]
PMS Trihexyphenidyl[9]
Procyclid[7]
Requip[8]
Trihexane[9]
Trihexy[9]

ANTIFUNGALS (Topical)

GENERIC NAMES
1. AMPHOTERICIN B
2. BUTENAFINE
3. CICLOPIROX
4. CLOTRIMAZOLE
5. ECONAZOLE
6. FLUCONAZOLE
7. HALOPROGIN
8. KETOCONAZOLE (Topical)
9. MICONAZOLE
10. NAFTIFINE
11. NYSTATIN
12. OXICONAZOLE (Topical)
13. SULCONAZOLE
14. TERBINAFINE
15. TOLNAFTATE
16. UNDECYLENIC ACID

BRAND NAMES
Aftate for Athlete's Foot Aerosol Spray Liquid[15]
Aftate for Athlete's Foot Aerosol Spray Powder[15]
Aftate for Athlete's Foot Gel[15]
Aftate for Athlete's Foot Sprinkle Powder[15]
Aftate for Jock Itch Aerosol Spray Powder[15]
Aftate for Jock Itch Gel[15]
Aftate for Jock Itch Sprinkle Powder[15]
Caldesene Medicated Powder[16]
Canesten Cream[4]
Canesten Solution[4]
Cruex Aerosol Powder[16]
Cruex Antifungal Cream[16]
Cruex Antifungal Powder[16]
Cruex Antifungal Spray Powder[16]
Cruex Cream[16]
Cruex Powder[16]
Decylenes[16]
Decylenes Powder[16]
Desenex Aerosol Powder[16]
Desenex Antifungal Cream[16]
Desenex Antifungal Liquid[16]
Desenex Antifungal Ointment[16]
Desenex Antifungal Penetrating Foam[16]
Desenex Antifungal Powder[16]
Desenex Antifungal Spray Powder[16]
Desenex Max Cream[16]
Desenex Ointment[16]
Desenex Powder[16]
Desenex Solution[16]
Ecostatin[5]
Exelderm[6]
Fungizone[3]
Genaspore Cream[15]
Gordochom Solution[16]
Halotex[7]
Lamisil[14]
Lamisil Solution 1%[14]
Loprox[3]
Lotriderm[4]
Lotrimin AF[4]
Lotrimin Cream[4]
Lotrimin Lotion[4]
Lotrimin Ointment[4]
Lotrisone[4]
Mentax[2]
Micatin[4]
Monistat-Derm[4]
Mycelex Cream[4]
Mycelex Solution[4]
Myclo Cream[4]
Myclo Solution[4]
Myclo Spray[4]
Mycostatin[11]
Nadostine[11]
Naftin[10]
Nilstat[11]
Nizoral A-D[8]
Nizoral Shampoo[8]
NP-27 Cream[15]
NP-27 Powder[15]
NP-27 Solution[15]
NP-27 Spray Powder[15]
Nyaderm[11]
Nystex[11]
Nystop[11]
Oxistat[12]
Penlac[3]
Pitrex Cream[15]
Spectazole[5]
Tinactin Aerosol Liquid[15]
Tinactin Aerosol Powder[15]
Tinactin Antifungal Deodorant Powder Aerosol[15]
Tinactin Cream[15]
Tinactin Jock Itch Aerosol Powder[15]
Tinactin Jock Itch Cream[15]
Tinactin Jock Itch Spray Powder[15]
Tinactin Plus Powder[15]

Tinactin Powder[15]
Tinactin Solution[15]
Ting Antifungal Cream[15]
Ting Antifungal Powder[15]
Ting Antifungal Spray Liquid[15]
Ting Antifungal Spray Powder[15]
Zeasorb-AF Powder[15]

ANTIFUNGALS (Vaginal)

GENERIC NAMES
1. BUTOCONAZOLE
2. CLOTRIMAZOLE
3. ECONAZOLE
4. GENTIAN VIOLET
5. MICONAZOLE
6. NYSTATIN
7. TERCONAZOLE
8. TIOCONAZOLE

BRAND NAMES
Canesten[2]
Canesten 1[2]
Canesten 3[2]
Canesten 10%[2]
Ecostatin[3]
FemCare[2]
Femizole Prefil[2]
Femizole-7[2]
Genapax[4]
Gyne-Lotrimin[2]
Gyne-Lotrimin 3[2]
Gyno-Trosyd[8]
Monistat[5]
Monistat 1[8]
Monistat 3[5]
Monistat 5[5]
Monistat 7[5]
Mycelex-7[2]
Mycelex-G[2]
Myclo[2]
Mycostatin[6]
Nadostine[6]
Nilstat[6]
Nyaderm[6]
Terazol 3[7]
Terazol 7[7]
Three Day Cream[2]
Vagistat[8]
Vagistat-1[8]

ANTIHISTAMINES

GENERIC NAMES
1. ACRIVASTINE
2. AZATADINE
3. BROMODIPHENHYDRAMINE
4. BROMPHENIRAMINE
5. CARBINOXAMINE
6. CHLORPHENIRAMINE
7. CLEMASTINE FUMARATE
8. CYPROHEPTADINE
9. DEXBROMPHENIRAMINE
10. DEXCHLORPHENIRAMINE
11. DIMENHYDRINATE
12. DIPHENHYDRAMINE
13. DIPHENYLPYRALINE
14. DOXYLAMINE
15. PHENINDAMINE
16. PHENIRAMINE
17. PHENYLTOLOXAMINE
18. PYRILAMINE
19. TRIPELENNAMINE
20. TRIPROLIDINE

BRAND NAMES
Aclophen[6]
Actacin[20]
Actagen[20]
Actagen-C Cough[20]
Actidil[18]
Actifed[20]
Actifed 12-Hour[20]
Actifed A[20]
Actifed Allergy Nighttime Caplets[20]
Actifed DM[20]
Actifed Plus[20]
Actifed Plus Caplets
Actifed with Codeine Cough[20]
AH-Chew[6]
Alamine-C Liquid[6]
Alersule[6]
Allent[5]
Alleract[18]
Aller-Chlor[6]
Allercon[20]
Allerdryl[12]
Allerest Maximum Strength[6]
Allerfrim[20]
Allerfrin[20]
Allerfrin with Codeine[20]
Allergy Cold[20]
Allergy Formula Sinutab[9]
AllerMax Caplets[12]
Aller-med[12]
Allerphed[20]
Allert[6]
All-Nite Cold Formula[14]
Ambay Cough[3]
Ambenyl Cough[3]
Ambophen Expectorant[3]
Ami-Drix[9]
Anamine[6]
Anamine HD[6]
Anamine T. D.[6]
Anaplex[6]
Anaplex HD[6]
Anaplex S.R.[6]
Apo-Dimenhydrinate[11]
Aprodrine[20]
Aprodrine with Codeine[20]
Atrofed[20]
Atrohist Pediatric[6]
Atrohist Pediatric Suspension Dye Free[6, 18]
Atrohist Sprinkle[6]
Banophen[12]
Banophen Caplets[12]
Baydec DM Drops[5]
Bayer Select Night Time Cold Caplets[20]
Bayhistine DH[6]
Beldin[12]
Belix[12]
Bena-D 10[12]
Bena-D 50[12]
Benadryl 25[12]
Benadryl Allergy/Sinus Headache Caplets[12]
Benadryl Cold[12]
Benadryl Cold Nighttime Liquid[12]
Benadryl Complete Allergy[12]
Benadryl Decongestant[12]
Benadryl Kapseals[12]
Benadryl Plus[12]
Benahist 10[12]
Benahist 50[12]
Ben-Allergin 50[12]
Benaphen[12]
Benoject-10[12]
Benoject-50[12]
Benylin Cold[12]
Benylin Cough[12]
Benylin Decongestant[12]
Brexin[6]
Brexin-L.A[6].
Brofed[5]
Bromanyl[3]
Bromarest DX Cough[5]
Bromatane DX Cough[5]
Bromfed[5]
Bromfed-AT[5]
Bromfed-DM[5]
Bromfed-PD[5]
Bromphen DX Cough[5]
Brompheril[9]
Bronkotuss Expectorant[6]
Brotane DX Cough[5]
Bydramine Cough[12]
Calm X[11]
Calmylin #4[12]
Calmylin with Codeine[10]
Carbinoxamine Compound[5]
Carbiset[5]
Carbiset-TR[5]
Carbodec[5]
Carbodec DM Drops[5]
Carbodec TR[5]
Cardec DM[5]
Cardec DM Drops[5]
Cardec DM Pediatric[5]
Cardec-S[5]
Cenafed Plus[20]
Cerose-DM[6]
Cheracol Sinus[5]
Children's Dramamine[11]
Children's Tylenol Cold[6]
Children's Tylenol Cold Multi-Symptom Plus Cough[6]
Chlo-Amine[6]
Chlor-100[6]
Chlorafed[6]
Chlorafed H.S. Timecelles[6]
Chlorafed Timecelles[6]
Chlorate[6]
Chlorgest-HD[6]
Chlor-Niramine[6]
Chlorphed[3]
Chlorphedrine SR[3]
Chlor-Pro[6]
Chlor-Pro 10[6]
Chlorspan-12[6]
Chlortab-4[6]
Chlortab-8[6]
Chlor-Trimeton[6]
Chlor-Trimeton 4 Hour Relief[6]
Chlor-Trimeton 12 Hour Relief[6]
Chlor-Trimeton Allergy[6]
Chlor-Trimeton Decongestant[6]
Chlor-Trimeton Repetabs[6]
Chlor-Tripolon[6]
Chlor-Tripolon Decongestant Extra Strength[6]
Chlor-Tripolon Decongestant Repetabs[6]
Citra Forte[6]
CoActifed[20]
CoActifed Expectorant[20]
Co-Apap[6]
Codehist DH[6]

Codimal[6]
Codimal DH[18]
Codimal DM[6]
Codimal PH[18]
Codimal-A[5]
Codimal-L.A.[6]
Codimal-L.A. Half[6]
Colfed-A[6]
Colrex Compound[6]
Colrex Cough[6]
Coltab Children's[6]
Comhist[6]
Comhist LA[6]
Compoz[12]
Comtrex A/S[6]
Comtrex A/S Caplets[5]
Comtrex Hot Flu Relief[6]
Comtrex Multi-Symptom Hot Flu Relief[6]
Comtrex Nighttime[6]
Comtrex Nighttime Maximum Strength Cold and Flu Relief[6]
Comtrex Nighttime Maximum[6] Strength Cold, Cough and Flu Relief[6]
Congestant D[6]
Conjec-B[5]
Contac 12-Hour[6]
Contac 12-Hour Allergy[7]
Contac Allergy/Sinus Night Caplets[7]
Contac Night Caplets[12]
Contac Severe Cold Formula[6]
Contac Severe Cold Formula Night Strength[6]
Cophene No. 2[6]
Cophene-B[5]
Co-Pyronil 2[6]
Coricidin with Codeine[6]
Cotridin[20]
Cotridin Expectorant[20]
CoTylenol Cold Medication[6]
D.A. Chewable[6]
Dallergy[6]
Dallergy Caplets[6]
Dallergy Jr[5].
Dallergy-D[6]
Decohistine DH[6]
Deconamine[6]
Deconamine SR[6]
Dexaphen SA[9]
Dexchlor[10]
Dexophed[9]
Diamine T.D.[5]
Dihistine[6]
Dihistine DH[6]
Dimetabs[11]
Dimetane[5]
Dimetane Decongestant Caplets[5]
Dimetane Extentabs[5]
Dimetane-DX Cough[5]
Dimetane-Ten[5]
Dimetapp Allergy[5]
Dimetapp Allergy Liqui-Gels[5]
Dimetapp Plus Caplets[5]
Dimetapp with Codeine[5]
Dimetapp-A[5]
Dimetapp-A Pediatric[5]
Dimetapp-DM[5]
Dimetapp-DM Cough and Cold[5]
Dimetapp-DM Elixir[5]
Dinate[11]
Diphen Cough[12]
Diphenacen-10[12]
Diphenacen-50[12]
Diphenadryl[12]
Disobrom[9]
Disophrol[9]
Disophrol Chronotabs[9]
Dommanate[11]
Donatussin[6]
Donatussin Drops[6]
Dondril[6]
Dorcol Children's Cold Formula[5]
Dormarex 2[12]
Dormin[12]
Dramamine[11]
Dramamine Chewable[11]
Dramamine Liquid[11]
Dramanate[11]
Dramocen[11]
Dramoject[11]
Dristan AF[6]
Dristan Cold and Flu[6]
Dristan Cold Maximum Strength Caplets[5]
Dristan Cold Multi-Symptom Formula[6]
Dristan Formula P[18]
Drixoral[9]
Drixoral Cold and Allergy[9]
Drixoral Cold and Flu[9]
Drixoral Plus[9]
Drixoral Sinus[9]
Drixtab[9]
Drize[6]
Duralex[6]
Dura-Tap PD[6]
Dura-Vent/DA[6]
Dymenate[11]
Ed A-Hist[6]
Effective Strength Cough Formula[6]
Efidac 24 Chlorpheniramine[6]
Endafed[5]
Endagen-HD[6]
Endal HD[6]
Endal-HD Plus[6]
Extendryl[6]
Extendryl JR[6]
Extendryl SR[6]
Father John's Medicine Plus[6]
Fedahist[6]
Fedahist Decongestant[6]
Fedahist Gyrocaps[6]
Fedahist Timecaps[6]
Fenylhist[12]
Fynex[12]
Genac[20]
Genahist[12]
GenAllerate[6]
Gendecon[6]
Gen-D-phen[12]
Gravol[11]
Gravol L/A[11]
Hayfebrol[6]
HHistafed C[18]
Histagesic Modified[6]
Histaject Modified[5]
Histalet[6]
Histalet-DM[6]
Histatab Plus[6]
Histatan[6]
Histatuss Pediatric[6]
Histor-D[6]
Histor-D Timecelles[6]
Histussin HC[6]
Hycomine Compound[6]
Hycomine-S Pediatric[6]
Hydramine[12]
Hydramine Cough[12]
Hydramyn[12]
Hydrate[11]
Hydril[12]
Hyrexin-50[12]
Improved Sino-Tuss[6]
Insomnal[12]
Isoclor[6]
Isoclor Timesules[6]
Klerist-D[6]
Kolephrin[6]
Kolephrin/DM Caplets[6]
Kronofed-A[6]
Kronofed-A Jr.[6]
Lodrane LD[5]
Mapap Cold Formula[6]
Marmine[11]
Maximum Strength Tylenol Allergy Sinus Caplets[6]
Meda Syrup Forte[6]
Medi-Flu[6]
Medi-Flu Caplets[6]
Midahist DH[6]
Motion-Aid[12]
Myfed[20]
Myhistine[22]
Myhistine DH[22]
Myidil[20]
Naldelate[6]
Nasahist B[5]
Nauseatol[11]
ND Clear T.D.[6]
ND Stat Revised[5]
ND-Gesic[6]
Neocitran A[16]
Neocitran Colds and Flu Calorie Reduced[16]
NeoCitran DM Coughs & Cold[16]
NeoCitran Extra Strength Colds and Flu[16]
Nervine Night-time Sleep-Aid[12]
Nico-Vert[11]
Nidryl[12]
Nisaval[17]
Nolahist[18]
Noradryl[12]
Norafed[18]
Nordryl[10]
Nordryl Cough[10]
Novafed A[6]
Novahistex[6]
Novahistine[6]
Novahistine DH Expectorant[6]
Novahistine DH Liquid[6]
Novodimenate[11]
Novopheniram[6]
NyQuil Liquicaps[12]
NyQuil Nighttime Colds Medicine[12]
Nytime Cold Medicine Liquid[14]
Nytol Maximum Strength[12]
Nytol with DPH[12]
Omnicol[6]
OMNIhist L.A.[6]
Omni-Tuss[6]
Optimine[3]
Oraminic II[5]
Par-Drix[9]
PBZ[19]

PBZ-SR[19]
PediaCare Allergy[6]
PediaCare Children's Cold Relief-Night Rest Cough-Cold Formula[6]
PediaCare Children's Cough-Cold Formula[6]
PediaCare Cold Formula[6]
PediaCare Cough-Cold[6]
Pediacof Cough[6]
Pelamine[19]
Periactin[8]
Pertussin All Night PM[14]
Pfeiffer's Allergy[6]
Phenapap Sinus Headache & Congestion[6]
Phendry[12]
Phendry Children's Allergy Medicine[12]
Phenetron[6]
Phenetron Lanacaps[6]
Phenhist DH with Codeine[6]
PMS-Dimenhydrinate[11]
Poladex T.D.[10]
Polaramine[10]
Polaramine Expectorant[10]
Polaramine Repetabs[10]
Prehist[6]
Prehist Cough Mixture 4[6]
Prehist D[6]
Promist HD Liquid[6]
Pseudo-Car DM[5]
Pseudo-Chlor[6]
Pseudodine C Cough[20]
Pseudo-gest Plus[6]
P-V-Tussin[6]
Pyribenzamine[19]
Pyrilamine Maleate Tablets[18]
Quelidrine Cough[6]
Remcol-C[6]
Rentamine Pediatric[6]
Rescon-DM[6]
Rescon-ED[6]
Rescon-JR[6]
Resporal TR[9]
Rhinatate[6]
Rhinogesic[6]
Rhinosyn[6]
Rhinosyn-DM[6]
Rhinosyn-PD[6]
Rinade B.I.D.[6]
Robitussin A-C[14]
Robitussin Allergy and Cough[4]
Robitussin Night Relief[18]
Robitussin Night Relief Colds Formula Liquid[18]
Robitussin with Codeine[16]
Rolatuss Expectorant[6]
Rolatuss Plain[6]
Rondamine-DM Drops[5]
Rondec[5]
Rondec Drops[5]
Rondec-DM[5]
Rondec-DM Drops[5]
Rondec-TR[5]
R-Tannamine[6]
R-Tannamine Pediatric[6]
R-Tannate[6]
R-Tannate Pediatric[6]
Ryna[6]
Ryna-C Liquid[6]
Rynatan[6]
Rynatan Pediatric[6]
Rynatan-S Pediatric[6]
Rynatuss[6]
Rynatuss Pediatric[6]
Salphenyl[6]
Scot-Tussin DM[6]
Scot-Tussin Original 5-Action Cold Medicine[14]
Semprex-D[1]
Siladryl[12]
Silphen[12]
Simplet[6]
Simply Sleep[12]
Sinarest Sinus[6]
Sine-Off Maximum Strength Allergy/Sinus Formula Caplets[6]
Singlet[6]
Sinutab[6]
Sinutab Extra Strength[6]
Sinutab Regular[6]
Sinutrex Extra Strength[6]
Sleep-Eze 3[12]
Sominex Formula 2[12]
Sudafed Plus[6]
Tanoral[6]
Tavist[7]
Tavist-1[7]
Tavist Allergy/Sinus/Headache[7]
T-Dry[6]
T-Dry Junior[6]
Tega-Vert[11]
Telachlor[6]
Teldrin[6]
TheraFlu Nighttime Maximum Strength[6]
TheraFlu/Flu & Cold[6]
TheraFlu/Flu, Cold & Cough[6]
Thera-Hist[6]
Touro A&H[5]
Travamine[11]
Triacin C Cough[20]
Triafed[20]
Triafed with Codeine[20]
Triaminic DM Nighttime For Children[6]
Triaminic Nite Light[6]
Tricodene Sugar Free[6]
Tricom Tablets[6]
Trifed[20]
Trifed-C Cough[20]
Trimedine Liquid[6]
Triminol Cough[6]
Trinalin Repetabs[3]
Tri-Nefrin Extra Strength[6]
Trinex[6]
Triofed[20]
Triotann[6]
Triotann Pediatric[6]
Tripodrine[20]
Triposed[20]
Trip-Tone[11]
Tritann Pediatric[6]
Tri-Tannate[6]
Tri-Tannate Plus Pediatric[6]
Trymegen[6]
Tussafed[5]
Tussanil Plain[6]
Tussar DM[6]
Tussionex[6]
Tussirex with Codeine Liquid[16]
Tusstat[12]
Twilite[12]
Ty-Cold Cold Formula[6]
Tylenol Allergy Sinus Gelcaps[12]
Tylenol Allergy Sinus NightTime Maximum Strength Caplets[12]
Tylenol Cold and Flu[6]
Tylenol Cold Medication[6]
Tylenol Cold Night Time[12]
ULTRAbrom PD[5]
Uni-Bent Cough[12]
Unisom Nighttime Sleep Aid[14]
Unisom SleepGels Maximum Strength[12]
Vanex Forte R[6]
Vanex-HD[6]
Veltane[5]
Vertab[11]
Vicks 44 Cold, Flu and Cough Liquid-Caps[17]
Vicks 44M Cough, Cold and Flu Relief[6]
Vicks 44M Cough, Cold and Flu Relief LiquiCaps[6]
Vicks Children's NyQuil Allergy/Head Cold[6]
Vicks NyQuil Multi-Symptom Cold/Flu Relief[14]
Vicks NyQuil Multi-Symptom LiquiCaps[14]
Vicks Pediatric Formula 44M Multi-Symptom Cough & Cold[6]
Viro-Med[6]
Wehamine[11]
Wehdryl[12]
Wehdryl-10[12]
Wehdryl-50[12]

ANTIHISTAMINES, PHENOTHIAZINE-DERIVATIVE

GENERIC NAMES
1. PROMETHAZINE
2. TRIMEPRAZINE

BRAND NAMES
Anergan 25[1]
Anergan 50[1]
Antinaus 50[1]
Histantil[1]
Mallergan-VC with Codeine[1]
Panectyl[2]
Penazine VC with Cough[1]
Pentazine[1]
Phenameth DM[1]
Phenameth VC with Codeine[1]
Phenazine 25[1]
Phenazine 50[1]
Phencen-50[1]
Phenergan[1]
Phenergan Fortis[1]
Phenergan Plain[1]
Phenergan VC[1]
Phenergan VC with Codeine[1]
Phenergan with Codeine[1]
Phenergan with Dextromethorphan[1]
Phenoject-50[1]
Pherazine DM[1]
Pherazine VC[1]
Pherazine VC with Codeine[1]
Pherazine with Codeine[1]
PMS Promethazine[1]
Pro-Med 50[1]
Promehist with Codeine[1]
Promerhegan[1]

Promet[1]
Prometh VC with Codeine[1]
Prometh VC Plain[1]
Prometh with Dextromethorphan[1]
Prometh-25[1]
Prometh-50[1]
Promethazine DM[1]
Promethazine VC[1]
Prorex-25[1]
Prorex-50[1]
Prothazine[1]
Prothazine Plain[1]
Shogan[1]
TV-Gan-25[1]
V-Gan-50[1]

ANTI-INFLAMMATORY DRUGS, NON-STEROIDAL (NSAIDs)

GENERIC NAMES
1. DICLOFENAC
2. DIFLUNISAL
3. ETODOLAC
4. FENOPROFEN
5. FLOCTAFENINE
6. FLURBIPROFEN
7. IBUPROFEN
8. INDOMETHACIN
9. KETOPROFEN
10. KETOROLAC
11. MECLOFENAMATE
12. MEFENAMIC ACID
13. NABUMETONE
14. NAPROXEN
15. OXAPROZIN
16. PHENYLBUTAZONE
17. PIROXICAM
18. SULINDAC
19. TENOXICAM
20. TIAPROFENIC ACID
21. TOLMETIN

BRAND NAMES
Aches-N-Pain[7]
Advil[7]
Advil Caplets[7]
Advil Chewable Tablets[7]
Advil Cold and Sinus Caplets[7]
Advil First[7]
Advil Flu & Body Ache[7]
Advil Migraine[7]
Albert Tiafen[20]
Aleve[14]
Aleve Cold & Sinus[7]
Alka-Butazolidin[16]
Alkabutazone[16]
Alka-Phenylbutazone[16]
Alrheumat[9]
Amersol[7]
Anaprox[14]
Anaprox DS[14]
Ansaid[6]
Apo-Diclo[1]
Apo-Diflunisal[2]
Apo-Flurbiprofen[6]
Apo-Ibuprofen[7]
Apo-Indomethacin[8]
Apo-Keto[9]
Apo-Keto-E[9]
Apo-Naproxen[14]
Apo-Phenylbutazone[16]
Apo-Piroxicam[17]
Apsifen[7]
Apsifen-F[7]
Arthrotec[1]
Bayer Select Ibuprofen Caplets[7]
Bayer Select Pain Relief Formula Caplets[7]
Brufen[7]
Butacote[16]
Butazone[16]
Cataflam[1]
Children's Advil[7]
Children's Motrin[7]
Clinoril[18]
CoAdvil Caplets[7]
Cotybutazone[16]
Cramp End[7]
Daypro[15]
Dimetapp Sinus Caplets[7]
Dolgesic[7]
Dolobid[2]
Dristan Sinus Caplets[7]
EC-Naprosyn[14]
Excedrin-IB Caplets[7]
Excedrin-IB Tablets[7]
Feldene[17]
Fenopron[4]
Froben[6]
Froben SR[6]
Genpril[7]
Genpril Caplets[7]
Haltran[7]
Ibifon-600 Caplets[7]
Ibren[7]
Ibu[7]
Ibu-4[7]
Ibu-6[7]
Ibu-8[7]
Ibu-200[7]
Ibumed[7]
Ibuprin[7]
Ibupro-600[7]
Ibu-Tab[7]
Ibutex[7]
Idarac[5]
Ifen[7]
Imbrilon[3]
Indameth[8]
Indocid[8]
Indocid SR[8]
Indocin SR[8]
Lodine[2]
Lodine XL[2]
Meclofen[11]
Meclomen[11]
Medipren[7]
Medipren Caplets[7]
Midol 200[7]
Midol-IB[7]
Mobiflex[19]
Motrin[7]
Motrin, Children's[7]
Motrin Cold and Flu[7]
Motrin, Infants[7]
Motrin-IB[7]
Motrin-IB Caplets[7]
Motrin-IB Sinus[7]
Motrin-IB Sinus Caplets[7]
Motrin Migraine[7]
Nalfon[4]
Nalfon 200[4]
Naprelan[14]
Naprosyn[14]
Naprosyn-E[14]
Naprosyn-SR[14]
Naxen[14]
Novobutazone[16]
Novo-Keto-EC[9]
Novomethacin[8]
Novonaprox[14]
Novopirocam[17]
Novoprofen[7]
Novo-Sundac[18]
Nu-Indo[8]
Nu-Pirox[17]
Nuprin[7]
Nuprin Caplets[7]
Orudis[9]
Orudis-E[9]
Orudis-KT[9]
Orudis-SR[9]
Oruvail[9]
Pamprin-IB[7]
Paxofen[7]
Pedia[7]
Phenylone Plus[16]
Ponstan[12]
Ponstel[12]
Progesic[4]
Relafen[12]
Rhodis[9]
Rhodis-EC[9]
Ro-Profen[7]
Rufen[7]
Saleto-200[7]
Saleto-400[7]
Saleto-600[7]
Saleto-800[7]
Sine-Aid IB[7]
Surgam[20]
Surgam SR[20]
Synflex[14]
Synflex DS[14]
Telectin DS[21]
Toradol[10]
Trendar[7]
Vicoprofen[6]
Voltaren[1]
Voltaren Rapide[1]
Voltaren SR[1]
Voltaren XR[1]
Voltarol[1]
Voltarol Retard[1]

ANTI-INFLAMMATORY DRUGS, STEROIDAL (Ophthalmic)

GENERIC NAMES
1. BETAMETHASONE
2. DEXAMETHASONE
3. FLUOROMETHOLONE
4. HYDROCORTISONE
5. LOTEPREDNOL
6. MEDRYSONE
7. PREDNISOLONE
8. RIMEXOLONE

BRAND NAMES
Ak-Pred[7]
AK-Tate[7]
Alrex[5]
Baldex[2]
Betnesol[1]
Cortamed[4]
Cortisol[4]
Decadron[2]

Dexair[2]
Dexotic[2]
Dexsone[2]
Diodex[2]
Econopred[7]
Econopred Plus[7]
Eflone[3]
Flarex[3]
Fluor-Op[3]
FML Forte[3]
FML Liquifilm[3]
FML S.O.P.[3]
HMS Liquifilm[6]
Inflamase Forte[7]
Inflamase-Mild[7]
I-Pred[7]
Life-Pred[7]
Lotemax[5]
Maxidex[2]
Ocu-Dex[2]
Ocu-Pred[7]
Ocu-Pred Forte[7]
Ocu-Pred-A[7]
PMS-Dexamethasone Sodium Phosphate[2]
Pred Forte[7]
Pred Mild[7]
Predair[7]
Predair Forte[7]
Predair-A[7]
Spersadex[2]
Storz-Dexa[2]
Tobradex[2]
Ultra Pred[7]
Vexol[8]

ANTISEBORRHEICS (Topical)

GENERIC NAMES

1. CHLOROXINE
2. PYRITHIONE
3. SALICYLIC ACID, SULFUR & COAL TAR
4. SELENIUM SULFIDE

BRAND NAMES

Capitrol[1]
Dan-Gard[2]
DHS Zinc Dandruff Shampoo[2]
Exsel[4]
Glo-Sel[4]
Head & Shoulders[2]
Head & Shoulders Antidandruff Cream Shampoo Normal to Dry Formula[2]
Head & Shoulders Antidandruff Cream Shampoo Normal to Oily Formula[2]
Head & Shoulders Antidandruff Lotion Shampoo 2 in 1 Formula[2]
Head & Shoulders Antidandruff Lotion Shampoo Normal to Dry Formula[2]
Head & Shoulders Antidandruff Lotion Shampoo Normal to Oily Formula[2]
Head & Shoulders Dry Scalp 2 in 1 Formula Lotion Shampoo[2]
Head & Shoulders Dry Scalp Conditioning Formula Lotion Shampoo[2]
Head & Shoulders Dry Scalp Regular Formula Lotion Shampoo[2]
Head & Shoulders Intensive Treatment 2 in 1 Formula Dandruff Lotion Shampoo[4]
Head & Shoulders Intensive Treatment Conditioning Formula Dandruff Lotion Shampoo[4]
Head & Shoulders Intensive Treatment Regular Formula Dandruff Lotion Shampoo[4]
Meted Maximum Strength Anti-Dandruff Shampoo with Conditioners[3]
Sebex-T Tar Shampoo[2]
Sebulex Conditioning Suspension Shampoo[3]
Sebulex Lotion Shampoo[3]
Sebulon[2]
Sebutone[3]
Selsun[4]
Selsun Blue[4]
Selsun Blue Dry Formula[4]
Selsun Blue Extra Conditioning Formula[4]
Selsun Blue Extra Medicated Formula[4]
Selsun Blue Oily Formula[4]
Selsun Blue Regular Formula[4]
Theraplex Z[2]
Vanseb Cream Dandruff Shampoo[3]
Vanseb Lotion Dandruff Shampoo[3]
Vanseb-T[3]
Zincon[2]
ZNP[2]

APPETITE SUPPRESSANTS

GENERIC NAMES

1. BENZPHETAMINE
2. DIETHYLPROPION
3. MAZINDOL
4. PHENDIMETRAZINE
5. PHENTERMINE

BRAND NAMES

Adipex-P[5]
Adipost[4]
Adphen[4]
Anorex SR[4]
Anoxine-AM[5]
Appecon[4]
Bontril PDM[4]
Bontril Slow Release[4]
Dapex-37.5[5]
Didrex[1]
Dital[4]
Dyrexan-OD[4]
Fastin[5]
Ionamin[5]
Mazanor[3]
Melfiat-105 Unicelles[4]
Metra[4]
M-Orexic[2]
Obalan[4]
Obe-Del[4]
Obe-Mar[5]
Obe-Nix[5]
Obephen[5]
Obermine[5]
Obestin-30[5]
Obezine[4]
Oby-Trim[5]
Panrexin M[4]
Panrexin MTP[4]
Panshape[5]
Parzine[4]
Phendiet[4]
Phendimet[4]
Phentercot[5]
Phentra[5]
Phentride[5]
Phentrol[5]
Phenzine[4]
Plegine[4]
Prelu-2[4]
Preludin-Endurets[4]
PT 105[4]
Rexigen[4]
Rexigen Forte[4]
Sanorex[3]
Slynn-LL[4]
Statobex[4]
T-Diet[5]
Tega-Nil[4]
Tenuate[2]
Tenuate Dospan[2]
Tepanil[2]
Tepanil Ten-Tab[2]
Teramin[5]
Trimstat[4]
Trimtabs[4]
Wehless[4]
Wehless Timecelles[4]
Weightrol[4]
X-Trozine[4]
X-Trozine LA[4]
Zantryl[5]

ASPIRIN

8-Hour Bayer Timed Release
217
217 Strong
Acetylsalicylic Acid
Alka-Seltzer Effervescent Pain Reliever & Antacid
Alka-Seltzer Morning Relief Medicine
Alpha-Phed
Anacin
APAC Improved
APF Arthritic Pain Formula
Arthrinol
Arthrisin
Arthritis Pain Formula
Artria S.R.
A.S.A.
A.S.A. Enseals
Ascriptin
Ascriptin A/D
Aspergum
Astrin
Axotal
Bayer
Bayer Extra Strength Aspirin
Bayer Timed-Release Arthritic Pain Formula
Buffaprin
Bufferin
Buffets II
Buffinol

Butalgen
Cama Arthritis Reliever
Coricidin with Codeine
Coryphen
Dristan Formula P
Duradyne
Easprin
Ecotrin
Empirin
Entrophen
Excedrin Extra Strength Caplets
Excedrin Extra Strength Tablets
Excedrin Migraine
Extra Strength Bayer PM
Fiorgen PF
Fiorinal
Fiormor
Fortabs
Gelpirin
Gemnisyn
Goody's Extra Strength Tablets
Goody's Headache Powders
Halfprin
Headstart
Isobutal
Isolin
Isollyl Improved
Laniroif
Lanorinal
Magnaprin
Magnaprin Arthritis Strength
Maprin
Marnal
Measurin
Nervine
Night-Time Effervescent Cold
Norwich Aspirin
Novasen
P-A-C Revised Formula
Presalin
Riphen
Robaxisal
Sal-Adult
Salatin
Saleto
Sal-Infant
Salocol
Soma Compound
St. Joseph Adult Chewable
  Aspirin
Supac
Supasa
Synalgos-DC
Tecnal
Tenol Plus
Therapy Bayer
Triaphen
Tri-Pain
Trigesic
Ursinus Inlay
Vanquis
Vibutal
Viro-Med
Zorprin

BARBITURATES

__GENERIC NAMES__

1. AMOBARBITAL
2. APROBARBITAL
3. BUTABARBITAL
4. BUTALBITAL
5. MEPHOBARBITAL
6. METHARBITAL
7. PENTOBARBITAL
8. PHENOBARBITAL
9. SECOBARBITAL
10. SECOBARBITAL & AMOBARBITAL
11. TALBUTAL

__BRAND NAMES__

Alurate[2]
Amaphen[4]
Amytal[1]
Ancalixir[8]
Anolor-300[4]
Anoquan[4]
Arcet[4]
Axotal[4]
Azma Aid[8]
Bancap[4]
Barbita[8]
Bronkolixir[8]
Bronkotabs[8]
Bucet[4]
Busodium[3]
Butace[4]
Butalan[3]
Butalgen[4]
Butisol[3]
Cafergot PB[7]
Dolmar[4]
Endolor[4]
Esgic[4]
Esgic-Plus4[1]
Ezol[4]
Femcet[4]
Fiorgen PF[4]
Fioricet[4]
Fiorinal[4]
Fiormor[4]
Fortabs[4]
G-1[4]
Gemonil[6]
Guaiphed[8]
Isobutal[4]
Isocet[4]
Isolin[4]
Isollyl Improved[4]
Isopap[4]
Laniroif[4]
Lanorinal[4]
Luminal[8]
Marnal[4]
Mebaral[5]
Medigesic[4]
Mudrane GG[8]
Nembutal[7]
Nova Rectal[7]
Novopentobarb[7]
Novosecobarb[9]
Pacaps[4]
Phedral-C.T.[8]
Phrenilin[4]
Phrenilin Forte[4]
Primatene "P" Formula[8]
Repan[4]
Sarisol No. 2[3]
Seconal[9]
Sedapap[4]
Solfoton[8]
Tecnal[4]
Tedral[8]
Tedral SA[8]
Tedrigen[8]
Tencet[4]
T.E.P.[8]
Theodrine[8]
Theodrine Pediatric[8]
Theofed[8]
Theofedral[8]
Triad[4]
Triaprin[4]
Tuinal[10]
Two-Dyne[4]
Vibutal[4]

BARBITURATES, ASPIRIN & CODEINE (Also contains caffeine)

__GENERIC NAMES__

1. BUTALBITAL, ASPIRIN & CODEINE
2. PHENOBARBITAL, ASPIRIN & CODEINE

__BRAND NAMES__

Ascomp with Codeine No. 3[1]
B-A-C with Codeine[1]
Butalbital Compound with
  Codeine[1]
Butinal with Codeine No. 3[1]
Fiorgen with Codeine[1]
Fiorinal with Codeine[1]
Fiorinal with Codeine No. 3[1]
Fiorinal-C1/4[1]
Fiorinal-C1/2[1]
Fiormor with Codeine[1]
Idenal with Codeine[1]
Isollyl with Codeine[1]
Phenaphen with Codeine No. 2[2]
Phenaphen with Codeine No. 3[2]
Phenaphen with Codeine No. 4[2]

BELLADONNA ALKALOIDS & BARBITURATES

__GENERIC NAMES__

1. ATROPINE & PHENOBARBITAL
2. ATROPINE, HYOSCYAMINE, SCOPOLAMINE & BUTABARBITAL
3. ATROPINE, HYOSCYAMINE, SCOPOLAMINE & PHENOBARBITAL
4. BELLADONNA & AMOBARBITAL
5. BELLADONNA & BUTABARBITAL
6. BELLADONNA & PHENOBARBITAL
7. HYOSCYAMINE & PHENOBARBITAL

__BRAND NAMES__

Antrocol[1]
Barbidonna[3]
Barbidonna 2[3]
Barophen[3]
Belladenal[7]
Belladenal Spacetabs[6]
Belladenal-S[7]
Bellalphen[3]
Butibel[5]
Chardonna-2[6]
Donnamor[3]

Donnapine[3]
Donna-Sed[6]
Donnatal[3]
Donnatal Extentabs[3]
Donnatal No. 2[3]
Donphen[3]
Hyosophen[3]
Kinesed[3]
Levsin with Phenobarbital[6]
Levsinex with Phenobarbital Timecaps[7]
Levsin-PB[7]
Malatal[3]
Pheno-Bella[6]
Relaxadon[3]
Spaslin[3]
Spasmolin[3]
Spasmophen[3]
Spasquid[3]
Susano[3]

BENZODIAZEPINES

GENERIC NAMES

1. ALPRAZOLAM
2. BROMAZEPAM
3. CHLORDIAZEPOXIDE
4. CLONAZEPAM
5. CLORAZEPATE
6. DIAZEPAM
7. ESTAZOLAM
8. FLURAZEPAM
9. HALAZEPAM
10. KETAZOLAM
11. LORAZEPAM
12. MIDAZOLAM
13. NITRAZEPAM
14. OXAZEPAM
15. PRAZEPAM
16. QUAZEPAM
17. TEMAZEPAM

BRAND NAMES

Alprazolam Intensol[1]
Apo-Alpraz[1]
Apo-Chlordiazepoxide[3]
Apo-Clorazepate[5]
Apo-Diazepam[6]
Apo-Flurazepam[8]
Apo-Lorazepam[11]
Apo-Oxazepam[14]
Ativan[17]
Centrax[15]
Clindex[3]
Clinoxide[3]
Dalmane[8]
Diastat[6]
Diazemuls[6]
Diazepam Intensol[6]
Doral[16]
Klonopin[4]
Lectopam[2]
Librax[3]
Libritabs[3]
Librium[3]
Lidoxide[3]
Limbitrol[3]
Limbitrol DS[3]
Lipoxide[3]
Loftran[16]
Lorazepam Intensol[11]
Medilium[3]
Meval[6]
Mogadon[15]
Novo-Alprazol[1]
Novoclopate[5]
Novodipam[6]
Novoflupam[8]
Novolorazem[11]
Novopoxide[3]
Novoxapam[14]
Nu-Alpraz[1]
Nu-Loraz[11]
Paxipam[9]
PMS Diazepam[6]
ProSom[7]
Restoril[17]
Rivotril[4]
Serax[14]
Solium[3]
Somnol[8]
T-Quil[6]
Tranxene[5]
Tranxene T-Tab[5]
Tranxene-SD[5]
Valium[6]
Valrelease[6]
Vivol[6]
Xanax[1]
Zapex[14]
Zebrax[3]
Zetran[6]

BENZOYL PEROXIDE

Acetoxyl 2.5 Gel
Acetoxyl 5 Gel
Acetoxyl 10 Gel
Acetoxyl 20 Gel
Acne-5 Lotion
Acne-10 Lotion
Acne-Aid 10 Cream
Acne-Mask
Acnomel B.P. 5 Lotion
Ben-Aqua 2½ Gel
Ben-Aqua 2½ Lotion
Ben-Aqua 5 Gel
Ben-Aqua 5 Lotion
Ben-Aqua 10 Gel
Ben-Aqua 10 Lotion
Ben-Aqua Masque 5
Benoxyl 5 Lotion
Benoxyl 5 Wash
Benoxyl 10 Lotion
Benoxyl 10 Wash
Benoxyl 20 Lotion
Benzac Ac 2½ Gel
Benzac Ac 5 Gel
Benzac Ac 10 Gel
Benzac W 2½ Gel
Benzac W 5 Gel
Benzac W 10 Gel
Benzaclin
Benzagel 5 Acne Lotion
Benzagel 5 Acne Wash
Benzagel 5 Gel
Benzagel 10 Gel
Benzamycin
BenzaShave 5 Cream
BenzaShave 10 Cream
Brevoxyl 4 Gel
Buf-Oxal 10
Clear By Design 2.5 Gel
Clearasil BP Plus 5 Cream
Clearasil BP Plus 5 Lotion
Clearasil Maximum Strength Medicated Anti-Acne 10 Tinted Cream
Clearasil Maximum Strength Medicated Anti-Acne 10 Vanishing Cream
Clearasil Medicated Anti-Acne 10 Vanishing Lotion
Cuticura Acne 5 Cream
Del-Aqua-5 Gel
Del-Aqua-10 Gel
Del-Ray
Dermoxyl 2.5 Gel
Dermoxyl 5 Gel
Dermoxyl 10 Gel
Dermoxyl 20 Gel
Dermoxyl Aqua
Desquam-E 2.5 Gel
Desquam-E 5 Gel
Desquam-E 10 Gel
Desquam-X 2.5 Gel
Desquam-X 5 Gel
Desquam-X 5 Wash
Desquam-X 10 Gel
Desquam-X 10 Wash
Dry and Clear 5 Lotion
Dry and Clear Double Strength 10 Cream
Dryox 5 Gel
Dryox 10 Gel
Dryox 20 Gel
Dryox Wash 5
Dryox Wash 10
Fostex 5 Gel
Fostex 10 Bar
Fostex 10 Cream
Fostex 10 Gel
Fostex 10 Wash
H_2Oxyl 2.5 Gel
H_2Oxyl 5 Gel
H_2Oxyl 10 Gel
H_2Oxyl 20 Gel
Loroxide 5 Lotion with Flesh Tinted Base
Loroxide 5.5 Lotion
Neutrogena Acne Mask 5
Noxzema Clear-Ups Maximum Strength 10
Noxzema Clear-Ups On-the-Spot 10 Lotion
Oxy 5 Tinted Lotion
Oxy 5 Vanishing Formula Lotion
Oxy 5 Vanishing Lotion
Oxy 10
Oxy 10 Daily Face Wash
Oxy 10 Tinted Lotion
Oxy 10 Vanishing Lotion
Oxyderm 5 Lotion
Oxyderm 10 Lotion
Oxyderm 20 Lotion
PanOxyl 5 Bar
PanOxyl 5 Gel
PanOxyl 10 Bar
PanOxyl 10 Gel
PanOxyl 15 Gel
PanOxyl 20 Gel
PanOxyl AQ 2½ Gel
PanOxyl AQ 5 Gel
Persa-Gel 5
Persa-Gel 10
Persa-Gel W 5
Persa-Gel W 10
pHisoAc BP 10

Propa P.H. 10 Acne Cover Stick
Propa P.H. 10 Liquid Acne Soap
Stri-Dex Maximum Strength Treatment 10 Cream
Theroxide 5 Lotion
Theroxide 10 Lotion
Theroxide 10 Wash
Topex 5 Lotion
Topex 10 Lotion
Vanoxide 5 Lotion
Xerac BP 5 Gel
Xerac BP 10 Gel
Zeroxin-5 Gel
Zeroxin-10 Gel

BETA-ADRENERGIC BLOCKING AGENTS

GENERIC NAMES
1. ACEBUTOLOL
2. ATENOLOL
3. BETAXOLOL
4. BISOPROLOL
5. CARTEOLOL
6. CARVEDILOL
7. LABETALOL
8. LEVOBETAXOLOL
9. METOPROLOL
10. NADOLOL
11. OXPRENOLOL
12. PENBUTOLOL
13. PINDOLOL
14. PROPRANOLOL
15. SOTALOL
16. TIMOLOL

BRAND NAMES
Apo-Atenolol[2]
Apo-Metoprolol[9]
Apo-Propranolol[14]
Apo-Timol[16]
Betaloc[9]
Betaxon[8]
Betapace[15]
Blocadren[16]
Cartrol[5]
Coreg[6]
Corgard[10]
Detensol[14]
Inderal[14]
Inderal LA[14]
Kerlone[3]
Levatol[12]
Lopressor[9]
Lopressor SR[9]
Monitan[1]
Normodyne[7]
Novo-Atenol[2]
Novometoprol[9]
Novo-Pindol[13]
Novopranol[14]
Novo-Timol[16]
NuMetop[9]
Sectral[1]
Slow-Trasicor[11]
Sotacor[15]
Syn-Nadolol[10]
Syn-Pindolol[13]
Tenormin[2]
Toprol[9]
Toprol XL[9]
Toprol XL-XR[9]
Trandate[7]
Trasicor[11]
Visken[13]
Zebeta[4]

BETA-ADRENERGIC BLOCKING AGENTS & THIAZIDE DIURETICS

GENERIC NAMES
1. ATENOLOL & CHLORTHALIDONE
2. BETAXOLOL & CHLORTHALIDONE
3. BISOPROLOL & HYDROCHLOROTHIAZIDE
4. LABETALOL & HYDROCHLOROTHIAZIDE
5. METOPROLOL & HYDROCHLOROTHIAZIDE
6. NADOLOL & BENDROFLUMETHIAZIDE
7. PINDOLOL & HYDROCHLOROTHIAZIDE
8. PROPRANOLOL & HYDROCHLOROTHIAZIDE
9. TIMOLOL & HYDROCHLOROTHIAZIDE

BRAND NAMES
Co-Betaloc[5]
Corzide[6]
Inderide[8]
Inderide LA[8]
Kerledex[2]
Lopressor HCT[5]
Normozide[4]
Tenoretic[1]
Timolide[9]
Trandate HCT[4]
Viskazide[7]
Ziac[3]

BRONCHODILATORS, ADRENERGIC

GENERIC NAMES
1. ALBUTEROL
2. BITOLTEROL
3. EPHEDRINE SULFATE
4. EPINEPHRINE
5. ETHYLNOREPINEPHRINE
6. FENOTEROL
7. FORMOTEROL
8. ISOPROTERENOL
9. LEVALBUTEROL
10. METAPROTERENOL
11. PIRBUTEROL
12. PROCATEROL
13. RACEPINEPHRINE
14. SALMETEROL
15. TERBUTALINE

BRAND NAMES
Accuneb[1]
Adrenalin[1]
Advair Diskus[13]
Alupent[10]
Ana-Guard[4]
Arm-a-Med Metaproterenol[10]
AsthmaHaler[4]
AsthmaNefrin[13]
Berotec[6]
Brethaire[15]
Brethine[15]
Bricanyl[15]
Bronkaid Mist[4]
Bronkaid Mist Suspension[4]
Bronkaid Mistometer[4]
Bronkephrine[5]
Combivent[1]
Dey-Dose Isoproterenol[8]
Dey-Dose Metaproterenol[10]
Dey-Dose Racepinephrine[13]
Dey-Lute Metaproterenol[10]
Dispos-a-Med Isoptroterenol[8]
Duoneb[1]
Ephed II[3]
EpiPen Auto-Injector[4]
EpiPen Jr. Auto-Injector[4]
Foradil Aerolizer[7]
Isuprel[8]
Isuprel Glossets[8]
Isuprel Mistometer[8]
Maxair[11]
Medihaler-Epi[4]
Medihaler-Iso[8]
microNEFRIN[13]
Nephron[13]
Norisodrine Aerotrol[8]
Novosalmol[1]
Primatene Mist[4]
Primatene Mist Suspension[4]
Pro-Air[12]
Prometa[10]
Proventil[1]
Proventil HFA[1]
Proventil Repetabs[1]
Serevent[14]
Sus-Phrine[4]
Tornalate[2]
Vapo-Iso[8]
Ventolin[1]
Ventolin HFA[1]
Ventolin Rotocaps[1]
Volmax[1]
Xopenex[9]

BRONCHODILATORS, XANTHINE

GENERIC NAMES
1. AMINOPHYLLINE
2. DYPHILLINE
3. OXTRIPHYLLINE
4. THEOPHYLLINE

BRAND NAMES
Accurbron[4]
Aerolate III[4]
Aerolate Jr.[4]
Aerolate Sr.[4]
Aerophyllin[1]
Aminophyllin[1]
Apo-Oxtriphylline[3]
Aquaphyllin[4]
Asmalix[4]
Bronkodyl[4]
Choledyl[3]
Choledyl Delayed-Release[3]
Choledyl SA[3]
Constant-T[4]
Corophyllin[1]
Dilor[2]
Dilor-400[2]
Duraphyl[4]
Dyflex 200[2]
Dyflex 400[2]

Elixicon[4]
Elixomin[1]
Elixophyllin[4]
Elixophyllin SR[4]
Lanophyllin[4]
Lixolin[4]
Lufyllin[4]
Lufyllin-400[2]
Neothylline[2]
Novotriphyl[3]
Palaron[1]
Phyllocontin[1]
Phyllocontin-350[1]
PMS Theophylline[4]
Protophylline[2]
Pulmophylline[4]
Quibron-T[4]
Quibron-T Dividose[4]
Quibron-T/SR[4]
Quibron-T/SR Dividose[4]
Respbid[4]
Slo-Bid[4]
Slo-bid Gyrocaps[4]
Slophyllin[4]
Slo-Phyllin[4]
Slo-Phyllin Gyrocaps[4]
Solu-Phyllin[4]
Somophyllin[1]
Somophyllin-12[1]
Somophyllin-CRT[1]
Somophyllin-DF[1]
Somophyllin-T[1]
Sustaire[4]
Synophylate[4]
Theo-24[4]
Theo-250[4]
Theobid Duracaps[4]
Theobid Jr. Duracaps[4]
Theochron[4]
Theoclear L.A. 130 Cenules[4]
Theoclear L.A. 260 Cenules[4]
Theoclear-80[4]
Theocot[4]
Theo-Dur[4]
Theo-Dur Sprinkle[4]
Theolair[4]
Theolair-SR[4]
Theomar[4]
Theon[4]
Theophylline SR[4]
Theo-Sav[4]
Theospan SR[4]
Theo-SR[4]
Theostat[4]
Theostat 80[4]
Theo-Time[4]
Theovent Long-acting[4]
Theox[4]
Thylline[2]
T-Phyl[4]
Truphylline[1]
Truxophyllin[4]
Uniphyl[4]

CAFFEINE

222
282
292
692
Actamin Super
Alka-Seltzer Morning Relief
Amaphen
Anacin
Anacin with Codeine
Anolor-300
Anoquan
A.P.C.
Aspirin Free Bayer Select
Maximum Strength Headache
Pain Relief Caplets
Aspirin-Free Excedrin Caplets
Cafergot
Cafergot PB
Cafertine
Cafetrate
Caffedrine
Caffefrine Caplets
Citrated Caffeine
Cotanal 65
Darvon-N Compound
Dexitac
Dristan AF
Dristan AF Plus
Dristan Formula P
Enerjets
Ercaf
Ergo-Caff
Esgic
Esgic-Plus
Excedrin Caplets
Excedrin Extra Strength Caplets
Excedrin Extra Strength Tablets
Excedrin Migraine
Fendol
Fiorinal
Gotamine
Keep Alert
Kolephrin
Migergot
Novo-AC and C
Omnicol
P-A-C Revised Formula
Pacaps
PC-Cap
Pep-Back
Propoxyphene Compound-65
Quick Pep
Repan
S-A-C
Salatin
Saleto
Saleto-D
Salocol
Scot-tussin Original 5-Action
Cold Medicine
Sinapils
Snap Back
Supac
Synalgos-DC
Tirend
Trigesic
Two-Dyne
Vanquish
Vivarin
Wake-Up
Wigraine

CALCIUM CHANNEL BLOCKERS

GENERIC NAMES
1. AMLODIPINE
2. BEPRIDIL
3. DILTIAZEM
4. FELODIPINE
5. FLUNARIZINE
6. ISRADIPINE
7. NICARDIPINE
8. NIFEDIPINE
9. NISOLDIPINE
10. VERAPAMIL

BRAND NAMES
Adalat[8]
Adalat CC[8]
Adalat FT[8]
Adalat P.A.[8]
Apo-Diltiaz[3]
Apo-Nifed[8]
Apo-Verap[10]
Bepadin[2]
Calan[10]
Calan SR[10]
Cardene[7]
Cardene SR[7]
Cardizem[3]
Cardizem CD[3]
Cardizem SR[3]
Chronovera[10]
Dilacor-XR[3]
Dyna Circ[6]
Isoptin[10]
Isoptin SR[10]
Lexxel[4]
Lotrel[1]
Norvasc[1]
Novo-Diltazem[3]
Novo-Nifedin[8]
Novo-Veramil[10]
Nu-Diltiaz[3]
Nu-Nifed[8]
Nu-Verap[10]
Plendil[4]
Procardia[8]
Procardia XL[8]
Renedil[4]
Sibelium[5]
Sular[9]
Syn-Diltiazem[3]
Tarka[10]
Teczem[3]
Tiazac[3]
Vascor[2]
Verelan[10]

CALCIUM SUPPLEMENTS

GENERIC NAMES
1. CALCIUM CARBONATE
2. CALCIUM CITRATE
3. CALCIUM GLUBIONATE
4. CALCIUM GLUCONATE
5. CALCIUM GLYCEROPHOSPHATE & CALCIUM LACTATE
6. CALCIUM LACTATE
7. DIBASIC CALCIUM PHOSPHATE
8. TRIBASIC CALCIUM PHOSPHATE

BRAND NAMES
Apo-Cal[1]
BioCal[1]
Calcarb 600[1]
Calci-Chew[1]
Calciday 667[1]
Calcilac[1]
Calcite 500[1]

Calcium Carbonate/600[1]
Calcium Stanley[4]
Calcium-600[1]
Calcium-Sandoz[3]
Calcium-Sandoz Forte[1,6]
Calglycine[1]
Calphosan[5]
Calsan[1]
Caltrate[1]
Caltrate-300[1]
Caltrate-600[1]
Caltrate Chewable[1]
Chooz[1]
Citracal[2]
Citracal Liquitabs[2]
Gencalc 600[1]
Gramcal[1,6]
Mallamint[1]
Neo-Calglucon[3]
Nephro-Calci[1]
Os-Cal[1]
Os-Cal 500[1]
Os-Cal Chewable[1]
Oysco[1]
Oysco 500 Chewable[1]
Oyst-Cal[1]
Oyst-Cal 500 Chewable[1]
Oystercal 500[1]
Posture[8]
Rolaids-Calcium Rich[1]
Titralac[1]
Tums[1]
Tums E-X[1]

COAL TAR (Topical)

Alphosyl
Aquatar
Balnetar
Balnetar Therapeutic Tar Bath
Cutar Water Dispersible Emollient Tar
Denorex
Denorex Extra Strength Medicated Shampoo
Denorex Extra Strength Medicated Shampoo with Conditioners
Denorex Medicated Shampoo
Denorex Medicated Shampoo and Conditioner
Denorex Mountain Fresh Herbal Scent Medicated Shampoo
DHS Tar Gel Shampoo
DHS Tar Shampoo
Doak Oil
Doak Oil Forte
Doak Oil Forte Therapeutic Bath Treatment
Doak Oil Therapeutic Bath Treatment For All-Over Body Care
Doak Tar Lotion
Doak Tar Shampoo
Doctar
Doctar Hair & Scalp Shampoo & Conditioner
Estar
Fototar
Ionil-T Plus
Lavatar
Liquor Carbonis Detergens
Medotar
Pentrax Extra-Strength Therapeutic Tar Shampoo
Pentrax Tar Shampoo
psoriGel
PsoriNail
Tar Doak
Taraphilic
Tarbonis
Tarpaste
Tarpaste Doak
T/Derm Tar Emollient
Tegrin Lotion for Psoriasis
Tegrin Medicated Cream Shampoo
Tegrin Medicated Shampoo Concentrated Gel
Tegrin Medicated Shampoo Extra Conditioning Formula
Tegrin Medicated Shampoo Herbal Formula
Tegrin Medicated Shampoo Original Formula
Tegrin Medicated Soap for Psoriasis
Tegrin Skin Cream for Psoriasis
Tersa-Tar Mild Therapeutic Shampoo with Protein and Conditioner
Tersa-Tar Soapless Tar Shampoo
Tersa-Tar Therapeutic Shampoo
T-Gel
T/Gel Therapeutic Conditioner
T/Gel Therapeutic Shampoo
Theraplex T Shampoo
Zetar
Zetar Emulsion
Zetar Medicated Antiseborrheic Shampoo

CONTRACEPTIVES, ORAL & SKIN

GENERIC NAMES

1. DESOGESTREL & ETHINYL ESTRADIOL
2. DROSPERINONE & ETHINYL ESTRADIOL
3. ETHYNODIOL DIACETATE & ETHINYL ESTRADIOL
4. LEVONORGESTREL & ETHINYL ESTRADIOL
5. NORELGESTROMIN & ETHINYL ESTRADIOL
6. NORETHINDRONE & ETHINYL ESTRADIOL
7. NORETHINDRONE & MESTRANOL
8. NORETHINDRONE ACETATE & ETHINYL ESTRADIOL
9. NORGESTIMATE & ETHINYL ESTRADIOL
10. NORGESTREL & ETHINYL ESTRADIOL

BRAND NAMES

Alesse[4]
Brevicon[6]
Brevicon 0.5/35[6]
Brevicon 1/35[6]
Cyclen[9]
Cyclessa[1]
Demulen 1/35[3]
Demulen 1/50[3]
Demulen 30[3]
Demulen 50[3]
Desogen 28[1]
Desogen Ortho-Cept[1]
Estrostep[6]
Estrostep Fe[6]
GenCept 0.5/35[6]
GenCept 1/35[6]
GenCept 10/11[6]
Genora 0.5/35[6]
Genora 1/35[6]
Genora 1/50[7]
Jenest-28[6]
Levlen[4]
Levlite[4]
Levora[4]
Loestrin 1/20[8]
Loestrin 1.5/30[8]
Lo/Ovral[10]
Marvelon[1]
Minestrin 1/20[8]
Min-Ovral[4]
ModiCon[6]
Necon 0.5/35-21[6]
Necon 0.5/35-28[6]
Necon 1/35-21[6]
Necon 1/35-28[6]
Necon 1/50-21[6]
Necon 1/50-28[6]
Necon 10/11-21[6]
Necon 10/11-28[6]
N.E.E. 1/35[6]
N.E.E. 1/50[6]
Nelova 0.5/35E[6]
Nelova 1/35E[6]
Nelova 1/50M[6]
Nelova 10/11[6]
Nelulen 1/35E[3]
Nelulen 1/50E[3]
Norcept-E 1/35[8]
Nordette[4]
Norethin 1/35E[6]
Norethin 1/50M[7]
Norinyl 1+35[6]
Norinyl 1+50[7]
Norinyl 1/50[7]
Norlestrin 1/50[8]
Norlestrin 2.5/50[8]
Ortho 0.5/35[6]
Ortho 1/35[6]
Ortho 7/7/7[6]
Ortho 10/11[6]
Ortho-Cept[1]
Ortho-Cyclen[9]
Orthro Evra[5]
Ortho-Novum 0.5[6]
Ortho-Novum 1/35[6]
Ortho-Novum 1/50[7]
Ortho-Novum 1/80[7]
Ortho-Novum 2[6]
Ortho-Novum 7/7/7[6]
Ortho-Novum 10/11[7]
Ortho-Tri-Cyclen 21[7]
Ortho-Tri-Cyclen 28[7]
Ovcon-35[6]
Ovcon-50[6]
Ovral[10]
Symphasic[6]
Tri-Cyclen[9]
Tri-Levlen[4]
Tri-Norinyl[6]
Triphasil[4]
Triquilar[4]

Trivora[4]
Yasmin[2]
Zovia 1/35E[3]
Zovia 1/50E[3]

CONTRACEPTIVES, VAGINAL

GENERIC NAMES
1. BENZALKONIUM CHLORIDE
2. ETONOGESTREL & ETHINYL ESTRADIOL
3. NONOXYNOL 9
4. OCTOXYNOL 9

BRAND NAMES
Advantage 24[3]
Because[3]
Conceptrol Gel[3]
Conceptrol-Contraceptive Inserts[3]
Delfen[3]
Emko[3]
Encare[3]
Gynol II Extra Strength[3]
Gynol II Original Formula[3]
Koromex Cream[3]
Koromex Crystal Gel[3]
Koromex Foam[3]
Koromex Jelly[3]
K-Y Plus[3]
NuvaRing[2]
Ortho-Creme[3]
Ortho-Gynol[4]
Pharmatex[1]
Pre-Fil[3]
Ramses Contraceptive Foam[3]
Ramses Contraceptive Vaginal Jelly[3]
Ramses Crystal Clear Gel[3]
Semicid[3]
Shur-Seal[3]
VCF[3]

DEXTROMETHORPHAN

2/G-DM Cough
Actifed DM
Alka-Seltzer Plus Nighttime Cold
All-Nite Cold Formula
Ambenyl-D Decongestant Cough Formula
Anatuss DM
Anti Tuss DM Expectorant
Balminil DM
Baydec DM Drops
Bayer Select Chest Cold Tablets
Bayer Select Flu Relief Caplets
Bayer Select Head and Chest Cold Caplets
Bayer Select Night Time Cold Caplets
Baytussin DM
Benylin DM-D
Benylin DM-D-E
Benylin DM-D-E Extra Strength
Benylin DM-E
Benylin Expectorant Cough Formula
Bromarest DX Cough
Bromatane DX Cough
Bromfed-AT
Bromfed-DM
Bromphen DX Cough
Broncho-Grippol-DM
Brotane DX Cough
Calmylin
Calmylin #1
Calmylin #2
Calmylin #3
Calmylin #4
Calmylin Cough & Cold
Calmylin Pediatric
Carbinoxamine Compound
Carbodec DM Drops
Cardec DM
Cardec DM Drops
Cardec DM Pediatric
Cerose-DM
Cheracol D Cough
Children's Benylin DM-D
Children's Formula Cough
Children's Hold
Children's Tylenol Cold Multi-Symptom Plus Cough
Co-Apap
Codimal DM
Codistan No. 1
Colrex Cough
Comtrex Cough Formula
Comtrex Daytime Caplets
Comtrex Daytime Maximum Strength Cold and Flu Relief
Comtrex Daytime Maximum Strength Cold, Cough and Flu Relief
Comtrex Hot Flu Relief
Comtrex Multi-Symptom Hot Flu Relief
Comtrex Multi-Symptom Non-Drowsy Caplets
Comtrex Nighttime
Comtrex Nighttime Maximum Strength Cold and Flu Relief
Comtrex Nighttime Maximum Strength Cold, Cough and Flu Relief
Conar
Conar Expectorant
Conar-A
Concentrin
Congespirin
Contac Jr. Children's Cold Medicine
Contac Night Caplets
Contac Severe Cold Formula
Contac Severe Cold Formula Night Strength
Coricidin Cough
CoTylenol Cold Medication
Cough X
Cremacoat 1
Cremacoat 3 Throat Coating Cough Medicine
Creo-Terpin
DayCare
DayQuil Liquicaps
DayQuil Non-Drowsy Cold/Flu
DayQuil Non-Drowsy Cold/Flu LiquiCaps
Delsym
Diabetic Tussin DM
Dimacol
Dimetane-DX Cough
DM Cough
DM Syrup
Donatussin
Dondril
Dorcol Children's Cough
Dristan Cold and Flu
Dristan Juice Mix-in Cold, Flu, & Cough
Drixoral Cough
Effective Strength Cough Formula
Effective Strength Cough Formula with Decongestant
Efficol Cough Whip (Cough Suppressant/Decongestant)
Efficol Cough Whip (Cough Suppressant/Expectorant)
Extra Action Cough
Father John's Medicine Plus
Genatuss DM
Genite
Glycotuss-dM
Guiamid D.M. Liquid
Guiatuss-DM
Guiatussin with Dextromethorphan
Halotussin-DM Expectorant
Histalet-DM
Hold
Humibid DM Sprinkle
Improved Sino-Tuss
Koffex
Kolephrin GG/DM
Kolephrin/DM Caplets
Kophane Cough and Cold Formula
Mapap Cold Formula
Maximum Strength Tylenol Flu Gelcaps
Meda Syrup Forte
Medatussin
Medi-Flu
Medi-Flu Caplets
Mediquell
Mediquell Decongestant Formula
Mytussin DM
Naldecon Senior DX
Naldecon-DX
NeoCitran DM Coughs & Colds
Neo-DM
Noratuss II Liquid
Novahistex DM
Novahistine Cough & Cold Formula Liquid
Novahistine DMX Liquid
NyQuil Hot Therapy
NyQuil Liquicaps
NyQuil Nighttime Colds Medicine
Nytcold Medicine
Nytime Cold Medicine Liquid
Omnicol
Ornex DM 15
Ornex DM 30
Ornex Severe Cold No Drowsiness Caplets
Orthoxicol Cough
Par Glycerol-DM
PediaCare 1
PediaCare Children's Cold Relief Night Rest Cough-Cold Formula
PediaCare Children's Cough-Cold
PediaCare Cough-Cold
Pertussin All Night CS
Pertussin All Night PM

Pertussin Cough Suppressant
Pertussin CS
Pertussin ES
Phanatuss
Phenameth DM
Phenergan with Dextromethorphan
Pherazine DM
Primatuss Cough Mixture 4
Primatuss Cough Mixture 4D
Prometh with Dextromethorphan
Promethazine DM
Prominicol Cough
Pseudo-Car DM
Quelidrine Cough
Queltuss
Remcol-C
Rescon-DM
Rhinosyn-DM
Rhinosyn-DMX Expectorant
Rhinosyn-X
Robafen DM
Robidex
Robitussin Allergy and Cough[4]
Robitussin Cold and Cough Liqui-Gels
Robitussin Cough Calmers
Robitussin Honey Flu
Robitussin Maximum Strength Cough and Cold
Robitussin Maximum Strength Cough Suppressant
Robitussin Night Relief
Robitussin Night Relief Colds Formula Liquid
Robitussin Pediatric Cough & Cold
Robitussin-DM
Robitussin-Pediatric
Rondamine-DM Drops
Rondec-DM
Rondec-DM Drops
Ru-Tuss Expectorant
SafeTussin 30
Scot-Tussin DM
Sedatuss
Silexin Cough
Snaplets-DM
Snaplets-Multi
St. Joseph Cough Suppressant for Children
Sucrets Cough Control
Sudafed Cold & Cough Liquid Caps
Sudafed Cough
Sudafed DM
Sudafed Severe Cold Formula Caplets
Terphan
Terpin-Dex
TheraFlu Maximum Strength Non-Drowsy Formula Flu, Cold & Cough Medicine
TheraFlu Nighttime Maximum Strength
TheraFlu/Flu, Cold & Cough
Tolu-Sed DM Cough
Touro DM
Triaminic DM Nighttime for Children
Triaminic Nite Light
Triaminic Sore Throat Formula
Tricodene Sugar Free
Trimedine Liquid
Triminol Cough
Trind DM Liquid
Trocal
Tussafed
Tussafed Drops
Tussar DM
Tuss-DM
Ty-Cold Cold Formula
Tylenol Cold and Flu
Tylenol Cold and Flu No Drowsiness Powder
Tylenol Cold Medication
Tylenol Cold Medication, Non-Drowsy
Tylenol Cold Night Time
Tylenol Cold No Drowsiness Formula Gelcaps
Tylenol Cough
Tylenol Cough with Decongestant
Tylenol Maximum Strength Cough
Tylenol Maximum Strength Flu Gelcaps
Uni-Tussin DM
Unproco
Vicks 44 Cold, Flu and Cough Liqui-Caps
Vicks 44 Cough and Cold Relief Liqui-Caps
Vicks 44 Non-Drowsy Cold and Cough LiquiCaps
Vicks 44D Dry Hacking Cough and Head Congestion
Vicks 44M Cough, Cold and Flu Relief
Vicks 44M Cough, Cold and Flu Relief LiquiCaps
Vicks Children's Cough
Vicks Dayquil Liquicaps
Vicks Formula 44D Decongestant Cough Mixture
Vicks Formula 44M Multi-Symptom Cough Mixture
Vicks NyQuil Multi-Symptom Cold/Flu Relief
Vicks NyQuil Multi-Symptom LiquiCaps
Vicks Pediatric Formula 44D Cough and Decongestant
Vicks Pediatric Formula 44E
Vicks Pediatric Formula 44M Multi-Symptom Cough & Cold
Viro-Med

DICYCLOMINE

Antispas
A-Spas
Bentyl
Bentylol
Byclomine
Dibent
Di-Cyclonex
Dilomine
Di-Spaz
Forulex
Lomine
Neoquess
Or-Tyl
Protylol
Spasmoban
Spasmoject
Viscerol

DIURETICS, THIAZIDE

GENERIC NAMES

1. BENDROFLUMETHIAZIDE
2. BENZTHIAZIDE
3. CHLOROTHIAZIDE
4. CHLORTHALIDONE
5. CYCLOTHIAZIDE
6. HYDROCHLOROTHIAZIDE
7. HYDROFLUMETHIAZIDE
8. METHYCLOTHIAZIDE
9. METOLAZONE
10. POLYTHIAZIDE
11. QUINETHAZONE
12. TRICHLORMETHIAZIDE

BRAND NAMES

Anhydron[5]
Apo-Chlorthalidone[4]
Apo-Hydro[6]
Aquatensen[8]
Diucardin[7]
Diuchlor H[6]
Diulo[9]
Diuril[3]
Duretic[8]
Enduron[8]
Esidrix[6]
Exna[2]
Hydrex[2]
Hydro-D[6]
HydroDIURIL[6]
Hydromox[1]
Hygroton[4]
Hyzaar[6]
Metahydrin[2]
Minizide[10]
Mykrox[9]
Naqua[12]
Naturetin[1]
Neo-Codema[6]
Novo-Hydrazide[6]
Novo-Thalidone[4]
Oretic[6]
Renese[10]
Saluron[7]
Teveten HCT[6]
Thalitone[4]
Uniretic[6]
Uridon[4]
Urozide[6]
Zaroxolyn[9]

EPHEDRINE

Ami Rax
Azma Aid
Broncholate
Bronkotabs
Bronkolixir
Bronkotuss Expectorant
Guaiphed
Histatuss Pediatric
Hydrophed
KIE
Marax
Mudrane GG
Omni-Tuss
Phedral-C.T.
Primatene "P" Formula
Quelidrine Cough
Rentamine Pediatric
Rynatuss
Rynatuss Pediatric

Tedral
Tedral SA
Tedrigen
T.E.H. Compound
T.E.P.
Theodrine
Theodrine Pediatric
Theofed
Theofedral
Theomax DF

ERYTHROMYCINS

GENERIC NAMES

1. ERYTHROMYCIN ESTOLATE
2. ERYTHROMYCIN ETHYLSUCCINATE
3. ERYTHROMYCIN GLUCEPTATE
4. ERYTHROMYCIN LACTOBIONATE
5. ERYTHROMYCIN STEARATE
6. ERYTHROMYCIN-BASE

BRAND NAMES

Apo-Erythro[6]
Apo-Erythro E-C[6]
Apo-Erythro ES[2]
Apo-Erythro-S[5]
E-Base[6]
E.E.S.[2]
E/Gel[6]
Emgel[6]
E-Mycin[6]
Erybid[6]
ERYC[6]
EryPed[2]
Ery-Tab[6]
Erythraderm[6]
Erythro[2]
Erythrocin[5]
Erythrocot[5]
Erythromid[6]
Eryzole[6]
Ilosone[1]
Ilotycin[3]
My-E[5]
Novorythro[5]
PCE Dispersatabs[5]
Pediazole[6]
Sulfimycin[6]
Wintrocin[5]

ESTROGENS

GENERIC NAMES

1. CONJUGATED ESTROGENS
2. DIETHYLSTILBESTROL
3. ESTERIFIED ESTROGENS
4. ESTRADIOL
5. ESTROGEN
6. ESTRONE
7. ESTROPIPATE
8. ETHINYL ESTRADIOL
9. QUINESTROL

BRAND NAMES

Activella[4]
Alora[4]
Cenestin[1]
C.E.S.[1]
Climara[5]
Clinagen LA 40[5]
Congest[1]
Deladiol-40[5]
Delestrogen[5]
depGynogen[5]
Depo Estradiol[4]
Depogen[5]
DES[2]
Dura-Estrin[5]
Duragen[5]
Duragen-20[5]
Duragen-40[5]
E-Cypionate[5]
Esclim[4]
Estinyl[8]
Estrace[5]
Estraderm[5]
Estragyn 5[6]
Estragyn LA 5[5]
Estra-L[5]
Estratab[3]
Estring[4]
Estro-A[6]
Estro-Cyp[5]
Estrofem[5]
Estroject-L.A.[5]
Estro-L.A.[5]
Estro-Span[5]
Estrovis[9]
Femhrt[8]
Femogex[5]
Gynogen L.A. 20[5]
Gynogen L.A. 40[6]
Honvol [3]
Kestrone-5[7]
Mannest[2]
Menaval-20[6]
Menest [4]
Neo-Estrone[4]
Ogen[8]
Ogen 1.25[8]
Ogen 2.5[8]
Ogen 6.25[8]
Ortho-Est[8]
Piperazine[7]
Premarin[1]
Premphase[1]
Prempro[1]
Stilbestrol[3]
Stilphostrol[2]
Valergen-10[5]
Valergen-20[5]
Valergen-40[5]
Vivelle[5]
Wehgen[6]

GUAIFENESIN

2/G-DM Cough
Adatuss D.C. Expectorant
Alamine Expectorant
Ambenyl-D Decongestant Cough Formula
Amonidrin
Anatuss DM
Anatuss LA
Anti-Tuss
Anti-Tuss DM Expectorant
Asbron G
Asbron G Inlay Tablets
Balminil Expectorant
Bayer Select Head and Chest Cold Caplets
Bayhistine Expectorant
Baytussin AC
Baytussin DM
Benylin DM-D-E
Benylin DM-D-E Extra Strength
Benylin DM-E
Benylin Expectorant Cough Formula
Benylin with Codeine
Benylin-E
Breonesin
Brexin
Bronchial
Broncholate
Broncomar GG
Bronkolixir
Bronkotabs
Bronkotuss Expectorant
Brontex
Calmylin
Calmylin #3
Calmylin Cough & Cold
Calmylin with Codeine
Cheracol
Cheracol D Cough
Children's Formula Cough
CoActifed Expectorant
Codiclear DH
Codimal Expectorant
Codistan No. 1
Colrex Expectorant
Comtrex Cough Formula
Conar Expectorant
Conar-A
Concentrin
Congess JR
Congess SR
Congestac Caplets
Cotridin Expectorant
Cremacoat 2
Cremacoat 3 Throat Coating Cough Medicine
C-Tussin Expectorant
DayCare
DayQuil Liquicaps
DayQuil Non-Drowsy Cold/Flu
DayQuil Non-Drowsy Cold/Flu LiquiCaps
Deconsal II
Deconsal Pediatric
Deconsal Sprinkle
Deproist Expectorant with Codeine
Detussin Expectorant
Diabetic Tussin DM
Diabetic Tussin EX
Dihistine Expectorant
Dilaudid Cough
Dimacol
Dimetane Expectorant-C
Donatussin
Donatussin DC
Donatussin Drops
Dorcol Children's Cough
Duratuss
Duratuss HD
Ed-Bron G
Elixophyllin-GG
Entex PSE
Entuss Expectorant
Entuss Pediatric Expectorant
Entuss-D
Equibron G
Extra Action Cough
Father John's Medicine Plus
Fedahist Expectorant

Fedahist Expectorant Pediatric Drops
Fendol
Fenesin
Gee-Gee
Genatuss
Genatuss DM
GG-CEN
Glyate
Glyceryl T
Glycofed
Glycotuss
Glycotuss-dM
Glydeine Cough
Glytuss
GP-500
Guaifed
Guaifed-PD
GuaiMAX-D
Guaitab
GuiaCough PE
Guiamid D.M. Liquid
Guaiphed
Guiatuss A.C.
Guiatuss PE
Guiatuss-DM
Guiatussin DAC
Guiatussin with Codeine Liquid
Guiatussin with Dextromethorphan
Halotussin
Halotussin-DM Expectorant
Histalet X
Humibid Guaifenesin Plus
Humibid L.A.
Humibid Sprinkle
Humibid-DM Sprinkle
Hycotuss Expectorant
Hytuss
Hytuss-2X
Isoclor Expectorant
Kolephrin GG/DM
Kwelcof Liquid
Malotuss
Meda Syrup Forte
Medatussin
Medatussin Plus
Mudrane GG
Mudrane GG2
Myhistine Expectorant
Mytussin AC
Mytussin DAC
Mytussin DM
Naldecon Senior DX
Naldecon Senior EX
Nasatab LA
NeoCitrin DM Coughs & Colds
Noratuss II Liquid
Nortussin
Nortussin with Codeine
Novagest Expectorant with Codeine
Novahistex DH Expectorant
Novahistine DH Expectorant
Novahistine DMX Liquid
Novahistine Expectorant
Nucochem Expectorant
Nucochem Pediatric Expectorant
Nucofed Expectorant
Nucofed Pediatric Expectorant
Organidin
Pertussin All Night CS
Phanatuss
Phenhist Expectorant
Pneumomist
Polaramine Expectorant
Poly-Histine Expectorant Plain
Pseudo-Bid
P-V-Tussin Tablets
Queltuss
Quibron
Quibron 300
Rescon-GG
Respaire-60 SR
Respaire-120 SR
Resyl
Rhinosyn-DMX Expectorant
Rhinosyn-X
Robafen AC Cough
Robafen DAC
Robafen DM
Robitussin
Robitussin A-C
Robitussin Cold & Cough Liqui-Gels
Robitussin Severe Congestion Liqui-Gels
Robitussin with Codeine
Robitussin-DAC
Robitussin-DM
Robitussin-PE
Ru-Tuss DE
Ru-Tuss Expectorant
Rymed
Rymed Liquid
Rymed-TR
Ryna-CX Liquid
SafeTussin 30
Scot-Tussin
Silexin Cough
Sinufed Timecelles
Sinumist-SR
Sinupan
Slo-Phyllin GG
SRC Expectorant
Stamoist E
Sudafed Cough
Sudafed Expectorant
Syncophylate-GG
Theolate
T-Moist
Tolu-Sed Cough
Tolu-Sed DM Cough
Touro DM
Touro Ex
Touro LA Caplets
Trinex
Tussafin Expectorant
Tussar SF
Tussar-2
Tuss-DM
Tuss-LA
Uni-Bronchial
Uni-Tussin
Uni-Tussin DM
Unproco
Vanex Expectorant
V-Dec-M
Versacaps
Vicks Children's Cough
Vicks Formula 44D Decongestant Cough Mixture
Vicks Formula 44M Multi-Symptom Cough Mixture
Vicks Pediatric Formula 44E
Vicodin-Tuss
Viro-Med
Zephrex
Zephrex-LA

INSULIN

Humulin BR
Humulin L
Humulin N
Humulin R
Humulin U
Insulatard NPH
Insulatard NPH Human
Lente
Lente Iletin I
Lente Iletin II
Mixtard
Mixtard Human
Novolin 70/30
Novolin 70/30 PenFill
Novolin 70/30 Prefilled
Novolin ge NPH PenFill
Novolin ge Toronto PenFill
Novolin L
Novolin N
Novolin N PenFill
Novolin N Prefilled
Novolin R
Novolin R PenFill
Novolin R Prefilled
NPH
NPH Iletin I
NPH Iletin II
Protamine Zinc & Iletin
Protamine Zinc & Iletin I
Protamine Zinc & Iletin II
PZI
Regular
Regular (Concentrated) Iletin
Regular (Concentrated) Iletin II, U-500
Regular Iletin I
Regular Iletin II
Regular Insulin
Semilente
Semilente Iletin
Semilente Iletin I
Ultralente
Ultralente Iletin I
Velosulin
Velosulin BR
Velosulin Human

IRON SUPPLEMENTS

GENERIC NAMES

1. FERROUS FUMARATE
2. FERROUS GLUCONATE
3. FERROUS SULFATE
4. IRON DEXTRAN
5. IRON POLYSACCHARIDE
6. IRON SORBITOL

BRAND NAMES

Apo-Ferrous Gluconate[2]
Apo-Ferrous Sulfate[3]
Femiron[1]
Feosol[3]
Feostat[1]
Feostat Drops[1]
Fergon[2]
Fer-In-Sol[3]
Fer-In-Sol Drops[3]
Fer-In-Sol Syrup[3]

Fer-Iron[3]
Fero-folic 500[3]
Fero-Grad[3]
Fero-Gradumet[3]
Ferralet[2]
Ferralyn[3]
Ferra-TD[3]
Fertinic[3]
Geritol Tablets[1]
Hemocyte[1]
Hytinic[5]
Ircon[1]
Jectofer[6]
Neo-Fer[1]
Niferex[5]
Niferex-150[5]
Novoferrogluc[5]
Novoferrosulfa[2]
Novofumar[3]
Nu-Iron[1]
Nu-Iron 150[5]
Palafer[1]
Palmiron[1]
PMS Ferrous Sulfate[3]
Simiron[2]
Slow Fe[3]
Span-FF[1]

KERATOLYTICS

GENERIC NAMES

1. RESORCINOL
2. RESORCINOL & SULFUR
3. SALICYLIC ACID
4. SALICYLIC ACID & SULFUR
5. SULFUR (Topical)

BRAND NAMES

Acne-Aid Gel[2]
AcnoAcnomel Cake[2]
Acnomel Cream[2]
Acnomel Vanishing Cream[2]
Acnomel-Acne Cream[2]
Acnotex[4]
Antinea[3]
Aveeno Acne Bar[4]
Aveeno Cleansing Bar[4]
Bensulfoid Cream[2]
Buf-Puf Acne Cleansing Bar with Vitamin E[3]
Buf-Puf Medicated Maximum Strength Pads[3]
Buf-Puf Medicated Regular Strength Pads[3]
Calicylic[3]
Clear Away[3]
Clear by Design Medicated Cleansing Pads[3]
Clearasil Adult Care Medicated Blemish Cream[2]
Clearasil Adult Care Medicated Blemish Stick[2]
Clearasil Clearstick Maximum[3] Strength Topical Solution[3]
Clearasil Clearstick Regular Strength Topical Solution[3]
Clearasil Double Textured Pads Maximum Strength[3]
Clearasil Double Textured Pads Regular Strength[3]
Clearasil Medicated Deep[3] Cleanser Topical Solution
Compound W Gel[3]
Compound W Liquid[3]
Creamy SS Shampoo[4]
Cuplex Gel[3]
Cuticura Ointment[5]
Diasporal Cream[4]
Duofilm[3]
Duoplant[3]
Duoplant Topical Solution[3]
Finac[5]
Fostex CM[4]
Fostex Medicated Cleansing Bar[4]
Fostex Medicated Cleansing Cream[4]
Fostex Medicated Cleansing Liquid[4]
Fostex Regular Strength Medicated Cleansing Bar[4]
Fostex Regular Strength Medicated Cleansing Cream[4]
Fostex Regular Strength Medicated Cover-Up[4]
Fostril Cream[5]
Fostril Lotion[5]
Freezone[3]
Gordofilm[3]
Hydrisalic[3]
Ionax Astringent Skin Cleanser Topical Solution[3]
Ionil Plus Shampoo[3]
Ionil Shampoo[3]
Keralyt[3]
Keratex Gel[3]
Lactisol[3]
Listerex Golden Scrub Lotion[3]
Listerex Herbal Scrub Lotion[3]
Lotio Asulfa[3]
Mediplast[3]
Meted Maximum Strength Anti-Dandruff Shampoo with Conditioners[4]
Night Cast R[4]
Night Cast Regular Formula Mask-Lotion[4]
Night Cast Special Formula Mask-Lotion[2]
Noxzema Anti-Acne Gel[3]
Noxzema Anti-Acne Pads Maximum Strength[3]
Noxzema Anti-Acne Pads Regular Strength[3]
Occlusal Topical Solution[3]
Occlusal-HP Topical Solution[3]
Off-Ezy Topical Solution Corn & Callus Removal Kit[3]
Off-Ezy Topical Solution Wart Removal Kit[3]
Oxy Clean Medicated Cleanser[3]
Oxy Clean Medicated Pads Maximum Strength[3]
Oxy Clean Medicated Pads Sensitive Skin[3]
Oxy Clean Regular Strength[3]
Oxy Clean Regular Strength Medicated Cleanser Topical Solution[3]
Oxy Clean Regular Strength Medicated Pads[3]
Oxy Clean Sensitive Skin Cleanser Topical Solution[3]
Oxy Clean Sensitive Skin Pads[3]
Oxy Night Watch Maximum Strength Lotion[3]
Oxy Night Watch Night Time Acne Medication Extra[3] Strength Lotion[3]
Oxy Night Watch Night Time Acne Medication Regular Strength Lotion[3]
Oxy Night Watch Sensitive Skin Lotion[3]
Oxy Sensitive Skin Vanishing Formula Lotion[3]
P&S[3]
Paplex[3]
Paplex Ultra[3]
Pernox Lemon Medicated Scrub Cleanser[4]
Pernox Lotion Lathering Abradant Scrub Cleanser[4]
Pernox Lotion Lathering Scrub Cleanser[4]
Pernox Regular Medicated Scrub Cleanser[4]
Propa pH Medicated Acne Cream Maximum Strength[3]
Propa pH Medicated Cleansing Pads Maximum Strength[3]
Propa pH Medicated Cleansing Pads Sensitive Skin[3]
Propa pH Perfectly Clear Skin Cleanser Topical Solution Oily Skin[3]
Propa pH Perfectly Clear Skin Cleanser Topical Solution Sensitive Skin Formula[3]
R.A.[1]
Rezamid Lotion[2]
Salac[3]
Salacid[3]
Sal-Acid Plaster[3]
Salactic Film Topical Solution[3]
Sal-Clens Plus Shampoo[3]
Sal-Clens Shampoo[3]
Saligel[3]
Salonil[3]
Sal-Plant Gel Topical Solution[3]
Sastid (AL) Scrub[4]
Sastid Plain[4]
Sastid Plain Shampoo and Acne Wash[4]
Sastid Soap[4]
Sebasorb Liquid[4]
Sebex[4]
Sebucare[3]
Sebulex Antiseborrheic Treatment and Conditioning Shampoo[4]
Sebulex Antiseborrheic Treatment Shampoo[4]
Sebulex Conditioning Shampoo[4]
Sebulex Cream Medicated Shampoo[4]
Sebulex Medicated Dandruff Shampoo with Conditioners[4]
Sebulex Medicated Shampoo[4]
Sebulex Regular Medicated Dandruff Shampoo[4]
Sebulex Shampoo[4]
Stri-Dex[3]
Stri-Dex Dual Textured Pads Maximum Strength[3]
Stri-Dex Dual Textured Pads Regular Strength[3]
Stri-Dex Dual Textured Pads Sensitive Skin[3]

Stri-Dex Maximum Strength Pads[3]
Stri-Dex Regular Strength Pads[3]
Stri-Dex Super Scrub Pads[3]
Sulforcin[2]
Sulsal Soap[4]
Tersac Cleansing Gel[3]
Therac Lotion[4]
Trans-Plantar[3]
Trans-Ver-Sal[3]
Vanseb Cream Dandruff Shampoo[4]
Vanseb Lotion Dandruff Shampoo[4]
Verukan Topical Solution[3]
Verukan-HP Topical Solution[3]
Viranol[3]
Viranol Ultra[3]
Wart-Off Topical Solution[3]
X-Seb[3]

LAXATIVES, BULK-FORMING

GENERIC NAMES

1. CALCIUM POLYCARBOPHIL
2. CARBOXYMETHYLCELLULOSE SODIUM
3. MALT SOUP EXTRACT
4. METHYLCELLULOSE
5. POLYCARBOPHIL
6. PSYLLIUM
7. SENNOSIDES

BRAND NAMES

Cillium[6]
Citrucel Orange Flavor[4]
Citrucel Sugar-Free Orange Flavor[4]
Cologel[4]
Disolan Forte[2]
Disoplex[2]
Effer-syllium[6]
Equalactin[5]
Ex-Lax Natural Source Bulk Laxative[7]
Fiberall[5]
Fibercon[5]
FiberNorm[5]
Fiberpur[6]
Hydrocil Instant[6]
Karacil[6]
Konsyl[5]
Konsyl Easy Mix Formula[6]
Konsyl-D[6]
Konsyl-Orange[6]
Maalox Daily Fiber Therapy[6]
Maalox Daily Fiber Therapy Citrus Flavor[6]
Maalox Daily Fiber Therapy Orange Flavor[6]
Maalox Sugar Free Citrus Flavor[6]
Maalox Sugar Free Orange Flavor[6]
Maltsupex[3]
Metamucil[6]
Metamucil Apple Crisp Fiber Wafers[6]
Metamucil Cinnamon Spice Fiber Wafers[6]
Metamucil Instant Mix, Orange Flavor[6]
Metamucil Smooth Citrus Flavor[6]
Metamucil Smooth Orange Flavor[6]
Metamucil Smooth, Sugar-Free Citrus Flavor[6]
Metamucil Smooth, Sugar-Free Orange Flavor[6]
Metamucil Smooth, Sugar-Free Regular Flavor[6]
Metamucil Sugar Free[6]
Metamucil Sugar Free Citrus Flavor[6]
Metamucil Sugar Free Lemon-Lime Flavor[6]
Metamucil Sugar Free Orange Flavor[6]
Mitrolan[5]
Modane Bulk[6]
Mylanta Natural Fiber Supplement[6]
Mylanta Sugar Free Natural Fiber Supplement[6]
Naturacil[6]
Natural Source Fibre Laxative[6]
Perdiem[6]
Perdiem Fiber[6]
Perdiem Plain[6]
Prodiem[6]
Prodiem Plain[6]
Prodiem Plus[6]
Pro-Lax[6]
Prompt[6]
Reguloid Natural[6]
Reguloid Orange[6]
Reguloid Orange Sugar Free[6]
Serutan[6]
Serutan Toasted Granules[6]
Siblin[6]
Syllact[6]
Syllamalt[3]
Versabran[6]
Vitalax Super Smooth Sugar Free Orange Flavor[6]
Vitalax Unflavored[6]
V-Lax[6]

LAXATIVES, OSMOTIC

GENERIC NAMES

1. GLYCERIN
2. LACTULOSE
3. MAGNESIUM CITRATE
4. MAGNESIUM HYDROXIDE
5. MAGNESIUM OXIDE
6. MAGNESIUM SULFATE
7. MILK OF MAGNESIA
8. MINERAL OIL
9. SODIUM BIPHOSPHATE
10. SODIUM PHOSPHATE

BRAND NAMES

Agarol Plain[7]
Agarol Strawberry[8]
Agarol Vanilla[8]
Bilagog[6]
Cholac[2]
Chronula[2]
Citroma[3]
Citro-Mag[3]
Citro-Nesia[3]
Constilac[2]
Constulose[2]
Duphalac[2]
Evalose[2]
Fleet Phospho-Soda[9]
Generlac[2]
Hayley's M-O[7]
Heptalac[2]
Lactulax[2]
Magnolax[7]
Mag-Ox 400[5]
Maox[5]
Phillips' Chewable[4]
Phillips' Concentrated[4]
Phillips' Magnesia Tablets[4]
Phillips' Milk of Magnesia[4]
Portalac[2]

LAXATIVES, SOFTENER/LUBRICANT

GENERIC NAMES

1. CASANTHRANOL & DOCUSATE
2. DOCUSATE
3. DOCUSATE CALCIUM
4. DOCUSATE POTASSIUM
5. DOCUSATE SODIUM
6. MINERAL OIL
7. POLOXAMER 188
8. SODIUM PHOSPHATE

BRAND NAMES

Afko-Lube[2]
Afko-Lube Lax[2]
Agarol Plain[6]
Agarol Marshmallow[6]
Agarol Raspberry[6]
Agarol Strawberry[6]
Agarol Vanilla[6]
Alaxin[7]
Bilax[2]
Colace[5]
Colace Microenema[5]
Correctol Extra Gentle[2]
Dialose[2]
Diocto[2]
Diocto-C[1]
Diocto-K[2]
Diocto-K Plus[1]
Dioeze[2]
Diosuccin[2]
Dio-Sul[2]
Diothron[1]
Disanthrol[1]
Disolan[2]
Disolan Forte[1]
Disonate[2]
Disoplex[2]
Di-Sosul[2]
Di-Sosul Forte[1]
Docu-K Plus[1]
DOK[2]
DOK Softgels[2]
Doss[2]
Doss Tablets[2]
Doxinate[2]
DSMC Plus[1]
Dulcodos[2]
Duosol[2]
Fleet Enema Mineral Oil[7]
Gentlax-S[2]
Kasof[2]
Kondremul[7]
Kondremul with Cascara[7]
Kondremul Plain[7]
Lansoyl[7]
Laxinate 100[2]

Liqui-Doss[7]
Milkinol[7]
Modane Plus[2]
Modane Soft[2]
Molatoc[2]
Molatoc-CST[2]
Neo-Cultol[7]
Neolax[2]
Nujol[7]
Peri-Colase[1]
Pertrogalar Plain[7]
PMS-Docusate Calcium[2]
PMS-Docusate Sodium[2]
PMS-Phosphates[8]
Pro-Cal-Sof[2]
Pro-Sof[1]
Pro-Sof Liquid Concentrate[1]
Pro-Sof Plus[1]
Regulace[2]
Regulax SS[2]
Regulex[2]
Regulex-D[2]
Regutol[2]
Senokot-S[2]
Stulex[2]
Sulfolax[2]
Surfak[2]
Therevac Plus[2]
Therevac-SB[2]
Trilax[2]
Zymenol[7]

LAXATIVES, STIMULANT

GENERIC NAMES
1. ALOE
2. BISACODYL
3. CASANTHRANOL
4. CASCARA
5. CASTOR OIL
6. DEHYDROCHOLIC ACID
7. SENNA
8. SENNOSIDES

BRAND NAMES
Afko-Lube Lax[3]
Alphamul[5]
Aromatic Cascara Fluidextract[4]
Bilax[6]
Bisac-Evac[2]
Bisacolax[2]
Bisco-Lax[2]
Black Draught[3]
Black-Draught Lax-Senna[7]
Caroid Laxative[2]
Carter's Little Pills[4]
Cascara Aromatic Fluidextract[4]
Cascara Sagrada[4]
Cholan-HMB[6]
Dacodyl[2]
Decholin[6]
Deficol[2]
Diocto-C[3]
Diocto-K Plus[1]
Diothron[3]
Disanthrol[3]
Disolan Forte[3]
Di-Sosul Forte[3]
Docu-K Plus[3]
Dosaflex[7]
Dr. Caldwell Senna Laxative[7]
DSMC Plus[3]
Dulcodos[2]
Dulcolax[2]
Emulsoil[5]
Ex-Lax Gentle Nature[8]
Fleet Bisacodyl[2]
Fleet Bisacodyl Prep[2]
Fleet Flavored Castor Oil[5]
Fleet Laxative[2]
Fletcher's Castoria[7]
Gentlax S[7]
Gentle Nature[8]
Glysennid[8]
Hepahydrin[6]
Herbal Laxative[8]
Kellogg's Castor Oil[5]
Kondremul with Cascara[4]
Laxit[2]
Molatoc-CST[3]
Mucinum Herbal[8]
Nature's Remedy[4]
Neolax[6]
Neoloid[5]
Nytilax[8]
Perdiem[7]
Peri-Colace[3]
PMS-Bisacodyl[2]
PMS-Sennosides[8]
Prodiem Plus[7]
Prompt[8]
Pro-Sof Plus[3]
Purge[5]
Regulace[3]
Senexon[7]
Senokot[7]
Senokot-S[7]
SenokotXTRA[7]
Senolax[7]
Theralax[2]
Trilax[6]
X-Prep Liquid[7]

MEPROBAMATE

Acabamate
Apo-Meprobamate
Equanil
Equanil Wyseals
Medi-Tran
Meprospan 200
Meprospan 400
Miltown
Neuramate
Novomepro
Novo-Mepro
Pax 400
Probate
Sedabamate
Trancot
Tranmep

NARCOTIC ANALGESICS

GENERIC NAMES
1. BUPRENORPHINE
2. CODEINE
3. CODEINE & TERPIN HYDRATE
4. DIHYDROCODEINE
5. FENTANYL
6. HYDROCODONE
7. HYDROCODONE & HOMATROPINE
8. HYDROCODONE & IBUPROFEN
9. HYDROMORPHONE
10. LEVORPHANOL
11. MEPERIDINE
12. METHADONE
13. MORPHINE
14. NALBUPHINE
15. OPIUM
16. OXYCODONE
17. OXYMORPHONE
18. PENTAZOCINE
19. PROPOXYPHENE

BRAND NAMES
642 [14]
Actagen-C Cough[2]
Actifed with Codeine Cough[2]
Actiq[5]
Adatuss D.C. Expectorant[6]
Allerfrin with Codeine[2]
Ambay Cough[2]
Ambenyl Cough[2]
Ambophen Expectorant[2]
Anamine HD[6]
Anaplex HD[6]
Aprodrine with Codeine[2]
Astramorph[13]
Astramorph-PF[13]
Baycodan[7]
Bayhistine DH[2]
Bayhistine Expectorant[2]
Baytussin AC[2]
Benylin with Codeine[2]
Bromanyl[2]
Brontex[2]
Buprenex[1]
Calcidrine[2]
Calmylin with Codeine[2]
Cheracol[2]
Chlorgest-HD[6]
Citra Forte[6]
CoActifed[2]
CoActifed Expectorant[2]
Codan[7]
Codehist DH[2]
Codeine Sulfate[2]
Codiclear DH[6]
Codimal DH[6]
Codimal PH[2]
Colrex Compound[2]
Coricidin with Codeine[2]
Coristex-DH [6]
Coristine-DH[6]
Cotanal-65[18]
Cotridin[2]
Cotridin Expectorant[2]
C-Tussin Expectorant[2]
Darvon[19]
Darvon-N[19]
Decohistine DH[2]
Demerol[11]
Deproist Expectorant with Codeine[2]
De-Tuss[6]
Detussin Expectorant[6]
Detussin Liquid[6]
Dihistine DH[2]
Dihistine Expectorant[2]
Dihydromorphinone[9]
Dilaudid[9]
Dilaudid Cough[9]
Dilaudid-HP[9]
Dolophine[12]
Donatussin DC[6]
Doxaphene[19]

Dromoran[10]
Duragesic[5]
Duramorph[13]
Duratuss HD[6]
Endagen-HD[6]
Endal-HD[6]
Endal-HD Plus[6]
Entuss Expectorant[6]
Entuss-D[6]
Epimorph[13]
Expectorant with Codeine[2]
Fortral[18]
Glydeine Cough[2]
Guiatuss A.C.[2]
Guiatussin DAC[2]
Guiatussin with Codeine Liquid[2]
Histafed C[2]
Histussin HC[6]
Hycodan[6]
Hycomine Compound[6]
Hycomine-S Pediatric[6]
Hycotuss Expectorant[6]
Hydromet[7]
Hydropane[7]
Hydrostal IR[8]
Isoclor Expectorant[2]
Kadian[13]
Kwelcof Liquid[6]
Laudanum[15]
Levo-Dromoran[10]
Levorphan[10]
Mallergan-VC with Codeine[2]
Methadose[12]
Midahist DH[2]
Morphitec[13]
M.O.S.[13]
M.O.S.-SR[13]
MS Contin[13]
MSIR[13]
MST Continus[13]
Mytussin AC[2]
Mytussin DAC[2]
Nortussin with Codeine [2]
Novagest Expectorant with Codeine[2]
Novahistex C[2]
Novahistex DH[6]
Novahistex DH Expectorant[6]
Novahistine DH Expectorant[2]
Novahistine DH Liquid[2]
Novahistine Expectorant[2]
Nubain[14]
Nucochem[2]
Nucochem Expectorant[2]
Nucochem Pediatric Expectorant[2]
Nucofed[2]
Nucofed Expectorant[2]
Nucofed Pediatric Expectorant[2]
Numorphan[17]
Omni-Tuss[2]
Oramorph[13]
Oramorph-SR[13]
Oxycontin SR[16]
Pantapon[15]
Paveral[2]
Pediacof Cough[2]
Pediatuss Cough[2]
Penazine VC with Cough[2]
Pethidine[11]
Phenameth VC with Codeine[2]
Phenergan VC with Codeine[2]
Phenergan with Codeine[2]
Phenhist DH with Codeine[2]
Phenhist Expectorant[2]
Pherazine VC with Codeine[2]
Pherazine with Codeine[2]
Physeptone[12]
Promehist with Codeine[2]
Prometh VC with Codeine[2]
Propoxycon[19]
Prunicodeine[2]
Pseudodine C Cough[2]
P-V-Tussin[6]
RMS Uniserts[13]
Robafen AC Cough[2]
Robafen DAC[2]
Robidone[6]
Robitussin A-C[2]
Robitussin-DAC[2]
Rolatuss Expectorant[2]
Rolatuss with Hydrocodone[6]
Roxanol[13]
Roxanol SR[13]
Roxicodone[16]
Ryna-C Liquid[2]
Ryna-CX Liquid[2]
Soma Compound[2]
SRC Expectorant[6]
Statex[13]
Statuss Expectorant[2]
Supeudol[16]
Talwin[18]
Talwin-NX[18]
Temgesic[1]
Terpin Hydrate and Codeine Syrup[2]
Tolu-Sed Cough[2]
Triacin C Cough[2]
Triafed with Codeine[2]
Tricodene #1[2]
Trifed-C Cough[2]
Tussafin Expectorant[6]
Tussanil DH[6]
Tussar SF[2]
Tussar-2[2]
Tussigon[7]
Tussionex[6]
Tussirex with Codeine Liquid[2]
Tyrodone[6]
Vanex Expectorant[6]
Vanex-HD[6]
Vicodin-Tuss[6]
Vicoprofen[8]

NARCOTIC ANALGESICS & ACETAMINOPHEN

GENERIC NAMES

1. ACETAMINOPHEN & CODEINE
2. DIHYDROCODEINE & ACETAMINOPHEN
3. HYDROCODONE & ACETAMINOPHEN
4. MEPERIDINE & ACETAMINOPHEN
5. OXYCODONE & ACETAMINOPHEN
6. PENTAZOCINE & ACETAMINOPHEN
7. PROPOXYPHENE & ACETAMINOPHEN

BRAND NAMES

Allay[3]
Anexsia[3]
Anolor-DH5[3]
APAP with Codeine [1]
Atasol-8[1]
Atasol-15[1]
Atasol-30[1]
Bancap-HC[3]
Capital with Codeine [1]
Co-Gesic[3]
Compal[3]
Darvocet-N 50[7]
Darvocet-N 100[7]
Demerol-APAP[4]
DHCplus[2]
Dolacet[3]
Dolagesic[3]
Dolene-AP 65[7]
Duocet[3]
E-Lor[7]
Empracet 30[1]
Empracet 60[1]
Emtec[1]
Endocet[5]
Exdol-8[1]
Exdol-15[1]
Exdol-30[1]
EZ III[1]
Hycomed[3]
Hyco-Pap[3]
Hydrocet[2]
Hydrocodone with APAP[3]
Hydrogesic[3]
HY-PHEN[3]
Lenoltec with Codeine No. 1[1]
Lenoltec with Codeine No. 2[1]
Lenoltec with Codeine No. 3[1]
Lenoltec with Codeine No. 4[1]
Lorcet[3]
Lorcet 10/650[3]
Lorcet Plus[3]
Lorcet-HD[3]
Lortab[3]
Lortab 5[3]
Lortab 7[3]
Margesic #3[1]
Margesic-H[3]
Novogesic[1]
Onset[3]
Oxycocet[5]
Panacet 5/500[3]
Panlor[3]
Percocet[5]
Percocet-Demi[5]
Phenaphen with Codeine[1]
Polygesic[3]
Pro Pox with APAP[7]
Propacet 100[7]
Pyregesic-C[1]
Roxicet[5]
Roxilox[5]
Stagesic[3]
Talacen[6]
T-gesic[3]
Tylaprin with Codeine[1]
Tylenol No.1[1]
Tylenol No.1 Forte[1]
Tylenol with Codeine[1]
Tylenol with Codeine No. 1[1]
Tylenol with Codeine No. 2[1]
Tylenol with Codeine No. 3[1]
Tylenol with Codeine No. 4[1]
Tylox[5]
Ugesic[3]
Ultragesic[3]
Vanacet[3]

Vapocet[3]
Veganin[1]
Vendone[3]
Vicodin[3]
Vicodin ES[3]
Wygesic[7]
Zydone[3]

NARCOTIC ANALGESICS & ASPIRIN

GENERIC NAMES
1. ASPIRIN & CODEINE
2. BUFFERED ASPIRIN & CODEINE
3. DIHYDROCODEINE & ASPIRIN
4. HYDROCODONE & ASPIRIN
5. OXYCODONE & ASPIRIN
6. PENTAZOCINE & ASPIRIN
7. PROPOXYPHENE & ASPIRIN

BRAND NAMES
222[1]
282[1]
292[1]
293[1]
692[7]
A.C.&C.[1]
Anacin with Codeine[1]
Azdone[1]
Cotanal 65[7]
Damason-P[4]
Darvon Compound[6]
Darvon Compound 65[6]
Darvon with A.S.A.[6]
Darvon-N Compound[7]
Darvon-N with A.S.A.[7]
Drocade and Aspirin[3]
Emcodeine No. 2[1]
Emcodeine No. 3[1]
Emcodeine No. 4[1]
Empirin with Codeine[1]
Empirin with Codeine No. 3[1]
Empirin with Codeine No. 4[1]
Endodan[5]
Lortab ASA[4]
Novo-AC and C[1]
Oxycodan[5]
Panasal 5/500[4]
PC-Cap[7]
Percodan[5]
Percodan-Demi[5]
Propoxyphene Compound-65[7]
Roxiprin[5]
Synalgos-DC[3]
Talwin Compound[6]
Talwin Compound-50[6]

NITRATES

GENERIC NAMES
1. ERYTHRITYL TETRANITRATE
2. ISOSORBIDE DINITRATE
3. ISOSORBIDE MONONITRATE
4. NITROGLYCERIN (GLYCERYL TRINITRATE)
5. PENTAERYTHRITOL TETRANITRATE

BRAND NAMES
Apo-ISDN[2]
Cardilate[1]
Cedocard-SR[2]
Coradur[2]
Coronex[2]
Deponit[4]
Dilatrate-SR[2]
Duotrate[5]
Glyceryl Trinitrate[4]
IMDUR[3]
ISMO[3]
Iso-Bid [2]
Isonate[2]
Isorbid[2]
Isordil[2]
Isotrate[2]
Klavikordal[4]
Minitran[4]
Monoket[3]
Niong[4]
Nitro-Bid[4]
Nitrocap[4]
Nitrocap T.D.[4]
Nitrocine[4]
Nitrodisc[4]
Nitro-Dur[4]
Nitro-Dur II[4]
Nitrogard-SR[4]
Nitroglyn[4]
Nitrol[4]
Nitrolin[4]
Nitrolingual[4]
Nitronet[4]
Nitrong[4]
Nitrong SR[4]
Nitrospan[4]
Nitrostat[4]
Novosorbide[2]
NTS[4]
Pentritol[5]
Pentylan[5]
Peritrate[5]
Peritrate Forte[5]
Peritrate SA[5]
P.E.T.N.[5]
Sorbitrate[2]
Sorbitrate SA[2]
Transderm-Nitro[4]
Tridil[4]

OXYMETAZOLINE (Nasal)

4-Way Long Acting Nasal Spray
12-Hour Nostrilla Nasal Decongestant
Afrin 12 Hour Nasal Spray
Afrin 12 Hour Nose Drops
Afrin Cherry Scented Nasal Spray
Afrin Children's Strength 12 Hour Nose Drops
Afrin Children's Strength Nose Drops
Afrin Extra Moisturizing Nasal Decongestant Spray
Afrin Menthol Nasal Spray
Afrin Nasal Spray
Afrin No-Drip Extra Moisturizing
Afrin No-Drip Nasal Decongestant, Severe Congestion with Menthol
Afrin No-Drip Nasal Decongestant Sinus with Vapornase
Afrin No-Drip Sinus
Afrin Nose Drops
Afrin Sinus
Afrin Spray Pump
Allerest 12 Hour Nasal Spray
Cheracol Nasal Spray
Cheracol Nasal Spray Pump Cherry Scented
Coricidin Nasal Mist
Dristan 12-Hour Nasal Spray
Dristan Long Lasting Menthol Nasal Spray
Dristan Long Lasting Nasal Pump Spray
Dristan Long Lasting Nasal Spray
Dristan Long Lasting Nasal Spray 12 Hour Metered Dose Pump
Dristan Mentholated
Drixoral
Duramist Plus Up To 12 Hours Decongestant Nasal Spray
Duration 12 Hour Nasal Spray Pump
Nasal Decongestant Spray
Nasal Relief
Nasal Spray 12-Hour
Nasal Spray Long Acting
Nasal-12 Hour
Neo-Synephrine 12 Hour Nasal Spray
Neo-Synephrine 12 Hour Nasal Spray Pump
Neo-Synephrine 12 Hour Nose Drops
Neo-Synephrine 12 Hour Vapor Nasal Spray
Nostril Nasal Decongestant Mild
Nostril Nasal Decongestant Regular
NTZ Long Acting Decongestant Nasal Spray
NTZ Long Acting Decongestant Nose Drops
Sinarest 12 Hour Nasal Spray
Vicks Sinex 12-Hour Formula Decongestant Nasal Spray
Vicks Sinex 12-Hour Formula Decongestant Ultra Fine Mist
Vicks Sinex Long-Acting 12 Hour Nasal Spray

PENICILLINS

GENERIC NAMES
1. AMOXICILLIN
2. AMPICILLIN
3. BACAMPICILLIN
4. CARBENICILLIN
5. CLOXACILLIN
6. DICLOXACILLIN
7. FLUCLOXACILLIN
8. NAFCILLIN
9. OXACILLIN
10. PENICILLIN G
11. PENICILLIN V
12. PIVAMPICILLIN
13. PIVMECILLINAM

BRAND NAMES
Amoxil[1]
Apo-Amoxi[1]
Apo-Ampi[2]
Apo-Cloxi[5]
Apo-Pen VK[11]
Bactocill[9]
Beepen-VK[11]
Betapen-VK[11]
Cloxapen[5]

Dycill[6]
Dynapen[6]
Fluclox[7]
Geocillin[4]
Geopen Oral[4]
Ledercillin-VK[11]
Megacillin[10]
Nadopen-V[11]
Nadopen-V 200[11]
Nadopen-V 400[11]
Novamoxin[1]
Novo-Ampicillin[2]
Novo-Cloxin[5]
Novo-Pen VK[11]
Nu-Amoxi[11]
Nu-Ampi[2]
Nu-Cloxi[5]
Nu-Pen-VK[11]
Omnipen[2]
Orbenin[5]
Pathocil[6]
Pen Vee[11]
Pen Vee K[11]
Penbritin[2]
Penglobe[3]
Pentids[10]
Polycillin[2]
Pondocillin[12]
Principen[2]
Prostaphlin[9]
PVF[11]
PVF K[11]
Selexid[13]
Spectrobid[3]
Tegopen[5]
Totacillin[2]
Trimox[1]
Unipen[8]
V-Cillin K[11]
Veetids[11]
Wymox[1]

PHENOTHIAZINES

GENERIC NAMES

1. ACETOPHENAZINE
2. CHLORPROMAZINE
3. FLUPHENAZINE
4. MESORIDAZINE
5. METHOTRIMEPRAZINE
6. PERICYAZINE
7. PERPHENAZINE
8. PIPOTIAZINE
9. PROCHLORPERAZINE
10. PROMAZINE
11. THIOPROPAZATE
12. THIOPROPERAZINE
13. THIORIDAZINE
14. TRIFLUOPERAZINE
15. TRIFLUPROMAZINE

BRAND NAMES

Apo-Fluphenazine[3]
Apo-Perphenazine[7]
Apo-Thioridazine[13]
Apo-Trifluoperazine[14]
Chlorpromanyl-5[2]
Chlorpromanyl-20[2]
Chlorpromanyl-40[2]
Compazine[9]
Compazine Spansule[9]
Dartal[11]
Duo-Medihaler
Elavil Plus[7]
Etrafon[7]
Etrafon-A[7]
Etrafon-D[7]
Etrafon-F[7]
Etrafon-Forte[7]
Largactil[2]
Largactil Liquid[2]
Largactil Oral Drops[2]
Levoprome[5]
Majeptil[12]
Mellaril[13]
Mellaril Concentrate[13]
Mellaril-S[13]
Modecate[3]
Modecate Concentrate[3]
Moditen Enanthate[3]
Moditen HCl[3]
Moditen HCl-H.P.[3]
Neuleptil[6]
Novo-Chlorpromazine[2]
Novo-Flurazine[14]
Novo-Ridazine[13]
Nozinan[5]
Nozinan Liquid[5]
Nozinan Oral Drops[5]
Permitil[3]
Permitil Concentrate[3]
Piportil L_4[8]
PMS Levazine[7]
PMS Thioridazine[13]
Prolixin[3]
Prolixin Concentrate[3]
Prolixin Decanoate[3]
Prolixin Enanthate[3]
Prorazin[9]
Prozine [10]
Serentil[4]
Serentil Concentrate[4]
Solazine[14]
Stelazine[14]
Stelazine Concentrate[14]
Stemetil[9]
Stemetil Liquid[9]
Suprazine[14]
Terfluzine[14]
Terfluzine Concentrate[14]
Thorazine[2]
Thorazine Concentrate[2]
Thorazine Spansule[2]
Thor-Prom[2]
Tindal[2]
Triavil[7]
Trilafon[7]
Trilafon Concentrate[7]
Ultrazine-10[9]
Vesprin[5]

PHENYLEPHRINE

Aclophen
Advanced Formula Dristan Caplets
AH-Chew
Alersule
Anamine HD
Anaplex HD
Atrohist Pediatric
Atrohist Pediatric Suspension Dye Free
Atrohist Sprinkle
Cerose-DM
Chlorgest-HD
Citra Forte
Codimal DH
Codimal DM
Codimal PH
Colrex Compound
Colrex Cough
Coltab Children's
Comhist
Comhist LA
Conar
Conar Expectorant
Conar-A
Congespirin for Children Cold Tablets
Coristex-DH
Coristine-DH
D.A. Chewable
Dallergy
Dallergy Caplets
Dallergy-D Syrup
Deconsal Sprinkle
Dihistine
Dimetane Decongestant Caplets
Doktors
Donatussin
Donatussin DC
Donatussin Drops
Dondril
Dristan Cold Multi-Symptom Formula
Dristan Formula P
Dristan-AF
Dristan-AF Plus
Dura-Vent/DA
Ed A-Hist
Endagen-HD
Endal-HD
Endal-HD Plus
Extendryl
Extendryl JR
Extendryl SR
Father John's Medicine Plus
Fendol
Gendecon
Histagesic Modified
Histatab Plus
Histatan
Histatuss Pediatric
Histor-D
Histor-D Timecelles
Histussin HC
Hycomine Compound
Improved Sino-Tuss
Kolephrin
Mallergan-VC with Codeine
Meda Syrup Forte
Myhistine
ND-Gesic
Neocitran A
Neocitran Colds & Flu Calorie Reduced
NeoCitran DM Coughs & Colds
NeoCitran Extra Strength Colds & Flu
NeoCitran Extra Strength Sinus
Neo-Synephrine Nasal Drops
Neo-Synephrine Pediatric Nasal Drops
Nostril Spray Pump
Novahistex C
Novahistex DH
Novahistex DH Expectorant
Novahistine

Novahistine DH
Novahistine DH Expectorant
Omnicol
OMNIhist L.A.
Pediacof Cough
Pediatuss Cough
Phenameth VC
Phenameth VC with Codeine
Phenergan VC
Phenergan VC with Codeine
Pherazine VC
Pherazine VC with Codeine
Prehist
Prehist D
Prometh VC Plain
Prometh VC with Codeine
Promethazine VC
Quelidrine Cough
Rentamine Pediatric
Rescon-GG
Rhinall
Rhinall Children's Flavored Nose Drops
Rhinatate
Rhinogesic
Robitussin Night Relief
Robitussin Night Relief Colds Formula Liquid
Rolatuss Expectorant
Rolatuss Plain
R-Tannamine
R-Tannamine Pediatric
R-Tannate
R-Tannate Pediatric
Rymed
Rymed Liquid
Rynatan
Rynatan Pediatric
Rynatan-S Pediatric
Rynatuss
Rynatuss Pediatric
Salphenyl
Scot-Tussin
Scot-Tussin Original 5-Action Cold Medicine
Sinupan
Statuss Expectorant
Tanoral
Trimedine Liquid
Triotann
Triotann Pediatric
Tritann Pediatric
Tri-Tannate
Tri-Tannate Plus Pediatric
Tussanil Plain
Tussirex with Codeine Liquid
Vanex-HD
Vicks Sinex

POTASSIUM SUPPLEMENTS

GENERIC NAMES

1. POTASSIUM ACETATE
2. POTASSIUM BICARBONATE
3. POTASSIUM BICARBONATE & POTASSIUM CHLORIDE
4. POTASSIUM BICARBONATE & POTASSIUM CITRATE
5. POTASSIUM CHLORIDE
6. POTASSIUM GLUCONATE
7. POTASSIUM GLUCONATE & POTASSIUM CHLORIDE
8. POTASSIUM GLUCONATE & POTASSIUM CITRATE
9. POTASSIUM TRIPLEX

BRAND NAMES

Apo-K[5]
Cena-K[5]
Effer-K[4]
Gen-K[5]
Glu-K[6]
K+10[5]
K-10[5]
K-8[5]
K+Care[5]
K+Care ET[2]
Kalium Durules[5]
Kaochlor[5]
Kaochlor S-F[5]
Kaochlor-10[5]
Kaochlor-20[5]
Kaochlor-Eff[5]
Kaon[6]
Kaon-Cl[5]
Kaon-Cl 10[5]
Kaon-Cl 20[5]
Kato[5]
Kay Ciel[5]
Kay Ciel Elixir[5]
Kaylixir[6]
KCL[5]
K-Dur[5]
K-Electrolyte[2]
K-G Elixir[6]
K-Lease[5]
K-Long[5]
K-Lor[5]
Klor-Con 8[5]
Klor-Con 10[5]
Klor-Con Powder[5]
Klor-Con/25[5]
Klor-Con/EF[2]
Klorvess[3]
Klorvess 10% Liquid[5]
Klorvess Effervescent Granules[5]
Klotrix[5]
K-Lyte[2]
K-Lyte DS[4]
K-Lyte/Cl[3]
K-Lyte/Cl 50[3]
K-Lyte/CL Powder[5]
K-Med 900[5]
K-Norm[5]
Kolyum[7]
K-Sol[5]
K-Tab[5]
K-Vescent[2]
Micro-K[5]
Micro-K 10[5]
Micro-K LS[5]
Neo-K[3]
Potasalan[5]
Potassium-Rougier[6]
Potassium-Sandoz[3]
Roychlor 10%[5]
Roychlor 20%[5]
Royonate[6]
Rum-K[5]
Slow-K[5]
Ten K[5]
Tri-K[9]
Twin-K[8]

PROGESTINS

GENERIC NAMES

1. HYDROXYPROGESTERONE
2. MEDROXYPROGESTERONE
3. MEGESTROL
4. NORETHINDRONE
5. NORGESTREL
6. PROGESTERONE

BRAND NAMES

Activella[4]
Amen[3]
Aygestin[5]
Crinone[6]
Curretab[3]
Cycrin[3]
Depo-Provera[3]
Duralutin[1]
Femhrt[4]
Gesterol 50[6]
Gesterol L.A.[1]
Hy/Gestrone[1]
Hylutin[1]
Hyprogest[1]
Hyproval P.A.[1]
Megace[4]
Megace Oral Suspension[4]
Micronor[4]
Norlutate[4]
Norlutin[4]
Nor-Q.D.[4]
Ovrette[5]
Premphase[2]
Prempro[2]
Pro-Depo[1]
Prodrox[1]
Progestaject[6]
Progestilin[6]
Provera[3]

PSEUDOEPHEDRINE

Actacin
Actagen
Actagen-C Cough
Actifed
Actifed 12-Hour
Actifed A
Actifed Allergy Nighttime Caplets
Actifed DM
Actifed Plus
Actifed Plus Caplets
Actifed with Codeine Cough
Advil Cold and Sinus Caplets
Advil Flu & Body Ache
Afrinol Repetabs
Alamine Expectorant
Alamine-C Liquid
Aleve Cold & Sinus
Allegra D
Allent
Allercon
Allerest Maximum Strength
Allerest No-Drowsiness
Allerfrin
Allerfrin with Codeine
Allergy Cold
Allergy Formula Sinutab
AlleRid
Allerphed
All-Nite Cold Formula
Alpha-Phed

Ambenyl-D Decongestant Cough Formula
Ami-Drix
Anamine
Anamine T.D.
Anaplex
Anaplex S.R.
Anatuss DM
Anatuss LA
Aprodrine
Aprodrine with Codeine
Atrofed
Balminil Decongestant
BayCotussend Liquid
Baydec DM Drops
Bayer Select Flu Relief Caplets
Bayer Select Head Cold Caplets
Bayer Select Maximum Strength Sinus Pain Relief Caplets
Bayer Select Night Time Cold Caplets
Bayhistine DH
Bayhistine Expectorant
Benadryl Allergy/Sinus Headache Caplets
Benadryl Cold
Benadryl Cold Nighttime Liquid
Benadryl Decongestant
Benadryl Plus
Benylin Cold
Benylin Decongestant
Benylin DM-D
Benylin DM-D-E
Benylin DM-D-E Extra Strength
Benylin with Codeine
Beta-Phed
Brexin
Brexin-L.A.
Brofed
Bromarest DX Cough
Bromatane DX Cough
Bromfed
Bromfed-AT
Bromfed-DM
Bromfed-PD
Bromphen DX Cough
Brompheril
Brotane DX Cough
Calmylin
Calmylin #2
Calmylin #3
Calmylin Cough & Cold
Calmylin Pediatric
Calmylin with Codeine
Carbinoxamine Compound
Carbiset
Carbiset-TR
Carbodec
Carbodec DM Drops
Carbodec TR
Cardec DM
Cardec DM Drops
Cardec DM Pediatric
Cardec-S
Cenafed
Cenafed Plus
Cheracol Sinus
Children's Benylin DM-D
Children's Motrin Cold
Children's Sudafed Liquid
Children's Tylenol Cold
Children's Tylenol Cold Multi Symptom Plus Cough
Chlorafed
Chlorafed H.S. Timecelles
Chlorafed Timecelles
Chlorphedrine SR
Chlor-Trimeton 4 Hour Relief
Chlor-Trimeton 12 Hour Relief
Chlor-Trimeton Decongestant
Chlor-Trimeton Decongestant Repetabs
Chlor-Trimeton Non-Drowsy Decongestant 4 Hour
Chlor-Tripolon Decongestant Extra Strength
Chlor-Tripolon Decongestant Repetabs
Chlor-Tripolon Decongestant Tablets
Claritin Extra
Claritin-D
Claritin-D 12 Hour
CoActifed
CoActifed Expectorant
CoAdvil Caplets
Co-Apap
Codehist DH
Codimal
Codimal-L.A.
Codimal-L.A. Half
Coldrine
Colfed-A
Comtrex A/S
Comtrex A/S Caplets
Comtrex Cough Formula
Comtrex Daytime Caplets
Comtrex Daytime Maximum Strength Cold and Flu Relief
Comtrex Daytime Maximum Strength Cold, Cough and Flu Relief
Comtrex Hot Flu Relief
Comtrex Multi-Symptom Hot Flu Relief
Comtrex Multi-Symptom Non-Drowsy Caplets
Comtrex Nighttime
Comtrex Nighttime Maximum Strength Cold & Flu Relief
Comtrex Nighttime Maximum Strength Cold, Cough & Flu Relief
Concentrin
Congess JR
Congess SR
Congestac Caplets
Contac Allergy/Sinus Day Caplets
Contac Allergy/Sinus Night Caplets
Contac Maximum Strength Sinus Caplets
Contac Night Caplets
Contac Non-Drowsy Formula Sinus Caplets
Contac Severe Cold Formula
Contac Severe Cold Formula Night Strength
Cophene No. 2
Cophene-XP
Co-Pyronil 2
Cotridin
Cotridin Expectorant
CoTylenol Cold Medication
Cremacoat 3 Throat Coating Cough Medicine
C-Tussin Expectorant
Dallergy Jr.
Dallergy-D
DayCare
DayQuil Liquicaps
DayQuil Non-Drowsy Cold/Flu
DayQuil Non-Drowsy Cold/Flu LiquiCaps
DayQuil Non-Drowsy Sinus Pressure and Pain Relief Caplets
Decofed
Decohistine DH
Deconamine
Deconamine SR
Deconsal II
Deconsal Pediatric
DeFed-60
Deproist Expectorant with Codeine
De-Tuss
Detussin Expectorant
Detussin Liquid
Dexaphen SA
Dexophed
Dihistine DH
Dihistine Expectorant
Dimacol
Dimetane-DX Cough
Dimetapp Sinus Caplets
Disobrom
Disophrol
Disophrol Chronotabs
Dorcol Children's Cold Formula
Dorcol Children's Cough
Dorcol Children's Decongestant
Dristan Cold and Flu
Dristan Cold Caplets
Dristan Cold Maximum Strength Caplets
Dristan Juice Mix-in Cold, Flu, & Cough
Dristan Sinus Caplets
Drixoral
Drixoral Cold & Allergy
Drixoral Cold & Flu
Drixoral Non-Drowsy Formula
Drixoral Plus
Drixoral Sinus
Drixtab
Duralex
Dura-Tap PD
Duratuss
Duratuss HD
Effective Strength Cough Formula with Decongestant
Efidec/24
Eltor-120
Endafed
Entex PSE
Entuss Pediatric Expectorant
Entuss-D
Fedahist
Fedahist Decongestant
Fedahist Expectorant
Fedahist Expectorant Pediatric Drops
Fedahist Gyrocaps
Fedahist Timecaps
Genac
Genaphed
Genite

Glycofed
GP-500
Guaifed
Guaifed-PD
GuaiMAX-D
Guaitab
GuiaCough PE
Guiatuss PE
Guiatussin DAC
Halofed
Halofed Adult Strength
Hayfebrol
Head & Chest
Histafed C
Histalet
Histalet X
Histalet-DM
Humibid Guaifenesin Plus
Isoclor
Isoclor Expectorant
Isoclor Timesules
Klerist-D
Kolephrin/DM Caplets
Kronofed-A
Kronofed-A Jr.
Lodrane LD
Mapap Cold Formula
Maxenal
Maximum Strength Tylenol Allergy Sinus Caplets
Maximum Strength Tylenol Flu Gelcaps
Medi-Flu
Medi-Flu Caplets
Mediquell Decongestant Formula
Midahist DH
Motrin-IB Sinus
Motrin-IB Sinus Caplets
Myfed
Myfedrine
Myhistine DH
Myhistine Expectorant
Mytussin DAC
Naldegesic
Nasatab LA
ND Clear T.D.
Neofed
Noratuss II Liquid
Novafed
Novafed A
Novagest Expectorant with Codeine
Novahistex
Novahistex DM
Novahistine Cough & Cold Formula Liquid
Novahistine DH Liquid
Novahistine DMX Liquid
Novahistine Expectorant
Nucochem
Nucochem Expectorant
Nucochem Pediatric Expectorant
Nucofed
Nucofed Expectorant
Nucofed Pediatric Expectorant
NyQuil Hot Therapy
NyQuil Liquicaps
NyQuil Nighttime Colds Medicine
Nytcold Medicine
Nytime Cold Medicine Liquid
Ornex Maximum Strength Caplets
Ornex No Drowsiness Caplets
Ornex Severe Cold No Drowsiness Caplets
Par-Drix
PediaCare Children's Cold Relief Night Rest Cough-Cold Formula
PediaCare Children's Cough-Cold Formula
PediaCare Cold Formula
PediaCare Cough-Cold
PediaCare Infants' Oral Decongestant Drops
Pertussin All Night PM
Phenapap Sinus Headache & Congestion
Phenergan-D
Phenhist DH with Codeine
Phenhist Expectorant
Polaramine Expectorant
Primatuss Cough Mixture 4D
Promist HD Liquid
Pseudo
Pseudo-Bid
Pseudo-Car DM
Pseudo-Chlor
Pseudodine C Cough
Pseudofrin
Pseudogest
Pseudogest Plus
P-V-Tussin
Rescon-DM
Rescon-ED
Rescon-JR
Respaire-60 SR
Respaire-120 SR
Resporal TR
Rhinosyn
Rhinosyn-DM
Rhinosyn-PD
Rhinosyn-X
Rinade B.I.D.
Robafen DAC
Robafen DM
Robidrine
Robitussin Allergy and Cough[4]
Robitussin Cold and Cough Liqui-Gels
Robitussin Honey Flu
Robitussin Maximum Strength Cough & Cold
Robitussin Night Relief
Robitussin Pediatric Cough & Cold
Robitussin Severe Congestion Liqui-Gels
Robitussin-DAC
Robitussin-PE
Rondamine-DM Drops
Rondec
Rondec Drops
Rondec-DM
Rondec-DM Drops
Rondec-TR
Ru-Tuss DE
Ru-Tuss Expectorant
Rymed-TR
Ryna
Ryna-C Liquid
Ryna-CX Liquid
Seldane D
Semprex-D
Simplet
Sinarest No-Drowsiness
Sinarest Sinus
Sine-Aid
Sine-Aid IB
Sine-Aid Maximum Strength
Sine-Aid Maximum Strength Allergy/Sinus Formula Caplets
Sine-Aid Maximum Strength Gelcaps
Sine-Off Maximum Strength Allergy/Sinus Formula Caplets
Sine-Off Maximum Strength No Drowsiness Formula Caplets
Singlet
Sinufed Timecelles
Sinus Excedrin Extra Strength
Sinus Excedrin Extra Strength Caplets
Sinus Excedrin No Drowsiness
Sinus Excedrin No Drowsiness Caplets
Sinus Relief
SinuStat
Sinutab
Sinutab Extra Strength
Sinutab II Maximum Strength
Sinutab Maximum Strength without Drowsiness
Sinutab Maximum Strength without Drowsiness Caplets
Sinutab No Drowsiness
Sinutab No Drowsiness Extra Strength
Sinutab Regular
Sinutrex Extra Strength
SRC Expectorant
Stamoist E
Sudafed
Sudafed 12 Hour
Sudafed 60
Sudafed Cold & Cough Liquid Caps
Sudafed Cough
Sudafed DM
Sudafed Expectorant
Sudafed Plus
Sudafed Severe Cold Formula Caplets
Sudafed Sinus Maximum Strength
Sudafed Sinus Maximum Strength Caplets
Sudrin
Sufedrin
Super-Anahist
Tavist Allergy/Sinus/Headache
T-Dry
T-Dry Junior
TheraFlu Maximum Strength Non-Drowsy Formula Flu, Cold & Cough Medicine
TheraFlu Nighttime Maximum Strength
TheraFlu/Flu & Cold
TheraFlu/Flu, Cold & Cough
Thera-Hist
T-Moist
Touro A&H
Touro LA Caplets
Triacin C Cough
Triafed
Triafed with Codeine
Triaminic DM Nighttime for Children

Triaminic Nite Light
Triaminic Sore Throat Formula
Tricom Caplets
Trifed
Trifed-C Cough
Triminol Cough
Trinalin Repetabs
Trinex
Triofed
Tripodrine
Triposed
Tussafed
Tussafed Drops
Tussafin Expectorant
Tussar DM
Tussar-2
Tussend
Tussend Expectorant
Tussend Liquid
Tussin
Tuss-LA
Ty-Cold Cold Formula
Tylenol Allergy Sinus Gelcaps
Tylenol Allergy Sinus Night Time Maximum Strength Caplets
Tylenol Cold & Flu
Tylenol Cold & Flu No Drowsiness Powder
Tylenol Cold Medication
Tylenol Cold Medication, Non-Drowsy
Tylenol Cold Night Time
Tylenol Cold No Drowsiness Formula Gelcaps
Tylenol Cough
Tylenol Cough with Decongestant
Tylenol Maximum Strength Flu Gelcaps
Tylenol Sinus Maximum Strength
Tylenol Sinus Maximum Strength Caplets
Tylenol Sinus Maximum Strength Gelcaps
Tylenol Sinus Medication
Tylenol Sinus Medication Extra Strength
Tyrodone
ULTRAbrom PD
Ursinus Inlay
Vanex Expectorant
V-Dec-M
Versacaps
Vicks 44 Cough and Cold Relief Liqui-Caps
Vicks 44 Non-Drowsy Cold and Cough Liqui-Caps
Vicks 44D Dry Hacking Cough & Head Congestion
Vicks 44M Cough, Cold and Flu Relief
Vicks 44M Cough, Cold and Flu Relief LiquiCaps
Vicks Children's NyQuil Allergy/Head Cold
Vicks Dayquil Liquicaps
Vicks Formula 44D Decongestant Cough Mixture
Vicks Formula 44M Multi-Symptom Cough Mixture
Vicks NyQuil Multi-Symptom Cold/Flu Relief
Vicks NyQuil Multi-Symptom LiquiCaps
Vicks Pediatric Formula 44D Cough and Decongestant
Vicks Pediatric Formula 44M Multi-Symptom Cough & Cold
Viro-Med
Zephrex
Zephrex-LA
Zyrtec-D

RAUWOLFIA ALKALOIDS

GENERIC NAMES

1. DESERPIDINE
2. DESERPIDINE & HYDROCHLOROTHIAZIDE
3. DESERPIDINE & METHYCLOTHIAZIDE
4. RAUWOLFIA SERPENTINA
5. RAUWOLFIA SERPENTINA & BENDROFLUMETHIAZIDE
6. RESERPINE
7. RESERPINE & CHLOROTHIAZIDE
8. RESERPINE & CHLORTHALIDONE
9. RESERPINE & HYDROCHLOROTHIAZIDE
10. RESERPINE & HYDROFLUMETHIAZIDE
11. RESERPINE & METHYCLOTHIAZIDE
12. RESERPINE & POLYTHIAZIDE
13. RESERPINE & QUINETHAZONE
14. RESERPINE & TRICHLORMETHIAZIDE

BRAND NAMES

Demi-Regroton[8]
Diupres[7]
Diurese R[14]
Diurigen with Reserpine[7]
Diutensen-R[11]
Dureticyl[3]
Enduronyl[3]
Enduronyl Forte[3]
Harmonyl[1]
Hydropine[10]
Hydropine H.P.[6]
Hydropres[9]
Hydrosine[9]
Hydrotensin[9]
Mallopres[9]
Metatensin[14]
Naquival[14]
Novoreserpine[6]
Oreticyl[2]
Oreticyl Forte[2]
Raudixin[4]
Rauval[4]
Rauverid[4]
Rauzide[6]
Regroton[8]
Renese-R[9]
Reserfia[6]
Salazide[10]
Salutensin[10]
Salutensin-Demi[10]
Serpalan[6]
Serpasil[6]
Wolfina[4]

SALICYLATES

GENERIC NAMES

1. CHOLINE MAGNESIUM SALICYLATES
2. CHOLINE SALICYLATE
3. MAGNESIUM SALICYLATE
4. SALICYLAMIDE
5. SALSALATE
6. SODIUM SALICYLATE

BRAND NAMES

Amigesic[5]
Arthropan[2]
Choline Magnesium Trisalicylate[1]
Citra Forte[4]
Diagen[5]
Disalcid[5]
Doan's Pills[3]
Dodd's Pills[6]
Duoprin
Fendol[4]
Improved Sino-Tuss[4]
Kolephrin[4]
Kolephrin NN Liquid[4]
Magan[3]
Mobidin[3]
Mono-Gesic[5]
Omnicol[4]
Presalin[4]
Rhinogesic[4]
Rid-A-Pain Compound[4]
S-A-C[4]
Salcylic Acid[4]
Saleto[4]
Saleto-D[4]
Salflex[5]
Salgesic[4]
Salphenyl[4]
Salsitab[5]
Scot-tussin Original 5-Action Cold Medicine[6]
Tricosal[1]
Trilisate[1]
Tri-Pain[4]
Tussanil DH Tablets[4]
Tussirex with Codeine Liquid[6]
Uracel[6]

SCOPOLAMINE (Hyoscine)

Barbidonna
Barbidonna 2
Buscopan
Kinesed
Transderm-Scop
Transderm-V

SULFONAMIDES

GENERIC NAMES

1. SULFACYTINE
2. SULFADIAZINE
3. SULFAMETHIZOLE
4. SULFAMETHOXAZOLE
5. SULFISOXAZOLE

BRAND NAMES

Apo-Sulfamethoxazole[4]
Apo-Sulfatrim[4]
Apo-Sulfatrim DS[4]
Apo-Sulfisoxizole[5]
Bactrim[4]
Bactrim DS[4]

Cotrim[4]
Cotrim DS[4]
Co-trimoxazole[4]
Eryzole[5]
Gantanol[4]
Gantrisin[5]
Novo-Soxazole[5]
Novotrimel[4]
Novotrimel DS[4]
Nu-Cotrimox[4]
Nu-Cotrimox DS[4]
Pediazole[5]
Protrin[4]
Renoquid[1]
Roubac[4]
Septra[4]
Septra DS[4]
SMZ-TMP[4]
Sulfamethoprim[4]
Sulfamethoprim DS[4]
Sulfaprim[4]
Sulfaprim DS[4]
Sulfatrim[4]
Sulfatrim DS[4]
Sulfimycin[5]
Sulfizole[5]
Sulfoxaprim[4]
Sulfoxaprim DS[4]
Sulmeprim[4]
Thiosulfil Forte[3]
Triazole[4]
Triazole DS[4]
Trimeth-Sulfa[4]
Trisulfam[4]
Urobak[4]
Uroplus DS[4]
Uroplus SS[4]

SULFONYLUREAS

GENERIC NAMES
1. ACETOHEXAMIDE
2. CHLORPROPAMIDE
3. GLIMEPIRIDE
4. GLIPIZIDE
5. GLYBURIDE
6. TOLAZAMIDE
7. TOLBUTAMIDE

BRAND NAMES
Albert Glyburide[5]
Amaryl[3]
Apo-Chlorpropamide[2]
Apo-Glyburide[5]
Apo-Tolbutamide[7]
DiaBeta[5]
Diabinese[2]
Dimelor[1]
Dymelor[1]
Euglucon[5]
Gen-Glybe[5]
Glucamide[2]
Glucotrol[4]
Glucotrol XL[4]
Glynase PresTab[6]
Micronase[5]
Novo-Butamide[7]
Novo-Glyburide[4]
Novo-Propamide[2]
Orinase[7]
Tolamide[6]
Tolinase[6]

TETRACYCLINES

GENERIC NAMES
1. DEMECLOCYCLINE
2. DOXYCYCLINE
3. MINOCYCLINE
4. OXYTETRACYCLINE
5. TETRACYCLINE

BRAND NAMES
Achromycin[5]
Achromycin V[5]
Adoxa[2]
Apo-Doxy[2]
Apo-Tetra[5]
Arestin[3]
Declomycin[1]
Doryx[2]
Doxy-Caps[2]
Doxycin[2]
Doxy-Tabs[2]
E.P. Mycin[4]
Helidac[5]
Minocin[3]
Monodox[2]
Novodoxlin[2]
Novotetra[5]
Nu-Tetra[5]
Panmycin[5]
Periostat[5]
Robitet[5]
Sumycin[5]
Terramycin[4]
Tetracyn[5]
Tija[4]
Vibramycin[2]

THEOPHYLLINE

Ami Rax
Asbron G
Asbron G Inlay Tablets
Azma Aid
Bronchial
Broncomar GG
Bronkolixir
Bronkotabs
Ed-Bron G
Elixophyllin-GG
Equibron G
Glyceryl T
Guaiphed
Hydrophed
Marax
Marax D.F.
Mudrane GG
Mudrane GG2
Phedral-C.T
Primatene "P" Formula
Quibron
Quibron 300
Slo-Phyllin GG
Syncophylate-GG
Tedral
Tedral SA
Tedrigen
T.E.H. Compound
T.E.P.
Theodrine
Theodrine Pediatric
Theofed
Theofedral
Theolate
Theomax DF
Uni-Bronchial

Additional Drug Interactions

The following lists of drugs and their interactions with other drugs are continuations of lists found in the alphabetized drug charts beginning on page 2. These lists are alphabetized by generic name or drug class name, shown in large capital letters. Only those lists too long for the drug charts are included in this section. For complete information about any generic drug, see the alphabetized charts.

ADRENOCORTICOIDS (Systemic)

GENERIC NAME OR DRUG CLASS	COMBINED EFFECT
Attenuated virus vaccines*	Possible viral infection.
Azoles	Decreased azole effect.
Barbiturates*	Decreased prednisone effect. Oversedation.
Carbamazepine	Decreased adreno-corticoid effect.
Carbonic anhydrase inhibitors	Increased loss of calcium.
Chloral hydrate	Decreased adreno-corticoid effect.
Chlorthalidone	Potassium depletion.
Cholestyramine	Decreased adreno-corticoid effect.
Cholinergics*	Decreased cholinergic effect.
Colestipol	Decreased adreno-corticoid effect.
Contraceptives, oral*	Increased adreno-corticoid effect.
Cyclosporine	Decreased adreno-corticoid effect. Increased cyclo-sporine effect.
Digitalis preparations*	Dangerous potassium depletion. Possible digitalis toxicity.
Diuretics	Potassium depletion.
Ephedrine	Decreased adreno-corticoid effect.
Estrogens*	Increased adreno-corticoid effect.
Foscarnet	Potassium depletion.
Glutethimide	Decreased adreno-corticoid effect.
Insulin	Decreased insulin effect.
Insulin lispro	May require increased dosage of insulin.
Isoniazid	Decreased isoniazid effect.
Mifepristone	Decreased effect of mifepristone.
Mitotane	Decreased adreno-corticoid effect.
Phenobarbital	Decreased adreno-corticoid effect.
Phenytoin	Decreased adreno-corticoid effect.
Potassium supplements*	Decreased potassium effect.
Primidone	Decreased adreno-corticoid effect.
Rifampin	Decreased adreno-corticoid effect.
Salicylates*	Decreased salicylate effect.
Sympathomimetics*	Possible glaucoma.
Thyroid hormones*	May require thyroid hormone dosage change.

ANDROGENS & ESTROGENS

GENERIC NAME OR DRUG CLASS	COMBINED EFFECT
Insulin	Unpredictable increase or decrease in blood sugar.
Nicotinic acid	Decreased nicotinic acid.
Oxyphenbutazone	Decreased androgen and estrogen effect.

*See Glossary

GENERIC NAME OR DRUG CLASS	COMBINED EFFECT	GENERIC NAME OR DRUG CLASS	COMBINED EFFECT

ANDROGENS & ESTROGENS continued

GENERIC NAME OR DRUG CLASS	COMBINED EFFECT
Phenobarbital	Decreased androgen and estrogen effect.
Phenylbutazone	Decreased estrogen and testosterone effect.
Primidone	Decreased estrogen and testosterone effect.
Rifampin	Decreased estrogen and testosterone effect.
Terazosin	Decreased effectiveness of terazosin.
Thyroid hormones*	Decreased thyroid effect.
Ursodiol	Decreased ursodiol effect.

ANGIOTENSIN-CONVERTING ENZYME (ACE) INHIBITORS

GENERIC NAME OR DRUG CLASS	COMBINED EFFECT
Pentamidine	May increase bone marrow depression or make kidney damage more likely.
Pentoxifylline	Increased anti-hypertensive effect.
Potassium	May raise potassium levels in blood to toxic levels.
Potassium supplements*	Possible increased potassium in blood.
Sotalol	Increased antihypertensive effects of both drugs. Dosages may require adjustment.
Spironolactone	Possible excessive potassium in blood.
Terazosin	Decreased effectiveness of terazosin.
Tiopronin	Increased risk of toxicity to kidneys.
Triamterene	Possible excessive potassium in blood.

ANGIOTENSIN-CONVERTING ENZYME (ACE) INHIBITORS & HYDROCHLOROTHIAZIDE

GENERIC NAME OR DRUG CLASS	COMBINED EFFECT
Diuretics*	Decreased blood pressure.
Lisinopril	Increased antihypertensive effect. Dosage of each may require adjustment.
Lithium	Increased lithium effect.
Monoamine oxidase (MAO) inhibitors*	Increased hydrochlorothiazide effect.
Nicardipine	Blood pressure drop. Dosages may require adjustment.
Nimodipine	Possible irregular heartbeat. May worsen congestive heart failure.
Nitrates*	Excessive blood pressure drop.
Potassium supplements*	Excessive potassium in blood.
Probenecid	Decreased probenecid effect.
Sotalol	Increased antihypertensive effects of both drugs. Dosages may require adjustment.
Spironolactone	Possible excessive potassium in blood.
Triamterene	Possible excessive potassium in blood.

*See Glossary

GENERIC NAME OR DRUG CLASS	COMBINED EFFECT	GENERIC NAME OR DRUG CLASS	COMBINED EFFECT

ANTICOAGULANTS (Oral)

GENERIC NAME OR DRUG CLASS	COMBINED EFFECT
Cholestyramine	Decreased effect of anticoagulant.
Citalopram	May lessen the effect of warfarin.
Clofibrate	Increased effect of anticoagulant.
Colestipol	Decreased effect of anticoagulant.
Contraceptives, oral*	Decreased effect of anticoagulant.
Danazol	Increased effect of anticoagulant.
Dextrothyroxine	Increased effect of anticoagulant.
Diclofenac	Increased risk of bleeding.
Diflunisal	Increased effect of anticoagulant.
Dipyridamole	Increased risk of hemorrhage.
Disulfiram	Increased effect of anticoagulant.
Erythromycins*	Increased effect of anticoagulant.
Estramustine	Decreased effect of anticoagulant.
Estrogens	Decreased effect of anticoagulant.
Fenoprofen	Increased effect of anticoagulant.
Fluoxetine	May cause confusion, agitation, convulsions and high blood pressure. Avoid combining.
Fluvoxamine	Increased effect of warfarin.
Gemfibrozil	Increased effect of anticoagulant.
Glutethimide	Decreased effect of anticoagulant.
Griseofulvin	Decreased effect of anticoagulant.
Indomethacin	Increased effect of anticoagulant.
Leukotriene modifiers	Increased effect of warfarin.
Levamisole	Increased risk of bleeding.
Meloxicam	Increased risk bleeding.
Methimazole	Increased effect of anticoagulant.
Metronidazole	Increased effect of anticoagulant.
Mifepristone	Increased risk of excessive bleeding.
Mineral Oil	Decreased absorption of anticoagulant.
Nalidixic acid	Increased effect of anticoagulant.
Nicardipine	Possible increased effect of anticoagulant.
Nimodipine	Possible increased effect of anticoagulant.
Nizatidine	Increased effect of anticoagulant.
Omeprazole	Increased effect of anticoagulant.
Orlistat	Increased anticoagulant effect.
Paroxetine	Increased effect of anticoagulant.
Phenylbutazone	Increased effect of anticoagulant.
Phenytoin	Decreased levels of phenytoin.
Plicamycin	Increased effect of anticoagulant.
Propafenone	May require adjustment of anticoagulant dosage.
Primadone	Decreased effect of anticoagulant.
Quinidine	Increased effect of anticoagulant.
Raloxifene	May lessen effect of warfarin.
Rifampin	Decreased effect of anticoagulant.
Salicylates	Increased effect of anticoagulant.

*See Glossary

ANTICOAGULANTS (Oral) continued

GENERIC NAME OR DRUG CLASS	COMBINED EFFECT
Sulfadoxine and pyrimethamine	Increased risk of toxicity.
Sulindac	Increased effect of anticoagulant.
Suprofen	Increased risk of bleeding.
Testolactone	Increased effect of anticoagulant.
Thyroid hormones*	Increased effect of anticoagulant.
Tolcapone	May require adjustment in dosage of warfarin.
Toremifene	May increase time it takes blood to clot.
Vitamin E	Increased risk of bleeding.
Vitamin K	Decreased effect of anticoagulant.
Zafirlukast	May increase effect of warfarin.
Zileuton	Increased warfarin effect.
Note: Any medicine	Unpredictable absorption.

ANTICONVULSANTS, HYDANTOIN

GENERIC NAME OR DRUG CLASS	COMBINED EFFECT
Central nervous system (CNS) depressants*	Oversedation.
Chloramphenicol	Increased anticonvulsant effect.
Cimetidine	Increased anticonvulsant toxicity.
Contraceptives, oral*	Increased seizures.
Cyclosporine	May decrease cyclosporine effect.
Digitalis preparations*	Decreased digitalis effect.
Disopyramide	Decreased disopyramide effect.
Disulfiram	Increased anticonvulsant effect.
Estrogens*	Increased estrogen effect.
Felbamate	Increased side effects and adverse reactions.
Furosemide	Decreased furosemide effect.
Gold compounds*	Increased anticonvulsant blood levels. Hydantoin dose may require adjustment.
Glutethimide	Decreased anticonvulsant effect.
Griseofulvin	Increased griseofulvin effect.
Hypoglycemics, oral*	Possible decreased hypoglycemic effect.
Hypoglycemics, other*	Possible decreased hypoglycemic effect.
Isoniazid	Increased anticonvulsant effect.
Lamotrigine	Decreased lamotrigine effect with phenytoin.
Leucovorin	May counteract the effect of phenytoin or any hydantoin anticonvulsant.
Leukotriene modifiers	Increased phenytoin effect.
Loxapine	Decreased anticonvulsant effect of phenytoin or any hydantoin anticonvulsant.
Methadone	Decreased methadone effect.
Methotrexate	Increased methotrexate effect.
Methylphenidate	Increased anticonvulsant effect.
Mifepristone	Decreased effect of mifepristone.
Modafinil	Anticonvulsant dose may need adjustment.
Molindone	Increased phenytoin effect.

ADDITIONAL DRUG INTERACTIONS

***See Glossary**

GENERIC NAME OR DRUG CLASS	COMBINED EFFECT

ANTICONVULSANTS, HYDANTOIN continued

GENERIC NAME OR DRUG CLASS	COMBINED EFFECT
Monoamine oxidase (MAO) inhibitors*	Increased polythiazide effect.
Nicardipine	Increased anticonvulsant effect.
Nimodipine	Increased anticonvulsant effect.
Nitrates*	Excessive blood pressure drop.
Nizatidine	Increased effect and toxicity of phenytoin.
Omeprazole	Delayed excretion of phenytoin causing increased amount of phenytoin in blood.
Oxyphenbutazone	Increased anti-convulsant effect.
Para-aminosalicylic acid (PAS)	Increased anti-convulsant effect.
Paroxetine	Decreased anti-convulsant effect.
Phenacemide	Increased risk of paranoid symptoms.
Phenothiazines*	Increased anti-convulsant effect.
Phenylbutazone	Increased anti-convulsant effect.
Potassium supplements*	Decreased potassium effect.
Probenecid	Decreased probenecid effect.
Propafenone	Increased effect of both drugs and increased risk of toxicity.
Propranolol	Increased propranolol effect.
Quetiapine	Decreased quetiapine effect with phenytoin.
Quinidine	Increased quinidine effect.
Rifampin	Decreased anti-convulsant effect.
Sedatives*	Increased sedative effect.
Sotalol	Decreased sotalol effect.
Sucralfate	Decreased anti-convulsant effect.
Sulfa drugs*	Increased anti-convulsant effect.
Theophylline	Reduced anticonvulsant effect.
Trimethoprim	Increased phenytoin effect.
Valproic acid	Breakthrough seizures.
Xanthines*	Decreased effects of both drugs.
Zafirlukast	May increase effect of phenytoin.
Zaleplon	Decreased zaleplon effect.

ANTIDEPRESSANTS, TRICYCLIC

GENERIC NAME OR DRUG CLASS	COMBINED EFFECT
Antihistamines*	Increased anti-histamine effect.
Barbiturates*	Decreased anti-depressant effect. Increased sedation.
Benzodiazepines*	Increased sedation.
Bupropion	Increased risk of seizures.
Central nervous system (CNS) depressants*	Excessive sedation.
Cimetidine	Possible increased tricyclic antidepres-sant effect and toxicity.
Citalopram	Increased tricyclic antidepressant effect and toxicity.
Clonidine	Blood pressure increase. Avoid combination.
Clozapine	Toxic effect on the central nervous system.

*See Glossary

ANTIDEPRESSANTS, TRICYCLIC continued

GENERIC NAME OR DRUG CLASS	COMBINED EFFECT
Contraceptives, oral*	Increased depression.
Dextrothyroxine	Increased antidepressant effect. Irregular heartbeat.
Disulfiram	Delirium.
Dofetilide	Increased risk of heart problems.
Ethchlorvynol	Delirium.
Fluoxetine	Increased effect of tricyclic antidepressant. Possible toxicity.
Fluvoxamine	Increased antidepressant effect.
Furazolidine	Sudden, severe increase in blood pressure.
Guanabenz	Decreased guanabenz effect.
Guanadrel	Decreased guanadrel effect.
Guanethidine	Decreased guanethidine effect.
Haloperidol	Decreased lamotrigine effect.
Leucovorin	High alcohol content of leucovorin may cause adverse effects.
Levodopa	May increase blood pressure. May decrease levodopa effect.
Lithium	Possible decreased seizure threshold.
Methyldopa	Possible decreased methyldopa effect.
Methylphenidate	Possible increased tricyclic antidepressant effect and toxicity.
Modafinil	Increased antidepressant effect.
Molindone	Increased molindone effect.
Monoamine oxidase (MAO) inhibitors*	Fever, delirium, convulsions.
Narcotics*	Oversedation.
Nicotine	Increased effect of antidepressant (with imipramine).
Phenothiazines*	Possible increased tricyclic antidepressant effect and toxicity.
Phenytoin	Decreased phenytoin effect.
Procainamide	Possible irregular heartbeat.
Quinidine	Possible irregular heartbeat.
Sertraline	Increased depressive effects of both drugs.
Sympathomimetics*	Increased sympathomimetic effect.
Thyroid hormones*	Irregular heartbeat.
Tolcapone	May increase incidence of adverse effects of tolcapone.
Zaleplon	Increased effect of either drug. Avoid.
Zolpidem	Increased sedative effect. Avoid.

ANTIDYSKINETICS

GENERIC NAME OR DRUG CLASS	COMBINED EFFECT
Imatinib	Increased effect of pimozide.
Levodopa	Possible increased levodopa effect.
Monoamine oxidase (MAO) inhibitors*	Increased antidyskinetic effect.

*See Glossary

GENERIC NAME OR DRUG CLASS	COMBINED EFFECT

ANTIFUNGALS, AZOLES

GENERIC NAME OR DRUG CLASS	COMBINED EFFECT
Isoniazid	Decreased azole effect.
Losartan	Decreased losartan effect.
Methscopolamine	Decreased azole effect.
Methylprednisolone	Increased effect of methylprednisolone.
Mifepristone	Decreased effect of mifepristone.
Nizatidine	Decreased azole effect.
Omeprazole	Decreased azole effect.
Phenytoin	May alter effect of both drugs.
Propantheline	Decreased azole effect.
Quietapine	Increased risk of quietapine toxicity.
Ranitidine	Decreased azole effect.
Rifampin	Decreased azole effect.
Ritonavir	Increased ritonavir effect.
Scopolamine	Decreased azole effect.
Sibutramine	Increased effect of sibutramine.
Sildenafil (Viagra)	Effects unknown. Consult doctor.
Sodium bicarbonate	Decreased azole effect.
Warfarin	Increased warfarin effect.

ANTIHISTAMINES

GENERIC NAME OR DRUG CLASS	COMBINED EFFECT
Procarbazine	May increase sedation.
QT interval prolongation-causing drugs*	Serious heart rhythm problems with astemizole. Avoid.
Sedatives*	Excess sedation. Avoid.
Sertraline	Increased depressive effects of both drugs.
Sleep inducers*	Excess sedation. Avoid.
Sotalol	Increased antihistamine effect.
Tranquilizers*	Excess sedation. Avoid.

ANTIHISTAMINES, PHENOTHIAZINE-DERIVATIVE

GENERIC NAME OR DRUG CLASS	COMBINED EFFECT
Dronabinol	Increased effects of both drugs. Avoid.
Epinephrine	Decreased epinephrine effect.
Ethinamate	Dangerous increased effects of ethinamate. Avoid combining.
Extrapyramidal reaction*-causing medicines	Increased frequency and severity of extrapyramidal reactions.
Fluoxetine	Increased depressant effects of both drugs.
Guanethidine	Decreased guanethidine effect.
Guanfacine	May increase depressant effects of either medicine.
Leucovorin	High alcohol content of leucovorin may cause adverse effects.
Levodopa	Decreased levodopa effect.
Methyprylon	May increase sedative effect to dangerous level. Avoid.
Metyrosine	Increased likelihood of toxic symptoms of each.

*See Glossary

GENERIC NAME OR DRUG CLASS	COMBINED EFFECT	GENERIC NAME OR DRUG CLASS	COMBINED EFFECT

ANTIHISTAMINES, PHENOTHIAZINE-DERIVATIVE continued

GENERIC NAME OR DRUG CLASS	COMBINED EFFECT
Mind-altering drugs*	Increased effect of mind-altering drugs.
Molindone	Increased sedative and antihistamine effect.
Monoamine oxidase (MAO) inhibitors*	Increased antihistamine effect.
Nabilone	Greater depression of central nervous system.
Narcotics*	Increased narcotic effect.
Sedatives*	Increased sedative effect.
Sertraline	Increased depressive effects of both drugs.
Sotalol	Increased antihistamine effect.
Tranquilizers*	Increased tranquilizer effect. Avoid.

ANTI-INFLAMMATORY DRUGS, NONSTEROIDAL (NSAIDs)

GENERIC NAME OR DRUG CLASS	COMBINED EFFECT
Diuretics*	May decrease diuretic effect.
Gold compounds*	Increased risk of kidney toxicity.
Lithium	Increased lithium effect.
Losartan	Decreased antihypertensive effect.
Meglitinides	Unknown effect. Avoid.
Meloxicam	Increased risk of side effects of meloxicam.
Methotrexate	Increased risk of side effects of methotrexate.
Minoxidil	Decreased minoxidil effect.
Probenecid	Increased pain relief.
Terazosin	Decreased effectiveness of terazosin. Causes sodium and fluid retention.
Thyroid hormones*	Rapid heartbeat, blood pressure rise.
Tiopronin	Increased risk of toxicity to kidneys.
Triamterene	Reduced triamterene effect.

ASPIRIN

GENERIC NAME OR DRUG CLASS	COMBINED EFFECT
Dextrothyroxine (large doses, continuous use)	Increased dextrothyroxine effect.
Diclofenac	Increased risk of stomach ulcer.
Ethacrynic acid	Possible aspirin toxicity.
Furosemide	Possible aspirin toxicity. May decrease furosemide effect.
Gold compounds*	Increased likelihood of kidney damage.
Indomethacin	Risk of stomach bleeding and ulcers.
Ketoprofen	Increased risk of stomach ulcer.
Levamisole	Increased risk of bleeding.
Meloxicam	Increased risk of stomach ulcer.
Methotrexate	Increased methotrexate effect.
Minoxidil	Decreased minoxidil effect.
Oxprenolol	Decreased antihypertensive effect of oxprenolol.
Para-aminosalicylic acid	Possible aspirin toxicity.

*See Glossary

GENERIC NAME OR DRUG CLASS	COMBINED EFFECT	GENERIC NAME OR DRUG CLASS	COMBINED EFFECT

ASPIRIN continued

GENERIC NAME OR DRUG CLASS	COMBINED EFFECT
Penicillins*	Increased effect of both drugs.
Phenobarbital	Decreased aspirin effect.
Phenytoin	Increased phenytoin effect.
Probenecid	Decreased probenecid effect.
Propranolol	Decreased aspirin effect.
Rauwolfia alkaloids*	Decreased aspirin effect.
Salicylates*	Likely aspirin toxicity.
Sotalol	Decreased anti-hypertensive effect of sotalol.
Spironolactone	Decreased spirono-lactone effect.
Sulfinpyrazone	Decreased sulfin-pyrazone effect.
Terazosin	Decreased effective-ness of terazosin. Causes sodium and fluid retention.
Ticlopidine	Increased effect of both drugs.
Vitamin C (large doses)	Possible aspirin toxicity.
Valproic acid	May increase valproic acid effect.

ATROPINE, HYOSCYAMINE, METHENAMINE, METHYLENE BLUE, PHENYLSALICYLATE & BENZOIC ACID

GENERIC NAME OR DRUG CLASS	COMBINED EFFECT
Diuretics, thiazide*	Decreased urine acidity.
Furosemide	Possible salicylate toxicity.
Gold compounds*	Increased likelihood of kidney damage.
Haloperidol	Increased internal eye pressure.
Indomethacin	Risk of stomach bleeding and ulcers.
Ketoconazole	Reduced ketoconazole effect.
Meperidine	Increased atropine and hyoscyamine effect.
Methylphenidate	Increased atropine and hyoscyamine effect.
Minoxidil	Decreased minoxidil effect.
Monoamine oxidase (MAO) inhibitors*	Increased belladonna and atropine effect.
Orphenadrine	Increased atropine and hyoscyamine effect.
Oxprenolol	Decreased anti-hypertensive effect of oxprenolol.
Para-aminosalicylic acid (PAS)	Possible salicylate toxicity.
Penicillins*	Increased effect of both drugs.
Phenobarbital	Decreased salicylate effect.
Phenothiazines*	Increased atropine and hyoscyamine effect.
Phenytoin	Increased phenytoin effect.
Pilocarpine	Loss of pilocarpine effect in glaucoma treatment.
Potassium supplements*	Possible intestinal ulcers with oral potassium tablets.
Probenecid	Decreased probenecid effect.
Propranolol	Decreased salicylate effect.
Rauwolfia alkaloids*	Decreased salicylate effect.

*See Glossary

GENERIC NAME OR DRUG CLASS	COMBINED EFFECT	GENERIC NAME OR DRUG CLASS	COMBINED EFFECT

ATROPINE, HYOSCYAMINE, METHENAMINE, METHYLENE BLUE, PHENYLSALICYLATE & BENZOIC ACID continued

Salicylates*	Likely salicylate toxicity.
Sedatives* or central nervous system (CNS) depressants*	Increased sedative effect of both drugs.
Sodium bicarbonate	Decreased methenamine effect.
Spironolactone	Decreased spironolactone effect.
Sulfa drugs*	Possible kidney damage.
Sulfinpyrazone	Decreased sulfinpyrazone effect.
Vitamin C (1 to 4 grams per day)	Increased effect of methenamine, contributing to urine acidity; decreased atropine effect; possible salicylate toxicity.

BARBITURATES

Lamotrigine	Decreased lamotrigine effect.
Leukotriene modifiers	Decreased montelukast effect.
Meglitinides	Increased blood level of meglitinides.
Mind-altering drugs*	Dangerous sedation. Avoid.
Modafinil	Increased modafinil effect.
Monoamine oxidase (MAO) inhibitors*	Increased barbiurate effect.
Mifepristone	Decreased effect of mifepristone.
Narcotics*	Dangerous sedation. Avoid.
Sertraline	Increased depressive effects of both drugs.
Sotalol	Increased barbiturate effect. Dangerous sedation.
Valproic acid	Increased barbiturate effect.
Zaleplon	Decreased zaleplon effect.

BARBITURATES, ASPIRIN & CODEINE (Also contains caffeine)

Anticonvulsants*	Changed seizure patterns.
Antidepressants*	Decreased antidepressant effect. Possible dangerous oversedation.
Antidiabetics, oral*	Increased butalbital effect. Low blood sugar.
Antihistamines*	Dangerous sedation. Avoid.
Anti-inflammatory drugs, nonsteroidal (NSAIDs)*	Risk of stomach bleeding and ulcers.
Aspirin, other	Likely aspirin toxicity.
Beta-adrenergic blocking agents*	Decreased effect of beta-adrenergic blocker.
Carteolol	Increased narcotic effect. Dangerous sedation.
Contraceptives, oral*	Decreased contraceptive effect.
Digitoxin	Decreased digitoxin effect.
Doxycycline	Decreased doxycycline effect.
Dronabinol	Increased effect of drugs.

*See Glossary

GENERIC NAME OR DRUG CLASS	COMBINED EFFECT	GENERIC NAME OR DRUG CLASS	COMBINED EFFECT

BARBITURATES, ASPIRIN & CODEINE (Also contains caffeine) continued

Furosemide	Possible aspirin toxicity.
Gold compounds*	Increased likelihood of kidney damage.
Griseofulvin	Decreased griseofulvin effect.
Indapamide	Increased indapamide effect.
Indomethacin	Risk of stomach bleeding and ulcers.
Lamotrigine	Decreased lamotrigine effect.
Methotrexate	Increased methotrexate effect.
Mind-altering drugs*	Dangerous sedation. Avoid.
Minoxidil	Decreased minoxidil effect.
Monoamine oxidase (MAO) inhibitors*	Increased butalbital effect.
Naltrexone	Decreased analgesic effect.
Narcotics*	Dangerous sedation. Avoid.
Nitrates*	Excessive blood pressure drop.
Pain relievers*	Dangerous sedation. Avoid.
Para-aminosalicylic acid	Possible aspirin toxicity.
Penicillins*	Increased effect of drugs.
Phenobarbital	Decreased aspirin effect.
Phenothiazines*	Increased phenothiazine effect.
Phenytoin	Increased phenytoin effect.
Probenecid	Decreased probenecid effect.
Propranolol	Decreased aspirin effect.
Rauwolfia alkaloids*	Decreased aspirin effect.
Salicylates*	Likely aspirin toxicity.
Sedatives*	Dangerous sedation. Avoid.
Sleep inducers*	Dangerous sedation. Avoid.
Sotalol	Increased narcotic effect. Dangerous sedation.
Spironolactone	Decreased spirono-lactone effect.
Sulfinpyrazone	Decreased sulfin-pyrazone effect.
Tranquilizers*	Dangerous sedation. Avoid.
Valproic acid	Increased phenobarbital effect.
Vitamin C (large doses)	Possible aspirin toxicity.
Zidovudine	Increased toxicity of both.

BELLADONNA ALKALOIDS & BARBITURATES

Attapulgite	Decreased belladonna effect.
Beta-adrenergic blocking agents*	Decreased effects of beta-adrenergic blocker.
Carteolol	Increased barbiturate effect. Dangerous sedation.
Central nervous system (CNS) depressants*	Dangerous sedation. Avoid.
Contraceptives, oral*	Decreased contra-ceptive effect.
Digitoxin	Decreased digitoxin effect.
Doxycycline	Decreased doxycycline effect.
Dronabinol	Increased effects of both drugs. Avoid.
Furosemide	Possible orthostatic hypotension.
Griseofulvin	Decreased griseofulvin effect.
Haloperidol	Increased internal eye pressure.

*See Glossary

GENERIC NAME OR DRUG CLASS	COMBINED EFFECT	GENERIC NAME OR DRUG CLASS	COMBINED EFFECT

BELLADONNA ALKALOIDS & BARBITURATES continued

GENERIC NAME OR DRUG CLASS	COMBINED EFFECT
Indapamide	Increased indapamide effect.
Ketoconazole	Decreased ketoconazole effect.
Meperidine	Increased belladonna effect.
Methylphenidate	Increased belladonna effect.
Metronidazole	Decreased metronidazole effect.
Mind-altering drugs*	Dangerous sedation. Avoid.
Monoamine oxidase (MAO) inhibitors*	Increased belladonna and barbiturate effect.
Narcotics*	Dangerous sedation. Avoid.
Nitrates*	Increased internal eye pressure.
Nizatidine	Increased nizatidine effect.
Orphenadrine	Increased belladonna effect.
Pain relievers*	Dangerous sedation. Avoid.
Phenothiazines*	Increased belladonna effect. Danger of oversedation.
Pilocarpine	Loss of pilocarpine effect in glaucoma treatment.
Potassium supplements*	Possible intestinal ulcers with oral potassium tablets.
Quinidine	Increased belladonna effect.
Sedatives*	Dangerous sedation. Avoid.
Sleep inducers*	Dangerous sedation. Avoid.
Sotalol	Increased barbiturate effect. Dangerous sedation.
Tranquilizers*	Dangerous sedation. Avoid.
Valproic acid	Increased barbiturate effect.
Vitamin C	Decreased belladonna effect. Avoid large doses of vitamin C.

BENZODIAZEPINES

GENERIC NAME OR DRUG CLASS	COMBINED EFFECT
Narcotics*	Increased sedative effect of both drugs.
Nefazodone	Increased effect of nefazodone and alprazolam.
Nicotine	Increased benzodiazepine effect.
Omeprazole	Delayed excretion of benzodiazepine causing increased amount of benzodiazepine in blood.
Probenecid	Increased benzodiazepine effect.
Sertraline	Increased depressive effects of both drugs.
Zidovudine	Increased toxicity of zidovudine.

BETA-ADRENERGIC BLOCKING AGENTS

GENERIC NAME OR DRUG CLASS	COMBINED EFFECT
Diazoxide	Additional blood pressure drop.
Estrogens*	May cause blood pressure problems.
Flecainide	Increased effect of toxicity on heart muscle.
Fluvoxamine	Increased beta blocker effect.

*See Glossary

GENERIC NAME OR DRUG CLASS	COMBINED EFFECT	GENERIC NAME OR DRUG CLASS	COMBINED EFFECT

BETA-ADRENERGIC BLOCKING AGENTS continued

GENERIC NAME OR DRUG CLASS	COMBINED EFFECT
Guanabenz	May cause blood pressure problems.
Insulin	Hypoglycemic effects may be prolonged.
Leukotriene modifiers	Increased beta blocker effect.
Meglitinides	Increased risk of low blood sugar.
Miglitol	Decreased effect of propranolol.
Molindone	Increased tranquilizer effect.
Monoamine oxidase (MAO) inhibitors*	High blood pressure following MAO discontinuation.
Nefazodone	Dosages of both drugs may require adjustment.
Nicotine	Increased effect of propanolol.
Nitrates*	Possible excessive blood pressure drop.
Phenothiazines	Increased effect of both drugs.
Phenytoin	Decreased beta blocker effect.
Propafenone	Increased beta blocker effect.
Quinidine	May cause heart problems.
Reserpine	Increased reserpine effect. Excessive sedation and depression. Additional blood pressure drop.
Sympathomimetics*	Decreased effects of both drugs.
Warfarin	Increased warfarin effect.
Xanthines (aminophylline, theophylline)	Decreased effects of both drugs.

BETA-ADRENERGIC BLOCKING AGENTS & THIAZIDE DIURETICS

GENERIC NAME OR DRUG CLASS	COMBINED EFFECT
Antidiabetics*	Increased anti-diabetic effect.
Antihistamines*	Decreased anti-histamine effect.
Antihypertensives*	Increased anti-hypertensive effect.
Anti-inflammatory drugs, nonsteroidal (NSAIDs)*	Decreased anti-inflammatory effect.
Barbiturates*	Increased barbiturate effect. Dangerous sedation.
Bumetanide	Increased diuretic effect.
Calcium channel blockers*	Increased antihypertensive effect. Dosages of both drugs may require adjustments.
Cholestyramine	Decreased hydro-chlorthiazide effect.
Diclofenac	Decreased anti-hypertensive effect.
Digitalis preparations*	Excessive potassium loss that causes dangerous heart rhythms. Can either increase or decrease heart rate. Improves irregular heartbeat.
Diuretics, thiazide*	Increased effect of other thiazide diuretics.
Ethacrynic acid	Increased diuretic effect.
Furosemide	Increased diuretic effect.
Guanfacine	Increased effect of both drugs.
Hypoglycemics, oral*	Decreased ability to lower blood glucose.
Indapamide	Increased diuretic effect.
Insulin	Decreased ability to lower blood glucose.

*See Glossary

GENERIC NAME OR DRUG CLASS	COMBINED EFFECT	GENERIC NAME OR DRUG CLASS	COMBINED EFFECT

BETA-ADRENERGIC BLOCKING AGENTS & THIAZIDE DIURETICS continued

GENERIC NAME OR DRUG CLASS	COMBINED EFFECT
Lisinopril	Increased anti-hypertensive effect. Dosage of each may require adjustment.
Metolazone	Increased diuretic effect.
Miglitol	Decreased effect of propranolol.
Monoamine oxidase (MAO) inhibitors*	Increased hydro chlorothiazide effect.
Narcotics*	Increased narcotic effect. Dangerous sedation.
Nicardipine	Possible irregular heartbeat and congestive heart failure.
Nicotine	Increased beta blocker effect.
Nitrates*	Excessive blood pressure drop.
Phenytoin	Increased beta adrenergic effect.
Potassium supplements*	Decreased potassium effect.
Probenecid	Decreased probenecid effect.
Propafenone	Increased beta blocker effect.
Quinidine	Slows heart excessively.
Reserpine	Increased reserpine effect. Excessive sedation and depression.
Sympathomimetics*	Decreased effectiveness of both.
Theophylline	Decreased effectiveness of both.
Tocainide	May worsen congestive heart failure.
Zinc supplements	Increased need for zinc.

BRONCHODILATORS, ADRENERGIC

GENERIC NAME OR DRUG CLASS	COMBINED EFFECT
Rauwolfia	Decreased rauwolfia effect.
Sympathomimetics*, other	Increased brochodilator effect.
Terazosin	Decreased effectiveness of terazosin.
Theophylline	Increased gastro-intestinal intolerance.
Thyroid hormones*	Increased bronchodilator effect.
Tolcapone	May require adjustment in dosage.

BRONCHODILATORS, XANTHINE

GENERIC NAME OR DRUG CLASS	COMBINED EFFECT
Tacrine	Increased bronchodilator effect.
Ticlopidine	Increased theophylline effect.
Troleandomycin	Increased bronchodilator effect.
Zafirlukast	May increase effect of zafirlukast.
Zileuton	Increased theophylline effect.

CALCIUM CHANNEL BLOCKERS

GENERIC NAME OR DRUG CLASS	COMBINED EFFECT
Metformin	Increased metformin effect.
Nicardipine	Possible increased effect and toxicity of each drug.
Nimodipine	Dangerous blood pressure drop.
Nitrates*	Reduced angina attacks.

*See Glossary

GENERIC NAME OR DRUG CLASS	COMBINED EFFECT
CALCIUM SUPPLEMENTS	
Quinidine	Increased quinidine effect.
Rifampin	Decreased effect of calcium channel blocker.
Salicylates*	Increased salicylate effect.
Sulfa drugs*	Decreased sulfa effect.
Tetracyclines*	Decreased tetracycline effect.
Theophylline	May increase effect and toxicity of theophylline.
Vitamin A	Decreased vitamin effect.
Vitamin D	Increased vitamin absorption, sometimes excessively; decreased effect of calcium channel blocker.
Zafirlukast	May increase calcium channel blocker effect.
CARBAMAZEPINE	
Clozapine	Toxic effect on bone marrow and central nervous system.
Contraceptives, oral*	Reduced contraceptive protection. Use barrier birth control method.
Desmopressin	May increase desmopressin effect.
Digitalis preparations*	Excessive slowing of heart.
Diltiazem	Increased effect of carbamzepine.
Doxepin (topical)	Increased risk of toxicity of both drugs.
Doxycycline	Decreased doxycycline effect.
Estrogens*	Decreased estrogen effect.
Erythromycins*	Increased carbamazepine effect.
Ethinamate	Dangerous increased effects of ethinamate. Avoid combining.
Felbamate	Increased side effects and adverse reactions.
Fluoxetine	Increased carbamazepine effect.
Fluvoxamine	Possible toxicity of carbamazepine.
Guanfacine	May increase depressant effects of either drug.
Isoniazid	Increased risk of liver damage.
Itraconazole	Decreased itraconazole effect.
Lamotrigine	Decreased lamotrigine effect. Increased risk of side effects.
Leucovorin	High alcohol content of leucovorin may cause adverse effects.
Leukotriene modifiers	Increased effect of carbamazepine.
Mebendazole	Decreased effect of mebendazole.
Meglitinides	Blood sugar problems.
Mifeprisone	Decreased effect of mifepristone.
Modafinil	Increased antidepressant effect.
Monoamine oxidase (MAO) Inhibitors*	Dangerous overstimulation. Avoid.
Nicardipine	May increase carbamazepine effect and toxicity.
Nimodipine	May increase carbamazepine effect and toxicity.

*See Glossary

GENERIC NAME OR DRUG CLASS	COMBINED EFFECT	GENERIC NAME OR DRUG CLASS	COMBINED EFFECT

CARBAMAZEPINE continued

GENERIC NAME OR DRUG CLASS	COMBINED EFFECT
Nizatidine	Increased carbamazepine effect and toxicity.
Olanzapine	Decreased effect of olanzapine.
Phenytoin	Decreased carbamazepine effect.
Phenobarbital	Decreased carbamazepine effect.
Primidone	Decreased carbamazepine effect.
Propoxyphene (Darvon)	Increased toxicity of both. Avoid.
Risperidone	Decreased risperidone effect.
Sertraline	Increased depressive effects of both drugs.
Tiopronin	Increased risk of toxicity to bone marrow.
Tramadol	Decreased tramadol effect.
Verapamil	Possible increased carbamazepine effect.
Zafirlukast	May increase effect of carbamazepine.
Zaleplon	Decreased zaleplon effect.

CHLORZOXAZONE & ACETAMINOPHEN

GENERIC NAME OR DRUG CLASS	COMBINED EFFECT
Tranquilizers*	Increased sedation.
Zidovudine	Increased toxicity of zidovudine.

CLONIDINE & CHLORTHALIDONE

GENERIC NAME OR DRUG CLASS	COMBINED EFFECT
Fenfluramine	Possible increased clonidine effect.
Guanfacine	Impaired blood pressure control.
Indapamide	Increased diuretic effect.
Lithium	Increased lithium effect.
Monoamine oxidase (MAO) inhibitors*	Increased chlorthalidone effect.
Nabilone	Greater depression of central nervous system.
Nicardipine	Blood pressure drop. Dosage may require adjustment.
Nitrates*	Possible excessive blood pressure drop.
Potassium supplements*	Decreased potassium effect.
Probenecid	Decreased probenecid effect.
Sedatives* or central nervous system (CNS) depressants*	Increased sedative effect of both drugs.
Sotalol	Decreased antihypertensive effect.
Terazosin	Decreased terazosin effect.

CONTRACEPTIVES, ORAL & SKIN

GENERIC NAME OR DRUG CLASS	COMBINED EFFECT
Meprobamate	Decreased contraceptive effect.
Mineral oil	Decreased contraceptive effect.
Non-nucleoside reverse transcriptase inhibitors	Decreased contraceptive effect. Use alternative birth control method.
Phenothiazines*	Increased phenothiazine effect.

ADDITIONAL DRUG INTERACTIONS

*See Glossary

GENERIC NAME OR DRUG CLASS	COMBINED EFFECT	GENERIC NAME OR DRUG CLASS	COMBINED EFFECT

CONTRACEPTIVES, ORAL & SKIN continued

Rifampin	Decreased contraceptive effect.	**Thiazolidinediones**	Decreased contraceptive effect.
Sulfadoxine and pyrimethamine	Reduced reliability of the pill.	**Ursodiol**	Decreased ursodiol effect.
Terazosin	Decreases terazosin effect.	**Vitamin A**	Vitamin A excess.
Tetracyclines*	Decreased contraceptive effect.	**Vitamin C**	Possible increased contraceptive effect.

CYCLOSPORINE

Nimodipine	Increased cyclosporine toxicity.	**Tiopronin**	Increased risk of toxicity to kidneys.
Orlistat	Unknown effect. Monitor closely.	**Vancomycin**	Increased chance of hearing loss or kidney damage.
Rifampin	Decreased effect of cyclosporine.	**Virus vaccines**	Increased adverse reactions to vaccine.
Terbinafine (oral)	Decreased effect of cyclosporine.	**Zafirlukast**	May increase effect of cyclosporine.
Thiazolidinediones	Decreased effect of cyclosporine.		

DIFENOXIN & ATROPINE

Nitrates*	Increased internal eye pressure.	**Potassium supplements***	Possible intestinal ulcers with oral potassium tablets.
Orphenadrine	Increased atropine effect.	**Procainamide**	Increased atropine effect.
Phenothiazines*	Increased atropine effect.	**Sertraline**	Increased depressive effects of both drugs.
Pilocarpine	Loss of pilocarpine effect in glaucoma treatment.	**Vitamin C**	Decreased atropine effect. Avoid large doses of vitamin C.

DIGITALIS PREPARATIONS (Digitalis Glycosides)

Metoclopramide	Decreased digitalis absorption.	**Oxyphenbutazone**	Decreased digitalis effect.
Mineral Oil	Decreased digitalis effect.	**Paroxetine**	Increased levels of paroxetine in blood.
Nefazodone	Increased effect of digoxin.	**Phenobarbital**	Decreased digitalis effect.
Nicardipine	Increased digitalis effect. May need to reduce dose.	**Phenylbutazone**	Decreased digitalis effect.
Nizatidine	Increased digitalis effect.		

*See Glossary

GENERIC NAME OR DRUG CLASS	COMBINED EFFECT	GENERIC NAME OR DRUG CLASS	COMBINED EFFECT

DIGITALIS PREPARATIONS (Digitalis Glycosides) continued

GENERIC NAME OR DRUG CLASS	COMBINED EFFECT
Potassium supplements*	Overdose of either drug may cause severe heartbeat irregularity.
Propafenone	Increased digitalis absorption. May require decreased digitalis dosage.
PTU/Metronidazole	Decreased digitalis effect.
Quinidine	Increased digitalis effect.
Rauwolfia alkaloids*	Increased digitalis effect.
Rifampin	Possible decreased digitalis effect.
Sotalol	Can either increase or decrease heart rate. Improves irregular heartbeat.
Spironolactone	Increased digitalis effect. May require digitalis dosage reduction.
Sulfasalazine	Decreased digitalis absorption.
Sympathomimetics*	Increased risk of heartbeat irregularities.
Tetracycline	May increase digitalis absorption.
Thyroid hormones*	Digitalis toxicity.
Ticlopidine	Slightly decreased digitalis effect (digoxin only).
Trazodone	Possible increased digitalis toxicity.
Triamterene	Possible decreased digitalis effect.
Verapamil	Increased digitalis effect.

DIURETICS, LOOP

GENERIC NAME OR DRUG CLASS	COMBINED EFFECT
Meloxicam	Decreased effect of diuretic .
Nephrotoxics*	Increased risk of toxicity.
Nimodipine	Dangerous blood pressure drop.
Nitrates*	Excessive blood pressure drop.
Phenytoin	Decreased diuretic effect.
Potassium supplements*	Decreased potassium effect.
Probenecid	Decreased probenecid effect.
Salicylates* (including aspirin)	Dangerous salicylate retention.
Sedatives*	Increased diuretic effect.

DIURETICS, POTASSIUM-SPARING & HYDROCHLOROTHIAZIDE

GENERIC NAME OR DRUG CLASS	COMBINED EFFECT
Colestipol	Decreased diuretic effect. Take 1 hour before diuretic.
Cyclosporine	Increased potassium levels.
Digitalis preparations*	Increased digitalis effect.
Diuretics*, other	Increased effect of both drugs.
Folic acid	Decreased effect of folic acid.
Lithium	Possible lithium toxicity.
Metformin	Increased metformin effect.
Potassium-containing medications	Increased potassium levels.

GENERIC NAME OR DRUG CLASS	COMBINED EFFECT	GENERIC NAME OR DRUG CLASS	COMBINED EFFECT

DIURETICS, THIAZIDE

GENERIC NAME OR DRUG CLASS	COMBINED EFFECT
Indapamide	Increased diuretic effect.
Indomethacin	Decreased anti-hypertensive effect.
Lithium	Increased effect of lithium.
Meglitinides	Increased blood sugar levels.
Monoamine oxidase (MAO) inhibitors*	Increased anti-hypertensive effect.
Nicardipine	Blood pressure drop. Dosages may require adjustment.
Nimodipine	Dangerous blood pressure drop.
Nitrates*	Excessive blood pressure drop.
Opiates*	Dizziness or weakness when standing up after sitting or lying down.
Pentoxifylline	Increased anti-hypertensive effect.
Potassium supplements*	Decreased potassium effect.
Probenecid	Decreased probenecid effect.
Sotalol	Increased anti-hypertensive effect.
Terazosin	Decreased terazosin effect.
Toremifene	Possible increased calcium.
Zinc supplements	Increased need for zinc.

ERGOTAMINE, BELLADONNA & PHENOBARBITAL

GENERIC NAME OR DRUG CLASS	COMBINED EFFECT
Ephedrine	Dangerous blood pressure rise.
Epinephrine	Dangerous blood pressure rise.
Erythromycin	Decreased ergotamine effect.
Griseofulvin	Decreased griseofulvin effect.
Guanethidine	Decreased belladonna effect.
Haloperidol	Increased internal eye pressure.
Indapamide	Increased indapamide effect.
Meperidine	Increased belladonna effect.
Methylphenidate	Increased belladonna effect.
Metoclopramide	May decrease metoclopramide effect.
Mind-altering drugs*	Dangerous sedation. Avoid.
Monoamine oxidase (MAO) inhibitors*	Increased belladonna and phenobarbital effect.
Narcotics*	Dangerous sedation. Avoid.
Nitrates*	Increased internal eye pressure.
Nitroglycerin	Decreased nitroglycerin effect.
Orphenadrine	Increased belladonna effect.
Pain relievers*	Dangerous sedation. Avoid.
Phenothiazines*	Increased belladonna effect.
Pilocarpine	Loss of pilocarpine effect in glaucoma treatment.
Potassium supplements*	Possible intestinal ulcers with oral potassium tablets.
Quinidine	Increased belladonna effect.
Reserpine	Decreased belladonna effect.
Sedatives*	Dangerous sedation. Avoid.
Sleep inducers*	Dangerous sedation. Avoid.
Sumatriptan	Increased vasoconstriction. Delay 24 hours between drugs.

*See Glossary

ERGOTAMINE, BELLADONNA & PHENOBARBITAL continued

GENERIC NAME OR DRUG CLASS	COMBINED EFFECT
Tranquilizers*	Dangerous sedation. Avoid.
Troleandomycin	Increased adverse reactions of ergotamine.
Valproic acid	Increased phenobarbital effect.
Vitamin C	Decreased belladonna effect. Avoid large doses of vitamin C.

ESTROGENS

GENERIC NAME OR DRUG CLASS	COMBINED EFFECT
Insulin lispro	May need increased dosage of insulin.
Meprobamate	Increased estrogen effect.
Phenobarbital	Decreased estrogen effect.
Primidone	Decreased estrogen effect.
Pyridoxine (vitamin B-6)	Decreased pyridoxine effect.
Raloxifene	Not recommended for use with estrogen.
Rifampin	Decreased estrogen effect.
Tamoxifen	Decreased tamoxifen effect.
Thyroid hormones*	Decreased thyroid effect.
Ursodiol	Decreased effect of ursodiol.
Vitamin C	Possible increased estrogen effect.

FLUOROQUINOLONES

GENERIC NAME OR DRUG CLASS	COMBINED EFFECT
Digoxin	Increased digoxin effect.
Cyclosporine	Increased cyclosporine effect.
Didanosine	Decreased fluoroquinolone effect.
Iron supplements	Decreased fluoroquinolone effect.
Oxtriphylline	Increased risk of oxtriphylline toxicity.
Phenytoin	Decreased effect of phenytoin with ciprofloxacin.
Probenecid	Increased effect of fluoroquinolone.
QT interval prolongation causing drugs*	Heart rhythm problems.
Sucralfate	Decreased fluoroquinolone effect.
Theophylline	Increased risk of theophylline toxicity.
Warfarin	Increased warfarin effect.
Zinc	Decreased fluoroquinolone effect.

GUANETHIDINE

GENERIC NAME OR DRUG CLASS	COMBINED EFFECT
Rauwolfia alkaloids*	Excessively slow heartbeat. Weakness and faintness upon rising from chair or bed.
Sotalol	Increased antihypertensive effect.
Terazosin	Decreased effectiveness of terazosin.
Thioxanthenes*	Decreased guanethidine effect.
Trimeprazine	Decreased guanethidine effect.

*See Glossary

GENERIC NAME OR DRUG CLASS	COMBINED EFFECT

GUANETHIDINE & HYDROCHLOROTHIAZIDE

GENERIC NAME OR DRUG CLASS	COMBINED EFFECT
Digitalis preparations*	Excessive potassium loss that causes dangerous heart rhythms.
Diuretics, thiazide*	Increased thiazide and guanethidine effects.
Haloperidol	Decreased guanethidine effect.
Indapamide	Possible increased effects of both drugs. When monitored carefully, combination may be beneficial in controlling hypertension.
Insulin	Increased insulin effect.
Lithium	Increased lithium effect.
Minoxidil	Dosage adjustments may be necessary to keep blood pressure at proper level.
Monoamine oxidase (MAO) inhibitors*	Increased hydrochlorothiazide effect.
Nicardipine	Blood pressure drop. Dosages may require adjustment.
Nimodipine	Dangerous blood pressure drop.
Nitrates*	Excessive blood pressure drop.
Oxprenolol	Increased antihypertensive effects. Dosages of both drugs may require adjustments.
Phenothiazines*	Decreased guanethidine effect.
Potassium supplements*	Decreased potassium effect.
Probenecid	Decreased probenecid effect.
Sotalol	Increased antihypertensive effect.
Terazosin	Decreased effectiveness of terazosin.

GUANFACINE

GENERIC NAME OR DRUG CLASS	COMBINED EFFECT
Sympathomimetics*	May decrease antihypertensive effects of guanfacine.
Terazosin	Decreased effectiveness of terazosin.

HALOPERIDOL

GENERIC NAME OR DRUG CLASS	COMBINED EFFECT
Fluoxetine	Increased depressant effects of both drugs.
Guanethidine	Decreased guanethidine effect.
Guanfacine	May increase depressant effects of either drug.
Leucovorin	High alcohol content of leucovorin may cause adverse effects.
Levodopa	Decreased levodopa effect.
Lithium	Increased toxicity.
Loxapine	May increase toxic effects of both drugs.
Methyldopa	Possible psychosis.
Narcotics*	Excessive sedation.
Nefazodone	Unknown effect. May require dosage adjustment.
Pergolide	Decreased pergolide effect.
Procarbazine	Increased sedation.
Sertraline	Increased depressive effects of both drugs.

***See Glossary**

HISTAMINE H_2 RECEPTOR ANTAGONISTS

GENERIC NAME OR DRUG CLASS	COMBINED EFFECT
Digitalis preparations*	Increased digitalis effect.
Dofetilide	Increased risk of heart problems.
Encainide	Increased effect of histamine H_2 receptor antagonist.
Flurazepam	Increased effect and toxicity of flurazepam.
Glipizide	Increased effect and toxicity of glipizide.
Itraconazole	Decreased absorption of itraconazole.
Ketoconazole	Decreased ketoconazole absorption.
Labetalol	Increased antihypertensive effects.
Metformin	Increased metformin effect.
Metoclopramide	Decreased absorption of histamine H_2 receptor antagonist.
Methadone	Increased effect and toxicity of methadone.
Metoclopramide	Decreased absorption of histamine H_2 receptor antagonist.
Methadone	Increased effect and toxicity of methadone.
Metoprolol	Increased effect and toxicity of metoprolol.
Metronidazole	Increased effect and toxicity of metronidazole.
Miglitol	Decreased effect of ranitidine.
Moricizine	Increased concentration of H_2 receptor antagonist in the blood.
Morphine	Increased effect and toxicity of morphine.
Nicardipine	Possible increased effect and toxicity of nicardipine.
Nimodipine	Possible increased effect and toxicity of nimodipine.
Paroxetine	Increased levels of paroxetine in blood.
Phenytoin	Increased effect and toxicity of phenytoin
Propafenone	Increased effect of both drugs and increased risk of toxicity.
Propranolol	Possible increased propranolol effect.
Quinidine	Increased quinidine effect.
Tacrine	Increased tacrine effect.
Tamoxifen	Decreased tamoxifen effect.
Terbinafine (oral)	Increased effect of terbinafine with cimetidine.
Theophylline	Increases theophylline effect.
Triazolam	Increased effect and toxicity of triazolam.
Venlafaxine	With cimetidine—Increased risk of adverse reactions.
Verapamil	Increased effect and toxicity of verapamil.
Zaleplon	Increases zaleplon effect.

HYDRALAZINE

GENERIC NAME OR DRUG CLASS	COMBINED EFFECT
Sotalol	Increased antihypertensive effect.
Terazosin	Decreased effectiveness of terazosin.

***See Glossary**

GENERIC NAME OR DRUG CLASS	COMBINED EFFECT

HYDRALAZINE & HYDROCHLOROTHIAZIDE

GENERIC NAME OR DRUG CLASS	COMBINED EFFECT
Antihypertensives*, other	Increased anti-hypertensive effect.
Antivirals, HIV/AIDS*	Increased risk of peripheral neuropathy.
Barbiturates*	Increased hydrochlorothiazide effect.
Carteolol	Decreased anti-hypertensive effect.
Cholestyramine	Decreased hydrochlorothiazide effect.
Cortisone drugs*	Excessive potassium loss that causes dangerous heart rhythms.
Diazoxide	Increased anti-hypertensive effect.
Digitalis preparations*	Excessive potassium loss that causes dangerous heart rhythms.
Diuretics*, oral	Increased effect of both drugs. When monitored carefully, combination may be beneficial in controlling hypertension.
Indapamide	Increased diuretic effect.
Lithium	Increased lithium effect.
Monoamine oxidase (MAO) inhibitors*	Increased effect of drugs.
Nimodipine	Dangerous blood pressure drop.
Nitrates*	Excessive blood pressure drop.
Potassium supplements*	Decreased potassium effect.
Probenecid	Decreased probenecid effect.

INDAPAMIDE

GENERIC NAME OR DRUG CLASS	COMBINED EFFECT
Opiates*	Weakness and faintness when arising from bed or chair.
Probenecid	Decreased probenecid effect.
Sotalol	Increased anti-hypertensive effect.
Terazosin	Decreased effectiveness of terazosin.

KAOLIN, PECTIN, BELLADONNA & OPIUM

GENERIC NAME OR DRUG CLASS	COMBINED EFFECT
Ketoconazole	Decreased ketoconazole effect.
Lincomycins*	Decreased absorption of lincomycin. Separate doses by at least 2 hours.
MAO inhibitors*	Increased belladonna effect.
Meperidine	Increased belladonna effect.
Methylphenidate	Increased belladonna effect.
Mind-altering drugs*	Increased sedative effect.
Narcotics, other*	Increased narcotic effect.
Nitrates*	Increased internal eye pressure.
Orphenadrine	Increased belladonna effect.
Phenothiazines*	Increased sedative effect of paregoric.
Pilocarpine	Loss of pilocarpine effect in glaucoma treatment.
Potassium supplements*	Possible intestinal ulcers with oral potassium tablets.
Sedatives*	Excessive sedation.
Sleep inducers*	Increased effect of sleep inducers.

*See Glossary

GENERIC NAME OR DRUG CLASS	COMBINED EFFECT

KAOLIN, PECTIN, BELLADONNA & OPIUM continued

GENERIC NAME OR DRUG CLASS	COMBINED EFFECT
Sotalol	Increased narcotic effect. Dangerous sedation.
Tranquilizers*	Increased tranquilizer effect.
Vitamin C	Decreased belladonna effect. Avoid large doses of vitamin C.
All other oral medicines	Decreased absorption of other medicines. Separate doses by at least 2 hours.

LITHIUM

GENERIC NAME OR DRUG CLASS	COMBINED EFFECT
Fluvoxamine	Increased risk of seizure.
Haloperidol	Increased toxicity of both drugs.
Indomethacin	Increased lithium effect.
Iodide salts	Increased lithium effects on thyroid function.
Ketoprofen	May increase lithium in blood.
Meloxicam	Increased lithium effect.
Methyldopa	Increased lithium effect.
Molindone	Brain changes.
Oxyphenbutazone	Increased lithium effect.
Phenothiazines*	Decreased lithium effect.
Phenylbutazone	Increased lithium effect.
Phenytoin	Increased lithium effect.
Potassium iodide	Increased potassium iodide effect.
Sodium bicarbonate	Decreased lithium effect.
Sumatriptan	Adverse effects unknown. Avoid.
Theophylline	Decreased lithium effect.
Tiopronin	Increased risk of toxicity to kidneys.

LOXAPINE

GENERIC NAME OR DRUG CLASS	COMBINED EFFECT
Rauwolfia	May increase toxic effects of both drugs.
Sertraline	Increased depressive effects of both drugs.
Thioxanthenes*	May increase toxic effects of both drugs

MAPROTILINE

GENERIC NAME OR DRUG CLASS	COMBINED EFFECT
Fluoxetine	Increased depressant effects of both drugs.
Guanethidine	Decreased guanethidine effect.
Guanfacine	May increase depressant effects of either drug.
Leucovorin	High alcohol content of leucovorin may cause adverse effects.
Levodopa	Decreased levodopa effect.
Lithium	Possible decreased seizure threshold.
Methyldopa	Decreased methyldopa effect.

ADDITIONAL DRUG INTERACTIONS

*See Glossary

GENERIC NAME OR DRUG CLASS	COMBINED EFFECT	GENERIC NAME OR DRUG CLASS	COMBINED EFFECT

MAPROLTILINE continued

GENERIC NAME OR DRUG CLASS	COMBINED EFFECT
Methylphenidate	Possible increased antidepressant effect and toxicity.
Molindone	Increased tranquilizer effect.
Monoamine oxidase (MAO) inhibitors*	Fever, delirium, convulsions.
Narcotics*	Dangerous oversedation.
Phenothiazines*	Possible increased antidepressant effect and toxicity.
Phenytoin	Decreased phenytoin effect.
Quinidine	Irregular heartbeat.
Selegiline	Fever, delirium, convulsions.
Sertraline	Increased depressive effects of both drugs.
Sympathomimetics*	Increased sympathomimetic effect.
Thyroid hormones*	Irregular heartbeat.

MEPROBAMATE & ASPIRIN

GENERIC NAME OR DRUG CLASS	COMBINED EFFECT
Ethacrynic acid	Possible aspirin toxicity.
Furosemide	Possible aspirin toxicity. May decrease furosemide effect.
Gold compounds*	Increased likelihood of kidney damage.
Indomethacin	Risk of stomach bleeding and ulcers.
Methotrexate	Increased methotrexate effect.
Minoxidil	Decreased minoxidil effect.
Monoamine oxidase (MAO) inhibitors*	Increased meprobamate effect.
Narcotics*	Increased narcotic effect.
Oxprenolol	Decreased antihypertensive effect of oxprenolol.
Para-aminosalicylic acid (PAS)	Possible aspirin toxicity.
Penicillins*	Increased effect of both drugs.
Phenobarbital	Decreased aspirin effect.
Phenytoin	Increased phenytoin effect.
Probenecid	Decreased probenecid effect.
Propranolol	Decreased aspirin effect.
Rauwolfia alkaloids*	Decreased aspirin effect.
Salicylates, other*	Likely aspirin toxicity.
Sedatives*	Increased sedative effect.
Sleep inducers*	Increased effect of sleep inducer.
Spironolactone	Decreased spironolactone effect.
Sulfinpyrazone	Decreased sulfinpyrazone effect.
Tranquilizers*	Increased tranquilizer effect.
Vancomycin	Increased chance of hearing loss.
Vitamin C (large doses)	Possible aspirin toxicity.

METFORMIN

GENERIC NAME OR DRUG CLASS	COMBINED EFFECT
Trimethoprim	Increased metformin effect.
Vancomycin	Increased metformin effect.

*See Glossary

METHOTREXATE

GENERIC NAME OR DRUG CLASS	COMBINED EFFECT
Sulfa drugs*	Possible methotrexate toxicity.
Sulfadoxine and pyrimethamine	Increased risk of toxicity.
Tetracyclines*	Possible methotrexate toxicity.
Tiopronin	Increased risk of toxicity to bone marrow and kidneys.
Vaccines, live or killed	Increased risk of toxicity or reduced effectiveness of vaccine.

METHYLDOPA

GENERIC NAME OR DRUG CLASS	COMBINED EFFECT
Methyprylon	Increased sedative effect, perhaps to dangerous level. Avoid.
Monoamine oxidase (MAO) inhibitors*	Dangerous blood pressure rise.
Nabilone	Greater depression of central nervous system.
Nicardipine	Blood pressure drop. Dosages may require adjustment.
Nimodipine	Dangerous blood pressure drop.
Norepinephrine	Decreased methyldopa effect.
Pergolide	Decreased pergolide effect.
Phenoxybenzamine	Urinary retention.
Phenylephrine	Decreased methyldopa effect.
Phenylpropanolamine	Decreased methyldopa effect.
Phenytoin	Possible increased methotrexate toxicity.
Probenecid	Possible methotrexate toxicity.
Propranolol	Increased blood pressure (rarely).
Pyrimethamine	Increased toxic effect of methotrexate.
Salicylates* (including aspirin)	Possible methotrexate toxicity.
Sertraline	Increased depressive effects of both drugs.
Sotalol	Increased antihypertensive effect.
Sympathomimetic drugs*	Increased risk of heart block and high blood pressure.
Terazosin	Decreased effectiveness of terazosin.
Tolbutamide	Increased tolbutamide effect.
Tolcapone	May require adjustment in dosage of methyldopa.

METHYLDOPA & THIAZIDE DIURETICS

GENERIC NAME OR DRUG CLASS	COMBINED EFFECT
Antihypertensives*	Increased antihypertensive effect.
Barbiturates*	Increased hydrochlorothiazide effect.
Carteolol	Increased antihypertensive effect.
Cholestyramine	Decreased hydrochlorothiazide effect.
Cortisone drugs*	Excessive potassium loss that causes dangerous heart rhythms.
Dapsone	Increased risk of adverse effect on blood cells.
Didanosine	Increased risk of pancreatitis.
Digitalis preparations*	Excessive potassium loss that causes dangerous heart rhythms.
Diuretics, thiazide*	Increased effect of both drugs.
Haloperidol	Increased sedation, possibly dementia.

ADDITIONAL DRUG INTERACTIONS

*See Glossary

GENERIC NAME OR DRUG CLASS	COMBINED EFFECT	GENERIC NAME OR DRUG CLASS	COMBINED EFFECT

METHYLDOPA & THIAZIDE DIURETICS continued

Indapamide	Increased diuretic effect.	**Phenoxybenzanine**	Urinary retention.
Levodopa	Increased effect of both drugs.	**Phenylephrine**	Decreased methyldopa effect.
Lithium	Increased lithium effect.	**Phenylpropanolamine**	Decreased methyldopa effect.
Monoamine oxidase (MAO) inhibitors*	Dangerous blood pressure changes.	**Potassium supplements***	Decreased potassium effect.
Nabilone	Greater depression of central nervous system.	**Propranolol**	Increased blood pressure (rarely).
Nicardipine	Blood pressure drop. Dosages may require adjustment.	**Sertraline**	Increased depressive effects of both drugs.
Nimodipine	Dangerous blood pressure drop.	**Sotalol**	Increased anti-hypertensive effect.
Nitrates*	Excessive blood pressure drop.	**Terazosin**	Decreased terazosin effect.
Norepinephrine	Decreased methyldopa effect.	**Tolbutamide**	Increased tolbutamide effect.
		Zinc supplements	Increased need for zinc.

METOCLOPRAMIDE

Narcotics*	Decreased metoclo-pramide effect.	**Sertraline**	Increased depressive effects of both drugs.
Nizatidine	Decreased nizatidine absorption.	**Tetracyclines***	Slow stomach emptying.
Pergolide	Decreased pergolide effect.	**Thiothixines***	Increased chance of muscle spasm and trembling.
Phenothiazines*	Increased chance of muscle spasm and trembling.		

MOLINDONE

Narcotics*	Increased narcotic effect.	**Sertraline**	Increased depressive effects of both drugs.
Phenytoin	Increased or decreased phenytoin effect.	**Sotalol**	Increased tranquilizer effect. Increased sotalol effect.

MONOAMINE OXIDASE (MAO) INHIBITORS

Central nervous system (CNS) depressants*	Excessive depressant action.	**Citalopram**	Can cause a life-threatening reaction. Avoid.

***See Glossary**

MONOAMINE OXIDASE (MAO) INHIBITORS continued

GENERIC NAME OR DRUG CLASS	COMBINED EFFECT
Clozapine	Toxic effect on the central nervous system.
Doxepin (topical)	Potentially life-threatening. Allow 14 days between use of the 2 drugs.
Dexfenfluramine	Potentially life-threatening. Allow 14 days between use of 2 drugs.
Dextromethorphan	Very high blood pressure.
Diuretics*	Excessively low blood pressure.
Ephedrine	Increased blood pressure.
Fluoxetine	Serotonin syndrome (muscle rigidity, confusion, high fever). Avoid. Increased risk and severity of side effects. Allow 4 weeks between use of the 2 drugs.
Fluvoxamine	Potentially life-threatening. Allow 14 days between use of the 2 drugs.
Furazolidine	Sudden, severe increase in blood pressure.
Guanadrel	High blood pressure.
Guanethidine	Blood pressure rise.
Guanfacine	May increase depressant effects of either drug.
Indapamide	Increased indapamide effect.
Insulin	Increased hypoglycemic effect.
Leucovorin	High alcohol content of leucovorin may cause adverse effects.
Levodopa	Sudden, severe blood pressure rise.
Maprotiline	Dangerous blood pressure rise.
Meglitinides	Increased risk of low blood sugar.
Methyldopa	Sudden, severe blood pressure rise.
Methylphenidate	Increased blood pressure.
Mirtazapine	Potentially life-threatening. Allow 14 days between use of 2 drugs.
Monoamine oxidase (MAO) inhibitors (others, when taken together)	High fever, convulsions, death.
Narcotics*	Severe high blood pressure.
Nefazodone	Potentially life-threatening. Allow 14 days between use of the 2 drugs.
Paroxetine	Can cause a life-threatening reaction. Avoid. Increased risk and severity of side effects. Allow 4 weeks between use of the 2 drugs.
Phenothiazines*	Possible increased phenothiazine toxicity.
Phenylpropanolamine	Increased blood pressure.
Pseudoephedrine	Increased blood pressure.
Sertraline	Serotonin syndrome (muscle rigidity, confusion, high fever). Avoid. Increased risk and severity of side effects. Allow 4 weeks between use of the 2 drugs.
Sympathomimetics*	Blood pressure rise to life-threatening level.
Tolcapone	May reduce effectiveness of MAO inhibitor.
Tramadol	Increased risk of seizures.

*See Glossary

GENERIC NAME OR DRUG CLASS	COMBINED EFFECT

MONOAMINE OXIDASE (MAO) INHIBITORS continued

GENERIC NAME OR DRUG CLASS	COMBINED EFFECT
Trazodone	Increased risk of mental status changes.
Venlafaxine	Increased risk and severity of side effects. Allow 4 weeks between use of the 2 drugs.

NARCOTIC ANALGESICS

GENERIC NAME OR DRUG CLASS	COMBINED EFFECT
Cimetidine	Possible increased narcotic effect and toxicity.
Clozapine	Toxic effect on the central nervous system.
Ethinamate	Dangerous increased effects of ethinamate. Avoid combining.
Fluoxetine	Increased depressant effects of both drugs.
Guanfacine	May increase depressant effects of either drug.
Leucovorin	High alcohol content of leucovorin may cause adverse effects.
Methyprylon	Increased sedative effect, perhaps to dangerous level. Avoid.
Metformin	Increased effect of metformin with morphine.
Mind-altering drugs*	Increased sedative effect.
Molindone	Increased narcotic effect.
Monoamine oxidase (MAO) inhibitors*	Serious toxicity (including death).
Nabilone	Greater depression of central nervous system.
Nalbuphine	Possibly precipitates withdrawal with chronic narcotic use.
Naltrexone	Precipitates withdrawal symptoms. May lead to respiratory arrest, coma and death.
Narcotics*, other	Increased narcotic effect.
Nicotine	Increased effect of pentazocine and propoxyphene.
Nitrates*	Excessive blood pressure drop.
Pentazocine	Possibly precipitates withdrawal with chronic narcotic use.
Phenothiazines*	Increased sedative effect.
Phenytoin	Possible decreased narcotic effect.
Rifampin	Possible decreased narcotic effect.
Sedatives*	Increased sedative effect.
Selegiline	Severe toxicity characterized by breathing difficulties, seizures, coma.
Sertraline	Increased depressive effects of both drugs.
Sleep inducers*	Increased sedative effect.
Sotalol	Increased narcotic effect. Dangerous sedation.
Tramadol	Increased sedation.
Tranquilizers*	Increased sedative effect.

*See Glossary

GENERIC NAME OR DRUG CLASS	COMBINED EFFECT	GENERIC NAME OR DRUG CLASS	COMBINED EFFECT

NARCOTIC ANALGESICS & ACETAMINOPHEN

GENERIC NAME OR DRUG CLASS	COMBINED EFFECT
Phenothiazines*	Increased phenothiazine effect.
Sedatives*	Increased sedative effect.
Selegiline	Severe toxicity characterized by breathing difficulty, seizures, coma.
Sertraline	Increased depressive effects of both drugs.
Sleep inducers*	Increased sedative effect.
Sotalol	Increased narcotic effect. Dangerous sedation.
Tetracyclines*	May slow tetracycline absorption. Space doses 2 hours apart.
Tramadol	Increased sedation.
Tranquilizers*	Increased sedative effect.
Zidovudine	Increased toxicity of zidovudine.

NARCOTIC ANALGESICS & ASPIRIN

GENERIC NAME OR DRUG CLASS	COMBINED EFFECT
Anti-inflammatory drugs, nonsteroidal (NSAIDs)*	Risk of stomach bleeding and ulcers.
Aspirin, other	Likely aspirin toxicity.
Bumetanide	Possible aspirin toxicity.
Carteolol	Increased narcotic effect. Dangerous sedation.
Ethacrynic acid	Possible aspirin toxicity.
Furosemide	Possible aspirin toxicity. May decrease furosemide effect.
Gold compounds*	Increased likelihood of kidney damage.
Indomethacin	Risk of stomach bleeding and ulcers.
Methotrexate	Increased metho-trexate effect.
Minoxidil	Decreased minoxidil effect.
Narcotics*, other	Increased narcotic effect.
Nitrates*	Excessive blood pressure drop.
Propranolol	Decreased aspirin effect.
Rauwolfia alkaloids*	Decreased aspirin effect.
Salicylates, other*	Likely aspirin toxicity.
Sedatives*	Increased sedative effect.
Selegiline	Severe toxicity characterized by breathing difficulties, seizures, coma.
Sleep inducers*	Increased sedative effect.
Sotalol	Increased narcotic effect. Dangerous sedation.
Spironolactone	Decreased spironolactone effect.
Sulfinpyrazone	Decreased sulfinpyrazone effect.
Ticlopidine	Decreased effects of both drugs.
Tramadol	Increased sedation.
Tranquilizers*	Increased sedative effect.
Valproic acid	May increase valproic acid effect.
Vitamin C (large doses)	Possible aspirin toxicity.

***See Glossary**

GENERIC NAME OR DRUG CLASS	COMBINED EFFECT	GENERIC NAME OR DRUG CLASS	COMBINED EFFECT

NEFAZODONE

GENERIC NAME OR DRUG CLASS	COMBINED EFFECT
Triazolam	Increased effects of both drugs.

NIMODIPINE

GENERIC NAME OR DRUG CLASS	COMBINED EFFECT
Theophylline	May increase theophylline effect and toxicity.
Timolol eye drops	May cause increased effect of nimodipine on heart function.
Tocainide	Increased likelihood of adverse reaction from either drug.
Vitamin D (large doses)	Decreased nimodipine effect.

NUCLEOSIDE REVERSE TRANSCRIPTASE INHIBITORS

GENERIC NAME OR DRUG CLASS	COMBINED EFFECT
Probenecid	Increased effect of zalcitabine and zidovudine.
Rifampin	Decreased zidovudine effect.
Tenofovir	Increased effect of didanosine. Take tenofovir 2 hours before or 1 hour after didanosine.
Tetracyclines	Decreased antibiotic effect.

ORPHENADRINE, ASPIRIN & CAFFEINE

GENERIC NAME OR DRUG CLASS	COMBINED EFFECT
Adrenocorticoids, systemic	Increased risk of ulcers. Increased adrenocorticoid effect.
Allopurinol	Decreased allopurinol effect.
Antacids*	Decreased aspirin effect.
Anticholinergics*	Increased anticholinergic effect.
Anticoagulants*	Increased anticoagulant effect. Abnormal bleeding.
Antidepressants, tricyclic*	Increased sedation.
Antidiabetics, oral*	Low blood sugar.
Anti-inflammatory drugs, nonsteroidal (NSAIDs)*	Risk of stomach bleeding and ulcers.
Aspirin, other	Likely aspirin toxicity.
Chlorpromazine	Hypoglycemia (low blood sugar).
Contraceptives, oral*	Increased caffeine effect.
Furosemide	Possible aspirin toxicity.
Gold compounds*	Increased likelihood of kidney damage.
Griseofulvin	Decreased griseofulvin effect.
Indomethacin	Risk of stomach bleeding and ulcers.
Isoniazid	Increased caffeine effect.
Levodopa	Increased levodopa effect. (Improves effectiveness in treating Parkinson's disease.)
Methotrexate	Increased methotrexate effect.
Minoxidil	Decreased minoxidil effect.
Monoamine oxidase (MAO) inhibitors*	Dangerous blood pressure rise.
Nitrates*	Increased internal eye pressure.

*See Glossary

GENERIC NAME OR DRUG CLASS	COMBINED EFFECT	GENERIC NAME OR DRUG CLASS	COMBINED EFFECT

ORPHENADRINE, ASPIRIN & CAFFEINE continued

Para-aminosalicylic acid (PAS)	Possible aspirin toxicity.
Penicillins*	Increased effect of drugs.
Phenobarbital	Decreased aspirin effect.
Potassium supplements*	Increased possibility of intestinal ulcers with oral potassium tablets.
Probenecid	Decreased probenecid effect.
Propoxyphene	Possible confusion, nervousness, tremors.
Propranolol	Decreased aspirin effect.
Rauwolfia alkaloids*	Decreased aspirin effect.
Salicylates, other*	Likely aspirin toxicity.
Sedatives*	Decreased sedative effect.
Sleep inducers*	Decreased sedative effect.
Spironolactone	Decreased spironolactone effect.
Sulfinpyrazone	Decreased sulfinpyrazone effect.
Sympathomimetics*	Overstimulation.
Thyroid hormones*	Increased thyroid effect.
Tranquilizers*	Decreased tranquilizer effect.
Valproic acid	May increase valproic acid effect.
Vitamin C (large doses)	Possible aspirin toxicity.

PANCREATIN, PEPSIN, BILE SALTS, HYOSCYAMINE, ATROPINE, SCOPOLAMINE & PHENOBARBITAL

Aspirin	Decreased aspirin effect.
Attapulgite	Decreased anticholinergic effect.
Beta-adrenergic blocking agents*	Decreased effect of beta-adrenergic blocker.
Buclizine	Increased scopolamine effect.
Central nervous system (CNS) depressants*	Increased CNS depression.
Contraceptives, oral*	Decreased contraceptive effect.
Digitalis	Possible decreased absorption of digitalis.
Disopyramide	Increased atropine effect.
Dronabinol	Increased phenobarbital effect.
Griseofulvin	Decreased griseofulvin effect.
Haloperidol	Increased internal eye pressure.
Indapamide	Increased indapamide effect.
Ketoconazole	Decreased ketoconazole effect.
Meperidine	Increased atropine effect.
Methylphenidate	Increased atropine effect.
Mind-altering drugs*	Dangerous sedation. Avoid.
Monoamine oxidase (MAO) inhibitors*	Increased atropine effect.
Narcotics*	Dangerous sedation. Avoid.
Nitrates*	Increased internal eye pressure.
Nizatidine	Increased nizatidine effect.
Orphenadrine	Increased atropine effect.
Phenothiazines*	Increased atropine effect.
Pilocarpine	Loss of pilocarpine effect in glaucoma treatment.

ADDITIONAL DRUG INTERACTIONS

*See Glossary

GENERIC NAME OR DRUG CLASS	COMBINED EFFECT	GENERIC NAME OR DRUG CLASS	COMBINED EFFECT

PANCREATIN, PEPSIN, BILE SALTS, HYOSCYAMINE, ATROPINE, SCOPOLAMINE & PHENOBARBITAL continued

GENERIC NAME OR DRUG CLASS	COMBINED EFFECT
Potassium supplements*	Possible intestinal ulcers with oral potassium tablets.
Quinidine	Increased quinidine and scopolamine effect.
Sedatives*	Dangerous sedation. Avoid.
Sleep inducers*	Dangerous sedation. Avoid.
Tranquilizers*	Dangerous sedation. Avoid.
Valproic acid	Increased phenobarbital effect.
Vitamin C	Decreased atropine effect. Avoid large doses of vitamin C.

PHENOTHIAZINES

GENERIC NAME OR DRUG CLASS	COMBINED EFFECT
Clozapine	Toxic effect on the central nervous system.
Dofetilide	Increased risk of heart problems.
Doxepin (topical)	Increased risk of toxicity of both drugs.
Guanethidine	Increased guanethidine effect.
Isoniazid	Increased risk of liver damage.
Levodopa	Decreased levodopa effect.
Lithium	Decreased lithium effect.
Mind-altering drugs*	Increased effect of mind-altering drug.
Molindone	Increased tranquilizer effect.
Narcotics*	Increased narcotic effect.
Procarbazine	Increased sedation.
Quetiapine	Decreased quetiapine effect with thioridazine.
Tramadol	Increased sedation.
Zolpidem	Increased sedation. Avoid.

POTASSIUM SUPPLEMENTS

GENERIC NAME OR DRUG CLASS	COMBINED EFFECT
Potassium-containing drugs*	Increased potassium levels.
Spironolactone	Dangerous rise in blood potassium.
Triamterene	Dangerous rise in blood potassium.
Vitamin B-12	Extended-release tablets may decrease vitamin B-12 absorption and increase vitamin B-12 requirements..

PRIMIDONE

GENERIC NAME OR DRUG CLASS	COMBINED EFFECT
Narcotics*	Increased narcotic effect.
Oxyphenbutazone	Decreased oxyphen-butazone effect.
Phenylbutazone	Decreased phenyl-butazone effect.
Phenytoin	Possible increased primidone toxicity.
Rifampin	Possible decreased primidone effect.
Sedatives*	Increased sedative effect.
Sertraline	Increased depressive effects of both drugs.

*See Glossary

GENERIC NAME OR DRUG CLASS	COMBINED EFFECT	GENERIC NAME OR DRUG CLASS	COMBINED EFFECT

PRIMIDONE continued

GENERIC NAME OR DRUG CLASS	COMBINED EFFECT	GENERIC NAME OR DRUG CLASS	COMBINED EFFECT
Sleep inducers*	Increased effect of sleep inducer.	**Tranquilizers***	Increased tranquilizer effect.

PROBENECID & COLCHICINE

GENERIC NAME OR DRUG CLASS	COMBINED EFFECT	GENERIC NAME OR DRUG CLASS	COMBINED EFFECT
Methotrexate	Increased methotrexate effect.	**Salicylates***	Decreased probenecid effect.
Mind-altering drugs*	Oversedation.	**Sedatives***	Oversedation.
Narcotics*	Oversedation.	**Sleep inducers***	Oversedation.
Nitrofurantoin	Increased nitro-furantoin effect.	**Sulfa drugs***	Slows elimination. May cause harmful accumulation of sulfa.
Para-aminosalicylic acid (PAS)	Increased effect of para-aminosalicylic acid.	**Thioguanine**	More likelihood of toxicity of both drugs.
Penicillins*	Enhanced penicillin effect.	**Tranquilizers***	Oversedation.
Phenylbutazone	Decreased antigout effect of colchicine.	**Valacyclovir**	Increased valacyclovir effect.
Pyrazinamide	Decreased probenecid effect.	**Vitamin B-12**	Decreased absorp-tion of vitamin B-12.
		Zidovudine	Increased risk of zidovudine toxicity.

PROCARBAZINE

GENERIC NAME OR DRUG CLASS	COMBINED EFFECT	GENERIC NAME OR DRUG CLASS	COMBINED EFFECT
Diuretics*	Excessively low blood pressure.	**Methyldopa**	Severe high blood pressure.
Doxapam	Increased blood pressure.	**Methylphenidate**	Excessive high blood pressure.
Ethinamate	Dangerous increased effects of ethinamate. Avoid combining.	**Methyprylon**	May increase seda-tive effect to danger-ous level. Avoid.
Fluoxetine	Increased depres-sant effects of both drugs.	**Monoamine oxidase (MAO) inhibitors, other***	High fever, convulsions, death.
Guanethidine	Blood pressure rise to life-threatening level.	**Nabilone**	Greater depression of central nervous system.
Guanfacine	May increase depressant effects of either medicine.	**Narcotics***	Increased sedation.
Leucovorin	High alcohol content of leucovorin may cause adverse effects.	**Phenothiazines***	Increased sedation.
Levamisole	Increased risk of bone marrow depression.	**Rauwolfia alkaloids***	Very high blood pressure.
Levodopa	Sudden, severe blood pressure rise.	**Reserpine**	Increased blood pressure, excitation.
		Sertraline	Increased depressive effects of both drugs.
		Sumatriptan	Adverse effects unknown. Avoid.

*See Glossary

GENERIC NAME OR DRUG CLASS	COMBINED EFFECT	GENERIC NAME OR DRUG CLASS	COMBINED EFFECT

PROCARBAZINE continued

GENERIC NAME OR DRUG CLASS	COMBINED EFFECT
Sympathomimetics*	Heartbeat abnormalities, severe high blood pressure.
Tiopronin	Increased risk of toxicity to bone marrow.

RAUWOLFIA ALKALOIDS

GENERIC NAME OR DRUG CLASS	COMBINED EFFECT
Lisinopril	Increased anti-hypertensive effect. Dosage of each may require adjustment.
Loxapine	May increase toxic effects of both drugs.
Methyprylon	May increase sedative effect to dangerous level. Avoid.
Mind-altering drugs*	Excessive sedation.
Monoamine oxidase (MAO) inhibitors*	Severe depression.
Nabilone	Greater depression of central nervous system.
Nicardipine	Blood pressure drop. Dosages may require adjustment.
Nimodipine	Dangerous blood pressure drop.
Pergolide	Decreased pergolide effect.
Sertraline	Increased depressive effects of both drugs.
Sotalol	Decreased anti-hypertensive effect.
Terazosin	Decreased effectiveness of terazosin.

RESERPINE, HYDRALAZINE & HYDROCHLOROTHIAZIDE

GENERIC NAME OR DRUG CLASS	COMBINED EFFECT
Allopurinol	Decreased allopurinol effect.
Amphetamines*	Decreased hydralazine effect.
Anticoagulants*, oral	Unpredictable increased or decreased effect of anticoagulant.
Anticonvulsants*	Serious change in seizure pattern.
Antidepressants, tricyclic*	Dangerous drop in blood pressure. Avoid combination unless under medical supervision.
Antihistamines*	Increased antihistamine effect.
Antihypertensives, other*	Increased anti-hypertensive effect.
Anti-inflammatory drugs, nonsteroidal (NSAIDs)*	Decreased hydralazine effect.
Aspirin	Decreased aspirin effect.
Barbiturates*	Increased hydrochlorothiazide effect.
Beta-adrenergic blocking agents*	Increased effect of rauwolfia alkaloids. Excessive sedation.
Carteolol	Increased anti-hypertensive effect.
Cholestyramine	Decreased hydrochlorothiazide effect.
Cortisone drugs*	Excessive potassium loss that causes dangerous heart rhythms.
Diazoxide	Increased anti-hypertensive effect.
Digitalis preparations*	Excessive potassium loss that causes dangerous heart rhythms.
Diuretics, oral*	Increased effects of drugs. When monitored carefully, combination may be beneficial in controlling hypertension.

*See Glossary

RESERPINE, HYDRALAZINE & HYDROCHLOROTHIAZIDE continued

GENERIC NAME OR DRUG CLASS	COMBINED EFFECT
Dronabinol	Increased effects of drugs.
Indapamide	Increased diuretic effect.
Levodopa	Decreased levodopa effect.
Lisinopril	Increased anti-hypertensive effect. Dosage of each may require adjustment.
Lithium	Increased lithium effect.
Mind-altering drugs*	Excessive sedation.
Monoamine oxidase (MAO) inhibitors*	Increased effects of both drugs. Severe depression.
Nicardipine	Blood pressure drop. Dosages may require adjustment.
Nimodipine	Dangerous blood pressure drop.
Nitrates*	Excessive blood pressure drop.
Oxprenolol	Increased anti-hypertensive effect. Dosages of drugs may require adjustments.
Pergolide	Decreased pergolide effect.
Potassium supplements*	Decreased potassium effect.
Probenecid	Decreased probenecid effect.
Sotalol	Decreased anti-hypertensive effect.
Terazosin	Decreased effectiveness of terazosin.

RETINOIDS (Oral)

GENERIC NAME OR DRUG CLASS	COMBINED EFFECT
Isotretinoin	Increased toxicity.
Medicated cosmetics	Excessive drying effect on skin.
Methotrexate	Increased toxicity to liver.
Tretinoin	Increased toxicity.
Vitamin A	Increased toxicity. Avoid.
Warfarin	Increased warfarin effect.

RIFAMYCINS

GENERIC NAME OR DRUG CLASS	COMBINED EFFECT
Non-nucleoside reverse transcriptase inhibitors	May require dosage adjustment of rifampin.
Phenytoin	Decreased phenytoin effect.
Probenecid	Possible toxicity to liver.
Protease inhibitors	Decreased protease inhibitor effect.
Quinidine	Decreased effect of both drugs.
Quinine	Decreased quinine effect.
Sildenafil	Decreased sildenafil effect.
Tacrolimus	Decreased tacrolimus effect.
Theophyllines*	Decreased theophylline effect.
Tocainide	Possible decreased blood cell production in bone marrow.
Trimethoprim	Decreased trimethoprim effect.
Zaleplon	Decreased zaleplon effect.
Zidovudine	Decreased zidovudine effect.

*See Glossary

GENERIC NAME OR DRUG CLASS	COMBINED EFFECT

SALICYLATES

GENERIC NAME OR DRUG CLASS	COMBINED EFFECT
Insulin lispro	May need decreased dosage of insulin.
Ketocanazole	With buffered salicylates—Decreased ketoconazole effect.
Methotrexate	Increased methotrexate effect and toxicity.
Para-aminosalicylic acid	Possible salicylate toxicity.
Penicillins*	Increased effect of both drugs.
Phenobarbital	Decreased salicylate effect.
Phenytoin	Increased phenytoin effect.
Probenecid	Decreased probenecid effect.
Rauwolfia alkaloids*	Decreased salicylate effect.
Salicylates*, other	Likely salicylate toxicity.
Sotalol	Decreased antihypertensive effect of sotalol.
Spironolactone	Decreased spironolactone effect.
Sulfinpyrazone	Decreased sulfinpyrazone effect.
Terazosin	Decreased effectiveness of terazosin. Causes sodium and fluid retention.
Urinary acidifiers*	Decreased excretion. Increased salicylate effect.
Urinary alkalizers*	Increased excretion. Decreased salicylate effect.
Valproic acid	Possible increased valproic acid toxicity.
Vitamin C (large doses)	Possible salicylate toxicity.
Zidovudine	increased zidovudine effect.

SCOPOLAMINE (Hyoscine)

GENERIC NAME OR DRUG CLASS	COMBINED EFFECT
Nabilone	Greater depression of central nervous system.
Nitrates*	Increased internal eye pressure.
Nizatidine	Increased nizatidine effect.
Orphenadrine	Increased scopolamine effect.
Phenothiazines*	Increased scopolamine effect.
Pilocarpine	Loss of pilocarpine effect in glaucoma treatment.
Potassium supplements*	Possible intestinal ulcers with oral potassium tablets.
Quinidine	Increased scopolamine effect.
Sedatives* or central nervous system (CNS) depressants*	Increased sedative effect of both drugs.
Sertraline	Increased depressive effects of both drugs.
Vitamin C	Decreased scopolamine effect. Avoid large doses of vitamin C.

SELECTIVE SEROTONIN REUPTAKE INHIBITORS (SSRIs)

GENERIC NAME OR DRUG CLASS	COMBINED EFFECT
Dextromethorphan	Increased risk of serotonin syndrome*.
Digoxin	Increased risk of side effects of both drugs.
Levodopa	Increased risk of serotonin syndrome*.
Lithium	Increased risk of serotonin syndrome*.

*See Glossary

SELECTIVE SEROTONIN REUPTAKE INHIBITORS (SSRIs) continued

GENERIC NAME OR DRUG CLASS	COMBINED EFFECT
Meperidine	Increased risk of serotonin syndrome*.
Moclobemide	Increased risk of side effects and serotonin syndrome*.
Monoamine oxidase (MAO) inhibitors*	Increased risk of adverse effects. May lead to convulsions and hypertensive crisis. Let 14 days elapse between taking the 2 drugs.
Nefazodone	Increased risk of serotonin syndrome*.
Pentazocine	Increased risk of serotonin syndrome*
Phenytoin	Increased effect of phenytoin.
Propranolol	Increased effect of propranolol.
Sumatriptan	Increased risk of serotonin syndrome*.
Theophylline	Increased effect of theophylline.
Tramadol	Increased risk of serotonin syndrome*.
Trazodone	Increased risk of serotonin syndrome*.
Tryptophan	Increased risk of serotonin syndrome*
Venlafaxine	Increased risk of serotonin syndrome*.

SELEGILINE

GENERIC NAME OR DRUG CLASS	COMBINED EFFECT
Sertraline	Increased depressive effects of both drugs.
Sumatriptan	Adverse effects unknown. Avoid.

SULFONYLUREAS

GENERIC NAME OR DRUG CLASS	COMBINED EFFECT
Insulin	Increased blood sugar lowering.
Insulin lispro	Increased anti-diabetic effect.
Isoniazid	Decreased blood sugar lowering.
Labetalol	Increased blood sugar lowering, may mask hypoglycemia.
Leukotriene modifiers	Increased effect of tolbutamide.
MAO inhibitors*	Increased blood sugar lowering.
Nicotinic acid	Decreased blood sugar lowering.
Oxyphenbutazone	Increased blood sugar lowering.
Phenothiazines*	Decreased blood sugar lowering.
Phenylbutazone	Increased blood sugar lowering.
Phenyramidol	Increased blood sugar lowering.
Phenytoin	Decreased blood sugar lowering.
Probenecid	Increased blood sugar lowering.
Pyrazinamide	Decreased blood sugar lowering.
Ranitidine	Increased blood sugar lowering.
Rifampin	Decreased blood sugar lowering.
Sulfa drugs*	Increased blood sugar lowering.
Sulfadoxine and pyrimethamine	Increased risk of toxicity.
Sulfaphenazole	Increased blood sugar lowering.
Thiazolidinediones*	May decrease plasma glucose concentrations.
Thyroid hormones*	Decreased blood sugar lowering.
Zafirlukast	May increase effect of tolbutamide.

*See Glossary

GENERIC NAME OR DRUG CLASS	COMBINED EFFECT	GENERIC NAME OR DRUG CLASS	COMBINED EFFECT

TETRACYCLINES

Vitamin A	Increased risk of intracranial hypertension.	**Zinc supplements**	Decreased tetracycline absorption if taken within 2 hours of each other.

THIOTHIXENE

Pergolide	Decreased pergolide effect.	**Sertraline**	Increased depressive effects of both drugs.
Quinidine	Increased risk of heartbeat irregularities.	**Tranquilizers***	Increased thiothixene effect. Excessive sedation.

TRIAZOLAM

Omeprazole	Delayed excretion of triazolam causing increased amount of triazolam in blood.	**Probenecid**	Increased triazolam effect.
		Zidovudine	Increased toxicity of zidovudine.

VALPROIC ACID

Sulfinpyrazone	Increased chance of bleeding.	**Tocainide**	Possible decreased blood cell production in bone marrow.

***See Glossary**

Glossary

Many of the following medical terms are found in the drug charts. Where drug names are listed, they indicate the generic or drug class and not the brand names.

A

ACE Inhibitors—See Angiotensin-Converting Enzyme (ACE) Inhibitors.

Acne Preparations—Creams, lotions and liquids applied to the skin to treat acne. These include adapalene; alcohol and acetone; alcohol and sulfur; azelaic acid; benzoyl peroxide; clindamycin; erythromycin; erythromycin and benzoyl peroxide; isotretinoin; meclocycline; resorcinol; resorcinol and sulfur; salicylic acid gel USP; salicylic acid lotion; salicylic acid ointment; salicylic acid pads; salicylic acid soap; salicylic acid and sulfur bar soap; salicylic acid and sulfur cleansing lotion; salicylic acid and sulfur cleansing suspension; salicylic acid and sulfur lotion; sulfurated lime; sulfur bar soap; sulfur cream; sulfur lotion; tetracycline, oral; tetracycline hydrochloride for topical solution; tretinoin.

Acridine Derivatives—Dyes or stains (usually yellow or orange) used for some medical tests and as antiseptic agents.

Acute—Having a short and relatively severe course.

Addiction—Psychological or physiological dependence upon a drug.

Addictive Drugs—Any drug that can lead to physiological dependence on the drug. These include alcohol, cocaine, marijuana, nicotine, opium, morphine, codeine, heroin (and other narcotics) and others.

Addison's Disease—Changes in the body caused by a deficiency of hormones manufactured by the adrenal gland. Usually fatal if untreated.

Adrenal Cortex—Center of the adrenal gland.

Adrenal Gland—Gland next to the kidney that produces cortisone and epinephrine (adrenalin).

Agranulocytosis—A symptom complex characterized by (1) a sharply decreased number of granulocytes (one of the types of white blood cells), (2) lesions of the throat and other mucous membranes, (3) lesions of the gastrointestinal tract and (4) lesions of the skin. Sometimes also called granulocytopenia.

Alkalizers—These drugs neutralize acidic properties of the blood and urine by making them more alkaline (or basic). Systemic alkalizers include potassium citrate and citric acid, sodium bicarbonate, sodium citrate and citric acid, and tricitrates. Urinary alkalizers include potassium citrate, potassium citrate and citric acid, potassium citrate and sodium citrate, sodium citrate and citric acid.

Alkylating Agent—Chemical used to treat malignant diseases.

Allergy—Excessive sensitivity to a substance that is ordinarily harmless. Reactions include sneezing, stuffy nose, hives, itching.

Alpha-Adrenergic Blocking Agents—A group of drugs used to treat hypertension. These drugs include prazosin, terazosin, doxazosin and labetalol (an alpha-adrenergic and beta-adrenergic combination drug). Also included are other drugs that produce an alpha-adrenergic blocking action such as haloperidol, loxapine, phenothiazines, thioxanthenes.

Amebiasis—Infection with amoebas, one-celled organisms. Causes diarrhea, fever and abdominal cramps.

Amenorrhea—Abnormal absence of menstrual periods.

Aminoglycosides—A family of antibiotics used for serious infections. Their usefulness is limited because of their relative toxicity compared to some other antibiotics. These drugs include amikacin, gentamicin, kanamycin, neomycin, netilmicin, streptomycin, tobramycin.

Amphetamines—A family of drugs that stimulates the central nervous system, prescribed to treat attention-deficit disorders in children and also for narcolepsy. They are habit-forming, are controlled under U.S. law and are no longer prescribed as appetite suppressants. These drugs include amphetamine, dextroamphetamine, methamphetamine. They may be ingredients of several combination drugs.

ANA Titers—A test to evaluate the immune system and to detect antinuclear antibodies (ANAs), substances that appear in the blood of some patients with autoimmune disease.

Analgesics—Agents that reduce pain without reducing consciousness.

Anaphylaxis—Severe allergic response to a substance. Symptoms are wheezing, itching, hives, nasal congestion, intense burning of hands and feet, collapse, loss of consciousness and cardiac arrest. Symptoms appear within a few seconds or minutes after exposure. Anaphylaxis is a severe medical emergency. Without appropriate treatment, it can cause death. Instructions for home treatment for anaphylaxis are on the front inside cover.

Androgens—Male hormones, including fluoxymesterone, methyltestosterone, testosterone, DHEA.

Anemia—Not enough healthy red blood cells in the bloodstream or too little hemoglobin in the red blood cells. Anemia is caused by an imbalance between blood loss and blood production.

Anemia, Aplastic—A form of anemia in which the bone marrow is unable to manufacture adequate numbers of blood cells of all types—red cells, white cells, and platelets.

Anemia, Hemolytic—Anemia caused by a shortened lifespan of red blood cells. The body can't manufacture new cells fast enough to replace old cells.

Anemia, Iron-Deficiency—Anemia caused when iron necessary to manufacture red blood cells is not available.

Anemia, Pernicious—Anemia caused by a vitamin B-12 deficiency. Symptoms include weakness, fatigue, numbness and tingling of the hands or feet and degeneration of the central nervous system.

Anemia, Sickle-Cell—Anemia caused by defective hemoglobin that deprives red blood cells of oxygen, making them sickle-shaped.

Anesthesias, General—Gases that are used in surgery to render patients unconscious and able to withstand the pain of surgical cutting and manipulation. They include enflurane, etomidate, fentanyl, halothane, isoflurane, ketamine, methohexital, methoxyflurane, nitrous oxide, propofol, thiamylal, thiopental, alfentanil, amobarbital, butabarbital, butorphanol, chloral hydrate, etomidate, fentanyl, tentanyl, hydroxyzine, ketamine, levorphanol, meperidine, midazolam, morphine parenteral, nalbuphine, oxymorphone, pentazocine, pentobarbital, phenobarbital, promethazine, propiomazine, scopolamine, secobarbital, sufentanil.

Anesthetics—Drugs that eliminate the sensation of pain.

Angina (Angina Pectoris)—Chest pain with a sensation of suffocation and impending death. Caused by a temporary reduction in the amount of oxygen to the heart muscle through diseased coronary arteries. The pain may also occur in the left shoulder, jaw or arm.

Angiotensin-Converting Enzyme (ACE) Inhibitors—A family of drugs used to treat hypertension and congestive heart failure. Inhibitors decrease the rate of conversion of angiotensin I into angiotensin II, which is the normal process for the angiotensin-converting enzyme. These drugs include benazepril, captopril, enalapril, fosinopril, lisinopril, moexipril, perindopril, quinapril, ramipril, trandolapril.

Antacids—A large family of drugs prescribed to treat hyperacidity, peptic ulcer, esophageal reflux and other conditions. These drugs include alumina and magnesia; alumina, magnesia and calcium carbonate; alumina, magnesia and simethicone; alumina and magnesium carbonate; alumina and magnesium trisilicate; alumina, magnesium trisilicate and sodium bicarbonate; aluminum carbonate; aluminum hydroxide; bismuth subsalicylate; calcium carbonate; calcium carbonate and magnesia; calcium carbonate, magnesia and simethicone; calcium and magnesium carbonates; calcium and magnesium carbonates and magnesium oxide; calcium carbonate and simethicone; dihydroxyaluminum aminoacetate; dihydroxyaluminum sodium carbonate; magaldrate; magaldrate and simethicone; magnesium carbonate and sodium bicarbonate; magnesium hydroxide; magnesium oxide; magnesium trisilicate, alumina and magnesia; simethicone, alumina, calcium carbonate and magnesia; simethicone, alumina, magnesium carbonate and magnesia; sodium bicarbonate.

Antacids, Calcium Carbonate—These antacids include calcium carbonate and magnesium, calcium carbonate and simethicone, calcium carbonate and magnesium carbonates.

Antacids, Magnesium-Containing—These antacids include magnesium carbonate, magnesium hydroxide, magnesium oxide and magnesium trisilicate. All these medicines are designed to treat excess stomach acidity. In addition to being an effective antacid, magnesium can sometimes cause unpleasant side effects and drug interactions. Look for the presence of magnesium in nonprescription drugs.

Anthelmintics—A family of drugs used to treat intestinal parasites. Names of these drugs include niclosamide, piperazine, pyrantel, pyrvinium, quinacrine, mebendazole, metronidazole, oxamniquine, praziquantel, thiabendazole.

Antiacne Topical Preparations—See Acne Preparations.

Antiadrenals—Medicines or drugs that prevent the effects of the hormones produced by the adrenal glands.

Antianginals—A group of drugs used to treat angina pectoris (chest pain that comes and goes, caused by coronary artery disease). These drugs include acebutolol, amlodipine, amyl nitrite, atenolol, bepridil, carteolol, diltiazem, felodipine, isosorbide dinitrate, labetalol, metoprolol, nadolol, nicardipine, nifedipine, nitroglycerin, oxprenolol, penbutolol, pindolol, propranolol, sotalol, timolol, verapamil.

Antianxiety Drugs—A group of drugs prescribed to treat anxiety. These drugs include alprazolam, bromazepam, buspirone, chlordiazepoxide, chlorpromazine, clomipramine, clorazepate, diazepam, halazepam, hydroxyzine, imipramine, ketazolam, lorazepam, meprobamate, oxazepam, prazepam, prochlorperazine, thioridazine, trifluoperazine, venlafaxine.

Antiarrhythmics—A group of drugs used to treat heartbeat irregularities (arrhythmias). These drugs include acebutolol, adenosine, amiodarone, atenolol, atropine, bretylium, deslanoside, digitalis, digitoxin, diltiazem, disopyramide, dofetilide, edrophonium, encainide, esmolol, flecainide, glycopyrrolate, hyoscyamine, lidocaine, methoxamine, metoprolol, mexiletine, moricizine, nadolol, oxprenolol, phenytoin, procainamide, propafenone, propranolol, quinidine, scopolamine, sotalol, timolol, tocainide, verapamil.

Antiasthmatics—Medicines used to treat asthma, which may be tablets, liquids or aerosols (to be inhaled to get directly to the bronchial tubes rather than through the bloodstream). These medicines include adrenocorticoids, glucocorticoid; albuterol; aminophylline; astemizole; beclomethasone; bitolterol; budesonide; cetirizine; corticotropin; cromolyn; dexamethasone; dyphylline; ephedrine; epinephrine; ethylnorepinephrine; fenoterol; flunisolide; fluticasone; ipratropium, isoetharine; isoproterenol; isoproterenol and phenylephrine; loratadine; metaproterenol; oxtriphylline; oxtriphylline and guaifenesin; pirbuterol; racepinephrine; terbutaline; theophylline; theophylline and guaifenesin; triamcinolone.

Antibacterials (Antibiotics)—A group of drugs prescribed to treat infections. These drugs include, amikacin, amoxicillin, amoxicillin and clavulanate, ampicillin, azlocillin, aztreonam, bacampicillin, carbenicillin, cefaclor, cefadroxil, cefamandole, cefazolin, cefonicid, cefoperazone, ceforanide, cefotaxime, cefotetan, cefoxitin, ceftazidime, ceftibuten, ceftizoxime, ceftriaxone, cefuroxime, cephalexin, cephalothin, cephapirin, cephradine, chloramphenicol, cinoxacin, clindamycin, cloxacillin, cyclacillin, cycloserine, demeclocycline, dicloxacillin, doxycycline, erythromycin, erythromycin and sulfisoxazole, flucloxacillin, fusidic acid, gentamicin, imipenem and cilastatin, kanamycin, lincomycin, methacycline, methenamine, methicillin, metronidazole, mezlocillin, minocycline, moxalactam, nafcillin, nalidixic acid, netilmicin, nitrofurantoin, norfloxacin, oxacillin, oxytetracycline, penicillin G, penicillin V, piperacillin, pivampicillin, rifabutin, rifampin, spectinomycin, streptomycin, sulfacytine, sulfadiazine and trimethoprim, sulfamethoxazole, sulfamethoxazole and trimethoprim, sulfisoxazole, tetracycline, ticarcillin, ticarcillin and clavulanate, tobramycin, trimethoprim, vancomycin.

Antibiotics—Chemicals that inhibit the growth of or kill germs. See Antibacterials.

Anticholinergics—Drugs that work against acetylcholine, a chemical found in many locations in the body, including connections between nerve cells and connections between muscle and nerve cells. Anticholinergic drugs include amantadine, anisotropine, atropine, belladonna, benztropine, clidinium, dicyclomine, glycopyrrolate, homatropine, hyoscyamine, ipratropium, isopropamide, mepenzolate, methantheline, methscopolamine, pirenzepine, propantheline, scopolamine, trihexphenidyl.

Anticoagulants—A family of drugs prescribed to slow the rate of blood clotting. These drugs include acenocoumarol, anisindione, dicumarol, dihydroergotamine and heparin, heparin, warfarin.

Anticonvulsants—A group of drugs prescribed to treat or prevent seizures (convulsions). These drugs include these families: barbiturates, carbonic anhydrase inhibitors, diones, hydantoins and succinimides. These are the names of the generic drugs in these families: acetazolamide, amobarbital, carbamazepine, carbonic anhydrase inhibitors, clobzamam, clonazepam, clorazepate, diazepam, dichlorphenamide, divalproex, ethosuximide, ethotoin, felbamate, fosphenytoin, gabapentin, lamotrigine, levetiracetam lorazepam, mephenytoin, mephobarbital, metharbital, methsuximide, nitrazepam, oxcarbazepine, paraldehyde, phenacemide, paramethadione, pentobarbital, phenobarbital, phenytoin, primidone, secobarbital, tiagabine, topiramate, trimethadione, valproic acid, zonisamide.

Antidepressants—A group of medicines prescribed to treat mental depression. These drugs include amitriptyline, amoxapine, bupropion, citalopram, clomipramine, desipramine, doxepin, fluoxetine, fluvoxamine, imipramine, isocarboxazid, lithium, maprotiline, mirtazapine, moclobemide, nefazodone, nortriptyline, paroxetine, phenelzine, protriptyline, sertraline, tranylcypromine, trazodone, trimipramine, venlafaxine.

Antidepressants, MAO (Monoamine Oxidase) Inhibitors—A special group of drugs prescribed for mental depression. These are not as popular as in years past because of a relatively high incidence of adverse effects. These drugs include isocarboxazid (Marplan), phenelzine (Nardil), tranylcypromine (Parnate).

Antidepressants, Tricyclic (TCAs)—A group of medicines with similar chemical structure and pharmacologic activity used to treat mental depression. These drugs include amitriptyline, amoxapine, clomipramine, desipramine, doxepin, imipramine, nortriptyline, protriptyline, trimipramine.

Antidiabetic Agents—A group of drugs used in the treatment of diabetes mellitus. These medicines all reduce blood sugar. These drugs include acarbose, acetohexamide, chlorpropamide, gliclazide, glimepiride, glipizide, glyburide, insulin, metformin, nateglinide, pioglitazone, repaglinide, rosiglitazone, tolazamide, tolbutamide, troglitazone.

Antidiarrheal Preparations—Medicines that treat diarrhea symptoms. Most do not cure the cause. Oral medicines include aluminum hydroxide; charcoal, activated; kaolin and pectin; loperamide; polycarbophil; psyllium hydrophilic mucilloid. Systemic medicines include carbohydrates; codeine; difenoxin and atropine; diphenoxylate and atropine; glucose and electrolytes; glycopyrrolate; kaolin, pectin, belladonna alkaloids and opium; kaolin, pectin and paregoric; opium tincture; paregoric.

Antidyskinetics—A group of drugs used for treatment of Parkinsonism (paralysis agitans) and drug-induced extrapyramidal reactions (see elsewhere in Glossary). These drugs include amantadine, benztropine, biperiden, bromocriptine, carbidopa and levodopa, diphenhydramine, entacapone, ethopropazine, levodopa, levodopa and benserazide, procyclidine, selegiline, trihexyphenidyl.

Antiemetics—A group of drugs used to treat nausea and vomiting. These drugs include buclizine, cyclizine, chlorpromazine, dimenhydrinate, diphenhydramine, diphenidol, domperidone, dronabinol, haloperidol, hydroxyzine, meclizine, metoclopramide, nabilone, ondansetron, perphenazine, prochlorperazine, promethazine, scopolamine, thiethylperazine, triflupromazine, trimethobenzamide.

Antifibrinolytic Drugs—Drugs that are used to treat serious bleeding. These drugs include aminocaproic acid and tranexamic acid.

Antifungals—A group of drugs used to treat fungus infections. Those listed as systemic are taken orally or given by injection. Those listed as topical are applied directly to the skin and include liquids, powders, creams, ointments and liniments. Those listed as vaginal are used topically inside the vagina and sometimes on the vaginal lips. These drugs include: Systemic—amphotericin B, miconazole, fluconazole, flucytosine, griseofulvin, itraconazole, ketoconazole, potassium iodide. Topical—amphotericin B; carbol-fuchsin; ciclopirox; clioquinol; clotrimazole; econazole; haloprogin; ketoconazole; mafenide; miconazole; naftifine; nystatin; oxiconazole; salicylic acid; silver sulfadiazine; sulconazole; sulfur and coal; terbinafine; tioconazole; tolnaftate; undecylenic acid. Vaginal—butoconazole, clotrimazole, econazole, gentian violet, miconazole, nystatin, terconazole, tioconazole.

Antifungals, Azole—Drugs used to treat certain types of fungal infections. These drugs include fluconazole, itraconazole, ketoconazole, miconazole.

Antiglaucoma Drugs—Medicines used to treat glaucoma. Those listed as systemic are taken orally or given by injection. Those listed as ophthalmic are for external use. These drugs include: Systemic—acetazolamide, dichlorphenamide, glycerin, mannitol, methazolamide, timolol, urea. Ophthalmic—apraclonidine, betaxolol, brimonidine, brinzolamide, carbachol ophthalmic solution, carteolol, demecarium, dipivefrin, dorzolamide, echothiophate, epinephrine, epinephrine bitartrate, epinephryl borate, isoflurophate, latanoprost, levobetaxolol, levobunolol, metipranolol, physostigmine, pilocarpine, timolol, unoprostone.

Antigout Drugs—Drugs to treat the metabolic disease called gout. Gout causes recurrent attacks of joint pain caused by deposits of uric acid in the joints. Antigout drugs include allopurinol, carprofen, colchicine, fenoprofen, ibuprofen, indomethacin, ketoprofen, naproxen, phenylbutazone, piroxicam, probenecid, probenecid and colchicine, sulfinpyrazone, sulindac.

Antihistamines—A family of drugs used to treat allergic conditions, such as hay fever, allergic conjunctivitis, itching, sneezing, runny nose, motion sickness, dizziness, sedation, insomnia and others. These drugs include astemizole, azatadine, brompheniramine, carbinoxamine, cetirizine, chlorpheniramine, clemastine, cyproheptadine, dexchlorpheniramine, dimenhydrinate, diphenhydramine, diphenylpyraline, doxylamine, fexofenadine, hydroxyzine, loratadine, phenindamine, promethazine, pyrilamine, trimeprazine, tripelennamine, triprolidine.

Antihyperammonemias—Medications that decrease the amount of ammonia in the blood. The ones with this pharmacological property that are available in the United States are lactulose, sodium benzoate and sodium phenylacetate.

Antihyperlipidemics—A group of drugs used to treat hyperlipidemia (high levels of lipids in the blood). These include atorvastatin, cerivastatin, cholestyramine, clofibrate, colesevelam, colestipol, fenofibrate, fluvastatin, gemfibrozil, lovastatin, niacin, pravastatin, probucol, simvastatin, sodium dichloroacetate.

Antihypertensives—Drugs used to help lower high blood pressure. These medicines can be used singly or in combination with other drugs. They work best if accompanied by a low-salt, low-fat diet plus an active exercise program. These drugs include acebutolol, amiloride, amiloride and hydrochlorothiazide, amlodipine, atenolol, atenolol and chlorthalidone, benazepril, bendroflumethiazide, benzthiazide, betaxolol, bisoprolol, bumetanide, candesartan, captopril, captopril and hydrochlorothiazide, carteolol, carvedilol, chlorothiazide, chlorthalidone, cilazapril, clonidine, clonidine and chlorthalidone, cyclothiazide, debrisoquine, deserpidine, deserpidine and hydrochlorothiazide, deserpidine and methyclothiazide, diazoxide, diltiazem, doxazosin, enalapril, enalapril and hydrochlorothiazide, eprosartan ethacrynic acid, felodipine, fosinopril, furosemide, guanabenz, guanadrel, guanethidine, guanethidine and hydrochlorothiazide, guanfacine, hydralazine, hydralazine and hydrochlorothiazide, hydrochlorothiazide, hydroflumethiazide, indapamide, irbesartan isradipine, labetalol, labetalol and hydrochlorothiazide, lisinopril, lisinopril and hydrochlorothiazide, losartan, losartan and hydrochlorothiazide, mecamylamine, methyclothiazide, methyldopa, methyldopa and chlorothiazide, methyldopa and hydrochlorothiazide, metolazone, metoprolol, metoprolol and hydrochlorothiazide, minoxidil, moexipril, nadolol, nadolol and bendroflumethiazide, nicardipine, nifedipine, nisoldipine, nitroglycerin, nitroprusside, oxprenolol, penbutolol, perindopril, pindolol, pindolol and hydrochlorothiazide, polythiazide, prazosin, prazosin and polythiazide, propranolol, propranolol and hydrochlorothiazide, quinapril, quinethazone, ramipril, rauwolfia serpentina, rauwolfia serpentina and bendroflumethiazide, reserpine, reserpine and chlorothiazide, reserpine and chlorthalidone, reserpine and hydralazine, reserpine, hydralazine and hydrochlorothiazide, reserpine and hydrochlorothiazide, reserpine and hydroflumethiazide, reserpine and methyclothiazide, reserpine and polythiazide, reserpine and quinethazone, reserpine and trichlormethiazide, sotalol, spironolactone, spironolactone and hydrochlorothiazide, telmisartan, terazosin, timolol, timolol and hydrochlorothiazide, torsemide, trandolapril, triamterene, triamterene and hydrochlorothiazide, trichlormethiazide, trimethaphan, valsartan, verapamil.

Anti-Inflammatory Drugs, Nonsteroidal (NSAIDs)—A family of drugs not related to cortisone or other steroids that decrease inflammation wherever it occurs in the body. Used for treatment of pain, fever, arthritis, gout, menstrual cramps and vascular headaches. These drugs include aspirin; aspirin, alumina and magnesia tablets; buffered aspirin; bufexamac; celecoxib; choline salicylate; choline and magnesium salicylates; diclofenac, diflunisal; fenoprofen; flurbiprofen, ibuprofen; indomethacin; ketoprofen; magnesium salicylate; meclofenamate; meloxicam; naproxen; piroxicam; rofecoxib; salsalate; sodium salicylate; sulindac; tolmetin.

Anti-Inflammatory Drugs, Steroidal—A family of drugs with pharmacologic characteristics similar to those of cortisone and cortisone-like drugs. They are used for many purposes to help the body deal with inflammation no matter what the cause. Steroidal drugs may be taken orally or by injection (systemic) or applied locally (topical) for the skin, eyes, ears, bronchial tubes and others. These drugs include: Nasal—beclomethasone, budesonide, dexamethasone, flunisolide, fluticasone, triamcinolone. Ophthalmic (eyes)—betamethasone, dexamethasone, fluorometholone, hydrocortisone, medrysone, prednisolone, rimexolone. Otic (ears)—betamethasone, desonide and acetic acid, dexamethasone, hydrocortisone, hydrocortisone and acetic acid, prednisolone. Systemic—betamethasone, corticotropin, cortisone, dexamethasone, hydrocortisone, methylprednisolone, paramethasone, prednisolone, prednisone, triamcinolone. Topical—alclometasone; amcinonide; beclomethasone; betamethasone; clobetasol; clobetasone; clocortolone; desonide; desoximetasone; dexamethasone; diflorasone; diflucortolone; flumethasone; fluocinolone; fluocinonide; fluocinonide; flurandrenolide; fluticasone; halcinonide; halobetasol; mometasone; procinonide and ciprocinonide; flurandrenolide; halcinonide; hydrocortisone; methylprednisolone; mometasone; triamcinolone.

Antimalarials (also called Antiprotozoals)—A group of drugs used to treat malaria. The choice depends on the precise type of malaria organism and its developmental state. These drugs include amphotericin B, atovaquone and proguanil, clindamycin, chloroquine, dapsone, demeclocycline, doxycycline, halofantrine; hydroxychloroquine, iodoquinol, methacycline, mefloquine, metronidazole, minocycline, oxytetracycline, pentamidine, primaquine, proguanil, pyrimethamine, quinacrine, quinidine, quinine, sulfadoxine and pyrimethamine, sulfamethoxazole, sulfamethoxazole and trimethoprim, sulfisoxazole, tetracycline.

Antimuscarines—Drugs that block the muscarinic action of acetylcholine and therefore decrease spasms of the smooth muscles. They are prescribed for peptic ulcers, dysmenorrhea, dizziness, seasickness, bedwetting, slow heart rate, toxicity from pesticides made from organophosphates and other medical problems. These drugs include anisotropine, atropine, belladonna, clidinium dicyclomine, glycopyrrolate, homatropine, hyoscyamine, hyoscyamine and scopolamine, isopropamide, mepenzolate, methantheline, methscopolamine, oxyphencyclimine, pirenzepine, propantheline, scopolamine, tridihexethyl.

Antimyasthenics—Medicines to treat myasthenia gravis, a muscle disorder (especially of the face and head) with increasing fatigue and weakness as muscles tire from use. These medicines include ambenonium, neostigmine, pyridostigmine.

Antineoplastics—Potent drugs used for malignant disease. Some of these are not described in this book, but they are listed here for completeness. These drugs include: Systemic—amifostine, altretamine, aminoglutethimide, amsacrine, anastrazole, antithyroid agents, asparaginase, azathioprine, bicalutamide, bleomycin, busulfan, capecitabine, carboplatin, carmustine, chlorambucil, chloramphenicol, chlorotrianisene, chromic phosphate, cisplatin, colchicine, cyclophosphamide, cyclosporine, cyproterone, cytarabine, dacarbazine, dactinomycin, daunorubicin, deferoxamine, diethylstilbestrol, docetaxel, doxorubicin, dromostanolone, epirubicin, estradiol, estradiol valerate, estramustine, estrogens (conjugated and esterified), estrone, ethinyl estradiol, etoposide, exemestane, floxuridine, flucytosine, fluorouracil, flutamide, fluoxymesterone, gemcitabine, gold compounds, goserelin, hexamethylmelamine, hydroxyprogesterone, hydroxyurea, ifosfamide, interferon alfa-2a and alfa-2b (recombinant), ketoconazole, letrozole, leucovorin, leuprolide, levamisole, levothyroxine, liothyronine, liotrix, lithium, lomustine, masoprocol, mechlorethamine, medroxyprogesterone, megestrol, melphalan, methyltestosterone, mercaptopurine, methotrexate, mitomycin, mitotane, mitoxantrone, nandrolone, paclitaxel, phenpropionate, penicillamine, plicamycin, porfimer, procarbazine, raltitrexed, sodium iodide I 131, sodium phosphate P 32, streptozocin, tamoxifen, temoporfin, teniposide, testolactone, testosterone, thioguanine, thiotepa, thyroglobulin, thyroid, thyrotropin, topotecan, toremifene, trastuzumab, trimetrexate, triptorelin, uracil mustard, valrubicin, vinblastine, vincristine, vindesine, vinorelbine, zidovudine. Topical—fluorouracil, mechlorethamine.

Antiparkisonism Drugs—Drugs used to treat Parkinson's disease. A disease of the central nervous system in older adults, it is characterized by gradual progressive muscle rigidity, tremors and clumsiness. These drugs include amantadine, benztropine, biperiden, bromocriptine, carbidopa and levodopa, diphenhydramine, entacapone, ethopropazine, levodopa, levodopa and benserazide, orphenadrine, pergolide, procyclidine, selegiline, trihexyphenidyl.

Antipsychotic Drugs—A group of drugs used to treat the mental disease of psychosis, including such variants as schizophrenia, manic-depressive illness, anxiety states, severe behavior problems and others. These drugs include acetophenazine, carbamazepine, chlorpromazine, chlorprothixene, fluphenazine, flupenthixol, fluspirilene, haloperidol, loxapine, mesoridazine, methotrimeprazine, molindone, pericyazine, perphenazine, pimozide, pipotiazine, prochlorperazine, promazine, risperidone, thioproperazine, thioridazine, thiothixene, trifluoperazine, triflupromazine.

Antithyroid Drugs—Drugs that decrease the amount of thyroid hormone produced by the thyroid gland.

Antitussives—A group of drugs used to suppress coughs. These drugs include benzonatate, chlophedianol, codeine (oral), dextromethorphan, diphenhydramine syrup, hydrocodone, hydromorphone, methadone, morphine.

Antiulcer Drugs—A group of medicines used to treat peptic ulcer in the stomach, duodenum or the lower end of the esophagus. These drugs include amitriptyline, antacids, anticholinergics, antispasmotics, bismuth subsalicylate, cimetidine, doxepin, famotidine, lansoprazole, misoprostol, nizatidine, omeprazole, ranitidine, sucralfate, trimipramine.

Antiurolithics—Medicines that prevent the formation of kidney stones.

Antiviral Drugs—A group of drugs used to treat viral infections. These drugs include: Ophthalmic (eye)—idoxuridine, trifluridine, vidarabine. Systemic—acyclovir, amantadine, didanosine, famciclovir, foscarnet, ganciclovir, oseltamivir, ribavirin, rimantadine, stavudine, zalcitabine, zanamivir, zidovudine. Topical—acyclovir, docosanol

Antivirals, HIV/AIDS—A group of drugs used to treat human immunodeficiency virus (HIV) and acquired immune deficiency syndrome (AIDS). They work by suppressing the replication of HIV. These drugs include abacavir, amprenavir, delavirdine, didanosine, efavirenz, indinavir, lamivudine, nelfinavir, nevirapine, ritonavir, saquinavir, stavudine, zalcitabine, zidovudine.

Appendicitis—Inflammation or infection of the appendix. Symptoms include loss of appetite, nausea, low-grade fever and tenderness in the lower right of the abdomen.

Appetite Suppressants—A group of drugs used to decrease the appetite as part of an overall treatment for obesity. These drugs include amphetamine and dextroamphetamine, benzphetamine, diethylpropion, fenfluramine, mazindol, phendimetrazine, phentermine, phenylpropanolamine, sibutramine.

Artery—Blood vessel carrying blood away from the heart.

Asthma—Recurrent attacks of breathing difficulty due to spasms and contractions of the bronchial tubes.

Attentuated Virus Vaccines—Liquid products of killed germs used for injections to prevent certain diseases.

B

Bacteria—Microscopic organisms. Some bacteria contribute to health; others (germs) cause disease and infection.

Barbiturates—Powerful drugs used for sedation, to help induce sleep and sometimes to prevent seizures. Except for use in seizures (phenobarbital), barbiturates are being used less and less because there are better, less hazardous drugs that produce the same or better effects. These drugs include amobarbital, aprobarbital, butabarbital, mephobarbital, metharbital, pentobarbital, phenobarbital, secobarbital, secobarbital and amobarbital, talbutal.

Basal Area of Brain—Part of the brain that regulates muscle control and tone.

Benzethonium Chloride—A compound used as a preservative in some drug preparations. It is also used in various concentrations for cleaning cooking and eating utensils and as a disinfectant.

Benzodiazepines—A family of drugs prescribed to treat anxiety and alcohol withdrawal and sometimes prescribed for sedation. These drugs include alprazolam, bromazepam, chlordiazepoxide, clonazepam, clorazepate, diazepam, estazolam, flurazepam, halazepam, ketazolam, lorazepam, nitrazepam, oxazepam, prazepam, quazepam, triazolam.

Beta Agonists—A group of drugs that act directly on cells in the body (beta-adrenergic receptors) to relieve spasms of the bronchial tubes and other organs consisting of smooth muscles. These drugs include albuterol, bitolterol, isoetharine, isoproterenol, methaproterenol, terbutaline.

Beta-Adrenergic Blocking Agents—A family of drugs with similar pharmacological actions with some variations. These drugs are prescribed for angina, heartbeat irregularities (arrhythmias), high blood pressure, hypertrophic subaortic stenosis, vascular headaches (as a preventative, not to treat once the pain begins) and others. Timolol is prescribed for treatment of open-angle glaucoma. These drugs include acebutolol, atenolol, betaxolol, bisoprolol, carteolol, labetalol, levobetaxolol, metoprolol, nadolol, oxprenolol, penbutolol, pindolol, propranolol, sotalol, timolol.

Bile Acids—Components of bile that are derived from cholesterol and formed in the liver. Bile acids aid the digestion of fat.

Blood Count—Laboratory studies to count white blood cells, red blood cells, platelets and other elements of the blood.

Blood Dyscrasia-Causing Medicines—Drugs which cause unpredictable damaging effects to human bone marrow. These effects occur in a small minority of patients and are not dependent upon dosage. These medicines include the following (some of which are not described in this book): ACE inhibitors, acetazolamide, aminopyrine, amodiaquine, anticonvulsants (dione, hydantoin, succinimide), antidepressants (tricyclic), antidiabetic agents (sulfonylurea), anti-inflammatory analgesics, antithyroid agents, captopril, carbamazepine, cephalosporins, chloramphenicol, cisplatin, clopidrogel, clozapine, dapsone, divalproex, felbamate, flecainide acetate, foscarnet, gold compounds, levamisole, loxapine, maprotiline, methicillin, methimazole, methsuximide, metronidazole, mirtazapine, pantoprazole, penicillins (some), penicillamine, pentamidine, phenacemide, phenothiazines, phensuximide, phenytoin, pimozide, primaquine, primidone, procainamide, propafenone, propylthiouracil, pyrimethamine (large doses), rabeprazole, rifampin, rifapentine, rituximab, sulfamethoxazole and trimethoprim, sulfasalazine, sulfonamides, thioxanthenes, ticlopidine, tiopronin, tocainide, topiramate, trastuzumab, trimethobenzamide, trimethoprim, valproic acid.

Blood Pressure, Diastolic—Pressure (usually recorded in millimeters of mercury) in the large arteries of the body when the heart muscle is relaxed and filling for the next contraction.

Blood Pressure, Systolic—Pressure (usually recorded in millimeters of mercury) in the large arteries of the body at the instant the heart muscle contracts.

Blood Sugar (Blood Glucose)—Necessary element in the blood to sustain life.

Bone Marrow Depressants—Medicines that affect the bone marrow to depress its normal function of forming blood cells. These medicines include the following (some of which are not described in this book): alcohol, aldesleukin, altretamine, amphotericin B (systemic), anticancer drugs, antithyroid drugs, azathioprine, bexarotene, busulfan, carboplatin, carmustine, chlorambucil, chloramphenicol, chromic phosphate, cisplatin, cladribine, clozapine, colchicine, cyclophosphamide, cyproterone, cytarabine, dacarbazine, dactinomycin, daunorubicin, didanosine, docetaxel, doxorubicin, eflornithine, epirubicin, etoposide, floxuridine, flucytosine, fludarabine, fluorouracil, ganciclovir, gemcitabine, hydroxyurea, idarubicin, ifosfamide, interferon, irinotecan, lomustine, mechlorethamine, melphalan, mercaptopurine, methotrexate, mitomycin, mitoxantrone, paclitaxel, pentostatin, plicamycin, procarbazine, sirolimus, streptozocin, sulfa drugs, temozolomide, teniposide, thioguanine, thiotepa, topotecan, trimetrexate, uracil mustard, valrubicin, vidarabine (large doses), vinblastine, vincristine, vindesine, vinorelbine, zidovudine.

Bone Marrow Depression—Reduction of the blood-producing capacity of human bone marrow. Can be caused by many drugs taken for long periods of time in high doses.

Brain Depressants—Any drug that depresses brain function, such as tranquilizers, narcotics, alcohol and barbiturates.

Bronchodilators—A group of drugs used to dilate the bronchial tubes to treat such problems as asthma, emphysema, bronchitis, bronchiectasis, allergies and others. These drugs include albuterol, aminophylline, bitolterol, cromolyn, dyphylline, ephedrine, epinephrine, ethylnorepinephrine, fenoterol, formoterol, ipratropium, isoetharine, isoproterenol, levalbuterol metaproterenol, nedocromil, oxtriphylline, oxtriphylline and guaifenesin, pirbuterol, procaterol, salmeterol, terbutaline, theophylline and guaifenesin.

Bronchodilators, Xanthine-Derivative—Drugs of similar chemical structure and pharmacological activity that are prescribed to dilate bronchial tubes in disorders such as asthma, bronchitis, emphysema and other chronic lung diseases. These drugs include aminophylline, dyphylline, oxtriphylline, theophylline.

BUN—Abbreviation for blood urea nitrogen. A test often used as a measurement of kidney function.

C

Calcium Channel Blockers—A group of drugs used to treat angina and heartbeat irregularities. These drugs include bepridil, diltiazem, felodipine, flunarizine, isradipine, nicardipine, nifedipine, nimodipine, verapamil.

Calcium Supplements—Supplements used to increase the calcium concentration in the blood in an attempt to make bones denser (as in osteoporosis). These supplements include calcium citrate, calcium glubionate, calcium gluconate, calcium glycerophosphate and calcium lactate, calcium lactate, dibasic calcium phosphate, tribasic calcium phosphate.

Carbamates—A group of drugs derived from carbamic acid and used for anxiety or as sedatives. They include meprobamate and ethinamate.

Carbonic Anhydrase Inhibitors—Drugs used to treat glaucoma and seizures and to prevent high altitude sickness. They include acetazolamide, brinzolamide, dichlorphenamide, dorzolamide, methazolamid.

Cataract—Loss of transparency in the lens of the eye.

Catecholamines—A group of drugs, also found naturally in the body, used to treat low blood pressure or shock. These drugs include dopamine, norepinephrine and epinephrine.

Cell—Unit of protoplasm, the essential living matter of all plants and animals.

Central Nervous System (CNS) Depressants—These drugs cause sedation or otherwise diminish brain activity and other parts of the nervous system. These drugs include alcohol, aminoglutethimide, anesthetics (general and injection-local), anticonvulsants, antidepressants (MAO inhibitors, tricyclic), antidyskinetics (except amantadine), antihistamines, apomorphine, azelastine, baclofen, barbiturates, benzodiazepines, beta-adrenergic blocking agents, brimonidine, buclizine, carbamazepine, chlophedianol, chloral hydrate, chlorzoxazone, clonidine, clozapine, cyclizine, cytarabine, difenoxin and atropine, diphenoxylate and atropine, disulfiram, donepezil, dronabinol, droperidol, ethchlorvynol, ethinamate, etomidate, fenfluramine, fluoxetine, glutethimide, guanabenz, guanfacine, haloperidol, hydroxyzine, ifosfamide, interferon, loxapine, magnesium sulfate (injection), maprotiline, meclizine, meprobamate, methyldopa, methyprylon, metoclopramide, metyrosine, mirtazapine, mitotane, molindone, nabilone, nefazodone, olanzapine, opioid (narcotic) analgesics, oxcarbazepine, oxybutynin, paraldehyde, paregoric, pargyline, paroxetine, phenothiazines, pimozide, procarbazine, promethazine, propiomazine, propofol, quetiapine, rauwolfia alkaloids, risperidone, scopolamine, sertraline, skeletal muscle relaxants (centrally acting), thalidomide, thioxanthenes, trazodone, trimeprazine, trimethobenzamide, zaleplon, zolpidem, zonisamide, zopiclone.

Central Nervous System (CNS) Stimulants—Drugs that cause excitation, anxiety and nervousness or otherwise stimulate the brain and other parts of the central nervous system. These drugs include amantadine, amphetamines, anesthetics (local), appetite suppressants (except fenfluramine), bronchodilators (xanthine-derivative), bupropion, caffeine, chlophedianol, cocaine, dextroamphetamine, diclofenac, doxapram, dronabinol, dyphylline, entacapone, ephedrine (oral), fluoroquinolones, fluoxetine, meropenem, methamphetamine, methylphenidate, moclobemide, modafanil, nabilone, pemoline, selegiline, sertraline, sympathomimetics, topiramate, tranylcypromine, zonisamide.

Cephalosporins—Antibiotics that kill many bacterial germs that penicillin and sulfa drugs can't destroy.

Cholinergics (Parasympathomimetics)—Chemicals that facilitate passage of nerve impulses through the parasympathetic nervous system.

Cholinesterase Inhibitors—Drugs that prevent the action of cholinesterase (an enzyme that breaks down acetylcholine in the body).

Chronic—Long-term, continuing. Chronic illnesses may not be curable, but they can often be prevented from becoming worse. Symptoms usually can be alleviated or controlled.

Cirrhosis—Disease that scars and destroys liver tissue resulting in abnormal function.

Citrates—Medicines taken orally to make urine more acid. Citrates include potassium citrate, potassium citrate and citric acid, potassium citrate and sodium citrate, sodium citrate and acid, tricitrates.

Coal Tar Preparations—Creams, ointments and lotions used on the skin for various skin ailments.

Cold Urticaria—Hives that appear in areas of the body exposed to the cold.

Colitis, Ulcerative—Chronic, recurring ulcers of the colon for unknown reasons.

Collagen—Support tissue of skin, tendon, bone, cartilage and connective tissue.

Colostomy—Surgical opening from the colon, the large intestine, to the outside of the body.

Coma—A sleeplike state from which a person cannot be aroused.

Compliance—The extent to which a person follows medical advice.

Congestive—Characterized by excess accumulation of fluid. In congestive heart failure, congestion occurs in the lungs, liver, kidneys and other parts of the body to cause shortness of breath, swelling of the ankles and feet, rapid heartbeat and other symptoms.

Constriction—Tightness or pressure.

Contraceptives, Oral (Birth Control Pills)—A group of hormones used to prevent ovulation, therefore preventing pregnancy. These hormones include drosperinone and ethinyl estradiol, ethynodiol diacetate and ethinyl estradiol, ethynodiol diacetate and mestranol, levonorgestrel and ethinyl estradiol, medroxyprogesterone, norethindrone tablets, norethindrone acetate and ethinyl estradiol, norethindrone and ethinyl estradiol, norethindrone and mestranol, norethynodrel and mestranol, norgestrel, norgestrel and ethinyl estradiol.

Contraceptives, Vaginal—Topical medications or devices applied inside the vagina to prevent pregnancy.

Convulsions—Violent, uncontrollable contractions of the voluntary muscles.

COPD (Chronic Obstructive Pulmonary Disease)—Lung conditions including emphysema and chronic bronchitis.

Corticosteroids (Adrenocorticosteroids)—Steroid hormones produced by the body's adrenal cortex or their synthetic equivalents.

Cortisone (Adrenocorticoids, Glucocorticoids) and Other Adrenal Steroids—Medicines that mimic the action of the steroid hormone cortisone, manufactured in the cortex of the adrenal gland. These drugs decrease the effects of inflammation within the body. They are available for injection, oral use, topical use for the skin, eyes and nose and inhalation for the bronchial tubes. These drugs include alclometasone; amcinonide; beclomethasone; benzyl benzoate; betamethasone; bismuth; clobetasol; clobetasone 17-butyrate; clocortolone; cortisone; desonide; desoximetasone; desoxycorticosterone; dexamethasone; diflorasone; diflucortolone; fludrocortisone; flumethasone; flunisolide; fluocinonide; fluocinonide, procinonide and ciprocinonide; fluorometholone; fluprednisolone, flurandrenolide; halcinonide; hydrocortisone; medrysone; methylprednisolone; mometasone; paramethasone; peruvian balsam; prednisolone; prednisone; triamcinolone; zinc oxide.

Cyclopegics—Eye drops that prevent the pupils from accommodating to varying degrees of light.

Cystitis—Inflammation of the urinary bladder.

D

Decongestants—Drugs used to open nasal passages by shrinking swollen membranes lining the nose. These drugs include:
Cough-suppressing—phenylephrine and dextromethorphan, phenylpropanolamine (phenylpropanolamine products are being discontinued) and caramiphen, phenylpropanolamine and dextromethorphan, phenylpropanolamine and hydrocodone, pseudoephedrine and codeine, pseudoephedrine and dextromethorphan, pseudoephedrine and hydrocodone. Cough-suppressing and pain-relieving—phenylpropanolamine, dextromethorphan and acetaminophen.
Cough-suppressing and sputum-thinning—phenylephrine, dextromethorphan and guaifenesin; phenylephrine, hydrocodone and guaifenesin; phenylpropanolamine, codeine and guaifenesin; phenylpropanolamine, dextromethorphan and guaifenesin; pseudoephedrine, codeine and guaifenesin; pseudoephedrine, dextromethorphan and guaifenesin; pseudoephedrine, hydrocodone and guaifenesin; phenylephrine, dextromethorphan, guaifenesin and acetaminophen; pseudoephedrine, dextromethorphan, guaifenesin and acetaminophen.
Sputum-thinning—ephedrine and guaifenesin;

ephedrine and potassium iodide; phenylephrine, phenylpropanolamine and guaifenesin; phenylpropanolamine and guaifenesin; pseudoephedrine and guaifenesin.
Nasal—ephedrine (oral), phenylpropanolamine, pseudoephedrine.
Ophthalmic (eye)—naphazoline, oxymetazoline, phenylephrine. Topical—oxymetazoline, phenylephrine, xylometazoline.

Delirium—Temporary mental disturbance characterized by hallucinations, agitation and incoherence.

Diabetes —Metabolic disorder in which the body can't use carbohydrates efficiently. This leads to a dangerously high level of glucose (a carbohydrate) in the blood.

Dialysis—Procedure to filter waste products from the bloodstream of patients with kidney failure.

Digitalis Preparations (Digitalis Glycosides)—Important drugs to treat heart disease, such as congestive heart failure, heartbeat irregularities and cardiogenic shock. These drugs include digitoxin, digoxin.

Digoxin—One of the digitalis drugs used to treat heart disease. All digitalis products were originally derived from the foxglove plant.

Dilation—Enlargement.

Disulfiram Reaction—Disulfiram (Antabuse) is a drug to treat alcoholism. When alcohol in the bloodstream interacts with disulfiram, it causes a flushed face, severe headache, chest pains, shortness of breath, nausea, vomiting, sweating and weakness. Severe reactions may cause death. A disulfiram reaction is the interaction of any drug with alcohol or another drug to produce these symptoms.

Diuretics—Drugs that act on the kidneys to prevent reabsorption of electrolytes, especially chlorides. They are used to treat edema, high blood pressure, congestive heart failure, kidney and liver failure and others. These drugs include amiloride, amiloride and hydrochlorothiazide, bendroflumethiazide, benzthiazide, bumetanide, chlorothiazide, chlorthalidone, cyclothiazide, ethacrynic acid, furosemide, glycerin, hydrochlorothiazide, hydroflumethiazide, indapamide, mannitol, methyclothiazide, metolazone, polythiazide, quinethazone, spironolactone, spironolactone and hydrochlorothiazide, triamterene, triamterene and hydrochlorothiazide, trichlormethiazide, urea.

Diuretics, Loop—Drugs that act on the kidneys to prevent reabsorption of electrolytes, especially sodium. They are used to treat edema, high blood pressure, congestive heart failure, kidney and liver failure and others. These drugs include bumetanide, ethacrynic acid, furosemide.

Diuretics, Potassium-Sparing—Drugs that act on the kidneys to prevent reabsorption of electrolytes, especially sodium. They are used to treat edema, high blood pressure, congestive heart failure, kidney and liver failure and others. This particular group of diuretics does not allow the unwanted side effect of low potassium in the blood to occur. These drugs include amiloride, spironolactone, triamterene.

Diuretics, Thiazide—Drugs that act on the kidneys to prevent reabsorption of electrolytes, especially chlorides. They are used to treat edema, high blood pressure, congestive heart failure, kidney and liver failure and others. These drugs include bendroflumethiazide, benzthiazide, chlorothiazide, chlorthalidone, cyclothiazide, hydrochlorothiazide, hydroflumethiazide, methyclothiazide, metolazone, polythiazide, quinethazone, trichlormethiazide.

Dopamine Agonists—Drugs that stimulate activity of dopamine (a brain chemical that helps control movement). These include bromocriptine, cabergoline, pergolide, ropinirole.

Dopamine Antagonists—Drugs that interfere with dopamine production (brain chemical that helps control movement). These drugs include haloperidol, metoclopramide, phenothiazines, thioxanthenes.

Duodenum—The first 12 inches of the small intestine.

E

ECG (or EKG)—Abbreviation for electrocardiogram or electrocardiograph. An ECG is a graphic tracing representing the electrical current produced by impulses passing through the heart muscle. This is a useful test in the diagnosis of heart disease, but used alone it usually can't make a complete diagnosis. An ECG is most useful in two areas:
(1) demonstrating heart rhythm disturbances and (2) demonstrating changes when there is a myocardial infarction (heart attack). It will detect enlargement of either heart chamber, but will not establish a diagnosis of heart failure or disease of the heart valves.

Eczema—Disorder of the skin with redness, itching, blisters, weeping and abnormal pigmentation.

EEG—Electroencephalogram or electroencephalograph. An EEG is a graphic recording of electrical activity generated spontaneously from nerve cells in the brain. This test is useful in the diagnosis of brain dysfunction, particularly in studying seizure disorders.

Electrolytes—Substances that can transmit electrical impulses when dissolved in body fluids. These include sodium, potassium, chloride, bicarbonate, and carbon dioxide.

Embolism—Sudden blockage of an artery by a clot or foreign material in the blood.

Emphysema—An irreversible disease in which the lung's air sacs lose elasticity and air accumulates in the lungs.

Endometriosis—Condition in which uterus tissue is found outside the uterus. Can cause pain, abnormal menstruation and infertility.

Enzyme Inducers—Drugs that increase the metabolism of another drug in the liver, resulting in a decrease of that drug's effect. These drugs include alcohol (chronic use), barbiturates (especially phenobarbital), carbamazepine, dexamethasone, efavirenz, glutethimide, griseofulvin, modafinil, nevirapine, phenylbutazone, phenytoin, primidone, rifabutin, rifampin, rifapentine, saquinavir, St. John's wort, troglitazone.

Enzyme Inhibitors—Drugs that decrease the metabolism of another drug in the liver, resulting in an increase of that drug's effect. These drugs include alcohol (high doses), allopurinol, amiodarone, amprenavir, azole antifungals, chloramphenicol, cimetidine, clarithromycin, clotrimazole, cyclosporine, danazol, diltiazem, disulfiram, divalproex, efavirenz, erythromycins, etomidate, fluoroquinolones, fluoxetine, fluvoxamine, indinavir, isoniazid, itraconazole, ketoconazole, letrozole, metoprolol, mibefradil, miconazole, modafinil, monoamine oxidase (MAO) inhibitors, nefazodone, nelfinavir, omeprazole, oral estrogen contraceptives, paroxetine, phenylbutazone, propranolol, quinidine, quinine, ritonavir, saquinavir, sertraline, tamoxifen, troleandomycin, valproic acid, venlafaxine, verapamil, zafirlukast.

Enzymes—Protein chemicals that can accelerate chemical reactions in the body.

Epilepsy—Episodes of brain disturbance that cause convulsions and loss of consciousness.

Ergot Preparations—Medicines used to treat migraine and other types of throbbing headaches. Also used after delivery of babies to make the uterus clamp down and reduce excessive bleeding.

Erythromycins—A group of drugs with similar structure used to treat infections. These drugs include erythromycin, erythromycin estolate, erythromycin ethylsuccinate, erthromycin gluceptate, erythromycin lactobionate, erythromycin stearate.

Esophagitis—Inflammation of the lower part of the esophagus, the tube connecting the throat and the stomach.

Estrogens—Female hormones used to replenish the body's stores after the ovaries have been removed or become nonfunctional after menopause. Also used with progesterone in some birth control pills and for other purposes. These drugs include:
Systemic— chlorotrianisene, diethylstilbestrol, estradiol, estrogens (conjugated and esterified), estrone, estropipate, ethinyl estradiol, quinestrol.
Vaginal—dienestrol, estradiol, estrogens (conjugated), estrone, estropipate.

Eustachian Tube—Small passage from the middle ear to the sinuses and nasal passages.

Extrapyramidal Reactions—Abnormal reactions in the power and coordination of posture and muscular movements. Movements are not under voluntary control. Some drugs associated with producing extrapyramidal reactions include amoxapine, antidepressants (tricyclic), droperidol, haloperidol, loxapine, metoclopramide, metyrosine, moclobemide, molindone, olanzapine, paroxetine, phenothiazines, pimozide, rauwolfia alkaloids, risperidone, tacrine, thioxanthenes.

Extremity—Arm, leg, hand or foot.

F

Fecal Impaction—Condition in which feces become firmly wedged in the rectum.

Fibrocystic Breast Disease—Overgrowth of fibrous tissue in the breast, producing non-malignant cysts.

Fibroid Tumors—Non-malignant tumors of the muscular layer of the uterus.

Flu (Influenza)—A virus infection of the respiratory tract that lasts three to ten days. Symptoms include headache, fever, runny nose, cough, tiredness and muscle aches.

Fluoroquinolones—A class of drugs used to treat bacterial infections, such as urinary tract infections and some types of bronchitis. These drugs include ciprofloxacin, enoxacin, gatifloxacin, levofloxacin, lomefloxacin, moxifloxacin, norfloxacin, ofloxacin, sparfloxacin.

Folate Antagonists—Drugs that impair the body's utilization of folic acid, which is necessary for cell growth. These drugs include dione anticonvulsants, hydantoin anticonvulsants, succinimide anticonvulsants, divalproex, methotrexate, oral contraceptives, phenobarbital (long-term use), pyrimethamine, sulfonamides, triamterene, trimethoprim, trimetrexate, valproic acid.

Folliculitis—Inflammation of a follicle.

Functional Dependence—The development of dependence on a drug for a normal body function. The primary example is the use of laxatives for a prolonged period so that there is a dependence on the laxative for normal bowel action.

G

G6PD—Deficiency of glucose 6-phosphate, which is necessary for glucose metabolism.

Ganglionic Blockers—Medicines that block the passage of nerve impulses through a part of the nerve cell called a ganglion. Ganglionic blockers are used to treat urinary retention and other medical problems. Bethanechol is one of the best ganglionic blockers.

Gastritis—Inflammation of the stomach.

Gastrointestinal—Of the stomach and intestinal tract.

Gland—Organ or group of cells that manufactures and excretes materials not required for its own metabolic needs.

Glaucoma—Eye disease in which increased pressure inside the eye damages the optic nerve, causes pain and changes vision.

Glucagon—Injectable drug that immediately elevates blood sugar by mobilizing glycogen from the liver.

Gold Compounds—Medicines which use gold as their base and are usually used to treat joint or arthritic disorders. These medicines include auranofin, aurothioglucose, gold sodium thiomalate.

H

H_2 Antagonists—Antihistamines that work against H_2 histamine. H_2 histamine may be liberated at any point in the body, but most often in the gastrointestinal tract.

Hangover Effect—The same feelings as a "hangover" after too much alcohol consumption. Symptoms include headache, irritability and nausea.

Hemochromatosis—Disorder of iron metabolism in which excessive iron is deposited in and damages body tissues, particularly of the liver and pancreas.

Hemoglobin—Pigment that carries oxygen in red blood cells.

Hemolytics—Drugs that can destroy red blood cells and separate hemoglobin from the blood cells. These include acetohydroxamic acid, antidiabetic agents (sulfonylurea), doxapram, furazolidone, mefenamic acid, menadiol, methyldopa, nitrofurans, primaquine, procainamide, quinidine, quinine, sulfonamides (systemic), sulfones, vitamin K.

Hemorrhage—Heavy bleeding.

Hemorrheologic Agents—Medicines to help control bleeding.

Hemosiderosis—Increase of iron deposits in body tissues without tissue damage.

Hepatitis—Inflammation of liver cells, usually accompanied by jaundice.

Hepatotoxics—Medications that can possibly cause toxicity or decreased normal function of the liver. These drugs include the following (some of which are not described in this book): acetaminophen (with long-term use); alcohol; amiodarone; anabolic steroids; androgens; angiotensin-converting enzyme (ACE) inhibitors; acitretin, anti-inflammatory drugs, nonsteroidal (NSAIDs), antithyroid agents, asparaginase, azlocillin, carbamazepine, carmustine; clindamycin; clofibrate; colestipol; cox 2 inhibitors; cyproterone; cytarabine; danazol; dantrolene; dapsone; daunorubicin; disulfiram; divalproex, dofetilide; erythromycins; estrogens; ethionamide; etretinate; felbamate; fenofibrate; fluconazole; flutamide; gold compounds; halothane; HMG-CoA reductase inhibitors; isoniazid; itraconazole; ketoconazole (oral); labetalol; mercaptopurine; methimazole, methotrexate; methyldopa; metronidazole, naltrexone; nevirapine, niacin (high doses); nilutamide, nitrofurans; pemoline; phenothiazines; phenytoin; piperacillin; plicamycin; pravastatin; probucol, rifampin; sulfamethoxazole and trimethoprim; sulfonamides; tacrine; testosterone; tizanidine; tolcapone; toremifene; tretinoin; troglitazone; valproic acid; zidovudine.

Hiatal Hernia—Section of the stomach that protrudes into the chest cavity.

Histamine—Chemical in body tissues that dilates the smallest blood vessels, constricts the smooth muscle surrounding the bronchial tubes and stimulates stomach secretions.

History—Past medical events in a patient's life.

Hives—Elevated patches on the skin that are redder or paler than surrounding skin and often itch severely.

Hoarseness—Husky, gruff, weak voice.

Hormone Replacement Therapy—A medication (estrogen) or combination of medications (estrogen and progestin or estrogen and androgen) used for treatment of premenopausal and menopausal symptoms and for prevention of diseases that affect women in their later years

Hormones—Chemical substances produced in the body to regulate other body functions.

Hypercalcemia—Too much calcium in the blood. This happens with some malignancies and in calcium overdose.

Hyperglycemia-Causing Medications—A group of drugs that may contribute to hyperglycemia (high blood sugar). These include oral estrogen-containing contraceptives, corticosteroids, estrogens, isoniazid, nicotinic acid, phenothiazines, phenytoin, sympathomimetics, thyroid hormones, thiazide diuretics.

Hyperkalemia-Causing Medications—Medicines that cause too much potassium in the bloodstream. These include ACE inhibitors; amiloride, anti-inflammatory drugs, nonsteroidal (NSAIDs); cyclosporine; digitalis glycosides; diuretics (potassium-sparing); pentamidine; spironolactone; succinylcholine chloride; tacrolimus; triamterene; trimethoprim; possibly any medicine that is combined with potassium.

Hypersensitivity—Serious reactions to many medications. The effects of hypersensitivity may be characterized by wheezing, shortness of breath, rapid heart rate, severe itching, faintness, unconsciousness and severe drop in blood pressure.

Hypertension—High blood pressure.

Hypervitaminosis—A condition due to an excess of one or more vitamins. Symptoms may include weakness, fatigue, loss of hair and changes in the skin.

Hypnotics—Drugs used to induce a sleeping state. See Barbiturates.

Hypocalcemia—Abnormally low level of calcium in the blood.

Hypoglycemia—Low blood sugar (blood glucose). A critically low blood sugar level will interfere with normal brain function and can damage the brain permanently.

Hypoglycemia-Causing Medications—A group of drugs that may contribute to hypoglycemia (low blood sugar). These include clofibrate, monoamine oxidase (MAO) inhibitors, probenecid, propranolol, rifabutin, rifampicin, salicylates, sulfonamides (long-acting), sulfonylureas.

Hypoglycemics—Drugs that reduce blood sugar. These include acetohexamide, chlorpropamide, gliclazide, glipizide, glyburide, insulin, metformin, tolazamide, tolbutamide.

Hypokalemia-Causing Medications—Medicines that cause a depletion of potassium in the bloodstream. These include adrenocorticoids (systemic), alcohol, amphotericin B (systemic), bronchodilators (adrenergic), capreomycin, carbonic anhydrase inhibitors, cisplatin, diuretics (loop and thiazide), edetate (long-term use), foscarnet, ifosfamide, indapamide, insulin, insulin lispro, laxatives (if dependent on), penicillins (some), salicylates, sirolimus, sodium bicarbonate, urea, vitamin D (overdose of).

Hypotension—Blood pressure decrease below normal. Symptoms may include weakness, lightheadedness and dizziness.

Hypotension-Causing Drugs—Medications that might cause hypotension (low blood pressure). These include alcohol, alpha adrenergic blocking agents, alprostadil, amantadine, anesthetics (general), angiotensin-converting enzyme inhibitors (ACE inhibitors), angiotensin II receptor antagonists, antidepressants (MAO inhibitors, tricyclic), antihypertensives, benzodiazepines used as preanesthetics, beta-adrenergic blocking agents, bromocriptine, cabergoline, calcium channel-blocking agents, carbidopa and levodopa, clonidine, clozapine, dipyridamole and aspirin, diuretics, docetaxel, droperidol, edetate calcium disodium, edetate disodium, haloperidol, hydralazine, levodopa, lidocaine (systemic), loxapine, magnesium sulfate, maprotiline, mirtazapine, molindone, nabilone (high doses), nefazodone, nitrates, olanzapine, opioid analgesics (including fentanil, fentanyl and sufentanil), oxcarbazepine, paclitaxel, pentamidine, phenothiazines, pimozide, pramipexole, procainamide, propofol, quinidine, radiopaques (materials used in x-ray studies), ranitidine risperidone, rituximab, ropinirole, sildenafil, thioxanthenes, tizanidine, tocainide, tolcapone, trazodone, vancomycin, venlafaxine. If you take any of these medications, be sure to tell a dentist, anesthesiologist or anyone else who intends to give you an anesthetic to put you to sleep.

Hypothermia-Causing Medications—Medicines that can cause a significant lowering of body temperature. These drugs include alcohol, alpha-adrenergic blocking agents (dihydroergotamine, ergotamine, labetalol, phenoxybenzamine, phentolamine, prazosin, tolazoline), barbiturates (large amounts), beta-adrenergic blocking agents, clonidine, insulin, minoxidil, narcotic analgesics (with overdose), phenothiazines, vasodilators.

I

Ichthyosis—Skin disorder with dryness, scaling and roughness.

Ileitis—Inflammation of the ileum, the last section of the small intestine.

Ileostomy—Surgical opening from the ileum, the end of the small intestine, to the outside of the body.

Immunosuppressants—Powerful drugs that suppress the immune system. Immuno-suppressants are used in patients who have had organ transplants or severe disease associated with the immune system. These drugs include the following (some of which are not described in this book): azathioprine, basiliximab, betamethasone, chlorambucil, corticotropin, cortisone, cyclophosphamide, cyclosporine, dacliximab, dexamethasone, hydrocortisone, mercaptopurine, methylprednisolone, muromonab, muromonab-CD3, mycophenolate, prednisolone, prednisone, sirolimus, tacrolimus, thalidomide, triamcinolone, ursodiol.

Impotence—Male's inability to achieve or sustain erection of the penis for sexual intercourse.

Insomnia—Sleeplessness.

Interaction—Change in the body's response to one drug when another is taken. Interaction may decrease the effect of one or both drugs, increase the effect of one or both drugs or cause toxicity.

Iron Supplements—Products that contain iron in a form that can be absorbed from the intestinal tract. Supplements include ferrous fumarate, ferrous gluconate, ferrous sulfate, iron dextran, iron-polysaccharide.

J

Jaundice—Symptoms of liver damage, bile obstruction or destruction of red blood cells. Symptoms include yellowed whites of the eyes, yellow skin, dark urine and light stool.

K

Keratosis—Growth that is an accumulation of cells from the outer skin layers.

Kidney Stones—Small, solid stones made from calcium, cholesterol, cysteine and other body chemicals.

L

Laxatives—Medicines prescribed to treat constipation. These medicines include bisacodyl; bisacodyl and docusate; casanthranol; casanthranol and docusate; cascara sagrada; cascara sagrada and aloe; cascara sagrada and phenolphthalein; castor oil; danthron; danthron and docusate; danthron and poloxamer 188; dehydrocholic acid; dehydrocholic acid and docusate; docusate; docusate and phenolphthalein; docusate and mineral oil; docusate and phenolphthalein; docusate, carboxymethylcellulose and casanthranol; glycerin; lactulose; magnesium citrate; magnesium hydroxide; magnesium hydroxide and mineral oil; magnesium oxide; magnesium sulfate; malt soup extract; malt soup extract and psyllium; methylcellulose; mineral oil; mineral oil and cascara sagrada; mineral oil and phenolphthalein; mineral oil, glycerin and phenolphthalein; phenolphthalein; poloxamer; polycarbophil; potassium bitartrate and sodium bicarbonate; psyllium; psyllium and senna; psyllium hydrophilic mucilloid; psyllium hydrophilic mucilloid and carboxymethyl-cellulose; psyllium hydrophilic mucilloid and sennosides; psyllium hydrophilic musilloid and senna; senna; senna and docusate; sennosides; sodium phosphate.

LDH—Abbreviation for lactate dehydrogenase. It is a measurement of cardiac enzymes used to confirm some heart conditions.

Lincomycins—A family of antibiotics used to treat certain infections.

Low-Purine Diet—A diet that avoids high-purine foods, such as liver, sweetbreads, kidneys, sardines, oysters and others. If you need a low-purine diet, request instructions from your doctor.

Lupus—Serious disorder of connective tissue that primarily affects women. Varies in severity with skin eruptions, joint inflammation, low white blood cell count and damage to internal organs, especially the kidneys.

Lymph Glands—Glands in the lymph vessels throughout the body that trap foreign and infectious matter and protect the bloodstream from infection.

M

Macrolides—A class of antibiotic (antibacterial) drugs. They include dirithromycin, erythromycin, lincomycin and vancomycin.

Male Hormones—Chemical substances secreted by the testicles, ovaries and adrenal glands in humans. Some male hormones used by humans are derived synthetically. Male hormones include testosterone cypionate and estradiol cypionate, testosterone enanthate and estradiol valerate.

Mania—A mood disturbance characterized by euphoria, agitation, elation, irritability, rapid and confused speech and excessive activity. Mania usually occurs as part of bipolar (manic-depressive) disorder.

Manic-Depressive Illness—Psychosis with alternating cycles of excessive enthusiasm and depression.

MAO Inhibitors—See Monoamine Oxidase (MAO) Inhibitors.

Mast Cell—Connective tissue cell.

Meglitinides—Drugs that stimulate the pancreas to produce insulin. Used to treat Type II (non-insulin dependent) diabetes. These drugs include repaglinide and nateglinide.

Menopause—The end of menstruation in the female, often accompanied by irritability, hot flashes, changes in the skin and bones and vaginal dryness.

Metabolism—Process of using nutrients and energy to build and break down wastes.

Migraine Headaches—Periodic headaches caused by constriction of arteries to the skull. Symptoms include severe pain, vision disturbances, nausea, vomiting and sensitivity to light.

Mind-Altering Drugs—Any drugs that decrease alertness, perception, concentration, contact with reality or muscular coordination.

Mineral Supplements—Mineral substances added to the diet to treat or prevent mineral deficiencies. They include iron, copper, magnesium, calcium, etc.

Monoamine Oxidase (MAO) Inhibitors—Drugs that prevent the activity of the enzyme monoamine oxidase (MAO) in brain tissue, thus affecting mood. MAO inhibitors include antidepressants, the use of which is frequently restricted because of severe side effects. These side effects may be interactions with other drugs (such as ephedrine or amphetamine) or foods containing tyramine (such as cheese) and may produce a sudden increase in blood pressure. MAOs include isocarboxazid, phenelzine, tranylcypromine.

Muscle Blockers—Same as muscle relaxants or skeletal muscle relaxants.

Muscle Relaxants—Medicines used to lessen painful contractions and spasms of muscles. These include atracurium, carisoprodol, chlorphenesin, chlorzoxazone, cyclobenzaprine, metaxalone, methocarbamol, metocurine, orphenadrine citrate, orphenadrine hydrochloride, pancuronium, phenytoin, succinylcholine, tubocurarine, vecuronium.

Myasthenia Gravis—Disease of the muscles characterized by fatigue and progressive paralysis. It is usually confined to muscles of the face, lips, tongue and neck.

Mydriatics—Eye drops that cause the pupils to dilate (become larger) to a marked degree.

N

Narcotics—A group of habit-forming, addicting drugs used for treatment of pain, diarrhea, cough, acute pulmonary edema and others. They are all derived from opium, a milky exudate in capsules of *papaver somniferum*. Law requires licensed physicians to dispense by prescription. These drugs include alfentanil, buprenorphine, butorphanol, codeine, fentanyl, hydrocodone, hydromorphone, levorphanol, meperidine, methadone, morphine, nalbuphine, opium, oxycodone, oxymorphone, paregoric, pentazocine, propoxyphene, sufentanil.

Nephrotoxic (Kidney-Poisoning) Medications—Under some circumstances, these medicines can be toxic to the kidneys. These medicines include acetaminophen (in high doses); acyclovir (injection of); aminoglycosides; amphotericin B (given internally); analgesic combinations containing acetaminophen and aspirin or other salicylates (with chronic high-dose use); anti-inflammatory analgesics (nonsteroidal); bacitracin (injection of); capreomycin; carmustine; chlorpropamide; cidofovir; ciprofloxacin; cisplatin; cox 2 inhibitors;

cyclosporine; deferoxamine (long-term use); edetate calcium disodium (with high doses); edetate disodium (with high dose); foscarnet; gold compounds; ifosfamide; imipenem; lithium; methicillin, methotrexate (with high dose therapy); methoxyflurane; nafcillin; neomycin (oral); pamidronate; penicillamine; pentamidine; pentostatin, phenacetin; plicamycin; polymyxins (injection of); radiopaques (materials used for special x-ray examinations); rifampin; streptozocin; sulfonamides; tacrolimus; tetracyclines (except doxycycline and minocycline); tiopronin; tretinoin; vancomycin (injection of).

Neuroleptic Malignant Syndrome—Ceaseless involuntary, jerky movements of the tongue, facial muscles and hands.

Neuromuscular Blocking Agents—A group of drugs prescribed to relax skeletal muscles. They are all given by injection, and descriptions are not included in this book. These drugs include atracurium, edrophonium, gallamine, neostigmine, metocurine, pancuronium, pyridostigmine, succinylcholine, tubocurarine, vecuronium.

Neurotoxic Medications—Medicines that cause toxicity to the nerve tissues in the body. These drugs include alcohol (chronic use), allopurinol; altretamine, amantadine; amiodarone; anticonvulsants (hydantoin), capreomycin, carbamazepine, chloramphenicol (oral), chloroquine, cilastatin, ciprofloxacin, cisplatin, cycloserine, cyclosporine, cytarabine, didanosine, disulfiram, docetaxel, ethambutol, ethionamide, fludarabine, hydroxychloroquine, imipenem, interferon, isoniazid, lincomycins, lindane (topical), lithium, meperidine, methotrexate, metronidazole, mexiletine, nitrofurantoin, oxcarbazepine, paclitaxel, pemoline, pentostatin, pyridoxine (large amounts), quinacrine, quinidine, quinine, stavudine, tacrolimus, tetracyclines, thalidomide, vinblastine, vincristine, vindesine, zalcitabine.

Nitrates—Medicines made from a chemical with a nitrogen base. Nitrates include erythrityl tetranitrate, isosorbide dinitrate, nitroglycerin, pentaerythritol tetranitrate.

Nonsteroidal Anti-Inflammatory Drugs (NSAIDs)—See Anti-Inflammatory Drugs, Nonsteroidal.

Nutritional Supplements—Substances used to treat and prevent deficiencies when the body is unable to absorb them by eating a well-balanced, nutritional diet. These supplements include: Vitamins—ascorbic acid, ascorbic acid and sodium ascorbate, calcifediol, calcitriol, calcium pantothenate, cyanocobalamin, dihydrotachysterol, ergocalciferol, folate sodium, folic acid, hydroxocobalamin, niacin, niacinamide, pantothenic, pyridoxine, riboflavin, sodium ascorbate, thiamine, vitamin A, vitamin E. Minerals—calcium carbonate, calcium citrate, calcium glubionate, calcium gluconate, calcium lactate, calcium phosphate (dibasic and tribasic), sodium fluoride. Other—levocarnitine, omega-3 polyunsaturated fatty acids.

O

Opiates—See Narcotics.

Orthostatic Hypotension—Excess drop in blood pressure when arising from a sitting or lying position.

Osteoporosis—Softening of bones caused by a loss of calcium usually found in bone. Bones become brittle and fracture easily.

Ototoxic Medications—These medicines may possibly cause hearing damage. They include aminoglycosides, 4-aminoquinolines, anti-inflammatory analgesics (nonsteroidal), bumetanide (injected), capreomycin, carboplatin, chloroquine, cisplatin, deferoxamine, erythromycins, ethacrynic acid, furosemide, hydroxychloroquine, quinidine, quinine, salicylates, vancomycin (injected).

Ovary—Female sexual gland where eggs mature and ripen for fertilization.

P

Pain Relievers—Non-narcotic medicines used to treat pain.

Palpitations—Rapid, forceful or throbbing heartbeat noticeable to the patient.

Pancreatitis—Serious inflammation or infection of the pancreas that causes upper abdominal pain.

Pancreatitis-associated Drugs—Medications associated with the development of pancreatitis. These include alcohol, asparaginase, azathioprine, didanosine, estrogens, furosemide, methyldopa, nitrofurantoin, sulfonamides, tetracyclines, thiazide diuretics, valproic acid.

Parkinson's Disease or Parkinson's Syndrome—Disease of the central nervous system. Characteristics are a fixed, emotionless expression of the face, tremor, slower muscle movements, weakness, changed gait and a peculiar posture.

Pellagra—Disease caused by a deficiency of the water-soluble vitamin thiamine (vitamin B-1). Symptoms include brain disturbance, diarrhea and skin inflammation.

Penicillin—Chemical substance (antibiotic) originally discovered as a product of mold, that can kill some bacterial germs.

Peripheral Neuropathy (Peripheral Neuritis)—Inflammation and degeneration of the nerve endings or of the terminal nerves. It most often occurs in the nerve tissue of the muscles of the extremities (arms and legs). Symptoms include pain of varying intensity and sensations of numbness, tingling and burning in the hands and feet. It can be caused by certain medications or chemicals, infections, chronic inflammation or nutritive disease.

Peripheral-neuropathy Associated Drugs—Medications that are associated with the development of peripheral neuropathy. These include chloramphenicol, cisplatin, dapsone, didanosine, ethambutol, ethionamide, hydralazine, isoniazid, lithium, metronidazole, nitrofurantoin, nitrous oxide, phenytoin, stavudine, vincristine, zalcitabine.

Phenothiazines—Drugs used to treat mental, nervous and emotional conditions. These drugs include acetophenazine, chlorpromazine, fluphenazine, mesoridazine, methotrimeprazine, pericyazine, perphenazine, prochlorperazine, promazine, thiopropazate, thioproperazine, thioridazine, trifluoperazine, triflupromazine.

Pheochromocytoma—A tumor of the adrenal gland that produces chemicals that cause high blood pressure, headache, nervousness and other symptoms.

Phlegm—Thick mucus secreted by glands in the respiratory tract.

Photophobia—Increased sensitivity to light as perceived by the human eye. Drugs that can cause photophobia include antidiabetic drugs, atropine, belladonna, bromides, chloroquine, ciprofloxacin, chlordiazepoxide, clidinium, clomiphene, dicyclomine, digitalis drugs, doxepin, ethambutol, ethionamide, ethosuximide, etretinate, glycopyrrolate, hydroxychloroquine, hydroxyzine, hyoscyamine, isopropamide, mephenytoin, methenamine, methsuximide, monoamine oxidase (MAO) inhibitors, nalidixic acid, norfloxacin, oral contraceptives, orphenadrine, paramethadione, phenothiazines, propantheline, quinidine, quinine, scopolamine, tetracyclines, tridihexethyl, trimethadione.

Photosensitizing Medications—Medicines that can cause abnormally heightened skin reactions to the effects of sunlight and ultraviolet light. These medicines include acetazolamide, acetohexamide, alprazolam, amantadine, amiloride, amiodarone, amitriptyline, amoxapine, antidiabetic agents (oral), barbiturates, bendroflumethiazide, benzocaine, benzoyl peroxide, benzthiazide, captopril, carbamazepine, chlordiazepoxide, chloroquine, chlorothiazide, chlorpromazine, chlorpropamide, chlortetracycline, chlorthalidone, ciprofloxacin, clindamycin, clofazimine, clofibrate, clomipramine, coal tar, contraceptives (estrogen-containing), cyproheptadine, dacarbazine, dapsone, demeclocycline, desipramine, desoximetasone, diethylstilbestrol, diflunisal, diltiazem, diphenhydramine, disopyramide, doxepin, doxycycline, enoxacin, estrogens, etretinate, flucytosine, fluorescein, fluorouracil, fluphenazine, flutamide, furosemide, glipizide, glyburide, gold preparations, griseofulvin, haloperidol, hexachlorophene, hydrochlorothiazide, hydroflumethiazide, ibuprofen, imipramine, indomethacin, isotretinoin, ketoprofen, lincomycin, lomefloxacin, maprotiline, mesoridazine, methacycline, methotrexate, methoxsalen, methyclothiazide, methyldopa, metolazone, minocycline, minoxidil, nabumetone, nalidixic acid, naproxen, nifedipine, norfloxacin, nortriptyline, ofloxacin, oral contraceptives, oxyphenbutazone, oxytetracycline, perphenazine, phenelzine, phenobarbital, phenylbutazone, phenytoin, piroxicam, polythiazide, prochlorperazine, promazine, promethazine, protriptyline, pyrazinamide, quinidine, quinine, sulfonamides, sulindac, tetracycline, thiabendazole, thioridazine, thiothixene, tolazamide, tolbutamide, tranylcypromine, trazodone, tretinoin, triamterene, trichlormethiazide, trifluoperazine, triflupromazine, trimeprazine, trimethoprim, trimipramine, triprolidine, vinblastine.

Pinworms—Common intestinal parasites that cause rectal itching and irritation.

Pituitary Gland—Gland at the base of the brain that secretes hormones to stimulate growth and other glands to produce hormones.

Platelet—Disc-shaped element of the blood, smaller than a red or white blood cell, necessary for blood clotting.

Polymyxins—A family of antibiotics that kill bacteria.

Polyp—Growth on a mucous membrane.

Porphyria—Inherited metabolic disorder characterized by changes in the nervous system and kidneys.

Post-Partum—Following delivery of a baby.

Potassium—Important chemical found in body cells.

Potassium Foods—Foods high in potassium content, including dried apricots and peaches, lentils, raisins, citrus and whole-grain cereals.

Potassium Supplements—Medicines needed by people who don't have enough potassium in their diets or by those who develop a deficiency due to illness or taking diuretics and other medicines. These supplements include chloride; potassium acetate; potassium bicarbonate; potassium bicarbonate and potassium chloride; potassium bicarbonate and potassium citrate; potassium chloride; potassium chloride, potassium bicarbonate and potassium citrate; potassium gluconate; potassium gluconate and potassium chloride; potassium gluconate and potassium citrate; potassium gluconate, potassium citrate and ammonium; trikates.

Premenstrual Dysphoric Disorder (PMDD)—A severe form of premenstrual syndrome which is characterized by severe monthly mood swings as well as physical symptoms that interfere with everyday life, especially a woman's relationships with her family and friends.

Progesterone—A female steroid sex hormone that is responsible for preparing the uterus for pregnancy.

Progestin—A synthetic hormone that is designed to mimic the actions of progesterone. These include hydroxyprogesterone, medroxyprogesterone, megestrol, norethindrone, norgestrel and progesterone.

Prostaglandins—A group of drugs used for a variety of therapeutic purposes. These drugs include alprostadil (treats newborns with congenital heart disease), carboprost and dinoprost (both used to induce labor) and dinoprostone (used to induce labor or to induce a late abortion).

Prostate—Gland in the male that surrounds the neck of the bladder and the urethra.

Protease Inhibitors—A class of anti-HIV drugs which inhibit the protease enzyme and stop virus replication. These drugs include: abacavir, amprenavir, indinavir, lopinavir and ritonavir; nelfinavir, ritonavir and saquinavir.

Protein Bound Drugs—Drugs that are firmly bound to protein in the blood serum, including clofibrate, diazepam, diazoxide, ibuprofen, indomethacin and naproxen.

Prothrombin—Blood substance essential in clotting.

Prothrombin Time (Pro Time)—Laboratory study used to follow prothrombin activity and keep coagulation safe.

Psoriasis—Chronic inherited skin disease. Symptoms are lesions with silvery scales on the edges.

Psychosis—Mental disorder characterized by deranged personality, loss of contact with reality and possible delusions, hallucinations or illusions.

Purine Foods—Foods that are metabolized into uric acid. Foods high in purines include anchovies, liver, brains, sweetbreads, sardines, kidneys, oysters, gravy and meat extracts.

Q

QT Interval Prolongation-Causing Drugs—A group of drugs that can cause serious heart rhythm problems. These drugs include amiodarone, astemizole, calcium channel blockers (especially bepridil),clarithyromycin, disopyramide, erythromycins, fluoroquinolones, maprotiline, pentamidine, phenothiazines, pimozide, procainamide, quinidine, thoridazole, tricyclic antidepressants.

R

Rauwolfia Alkaloids—Drugs that belong to the family of antihypertensives (drugs that lower blood pressure). Rauwolfia alkaloids are not used as extensively as in years past. They include alseroxylon, deserpidine, rauwolfia serpentina, reserpine.

RDA—Recommended daily allowance of a vitamin or mineral.

Rebound Effect—Return of a condition, often with increased severity, once the prescribed drug is withdrawn.

Renal—Pertaining to the kidney.

Retina—Innermost covering of the eyeball on which the image is formed.

Retinoids—A group of drugs that are synthetic vitamin A-like compounds used to treat skin conditions. These drugs include etretinate, isotretinoin and retinoic acid.

Retroperitoneal Imaging—Special x-rays or CT scans of the organs attached to the abdominal wall behind the peritoneum (the covering of the intestinal tract and lining of the walls of the abdominal and pelvic cavities).

Reye's Syndrome—Rare, sometimes fatal, disease of children that causes brain and liver damage.

Rickets—Bone disease caused by vitamin D deficiency. Bones become bent and distorted during infancy or childhood.

S

Salicylates—Medicines to relieve pain and reduce fever. These include aspirin, aspirin and caffeine, buffered aspirin, choline salicylate, choline and magnesium salicylates, magnesium salicylate, salicylamide, salsalate, sodium salicylate.

Sedatives—Drugs that reduce excitement or anxiety. They are used to produce sedation (calmness). These include alprazolam, amobarbital, aprobarbital, bromazepam, butalbital, chloral hydrate, clonazepam, clorazepate, chlordiazepoxide, diazepam, diphenhydramine, doxylamine, estazolam, ethchlorvynol, ethinamate, flurazepam, glutethimide, halazepam, hydroxyzine, ketazolam, lorazepam, methotrimeprazine, midazolam, nitrazepam, oxazepam, pentobarbital, phenobarbital, prazepam, promethazine, propiomazine, propofol, quazepam, secobarbital, temazepam, triazolam, trimeprazine, zaleplon, zolpidem, zopiclone.

Seizure—A sudden attack as of epilepsy or some other disease can cause changes of consciousness or convulsions.

Selective Serotonin Reuptake Inhibitors (SSRIs)—Medications used for treatment of depression that work by increasing the serotonin levels in the brain. Serotonin is a neurotransmitter (brain chemical) having to do with mood and behavior. These drugs include fluoxetine, fluvoxamine, paroxetine, sertraline. More information can be found on the individual drug chart for each drug.

Serotonergics—Medications or drugs that affect the levels of serotonin (a brain chemical) concerned with conscious processes. These drugs include clomipramine, fluoxetine, fluvoxamine, moclobemide, MAO inhibitors, nefazodone, paroxetine, sertraline, tryptophan, venlafaxine and some drugs of abuse.

Serotonin Syndrome—A potentially very serious interaction between certain drugs. Symptoms include confusion, irritability, muscle rigidity, chills, high fever, poor coordination, restlessness, sweating, trembling or shaking, twitching.

SGOT—Abbreviation for serum glutamic-oxaloacetic transaminase. Measuring the level in the blood helps demonstrate liver disorders and diagnose recent heart damage.

SGPT—Abbreviation for a laboratory study measuring the blood level of serum glutamic-pyruvic transaminase. Deviations from a normal level may indicate liver disease.

Sick Sinus Syndrome—A complicated, serious heartbeat rhythm disturbance characterized by a slow heart rate alternating with a fast or slow heart rate with heart block.

Sinusitis—Inflammation or infection of the sinus cavities in the skull.

Skeletal Muscle Relaxants (same as Skeletal Muscle Blockers)—A group of drugs prescribed to treat spasms of the skeletal muscles. These drugs include carisoprodol, chlorphenesin, chlorzoxazone, cyclobenzaprine, diazepam, lorazepam, metaxalone, methocarbamol, orphenadrine, phenytoin.

Sleep Inducers—Night-time sedatives to aid in falling asleep.

Streptococci—A bacteria that can cause infections in the throat, respiratory system and skin. Improperly treated, can lead to disease in the heart, joints and kidneys.

Stroke—Sudden, severe attack, usually sudden paralysis, from injury to the brain or spinal cord caused by a blood clot or hemorrhage in the brain.

Stupor—Near unconsciousness.

Sublingual—Under the tongue. Some drugs are absorbed almost as quickly this way as by injection.

Sulfa Drugs—Shorthand for sulfonamide drugs, which are used to treat infections.

Sulfonamides—Sulfa drugs prescribed to treat infections. They include sulfacytine, sulfamethoxazole, sulfamethoxazole and trimethoprim, sulfasalazine, sulfisoxazole.

Sulfonylureas—A family of drugs that lower blood sugar (hypoglycemic agents). Used in the treatment of some forms of diabetes.

Sympatholytics—A group of drugs that blocks the action of the sympathetic nervous system. These drugs include beta-blockers, guanethidine, hydralazine and prazosin.

Sympathomimetics—A large group of drugs that mimic the effects of stimulation of the sympathetic part of the autonomic nervous system. These drugs include albuterol, amphetamine, benzphetamine, bitolterol, cocaine, dextroamphetamine, diethylpropion, dobutamine, ephedrine, epinephrine, ethylnorepinephrine, fenfluramine, ipratropium, isoproterenol, isoetharine, mazindol, mephentermine, metaproterenol, metaraminol, methoxamine, norepinephrine, phendimetrazine, phentermine, phenylephrine, phenylpropanolamine, pirbuterol, pseudoephedrine, ritodrine, terbutaline.

T

Tardive Dyskinesia—Slow, involuntary movements of the jaw, lips and tongue caused by an unpredictable drug reaction. Drugs that can cause this include haloperidol, phenothiazines, thiothixene.

Tartrazine Dye—A dye used in foods and medicine preparations that may cause an allergic reaction in some people.

Tetracyclines—A group of medicines with similar chemical structure used to treat infections. These drugs include demeclocycline, doxycycline, methacycline, minocycline, oxytetracycline, tetracycline.

Thiazides—A group of chemicals that cause diuresis (loss of water through the kidneys). Frequently used to treat high blood pressure and congestive heart failure. Thiazides include bendroflumethiazide, benzthiazide, chlorothiazide, chlorthalidone, cyclothiazide, hydrochlorothiazide, hydroflumethiazide, methyclothiazide, metolazone, polythiazide, quinethazone, trichlormethiazide.

Thiothixines—See Thioxanthenes.

Thioxanthenes—Drugs used to treat emotional, mental and nervous conditions. These drugs include chlorprothixene, flupenthixol, thiothixene.

Thrombocytopenias—Diseases characterized by inadequate numbers of blood platelets circulating in the bloodstream.

Thrombolytic Agents—Drugs that help to dissolve blood clots. They include alteplase, anistreplase, streptokinase, urokinase.

Thrombophlebitis—Inflammation of a vein caused by a blood clot in the vein.

Thyroid—Gland in the neck that manufactures and secretes several hormones.

Thyroid Hormones—Medications that mimic the action of the thyroid hormone made in the thyroid gland. They include dextrothyroxine, levothyroxine, liothyronine, liotrix, thyroglobulin, thyroid.

Tic Douloureux—Painful condition caused by inflammation of a nerve in the face.

Tolerance–A decreasing response to repeated constant doses of a drug or a need to increase doses to produce the same physical or mental response.

Toxicity—Poisonous reaction to a drug that impairs body functions or damages cells.

Tranquilizers—Drugs that calm a person without clouding consciousness.

Transdermal Patches—Medicated patches that stick to the skin. There are more and more medications in this form. This method produces a prolonged systemic effect. If you are using this form, follow these instructions: Choose an area of skin without cuts, scars or hair, such as the upper arm, chest or behind the ear. Thoroughly clean area where patch is to be applied. If patch gets wet and loose, cover with an additional piece of plastic. Apply a fresh patch if the first one falls off. Apply each dose to a different area of skin if possible.

Tremor—Involuntary trembling.

Trichomoniasis—Infestation of the vagina by *trichomonas*, an infectious organism. The infection causes itching, vaginal discharge and irritation.

Triglyceride—Fatty chemical manufactured from carbohydrates for storage in fat cells.

Tyramine—Normal chemical component of the body that helps sustain blood pressure. Can rise to fatal levels in combination with some drugs. Tyramine is found in many foods:

Beverages—Alcohol beverages, especially Chianti or robust red wines, vermouth, ale, beer.

Breads—Homemade bread with a lot of yeast and breads or crackers containing cheese.

Fats—Sour cream.

Fruits—Bananas, red plums, avocados, figs, raisins, raspberries.

Meats and meat substitutes—Aged game, liver (if not fresh), canned meats, salami, sausage, aged cheese, salted dried fish, pickled herring, meat tenderizers.

Vegetables—Italian broad beans, green bean pods, eggplant.

Miscellaneous—Yeast concentrates or extracts, marmite, soup cubes, commercial gravy, soy sauce, any protein food that has been stored improperly or is spoiled.

U

Ulcer, Peptic—Open sore on the mucous membrane of the esophagus, stomach or duodenum caused by stomach acid.

Urethra—Hollow tube through which urine (and semen in men) is discharged.

Urethritis—Inflammation or infection of the urethra.

Uricosurics—A group of drugs that promotes excretion of uric acid in the urine. These drugs include probenecid and sulfinpyrazone.

Urinary Acidifiers—Medications that cause urine to become acid. These include ascorbic acid, potassium phosphate, potassium and sodium phosphates, racemethionine.

Urinary Alkalizers—Medications that cause urine to become alkaline. These include potassium citrate, potassium citrate and citric acid, potassium citrate and sodium citrate, sodium bicarbonate, sodium citrate and citric acid, tricitrate.

Uterus—Also called the womb. A hollow muscular organ in the female in which the embryo develops into a fetus.

V

Vascular—Pertaining to blood vessels.

Vascular Headache Preventatives—Medicines prescribed to prevent the occurrence of or reduce the frequency and severity of vascular headaches such as migraines. These drugs include atenolol; clonidine; ergotamine, belladonna alkaloids and phenobarbital; fenoprofen; flunarizine; ibuprofen; indomethacin; isocarboxazid, lithium; mefenamic acid; methysergide; metoprolol; nadolol; naproxen; phenelzine; pizotyline; propranolol; timolol, tranylcypromine, verapamil.

Vascular Headache Treatment—Medicine prescribed to treat vascular headaches such as migraines. These drugs include butalbital (combined with acetaminophen, aspirin, caffeine or codeine); cyproheptadine; diclofenac; diflunisal; dihydroergotamine; ergotamine; ergotamine and caffeine; ergotamine, caffeine, belladonna alkaloids and pentobarbital; etodolac; fenoprofen; ibuprofen; indomethacin (capsules, oral suspension, rectal); isometheptene, dichloralphenazone and acetaminophen; ketoprofen; meclofenamate; mefenamic acid; metoclopramide; naproxen; phenobarbital; sumatriptan.

Vasoconstrictor—Any agent that causes a narrowing of the blood vessels.

Vasodilator—Any agent that causes a widening of the blood vessels.

Vertigo—A sensation of motion, usually dizziness or whirling either of oneself or one's surroundings.

Virus—Infectious organism that reproduces in the cells of the infected host. Viruses cause many diseases in humans including the common cold.

X

Xanthines—Substances that stimulate muscle tissue, especially that of the heart. Types of xanthines include aminophylline, caffeine, dyphylline, oxtriphylline, theophylline.

Y

Yeast—A single-cell organism that can cause infections of the mouth, vagina, skin and parts of the gastrointestinal system.

GUIDE TO INDEX

Alphabetical entries in the index include three categories—1) drug generic names or drug family names, 2) drug brand names, and 3) drug therapeutic class names.

1. Generic names and drug family names (a group of similar generic drugs such as antihistamines) appear in capital letters, followed by their chart page number:

   ASPIRIN 146

   NARCOTIC ANALGESICS 586

2. Brand names appear in ***bold italic***, followed by their generic ingredient and chart page number or their drug family name and chart page number:

   Bayer - See ASPIRIN 146

   Some brand names contain two or more generic ingredients. These generic ingredients and chart page number or drug family and chart page number are listed in capital letters, following the brand name:

   Allent - See
   ANTIHISTAMINES 108
   PSEUDOEPHEDRINE 706

3. Drug therapeutic class (treatment) names appear in regular type, capital and lower-case letters. The generic drug names or drug family names in this book that fall into a particular therapeutic drug class are listed after the class name:

   Antifungal - See
   ANTIFUNGALS, AZOLES 90
   CLOTRIMAZOLE (Oral-Local) 254
   GRISEOFULVIN 392
   NYSTATIN 618

INDEX

B

C

INDEX

D

INDEX

E

F

G

H

J

K

L

N

INDEX

O

INDEX

P

Q

R

T

U

INDEX

V

INDEX

W

X

Y

Z

OTHER BOOKS OF INTEREST

Complete Guide to Symptoms, Illness & Surgery

H. Winter Griffith, M.D., Revised and Updated by Stephen Moore, M.D. and Kenneth Yoder, M.D. 0-399-52609-9/$17.95
The definitive reference source for diagnosing, understanding and seeking treatment for any illness—from the common cold to life-threatening cancer or heart disease.
A Perigee Trade Paperback

Complete Guide to Symptoms, Illness & Sugery for People over 50

H. Winter Griffith, M.D. 0-399-51749-9/$19.95
This complete guide to symptoms, illness and surgery for older Americans provides information on hundreds of symptoms; the details, causes and risk factors for illnesses, injuries and disorders; numerous illustrated surgeries, information on medication, and more.
A Perigee Trade Paperback

Complete Guide to Sports Injuries

H. Winter Griffith, M.D. 0-399-52305-7/$16.95
One of America's most trusted family physicians tell readers how to treat, avoid and rehabilitate nearly 200 of the most common sports injuries, including fractures, bruises, sprains, strains, dislocations and head injuries.
A Perigee Trade Paperback

TO ORDER CALL 1-800-788-6262, ext. 1. Refer to Ad #917

Perigee
The Berkley Publishing Group
A division of Penguin Putnam Inc.
375 Hudson Street
New York, NY 10014

* Prices subject to change

EMERGENCY GUIDE FOR OVERDOSE VICTIMS

This section lists *basic* steps in recognizing and treating immediate effects of drug overdose.

Study the information before you need it. If possible, take a course in first aid and learn external cardiac massage and mouth-to-mouth breathing techniques, called *cardiopulmonary resuscitation* (CPR).

For quick reference, list emergency telephone numbers in the spaces provided on the inside back cover for fire department paramedics, ambulance, poison control center and your doctor. These numbers, except for that of a doctor, are usually listed on the inside cover of your telephone directory.

IF VICTIM IS UNCONSCIOUS, NOT *BREATHING:*

1. Yell for help. Don't leave victim.
2. Dial 911 (emergency) or 0 (operator) for an ambulance or medical help. If the victim is a child, give mouth-to-mouth breathing for one minute, then dial 911 or 0.
3. Begin mouth-to-mouth breathing immediately.
4. If there is no heartbeat, give external cardiac massage.
5. Don't stop CPR until help arrives.
6. Don't try to make victim vomit.
7. If vomiting occurs, save vomit to take to emergency room for analysis.
8. Take medicine or empty bottles with you to emergency room.

IF VICTIM IS UNCONSCIOUS AND *BREATHING:*

1. Dial 911 (emergency) or 0 (operator) for an ambulance or medical help.
2. If you can't get help immediately, take victim to the nearest emergency room.
3. Don't try to make victim vomit.
4. If vomiting occurs, save vomit to take to emergency room for analysis.
5. Watch victim carefully on the way to the emergency room. If heart or breathing stops, use cardiac massage and mouth-to-mouth breathing (CPR).
6. Take medicine or empty bottles with you to emergency room.